A great package of resources for students and instructors—test banks, learning activities, client education guides, and other supplementary material

W9-BOB-691

ADDITIONAL BONUS MATERIAL

To help you and your students in your commitment to psychiatric nursing, we have provided a host of ancillary material. Students can find helpful easy-access learning and teaching aids on the **Student CD-ROM** attached inside the back cover and the FREE **Student Online Resource** at www.fadavis.com/townsend. Educators who adopt this book can receive an **Instructor's Resource Disk** with teaching aids to assist with your lessons.

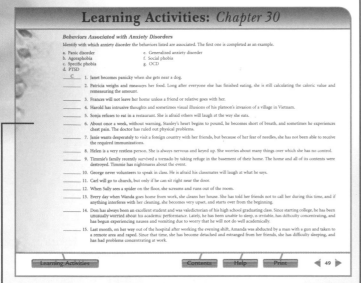

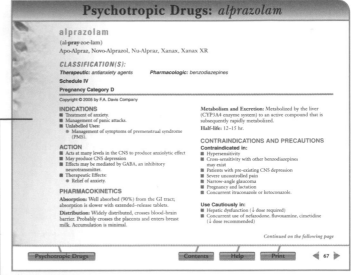

STUDENT CD-ROM

Electronic Test Bank
• **Nearly 300 Questions** to help the student with the course and prepare for the NCLEX® exam
  - **50 alternate item format NCLEX®-style questions**
  - More than **100 NCLEX®-style multiple-choice questions**
  - **135+** multiple-choice review questions
  - **Rationales** for Correct and Incorrect Answers

Electronic Student Workbook
• **More than 400** Helpful Learning Activities
• 55 **Psychotropic Drug Monographs** that can be printed and carried to clinicals
• 23 Sample **Client Education Teaching Guides** that can be reproduced as client/family handouts
• **Care Plans** and **Critical Pathways**
• **Medication Assessment Tool**
• **Levels of Anxiety**
• **Assigning Nursing Diagnoses to Client Behaviors**

FREE STUDENT ONLINE RESOURCE
www.fadavis.com/townsend

• 5 printable **Concept Map Care Plans** from the text plus 3 preformatted templates for customizing plans of care
• 16 Conventional Nursing **Care Plans**
• **Psychotropic Drug Monographs**
• 5 Schematic **Brain Illustrations**
• Meet the author/Contact the author

INSTRUCTOR'S RESOURCE DISK

Electronic Test Bank
• Updated and expanded to reflect **the latest NCLEX® test plan**
• **More than 800 NCLEX®-style questions** with **50 additional questions in new alternate item formats**. These are not duplicates of the 50 alternate item format NCLEX®-style questions found on the Student CD-ROM.
• **Page and chapter references**
• **Rationales for all correct and incorrect answers**

Complete PowerPoint Presentation covering all 45 chapters

Client Education Teaching Guides that can be reproduced as handouts

Instructor's Guide
• Chapter Focus/Objectives; Key Terms; Chapter Outline/Lecture Notes
• Case Studies for Use with Student Learning

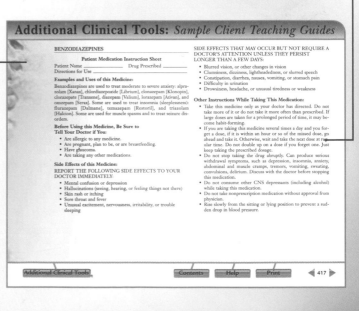

EVIDENCE-BASED

The book's evidence-based approach is reflected throughout the text

IMPLICATIONS OF RESEARCH FOR EVIDENCE-BASED PRACTICE

Dunn, A.L., Trivedi, M.H., Kampert, J.B., Clark, C.G., & Chambliss, H.O. (2005). Exercise treatment for depression: Efficacy and dose response. *American Journal of Preventive Medicine, 28*(1), 1–8.

Description of the Study: The purpose of this study was to examine (1) whether exercise is an efficacious treatment for mild to moderate major depressive disorder (MDD), and (2) the dose-response relation of exercise and reduction in depressive symptoms. Subjects included 80 men and women ages 20 to 45 years who had been diagnosed with mild to moderate MDD. Subjects were screened and eliminated from the study if they were 160 percent over ideal weight, consumed more than 21 drinks per week, had attempted suicide in the last 2 years or were assessed as a suicide risk, had been hospitalized for a psychiatric disorder in the last 5 years, were unable to exercise because of a medical condition, or were pregnant or planned to become pregnant. Measurement of depression was determined using the Hamilton Rating Scale for Depression (HRSD) at baseline and after 12 weeks of exercise intervention. Subjects were randomly assigned to 1 of 4 study groups: low-dose (7 kcal/kg per week) exercise 3 times a week (LD/3), public health recommended dose (17.5 kcal/kg per week) exercise 3 times a week (PHD/3), low-dose exercise 5 times a week (LD/5), public health dose exercise 5 times a week (PHD/5), or the control group, which was defined as 3 days per week of stretching flexibility exercise for 15 to 20 minutes per

session. The exercise groups received aerobic training on a treadmill or stationary bicycle.

Results of the Study: Forty-six percent of participants in the PHD group had a therapeutic response to treatment, defined as a 50 percent reduction in baseline HRSD score, and 42 percent of the PHD group had remission of symptoms, defined as an HRSD ___ group did not respond any bet___ control group, although both ___ depressive symptoms. The find___ for the 3-day/week and the 5-___ that the determining factor fo___ symptoms is total energy exp___ remission rates in the PHD gr___ depression treatments, such ___ behavioral therapy.

Implications for Nursing Prac___ amount recommended by c___ recommendations was found to be an effective monotherapy in treating mild to moderate MDD. This is important information for nurses who work in all types of practice settings. Many depressed clients do not seek therapy from psychiatric professionals, and many do not want to take antidepressant medication. Nurses can educate clients about the positive effects of exercise for relief from mild to moderate depression.

> Updated studies on **Implications of Research for Evidence-Based Practice** throughout the major clinical chapters provide research-based evidence for specific nursing interventions

ANGER AND AGGRESSION, DEFINED

Core Concept

Anger

Anger is an emotional state that varies in intensity from mild irritation to intense fury and rage. It is accompanied by physiological and biological changes, such as increases in heart rate, blood pressure, and levels of the hormones epinephrine and norepinephrine (American Psychological Association, 2005a).

Anger is a normal, healthy emotion that serves as a warning signal and alerts us to potential threat or trauma. It tri___rs energy that sets us up for a good fight or quick ___d can range from mild irritation to hot, fiery ___utterfield, 2000). Warren (1990) outlines some ___tal points about anger:

> New **Core Concept boxes** emphasize terms and ideas central to understanding the content

___ is not a primary emotion, but it is typically ___ienced as an almost automatic inner response to hurt, frustration, or fear.
2. Anger is physiological arousal. It instills feelings of power and generates preparedness.
3. Anger and aggression are significantly different.
4. The expression of anger is learned.
5. The expression of anger can come under personal control.

Anger is a very powerful emotion. When it is denied or buried, it can precipitate a number of physical problems such as migraine headaches, ulcers, colitis, and even coronary heart disease. When turned inward on oneself, anger can result in depression and low self-esteem. When it is expressed inappropriately, it commonly interferes with relationships. When suppressed, anger may turn into resentment, which often manifests itself in negative, passive-aggressive behavior.

Anger creates a state of preparedness by arousing the sympathetic nervous system. The activation of this system results in increased heart rate and blood pressure, increased secretion of epinephrine (resulting in additional physiological arousal), and increased levels of serum glucose, among others. Anger prepares the body, physiologically, to fight. When anger goes unresolved, this physiological arousal can be the predisposing factor to a number of health problems. Even if the situation that created the anger is removed by miles or years, it can be replayed through the memory, reactivating the sympathetic arousal when this occurs.

Table 17-1 lists positive and negative functions of anger.

Core Concept

Aggression

Aggression is a behavior intended to threaten or injure the victim's security or self-esteem. It means "to go against," "to assault," or "to attack." It is a response that aims at inflicting pain or injury on objects or persons. Whether the damage is caused by words, fists, or weapons, the behavior is virtually always designed to punish. It is frequently accompanied by bitterness, meanness, and ridicule. An aggressive person is often vengeful (Warren, 1990, p. 81).

The term *anger* often takes on a negative connotation because of its link with aggression. Aggression is one way individuals express anger. It is sometimes used to try to force someone into compliance with the aggressor's wishes, but at other times the only objective seems to be the infliction of punishment and pain. In virtually all instances, aggression is a negative function or destructive use of anger.

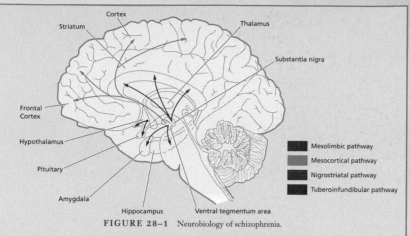

FIGURE 28-1 Neurobiology of schizophrenia.

Legend:
- Mesolimbic pathway
- Mesocortical pathway
- Nigrostriatal pathway
- Tuberoinfundibular pathway

NEW NEUROBIOLOGICAL CONTENT

New to this edition is an increased focus on the biological and behavioral components of mental illness

■ **New! Emphasis on biological causes** of disease, including anxiety disorders, bipolar disorder, dementia, depression, schizophrenia, and other DSM disorders

New! Unique color brain schematic illustrations show neurotransmitter pathways, identify the areas of the brain affected by specific diseases, and presents information on related psychotropics and their possible side effects

Neurotransmitters

A number of neurotransmitters have been implicated in the etiology of schizophrenia. These include dopamine, tamate, and GABA. The dopaminergic system has been most widely studied and closely linked to the symp

Areas of the Brain Affected

- Four major dopaminergic pathways have been identified:
  - *Mesolimbic pathway:* Originates in the ventral tegmentum area and projects to areas of the limbic syst amygdala, and hippocampus. The mesolimbic pathway is associated with functions of memory, er activity in the mesolimbic tract has been implicated in the positive symptoms of schizophrenia (e.g.,
  - *Mesocortical pathway:* originates in the ventral tegmentum area and has projections into the cortex. T with cognition, social behavior, planning, problem solving, motivation, and reinforcement in lear phrenia (e.g., flat affect, apathy, lack of motivation, and anhedonia) have been associated with diminish
  - *Nigrostriatal pathway:* originates in the substantia nigra and terminates in the striatum of the basal ganglia. This pathway is associated with the function of motor control. Degeneration in this pathway is associated with Parkinson's disease and involuntary psychomotor symptoms of schizophrenia.
  - *Tuberoinfundibular pathway:* originates in the hypothalamus and projects to the pituitary gland. It is associated with endocrine function, digestion, metabolism, hunger, thirst, temperature control, and sexual arousal. Implicated in certain endocrine abnormalities associated with schizophrenia.
- Two major groups of dopamine receptors and their highest tissue locations include:
  - The D_1 Family:
    - D_1 receptors: basal ganglia, nucleus accumbens, and cerebral cortex
    - D_5 receptors: hippocampus and hypothalamus, with lower concentrations in the cerebral cortex and basal ganglia
  - The D_2 Family:
    - D_2 receptors: basal ganglia, anterior pituitary, cerebral cortex, limbic structures
    - D_3 receptors: limbic regions, with lower concentrations in basal ganglia
    - D_4 receptors: frontal cortex, hippocampus, amygdala

Antipsychotic Medications

Type	Receptor Affinity	Associated Side Effects
Conventional (typical) antipsychotics:	Strong D_2 (dopamine)	EPS, hyperprolactinemia, Neuroleptic Malignant
Phenothiazines	Varying degrees of affinity for:	Syndrome
Haloperidol	(cholinergic) Ach	Anticholinergic effects
Provide relief of psychosis, improvement in	α_1 (norepinephrine)	Tachycardia, tremors, insomnia, postural hypotension
positive symptoms, worsening of negative	H (histamine)	Weight gain, sedation

UNIQUE AND USEFUL TOOLS

A wide range of resources will help students with their understanding of how to care for their clients

New! Two dozen Concept Map Care Plans—which are innovative visual care maps—offer students a way to succinctly visualize client problems and interventions

■ Care plans, critical pathways, and case studies
■ Ancillary material includes **23 Client Education Teaching Guides** for patient teaching and quick review of select psychiatric illnesses and psychotropic medications

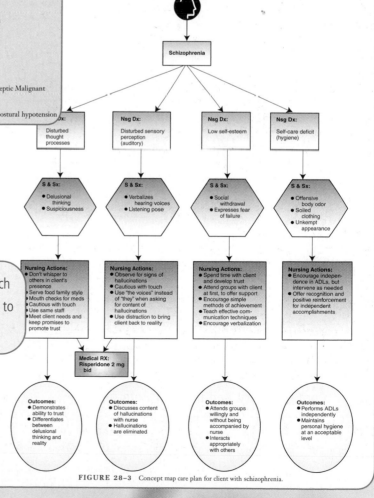

FIGURE 28-3 Concept map care plan for client with schizophrenia.

Schizophrenia

| Nsg Dx: Disturbed thought processes | Nsg Dx: Disturbed sensory perception (auditory) | Nsg Dx: Low self-esteem | Nsg Dx: Self-care deficit (hygiene) |

S & Sx:
- Delusional thinking
- Suspiciousness

S & Sx:
- Verbalizes hearing voices
- Listening pose

S & Sx:
- Social withdrawal
- Expresses fear of failure

S & Sx:
- Offensive body odor
- Soiled clothing
- Unkempt appearance

Nursing Actions:
- Don't whisper to others in client's presence
- Serve food family style
- Mouth checks for meds
- Cautious with touch
- Use same staff
- Meet client needs and keep promises to promote trust

Nursing Actions:
- Observe for signs of hallucinations
- Cautious with touch
- Use "the voices" instead of "they" when asking for content of hallucinations
- Use distraction to bring client back to reality

Nursing Actions:
- Spend time with client and develop trust
- Attend groups with client at first, to offer support
- Encourage simple methods of achievement
- Teach effective communication techniques
- Encourage verbalization

Nursing Actions:
- Encourage independence in ADLs, but intervene as needed
- Offer recognition and positive reinforcement for independent accomplishments

Medical RX: Risperidone 2 mg bid

Outcomes:
- Demonstrates ability to trust
- Differentiates between delusional thinking and reality

Outcomes:
- Discusses content of hallucinations with nurse
- Hallucinations are eliminated

Outcomes:
- Attends groups willingly and without being accompanied by nurse
- Interacts appropriately with others

Outcomes:
- Performs ADLs independently
- Maintains personal hygiene at an acceptable level

UP TO DATE

The full color, fifth edition of Mary Townsend's *Psychiatric Mental Health Nursing: Concepts of Care in Evidence-Based Practice* has been updated with new chapters, insets, and special features while retaining the clear reader-friendly structure students and educators appreciate.

21
CHAPTER

PSYCHOPHARMACOLOGY

Chapters begin with a **Chapter Outline, Key Terms, Objectives, and Core Concepts**

CHAPTER OUTLINE

OBJECTIVES
HISTORICAL PERSPECTIVES
HOW DO PSYCHOTROPICS WORK?

APPLYING THE NURSING PROCESS IN
PSYCHOPHARMACOLOGICAL THERAPY
SUMMARY
REVIEW QUESTIONS

■ New Medication tables and **updated drug coverage** in the Psychopharmacology chapter and throughout the text and CD-ROM

KEY TERMS

agranulocytosis
akathisia
akinesia
amenorrhea
dystonia
extrapyramidal
  symptoms
gynecomastia

hypertensive crisis
neuroleptic malignant
  syndrome
oculogyric crisis
priapism
retrograde ejaculation
serotonin syndrome
tardive dyskinesia

CORE CONCEPTS

neurotransmitter
psychotropic
  medication
receptor

OBJECTIVES

After reading this chapter, the student will be able to:

1. Discuss historical perspectives related to psychopharmacology.
2. Describe indications, actions, contraindications, precautions, side effects, and nursing implications for the following classifications of drugs:
   a. Antianxiety agents
   b. Antidepressants

c. Mood-stabilizing agents
d. Antipsychotics
e. Antiparkinsonian agents

■ Addresses the themes of the APA's focus on the Decade of Behavior (2000-2010) initiative

8. If the foregoing extrapyramidal symptoms should occur, which of the following would be a priority nursing intervention?
   a. Notify the physician immediately.
   b. Administer p.r.n. trihexyphenidyl (Artane).
   c. Withhold the next dose of antipsychotic medication.
   d. Explain to the client that these symptoms are only temporary and will disappear shortly.

9. A concern with children on long-term therapy with CNS stimulants for ADHD is:
   a. Addiction
   b. Weight gain
   c. Substance abuse
   d. Growth suppression

10. Doses of bupropion should be administered at least 8 hours apart and never doubled when a dose is missed. The reason for this is:
    a. To prevent orthostatic hypotension.
    b. To prevent seizures.
    c. To prevent hypertensive crisis.
    d. ...event extrapyramidal symptoms.

Chapters end with a summary, **NCLEX®-style chapter review questions**, and updated **Classical, Contemporary, and Internet References**

REFERENCES

...5). *Handbook of drug therapy in psychiatry* ...is: C.V. Mosby.
...deline Panel. (1993). *Depression in primary care: Volume 2. Treatment of major depression. Clinical practice guideline*, No. 5. Rockville, MD: U.S. Department of Health and Human Services, Public Health Service, Agency for Health Care Policy and Research. AHCPR Pub. No. 93-0551.
Drug facts and comparison (59th ed.). (2005). St. Louis: Wolters Kluwer.
Glod, C.A., & Levy, S. (1998). Psychopharmacology. In C.A. Glod (Ed.). *Contemporary psychiatric-mental health nursing: The brain-behavior connection*. Philadelphia: F.A. Davis.
Haddad, P.M. (2001). Antidepressant discontinuation syndromes: Clinical relevance, prevention, and management. *Drug Safety*, 24(3), 183-197.

Marangell, L.B., Silver, J.M., Goff, D.C., & Yudofsky, S.C. (2003). Psychopharmacology and electroconvulsive therapy. In R.E. Hales & S.C. Yudofsky (Eds.). *Textbook of clinical psychiatry* (4th ed.). Washington, DC: American Psychiatric Publishing.
Sadock, B.J., & Sadock, V.A. (2003). *Synopsis of psychiatry: Behavioral sciences/clinical psychiatry* (9th ed.). Philadelphia: Lippincott Williams & Wilkins.
Sage, D.L. (Producer) (1984). *The Brain: Madness*. Washington, DC: Public Broadcasting Company.
Schatzberg, A.F., Cole, J.O., & DeBattista, C. (2005). *Manual of clinical psychopharmacology* (5th ed.). Washington, DC: American Psychiatric Publishing.
Tandon, R., & Jibson, M.D. (2003). Safety and tolerability: How do second-generation atypical antipsychotics compare? *Current Psychosis & Therapeutic Reports, 1,* 15-21.

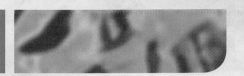

Still the most clearly written comprehensive source of information on psychiatric and mental health nursing

---

TEST YOUR CRITICAL THINKING SKILLS

Jimmy, age 9, has been admitted to the child psychiatric unit with a diagnosis of attention-deficit/hyperactivity disorder. He has been unmanageable at school and at home, and was recently suspended from school for continuous disruption of his class. He refuses to sit in his chair or do his work. He yells out in class, interrupts the teacher and the other students, and lately has become physically aggressive when he cannot have his way. He was suspended after hitting his teacher when she asked him to return to his seat.

Jimmy's mother describes him as a restless and demanding baby, who grew into a restless and demanding toddler. He has never gotten along well with his peers. Even as a small child, he would take his friends' toys away from them or bite them if they tried to hold their own with him. His 5-year-old sister is afraid of him and refuses to be alone with him.

During the nurse's intake assessment, Jimmy paced the

room or rocked in his chair. He talked incessantly on a superficial level and jumped from topic to topic. He told the nurse that he did not know why he was there. He acknowledged that he had some problems at school but said that was only because the other kids picked on him and the teacher did not like him. He said he got into trouble at home sometimes but that was because his parents liked his little sister better than they liked him.

The physician has ordered methylphenidate, 5 mg twice a day for Jimmy. His response [...] not going to take drugs. I'm not si[...]

Answer the following questions rela[...]

1. What are the pertinent assessme[...] the nurse?
2. What is the primary nursing diagnosis for Jimmy?
3. Aside from client safety, to what problems would the nurse want to direct intervention with Jimmy?

> **Test Your Critical Thinking Skills**
> boxes offer case studies and exercises

---

how he or she will respond in the future. A determination is made regarding follow-up therapy; if needed, the nurse provides referral information.

DISASTER NURSING

Although there are many definitions of **disaster**, a common feature is that the event overwhelms local resources and threatens the function and safety of the community (Norwood, Ursano, & Fullerton, 2004). A violent disaster, whether natural or manmade, may leave devastation of property or life. Such tragedies also leave victims with a damaged sense of safety and well-being, and varying degrees of emotional trauma (Oklahoma State Department of Health [OSDH], 2001). Children, who lack life experiences and coping skills, are particularly vulnerable. Their sense of order and security has been seriously disrupted, and they are unable to understand that the disruption is time limited and that their world will eventually return to normal.

APPLICATION OF THE NURSING PROCESS

Background Assessment Data

Individuals respond to traumatic events in many ways. Grieving is a natural response following any loss, and it may be more extreme if the disaster is directly experienced or witnessed (OSDH, 2001). The emotional effects of loss and disruption may show up immediately or may appear weeks or months later.

Psychological and behavioral responses common in adults following trauma and disaster include anger; disbelief; sadness; anxiety; fear; irritability; arousal; numbing; sleep disturbance; and increases in alcohol, caffeine, and tobacco use (Norwood, Ursano, & Fullerton, 2004). Preschool children commonly experience separation anxiety, regressive behaviors, nightmares, and hyperactive or withdrawn behaviors. Older children may have difficulty concentrating, somatic complaints, sleep disturbances, and concerns about safety. Adolescents' responses are often similar to those of adults.

Norwood, Ursano, and Fullerton (2004) state:

Nursing Diagnoses/Outcome Identification

Information from the assessment is analyzed, and appropriate nursing diagnoses reflecting the immediacy of the situation are identified. Some nursing diagnoses that may be relevant include:

- Risk for injury (trauma, suffocation, poisoning)
- Risk for infection
- Anxiety (panic)
- Fear
- Spiritual distress
- Risk for post-trauma syndrome
- Ineffective community coping

The following criteria may be used for measur[...] outcomes in the care of the client having experi[...] traumatic event.

The client:

1. Experiences minimal/no injury to self.
2. Demonstrates behaviors necessary to protect self from further injury.
3. Identifies interventions to prevent/reduce risk of infection.
4. Is free of infection.
5. Maintains anxiety at manageable level.
6. Expresses beliefs and values about spiritual issues.
7. Demonstrates ability to deal with emotional reactions in an individually appropriate manner.
8. Demonstrates an increase in activities to improve community functioning.

Planning/Implementation

Table 13–1 provides a plan of care for the client who has experienced a traumatic event. Selected nursing diagnoses are presented, along with outcome criteria, appropriate nursing interventions, and rationales for each.

Evaluation

In the final step of the nursing process, a reassessment is conducted to determine if the nursing actions have been successful in achieving the objectives of care. Evaluation of the nursing actions for the client who has experienced

> New and updated sections on **Disaster Nursing** (in Chapter 13), **Culture-bound syndrome** (in Chapter 6), and **Anger Management (in Chapter 17)**, with care plans, interventions, outcomes, and rationales

■ New Chapter on caring for **The Bereaved Individual** (Chapter 45)

■ The latest NANDA Taxonomy II (2005-2006) is used throughout the text

Be sure to visit www.fadavis.com/townsend for more resources

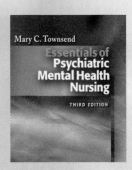
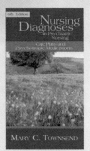
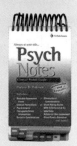

PSYCHIATRIC MENTAL HEALTH NURSING

CONCEPTS OF CARE IN EVIDENCE-BASED PRACTICE

FIFTH EDITION

MARY C. TOWNSEND, MN, APRN, BC

Clinical Specialist/Nurse Consultant
Adult Psychiatric Mental Health Nursing

Former Assistant Professor and
Coordinator, Mental Health Nursing
Kramer School of Nursing
Oklahoma City University
Oklahoma City, OK

F. A. DAVIS COMPANY / PUBLISHERS • PHILADELPHIA

F. A. Davis Company
1915 Arch Street
Philadelphia, PA 19103
www.fadavis.com

Printed in the United States of America

Last digit indicates print number: 10 9 8 7 6 5 4 3 2 1

Publisher, Nursing: Robert G. Martone
Project Editor, Nursing: Tom Ciavarella
Interior Design: Paul Fry
Cover Design: Emily Betsch

As new scientific information becomes available through basic and clinical research, recommended treatments and drug therapies undergo changes. The author(s) and publisher have
done everything possible to make this book accurate, up to date, and in accord with accepted
standards at the time of publication. The author(s), editors, and publisher are not responsible
for errors or omissions or for consequences from application of the book, and make no war-
ranty, expressed or implied, in regard to the contents of the book. Any practice described in
this book should be applied by the reader in accordance with professional standards of care
used in regard to the unique circumstances that may apply in each situation. The reader is advised always to check product information (package inserts) for changes and new information
regarding dose and contraindications before administering any drug. Caution is especially
urged when using new or infrequently ordered drugs.

Library of Congress Cataloging-in-Publication Data

Townsend, Mary C., 1941–
Psychiatric mental health nursing: concepts of care in evidence-based practice/Mary C.
Townsend–5th ed.
   p. ; cm.
 Includes bibliographical references and index.
 ISBN 0-8036-1451-9
 1. Psychiatric nursing.
[DNLM: 1. Psychiatric Nursing–methods. 2. Evidence-Based Medicine. 3. Mental
Disorders– nursing. 4. Psychotherapy–methods. WY 160 T749p 2006] I. Title.
RC440.T693 2006
616.89'0231–dc22

                          2005053758

THIS BOOK IS DEDICATED TO:

FRANCIE

GOD MADE SISTERS FOR SHARING LAUGHTER AND WIPING TEARS

ACKNOWLEDGMENTS

I owe a great deal of thanks to many people who supported me with their time and encouragement throughout this revision. To name a few, I thank:

ROBERT G. MARTONE, Publisher, Nursing, F. A. Davis Company, for your sense of humor and continuous optimistic outlook about the outcome of this project.

TOM CIAVARELLA, Project Editor, Nursing, F. A. Davis Company, for all your help and support in preparing the manuscript for publication.

JANE K. BRODY, Associate Professor, Nursing Department, Nassau Community College, and GOLDEN M. TRADEWELL, Chair, Department of Nursing, Southern Arkansas University for your assistance in preparing the test bank to accompany this textbook.

SANDRA MITCHELL, Assistant Professor of Nursing, and MATILDA KIRBY-SMITH, Coordinator of Instructional Technologies, Guilford Technical Community College, for your assistance in preparing the PowerPoint presentation to accompany this textbook.

THE NURSING EDUCATORS AND CLINICIANS who provide input and help keep me informed about current clinical and state-of-the-discipline issues.

MY DAUGHTERS, KERRY AND TINA, for all the joy you have provided me and all the hope that you instill in me. I'm so thankful that I have you.

MY GRANDDAUGHTER, MEGHAN, for showing me what life is truly all about. I am blessed by your very presence.

MY FURRY FRIENDS, BUCKY, CHIRO, AND ANGEL, for the pure pleasure you bring into my life every day that you live.

MY HUSBAND, JIM, who gives meaning to my life in so many ways. You are the one whose encouragement keeps me motivated, whose support gives me strength, and whose gentleness gives me comfort.

CONSULTANTS

ANGELINE CURTIS, BSN, MS, APRN-BC
Clinical Nurse Specialist, Mental Health Service Line
VA Medical Center
Decatur, GA

JANINE GRAF-KIRK, RN, BC, MA
Professor and Course Coordinator
for Psychiatric Mental Health Nursing
Trinitas School of Nursing
Elizabeth, New Jersey

DOTTIE IRVIN, DNS, APRN, BC
Associate Professor
St. John's College
Springfield, Illinois

PHYLLIS M. JACOBS, RN, MSN
Assistant Professor; Director, Undergraduate
Nursing Program
Wichita State University School of Nursing
Wichita, Kansas

CAROL T. MILLER, APRN-PMH, BC
Assistant Professor
Frederick Community College
Frederick, Maryland

PATRICIA NUTZ, RN, MSN, MEd
Professional Nurse Educator
School of Nursing
Jameson Memorial Hospital
New Castle, Pennsylvania

DARLENE D. PEDERSEN, MSN, APRN, BC
Director and Psychotherapist, PsychOptions
Glen Mills, Pennsylvania

KATHY WHITLEY, RN, MSN, FNP-C
Associate Professor, Nursing
Patrick Henry Community College
Martinsville, Virginia

MARA LYNN WILLIAMS, RN, BC
Program Director, Psychiatry
Intrepid USA Healthcare Services
Montgomery, Alabama

TO THE INSTRUCTOR

There is a saying that captures the spirit of our times—the only constant is change. The twenty-first century continues to bring about a great deal of change in the health care system in general and to nursing in particular. The body of knowledge in nursing continues to grow and expand as rapidly as nursing undergoes change. Nurses must draw upon this research base to support the care that they provide for their clients. This fifth edition of *Psychiatric Mental Health Nursing: Concepts of Care in Evidence-Based Practice* strives to present a holistic approach to evidence-based psychiatric nursing practice.

Just what does this mean? Research in nursing has been alive for decades. But over the years there has always existed a significant gap between research and practice. Evidence-based nursing has become a common theme within the nursing community. It has been defined as a process by which nurses make clinical decisions using the best available research evidence, their clinical expertise, and client preferences. Nurses are accountable to their clients to provide the highest quality of care based on knowledge of what is considered best practice. Change occurs so rapidly that what is considered best practice today may not be considered so tomorrow, based on newly acquired scientific data.

Included in this fifth edition are a number of new research studies that support psychiatric nursing interventions. As nurses, we are bombarded with new information and technological content on a daily basis. Not all of this information yields knowledge that can be used in clinical practice. It is our hope that the information in this new edition will serve to further the movement toward evidence-based practice in psychiatric nursing. There is still a long way to go, and research utilization is the foundation from which to advance the progression.

Well into the first decade of the new century, there are many new challenges to be faced. In 2002, President George W. Bush established the New Freedom Commission on Mental Health. This commission was charged with the task of conducting a comprehensive study of the United States mental health service delivery system. They were to identify unmet needs and barriers to services and recommend steps for improvement in services and support for individuals with serious mental illness. In July 2003, the commission presented its final report to the President. The Commission identified the following barriers: fragmentation and gaps in mental health care for children, adults with serious mental illness, and the elderly; and high unemployment and disability for people with serious mental illness. The report also pointed out that the fact that the U.S. has failed to identify mental health and suicide prevention as national priorities has put many lives at stake. The Commission outlined the following goals and recommendations for mental health reform:

- To address mental health with the same urgency as physical health
- To align relevant Federal programs to improve access and accountability for mental health services
- To ensure appropriate care is available for every child with a serious emotional disturbance and every adult with a serious mental illness
- To protect and enhance the rights of people with mental illness
- To improve access to quality care that is culturally competent
- To improve access to quality care in rural and geographically remote areas
- To promote mental health screening, assessment, and referral services
- To accelerate research to promote recovery and resilience, and ultimately to cure and prevent mental illness
- To advance evidence-based practices using dissemination and demonstration projects, and create a public-private partnership to guide their implementation
- To improve and expand the workforce providing evidence-based mental health services and supports
- To promote the use of technology to access mental health care and information

If these proposals become reality, it would surely mean improvement in the promotion of mental health and the care of mentally ill individuals. Many nurse leaders see this period of health care reform as an opportunity for nurses to expand their roles and assume key positions in education, prevention, assessment, and referral. Nurses are, and will continue to be, in key positions to assist individuals with mental illness to remain as independent as possible, to manage their illness within the community setting, and to strive to minimize the number of hospitalizations required.

In 2020, the ten leading causes of mortality throughout the world are projected to include heart disease; cerebrovascular disease; pulmonary disease; lower respiratory infections; tracheal, bronchial and lung cancers; traffic accidents; tuberculosis; stomach cancer; HIV/AIDS; and suicide. Behavior is an important element in prevention of these causes of mortality and in their treatment. In 2020, the three leading causes of disability throughout the world are projected to include heart disease, major depression, and traffic accidents. Behavior is once again an important underpinning of these three contributors of disability, and behavioral and social science research can lower the impact of these causes of morbidity and mortality. Many of these issues are addressed in this new edition.

CONTENT AND FEATURES NEW TO THIS EDITION

New chapter on caring for The Bereaved Individual (Chapter 45). This chapter identifies various theoretical perspectives of grieving. Normal and maladaptive responses to loss are described. Grieving behaviors common to individuals of various ages and cultures are discussed. The nursing process, including a nursing care plan, is applied to bereaved individuals. The concepts of hospice care and advanced directives are presented.

New content on Culture-Bound Syndromes (Chapter 6).

New content related to Neurobiological processes (Chapters 26, 28, 29, 30, and 40). The neurobiology of dementia, schizophrenia, depression, anxiety disorders, and violence is presented in the chapters that deal with these disorders. Illustrations of the neurotransmitter pathways and discussion of areas of the brain affected and the medications that target those areas are presented.

New medication tables (in addition to the chapter on Psychopharmacology) (Chapters 26, 28, and 29). New medication tables have been added to provide convenient, easy access to information related to medications that are relevant to specific psychiatric disorders (dementia, schizophrenia, depression, mania).

New content on Concept Mapping. Concept mapping is discussed in Chapter 9. Concept mapping is a diagrammatic teaching and learning strategy that allows students and faculty to visualize interrelationships between medical diagnoses, nursing diagnoses, assessment data, and treatments. The **concept map care plan** is an innovative approach to planning and organizing nursing care. Basically, it is a diagram of client problems and interventions. Compared to the commonly used column format care plans, concept map care plans are more succinct. They are practical, realistic, and time saving, and they serve to enhance critical-thinking skills and clinical

reasoning ability. Twenty-four (24) concept map care plans have been included with the diagnostic categories in this textbook.

New boxes that define core concepts (all chapters). Core concepts have been identified at the beginning of each chapter. Boxes with the definitions of these core concepts appear at the appropriate point within the text.

NANDA Taxonomy II (2005) from the *NANDA Nursing Diagnoses: Definitions & Classification 2005–2006* (NANDA International). Used throughout the text.

New and updated psychotropic medication information (Chapter 21 and in relevant clinical chapters).

New research studies with implications for evidence-based practice. (In all relevant clinical chapters.)

A new Student CD-ROM.

FEATURES THAT HAVE BEEN RETAINED

The major conceptual framework of stress-adaptation has been retained for its ease of comprehensibility and workability in the realm of psychiatric nursing. This framework continues to emphasize the multiple causation of mental illness while accepting the increasing biological implications in the etiology of certain disorders.

The concept of holistic nursing is retained in the fifth edition. The author has attempted to ensure that the physical aspects of psychiatric/mental health nursing are not overlooked. Both physical and psychosocial nursing diagnoses are included for physiological disorders (such as asthma, migraine headache, and HIV disease) and for psychological disorders (such as depression and anxiety). In all relevant situations, the mind/body connection is addressed.

Nursing process is retained in the fifth edition as the tool for delivery of care to the individual with a psychiatric disorder or to assist in the primary prevention or exacerbation of mental illness symptoms. The six steps of the nursing process, as described in the *ANA Standards of Clinical Nursing Practice, 2nd Ed.* (1998), are used to provide guidelines for the nurse. These standards of care are included for the *DSM-IV-TR* diagnoses, as well as the aging individual, the individual with HIV disease, and as examples in several of the therapeutic approaches. The six steps include:

Assessment: Data collection, under the format of *Background Assessment Data: Symptomatology*, which provides extensive assessment data for the nurse to draw upon when performing an assessment. Several assessment tools are also included.

Diagnosis: Analysis of the data is included from which nursing diagnoses common to specific psychiatric disorders are derived.

Outcome Identification: Outcomes are derived from the nursing diagnoses and stated as measurable goals.

Planning: A plan of care is presented with selected nursing diagnoses for all *DSM-IV-TR* diagnoses, as well as for the elderly client, the client with HIV disease, the elderly homebound client, the primary caregiver of the client with a chronic mental illness, and the bereaved individual. *Critical Pathways of Care* are included for clients in alcohol withdrawal, schizophrenic psychosis, depression, manic episode, PTSD, and anorexia nervosa. The planning standard also includes tables that list topics for educating clients and families about mental illness. **New to this edition: Concept map care plans for all major psychiatric diagnoses.**

Implementation: The interventions that have been identified in the plan of care are included along with rationale for each. Case studies at the end of each *DSM-IV-TR* chapter assist the student in the practical application of theoretical material. Also included as a part of this particular standard is Unit III of the textbook: *Therapeutic Approaches in Psychiatric Nursing Care.* This section of the textbook addresses psychiatric nursing intervention in depth, and frequently speaks to the differentiation in scope of practice between the basic level psychiatric nurse and the advanced practice level psychiatric nurse. Advanced practice nurses with prescriptive authority will find the extensive chapter on psychopharmacology particularly helpful.

Evaluation: The evaluation standard includes a set of questions that the nurse may use to assess whether the nursing actions have been successful in achieving the objectives of care.

Tables that list topics for client education (Clinical chapters).

Assigning nursing diagnoses to client behaviors (Appendix E).

Internet references with web site listings for information related to psychiatric disorders (Clinical chapters).

Taxonomy and diagnostic criteria from the *DSM-IV-TR (2000).* Used throughout the text.

Web site. The F. A. Davis/Townsend web site with additional nursing care plans that do not appear in the text, links to psychotropic medications, concept map care plans, and neurobiological content and illustrations.

ADDITIONAL EDUCATIONAL RESOURCES

Faculty may also find the following teaching aids that accompany this textbook helpful:

Instructor's Resource Disk (IRD). This IRD contains:

- **Approximately 800 multiple choice questions** (including new format questions reflecting the latest NCLEX blueprint). The greatest number of these questions has been written at the analysis and synthesis levels.
- **Lecture outlines** for all chapters
- **Learning activities** for all chapters (including answer key)
- **Answers to the Critical Thinking Exercises** from the textbook
- **PowerPoint Presentation** to accompany **all** chapters in the textbook

All chapters throughout the text have been updated and revised to reflect today's health care reformation and to provide information based on the latest current state of the discipline of nursing. It is my hope that the revisions and additions to this fifth edition continue to satisfy a need within psychiatric/mental health nursing practice. Many of the changes reflect feedback that I have received from users of the previous editions. To those individuals I express a heartfelt thanks. I welcome comments in an effort to retain what some have called the "user friendliness" of the text. I hope that this fifth edition continues to promote and advance the commitment to psychiatric/mental health nursing.

MARY C. TOWNSEND

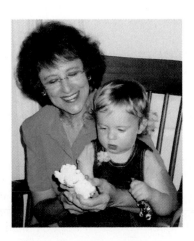

CONTENTS

CHAPTER 12
Milieu Therapy—The Therapeutic Community 184

CHAPTER 13
Crisis Intervention 193

CHAPTER 14
Relaxation Therapy 207

CHAPTER 15
Assertiveness Training 217

CHAPTER 28
Schizophrenia and Other Psychotic Disorders   453

CHAPTER 29
Mood Disorders   483

CHAPTER 30
Anxiety Disorders   523

CHAPTER 31

Somatoform and Sleep Disorders 560

CHAPTER 32

Dissociative Disorders 596

CHAPTER 33

Sexual and Gender Identity Disorders 623

CHAPTER 34

Eating Disorders 653

UNIT FIVE
PSYCHIATRIC/MENTAL HEALTH NURSING OF SPECIAL POPULATIONS

−8 For this thing I besought the LORD thrice...

I Corinthians 12 −9− "My grace is sufficient for thee: for my strength is made perfect in weakness"

10 −− for when I am weak then I am strong.

PSALM 5:4 For thou art not a God that hath pleasure in wickedness: neither shall evil dwell with thee. ↓ it cannot exist in Gods presence.

UNIT ONE

BASIC CONCEPTS IN PSYCHIATRIC/MENTAL HEALTH NURSING

PSALM 14:1
the fool hath said in his heart, There is no God.
They are corrupt, they have done abominable works,
There is none that doeth good −

Ps 5:5
The foolish shall not stand in thy sight: thou hatest all workers of iniquity

Ps 7:11 God judgeth the righteous, and God is angry with the wicked every day.

Psalm 1
− Blessed is the man that walketh not in the counsel of the ungodly, nor standeth in the way of sinners, nor sitteth in the seat of the scornful.
− But his delight is in the law of the LORD; and in his law doth he meditate day and night.
− And he shall be like a tree planted by the rivers of water, that bringeth fruit in season; his leaf also shall not wither; and whatsoever he doeth shall prosper.
− The ungodly are not so: but are like the chaff which the wind driveth away.
− Therefore the ungodly shall not stand in the judgment, nor sinners in the congregation of the righteous
− For the LORD knoweth the way of the righteous; but the way of the ungodly shall perish

THE CONCEPT OF STRESS ADAPTATION

CHAPTER OUTLINE

OBJECTIVES

STRESS AS A BIOLOGICAL RESPONSE ①

STRESS AS AN ENVIRONMENTAL EVENT ②

STRESS AS A TRANSACTION BETWEEN THE ③
INDIVIDUAL AND THE ENVIRONMENT

STRESS MANAGEMENT

SUMMARY

REVIEW QUESTIONS

KEY TERMS

"fight or flight"
   syndrome
general adaptation
   syndrome

precipitating event
predisposing factors

CORE CONCEPTS

adaptation
maladaptation
stressor

OBJECTIVES

After reading this chapter, the student will be able to:

1. Define *adaptation* and *maladaptation*.
2. Identify physiological responses to stress.
3. Explain the relationship between stress and "diseases of adaptation."
4. Describe the concept of stress as an environmental event.
5. Explain the concept of stress as a transaction between the individual and the environment.
6. Discuss adaptive coping strategies in the management of stress.

 sychologists and others have struggled for many years to establish an effective definition of **stress**. This term is used loosely today and still lacks a definitive explanation. Stress may be viewed as an individual's reaction to any change that requires an adjustment or response, which can be physical, mental, or emotional. Responses directed at stabilizing internal biological processes and preserving self-esteem could be viewed as healthy **adaptations to stress**.

Roy (1976) defined adaptive response as behavior that maintains the integrity of the individual. Adaptation is viewed as positive and is correlated with a healthy response. When behavior disrupts the integrity of the individual, it is perceived as **maladaptive**. Maladaptive responses by the individual are considered to be negative or unhealthy.

Various twentieth-century researchers have contributed to several different concepts of stress. Three of these concepts include stress as a biological response, stress as an environmental event, and stress as a transaction between the individual and the environment. This

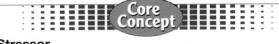

Stressor
A biological, psychological, social, or chemical factor that causes physical or emotional tension and may be a factor in the etiology of certain illnesses.

3

chapter includes an explanation of each of these concepts.

✓ STRESS AS A BIOLOGICAL RESPONSE

In 1956, Hans Selye published the results of his research concerning the physiological response of a biological system to a change imposed on it. Since his initial publication, he has revised his definition of stress, calling it "the state manifested by a specific syndrome which consists of all the nonspecifically-induced changes within a biologic system" (Selye, 1976). This syndrome of symptoms has come to be known as the **"fight or flight syndrome."** Schematics of these biological responses, both initially and with sustained stress, are presented in Figures 1–1 and 1–2. Selye called this general reaction of the body to stress the **general adaptation syndrome**. He described the reaction as a sequence of three distinct stages:

✓1. **Alarm Reaction Stage.** During this stage, the physi-

ological responses of the "fight or flight syndrome" are initiated.

2. **Stage of Resistance.** The individual uses the physiological responses of the first stage as a defense in the attempt to adapt to the stressor. If adaptation occurs, the third stage is prevented or delayed. Physiological symptoms may disappear.

3. **Stage of Exhaustion.** This stage occurs when there is a prolonged exposure to the stressor to which the body has become adjusted. The adaptive energy is depleted, and the individual can no longer draw from the resources for adaptation described in the first two stages. Diseases associated with adaptation (e.g., headaches, mental disorders, coronary artery disease, ulcers, colitis) may occur. Without intervention for reversal, exhaustion ensues, and in some cases even death (Selye, 1956, 1974).

This "fight or flight" response undoubtedly served our

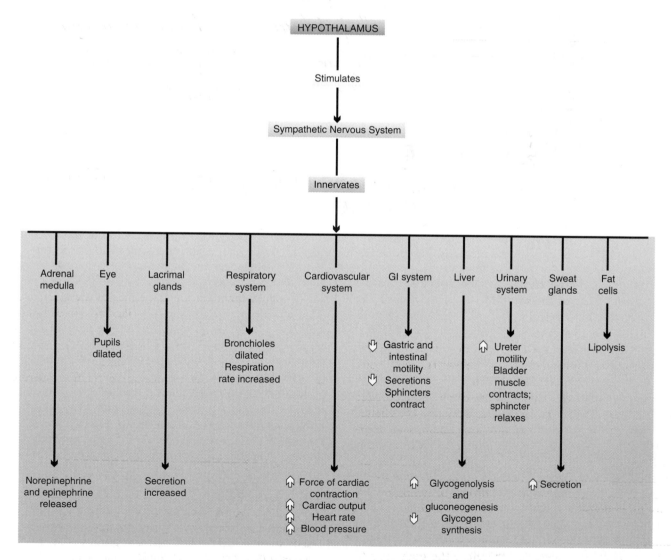

FIGURE 1–1   The "fight or flight" syndrome: the initial stress response.

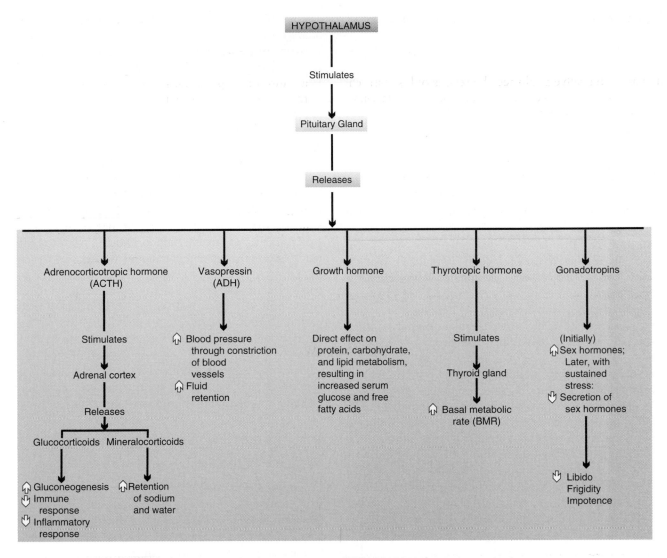

FIGURE 1-2   The "fight or flight" syndrome: the sustained stress response.

ancestors well. Those *Homo sapiens* who had to face the giant grizzly bear or the saber-toothed tiger as a part of their struggle for survival must have used these adaptive resources to their advantage. The response was elicited in emergency situations, used in the preservation of life, and followed by restoration of the compensatory mechanisms to the preemergent condition (homeostasis).

Selye performed his extensive research in a controlled setting with laboratory animals as subjects. He elicited physiological responses with physical stimuli, such as exposure to heat or extreme cold, electric shock, injection of toxic agents, restraint, and surgical injury. Since the publication of his original research, it has become apparent that the "fight or flight" syndrome of symptoms occurs in response to psychological or emotional stimuli, just as it does to physical stimuli. The psychological or emotional stressors are often not resolved as rapidly as some physical stressors, and therefore the body may be depleted of its adaptive energy more readily than it is

from physical stressors. The "fight or flight" response may be inappropriate, even dangerous, to the lifestyle of today, wherein stress has been described as a psychosocial state that is pervasive, chronic, and relentless. It is this chronic response that maintains the body in the aroused condition for extended periods of time that promotes susceptibility to diseases of adaptation (Hafen, Karren, Frandsen, & Smith, 1996).

Core Concept

Adaptation
Adaptation is said to occur when an individual's physical or behavioral response to any change in his or her internal or external environment results in preservation of individual integrity or timely return to equilibrium.

[handwritten: Cognitive Appraisal - individuals evaluation]

[handwritten: Cognitive Response]

STRESS AS AN ENVIRONMENTAL EVENT

A second concept defines stress as the "thing" or "event" that triggers the adaptive physiological and psychological responses in an individual. The event creates change in the life pattern of the individual, requires significant adjustment in lifestyle, and taxes available personal resources. The change can be either positive, such as outstanding personal achievement, or negative, such as being fired from a job. The emphasis here is on *change* from the existing steady state of the individual's life pattern.

Miller and Rahe (1997) have updated the original Social Readjustment Rating Scale devised by Holmes and Rahe in 1967. Just as in the earlier version, numerical values are assigned to various events, or changes, that are common in people's lives. The updated version reflects an increased number of stressors not identified in the original version. In the new study, Miller and Rahe found that women react to life stress events at higher levels of response than men, and unmarried people gave higher scores than married people for most of the events. Younger subjects rated more events at a higher stress level than older subjects. A high score on the Recent Life Changes Questionnaire (RLCQ) places the individual at greater susceptibility to physical or psychological illness. The questionnaire may be completed considering life stressors within either a 6-month or a 1-year period. Six-month totals equal to or greater than 300 life change units (LCUs) or 1-year totals equal to or greater than 500 LCU are considered indicative of a high level of recent life stress, thereby increasing the risk of illness for the individual. The RLCQ is presented in Table 1–1.

[handwritten: 1992]

It is unknown whether stress overload merely predisposes a person to illness or actually precipitates it, but there does appear to be a causal link (Pelletier, 1992). Life changes questionnaires have been criticized because they do not consider the individual's perception of the event. Individuals differ in their reactions to life events, and these variations are related to the degree to which the change is perceived as stressful. These types of instruments also fail to consider the individual's coping strategies and available support systems at the time when the life change occurs. Positive coping mechanisms and strong social or familial support can reduce the intensity of the stressful life change and promote a more adaptive response.

STRESS AS A TRANSACTION BETWEEN THE INDIVIDUAL ✓ AND THE ENVIRONMENT ✓

This definition of stress emphasizes the *relationship* between the individual and the environment. Personal characteristics and the nature of the environmental event

are considered. This illustration parallels the modern concept of the etiology of disease. No longer is causation viewed solely as an external entity; whether or not illness occurs depends also on the receiving organism's susceptibility. Similarly, to predict psychological stress as a reaction, the characteristics of the person in relation to the environment must be considered.

Precipitating Event

Lazarus and Folkman (1984) define *stress* as a relationship between the person and the environment that is appraised by the person as taxing or exceeding his or her resources and endangering his or her well being. A **precipitating event** is a stimulus arising from the internal or external environment and is perceived by the individual in a specific manner. Determination that a particular person/environment relationship is stressful depends on the individual's cognitive appraisal of the situation. *Cognitive appraisal* is an individual's evaluation of the personal significance of the event or occurrence. The event "precipitates" a response on the part of the individual, and the response is influenced by the individual's perception of the event. The *cognitive response* consists of a primary appraisal and a secondary appraisal.

Individual's Perception of the Event

Primary Appraisal *[handwritten: irrelevant benign→positive stressful]*

Lazarus and Folkman (1984) identify three types of primary appraisal: irrelevant, benign-positive, and stressful. An event is judged *irrelevant* when the outcome holds no significance for the individual. A *benign-positive* outcome is one that is perceived as producing pleasure for the individual. *Stress* appraisals include harm/loss, threat, and challenge. *Harm/loss* appraisals refer to damage or loss already experienced by the individual. Appraisals of a *threatening* nature are perceived as anticipated harms or losses. When an event is appraised as *challenging*, the individual focuses on potential for gain or growth, rather than on risks associated with the event. Challenge produces stress even though the emotions associated with it (eagerness and excitement) are viewed as positive, and coping mechanisms must be called on to face the new encounter. Challenge and threat may occur together when an individual experiences these positive emotions along with fear or anxiety over possible risks associated with the challenging event.

When stress is produced in response to harm/loss, threat, or challenge, a secondary appraisal is made by the individual.

Secondary Appraisal

This secondary appraisal is an assessment of skills, resources, and knowledge that the person possesses to deal

TABLE 1–1	The Recent Life Changes Questionnaire		
LIFE CHANGE EVENT	**LCU**	**LIFE CHANGE EVENT**	**LCU**
Health		**Home and Family**	
An injury or illness which:		Major change in living conditions	42
Kept you in bed a week or more, or sent you to the hospital	74	Change in residence:	
Was less serious than above	44	Move within the same town or city	25
Major dental work	26	Move to a different town, city, or state	47
Major change in eating habits	27	Change in family get-togethers	25
Major change in sleeping habits	26	Major change in health or behavior of family member	55
Major change in your usual type/amount of recreation	28	Marriage	50
		Pregnancy	67
Work		Miscarriage or abortion	65
Change to a new type of work	51	Gain of a new family member:	
Change in your work hours or conditions	35	Birth of a child	66
Change in your responsibilities at work:		Adoption of a child	65
More responsibilities	29	A relative moving in with you	59
Fewer responsibilities	21	Spouse beginning or ending work	46
Promotion	31	Child leaving home:	
Demotion	42	To attend college	41
Transfer	32	Due to marriage	41
Troubles at work:		For other reasons	45
With your boss	29	Change in arguments with spouse	50
With coworkers	35	In-law problems	38
With persons under your supervision	35	Change in the marital status of your parents:	
Other work troubles	28	Divorce	59
Major business adjustment	60	Remarriage	50
Retirement	52	Separation from spouse:	
Loss of job:		Due to work	53
Laid off from work	68	Due to marital problems	76
Fired from work	79	Divorce	96
Correspondence course to help you in your work	18	Birth of grandchild	43
		Death of spouse	119
Personal and Social		Death of other family member:	
Change in personal habits	26	Child	123
Beginning or ending school or college	38	Brother or sister	102
Change of school or college	35	Parent	100
Change in political beliefs	24		
Change in religious beliefs	29	**Financial**	
Change in social activities	27	Major change in finances:	
Vacation	24	Increased income	38
New, close, personal relationship	37	Decreased income	60
Engagement to marry	45	Investment and/or credit difficulties	56
Girlfriend or boyfriend problems	39	Loss or damage of personal property	43
Sexual difficulties	44	Moderate purchase	20
"Falling out" of a close personal relationship	47	Major purchase	37
An accident	48	Foreclosure on a mortgage or loan	58
Minor violation of the law	20		
Being held in jail	75		
Death of a close friend	70		
Major decision regarding your immediate future	51		
Major personal achievement	36		

LCU, life change unit.
SOURCE: Miller and Rahe (1997), with permission.

with the situation. The individual evaluates by considering the following:

● What coping strategies are available to me?
● Will the option I choose be effective in this situation?
● Do I have the ability to use that strategy in an effective manner?

The interaction between the primary appraisal of the event that has occurred and the secondary appraisal of available coping strategies determines the quality of the individual's adaptation response to stress.

Predisposing Factors

A variety of elements influence how an individual perceives and responds to a stressful event. These **predisposing factors** strongly influence whether the response is adaptive or maladaptive. Types of predisposing factors include genetic influences, past experiences, and existing conditions.

Genetic influences are those circumstances of an individual's life that are acquired through heredity. Examples include family history of physical and psychological conditions (strengths and weaknesses) and temperament (behavioral characteristics present at birth that evolve with development).

Past experiences are occurrences that result in learned patterns that can influence an individual's adaptation response. They include previous exposure to the stressor or other stressors, learned coping responses, and degree of adaptation to previous stressors.

Existing conditions incorporate vulnerabilities that influence the adequacy of the individual's physical, psychological, and social resources for dealing with adaptive demands. Examples include current health status, motivation, developmental maturity, severity and duration of the stressor, financial and educational resources, age, existing coping strategies, and a support system of caring others.

This transactional model of stress/adaptation will serve as a framework for the process of nursing in this text. A graphic display of the model is presented in Figure 1–3.

> ### Core Concept
>
> **Maladaptation**
> Maladaptation occurs when an individual's physical or behavioral response to any change in his or her internal or external environment results in disruption of individual integrity or in persistent disequilibrium.

STRESS MANAGEMENT*

The growth of stress management into a multimillion-dollar-a-year business attests to its importance in our society. Stress management involves the use of coping strategies in response to stressful situations. Coping strategies are adaptive when they protect the individual from harm (or additional harm) or strengthen the individual's ability to meet challenging situations. Adaptive responses help restore homeostasis to the body and impede the development of diseases of adaptation.

Coping strategies are considered maladaptive when the conflict being experienced goes unresolved or intensifies. Energy resources become depleted as the body struggles to compensate for the chronic physiological and psychological arousal being experienced. The effect is a significant vulnerability to physical or psychological illness. (A detailed discussion of the types of diseases of adaptation can be found in Chapter 36.)

---

*Techniques of stress management are discussed at greater length in Unit 3 of this text.

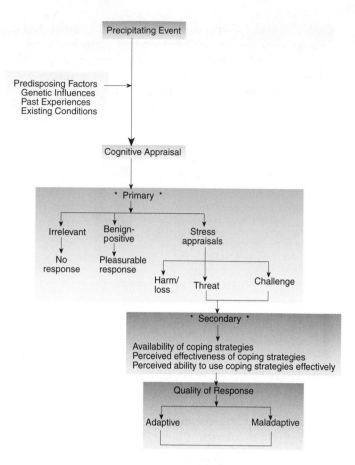

FIGURE 1–3 Transactional model of stress/adaptation.

Adaptive Coping Strategies

Awareness

The initial step in managing stress is awareness—to become aware of the factors that create stress and the feelings associated with a stressful response. Stress can be controlled only when one recognizes that it is being experienced. As one becomes aware of stressors, he or she can omit, avoid, or accept them.

Relaxation

Individuals experience relaxation in different ways. Some individuals relax by engaging in large-motor activities, such as sports, jogging, and physical exercise. Still others use techniques such as breathing exercises and progressive relaxation to relieve stress. (A discussion of relaxation therapy can be found in Chapter 14.)

Meditation *Spiritual*

Practiced for 20 minutes once or twice daily, meditation has been shown to produce a lasting reduction in blood pressure and other stress-related symptoms (Davis, Eshelman, & McKay, 2000). Meditation involves assuming a comfortable position, closing the eyes, casting off all other thoughts, and concentrating on a single word, sound, or phrase that has positive meaning to the individual. The technique is described in detail in Chapter 14.

Interpersonal Communication With a Caring Other *Spiritual*

As previously mentioned, the strength of one's available support systems is an existing condition that significantly influences the adaptiveness of coping with stress. Sometimes just "talking the problem out" with an individual who is empathetic is sufficient to interrupt escalation of the stress response. Writing about one's feelings in a journal or diary can also be therapeutic.

Problem Solving

An extremely adaptive coping strategy is to view the situation objectively (or to seek assistance from another individual to accomplish this if the anxiety level is too high to concentrate). After an objective assessment of the situation, the problem-solving/decision-making model can be instituted as follows:

1. Assess the facts of the situation.
2. Formulate goals for resolution of the stressful situation.
3. Study the alternatives for dealing with the situation.
4. Determine the risks and benefits of each alternative.
5. Select an alternative.
6. Implement the alternative selected.
7. Evaluate the outcome of the alternative implemented.
8. If the first choice is ineffective, select and implement a second option.

Pets

Recent psychological studies have begun to uncover evidence that those who care for pets, especially dogs and cats, are better able to cope with the stressors of life (Allen, Blascovich, & Mendes, 2002). The physical act of stroking or petting a dog or cat can be therapeutic. It gives the animal an intuitive sense of being cared for and at the same time gives the individual the calming feeling of warmth, affection, and interdependence with a reliable, trusting being. One study showed that among people who had had heart attacks, pet owners had one fifth the death rate of those who did not have pets (Friedmann & Thomas, 1995). Another study revealed evidence that individuals experienced a statistically significant drop in blood pressure in response to petting a dog or cat (Whitaker, 2000).

Music

It is true that music can "soothe the savage beast." Creating and listening to music stimulate motivation, enjoyment, and relaxation. Music can reduce depression and bring about measurable changes in mood and general activity.

SUMMARY

Stress has become a chronic and pervasive condition in the United States today. We live in a world of uncertainties, with a sophisticated media that keeps us informed and knowledgeable about the upheavals occurring around the world. In our own country, "life in the fast lane," a continuous drive for advancement, competitiveness, and the search for "the good life" have created a stress epidemic that has individuals, corporations, and health professionals searching for ways to calm the collective masses.

Only in recent years has the term *stress* come into vogue, partly because of the continuing lack of an adequate definition for the concept. Selye, who has become known as the founding father of stress research, defined stress as "the state manifested by a specific syndrome which consists of all the nonspecifically-induced changes within a biologic system." He determined that physical beings respond to stressful stimuli with a predictable set of physiological changes. He described the response in three distinct stages: (1) the alarm reaction stage, (2) the stage of resistance, and (3) the stage of exhaustion. Many illnesses, or diseases of adaptation, have their origin in this aroused state—this preparation for "fight or flight."

Miller and Rahe viewed stress not as the physiological response but as the environmental event that produced the physiological response. Their research centered on the study of life changes, or "events," that trigger the adaptive physiological and psychological responses in an individual. From their research, they devised the Recent Life Changes Questionnaire, which is used to determine an individual's vulnerability to stress-related illness. This concept of stress has received criticism based on its lack of consideration of the individual's personal perception of the event, potential for coping, and available support systems at the time of the life change.

Lazarus and others have expanded the concept of stress to encompass more than just change in an individual's existing steady state or the physiological response it produces. They define stress as a relationship between the person and the environment that is appraised by the person as taxing or exceeding his or her resources and endangering his or her well-being. Response to stimuli from the internal or external environment is determined by the individual's perception of the event through cognitive appraisal. A primary appraisal is made, during which the individual determines the personal significance of the event. If the event is perceived as threatening, the individual then makes a secondary appraisal to determine the availability and effectiveness of coping strategies to manage the stressful situation. The predisposing factors that influence how an individual perceives and responds to a stressful event also need to be considered. Genetic influences, past experiences, and existing conditions strongly influence whether the response is adaptive or maladaptive.

Adaptive responses protect the individual from harm (or additional harm) and help restore homeostasis to the body. They impede the development of diseases of adaptation. With maladaptive responses, conflict goes unresolved, energy resources become depleted, and the individual becomes vulnerable to physical or psychological illness.

Adaptive coping strategies for management of stress are varied and individual. Becoming aware of situations that create stress and the feelings associated with the stress response is an essential foundation in successful stress management.

Relaxation can be achieved by practicing breathing exercises or progressive relaxation techniques. Some individuals relax by exercising, playing sports, or participating in other large-motor activities. *Meditation* for 20 minutes once or twice daily has been shown to be an effective stress-reduction technique for some people. *Interpersonal communication with a caring other* or writing one's feelings in a journal or diary often interrupts escalation of the stress response. Using the *problem-solving/decision-making model* in an objective manner (or seeking assistance in doing so during a crisis situation) is adaptive and gives the individual a feeling of control over his or her life situation. *Pet ownership* has been shown to help individuals better cope with the stressors of life. The reliability and loyalty experienced, along with the giving and receiving of warmth and affection, produce a feeling of security as well as a unique and therapeutic coping strategy for an individual. *Music* is an adaptive coping strategy that has the capacity for stimulating motivation, enjoyment, and relaxation in some people. Additional therapies for assisting individuals to cope adaptively are presented in Unit 3 of this text.

Individual requirements for stress reduction vary widely. Nurses are in a unique position to assist individuals in identifying adaptive coping strategies. Stress has reached epidemic proportions in today's society, and efforts aimed at its control are essential.

REVIEW QUESTIONS

SELF-EXAMINATION/LEARNING EXERCISE

Select the answer that is *most* appropriate for questions 1 through 4.

1. Sondra, who lives in Maine, hears on the evening news that 25 people were killed in a tornado in south Texas. Sondra experiences no anxiety on hearing of this stressful situation. The most likely reason is that Sondra:
   a. Is selfish and does not care what happens to other people.
   b. Appraises the event as irrelevant to her own situation.
   c. Assesses that she has the skills to cope with the stressful situation.
   d. Uses suppression as her primary defense mechanism.

2. Cindy regularly develops nausea and vomiting when she is faced with a stressful situation. Which of the following is most likely a predisposing factor to this maladaptive response by Cindy?
   a. Cindy inherited her mother's "nervous" stomach.
   b. Cindy is fixed in a lower level of development.
   c. Cindy has never been motivated to achieve success.
   d. When Cindy was a child, her mother pampered her and kept her home from school when she was ill.

3. When an individual's stress response is sustained over a long period, the endocrine system involvement results in which of the following?
   a. Decreased resistance to disease
   b. Increased libido
   c. Decreased blood pressure
   d. Increased inflammatory response

4. Management of stress is extremely important in today's society because:
   a. Evolution has diminished human capability for "fight or flight."
   b. The stressors of today tend to be ongoing, resulting in a sustained response.
   c. We have stress disorders that did not exist in the days of our ancestors.
   d. One never knows when one will have to face a grizzly bear or saber-toothed tiger in today's society.

5. Match each of the following situations to its correct component of the Transactional Model of Stress/Adaptation.

   _____ 1. Mr. T is fixed in a lower level of development.   a. Precipitating stressor

   _____ 2. Mr. T's father had diabetes mellitus.   b. Past experiences

   _____ 3. Mr. T has been fired from his last five jobs.   c. Existing conditions

   _____ 4. Mr. T's baby was stillborn last month.   d. Genetic influences

6. Match the following types of primary appraisals to their correct definition of the event as perceived by the individual.

   _____ 1. Irrelevant   a. Perceived as producing pleasure

   _____ 2. Benign-positive   b. Perceived as anticipated harms or losses

   _____ 3. Harm/loss   c. Perceived as potential for gain or growth

   _____ 4. Threat   d. Perceived as having no significance to the individual.

   _____ 5. Challenge   e. Perceived as damage or loss already experienced

REFERENCES

Allen, K., Blascovich, J., & Mendes, W.B. (2002). Cardiovascular reactivity and the presence of pets, friends, and spouses: The truth about cats and dogs. *Psychosomatic Medicine, 64,* 727–739.

Davis, M.D., Eshelman, E.R., & McKay, M. (2000). *The relaxation and stress reduction workbook* (5th ed.). Oakland, CA: New Harbinger Publications.

Friedmann, E., & Thomas, S.A. (1995). Pet ownership, social support, and one-year survival after acute myocardial infarction in the cardiac arrhythmia suppression trial. *American Journal of Cardiology, 76*(17), 1213.

Hafen, B.Q., Karren, K.J., Frandsen, K.J., & Smith, N.L. (1996). *Mind/body health: The effects of attitudes, emotion, and relationships.* Boston: Allyn & Bacon.

Miller, M.A., & Rahe, R.H. (1997). Life changes scaling for the 1990s. *Journal of Psychosomatic Research, 43*(3), 279–292.

Pelletier, K.R. (1992). *Mind as healer, mind as slayer: A holistic approach to preventing stress disorders.* New York: Dell.

Whitaker, J. (2000). Pet owners are a healthy breed. *Health & Healing, 10*(10), 1–8.

CLASSICAL REFERENCES

Holmes, T., & Rahe, R. (1967). The Social Readjustment Rating Scale. *Journal of Psychosomatic Research, 11,* 213–218.

Lazarus, R.S., & Folkman, S. (1984). *Stress, appraisal and coping.* New York: Springer Publishing.

Roy, C. (1976). *Introduction to nursing: An adaptation model.* Englewood Cliffs, NJ: Prentice-Hall.

Selye, H. (1956). *The stress of life.* New York: McGraw-Hill.

Selye, H. (1974). *Stress without distress.* New York: Signet Books.

Selye, H. (1976). *The stress of life (rev. ed.).* New York: McGraw Hill.

MENTAL HEALTH/ MENTAL ILLNESS: HISTORICAL AND THEORETICAL CONCEPTS

CHAPTER OUTLINE

OBJECTIVES

HISTORICAL OVERVIEW OF PSYCHIATRIC CARE

MENTAL HEALTH

MENTAL ILLNESS

PSYCHOLOGICAL ADAPTATION TO STRESS

MENTAL HEALTH/MENTAL ILLNESS CONTINUUM

THE *DSM-IV-TR* MULTIAXIAL EVALUATION SYSTEM

SUMMARY

REVIEW QUESTIONS

KEY TERMS

anticipatory grieving
bereavement overload
defense mechanisms
    compensation
    denial
    displacement
    identification
    intellectualization
    introjection
    isolation
    projection
    rationalization
reaction formation
regression
repression
sublimation
suppression
undoing
humors
mental health
mental illness
neurosis
psychosis
"ship of fools"

CORE CONCEPTS

anxiety
grief

OBJECTIVES

After reading this chapter, the student will be able to:

1. Discuss the history of psychiatric care.
2. Define mental health and mental illness.
3. Discuss cultural elements that influence attitudes toward mental health and mental illness.
4. Describe psychological adaptation responses to stress.
5. Identify correlation of adaptive/maladaptive behaviors to the mental health/mental illness continuum.

he consideration of mental health and mental illness has its basis in the cultural beliefs of the society in which the behavior takes place. Some cultures are quite liberal in the range of behaviors that are considered acceptable, whereas others have very little tolerance for behaviors that deviate from the cultural norms.

A study of the history of psychiatric care reveals some shocking truths about past treatment of mentally ill individuals. Many were kept in control by means that today could be considered less than humane.

This chapter deals with the evolution of psychiatric care from ancient times to the present. **Mental health** and **mental illness** are defined, and the psychological adaptation to stress is explained in terms of the two major responses: **anxiety** and **grief**. A mental health/mental illness continuum and the *Diagnostic and Statistical Manual of Mental Disorders, 4th edition, Text Revision (DSM-IV-TR)*, multiaxial evaluation system are presented.

HISTORICAL OVERVIEW OF PSYCHIATRIC CARE

Primitive beliefs regarding mental disturbances took several views. Some thought that an individual with mental illness had been dispossessed of his or her soul and that the only way wellness could be achieved was if the soul returned. Others believed that evil spirits or supernatural or magical powers had entered the body. The "cure" for these individuals involved a ritualistic exorcism to purge the body of these unwanted forces. This often consisted of brutal beatings, starvation, or other torturous means. Still others considered that the mentally ill individual may have broken a taboo or sinned against another individual or God, for which ritualistic purification was required or various types of retribution were demanded. The correlation of mental illness to demonology or witchcraft led to some mentally ill individuals being burned at the stake.

The position of these ancient beliefs evolved with increasing knowledge about mental illness and changes in cultural, religious, and sociopolitical attitudes. The work of Hippocrates, about 400 B.C., began the movement away from belief in the supernatural. Hippocrates associated insanity and mental illness with an irregularity in the interaction of the four body fluids—blood, black bile, yellow bile, and phlegm. He called these body fluids **humors**, and associated each with a particular disposition. Disequilibrium among these four humors was thought to cause mental illness, and it was often treated by inducing vomiting and diarrhea with potent cathartic drugs.

During the Middle Ages (A.D. 500 to 1500), the association of mental illness with witchcraft and the supernatural continued to prevail in Europe. During this period, many severely mentally ill people were sent out to sea on sailing boats with little guidance to search for their lost rationality. The expression **"ship of fools"** was derived from this operation.

During the same period in the Middle Eastern Islamic countries, however, a change in attitude began to occur, from the perception of mental illness as the result of witchcraft or the supernatural to the idea that these individuals were actually ill. This notion gave rise to the establishment of special units for the mentally ill within general hospitals, as well as institutions specifically designed to house the insane. They can likely be considered the first asylums for the mentally ill.

Colonial Americans tended to reflect the attitudes of the European communities from which they had immigrated. Particularly in the New England area, individuals were punished for behavior attributed to witchcraft. In the 16th and 17th centuries, institutions for the mentally ill did not exist in the United States, and care of these individuals became a family responsibility. Those without family or other resources became the responsibility of the communities in which they lived and were incarcerated in places where they could do no harm to themselves or others.

The first hospital in America to admit mentally ill clients was established in Philadelphia in the middle of the 18th century. Benjamin Rush, often called the father of American psychiatry, was a physician at the hospital. He initiated the provision of humanistic treatment and care for the mentally ill. Although he included kindness, exercise, and socialization, he also employed harsher methods such as bloodletting, purging, various types of physical restraints, and extremes of temperatures, reflecting the medical therapies of that era.

The 19th century brought the establishment of a system of state asylums, largely the result of the work of Dorothea Dix, a former New England schoolteacher, who lobbied tirelessly on behalf of the mentally ill population. She was unfaltering in her belief that mental illness was curable and that state hospitals should provide humanistic therapeutic care. This system of hospital care for the mentally ill grew, but the mentally ill population grew faster. The institutions became overcrowded and understaffed, and conditions deteriorated. Therapeutic care reverted to custodial care. These state hospitals provided the largest resource for the mentally ill until the initiation of the community health movement of the 1960s (see Chapter 42).

The emergence of psychiatric nursing began in 1873 with the graduation of Linda Richards from the nursing program at the New England Hospital for Women and Children in Boston. She has come to be known as the first American psychiatric nurse. During her career, Richards was instrumental in the establishment of a number of psychiatric hospitals and the first school of psychiatric nursing at the McLean Asylum in Waverly, Massachusetts, in 1882. The focus in this school, and those that followed, was "training" in how to provide custodial care for clients in psychiatric asylums—training that did not include the study of psychological concepts. Significant change did not occur until 1955, when incorporation of psychiatric nursing into their curricula became a requirement for all undergraduate schools of nursing.

Nursing curricula emphasized the importance of the nurse–patient relationship and therapeutic communication techniques. Nursing intervention in the somatic therapies (e.g., insulin and electroconvulsive therapy) provided impetus for the incorporation of these concepts into nursing's body of knowledge.

With the apparently increasing need for psychiatric care in the aftermath of World War II, the government passed the National Mental Health Act of 1946. This legislation provided funds for the education of psychiatrists, psychologists, social workers, and psychiatric nurses. Graduate-level education in psychiatric nursing was established during this period. Also significant at this time was the introduction of antipsychotic medications, which made it possible for psychotic clients to more readily participate in their treatment, including nursing therapies.

Knowledge of the history of psychiatric/mental health care contributes to the understanding of the concepts presented in this chapter and those in Chapter 3, which describe the theories of personality development according to various 19th-century and 20th-century leaders in the psychiatric/mental health movement. Modern American psychiatric care has its roots in ancient times. A great deal of opportunity exists for continued advancement of this specialty within the practice of nursing.

MENTAL HEALTH

A number of theorists have attempted to define the concept of mental health. Many of these concepts deal with various aspects of individual functioning. Maslow (1970) emphasized an individual's motivation in the continuous quest for self-actualization. He identified a "hierarchy of needs," the lower ones requiring fulfillment before those at higher levels can be achieved, with self-actualization being fulfillment of one's highest potential. An individual's position within the hierarchy may reverse from a higher level to a lower level based on life circumstances. For example, an individual facing major surgery who has been working on tasks to achieve self-actualization may become preoccupied, if only temporarily, with the need for physiological safety. A representation of this needs hierarchy is presented in Figure 2–1.

Maslow described self-actualization as being "psychologically healthy, fully human, highly evolved, and fully mature." He believed that "healthy," or "self-actualized," individuals possessed the following characteristics:

1. An appropriate perception of reality
2. The ability to accept oneself, others, and human nature
3. The ability to manifest spontaneity
4. The capacity for focusing concentration on problem solving
5. A need for detachment and desire for privacy
6. Independence, autonomy, and a resistance to enculturation
7. An intensity of emotional reaction
8. A frequency of "peak" experiences that validates the worthwhileness, richness, and beauty of life
9. An identification with humankind
10. The ability to achieve satisfactory interpersonal relationships
11. A democratic character structure and strong sense of ethics
12. Creativity
13. A degree of nonconformance

Jahoda (1958) has identified a list of six indicators that she suggests are a reflection of mental health:

1. **A Positive Attitude Toward Self.** This includes an objective view of self, including knowledge and acceptance of strengths and limitations. The individual feels a strong sense of personal identity and a security within the environment.
2. **Growth, Development, and the Ability to Achieve Self-actualization.** This indicator correlates with whether the individual successfully achieves the tasks associated with each level of development (see Erikson, Chapter 3). With successful achievement in each level the individual gains motivation for advancement to his or her highest potential.
3. **Integration.** The focus here is on maintaining an equilibrium or balance among various life processes. Integration includes the ability to adaptively respond to the environment and the development of a philosophy of life, both of which help the individual maintain anxiety at a manageable level in response to stressful situations.
4. **Autonomy.** This refers to the individual's ability to perform in an independent, self-directed manner. The individual makes choices and accepts responsibility for the outcomes.
5. **Perception of Reality.** Accurate reality perception is a positive indicator of mental health. This includes perception of the environment without distortion, as well as the capacity for empathy and social sensitivity—a respect and concern for the wants and needs of others.
6. **Environmental Mastery.** This indicator suggests that the individual has achieved a satisfactory role within the group, society, or environment. It suggests that he or she is able to love and accept the love of others. When faced with life situations, the individual

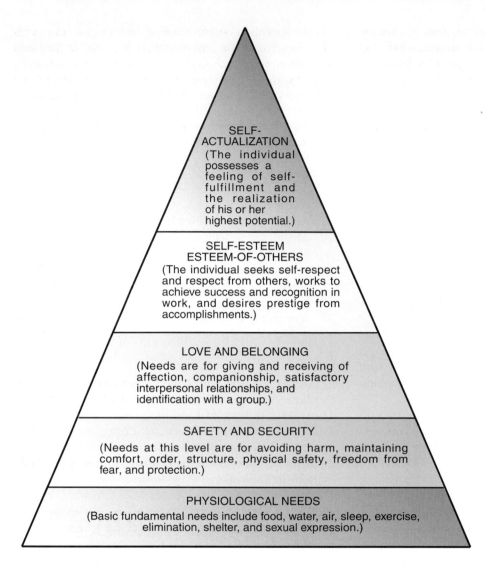

FIGURE 2–1   Maslow's hierarchy of needs.

is able to strategize, make decisions, change, adjust, and adapt. Life offers satisfaction to the individual who has achieved environmental mastery.

The American Psychiatric Association (APA) (2003) defines mental health as:

> A state of being that is relative rather than absolute. The successful performance of mental functions shown by productive activities, fulfilling relationships with other people, and the ability to adapt to change and to cope with adversity.

Robinson (1983) has offered the following definition of mental health:

> a dynamic state in which thought, feeling, and behavior that is age-appropriate and congruent with the local and cultural norms is demonstrated. (p. 74)

For purposes of this text, and in keeping with the framework of stress/adaptation, a modification of Robinson's definition of mental health is considered. Thus, *mental health* is viewed as the successful adaptation to stressors from the internal or external environment, evidenced by thoughts, feelings, and behaviors that are age appropriate and congruent with local and cultural norms.

MENTAL ILLNESS

A universal concept of mental illness is difficult because of the cultural factors that influence such a definition. Certain elements are associated with individuals' perceptions of mental illness, regardless of cultural origin, however. Horwitz (2002) identifies two of these elements as (1) incomprehensibility and (2) cultural relativity.

Incomprehensibility relates to the inability of the general population to understand the motivation behind the behavior. When observers are unable to find meaning or comprehensibility in behavior, they are likely to label that behavior as mental illness. Horwitz states, "Observers attribute labels of mental illness when the rules, conventions, and understandings they use to interpret behavior fail to find any intelligible motivation behind an action." The element of *cultural relativity* considers that these rules, conventions, and understandings are conceived within an individual's own particular culture. Behavior that is considered "normal" and "abnormal" is defined by one's cultural or societal norms. Therefore, a behavior that is recognized as mentally ill in one society may be viewed as "normal" in another society, and vice versa. Horwitz identified a number of cultural aspects of mental illness, which are presented in Table 2–1.

In the *DSM-IV-TR* (American Psychiatric Association [APA], 2000), the APA defined mental illness or a mental disorder as

> a clinically significant behavioral or psychological syndrome or pattern that occurs in a person and that is associated with present distress (e.g., a painful symptom) or disability (i.e., impairment in one or more important areas of functioning), or with a significantly increased risk of suffering death, pain, disability, or an important loss of freedom ... and is not merely an expectable and culturally sanctioned response to a particular event (e.g., the death of a loved one)." (p. xxxi)

TABLE 2–1	Cultural Aspects of Mental Illness

1. Usually members of the lay community, rather than a psychiatric professional, initially recognize that an individual's behavior deviates from societal norms.
2. People who are related to an individual or who are of the same cultural or social group are less likely to label that individual's behavior as mental illness than is someone who is relationally or culturally distant. Relatives (or people of the same cultural or social group) try to "normalize" the behavior; that is, they try to find an explanation for the behavior.
3. Psychiatrists see a person with mental illness most often when the family members can no longer deny the illness and often when the behavior is at its worst. The local or cultural norms define pathological behavior.
4. Individuals in the lowest social class usually display the highest amount of mental illness symptoms. However, they tend to tolerate a wider range of behaviors that deviate from societal norms and are less likely to consider these behaviors as indicative of mental illness. Mental illness labels are most often applied by psychiatric professionals.
5. The higher the social class, the greater the recognition of mental illness behaviors. Members of the higher social classes are likely to be self labeled or labeled by family members or friends. Psychiatric assistance is sought near the first signs of emotional disturbance.
6. The more highly educated the person, the greater the recognition of mental illness behaviors. However, even more relevant than the *amount* of education is the *type* of education. Individuals in the more humanistic types of professions (lawyers, social workers, artists, teachers, nurses) are more likely to seek psychiatric assistance than professionals such as business executives, computer specialists, accountants, and engineers.
7. In terms of religion, Jewish people are more likely to seek psychiatric assistance than are Catholics or Protestants.
8. Women are more likely than men to recognize the symptoms of mental illness and seek assistance.
9. The greater the cultural distance from the *mainstream* of society (i.e., the fewer the ties with *conventional* society), the greater the likelihood of a negative response by society to mental illness. For example, immigrants have a greater distance from the mainstream than the native born, blacks greater than whites, and "bohemians" greater than bourgeoisie. They are more likely to be subjected to coercive treatment, and involuntary psychiatric commitments are more common.

SOURCE: Adapted from Horwitz (2002).

For purposes of this text, and in keeping with the framework of stress/adaptation, *mental illness* is characterized as maladaptive responses to stressors from the internal or external environment, evidenced by thoughts, feelings, and behaviors that are incongruent with the local and cultural norms and that interfere with the individual's social, occupational, and/or physical functioning.

PSYCHOLOGICAL ADAPTATION TO STRESS

All individuals exhibit some characteristics associated with both mental health and mental illness at any given point in time. Chapter 1 described how an individual's response to stressful situations was influenced by his or her personal perception of the event and a variety of predisposing factors, such as heredity, temperament, learned response patterns, developmental maturity, existing coping strategies, and support systems of caring others.

Anxiety and grief have been described as two major, primary psychological response patterns to stress. A variety of thoughts, feelings, and behaviors are associated with each of these response patterns. Adaptation is determined by the degree to which the thoughts, feelings, and behaviors interfere with an individual's functioning.

Core Concept

Anxiety
A diffuse apprehension that is vague in nature and is associated with feelings of uncertainty and helplessness.

Anxiety

Feelings of anxiety are so common in our society that they are almost considered universal. Low levels of anxiety are adaptive and can provide the motivation required for survival. Anxiety becomes problematic when the individual is unable to prevent the anxiety from escalating to a level that interferes with the ability to meet basic needs.

Peplau (1963) described four levels of anxiety: mild, moderate, severe, and panic. It is important for nurses to be able to recognize the symptoms associated with each level to plan for appropriate intervention with anxious individuals.

1. **Mild Anxiety.** This level of anxiety is seldom a problem for the individual. It is associated with the tension experienced in response to the events of day-to-day living. Mild anxiety prepares people for action. It sharpens the senses, increases motivation for productivity, increases the perceptual field, and results in a

heightened awareness of the environment. Learning is enhanced and the individual is able to function at his or her optimal level.

2. **Moderate Anxiety.** As the level of anxiety increases, the extent of the perceptual field diminishes. The moderately anxious individual is less alert to events occurring in the environment. The individual's attention span and ability to concentrate decrease, although he or she may still attend to needs with direction. Assistance with problem solving may be required. Increased muscular tension and restlessness are evident.

3. **Severe Anxiety.** The perceptual field of the severely anxious individual is so greatly diminished that concentration centers on one particular detail only or on many extraneous details. Attention span is extremely limited, and the individual has much difficulty completing even the most simple task. Physical symptoms (e.g., headaches, palpitations, insomnia) and emotional symptoms (e.g., confusion, dread, horror) may

be evident. Discomfort is experienced to the degree that virtually all overt behavior is aimed at relieving the anxiety.

4. **Panic Anxiety.** In this most intense state of anxiety, the individual is unable to focus on even one detail in the environment. Misperceptions are common, and a loss of contact with reality may occur. The individual may experience hallucinations or delusions. Behavior may be characterized by wild and desperate actions or extreme withdrawal. Human functioning and communication with others is ineffective. Panic anxiety is associated with a feeling of terror, and individuals may be convinced that they have a life-threatening illness or fear that they are "going crazy" or losing control (APA, 2000). Prolonged panic anxiety can lead to physical and emotional exhaustion and can be a life-threatening situation.

A synopsis of the characteristics associated with each of the four levels of anxiety is presented in Table 2–2.

TABLE 2–2	**Levels of Anxiety**			
LEVEL	**PERCEPTUAL FIELD**	**ABILITY TO LEARN**	**PHYSICAL CHARACTERISTICS**	**EMOTIONAL/BEHAVIORAL CHARACTERISTICS**
Mild	Heightened perception (e.g., noises may seem louder; details within the environment are clearer) Increased awareness Increased alertness	Learning is enhanced.	Restlessness Irritability	May remain superficial with others. Rarely experienced as distressful. Motivation is increased.
Moderate	Reduction in perceptual field. Reduced alertness to environmental events (e.g., someone talking may not be heard; part of the room may not be noticed)	Learning still occurs, but not at optimal ability. Decreased attention span Decreased ability to concentrate	Increased restlessness Increased heart and respiration rate Increased perspiration Gastric discomfort Increased muscular tension Increase in speech rate, volume, and pitch	A feeling of discontent May lead to a degree of impairment in interpersonal relationships as individual begins to focus on self and the need to relieve personal discomfort.
Severe	Greatly diminished; only extraneous details are perceived, or fixation on a single detail may occur. May not take notice of an event even when attention is directed by another.	Extremely limited attention span. Unable to concentrate or problem-solve. Effective learning cannot occur.	Headaches Dizziness Nausea Trembling Insomnia Palpitations Tachycardia Hyperventilation Urinary frequency Diarrhea	Feelings of dread, loathing, horror Total focus on self and intense desire to relieve the anxiety
Panic	Unable to focus on even one detail within the environment. Misperceptions of the environment are common (e.g., a perceived detail may be elaborated and out of proportion).	Learning cannot occur. Unable to concentrate. Unable to comprehend even simple directions.	Dilated pupils Labored breathing Severe trembling Sleeplessness Palpitations Diaphoresis and pallor Muscular incoordination Immobility or purposeless hyperactivity Incoherence or inability to verbalize	Sense of impending doom. Terror Bizarre behavior, including shouting, screaming, running about wildly, clinging to anyone or anything from which a sense of safety and security is derived. Hallucinations; delusions Extreme withdrawal into self

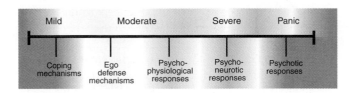

FIGURE 2–2 ● Adaptation responses on a continuum of anxiety.

Behavioral Adaptation Responses to Anxiety

A variety of behavioral adaptation responses occur at each level of anxiety. Figure 2–2 depicts these behavioral responses on a continuum of anxiety ranging from mild to panic.

Mild Anxiety. At the mild level, individuals employ any of a number of coping behaviors that satisfy their needs for comfort. Menninger (1963) described the following types of coping mechanisms that individuals use to relieve anxiety in stressful situations:

- Sleeping
- Eating
- Physical exercise
- Smoking
- Crying
- Pacing
- Yawning
- Drinking
- Daydreaming
- Laughing
- Cursing
- Nail biting

- Foot swinging
- Fidgeting
- Finger tapping
- Talking to someone with whom one feels comfortable

Undoubtedly there are many more responses too numerous to mention here, considering that each individual develops his or her own unique ways to relieve anxiety at the mild level. Some of these behaviors are more adaptive than others.

Mild-to-Moderate Anxiety. Sigmund Freud (1961) identified the ego as the reality component of the personality that governs problem solving and rational thinking. As the level of anxiety increases, the strength of the ego is tested, and energy is mobilized to confront the threat. Anna Freud (1953) identified a number of **defense mechanisms** employed by the ego in the face of threat to biological or psychological integrity. Some of these ego defense mechanisms are more adaptive than others, but all are used either consciously or unconsciously as a protective device for the ego in an effort to relieve mild to moderate anxiety. They become maladaptive when they are used by an individual to such a degree that there is interference with the ability to deal with reality, with effective interpersonal relationships, or with occupational performance. Maladaptive use of defense mechanisms promotes disintegration of the ego. The major ego defense mechanisms identified by Anna Freud are discussed here and summarized in Table 2–3.

TABLE 2–3   Ego Defense Mechanisms

DEFENSE MECHANISM	EXAMPLE	DEFENSE MECHANISM	EXAMPLE
Compensation Covering up a real or perceived weakness by emphasizing a trait one considers more desirable	A physically handicapped boy is unable to participate in football, so he compensates by becoming a great scholar.	**Rationalization** Attempting to make excuses or formulate logical reasons to justify unacceptable feelings or behaviors.	John tells the rehab nurse, "I drink because it's the only way I can deal with my bad marriage and my worse job."
Denial Refusing to acknowledge the existence of a real situation or the feelings associated with it	A woman drinks alcohol every day and cannot stop, failing to acknowledge that she has a problem.	**Reaction Formation** Preventing unacceptable or undesirable thoughts or behaviors from being expressed by exaggerating opposite thoughts or types of behaviors	Jane hates nursing. She attended nursing school to please her parents. During career day, she speaks to prospective students about the excellence of nursing as a career.
Displacement The transfer of feelings from one target to another that is considered less threatening or that is neutral	A client is angry with his physician, does not express it, but becomes verbally abusive with the nurse.	**Regression** Retreating in response to stress to an earlier level of development and the comfort measures associated with that level of functioning.	When 2-year-old Jay is hospitalized for tonsillitis he will drink only from a bottle, even though his mom states he has been drinking from a cup for 6 months.

(Continued on following page)

TABLE 2–3	Ego Defense Mechanisms (Continued)		
DEFENSE MECHANISM	**EXAMPLE**	**DEFENSE MECHANISM**	**EXAMPLE**
Identification An attempt to increase self-worth by acquiring certain attributes and characteristics of an individual one admires	A teenager who required lengthy rehabilitation after an accident decides to become a physical therapist as a result of his experiences.	**Repression** Involuntarily blocking unpleasant feelings and experiences from one's awareness	An accident victim can remember nothing about his accident.
Intellectualization An attempt to avoid expressing actual emotions associated with a stressful situation by using the intellectual processes of logic, reasoning, and analysis	S's husband is being transferred with his job to a city far away from her parents. She hides anxiety by explaining to her parents the advantages associated with the move.	**Sublimation** Rechanneling of drives or impulses that are personally or socially unacceptable into activities that are constructive	A mother whose son was killed by a drunk driver channels her anger and energy into being the president of the local chapter of Mothers Against Drunk Drivers.
Introjection Integrating the beliefs and values of another individual into one's own ego structure	Children integrate their parents' value system into the process of conscience formation. A child says to friend, "Don't cheat. It's wrong."	**Suppression** The voluntary blocking of unpleasant feelings and experiences from one's awareness	Scarlett O'Hara says, "I don't want to think about that now. I'll think about that tomorrow."
Isolation Separating a thought or memory from the feeling tone or emotion associated with it	A young woman describes being attacked and raped, without showing any emotion.	**Undoing** Symbolically negating or canceling out an experience that one finds intolerable	Joe is nervous about his new job and yells at his wife. On his way home he stops and buys her some flowers.
Projection Attributing feelings or impulses unacceptable to one's self to another person	Sue feels a strong sexual attraction to her track coach and tells her friend, "He's coming on to me!"		

1. **Compensation** is the covering up of a real or perceived weakness by emphasizing a trait one considers more desirable.

EXAMPLE:

(a) A handicapped boy who is unable to participate in sports compensates by becoming a great scholar. (b) A young man who is the shortest among members of his peer group views this as a deficiency and compensates by being overly aggressive and daring.

2. **Denial** is the refusal to acknowledge the existence of a real situation or the feelings associated with it.

EXAMPLE:

(a) A woman has been told by her family doctor that she has a lump in her breast. An appointment is made for her with a surgeon; however, she does not keep the appointment and goes about her activities of daily living with no evidence of concern. (b) Individuals continue to smoke cigarettes even though they have been told of the health risk involved.

3. **Displacement** is the transferring of feelings from one target to another that is considered less threatening or neutral.

EXAMPLE:

(a) A man who is passed over for promotion on his job says nothing to his boss but later belittles his son for not making the basketball team. (b) A boy who is teased and hit by the class bully on the playground comes home after school and kicks his dog.

4. **Identification** is an attempt to increase self-worth by acquiring certain attributes and characteristics of an individual one admires.

EXAMPLE:

(a) A teenage girl emulates the mannerisms and style of dress of a popular female rock star. (b) The young son of a famous civil rights worker adopts his father's attitudes and behaviors with the intent of pursuing similar aspirations.

5. **Intellectualization** is an attempt to avoid expressing actual emotions associated with a stressful situation by

using the intellectual processes of logic, reasoning, and analysis.

> **EXAMPLE:**

(a) A man whose brother is in a cardiac intensive care unit following a severe myocardial infarction (MI) spends his allotted visiting time in discussion with the nurse, analyzing test results and making a reasonable determination about the pathophysiology that may have occurred to induce the MI. (b) A young psychology professor receives a letter from his fiancée breaking off their engagement. He shows no emotion when discussing this with his best friend. Instead he analyzes his fiancée's behavior and tries to reason why the relationship failed.

6. **Introjection** is the internalization of the beliefs and values of another individual such that they symbolically become a part of the self to the extent that the feeling of separateness or distinctness is lost.

> **EXAMPLE:**

(a) A small child develops her conscience by internalizing what the parents believe is right and wrong. The parents literally become a part of the child. The child says to a friend while playing, "Don't hit people. It's not nice!" (b) A psychiatric client claims to be the Son of God, drapes himself in a sheet and blanket, "performs miracles" on other clients, and refuses to respond unless addressed as Jesus Christ.

7. **Isolation** is the separation of a thought or a memory from the feeling tone or emotions associated with it (sometimes called emotional isolation).

> **EXAMPLE:**

(a) A young woman describes being attacked and raped by a street gang. She displays an apathetic expression and no emotional tone. (b) A physician is able to isolate her feelings about the eventual death of a terminally ill cancer client by focusing her attention instead on the chemotherapy that will be given.

8. **Projection** is the attribution of feelings or impulses unacceptable to one's self to another person. The individual "passes the blame" for these undesirable feelings or impulses to another, thereby providing relief from the anxiety associated with them.

> **EXAMPLE:**

(a) A young soldier who has an extreme fear of participating in military combat tells his sergeant that the others in his unit are "a bunch of cowards." (b) A businessperson who values punctuality is late for a meeting and states, "Sorry I'm late. My assistant forgot to remind me of the time. It's so hard to find good help these days."

9. **Rationalization** is the attempt to make excuses or formulate logical reasons to justify unacceptable feelings or behaviors.

> **EXAMPLE:**

(a) A young woman is turned down for a secretarial job after a poor performance on a typing test. She claims, "I'm sure I could have done a better job on a word processor. Hardly anyone uses an electric typewriter anymore!" (b) A young man is unable to afford the sports car he wants so desperately. He tells the salesperson, "I'd buy this car but I'll be getting married soon. This is really not the car for a family man."

10. **Reaction formation** is the prevention of unacceptable or undesirable thoughts or behaviors from being expressed by exaggerating opposite thoughts or types of behaviors.

> **EXAMPLE:**

(a) The young soldier who has an extreme fear of participating in military combat volunteers for dangerous frontline duty. (b) A secretary is sexually attracted to her boss and feels an intense dislike toward his wife. She treats her boss with detachment and aloofness while performing her secretarial duties and is overly courteous, polite, and flattering to his wife when she comes to the office.

11. **Regression** is the retreating to an earlier level of development and the comfort measures associated with that level of functioning.

> **EXAMPLE:**

(a) When his mother brings his new baby sister home from the hospital, 4-year-old Tommy, who had been toilet trained for more than a year, begins to wet his pants, cry to be held, and suck his thumb. (b) A person who is depressed may withdraw to his or her room, curl up in a fetal position on the bed, and sleep for long periods of time.

12. **Repression** is the involuntary blocking of unpleasant feelings and experiences from one's awareness.

> **EXAMPLE:**

(a) A woman cannot remember being sexually assaulted when she was 15 years old. (b) A teenage boy cannot remember driving the car that was involved in an accident in which his best friend was killed.

13. **Sublimation** is the rechanneling of drives or impulses that are personally or socially unacceptable (e.g., aggressiveness, anger, sexual drives) into activities that are more tolerable and constructive.

EXAMPLE:

(a) A teenage boy with strong competitive and aggressive drives becomes the star football player on his high school team. (b) A young unmarried woman with a strong desire for marriage and a family achieves satisfaction and success in establishing and operating a daycare center for preschool children.

14. **Suppression** is the voluntarily blocking of unpleasant feelings and experiences from one's awareness.

EXAMPLE:

(a) Scarlett O'Hara says, "I'll think about that tomorrow." (b) A young woman who is depressed about a pending divorce proceeding tells the nurse, "I just don't want to talk about the divorce. There's nothing I can do about it anyway."

15. **Undoing** is the act of symbolically negating or canceling out a previous action or experience that one finds intolerable.

EXAMPLE:

(a) A man spills some salt on the table, and then sprinkles some over his left shoulder to "prevent bad luck." (b) A man who is anxious about giving a presentation at work yells at his wife during breakfast. He stops on his way home from work that evening to buy her a dozen red roses.

Moderate-to-Severe Anxiety. Anxiety at the moderate-to-severe level that remains unresolved over an extended period of time can contribute to a number of physiological disorders. The *DSM-IV-TR* (APA, 2000) describes these disorders as "the presence of one or more specific psychological or behavioral factors that adversely affect a general medical condition." The psychological factors may exacerbate symptoms of, delay recovery from, or interfere with treatment of the medical condition. The condition may be initiated or exacerbated by an environmental situation that the individual perceives as stressful. Measurable pathophysiology can be demonstrated. The *DSM-IV-TR* states:

> Psychological and behavioral factors may affect the course of almost every major category of disease, including cardiovascular conditions, dermatological conditions, endocrinological conditions, gastrointestinal conditions, neoplastic conditions, neurological conditions, pulmonary conditions, renal conditions, and rheumatological conditions. (p. 732)

A more comprehensive discussion of specific psychophysiological disorders is presented in Chapter 36.

Severe Anxiety. Extended periods of repressed severe anxiety can result in psychoneurotic patterns of behaving. **Neurosis** is no longer a separate category of disorders in the *DSM-IV-TR* (APA, 2000). However, the term is still used in the literature to further describe the symptomatology of certain disorders. Neuroses are psychiatric disturbances, characterized by excessive anxiety that is expressed directly or altered through defense mechanisms. It appears as a symptom, such as an obsession, a compulsion, a phobia, or a sexual dysfunction (Sadock & Sadock, 2003). The following are common characteristics of people with neuroses:

1. They are aware that they are experiencing distress.
2. They are aware that their behaviors are maladaptive.
3. They are unaware of any possible psychological causes of the distress.
4. They feel helpless to change their situation.
5. They experience no loss of contact with reality.

The following disorders are examples of psychoneurotic responses to anxiety as they appear in the *DSM-IV-TR*. They are discussed in this text in Chapters 30, 31, and 32.

1. **Anxiety Disorders.** Disorders in which the characteristic features are symptoms of anxiety and avoidance behavior (e.g., phobias, obsessive–compulsive disorder, panic disorder, generalized anxiety disorder, and posttraumatic stress disorder).
2. **Somatoform Disorders.** Disorders in which the characteristic features are physical symptoms for which there is no demonstrable organic pathology. Psychological factors are judged to play a significant role in the onset, severity, exacerbation, or maintenance of the symptoms (e.g., hypochondriasis, conversion disorder, somatization disorder, pain disorder).
3. **Dissociative Disorders.** Disorders in which the characteristic feature is a disruption in the usually integrated functions of consciousness, memory, identity, or perception of the environment (e.g., dissociative amnesia, dissociative fugue, dissociative identity disorder, and depersonalization disorder).

Panic Anxiety. At this extreme level of anxiety, an individual is not capable of processing what is happening in the environment, and may lose contact with reality. **Psychosis** is defined as a loss of ego boundaries or a gross impairment in reality testing (APA, 2000). Psychoses are serious psychiatric disturbances characterized by the presence of delusions or hallucinations and the impairment of interpersonal functioning and relationship to the external world. The following are common characteristics of people with psychoses:

1. They experience minimal distress (emotional tone is flat, bland, or inappropriate).
2. They are unaware that their behavior is maladaptive.
3. They are unaware of any psychological problems.

4. They are exhibiting a flight from reality into a less stressful world or into one in which they are attempting to adapt.

Examples of psychotic responses to anxiety include the schizophrenic, schizoaffective, and delusional disorders. They are discussed at length in Chapter 28.

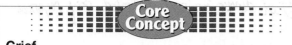

Core Concept

Grief

Grief is a subjective state of emotional, physical, and social responses to the loss of a valued entity.

Grief

Losses may be real, in which case they can be substantiated by others (e.g., death of a loved one, loss of personal possessions), or they may be perceived by the individual alone, unable to be shared or identified by others (e.g., loss of the feeling of femininity following mastectomy). Any situation that creates change for an individual can be identified as a loss. Failure (either real or perceived) can be viewed as a loss.

The loss, or anticipated loss, of anything of value to an individual can trigger the grief response. This period of characteristic emotions and behaviors is called *mourning*. The "normal" mourning process is adaptive and is characterized by feelings of sadness, guilt, anger, helplessness, hopelessness, and despair. Indeed, an absence of mourning may be considered maladaptive.

absence of mourning is maladaptive

Stages of Grief

Kübler-Ross (1969), in extensive research with terminally ill patients, identified five stages of feelings and behaviors that individuals experience in response to a real, perceived, or anticipated loss:

5 Stages

Stage 1—Denial. This is a stage of shock and disbelief. The response may be one of "No, it can't be true!" The reality of the loss is not acknowledged. Denial is a protective mechanism that allows the individual to cope in an immediate time frame while organizing more effective defense strategies.

Stage 2—Anger. "Why me?" and "It's not fair!" are comments often expressed during the anger stage. Envy and resentment toward individuals not affected by the loss are common. Anger may be directed at the self or displaced on loved ones, caregivers, and even God. There may be a preoccupation with an idealized image of the lost entity.

Stage 3—Bargaining. During this stage, which is usually not visible or evident to others, a "bargain" is made with God in an attempt to reverse or postpone the loss. "If God will help me through this, I promise I will go to church every Sunday and volunteer my time to help others." Sometimes the promise is associated with feelings of guilt for not having performed satisfactorily, appropriately, or sufficiently.

Stage 4—Depression. During this stage, the full impact of the loss is experienced. The sense of loss is intense, and feelings of sadness and depression prevail. This is a time of quiet desperation and disengagement from all association with the lost entity. This stage differs from pathological depression in that it represents advancement toward resolution rather than the fixation in an earlier stage of the grief process.

Stage 5—Acceptance. The final stage brings a feeling of peace regarding the loss that has occurred. It is a time of quiet expectation and resignation. The focus is on the reality of the loss and its meaning for the individuals affected by it.

All individuals do not experience each of these stages in response to a loss, nor do they necessarily experience them in this order. Some individuals' grieving behaviors may fluctuate, and even overlap, between stages.

Anticipatory Grief

When a loss is anticipated, individuals often begin the work of grieving before the actual loss occurs. Most people re-experience the grieving behaviors once the loss occurs, but having this time to prepare for the loss can facilitate the process of mourning, actually decreasing the length and intensity of the response. Problems arise, particularly in anticipating the death of a loved one, when family members experience **anticipatory grieving** and the mourning process is completed prematurely. They disengage emotionally from the dying person, who may then experience feelings of being rejected by loved ones at a time when this psychological support is so necessary.

Resolution

The grief response can last from weeks to years. It cannot be hurried, and individuals must be allowed to progress at their own pace. In the loss of a loved one, grief work usually lasts for at least a year, during which the grieving person experiences each significant "anniversary" date for the first time without the loved one present.

Length of the grief process may be prolonged by a number of factors. If the relationship with the lost entity had been marked by ambivalence or if there had been an enduring "love–hate" association, reaction to the loss may be burdened with guilt. Guilt lengthens the grief reaction by promoting feelings of anger toward the self for having committed a wrongdoing or behaved in an unacceptable manner toward that which is now lost, and perhaps the grieving person may even feel that his or her behavior has contributed to the loss.

Anticipatory grieving is thought to shorten the grief response in some individuals who are able to work through some of the feelings before the loss occurs. If the loss is sudden and unexpected, mourning may take longer than it would if individuals were able to grieve in anticipation of the loss.

Length of the grieving process is also affected by the number of recent losses experienced by an individual and whether he or she is able to complete one grieving process before another loss occurs. This is particularly true for elderly individuals who may be experiencing numerous losses, such as spouse, friends, other relatives, independent functioning, home, personal possessions, and pets, in a relatively short time. Grief accumulates, and this represents a type of **bereavement overload**, which for some individuals presents an impossible task of grief work.

Resolution of the process of mourning is thought to have occurred when an individual can look back on the relationship with the lost entity and accept both the pleasures and the disappointments (both the positive and the negative aspects) of the association (Bowlby and Parkes, 1970). Disorganization and emotional pain have been experienced and tolerated. Preoccupation with the lost entity has been replaced with energy and the desire to pursue new situations and relationships.

Maladaptive Grief Responses

Maladaptive responses to loss occur when an individual is not able to satisfactorily progress through the stages of grieving to achieve resolution. Usually in these cases an individual becomes fixed in the denial or anger stage of the grief process. Several types of grief responses have been identified as pathological. They include responses that are prolonged, delayed or inhibited, or distorted. The *prolonged* response is characterized by an intense preoccupation with memories of the lost entity for *many years after the loss has occurred*. Behaviors associated with the stages of denial or anger are manifested, and disorganization of functioning and intense emotional pain related to the lost entity are evidenced.

In the *delayed or inhibited* response, the individual becomes fixed in the denial stage of the grieving process. The emotional pain associated with the loss is not experienced, but anxiety disorders (e.g., phobias, hypochondriasis) or sleeping and eating disorders (e.g., insomnia, anorexia) may be evident. The individual may remain in denial for many years until the grief response is triggered by a reminder of the loss or even by another, unrelated loss.

The individual who experiences a *distorted* response is fixed in the anger stage of grieving. In the distorted response, all the normal behaviors associated with grieving, such as helplessness, hopelessness, sadness, anger, and guilt, are exaggerated out of proportion to the situation. The individual turns the anger inward on the self, is consumed with overwhelming despair, and is unable to function in normal activities of daily living. Pathological depression is a distorted grief response (see Chapter 29).

Pathological depression is a distorted grief response

MENTAL HEALTH/MENTAL ILLNESS CONTINUUM

Anxiety and grief have been described as two major, primary responses to stress. In Figure 2–3, both of these responses are presented on a continuum according to degree of symptom severity. Disorders as they appear in the *DSM-IV-TR* are identified at their appropriate placement along the continuum.

THE *DSM-IV-TR* MULTIAXIAL EVALUATION SYSTEM

The APA endorses case evaluation on a multiaxial system, "to facilitate comprehensive and systematic evaluation with attention to the various mental disorders and general medical conditions, psychosocial and environmental problems, and level of functioning that might be overlooked if the focus were on assessing a single presenting problem." Each individual is evaluated on five axes. They are defined by the *DSM-IV-TR* in the following manner:

Axis I—Clinical Disorders and Other Conditions That May Be a Focus of Clinical Attention. This includes all mental disorders (except personality disorders and mental retardation).

Axis II—Personality Disorders and Mental Retardation. These disorders usually begin in childhood or adolescence and persist in a stable form into adult life.

Axis III—General Medical Conditions. These include any current general medical condition that is potentially relevant to the understanding or management of the individual's mental disorder.

Axis IV—Psychosocial and Environmental Problems. These are problems that may affect the diagnosis, treatment, and prognosis of mental disorders named on axes I and II. These include problems related to primary support group, social environment, education, occupation, housing, economics, access to health care services, interaction with the legal system or crime, and other types of psychosocial and environmental problems.

Axis V—Global Assessment of Functioning. This allows the clinician to rate the individual's overall functioning on the Global Assessment of Functioning (GAF) Scale. This scale represents in global terms a single measure of the individual's psychological, social, and occupational functioning. A copy of the GAF Scale appears in

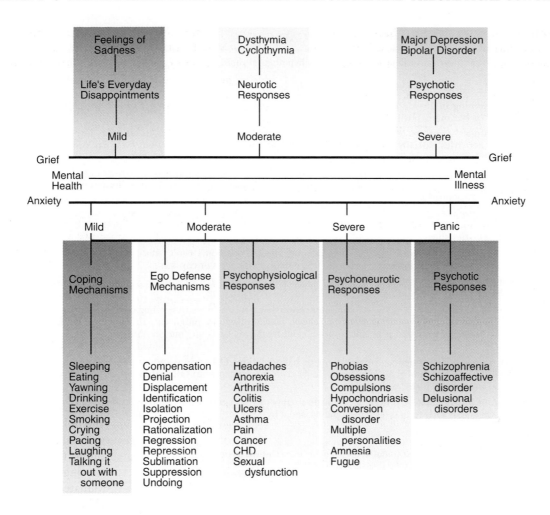

FIGURE 2–3   Conceptualization of anxiety and grief responses along the mental health/mental illness continuum.

Table 2–4. The *DSM-IV-TR* outline of axes I and II categories and codes is presented in Appendix C.

EXAMPLE OF A PSYCHIATRIC DIAGNOSIS

Axis I	300.4	Dysthymic Disorder
Axis II	301.6	Dependent Personality Disorder
Axis III	244.9	Hypothyroidism
Axis IV		Unemployed
Axis V	GAF = 65	
	(current)	

EVIDENCED
BY

SUMMARY

The history of psychiatric care has an unquestionable influence on the manner in which individuals with mental illness are treated today. Psychiatric care has its roots in ancient times, when etiology was based in superstition and ideas related to the supernatural. Treatment was inhumane, and accounts of torturous methods abound in the literature. Conditions have improved, largely because of the influence of leaders such as Benjamin Rush,

Dorothea Dix, and Linda Richards, whose endeavors provided a model for humanistic treatment of individuals with mental illness.

Various definitions of mental health and mental illness from the literature were presented. For purposes of this text, *mental health* is defined as "the successful adaptation to stressors from the internal or external environment, evidenced by thoughts, feelings, and behaviors that are age-appropriate and congruent with local and cultural norms." *Mental illness* is defined as "maladaptive responses to stressors from the internal or external environment, evidenced by thoughts, feelings, and behaviors that are incongruent with the local and cultural norms, and interfere with the individual's social, occupational, or physical functioning."

Most cultures label behavior as mental illness on the basis of *incomprehensibility* and *cultural relativity*. When observers are unable to find meaning or comprehensibility in behavior, they are likely to label that behavior as a symptom of mental illness. The meaning of behaviors is determined within individual cultures.

Anxiety and *grief* have been identified as the two major,

| TABLE 2–4 | Global Assessment of Functioning (GAF) Scale |

Consider psychological, social, and occupational functioning on a hypothetical continuum of mental health–illness. Do not include impairment in functioning due to physical (or environmental) limitations.

Code	(Note: Use intermediate codes when appropriate, e.g., 45, 68, 72)
100 91	**Superior functioning in a wide range of activities, life's problems never seem to get out of hand, is sought out by others because of his or her many positive qualities. No symptoms.**
90 | 81	Absent or minimal symptoms (e.g., mild anxiety before an exam), **good functioning in all areas interested and involved in a wide range of activities, socially effective, generally satisfied with life, no more than everyday problems or concerns** (e.g., an occasional argument with family members).
80 | 71	**If symptoms are present, they are transient and expectable reactions to psychosocial stressors** (e.g., difficulty concentrating after family argument); **no more than slight impairment in social, occupational, or school functioning** (e.g., temporarily falling behind in schoolwork).
70 | 61	**Some mild symptoms** (e.g., depressed mood and mild insomnia) **OR some difficulty in social, occupational, or school functioning** (e.g., occasional truancy, or theft within the household), **but generally functioning pretty well, has some meaningful interpersonal relationships.**
60 51	**Moderate symptoms** (e.g., flat affect and circumstantial speech, occasional panic attacks) **OR moderate difficulty in social, occupational, or school functioning** (e.g., few friends, conflicts with peers or coworkers).
50 41	**Serious symptoms** (e.g., suicidal ideation, severe obsessional rituals, frequent shoplifting) **OR any serious impairment in social, occupational, or school functioning** (e.g., no friends, unable to keep a job).
40 | | 31	**Some impairment in reality testing or communication** (e.g., speech is at times illogical, obscure, or irrelevant) **OR major impairment in several areas, such as work or school, family relations, judgment, thinking, or mood** (e.g., depressed man avoids friends, neglects family, and is unable to work; child frequently beats up younger children, is defiant at home, and is failing at school).
30 | 21	**Behavior is considerably influenced by delusions or hallucinations OR serious impairment in communication or judgment** (e.g., sometimes incoherent, acts grossly inappropriately, suicidal preoccupation) **OR inability to function in almost all areas** (e.g., stays in bed all day; no job, home, or friends).
20 | 11	**Some degree of hurting self or others** (e.g., suicide attempts without clear expectation of death; frequently violent; manic excitement) **OR occasionally fails to maintain minimal personal hygiene** (e.g., smears feces) **OR gross impairment in communication** (e.g., largely incoherent or mute).
10 1	**Persistent danger of severely hurting self or others** (e.g., recurrent violence) **OR persistent inability to maintain minimal personal hygiene OR serious suicidal act with clear expectation of death.**
0	**Inadequate information.**

SOURCE: *Diagnostic and Statistical Manual of Mental Disorders* (4th ed.). *Text Revision.* Washington, DC: American Psychiatric Association (2000). With permission.

primary responses to stress. Peplau (1963) defined anxiety by levels of symptom severity: mild, moderate, severe, and panic. Behaviors associated with levels of anxiety include coping mechanisms, ego defense mechanisms, psychophysiological responses, psychoneurotic responses, and psychotic responses.

Grief is described as a response to loss of a valued entity. Stages of normal mourning as identified by Kübler-Ross (1969) are denial, anger, bargaining, depression, and acceptance. Anticipatory grief is grief work that is begun, and sometimes completed, before the loss occurs. Resolution is thought to occur when an individual is able to remember and accept both the positive and negative aspects associated with the lost entity. Grieving is thought to be maladaptive when the mourning process is prolonged, delayed or inhibited, or becomes distorted and exaggerated out of proportion to the situation. Pathological depression is considered to be a distorted reaction. The behaviors and associated disorders of anxiety and grief were presented on the mental health/mental illness continuum.

The *DSM-IV-TR* multiaxial system of diagnostic classification was explained and the Global Assessment of Functioning (GAF) Scale was presented.

REVIEW QUESTIONS

SELF-EXAMINATION

Situation: Anna is 72 years old. She has been a widow for 20 years. When her husband had been dead for a year, her daughter gave Anna a puppy, which she named Lucky. Lucky was a happy, lively mutt of unknown origin, and he and Anna soon became inseparable. Lucky lived to a ripe old age of 16, dying in Anna's arms 3 years ago. Anna's daughter has consulted the community mental health nurse practitioner about her mother, stating, "She doesn't do a thing for herself anymore, and all she wants to talk about is Lucky. She visits his grave every day! She still cries when she talks about him. I don't know what to do!"

Select the answer that is *most* appropriate for this situation.

1. Anna's behavior would be considered maladaptive because:
   a. It has been more than 3 years since Lucky died.
   b. Her grief is too intense just over the loss of a dog.
   c. Her grief is interfering with her functioning.
   d. People in this culture would not comprehend such behavior over the loss of a pet.

2. Anna's grieving behavior would most likely be considered to be:
   a. Delayed
   b. Inhibited
   c. Prolonged
   d. Distorted

3. Anna is most likely fixed in which stage of the grief process?
   a. Denial
   b. Anger
   c. Depression
   d. Acceptance

4. Anna is of the age when she may have experienced many losses coming close together. What is this called?
   a. Bereavement overload
   b. Normal mourning
   c. Isolation
   d. Cultural relativity

5. Anna's daughter has likely put off seeking help for Anna because:
   a. Women are less likely to seek help for emotional problems than men.
   b. Relatives often try to "normalize" the behavior, rather than label it mental illness.
   c. She knows that all old people are expected to be a little depressed.
   d. She is afraid that the neighbors "will think her mother is crazy."

6. On the day that Lucky died, he got away from Anna while they were taking a walk. He ran into the street and was hit by a car. Anna cannot remember any of these circumstances of his death. This is an example of what defense mechanism?
   a. Rationalization
   b. Suppression
   c. Denial
   d. Repression

7. Lucky sometimes refused to obey Anna, and indeed did not come back to her when she called to him on the day he was killed. But Anna continues to insist, "He was the very best dog. He always minded me. He always did everything I told him to do." This represents the defense mechanism of:
   a. Sublimation
   b. Compensation

    c. Reaction formation

    d. Undoing

8. Anna's maladaptive grief response may be attributed to:
   a. Unresolved grief over loss of her husband.
   b. Loss of several relatives and friends over the last few years.
   c. Repressed feelings of guilt over the way in which Lucky died.
   d. Any or all of the above.

9. For what reason would Anna's illness be considered a neurosis rather than a psychosis?
   a. She is unaware that her behavior is maladaptive.
   b. She exhibits inappropriate affect (emotional tone).
   c. She experiences no loss of contact with reality.
   d. She tells the nurse, "There is nothing wrong with me!"

10. Which of the following statements by Anna might suggest that she is achieving resolution of her grief over Lucky's death?
    a. "I don't cry anymore when I think about Lucky."
    b. "It's true. Lucky didn't always mind me. Sometimes he ignored my commands."
    c. "I remember how it happened now. I should have held tighter to his leash!"
    d. "I won't ever have another dog. It's just too painful to lose them."

Match the following defense mechanisms to the appropriate situation:

_____ 11. Compensation

    a. Tommy, who is small for his age, is teased at school by the older boys. When he gets home from school, he yells at and hits his little sister.

_____ 12. Denial

    b. Johnny is in a wheelchair as a result of paralysis of the lower limbs. Before his accident, he was the star athlete on the football team. Now he obsessively strives to maintain a 4.0 grade point average in his courses.

_____ 13. Displacement

    c. Nancy and Sally are 4 years old. While playing with their dolls, Nancy says to Sally, "Don't hit your dolly. It's not nice to hit people!"

_____ 14. Identification

    d. Jackie is 4 years old. He has wanted a baby brother very badly, yet when his mother brings the new sibling home from the hospital, Jackie cries to be held when the baby is being fed and even starts to soil his clothing, although he has been toilet trained for 2 years.

_____ 15. Intellectualization

    e. A young man is late for class. He tells the professor, "Sorry I'm late, but my stupid wife forgot to set the alarm last night!"

_____ 16. Introjection

    f. Nancy was emotionally abused as a child and hates her mother. However, when she talks to others about her mother, she tells them how wonderful she is and how much she loves her.

_____ 17. Isolation

    g. Pete grew up in a rough neighborhood where fighting was a way of coping. He is tough and aggressive and is noticed by the football coach, who makes him a member of the team. Within the year he becomes the star player.

_____ 18. Projection

    h. Fred stops at the bar every night after work and has several drinks. During the last 6 months he has been charged twice with driving under the influence, both times while driving recklessly after leaving the bar. Last night, he was stopped again. The judge ordered rehabilitation services. Fred responded, "I don't need rehab. I can stop drinking anytime I want to!"

_____ 19. Rationalization

i. Mary tries on a beautiful dress she saw in the store window. She discovers that it costs more than she can afford. She says to the salesperson, "I'm not going to buy it. I really don't look good in this color."

_____ 20. Reaction formation

j. Janice is extremely upset when her boyfriend of 2 years breaks up with her. Her best friend tries to encourage her to talk about the breakup, but Janice says, "No need to talk about him anymore. He's history!"

_____ 21. Regression

k. While jogging in the park, Linda was kidnapped and taken as a hostage by two men who had just robbed a bank. She was held at gunpoint for 2 days until she was able to escape from the robbers. In her account to the police, she speaks of the encounter with no display of emotion whatsoever.

_____ 22. Repression

l. While Mark is on his way to work a black cat runs across the road in front of his car. Mark turns the car around, drives back in the direction from which he had come, and takes another route to work.

_____ 23. Sublimation

m. Fifteen-year-old Zelda has always wanted to be a teacher. Ms. Fry is Zelda's history teacher. Zelda admires everything about Ms. Fry and wants to be just like her. She changes her hair and dress style to match that of Ms. Fry.

_____ 24. Suppression

n. Bart is turned down for a job he desperately wanted. He shows no disappointment when relating the situation to his girlfriend. Instead, he reviews the interview and begins to analyze systematically why the interaction was ineffective for him.

_____ 25. Undoing

o. Eighteen-year-old Jennifer can recall nothing related to an automobile accident in which she was involved 8 years ago and in which both of her parents were killed.

R E F E R E N C E S

American Psychiatric Association. (2003). *American psychiatric glossary* (8th ed.). Washington, DC: American Psychiatric Publishing.

American Psychiatric Association. (2000). *Diagnostic and statistical manual of mental disorders* (4th ed.) Text revision. Washington, DC: American Psychiatric Association.

Horwitz, A.V. (2002). *The social control of mental illness.* Clinton Corners, NY: Percheron Press.

Sadock, B.J., & Sadock, V.A. (2003). *Synopsis of psychiatry: Behavioral sciences/clinical psychiatry* (9th ed.). Baltimore: Lippincott Williams & Wilkins.

Robinson, L. (1983). *Psychiatric nursing as a human experience* (3rd ed.). Philadelphia: WB Saunders.

C L A S S I C A L   R E F E R E N C E S

Bowlby, J., & Parkes, C.M. (1970). Separation and loss. In E.J. Anthony, & C. Koupernik (Eds.). *International yearbook for child psychiatry and allied disciplines: The child and his family,* (Vol. 1). New York: John Wiley & Sons.

Freud, A. (1953). *The ego and mechanisms of defense.* New York: International Universities Press.

Freud, S. (1961). The ego and the id. In *Standard edition of the complete psychological works of Freud,* Vol. XIX. London: Hogarth Press.

Jahoda, M. (1958). *Current concepts of positive mental health.* New York: Basic Books.

Kübler-Ross, E. (1969). *On death and dying.* New York: Macmillan.

Maslow, A. (1970). *Motivation and personality* (2nd ed.). New York: Harper & Row.

Menninger, K. (1963). *The vital balance.* New York: Viking Press.

Peplau, H. (1963). A working definition of anxiety. In S. Burd & M. Marshall (Eds.). *Some clinical approaches to psychiatric nursing.* New York: Macmillan.

UNIT TWO

FOUNDATIONS FOR PSYCHIATRIC/MENTAL HEALTH NURSING

THEORETICAL MODELS OF PERSONALITY DEVELOPMENT

CHAPTER OUTLINE

OBJECTIVES

PSYCHOANALYTIC THEORY

INTERPERSONAL THEORY

THEORY OF PSYCHOSOCIAL DEVELOPMENT

THEORY OF OBJECT RELATIONS

COGNITIVE DEVELOPMENT THEORY

THEORY OF MORAL DEVELOPMENT

A NURSING MODEL—HILDEGARD E. PEPLAU

SUMMARY

REVIEW QUESTIONS

KEY TERMS

cognitive development
cognitive maturity
counselor
ego
id
libido

psychodynamic
    nursing
superego
surrogate
symbiosis
technical expert
temperament

CORE CONCEPT

personality

OBJECTIVES

After reading this chapter, the student will be able to:

1. Define *personality*.
2. Identify the relevance of knowledge associated with personality development to nursing in the psychiatric/mental health setting.
3. Discuss the major components of the following developmental theories:
   a. Psychoanalytic theory—Freud
   b. Interpersonal theory—Sullivan
   c. Theory of psychosocial development—Erikson

   d. Theory of object relations development—Mahler
   e. Cognitive development theory—Piaget
   f. Theory of moral development—Kohlberg
   g. A nursing model of interpersonal development—Peplau

*T*he *DSM-IV-TR* (American Psychiatric Association [APA], 2000) defines **personality** traits as "enduring patterns of perceiving, relating to, and thinking about the environment and oneself that are exhibited in a wide range of social and personal contexts" (p. 686).

Nurses must have a basic knowledge of human per-

sonality development to understand maladaptive behavioral responses commonly seen in psychiatric clients. Developmental theories identify behaviors associated with various *stages* through which individuals pass, thereby specifying what is appropriate or inappropriate at each developmental level.

Specialists in child development believe that infancy

and early childhood are the major life periods for the origination and occurrence of developmental change. Specialists in life-cycle development believe that people continue to develop and change throughout life, thereby suggesting the possibility for renewal and growth in adults.

Developmental stages are identified by age. Behaviors can then be evaluated by whether or not they are recognized as age appropriate. Ideally, an individual successfully fulfills all the tasks associated with one stage before moving on to the next stage (at the appropriate age). Realistically, however, this seldom happens. One reason is related to **temperament**, or the inborn personality characteristics that influence an individual's manner of reacting to the environment, and ultimately his or her developmental progression (Chess & Thomas, 1986). The environment may also influence one's developmental pattern. Individuals who had been reared in a dysfunctional family system often have retarded ego development. According to specialists in life-cycle development, behaviors from an unsuccessfully completed stage can be modified and corrected in a later stage.

Stages overlap, and an individual may be working on tasks associated with several stages at one time. When an individual becomes fixed in a lower level of development, with age-inappropriate behaviors focused on fulfillment of those tasks, psychopathology may become evident. Only when personality traits are inflexible and maladaptive and cause either significant functional impairment or subjective distress do they constitute "personality disorders" (APA, 2000). These disorders are discussed in Chapter 37.

> ### Core Concept
>
> **Personality**
> The combination of character, behavioral, temperamental, emotional, and mental traits that are unique to each specific individual.

PSYCHOANALYTIC THEORY

Freud (1961), who has been called the father of psychiatry, is credited as the first to identify development by stages. He considered the first 5 years of a child's life to be the most important, because he believed that an individual's basic character had been formed by the age of 5.

Freud's personality theory can be conceptualized according to structure and dynamics of the personality, topography of the mind, and stages of personality development.

Structure of the Personality

Freud organized the structure of the personality into three major components: the **id, ego,** and **superego.**

They are distinguished by their unique functions and different characteristics.

Id

The *id* is the locus of instinctual drives—the "pleasure principle." Present at birth, it endows the infant with instinctual drives that seek to satisfy needs and achieve immediate gratification. Id-driven behaviors are impulsive and may be irrational.

Ego

The *ego,* also called the *rational self* or the "reality principle," begins to develop between the ages of 4 and 6 months. The ego experiences the reality of the external world, adapts to it, and responds to it. As the ego develops and gains strength, it seeks to bring the influences of the external world to bear upon the id, to substitute the reality principle for the pleasure principle (Marmer, 2003). A primary function of the ego is one of mediator; that is, to maintain harmony among the external world, the id, and the superego.

Superego

If the id is identified as the pleasure principle, and the ego the reality principle, the *superego* might be referred to as the "perfection principle." The superego, which develops between ages 3 and 6 years, internalizes the values and morals set forth by primary caregivers. Derived out of a system of rewards and punishments, the superego is composed of two major components: the *ego-ideal* and the *conscience.* When a child is consistently rewarded for "good" behavior, self-esteem is enhanced, and the behavior becomes part of the ego-ideal; that is, it is internalized as part of his or her value system. The conscience is formed when the child is punished consistently for "bad" behavior. The child learns what is considered morally right or wrong from feedback received from parental figures and from society or culture. When moral and ethical principles or even internalized ideals and values are disregarded, the conscience generates a feeling of guilt within the individual. The superego is important in the socialization of the individual because it assists the ego in the control of id impulses. When the superego becomes rigid and punitive, problems with low self-confidence and low self-esteem arise.

Topography of the Mind

Freud classified all mental contents and operations into three categories: the conscious, the preconscious, and the unconscious.

- The *conscious* includes all memories that remain within an individual's awareness. It is the smallest of the three categories. Events and experiences that are easily remembered or retrieved are considered to be within one's conscious awareness. Examples include telephone numbers, birthdays of self and significant others, the dates of special holidays, and what one had for lunch this noon. The conscious mind is thought to be under the control of the ego, the rational and logical structure of the personality.
- The *preconscious* includes all memories that may have been forgotten or are not in present awareness but with attention can be readily recalled into consciousness. Examples include telephone numbers or addresses once known but little used and feelings associated with significant life events that may have occurred at sometime in the past. The preconscious enhances awareness by helping to *suppress* unpleasant or nonessential memories from consciousness. It is thought to be partially under the control of the superego, which helps to suppress unacceptable thoughts and behaviors.
- The *unconscious* includes all memories that one is unable to bring to conscious awareness. It is the largest of the three topographical levels. Unconscious material consists of unpleasant or nonessential memories that have been *repressed* and can be retrieved only through therapy, hypnosis, and with certain substances that alter the awareness and have the capacity to restructure repressed memories. Unconscious material may also emerge in dreams and in seemingly incomprehensible behavior.

Dynamics of the Personality

Freud believed that *psychic energy* is the force or impetus required for mental functioning. Originating in the id, it instinctually fulfills basic physiological needs. Freud called this psychic energy (or the drive to fulfill basic physiological needs such as hunger, thirst, and sex) the **libido**. As the child matures, psychic energy is diverted from the id to form the ego and then from the ego to form the superego. Psychic energy is distributed within these three components, with the ego retaining the largest share to maintain a balance between the impulsive behaviors of the id and the idealistic behaviors of the superego. If an excessive amount of psychic energy is stored in one of these personality components, behavior will reflect that part of the personality. For instance, impulsive behavior prevails when excessive psychic energy is stored in the id. Over investment in the ego reflects self-absorbed, or narcissistic, behaviors; an excess within the superego results in rigid, self-deprecating behaviors.

Freud used the terms *cathexis* and *anticathexis* to describe the forces within the id, ego, and superego that are used to invest psychic energy in external sources to satisfy needs. Cathexis is the process by which the id invests energy into an object in an attempt to achieve gratification. An example is the individual who instinctively turns to alcohol to relieve stress. Anticathexis is the use of psychic energy by the ego and the superego to control id impulses. In the example cited, the ego would attempt to control the use of alcohol with rational thinking, such as, "I already have ulcers from drinking too much. I will call my AA counselor for support. I will not drink." The superego would exert control with such thinking as "I shouldn't drink. If I drink, my family will be hurt and angry. I should think of how it affects them. I'm such a weak person." Freud believed that an imbalance between cathexis and anticathexis resulted in internal conflicts, producing tension and anxiety within the individual. Freud's daughter Anna devised a comprehensive list of defense mechanisms believed to be used by the ego as a protective device against anxiety in mediating between the excessive demands of the id and the excessive restrictions of the superego (see Chapter 2).

Freud's Stages of Personality Development

Freud described formation of the personality through five stages of *psychosexual* development. He placed much emphasis on the first 5 years of life and believed that characteristics developed during these early years bore heavily on one's adaptation patterns and personality traits in adulthood. Fixation in an early stage of development will almost certainly result in psychopathology. An outline of these five stages is presented in Table 3–1.

TABLE 3–1	Freud's Stages of Psychosexual Development	
AGE	**STAGE**	**MAJOR DEVELOPMENTAL TASKS**
Birth–18 months	Oral	Relief from anxiety through oral gratification of needs
18 months–3 years	Anal	Learning independence and control, with focus on the excretory function
3–6 years	Phallic	Identification with parent of same sex; development of sexual identity; focus on genital organs
6–12 years	Latency	Sexuality repressed; focus on relationships with same-sex peers
13–20 years	Genital	Libido reawakened as genital organs mature; focus on relationships with members of the opposite sex

Oral Stage: Birth to 18 Months

During the oral stage, behavior is directed by the id, and the goal is immediate gratification of needs. The focus of energy is the mouth, with behaviors that include sucking, chewing, and biting. The infant feels a sense of attachment and is unable to differentiate the self from the person who is providing the mothering. This includes feelings such as anxiety. Because of this lack of differentiation, a pervasive feeling of anxiety on the part of the mother may be passed on to her infant, leaving the child vulnerable to similar feelings of insecurity. With the beginning of development of the ego at age 4 to 6 months, the infant starts to view the self as separate from the mothering figure. A sense of security and the ability to trust others is derived from the gratification of fulfilling basic needs during this stage.

Anal Stage: 18 Months to 3 Years

The major tasks in the anal stage are gaining independence and control, with particular focus on the excretory function. Freud believed that the manner in which the parents and other primary caregivers approach the task of toilet training may have far-reaching effects on the child in terms of values and personality characteristics. When toilet training is strict and rigid, the child may choose to retain the feces, becoming constipated. Adult retentive personality traits influenced by this type of training include stubbornness, stinginess, and miserliness. An alternate reaction to strict toilet training is for the child to expel feces in an unacceptable manner or at inappropriate times. Far-reaching effects of this behavior pattern include malevolence, cruelty to others, destructiveness, disorganization, and untidiness.

Toilet training that is more permissive and accepting attaches the feeling of importance and desirability to feces production. The child becomes extroverted, productive, and altruistic.

Phallic Stage: 3 to 6 Years

In the phallic stage, the focus of energy shifts to the genital area. Discovery of differences between genders results in a heightened interest in the sexuality of self and others. This interest may be manifested in sexual self-exploratory or group-exploratory play. Freud proposed that the development of the *Oedipus complex* (males) or *Electra complex* (females) occurred during this stage of development. He described this as the child's unconscious desire to eliminate the parent of the same sex and to possess the parent of the opposite sex for himself or herself. Guilt feelings result with the emergence of the superego during these years. Resolution of this internal conflict occurs when the child develops a strong identification with the parent of the same sex and that parent's attitudes, beliefs, and value systems are subsumed by the child.

Latency Stage: 6 to 12 Years

During the elementary school years, the focus changes from egocentrism to more interest in group activities, learning, and socialization with peers. Sexuality is not absent during this period but remains obscure and imperceptible to others. The preference is homosexual; children of this age show a distinct preference for same-sex relationships, even rejecting members of the opposite sex.

Genital Stage: 13 to 20 Years

In the genital stage, the maturing of the genital organs results in a reawakening of the libidinal drive. The focus is on relationships with members of the opposite sex and preparations for selecting a mate. The development of sexual maturity evolves from self-gratification to behaviors deemed acceptable by societal norms. Interpersonal relationships are based on genuine pleasure derived from the interaction rather than from the more self-serving implications of childhood associations.

Relevance of Psychoanalytic Theory to Nursing Practice

Knowledge of the structure of the personality can assist nurses who work in the mental health setting. The ability to recognize behaviors associated with the id, the ego, and the superego assists in the assessment of developmental level. Understanding the use of ego defense mechanisms is important in making determinations about maladaptive behaviors, in planning care for clients to assist in creating change (if desired), or in helping clients accept themselves as unique individuals.

INTERPERSONAL THEORY

Sullivan (1953) believed that individual behavior and personality development are the direct result of interpersonal relationships. Before the development of his own theoretical framework, Sullivan embraced the concepts of Freud. Later, he changed the focus of his work from the *intrapersonal* view of Freud to one with more *interpersonal* flavor in which human behavior could be observed in social interactions with others. His ideas, which were not universally accepted at the time, have been integrated into the practice of psychiatry through publication only since his death in 1949. Sullivan's major concepts include the following:

Anxiety is a feeling of emotional discomfort, toward the relief or prevention of which all behavior is aimed. Sullivan believed that anxiety is the "chief disruptive force in interpersonal relations and the main factor in the development of serious difficulties in living." It arises out of one's inability to satisfy needs or to achieve interpersonal security.

Satisfaction of needs is the fulfillment of all requirements associated with an individual's physicochemical environment. Sullivan identified examples of these requirements as oxygen, food, water, warmth, tenderness, rest, activity, sexual expression—virtually anything that, when absent, produces discomfort in the individual.

Interpersonal security is the feeling associated with relief from anxiety. When all needs have been met, one experiences a sense of total well-being, which Sullivan termed *interpersonal security*. He believed individuals have an innate need for interpersonal security.

Self-system is a collection of experiences, or security measures, adopted by the individual to protect against anxiety. Sullivan identified three components of the self-system, which are based on interpersonal experiences early in life:

● The "*good me*" is the part of the personality that develops in response to positive feedback from the primary caregiver. Feelings of pleasure, contentment, and gratification are experienced. The child learns which behaviors elicit this positive response as it becomes incorporated into the self-system.

● The "*bad me*" is the part of the personality that develops in response to negative feedback from the primary caregiver. Anxiety is experienced, eliciting feelings of discomfort, displeasure, and distress. The child learns to avoid these negative feelings by altering certain behaviors.

● The "*not me*" is the part of the personality that develops in response to situations that produce intense anxiety in the child. Feelings of horror, awe, dread, and loathing are experienced in response to these situations, leading the child to deny these feelings in an effort to relieve anxiety. These feelings, having then been denied, become "not me," but someone else. This withdrawal from emotions has serious implications for mental disorders in adult life.

Sullivan's Stages of Personality Development

Infancy: Birth to 18 Months

During the beginning stage, the major developmental task for the child is the gratification of needs. This is accomplished through activity associated with the mouth, such as crying, nursing, and thumb sucking.

Childhood: 18 Months to 6 Years

At ages 18 months to 6 years, the child learns that interference with fulfillment of personal wishes and desires may result in delayed gratification. He or she learns to accept this and feel comfortable with it, recognizing that delayed gratification often results in parental approval, a more lasting type of reward. Tools of this stage include the mouth, the anus, language, experimentation, manipulation, and identification.

Juvenile: 6 to 9 Years

The major task of the juvenile stage is formation of satisfactory relationships within peer groups. This is accomplished through the use of competition, cooperation, and compromise.

Preadolescence: 9 to 12 Years

The tasks at the preadolescence stage focus on developing relationships with persons of the same sex. One's ability to collaborate with and show love and affection for another person begins at this stage.

Early Adolescence: 12 to 14 Years

During early adolescence, the child is struggling with developing a sense of identity that is separate and independent from the parents. The major task is formation of satisfactory relationships with members of the opposite sex. Sullivan saw the emergence of lust in response to biological changes as a major force occurring during this period.

Late Adolescence: 14 to 21 Years

The late adolescent period is characterized by tasks associated with the attempt to achieve interdependence within the society and the formation of a lasting, intimate relationship with a selected member of the opposite sex. The genital organs are the major developmental focus of this stage.

An outline of the stages of personality development according to Sullivan's interpersonal theory is presented in Table 3–2.

Relevance of Interpersonal Theory to Nursing Practice

The interpersonal theory has significant relevance to nursing practice. Relationship development, which is a

TABLE 3–2	Stages of Development in Sullivan's Interpersonal Theory	
AGE	**STAGE**	**MAJOR DEVELOPMENTAL TASKS**
Birth–18 months	Infancy	Relief from anxiety through oral gratification of needs
18 months–6 years	Childhood	Learning to experience a delay in personal gratification without undue anxiety
6–9 years	Juvenile	Learning to form satisfactory peer relationships
9–12 years	Preadolescence	Learning to form satisfactory relationships with persons of same sex; initiating feelings of affection for another person
12–14 years	Early adolescence	Learning to form satisfactory relationships with persons of the opposite sex; developing a sense of identity
14–21 years	Late adolescence	Establishing self-identity; experiencing satisfying relationships; working to develop a lasting, intimate opposite-sex relationship

major concept of this theory, is a major psychiatric nursing intervention. Nurses develop therapeutic relationships with clients in an effort to help them generalize this ability to interact successfully with others.

Knowledge about the behaviors associated with all levels of anxiety and methods for alleviating anxiety helps nurses to assist clients achieve interpersonal security and a sense of well-being. Nurses use the concepts of Sullivan's theory to help clients achieve a higher degree of independent and interpersonal functioning.

THEORY OF PSYCHOSOCIAL DEVELOPMENT

Erikson (1963) studied the influence of social processes on the development of the personality. He described eight stages of the life cycle during which individuals struggle with developmental "crises." Specific tasks associated with each stage must be completed for resolution of the crisis and for emotional growth to occur. An out-

line of Erikson's stages of psychosocial development is presented in Table 3–3.

Erikson's Stages of Personality Development

Trust versus Mistrust: Birth to 18 Months

Major Developmental Task. From birth to 18 months, the major task is to develop a basic trust in the mothering figure and learn to generalize it to others.

● Achievement of the task results in self-confidence, optimism, faith in the gratification of needs and desires, and hope for the future. The infant learns to trust when basic needs are met consistently.
● Nonachievement results in emotional dissatisfaction with the self and others, suspiciousness, and difficulty with interpersonal relationships. The task remains unresolved when primary caregivers fail to respond to the infant's distress signals promptly and consistently.

TABLE 3–3	Stages of Development in Erikson's Psychosocial Theory	
AGE	**STAGE**	**MAJOR DEVELOPMENTAL TASKS**
Infancy (Birth–18 months)	Trust vs. mistrust	To develop a basic trust in the mothering figure and learn to generalize it to others
Early childhood (18 months–3 years)	Autonomy vs. shame and doubt	To gain some self-control and independence within the environment
Late childhood (3–6 years)	Initiative vs. guilt	To develop a sense of purpose and the ability to initiate and direct own activities
School age (6–12 years)	Industry vs. inferiority	To achieve a sense of self-confidence by learning, competing, performing successfully, and receiving recognition from significant others, peers, and acquaintances
Adolescence (12–20 years)	Identity vs. role confusion	To integrate the tasks mastered in the previous stages into a secure sense of self
Young adulthood (20–30 years)	Intimacy vs. isolation	To form an intense, lasting relationship or a commitment to another person, cause, institution, or creative effort
Adulthood (30–65 years)	Generativity vs. stagnation	To achieve the life goals established for oneself, while also considering the welfare of future generations
Old age (65 years–death)	Ego integrity vs. despair	To review one's life and derive meaning from both positive and negative events, while achieving a positive sense of self-worth

Autonomy versus Shame and Doubt: 18 Months to 3 Years

Major Developmental Task. The major task during the ages of 18 months to 3 years is to gain some self-control and independence within the environment.

- Achievement of the task results in a sense of self-control and the ability to delay gratification, and a feeling of self-confidence in one's ability to perform. Autonomy is achieved when parents encourage and provide opportunities for independent activities.
- Nonachievement results in a lack of self-confidence, a lack of pride in the ability to perform, a sense of being controlled by others, and a rage against the self. The task remains unresolved when primary caregivers restrict independent behaviors, both physically and verbally, or set the child up for failure with unrealistic expectations.

Initiative versus Guilt: 3 to 6 Years

Major Developmental Task. During the ages of 3 to 6 years, the goal is to develop a sense of purpose and the ability to initiate and direct one's own activities.

- Achievement of the task results in the ability to exercise restraint and self-control of inappropriate social behaviors. Assertiveness and dependability increase, and the child enjoys learning and personal achievement. The conscience develops, thereby controlling the impulsive behaviors of the id. Initiative is achieved when creativity is encouraged and performance is recognized and positively reinforced.
- Nonachievement results in feelings of inadequacy and a sense of defeat. Guilt is experienced to an excessive degree, even to the point of accepting liability in situations for which one is not responsible. The child may view himself or herself as evil and deserving of punishment. The task remains unresolved when creativity is stifled and parents continually expect a higher level of achievement than the child produces.

Industry versus Inferiority: 6 to 12 Years

Major Developmental Task. The major task for 6- to 12-year-olds is to achieve a sense of self-confidence by learning, competing, performing successfully, and receiving recognition from significant others, peers, and acquaintances.

- Achievement of the task results in a sense of satisfaction and pleasure in the interaction and involvement with others. The individual masters reliable work habits and develops attitudes of trustworthiness. He or she is conscientious, feels pride in achievement, and enjoys play but desires a balance between fantasy and "real world" activities. Industry is achieved when encouragement is given to activities and responsibilities in the school and community, as well as those within the home, and recognition is given for accomplishments.
- Nonachievement results in difficulty in interpersonal relationships because of feelings of personal inadequacy. The individual can neither cooperate and compromise with others in group activities nor problem solve or complete tasks successfully. He or she may become either passive and meek or overly aggressive to cover up for feelings of inadequacy. If this occurs, the individual may manipulate or violate the rights of others to satisfy his or her own needs or desires; he or she may become a workaholic with unrealistic expectations for personal achievement. This task remains unresolved when parents set unrealistic expectations for the child, when discipline is harsh and tends to impair self-esteem, and when accomplishments are consistently met with negative feedback.

Identity versus Role Confusion: 12 to 20 Years

Major Developmental Task. At 12 to 20 years, the goal is to integrate the tasks mastered in the previous stages into a secure sense of self.

- Achievement of the task results in a sense of confidence, emotional stability, and a view of the self as a unique individual. Commitments are made to a value system, to the choice of a career, and to relationships with members of both genders. Identity is achieved when adolescents are allowed to experience independence by making decisions that influence their lives. Parents should be available to offer support when needed but should gradually relinquish control to the maturing individual in an effort to encourage the development of an independent sense of self.
- Nonachievement results in a sense of self-consciousness, doubt, and confusion about one's role in life. Personal values or goals for one's life are absent. Commitments to relationships with others are nonexistent, but instead are superficial and brief. A lack of self-confidence is often expressed by delinquent and rebellious behavior. Entering adulthood, with its accompanying responsibilities, may be an underlying fear. This task can remain unresolved for many reasons. Examples include the following:
  - When independence is discouraged by the parents, and the adolescent is nurtured in the dependent position
  - When discipline within the home has been overly harsh, inconsistent, or absent
  - When there has been parental rejection or frequent shifting of parental figures

Intimacy versus Isolation: 20 to 30 Years

Major Developmental Task. The objective for 20- to 30-year-olds is to form an intense, lasting relationship or a commitment to another person, a cause, an institution, or a creative effort (Murray & Zentner, 2001).

● Achievement of the task results in the capacity for mutual love and respect between two people and the ability of an individual to pledge a total commitment to another. The intimacy goes far beyond the sexual contact between two people. It describes a commitment in which personal sacrifices are made for another, whether it be another person or, if one chooses, a career or other type of cause or endeavor to which an individual elects to devote his or her life. Intimacy is achieved when an individual has developed the capacity for giving of oneself to another. This is learned when one has been the recipient of this type of giving within the family unit.

● Nonachievement results in withdrawal, social isolation, and aloneness. The individual is unable to form lasting, intimate relationships, often seeking intimacy through numerous superficial sexual contacts. No career is established; he or she may have a history of occupational changes (or may fear change and thus remain in an undesirable job situation). The task remains unresolved when love in the home has been deprived or distorted through the younger years (Murray & Zentner, 2001). One fails to achieve the ability to give of the self without having been the recipient early on from primary caregivers.

Generativity versus Stagnation or Self-Absorption: 30 to 65 Years

Major Developmental Task. The major task here is to achieve the life goals established for oneself while also considering the welfare of future generations.

● Achievement of the task results in a sense of gratification from personal and professional achievements, and from meaningful contributions to others. The individual is active in the service of and to society. Generativity is achieved when the individual expresses satisfaction with this stage in life and demonstrates responsibility for leaving the world a better place in which to live.

● Nonachievement results in lack of concern for the welfare of others and total preoccupation with the self. He or she becomes withdrawn, isolated, and highly self-indulgent, with no capacity for giving of the self to others. The task remains unresolved when earlier developmental tasks are not fulfilled and the individual does not achieve the degree of maturity required to derive gratification out of a personal concern for the welfare of others.

Ego Integrity versus Despair: 65 Years to Death

Major Developmental Task. Between the age of 65 years and death, the goal is to review one's life and derive meaning from both positive and negative events, while achieving a positive sense of self.

● Achievement of the task results in a sense of self-worth and self-acceptance as one reviews life goals, accepting that some were achieved and some were not. The individual derives a sense of dignity from his or her life experiences and does not fear death, rather viewing it as another phase of development. Ego integrity is achieved when individuals have successfully completed the developmental tasks of the other stages and have little desire to make major changes in how their lives have progressed.

● Nonachievement results in a sense of self-contempt and disgust with how life has progressed. The individual would like to start over and have a second chance at life. He or she feels worthless and helpless to change. Anger, depression, and loneliness are evident. The focus may be on past failures or perceived failures. Impending death is feared or denied, or ideas of suicide may prevail. The task remains unresolved when earlier tasks are not fulfilled: self-confidence, a concern for others, and a strong sense of self-identity were never achieved.

Relevance of Psychosocial Development Theory to Nursing Practice

Erikson's theory is particularly relevant to nursing practice in that it incorporates sociocultural concepts into the development of personality. Erikson provides a systematic, stepwise approach and outlines specific tasks that should be completed during each stage. This information can be used quite readily in psychiatric/mental health nursing. Many individuals with mental health problems are still struggling to achieve tasks from a number of developmental stages. Nurses can plan care to assist these individuals to fulfill these tasks and move on to a higher developmental level.

THEORY OF OBJECT RELATIONS

Mahler (Mahler, Pine, & Bergman, 1975) formulated a theory that describes the separation-individuation process of the infant from the maternal figure (primary caregiver). She describes this process as progressing through three major phases. She further delineates phase III, the separation-individuation phase, into four subphases. Mahler's developmental theory is outlined in Table 3–4.

	TABLE 3–4	**Stages of Development in Mahler's Theory of Object Relations**	

AGE	PHASE/SUBPHASE	MAJOR DEVELOPMENTAL TASKS
Birth–1 month	I. Normal autism	Fulfillment of basic needs for survival and comfort
1–5 months	II. Symbiosis	Development of awareness of external source of need fulfillment
	III. Separation–Individuation	
5–10 months	a. Differentiation	Commencement of a primary recognition of separateness from the mothering figure
10–16 months	b. Practicing	Increased independence through locomotor functioning; increased sense of separateness of self
16–24 months	c. Rapprochement	Acute awareness of separateness of self; learning to seek "emotional refueling" from mothering figure to maintain feeling of security
24–36 months	d. Consolidation	Sense of separateness established; on the way to object constancy (i.e., able to internalize a sustained image of loved object/person when it is out of sight); resolution of separation anxiety

Phase I: The Autistic Phase (Birth to 1 Month)

In the autistic phase, also called *normal autism*, the infant exists in a half-sleeping, half-waking state and does not perceive the existence of other people or an external environment. The fulfillment of basic needs for survival and comfort is the focus and is merely accepted as it occurs.

Phase II: The Symbiotic Phase (1 to 5 Months)

Symbiosis is a type of "psychic fusion" of mother and child. The child views the self as an extension of the mother, but with a developing awareness that it is she who fulfills his or her every need. Mahler suggests that absence of, or rejection by, the maternal figure at this phase can lead to symbiotic psychosis.

Phase III: Separation-Individuation (5 to 36 Months)

This third phase represents what Mahler calls the "psychological birth" of the child. *Separation* is defined as the physical and psychological attainment of a sense of personal distinction from the mothering figure. *Individuation* occurs with a strengthening of the ego and an acceptance of a sense of "self," with independent ego boundaries. Four subphases through which the child evolves in his or her progression from a symbiotic extension of the mothering figure to a distinct and separate being are described.

Subphase 1: Differentiation (5 to 10 Months)

The differentiation phase begins with the child's initial physical movements away from the mothering figure. A primary recognition of separateness commences.

Subphase 2: Practicing (10 to 16 Months)

With advanced locomotor functioning, the child experiences feelings of exhilaration from increased independence. He or she is now able to move away from, and return to, the mothering figure. A sense of omnipotence is manifested.

Subphase 3: Rapprochement (16 to 24 Months)

This third subphase, rapprochement, is extremely critical to the child's healthy ego development. During this time, the child becomes increasingly aware of his or her separateness from the mothering figure, while the sense of fearlessness and omnipotence diminishes. The child, now recognizing the mother as a separate individual, wishes to reestablish closeness with her but shuns the total reengulfment of the symbiotic stage. The need is for the mothering figure to be available to provide "emotional refueling" on demand.

Critical to this subphase is the mothering figure's response to the child. If she is available to fulfill emotional needs, as they are required, the child develops a sense of security in the knowledge that he or she is loved and will not be abandoned. However, if emotional needs are inconsistently met or if the mother rewards clinging, dependent behaviors and withholds nurturing when the child demonstrates independence, feelings of rage and a fear of abandonment develop and often persist into adulthood.

Subphase 4: Consolidation (24 to 36 Months)

With achievement of the consolidation subphase, a definite individuality and sense of separateness of self are established. Objects are represented as whole, with the child having the ability to integrate both "good" and "bad." A degree of object constancy is established, as the child is able to internalize a sustained image of the mothering figure as enduring and loving, while maintaining the perception of her as a separate person in the outside world.

Relevance of Object Relations Theory to Nursing Practice

Understanding of the concepts of Mahler's theory of object relations assists the nurse to assess the client's level of individuation from primary caregivers. The emotional problems of many individuals can be traced to lack of fulfillment of the tasks of separation/individuation. Examples include problems related to dependency and excessive anxiety. The individual with borderline personality disorders is thought to be fixed in the rapprochement phase of development, harboring fears of abandonment and underlying rage. This knowledge is important in the provision of nursing care to these individuals.

COGNITIVE DEVELOPMENT THEORY

Piaget (Piaget & Inhelder, 1969) has been called the father of child psychology. His work concerning **cognitive development** in children is based on the premise that human intelligence is an extension of biological adaptation, or one's ability to adapt psychologically to the environment. He believed that human intelligence progresses through a series of stages that are related to age, demonstrating at each successive stage a higher level of logical organization than at the previous stages.

From his extensive studies of cognitive development in children, Piaget discovered four major stages, each of which he believed to be a necessary prerequisite for the one that follows. An outline is presented in Table 3–5.

Stage 1: Sensorimotor (Birth to 2 Years)

From the beginning, the child is concerned only with satisfying basic needs and comforts. The self is not differentiated from the external environment. As the sense of differentiation occurs, with increasing mobility and awareness, the mental system is expanded. The child develops a greater understanding regarding objects within the external environment and their effects upon him or her. Knowledge is gained regarding the ability to manipulate objects and experiences within the environment. The sense of *object permanence*—the notion that an object will continue to exist when it is no longer present to the senses—is initiated.

Stage 2: Preoperational (2 to 6 Years)

Piaget believed that preoperational thought is characterized by egocentrism. Personal experiences are thought to be universal, and the child is unable to accept the differing viewpoints of others. Language development progresses, as does the ability to attribute special meaning to symbolic gestures (e.g., bringing a story book to mother is a symbolic invitation to have a story read). Reality is often given to inanimate objects. Object permanence culminates in the ability to conjure up mental representations of objects or people.

Stage 3: Concrete Operations (6 to 12 Years)

The ability to apply logic to thinking begins in this stage; however, "concreteness" still predominates. An understanding of the concepts of reversibility and spatiality is developed. For example, the child recognizes that changing the shape of objects does not necessarily change the amount, weight, volume, or the ability of the object to return to its original form. Another achievement of this stage is the ability to classify objects by any of their several characteristics. For example, he or she can classify all poodles as dogs but recognizes that all dogs are not poodles.

The concept of a lawful self is developed at this stage as the child becomes more socialized and rule conscious. Egocentrism decreases, the ability to cooperate in inter-

TABLE 3–5	Piaget's Stages of Cognitive Development	
AGE	**STAGE**	**MAJOR DEVELOPMENTAL TASKS**
Birth–2 years	Sensorimotor	With increased mobility and awareness, development of a sense of self as separate from the external environment; the concept of object permanence emerges as the ability to form mental images evolves
2–6 years	Preoperational	Learning to express self with language; development of understanding of symbolic gestures; achievement of object permanence
6–12 years	Concrete operations	Learning to apply logic to thinking; development of understanding of reversibility and spatiality; learning to differentiate and classify; increased socialization and application of rules
12–15+ years	Formal operations	Learning to think and reason in abstract terms; making and testing hypotheses; capability of logical thinking and reasoning expand and are refined; cognitive maturity achieved

actions with other children increases, and understanding and acceptance of established rules grow.

Stage 4: Formal Operations (12 to 15+ Years)

At this stage, the individual is able to think and reason in abstract terms. He or she can make and test hypotheses using logical and orderly problem solving. Current situations and reflections of the future are idealized, and a degree of egocentrism returns during this stage. There may be some difficulty reconciling idealistic hopes with more rational prospects. Formal operations, however, enable individuals to distinguish between the ideal and the real. Piaget's theory suggests that most individuals achieve **cognitive maturity**, the capability to perform all mental operations needed for adulthood, in middle to late adolescence.

Relevance of Cognitive Development Theory to Nursing Practice

Nurses who work in psychiatry are likely to be involved in helping clients, particularly depressed clients, with techniques of cognitive therapy. In cognitive therapy, the individual is taught to control thought distortions that are considered to be a factor in the development and maintenance of mood disorders. In the cognitive model, depression is characterized by a triad of negative distortions related to expectations of the environment, self, and future. In this model, depression is viewed as a distortion in cognitive development, the self is unrealistically devalued, and the future is perceived as hopeless. Therapy focuses on changing "automatic thoughts" that occur spontaneously and contribute to the distorted affect. Nurses who assist with this type of therapy must have knowledge of how cognition develops in order to help clients identify the distorted thought patterns and make the changes required for improvement in affective functioning.

THEORY OF MORAL DEVELOPMENT

Kohlberg's (1968) stages of moral development are not closely tied to specific age groups. Research was conducted with males ranging in age from 10 to 28 years. Kohlberg believed that each stage is necessary and basic to the next stage and that all individuals must progress through each stage sequentially. He defined three major levels of moral development, each of which is further subdivided into two stages each. An outline of Kohlberg's developmental stages is presented in Table 3–6. Most people do not progress through all six stages.

Level I: Preconventional Level (Prominent from Ages 4 to 10 Years)

Stage 1: Punishment and Obedience Orientation. At the punishment and obedience orientation stage, the individual is responsive to cultural guidelines of good or bad and right or wrong, but primarily in terms of the known related consequences. Fear of punishment is likely to be the incentive for conformity (e.g., "I'll do it, because if I don't I can't watch TV for a week.")

Stage 2: Instrumental Relativist Orientation. Behaviors at the instrumental relativist orientation stage are guided by egocentrism and concern for self. There is an intense desire to satisfy one's own needs, but occasionally the needs of others are considered. For the most part, decisions are based on personal benefits derived (e.g., "I'll do it if I get something in return," or occasionally, "... because you asked me to").

LEVEL/AGE*	STAGE	DEVELOPMENTAL FOCUS
I. Preconventional (common from age 4 to 10 years)	1. Punishment and obedience orientation	Behavior motivated by fear of punishment
	2. Instrumental relativist orientation	Behavior motivated by egocentrism and concern for self.
II. Conventional (common from age 10 to 13 years, and into adulthood)	3. Interpersonal concordance orientation	Behavior motivated by expectations of others; strong desire for approval and acceptance
	4. Law and order orientation	Behavior motivated by respect for authority
III. Postconventional (can occur from adolescence on)	5. Social contract legalistic orientation	Behavior motivated by respect for universal laws and moral principles; guided by internal set of values
	6. Universal ethical principle orientation	Behavior motivated by internalized principles of honor, justice, and respect for human dignity; guided by the conscience

TABLE 3–6 Kohlberg's Stages of Moral Development

*Ages in Kohlberg's theory are not well defined. The stage of development is determined by the motivation behind the individual's behavior.

Level II: Conventional Level (Prominent from Ages 10 to 13 Years and into Adulthood)*

Stage 3: Interpersonal Concordance Orientation. Behavior at the interpersonal concordance orientation stage is guided by the expectations of others. Approval and acceptance within one's societal group provide the incentive to conform (e.g., "I'll do it because you asked me to," "… because it will help you," or "… because it will please you").

Stage 4: Law and Order Orientation. In the law and order orientation stage, there is a personal respect for authority. Rules and laws are required and override personal principles and group mores. The belief is that all individuals and groups are subject to the same code of order, and no one shall be exempt (e.g., "I'll do it because it is the law").

Level III: Postconventional Level (Can Occur from Adolescence Onward)

Stage 5: Social Contract Legalistic Orientation. Individuals who reach stage 5 have developed a system of values and principles that determine for them what is right or wrong; behaviors are acceptably guided by this value system, provided they do not violate the human rights of others. They believe that all individuals are entitled to certain inherent human rights, and they live according to universal laws and principles. However, they hold the idea that the laws are subject to scrutiny and change as needs within society evolve and change (e.g., "I'll do it because it is the moral and legal thing to do, even though it is not my personal choice").

Stage 6: Universal Ethical Principle Orientation. Behavior at stage 6 is directed by internalized principles of honor, justice, and respect for human dignity. Laws are abstract and unwritten, such as the "Golden Rule," "equality of human rights," and "justice for all." They are not the concrete rules established by society. The conscience is the guide, and when one fails to meet the self-expected behaviors, the personal consequence is intense guilt. The allegiance to these ethical principles is so strong that the individual will stand by them even knowing that negative consequences will result (e.g., "I'll do it because I believe it is the right thing to do, even though it is illegal and I will be imprisoned for doing it").

Relevance of Moral Development Theory to Nursing Practice

Moral development has relevance to psychiatric nursing in that it affects critical thinking about how individuals ought to behave and treat others. Moral behavior reflects the way a person interprets basic respect for other persons, such as the respect for human life, freedom, justice, or confidentiality. Psychiatric nurses must be able to assess the level of moral development of their clients in order to be able to help them in their effort to advance in their progression toward a higher level of developmental maturity.

A NURSING MODEL— HILDEGARD E. PEPLAU

Peplau (1991) applied interpersonal theory to nursing practice and, most specifically, to nurse-client relationship development. She provides a framework for "psychodynamic nursing," the interpersonal involvement of the nurse with a client in a given nursing situation. Peplau states, "Nursing is helpful when both the patient and the nurse grow as a result of the learning that occurs in the nursing situation."

Peplau correlates the stages of personality development in childhood to stages through which clients advance during the progression of an illness. She also views these interpersonal experiences as learning situations for nurses to facilitate forward movement in the development of personality. She believes that when there is fulfillment of psychological tasks associated with the nurse-client relationship, the personalities of both can be strengthened. Key concepts include the following:

- *Nursing* is a human relationship between an individual who is sick, or in need of health services, and a nurse especially educated to recognize and to respond to the need for help.
- **Psychodynamic nursing** is being able to understand one's own behavior, to help others identify felt difficulties, and to apply principles of human relations to the problems that arise at all levels of experience.
- *Roles* are sets of values and behaviors that are specific to functional positions within social structures. Peplau identifies the following *nursing roles*:
  - A *resource person* provides specific, needed information that helps the client understand his or her problem and the new situation.
  - A **counselor** listens as the client reviews feelings related to difficulties he or she is experiencing in any aspect of life. "Interpersonal techniques" have been identified to facilitate the nurse's interaction in the process of helping the client solve problems and make decisions concerning these difficulties.
  - A *teacher* identifies learning needs and provides information to the client or family that may aid in improvement of the life situation.
  - A *leader* directs the nurse-client interaction and ensures that appropriate actions are undertaken to facilitate achievement of the designated goals.

---

*Eighty percent of adults are fixed in level II, with a majority of women in Stage 3 and a majority of men in Stage 4.

- A **technical expert** understands various professional devices and possesses the clinical skills necessary to perform the interventions that are in the best interest of the client.
- A **surrogate** serves as a substitute figure for another.

Phases of nurse-client relationship are stages of overlapping roles or functions in relation to health problems, during which the nurse and client learn to work cooperatively to resolve difficulties. Peplau identifies four phases:

- *Orientation* is the phase during which the client, nurse, and family work together to recognize, clarify, and define the existing problem.
- *Identification* is the phase after which the client's initial impression has been clarified and when he or she begins to respond selectively to those who seem to offer the help that is needed. Clients may respond in one of three ways: (1) on the basis of participation or interdependent relationship with the nurse; (2) on the basis of independence or isolation from the nurse; or (3) on the basis of helplessness or dependence on the nurse (Peplau, 1991).
- *Exploitation* is the phase during which the client proceeds to take full advantage of the services offered to him or her. Having learned which services are available, feeling comfortable within the setting, and serving as an active participant in his or her own health care, the client exploits the services available and explores all possibilities of the changing situation.
- *Resolution* occurs when the client is freed from identification with helping persons and gathers strength to assume independence. Resolution is the direct result of successful completion of the other three phases.

Peplau's Stages of Personality Development

Psychological tasks are developmental lessons that must be learned on the way to achieving maturity of the personality. Peplau identifies four psychological tasks that she associates with the stages of infancy and childhood described by Freud and Sullivan. She states:

> When psychological tasks are successfully learned at each era of development, biological capacities are used productively and relations with people lead to productive living. When they are not successfully learned they carry over into adulthood and attempts at learning continue in devious ways, more or less impeded by conventional adaptations that provide a superstructure over the baseline of actual learning. (Peplau, 1991, p. 166)

In the context of nursing, Peplau (1991) relates these four psychological tasks to the demands made on nurses in their relationships with clients. She maintains the following:

> Nursing can function as a maturing force in society. Since illness is an event that is experienced along with feelings that derive from older experiences but are reenacted in the relationship of nurse to patient, the nurse-patient relationship is seen as an opportunity for nurses to help patients to complete the unfinished psychological tasks of childhood in some degree. (p. 159)

Peplau's psychological tasks of personality development include the four stages outlined in the following paragraphs. An outline of the stages of personality development according to Peplau's theory is presented in Table 3–7.

Learning to Count on Others

Nurses and clients first come together as strangers. Both bring to the relationship certain "raw materials," such as inherited biological components, personality characteristics (*temperament*), individual intellectual capacity, and specific cultural or environmental influences. Peplau relates these to the same "raw materials" with which an infant comes into this world. The newborn is capable of experiencing *comfort* and *discomfort*. He or she soon learns to communicate feelings in a way that results in the fulfillment of comfort needs by the mothering figure who provides love and care unconditionally. However, fulfillment of these dependency needs is inhibited when goals of the mothering figure become the focus, and love and

AGE	STAGE	MAJOR DEVELOPMENTAL TASKS
Infancy	Learning to count on others	Learning to communicate in various ways with the primary caregiver in order to have comfort needs fulfilled
Toddlerhood	Learning to delay satisfaction	Learning the satisfaction of pleasing others by delaying self-gratification in small ways
Early childhood	Identifying oneself	Learning appropriate roles and behaviors by acquiring the ability to perceive the expectations of others
Late childhood	Developing skills in participation	Learning the skills of compromise, competition, and cooperation with others; establishment of a more realistic view of the world and a feeling of one's place in it

TABLE 3–7   Stages of Development in Peplau's Interpersonal Theory

care are contingent on meeting the needs of the caregiver rather than the infant.

Clients with unmet dependency needs regress during illness and demonstrate behaviors that relate to this stage of development. Other clients regress to this level because of physical disabilities associated with their illness. Peplau believes that when nurses provide unconditional care, they help these clients progress toward more mature levels of functioning. This may involve the role of "surrogate mother," in which the nurse fulfills needs for the client with the intent of helping him or her grow, mature, and become more independent.

Learning to Delay Satisfaction

Peplau relates this stage to that of toddlerhood, or the first step in the development of interdependent social relationships. Psychosexually, it is compared to the anal stage of development, when a child learns that, because of cultural mores, he or she cannot empty the bowels for relief of discomfort at will, but must delay to use the toilet, which is considered more culturally acceptable. When toilet training occurs too early or is very rigid, or when appropriate behavior is set forth as a condition for love and caring, tasks associated with this stage remain unfulfilled. The child feels powerless and fails to learn the satisfaction of pleasing others by delaying self-gratification in small ways. He or she may also exhibit rebellious behavior by failing to comply with demands of the mothering figure in an effort to counter the feelings of powerlessness. The child may accomplish this by withholding the fecal product or failing to deposit it in the culturally acceptable manner.

Peplau cites Fromm (1949) in describing the following potential behaviors of individuals who have failed to complete the tasks of the second stage of development:

- Exploitation and manipulation of others to satisfy their own desires because they are unable to do so independently
- Suspiciousness and envy of others, directing hostility toward others in an effort to enhance their own self-image
- Hoarding and withholding possessions from others; miserliness
- Inordinate neatness and punctuality
- Inability to relate to others through sharing of feelings, ideas, or experiences
- Ability to vary the personality characteristics to those required to satisfy personal desires at any given time

When nurses observe these types of behaviors in clients, it is important to encourage full expression and to convey unconditional acceptance. When the client learns to feel safe and unconditionally accepted, he or she is more likely to let go of the oppositional behavior and

advance in the developmental progression. Peplau (1991) states:

> Nurses who aid patients to feel safe and secure, so that wants can be expressed and satisfaction eventually achieved, also help them to strengthen personal power that is needed for productive social activities. (p. 207)

Identifying Oneself

"A concept of self develops as a product of interaction with adults" (Peplau, 1991, p. 211). A child learns to structure self-concept by observing how others interact with him or her. Roles and behaviors are established out of the child's perception of the expectations of others. When children perceive that adults expect them to maintain more-or-less permanent roles as infants, they perceive themselves as helpless and dependent. When the perceived expectation is that the child must behave in a manner beyond his or her maturational level, the child is deprived of the fulfillment of emotional and growth needs at the lower levels of development. Children who are given freedom to respond to situations and experiences unconditionally (i.e., with behaviors that are appropriate to their feelings) learn to improve on and reconstruct behavioral responses at their own individual pace. Peplau (1991) states, "The ways in which adults appraise the child and the way he functions in relation to his experiences and perceptions are taken in or introjected and become the child's view of himself" (p. 213).

In nursing, it is important for the nurse to recognize cues that communicate how the client feels about himself or herself and about the presenting medical problem. In the initial interaction, it is difficult for the nurse to perceive the "wholeness" of the client, because the focus is on the condition that has caused him or her to seek help. Likewise, it is difficult for the client to perceive the nurse as a "mother (or father)" or "somebody's wife (or husband)" or as having a life aside from being there to offer assistance with the immediate presenting problem. As the relationship develops, nurses must be able to recognize client behaviors that indicate unfulfilled needs and provide experiences that promote growth. For example, the client who very proudly announces that she has completed activities of daily living independently and wants the nurse to come and inspect her room may still be craving the positive reinforcement associated with lower levels of development.

Nurses must also be aware of the predisposing factors that they bring to the relationship. Attitudes and beliefs about certain issues can have a deleterious effect on the client and interfere not only with the therapeutic relationship but also with the client's ability for growth and development. For example, a nurse who has strong beliefs against abortion may treat a client who has just undergone an abortion with disapproval and disrespect. The nurse may respond in this manner without even realizing he or she is doing so. Attitudes and values are introjected during early development and can be integrated so completely as to become a part of the self-system. Nurses must have knowledge and appreciation of their own concept of self in order to develop the flexibility required to accept all clients as they are, unconditionally. Effective resolution of problems that arise in the interdependent relationship can be the means for both client and nurse to reinforce positive personality traits and modify those more negative views of self.

Developing Skills in Participation

Peplau cites Sullivan's (1953) description of the "juvenile" stage of personality development (ages 6 through 9). During this stage, the child develops the capacity to "compromise, compete, and cooperate" with others. These skills are considered basic to one's ability to participate collaboratively with others. If a child tries to use the skills of an earlier level of development (e.g., crying, whining, demanding), he or she may be rejected by peers of this juvenile stage. As this stage progresses, children begin to view themselves through the eyes of their peers. Sullivan (1953) called this "consensual validation." Preadolescents take on a more realistic view of the world and a feeling of their place in it. The capacity to love others (besides the mother figure) develops at this time and is expressed in relation to one's self-acceptance.

Failure to develop appropriate skills at any point along the developmental progression results in an individual's difficulty with participation in confronting the recurring problems of life. It is not the responsibility of the nurse to teach solutions to problems, but rather to help clients improve their problem-solving skills so that they may achieve their own resolution. This is accomplished through development of the skills of competition, compromise, cooperation, consensual validation, and love of self and others. Nurses can assist clients to develop or refine these skills by helping them to identify the problem, define a goal, and take the responsibility for performing the actions necessary to reach that goal. Peplau (1991) states:

> Participation is required by a democratic society. When it has not been learned in earlier experiences, nurses have an opportunity to facilitate learning in the present and thus to aid in the promotion of a democratic society. (p. 259)

Relevance of Peplau's Model to Nursing Practice

Peplau's model provides nurses with a framework to interact with clients, many of whom are fixed in—or because of illness have regressed to—an earlier level of development. She suggests roles that nurses may assume to assist clients to progress, thereby achieving or resuming their appropriate developmental level. Appropriate developmental progression arms the individual with the ability to confront the recurring problems of life. Nurses serve to facilitate learning of that which has not been learned in earlier experiences.

SUMMARY

Growth and development are unique with each individual and continue throughout the life span. With each stage, there evolves an increasing complexity in the growth of the personality. This chapter has provided a description of the theories of Freud, Sullivan, Erikson, Mahler, Piaget, and Kohlberg. In addition, the theoretical concepts of Peplau, and their application to interpersonal relations in nursing, were presented. These theorists together provide a multifaceted approach to personality development, encompassing cognitive, psychosocial, and moral aspects.

Nurses must have a basic knowledge of human personality development to understand maladaptive behavioral responses commonly seen in psychiatric clients. Knowledge of the appropriateness of behaviors at each developmental level is vital to the planning and implementation of quality nursing care.

REVIEW QUESTIONS

SELF-EXAMINATION/LEARNING EXERCISE

Situation: Mr. J. is 35 years old. He has been admitted to the psychiatric unit for observation and evaluation following his arrest on charges that he robbed a convenience store and sexually assaulted the store clerk. Mr. J. was the illegitimate child of a teenage mother who deserted him when he was 6 months old. He was shuffled from one relative to another until it was clear that no one wanted him. Social Services placed him in foster homes, from which he continuously ran away. During his teenage years he was arrested a number of times for stealing, vandalism, arson, and various other infractions of the law. He was shunned by his peers and to this day has little interaction with others. On the unit, he appears very anxious, paces back and forth, and darts his head from side to side in a continuous scanning of the area. He is unkempt and unclean. He has refused to eat, making some barely audible comment related to "being poisoned." He has shown no remorse for his misdeeds.

Select the answer that is *most* appropriate for this situation.

1. Theoretically, in which level of psychosocial development (according to Erikson) would you place Mr. J.?
   a. Intimacy vs. isolation
   b. Generativity vs. self-absorption
   c. Trust vs. mistrust
   d. Autonomy vs. shame and doubt

2. According to Erikson's theory, where would you place Mr. J. based on his behavior?
   a. Intimacy vs. isolation
   b. Generativity vs. self-absorption
   c. Trust vs. mistrust
   d. Autonomy vs. shame and doubt

3. According to Mahler's theory, Mr. J. did not receive the critical "emotional refueling" required during the rapprochement phase of development. What are the consequences of this deficiency?
   a. He has not yet learned to delay gratification.
   b. He does not feel guilt about wrongdoings to others.
   c. He is unable to trust others.
   d. He has internalized rage and fears of abandonment.

4. In what stage of development is Mr. J. fixed according to Sullivan's interpersonal theory?
   a. Infancy. He relieves anxiety through oral gratification.
   b. Childhood. He has not learned to delay gratification.
   c. Early adolescence. He is struggling to form an identity.
   d. Late adolescence. He is working to develop a lasting relationship.

5. Which of the following describes the psychoanalytical structure of Mr. J.'s personality?
   a. Weak id, strong ego, weak superego
   b. Strong id, weak ego, weak superego
   c. Weak id, weak ego, punitive superego
   d. Strong id, weak ego, punitive superego

6. In which of Peplau's stages of development would you assess Mr. J.?
   a. Learning to count on others
   b. Learning to delay gratification
   c. Identifying oneself
   d. Developing skills in participation

7. In planning care for Mr. J., which of the following would be the primary focus for nursing?
   a. To decrease anxiety and develop trust
   b. To set limits on his behavior
   c. To ensure that he gets to group therapy
   d. To attend to his hygiene needs

Match the nursing role as described by Peplau with the nursing care behaviors listed on the right:

_____ 8. Surrogate

_____ 9. Counselor

_____ 10. Resource person

A. "Mr. J., please tell me what it was like when you were growing up."

B. "What questions do you have about being here on this unit?"

C. "Some changes will have to be made in in your behavior. I care about what happens to you."

REFERENCES

American Psychiatric Association (2000). *Diagnostic and statistical manual of mental disorders* (4th ed.) Text Revision. Washington, DC: American Psychiatric Publishing.

Marmer, S.S. (2003). Theories of the mind and psychopathology. In R.E. Hales & S.C. Yudofsky (Eds.). *Textbook of clinical psychiatry* (4th ed.). Washington, DC: American Psychiatric Publishing.

Murray, R., & Zentner, J. (2001). *Health promotion strategies through the life span* (7th ed.). Upper Saddle River, NJ: Prentice Hall.

Peplau, H.E. (1991). *Interpersonal relations in nursing*. New York: Springer.

CLASSICAL REFERENCES

Chess, S., & Thomas, A. (1986). *Temperament in clinical practice*. New York: Guilford Press.

Erikson, E. (1963). *Childhood and society* (2nd ed.). New York: WW Norton.

Freud, S. (1961). The ego and the id. *Standard edition of the complete psychological works of Freud*, Vol XIX. London: Hogarth Press.

Fromm, E. (1949). *Man for himself*. New York: Farrar & Rinehart.

Kohlberg, L. (1968). Moral development. In *International encyclopedia of social science*. New York: Macmillan.

Mahler, M., Pine, F., & Bergman, A. (1975). *The psychological birth of the human infant*. New York: Basic Books.

Piaget, J., & Inhelder, B. (1969). *The psychology of the child*. New York: Basic Books.

Sullivan, H.S. (1953). *The interpersonal theory of psychiatry*. New York: WW Norton.

4
CHAPTER

CONCEPTS OF
PSYCHOBIOLOGY

CHAPTER OUTLINE

OBJECTIVES

THE NERVOUS SYSTEM: AN ANATOMICAL
REVIEW

NEUROENDOCRINOLOGY

GENETICS

PSYCHOIMMUNOLOGY

IMPLICATIONS FOR NURSING

SUMMARY

REVIEW QUESTIONS

KEY TERMS

axon
cell body
circadian rhythms
dendrites
genotype
limbic system

neuron
neurotransmitter
phenotype
receptor sites
synapse

CORE CONCEPTS

genetics
neuroendocrinology
psychobiology
psychoimmunology

OBJECTIVES

After reading this chapter, the student will be able to:

1. Identify gross anatomical structures of the brain and describe their functions.
2. Discuss the physiology of neurotransmission in the central nervous system.
3. Describe the role of neurotransmitters in human behavior.
4. Discuss the association of endocrine functioning to the development of psychiatric disorders.
5. Describe the role of genetics in the development of psychiatric disorders.

6. Discuss the correlation of alteration in brain functioning to various psychiatric disorders.
7. Identify various diagnostic procedures used to detect alteration in biological functioning that may be contributing to psychiatric disorders.
8. Discuss the influence of psychological factors on the immune system.
9. Discuss the implications of psychobiological concepts to the practice of psychiatric/mental health nursing.

 n recent years, a greater emphasis has been placed on the study of the organic basis for psychiatric illness. This "neuroscientific revolution" began in earnest when the 101st legislature of the United States designated the 1990s as the "decade of the brain." With this legislation came the challenge of studying the biological basis of behavior.

Several mental illnesses are now being considered as physical disorders that are the result of malfunctions and/or malformations of the brain.

This is not to imply that psychosocial and sociocultural influences are totally discounted. Such a notion would negate the transactional model of stress/adaptation on which the framework of this textbook is conceptualized.

The systems of biology, psychology, and sociology are not mutually exclusive—they are interacting systems. This is clearly indicated by the fact that individuals experience biological changes in response to various environmental events. Indeed, each of these disciplines may be, at various times, most appropriate for explaining behavioral phenomena.

This chapter focuses on the role of neurophysiological, neurochemical, genetic, and endocrine influences on psychiatric illness. Various diagnostic procedures used to detect alteration in biological function that may contribute to psychiatric illness are identified, and the implications to psychiatric/mental health nursing are discussed.

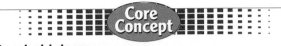

Core Concept

Psychobiology
The study of the biological foundations of cognitive, emotional, and behavioral processes.

THE NERVOUS SYSTEM: AN ANATOMICAL REVIEW

The Brain

The brain has three major divisions, subdivided into six major parts:

1. Forebrain
   a. Cerebrum
   b. Diencephalon
2. Midbrain
   a. Mesencephalon
3. Hindbrain
   a. Pons
   b. Medulla
   c. Cerebellum

Each of these structures is discussed individually. A summary is presented in Table 4–1.

Cerebrum

The cerebrum consists of a right and a left hemisphere and constitutes the largest part of the human brain. The right and left hemispheres are connected by a deep groove, which houses a band of 200 million **neurons** (nerve cells) called the corpus callosum. Because each hemisphere controls different functions, information is processed through the corpus callosum so that each hemisphere is aware of the activity of the other.

The surface of the cerebrum consists of gray matter and is called the cerebral cortex. The gray matter is so called because the neuron cell bodies of which it is composed look gray to the eye. These gray matter cell bodies are thought to be the actual thinking structures of the brain. Another pair of masses of gray matter called basal

TABLE 4–1	Structure and Function of the Brain
STRUCTURE	**PRIMARY FUNCTION**
I. The Forebrain A. Cerebrum	Composed of two hemispheres separated by a deep groove that houses a band of 200 million neurons called the corpus callosum. The outer shell is called the cortex. It is extensively folded and consists of billions of neurons. The left hemisphere appears to be dominant in most people. The right hemisphere may be called the "creative" brain and is associated with affect and spatial-perceptual functions. Each hemisphere is divided into four lobes.
1. Frontal lobes	Voluntary body movement, including movements that permit speaking, thinking and judgment formation, and expression of feelings.
2. Parietal lobes	Perception and interpretation of most sensory information (including touch, pain, taste, and body position).
3. Temporal lobes	Hearing, short-term memory, and sense of smell; expression of emotions through connection with limbic system.
4. Occipital lobes	Visual reception and interpretation.
B. Diencephalon	Connects cerebrum with lower brain structures.
1. Thalamus	Integrates all sensory input (except smell) on way to cortex; some involvement with emotions and mood.
2. Hypothalamus	Regulates anterior and posterior lobes of pituitary gland; exerts control over actions of the autonomic nervous system; regulates appetite and temperature.
3. Limbic system	Consists of medially placed cortical and subcortical structures and the fiber tracts connecting them with one another and with the hypothalamus. It is sometimes called the "emotional brain"—associated with feelings of fear and anxiety; anger and aggression; love, joy, and hope; and with sexuality and social behavior.
II. The Midbrain A. Mesencephalon	Responsible for visual, auditory, and balance ("righting") reflexes.
III. The Hindbrain A. Pons	Regulation of respiration and skeletal muscle tone; ascending and descending tracts connect brain stem with cerebellum and cortex.
B. Medulla	Pathway for all ascending and descending fiber tracts; contains vital centers that regulate heart rate, blood pressure, and respiration; reflex centers for swallowing, sneezing, coughing, and vomiting.
C. Cerebellum	Regulates muscle tone and coordination and maintains posture and equilibrium.

ganglia is found deep within the cerebral hemispheres. The basal ganglia are responsible for certain subconscious aspects of voluntary movement, such as swinging the arms when walking, gesturing while speaking, and regulating muscle tone (Scanlon & Sanders, 2003).

The cerebral cortex is identified by numerous folds, called gyri, and deep grooves between the folds, called sulci. This extensive folding extends the surface area of the cerebral cortex, and thus permits the presence of millions more neurons than would be possible without it (as is the case in the brains of some animals, such as dogs and cats). Each hemisphere of the cerebral cortex is divided into the frontal lobe, parietal lobe, temporal lobe, and occipital lobe. These lobes, which are named for the overlying bones in the cranium, are identified in Figure 4–1.

The Frontal Lobes. Voluntary body movement is controlled by the impulses through the frontal lobes. The right frontal lobe controls motor activity on the left side of the body and the left frontal lobe controls motor activity on the right side of the body. Movements that permit speaking are also controlled by the frontal lobe, usually only on the left side (Scanlon & Sanders, 2003). The frontal lobe may also play a role in the emotional experience, as evidenced by changes in mood and character after damage to this area. The alterations include fear,

aggressiveness, depression, rage, euphoria, irritability, and apathy and are likely related to a frontal lobe connection to the **limbic system**. The frontal lobe may also be involved (indirectly through association fibers linked to primary sensory areas) in thinking and perceptual interpretation of information.

The Parietal Lobes. Somatosensory input occurs in the parietal lobe area of the brain. These include touch, pain and pressure, taste, temperature, perception of joint and body position, and visceral sensations. The parietal lobes also contain association fibers linked to the primary sensory areas through which sensory–perceptual information is interpreted. Language interpretation is associated with the left hemisphere of the parietal lobe.

The Temporal Lobes. The upper anterior temporal lobe is concerned with auditory functions, while the lower part is dedicated to short-term memory. The sense of smell has a connection to the temporal lobes, as the impulses carried by the olfactory nerves end in this area of the brain (Scanlon & Sanders, 2003). The temporal lobes also play a role in the expression of emotions through an interconnection with the limbic system. The left temporal lobe, along with the left parietal lobe, is involved in language interpretation.

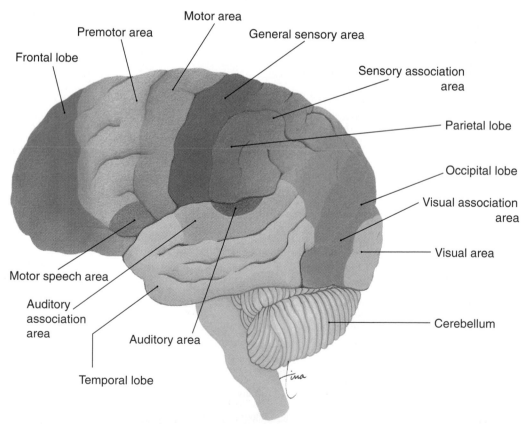

FIGURE 4–1 Left cerebral hemisphere showing some of the functional areas that have been mapped. (From Scanlon, V.C., & Sanders, T. *Essentials of anatomy and physiology*, 4th ed. F.A. Davis, Philadelphia, 2003.)

The Occipital Lobes. The occipital lobes are the primary area of visual reception and interpretation. Visual perception, which gives individuals the ability to judge spatial relationships such as distance and to see in three dimensions, is also processed in this area (Scanlon & Sanders, 2003). Language interpretation is influenced by the occipital lobes through an association with the visual experience.

Diencephalon

The second part of the forebrain is the diencephalon, which connects the cerebrum with lower structures of the brain. The major components of the diencephalon include the thalamus, the hypothalamus, and the limbic system. These structures may be identified in Figures 4–2 and 4–3.

Thalamus. The thalamus integrates all sensory input (except smell) on its way to the cortex. This helps the cerebral cortex interpret the whole picture very rapidly, rather than experiencing each sensation individually. The thalamus is also involved in temporarily blocking minor sensations, so that an individual can concentrate on one important event when necessary. For example, an individual who is studying for an examination may be unaware of the clock ticking in the room, or even of another person walking into the room, because the thalamus has temporarily blocked these incoming sensations from the cortex (Scanlon & Sanders, 2003).

Hypothalamus. The hypothalamus is located just below the thalamus and just above the pituitary gland and has a number of diverse functions.

1. **Regulation of the Pituitary Gland.** The pituitary gland consists of two lobes: the posterior lobe and the anterior lobe.
   a. *The posterior lobe* of the pituitary gland is actually extended tissue from the hypothalamus. The posterior lobe stores antidiuretic hormone (which helps to maintain blood pressure through regulation of water retention) and oxytocin (the hormone

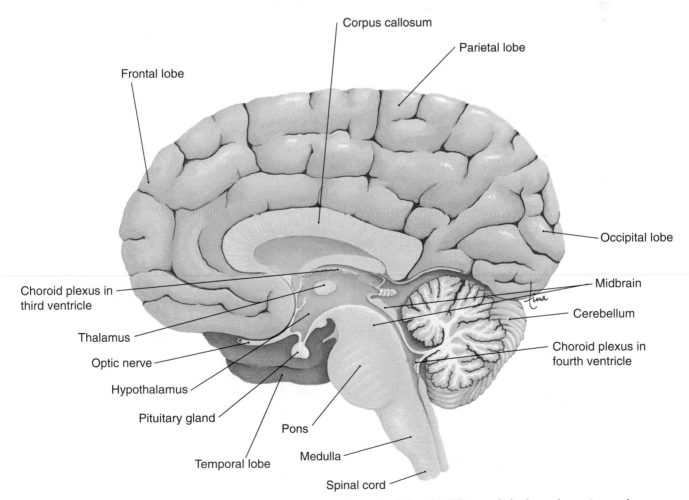

FIGURE 4–2 Midsagittal section of the brain as seen from the left side. This medial plane shows internal anatomy as well as the lobes of the cerebrum. (From Scanlon, V.C., & Sanders, T. *Essentials of anatomy and physiology*, 4th ed. F.A. Davis, Philadelphia, 2003.)

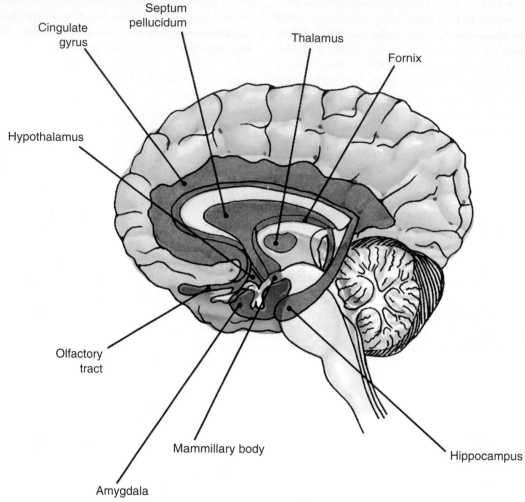

FIGURE 4–3 Structures of the limbic system. (Adapted from Scanlon, V.C., & Sanders, T. *Essentials of anatomy and physiology*, 4th ed. F.A. Davis, Philadelphia, 2003.)

responsible for stimulation of the uterus during labor, and the release of milk from the mammary glands). Both of these hormones are produced in the hypothalamus. When the hypothalamus detects the body's need for these hormones, it sends nerve impulses to the posterior pituitary for their release.

b. *The anterior lobe* of the pituitary gland consists of glandular tissue that produces a number of hormones used by the body. These hormones are regulated by "releasing factors" from the hypothalamus. When the hormones are required by the body, the releasing factors stimulate the release of the hormone from the anterior pituitary and the hormone in turn stimulates its target organ to carry out its specific functions.

2. **Direct Neural Control Over the Actions of the Autonomic Nervous System**. The hypothalamus regulates the appropriate visceral responses during

various emotional states. The actions of the autonomic nervous system are described later in this chapter.

3. **Regulation of Appetite**. Appetite is regulated through response to blood nutrient levels.

4. **Regulation of Temperature**. The hypothalamus senses internal temperature changes in the blood that flows through the brain. It receives information through sensory input from the skin about external temperature changes. The hypothalamus then uses this information to promote certain types of responses (e.g., sweating or shivering) that help to maintain body temperature within the normal range (Scanlon & Sanders, 2003).

Limbic System. The part of the brain known as the limbic system consists of portions of the cerebrum and the diencephalon. The major components include the medially placed cortical and subcortical structures and the fiber tracts connecting them with one another and with the hypothalamus. The system is composed of the amygdala, mammillary body, olfactory tract, hypothalamus, cingulate gyrus, septum pellucidum, thalamus, hippocampus, and neuronal connecting pathways, such as the fornix and others. This system has been called "the emotional brain" and is associated with feelings of fear and anxiety; anger, rage, and aggression; love, joy, and hope; and with sexuality and social behavior.

Mesencephalon

Structures of major importance in the mesencephalon, or midbrain, include nuclei and fiber tracts. The mesencephalon extends from the pons to the hypothalamus and is responsible for integration of various reflexes, including visual reflexes (e.g., automatically turning away from a dangerous object when it comes into view), auditory reflexes (e.g., automatically turning toward a sound that is heard), and righting reflexes (e.g., automatically keeping the head upright and maintaining balance) (Scanlon & Sanders, 2003). The mesencephalon may be identified in Figure 4–2.

Pons

The pons is a bulbous structure that lies between the midbrain and the medulla (Figure 4–2). It is composed of large bundles of fibers and forms a major connection between the cerebellum and the brainstem. It also contains the central connections of cranial nerves V through VIII and centers for respiration and skeletal muscle tone.

Medulla

The medulla is the connecting structure between the spinal cord and the pons and all of the ascending and descending fiber tracts pass through it. The vital centers are contained in the medulla, and it is responsible for regulation of heart rate, blood pressure, and respiration. Also in the medulla are reflex centers for swallowing, sneezing, coughing, and vomiting (Scanlon & Sanders, 2003). It also contains nuclei for cranial nerves IX through XII. The medulla, pons, and midbrain form the structure known as the brainstem. These structures may be identified in Figure 4–2.

Cerebellum

The cerebellum is separated from the brainstem by the fourth ventricle but has connections to the brainstem through bundles of fiber tracts. It is situated just below the occipital lobes of the cerebrum (Figures 4–1 and 4–2). The functions of the cerebellum are concerned with involuntary movement, such as muscular tone and coordination and the maintenance of posture and equilibrium.

Nerve Tissue

The tissue of the central nervous system (CNS) consists of nerve cells, called neurons, that generate and transmit electrochemical impulses. The structure of a neuron is composed of a cell body, an axon, and dendrites. The **cell body** contains the nucleus and is essential for the continued life of the neuron. The **dendrites** are processes that transmit impulses toward the cell body, and the **axon** transmits impulses away from the cell body. The axons and dendrites are covered by layers of cells called *neuroglia* that form a coating, or "sheath," of myelin. *Myelin* is a phospholipid that provides insulation against short-circuiting of the neurons during their electrical activity and increases the velocity of the impulse. The white matter of the brain and spinal cord is so called because of the whitish appearance of the myelin sheath over the axons and dendrites. The gray matter is composed of cell bodies that contain no myelin.

The three classes of neurons include afferent (sensory), efferent (motor), and interneurons. The *afferent neurons* carry impulses from receptors in the internal and external periphery to the CNS, where they are then interpreted into various sensations. The *efferent neurons* carry impulses from the CNS to *effectors* in the periphery, such as muscles (that respond by contracting) and glands (that respond by secreting). A schematic of afferent and efferent neurons is presented in Figure 4–4.

Interneurons exist entirely within the CNS, and 99 percent of all nerve cells belong to this group. They may carry only sensory or motor impulses, or they may serve as integrators in the pathways between afferent and efferent neurons. They account in large part for thinking, feelings, learning, language, and memory. The directional pathways of afferent, efferent, and interneurons are presented in Figure 4–5.

Synapses

Information is transmitted through the body from one neuron to another. Some messages may be processed through only a few neurons, while others may require thousands of neuronal connections. The neurons that transmit the impulses do not actually touch each other. The junction between two neurons is called a **synapse**. The small space between the axon terminals of one neuron and the cell body or dendrites of another is called the *synaptic cleft*. Neurons conducting impulses toward the synapse are called *presynaptic neurons* and those conducting impulses away are called *postsynaptic neurons*.

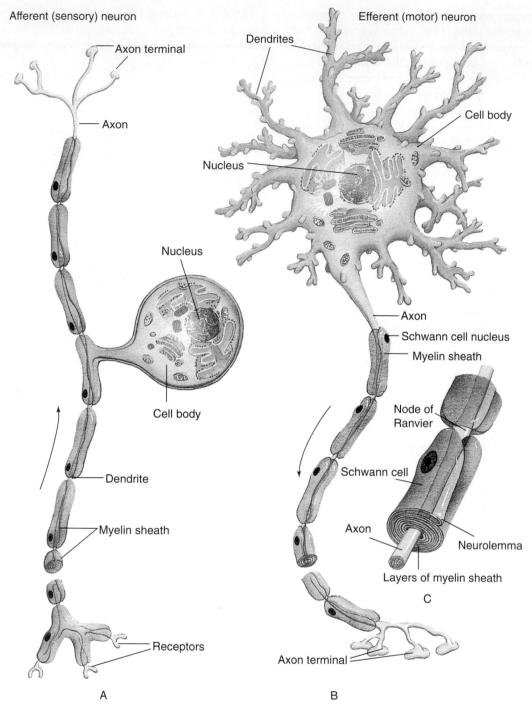

FIGURE 4–4 Neuron structure. *(A)* A typical sensory neuron. *(B)* A typical motor neuron. The arrows indicate the direction of impulse transmission. *(C)* Details of the myelin sheath and neurolemma formed by Schwann cells. (From Scanlon, V.C., & Sanders, T. *Essentials of anatomy and physiology*, 4th ed. F.A. Davis, Philadelphia, 2003.)

A chemical, called a **neurotransmitter**, is stored in the axon terminals of the presynaptic neuron. An electrical impulse through the neuron causes the release of this neurotransmitter into the synaptic cleft. The neurotransmitter then diffuses across the synaptic cleft and combines with **receptor sites** that are situated on the cell membrane of the postsynaptic neuron. The result of the combination of neurotransmitter–receptor site is the determination of whether or not another electrical impulse is generated. If one is generated, the result is called an *excitatory response* and the electrical impulse moves on to the next synapse, where the same process recurs. If another electrical impulse is not generated by the neurotransmitter–receptor site combination, the

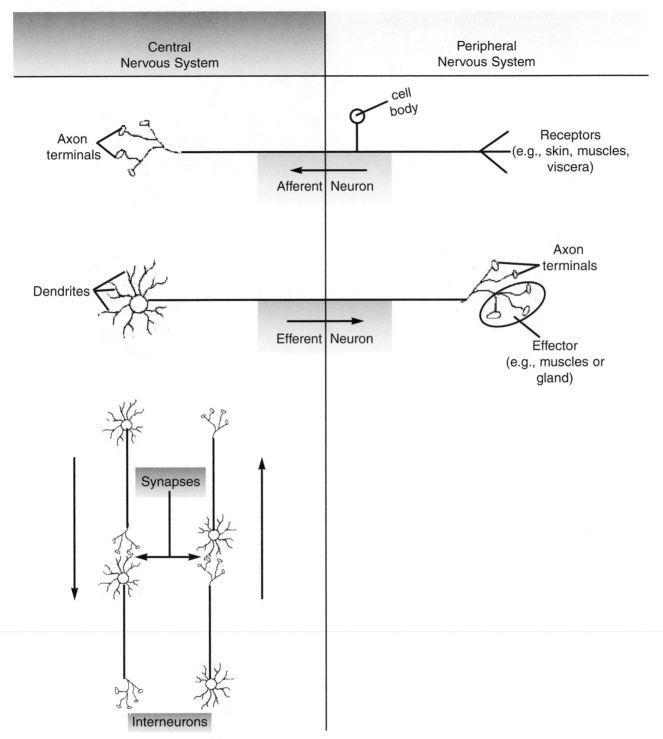

FIGURE 4–5   Directional pathways of neurons

result is called an *inhibitory response*, and synaptic transmission is terminated.

The cell body or dendrite of the postsynaptic neuron also contains a chemical *inactivator* that is specific to the neurotransmitter that has been released by the presynaptic neuron. When the synaptic transmission has been completed, the chemical inactivator quickly inactivates the neurotransmitter to prevent unwanted, continuous impulses, until a new impulse from the presynaptic neuron releases more neurotransmitter. A schematic representation of a synapse is presented in Figure 4–6.

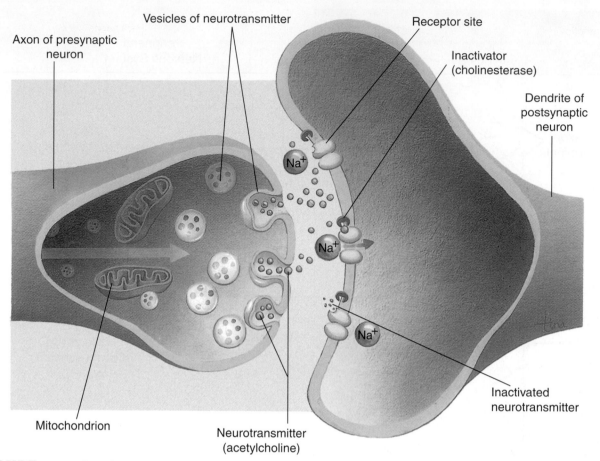

FIGURE 4–6 Impulse transmission at a synapse. The arrow indicates the direction of electrical impulses. (From Scanlon, V.C., & Sanders, T. *Essentials of anatomy and physiology,* 4th ed. F.A. Davis, Philadelphia, 2003.)

Autonomic Nervous System

The autonomic nervous system (ANS) is actually considered part of the peripheral nervous system. Its regulation is integrated by the hypothalamus, however, and therefore the emotions exert a great deal of influence over its functioning. For this reason, the ANS has been implicated in the etiology of a number of psychophysiological disorders. These diseases of adaptation are discussed in detail in Chapter 36.

The ANS has two divisions: the sympathetic and the parasympathetic. The sympathetic division is dominant in stressful situations and prepares the body for the "fight or flight" response that was discussed in Chapter 1. The neuronal cell bodies of the sympathetic division originate in the thoracolumbar region of the spinal cord. Their axons extend to the chains of sympathetic ganglia, where they synapse with other neurons that subsequently innervate the visceral effectors. This results in an increase in heart rate and respirations and a decrease in digestive secretions and peristalsis. Blood is shunted to the vital organs and to skeletal muscles to ensure adequate oxygenation.

The neuronal cell bodies of the parasympathetic division originate in the brainstem and the sacral segments of the spinal cord, and extend to the parasympathetic ganglia where the synapse takes place either very close to or actually in the visceral organ being innervated. In this way, a very localized response is possible. The parasympathetic division dominates when an individual is in a relaxed, nonstressful condition. The heart and respirations are maintained at a normal rate, and secretions and peristalsis increase for normal digestion. Elimination functions are promoted. A schematic representation of the autonomic nervous system is shown in Figure 4–7.

Neurotransmitters

Neurotransmitters were described earlier in the explanation of synaptic activity. They are discussed separately and in detail here because of the essential function they play in the role of human emotion and behavior and because they are the target for mechanism of action of many of the psychotropic medications.

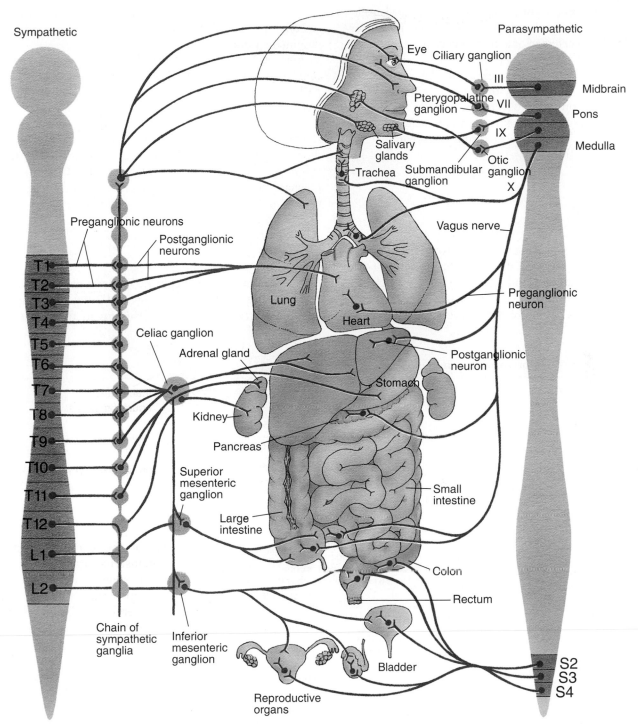

FIGURE 4–7 The autonomic nervous system. The sympathetic division is shown on the left, and the parasympathetic division is shown on the right (both divisions are bilateral). (From Scanlon, V.C., & Sanders, T. *Essentials of anatomy and physiology*, 4th ed. F.A. Davis, Philadelphia, 2003).

Neurotransmitters are chemicals that convey information across synaptic clefts to neighboring target cells. They are stored in small vesicles in the axon terminals of neurons. When the action potential, or electrical impulse, reaches this point, the neurotransmitters are released from the vesicles. They cross the synaptic cleft and bind with receptor sites on the cell body or dendrites of the adjacent neuron to allow the impulse to continue its course or to prevent the impulse from continuing. After the neurotransmitter has performed its function in the synapse, it either returns to the vesicles to be stored and used again, or it is inactivated and dissolved by enzymes. The process of being stored for reuse is called *reuptake*, a function that holds significance for understanding the mechanism of action of certain psychotropic medications.

Many neurotransmitters exist in the central and peripheral nervous systems, but only a limited number have implications for psychiatry. Major categories include cholinergics, monoamines, amino acids, and neuropeptides. Each of these is discussed separately and summarized in Table 4–2.

Cholinergics

Acetylcholine. Acetylcholine was the first chemical to be identified and proven as a neurotransmitter. It is a major effector chemical in the ANS, producing activity at all sympathetic and parasympathetic presynaptic nerve terminals and all parasympathetic postsynaptic nerve terminals. It is highly significant in the neurotrans-

mission that occurs at the junctions of nerve and muscles. Acetylcholinesterase is the enzyme that destroys acetylcholine or inhibits its activity.

In the CNS, acetylcholine neurons innervate the cerebral cortex, hippocampus, and limbic structures. The pathways are especially dense through the area of the basal ganglia in the brain.

Functions of acetylcholine are manifold and include sleep, arousal, pain perception, modulation and coordination of movement, and memory acquisition and retention (Murphy & Deutsch, 1991). Cholinergic mechanisms may have some role in certain disorders of motor behavior and memory, such as Parkinson's, Huntington's, and Alzheimer's diseases.

Monoamines

Norepinephrine. Norepinephrine is the neurotransmitter that produces activity at the sympathetic postsynaptic nerve terminals in the ANS resulting in the "fight or

TABLE 4–2 Neurotransmitters in the CNS

NEUROTRANSMITTER	LOCATION/FUNCTION	POSSIBLE IMPLICATIONS FOR MENTAL ILLNESS
I. Cholinergics		
A. Acetylcholine	ANS: Sympathetic and parasympathetic presynaptic nerve terminals; parasympathetic postsynaptic nerve terminals CNS: Cerebral cortex, hippocampus, limbic structures, and basal ganglia Functions: Sleep, arousal, pain perception, movement, memory	Increased levels: Depression Decreased levels: Alzheimer's disease, Huntington's disease, Parkinson's disease
II. Monoamines		
A. Norepinephrine	ANS: Sympathetic postsynaptic nerve terminals CNS: Thalamus, hypothalamus, limbic system, hippocampus, cerebellum, cerebral cortex Functions: Mood, cognition, perception, locomotion, cardiovascular functioning, and sleep and arousal	Decreased levels: Depression Increased levels: Mania, anxiety states, schizophrenia
B. Dopamine	Frontal cortex, limbic system, basal ganglia, thalamus, posterior pituitary, and spinal cord Functions: Movement and coordination, emotions, voluntary judgment, release of prolactin	Decreased levels: Parkinson's disease and depression Increased levels: Mania and schizophrenia
C. Serotonin	Hypothalamus, thalamus, limbic system, cerebral cortex, cerebellum, spinal cord Functions: Sleep and arousal, libido, appetite, mood, aggression, pain perception, coordination, judgment	Decreased levels: Depression Increased levels: Anxiety states
D. Histamine	Hypothalamus	Decreased levels: Depression
III. Amino Acids		
A. Gamma-aminobutyric acid (GABA)	Hypothalamus, hippocampus, cortex, cerebellum, basal ganglia, spinal cord, retina Functions: Slowdown of body activity	Decreased levels: Huntington's disease, anxiety disorders, schizophrenia, and various forms of epilepsy
B. Glycine	Spinal cord and brain stem Functions: Recurrent inhibition of motor neurons	Toxic levels: "glycine encephalopathy," decreased levels are correlated with spastic motor movements
C. Glutamate and aspartate	Pyramidal cells of the cortex, cerebellum, and the primary sensory afferent systems; hippocampus, thalamus, hypothalamus, spinal cord Functions: Relay of sensory information and in the regulation of various motor and spinal reflexes	Increased levels: Huntington's disease, temporal lobe epilepsy, spinal cerebellar degeneration

(Continued on opposite page)

NEUROTRANSMITTER	LOCATION/FUNCTION	POSSIBLE IMPLICATIONS FOR MENTAL ILLNESS
IV. Neuropeptides		
A. Endorphins and enkephalins	Hypothalamus, thalamus, limbic structures, midbrain, and brain stem; enkephalins are also found in the gastrointestinal tract Functions: Modulation of pain and reduced peristalsis (enkephalins)	Modulation of dopamine activity by opioid peptides may indicate some link to the symptoms of schizophrenia
B. Substance P	Hypothalamus, limbic structures, midbrain, brain stem, thalamus, basal ganglia, and spinal cord; also found in gastrointestinal tract and salivary glands Function: Regulation of pain	Decreased levels: Huntington's disease and Alzheimer's disease Increased levels: Depression
C. Somatostatin	Cerebral cortex, hippocampus, thalamus, basal ganglia, brain stem, and spinal cord Function: Inhibits release of norepinephrine; stimulates release of serotonin, dopamine, and acetylcholine	Decreased levels: Alzheimer's disease Increased levels: Huntington's disease

flight" responses in the effector organs. In the CNS, norepinephrine pathways originate in the pons and medulla and innervate the thalamus, dorsal hypothalamus, limbic system, hippocampus, cerebellum, and cerebral cortex. When norepinephrine is not returned for storage in the vesicles of the axon terminals, it is metabolized and inactivated by the enzymes monoamine oxidase (MAO) and catechol-O-methyl-transferase (COMT).

The functions of norepinephrine include the regulation of mood, cognition, perception, locomotion, cardiovascular functioning, and sleep and arousal (Murphy & Deutsch, 1991). The activity of norepinephrine also has been implicated in certain mood disorders such as depression and mania, in anxiety states, and in schizophrenia (Sadock & Sadock, 2003).

Dopamine. Dopamine pathways arise from the midbrain and hypothalamus and terminate in the frontal cortex, limbic system, basal ganglia, and thalamus. Dopamine neurons in the hypothalamus innervate the posterior pituitary and those from the posterior hypothalamus project to the spinal cord. As with norepinephrine, the inactivating enzymes for dopamine are MAO and COMT.

Dopamine functions include regulation of movements and coordination, emotions, voluntary decision-making ability, and because of its influence on the pituitary gland, it inhibits the release of prolactin (Sadock & Sadock, 2003). Increased levels of dopamine are associated with mania (Dubovsky, Davies, & Dubovsky, 2003) and schizophrenia (Ho, Black, & Andreasen, 2003).

Serotonin. Serotonin pathways originate from cell bodies located in the pons and medulla and project to areas including the hypothalamus, thalamus, limbic system, cerebral cortex, cerebellum, and spinal cord. Serotonin that is not returned to be stored in the axon terminal vesicles is catabolized by the enzyme MAO.

Serotonin may play a role in sleep and arousal, libido, appetite, mood, aggression, and pain perception. The serotoninergic system has been implicated in the etiology of certain psychopathological conditions including anxiety states, mood disorders, and schizophrenia (Sadock & Sadock, 2003).

Histamine. The role of histamine in mediating allergic and inflammatory reactions has been well documented. Its role in the CNS as a neurotransmitter has only recently been confirmed, and the availability of information is limited. The highest concentrations of histamine are found within various regions of the hypothalamus. The enzyme that catabolizes histamine is MAO. Although the exact processes mediated by histamine with the CNS are uncertain, some data suggest that histamine may play a role in depressive illness.

Amino Acids

Inhibitory Amino Acids

Gamma-Aminobutyric Acid. Gamma-aminobutyric acid (GABA) has a widespread distribution in the CNS, with high concentrations in the hypothalamus, hippocampus, cortex, cerebellum, and basal ganglia of the brain, in the gray matter of the dorsal horn of the spinal cord, and in the retina. Most GABA is associated with short inhibitory interneurons, although some long-axon pathways within the brain also have been identified. GABA is catabolized by the enzyme GABA transaminase.

Inhibitory neurotransmitters, such as GABA, prevent postsynaptic excitation, interrupting the progression of the electrical impulse at the synaptic junction. This function is significant when slowdown of body activity is advantageous. Enhancement of the GABA system is the mechanism of action by which the benzodiazepines produce their calming effect.

Alterations in the GABA system have been implicated in the etiology of anxiety disorders, movement disorders (e.g., Huntington's disease), and various forms of epilepsy.

Glycine. The highest concentrations of glycine in the CNS are found in the spinal cord and brainstem. Little is known about the possible enzymatic metabolism of glycine.

Glycine appears to be the neurotransmitter of recurrent inhibition of motor neurons within the spinal cord, and is possibly involved in the regulation of spinal and brainstem reflexes. It has been implicated in the pathogenesis of certain types of spastic disorders and in "glycine encephalopathy," which is known to occur with toxic accumulation of the neurotransmitter in the brain and cerebrospinal fluid (Murphy & Deutsch, 1991).

Excitatory Amino Acids

Glutamate and Aspartate. Glutamate and aspartate appear to be primary excitatory neurotransmitters in the pyramidal cells of the cortex, the cerebellum, and the primary sensory afferent systems. They are also found in the hippocamus, thalamus, hypothalamus, and spinal cord. Glutamate and aspartate are inactivated by uptake into the tissues and through assimilation in various metabolic pathways.

Glutamate and aspartate function in the relay of sensory information and in the regulation of various motor and spinal reflexes. Alteration in these systems has been implicated in the etiology of certain neurodegenerative disorders, such as Huntington's disease, temporal lobe epilepsy, and spinal cerebellar degeneration.

Neuropeptides

Numerous neuropeptides have been identified and studied. They are classified by the area of the body in which they are located or by their pharmacological or functional properties. Although their role as neurotransmitters has not been clearly established, it is known that they often coexist with the classic neurotransmitters within a neuron; however, the functional significance of this coexistence still requires further study. Hormonal neuropeptides are discussed in the section of this chapter on psychoendocrinology.

Opioid Peptides. Opioid peptides, which include the endorphins and enkephalins, have been widely studied. Opioid peptides are found in various concentrations in the hypothalamus, thalamus, limbic structures, midbrain, and brain stem. Enkephalins are also found in the gastrointestinal (GI) tract. Opioid peptides are thought to have a role in pain modulation, with their natural morphine-like properties. They are released in response to painful stimuli, and may be responsible for producing the analgesic effect following acupuncture. Opioid peptides alter the release of dopamine and affect the spontaneous activity of the dopaminergic neurons. These findings may have some implication for opioid peptide–dopamine interaction in the etiology of schizophrenia.

Substance P. Substance P was the first neuropeptide to be discovered. It is present in high concentrations in the hypothalamus, limbic structures, midbrain, and brainstem, and is also found in the thalamus, basal ganglia, and spinal cord. Substance P has been found to be highly concentrated in sensory fibers, and for this reason is thought to play a role in sensory transmission, particularly in the regulation of pain. Substance P abnormalities have been associated with Huntington's disease, dementia of the Alzheimer's type, and mood disorders (Sadock & Sadock, 2003).

Somatostatin. Somatostatin (also called growth hormone-inhibiting hormone) is found in the cerebral cortex, hippocampus, thalamus, basal ganglia, brainstem, and spinal cord, and has multiple effects on the CNS. It exerts inhibitory effects on the release of norepinephrine and stimulatory effects on serotonin. It stimulates the turnover and release of dopamine in the basal ganglia and acetylcholine in the brainstem and hippocampus. Postmortem examinations have revealed high concentrations of somatostatin in brain specimens of clients with Huntington's disease, and low concentrations in those with Alzheimer's disease.

> **Core Concept**
>
> **Neuroendocrinology**
> The study of the interaction between the nervous system and the endocrine system, and the effects of various hormones on cognitive, emotional, and behavioral functioning.

NEUROENDOCRINOLOGY

Human endocrine functioning has a strong foundation in the CNS, under the direction of the hypothalamus, which has direct control over the pituitary gland. The pituitary gland has two major lobes—the anterior lobe (also called the *adenohypophysis*) and the posterior lobe (also called the *neurohypophysis*). The pituitary gland is only about the size of a pea, but despite its small size and because of the powerful control it exerts over endocrine functioning in humans, it is sometimes called the "master gland" (Figure 4–8 shows the hormones of the pituitary gland and their target organs.) Many of the hormones subject to hypothalamus–pituitary regulation may have implications for behavioral functioning. Discussion of these hormones is summarized in Table 4–3.

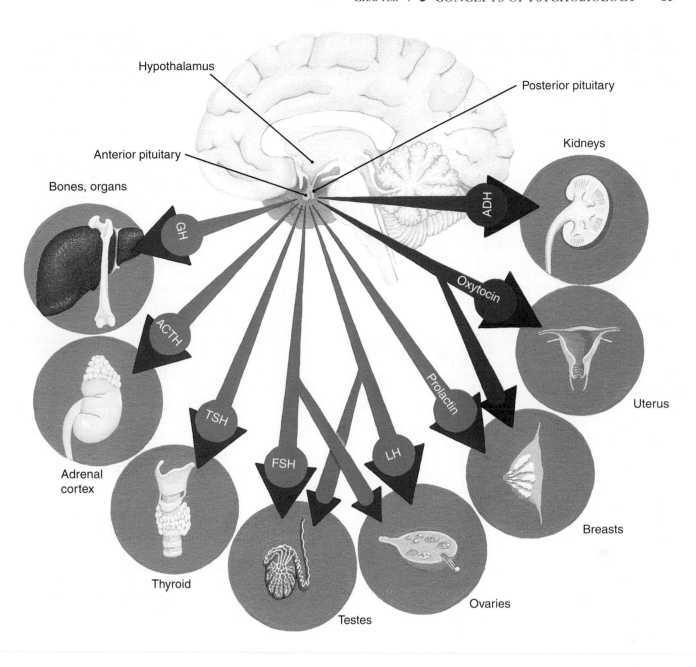

Anterior pituitary hormones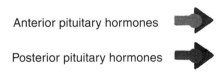

Posterior pituitary hormones

FIGURE 4–8 Hormones of the pituitary gland and their target organs. (From Scanlon, V.C., & Sanders, T. *Essentials of anatomy and physiology*, 4th ed. F.A. Davis, Philadelphia, 2003.)

Pituitary Gland

The Posterior Pituitary (Neurohypophysis)

The hypothalamus has direct control over the posterior pituitary through efferent neural pathways. Two hormones are found in the posterior pituitary: vasopressin (antidiuretic hormone) and oxytocin. They are actually produced by the hypothalamus and stored in the posterior pituitary. Their release is mediated by neural impulses from the hypothalamus (Figure 4–9).

Antidiuretic Hormone. The main function of antidiuretic hormone (ADH) is to conserve body water and

TABLE 4–3	Hormones of the Neuroendocrine System			
HORMONE	LOCATION AND STIMULATION OF RELEASE	TARGET ORGAN	FUNCTION	POSSIBLE BEHAVIORAL CORRELATION TO ALTERED SECRETION
Antidiuretic hormone (ADH)	Posterior pituitary; release stimulated by dehydration, pain, stress	Kidney (causes increased reabsorption)	Conservation of body water and maintenance of blood pressure	Polydipsia; altered pain response; modified sleep pattern
Oxytocin	Posterior pituitary; release stimulated by end of pregnancy; stress; during sexual arousal	Uterus; breasts	Contraction of the uterus for labor; release of breast milk	May play role in stress response by stimulation of ACTH
Growth hormone (GH)	Anterior pituitary; release stimulated by growth hormone-releasing hormone from hypothalamus	Bones and tissues	Growth in children; protein synthesis in adults	Anorexia nervosa
Thyroid-stimulating hormone (TSH)	Anterior pituitary; release stimulated by thyrotropin-releasing hormone from hypothalamus	Thyroid gland	Stimulation of secretion of needed thyroid hormones for metabolism of food and regulation of temperature	Increased levels: insomnia, anxiety, emotional lability Decreased levels: fatigue, depression
Adrenocorticotropic hormone (ACTH)	Anterior pituitary; release stimulated by corticotropin-releasing hormone from hypothalamus	Adrenal cortex	Stimulation of secretion of cortisol, which plays a role in response to stress	Increased levels: mood disorders, psychosis Decreased levels: depression, apathy, fatigue
Prolactin	Anterior pituitary; release stimulated by prolactin-releasing hormone from hypothalamus	Breasts	Stimulation of milk production	Increased levels: depression, anxiety, decreased libido, irritability
Gonadotropic hormones	Anterior pituitary; release stimulated by gonadotropin-releasing hormone from hypothalamus	Ovaries and testes	Stimulation of secretion of estrogen, progesterone, and testosterone; role in ovulation and sperm production	Decreased levels: depression and anorexia nervosa Increased testosterone: increased sexual behavior and aggressiveness
Melanocyte-stimulating hormone (MSH)	Anterior pituitary; release stimulated by onset of darkness	Pineal gland	Stimulation of secretion of melatonin	Increased levels: depression

maintain normal blood pressure. The release of ADH is stimulated by pain, emotional stress, dehydration, increased plasma concentration, and decreases in blood volume. An alteration in the secretion of this hormone may be a factor in the polydipsia observed in about 10 to 15 percent of hospitalized psychiatric patients. Other factors correlated with this behavior include adverse effects of psychotropic medications and features of the behavioral disorder itself. ADH also may play a role in learning and memory, in alteration of the pain response, and in the modification of sleep patterns.

Oxytocin. Oxytocin stimulates contraction of the uterus at the end of pregnancy and stimulates release of milk from the mammary glands (Scanlon & Sanders, 2003). It is also released in response to stress and during sexual arousal. Its role in behavioral functioning is unclear, although it is possible that oxytocin may act in certain situations to stimulate the release of adrenocorticotropic hormone (ACTH), thereby playing a key role in the overall hormonal response to stress.

The Anterior Pituitary (Adenohypophysis)

The hypothalamus produces *releasing hormones* that pass through capillaries and veins of the hypophyseal portal system to capillaries in the anterior pituitary, where they stimulate secretion of specialized hormones. This pathway is presented in Figure 4–9. The hormones of the anterior pituitary gland regulate multiple body functions and include growth hormone, thyroid-stimulating hormone, ACTH, prolactin, gonadotropin-stimulating hormone, and melanocyte-stimulating hormone. Most of these hormones are regulated by a *negative feedback mechanism*. Once the hormone has exerted its effects, the

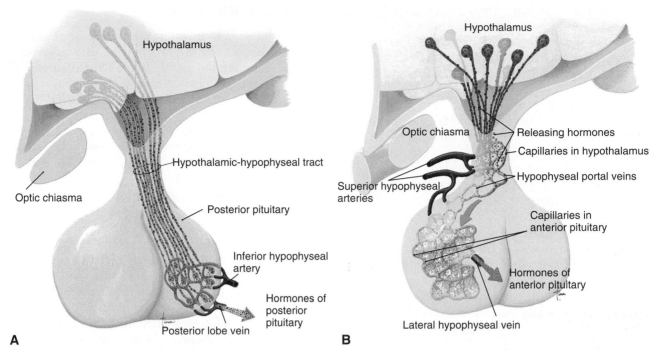

FIGURE 4–9   Structural relationships of hypothalamus and pituitary gland. *(A)* Posterior pituitary stores hormones produced in the hypothalamus. *(B)* Releasing hormones of the hypothalamus circulate directly to the anterior pituitary and influence its secretions. Notice the two networks of capillaries. (From Scanlon, V.C., & Sanders, T. *Essentials of anatomy and physiology*, 4th ed. F.A. Davis, Philadelphia, 2003.)

information is "fed back" to the anterior pituitary, which inhibits the release, and ultimately decreases the effects, of the stimulating hormones.

Growth Hormone. The release of growth hormone (GH), also called somatotropin, is stimulated by growth hormone-releasing hormone (GHRH) from the hypothalamus. Its release is inhibited by growth hormone-inhibiting hormone (GHIH), or somatostatin, also from the hypothalamus. It is responsible for growth in children, as well as continued protein synthesis throughout life. During periods of fasting, it stimulates the release of fat from the adipose tissue to be used for increased energy. The release of GHIH is stimulated in response to periods of hyperglycemia. GHRH is stimulated in response to hypoglycemia and to stressful situations. During prolonged stress, GH has a direct effect on protein, carbohydrate, and lipid metabolism, resulting in increased serum glucose and free fatty acids to be used for increased energy. There has been some indication of a possible correlation between abnormal secretion of growth hormone and anorexia nervosa.

Thyroid-Stimulating Hormone. Thyrotropin-releasing hormone (TRH) from the hypothalamus stimulates the release of thyroid-stimulating hormone (TSH), or thyrotropin, from the anterior pituitary. TSH stimulates the thyroid gland to secrete triiodothyronine (T_3)

and thyroxine (T_4). Thyroid hormones are integral to the metabolism of food and the regulation of temperature.

A correlation between thyroid dysfunction and altered behavioral functioning has been studied. Early reports in the medical literature associated hyperthyroidism with irritability, insomnia, anxiety, restlessness, weight loss, and emotional lability, and in some instances with progressing to delirium or psychosis. Symptoms of fatigue, decreased libido, memory impairment, depression, and suicidal ideations have been associated with chronic hypothyroidism. Studies have correlated various forms of thyroid dysfunction with mood disorders, anxiety, eating disorders, schizophrenia, and dementia.

Adrenocorticotropic Hormone. Corticotropin-releasing hormone (CRH) from the hypothalamus stimulates the release of ACTH from the anterior pituitary. ACTH stimulates the adrenal cortex to secrete cortisol. The role of cortisol in human behaviors is not well understood, although it seems to be secreted under stressful situations. Disorders of the adrenal cortex can result in hyposecretion or hypersecretion of cortisol.

Addison's disease is the result of hyposecretion of the hormones of the adrenal cortex. Behavioral symptoms of hyposecretion include mood changes with apathy, social withdrawal, impaired sleep, decreased concentration, and fatigue. Hypersecretion of cortisol results in Cushing's disease and is associated with behaviors that include depression, mania, psychosis, and suicidal ideation. Cognitive impairments also have been commonly observed.

Prolactin. Serum prolactin levels are regulated by prolactin-releasing hormone (PRH) and prolactin-inhibiting hormone (PIH) from the hypothalamus. Prolactin stimulates milk production by the mammary glands in the presence of high levels of estrogen and progesterone during pregnancy. Behavioral symptoms associated with hypersecretion of prolactin include depression, decreased libido, stress intolerance, anxiety, and increased irritability.

Gonadotropic Hormones. The gonadotropic hormones are so called because they produce an effect on the gonads—the ovaries and the testes. The gonadotropins include follicle-stimulating hormone (FSH) and luteinizing hormone (LH), and their release from the anterior pituitary is stimulated by gonadotropin-releasing hormone (GnRH) from the hypothalamus. In women, FSH initiates maturation of ovarian follicles into the ova and stimulates their secretion of estrogen. LH is responsible for ovulation and the secretion of progesterone from the corpus luteum. In men, FSH initiates sperm production in the testes, and LH increases secretion of testosterone by the interstitial cells of the testes (Scanlon & Sanders, 2003). The gonadotropins are regulated by a negative feedback of gonadal hormones at the hypothalamic or pituitary level.

Limited evidence exists to correlate gonadotropins to behavioral functioning, although some observations have been made to warrant hypothetical consideration. Studies have indicated decreased levels of testosterone, LH, and FSH in depressed men. Increased sexual behavior and aggressiveness have been linked to elevated testosterone levels in both men and women. Decreased plasma levels of LH and FSH commonly occur in patients with anorexia nervosa. Supplemental estrogen therapy has resulted in improved mentation and mood in some depressed women.

Melanocyte-Stimulating Hormone. Melanocyte-stimulating hormone (MSH) from the hypothalamus stimulates the pineal gland to secrete melatonin. The release of melatonin appears to depend on the onset of darkness and is suppressed by light. Studies of this hormone have indicated that environmental light can affect neuronal activity and influence *circadian rhythms*. Correlation between abnormal secretion of melatonin and symptoms of depression has led to the recent implication of melatonin in the etiology of seasonal affective disorder (SAD), in which individuals become depressed only during the fall and winter months when the amount of daylight decreases.

Circadian Rhythms

Human biological rhythms are largely determined by genetic coding, with input from the external environment influencing the cyclic effects. **Circadian rhythms** in humans follow a near-24-hour cycle and may influence a variety of regulatory functions, including the sleep–wake cycle, body temperature regulation, patterns of activity such as eating and drinking, and hormone secretion. The 24-hour rhythms in humans are affected to a large degree by the cycles of lightness and darkness. This occurs because of a "pacemaker" in the brain that sends messages to other systems in the body and maintains the 24-hour rhythm. This endogenous pacemaker appears to be the suprachiasmatic nuclei of the hypothalamus. These nuclei receive projections of light through the retina, and in turn stimulate electrical impulses to various other systems in the body, mediating the release of neurotransmitters or hormones that regulate bodily functioning.

Most of the biological rhythms of the body operate over a period of about 24 hours, but cycles of longer lengths have been studied. For example, women of menstruating age show monthly cycles of progesterone levels in the saliva, of skin temperature over the breasts, and of prolactin levels in the plasma of the blood (Hughes, 1989).

Some rhythms may even last as long as a year. These circannual rhythms are particularly relevant to certain medications, such as cyclosporine, that appears to be more effective at some times than others during the period of about a year (Hughes, 1989). Recently, clinical studies have shown that administration of chemotherapy during the appropriate circadian phase can significantly increase the efficacy and decrease the toxic effects of certain cytotoxic agents (Lis et al., 2003).

The Role of Circadian Rhythms in Psychopathology

Circadian rhythms may play a role in psychopathology. Because many hormones have been implicated in behavioral functioning, it is reasonable to believe that peak secretion times could be influential in predicting certain behaviors. The association of depression to increased secretion of melatonin during darkness hours has already been discussed. External manipulation of the light–dark cycle and removal of external time cues often have beneficial effects on mood disorders.

Symptoms that occur in the premenstrual cycle have also been linked to disruptions in biological rhythms. A number of the symptoms associated with this syndrome strongly resemble those attributed to depression, and hormonal changes have been implicated in the etiology. Some of these changes include progesterone–estrogen imbalance, increase in prolactin and mineralocorticoids, high level of prostaglandins, decrease in endogenous opiates, changes in metabolism of biogenic amines (serotonin, dopamine, norepinephrine, acetylcholine), and variations in secretion of glucocorticoids or melatonin.

Sleep disturbances are common in both depression and premenstrual dysphoric disorder. Because the sleep–wakefulness cycle is probably the most fundamental of biological rhythms, it is discussed in greater detail.

A representation of bodily functions affected by 24-hour biological rhythms is presented in Figure 4–10.

Sleep

The sleep–wake cycle is genetically determined rather than learned and is established some time after birth. Even when environmental cues such as the ability to detect light and darkness are removed, the human sleep–wake

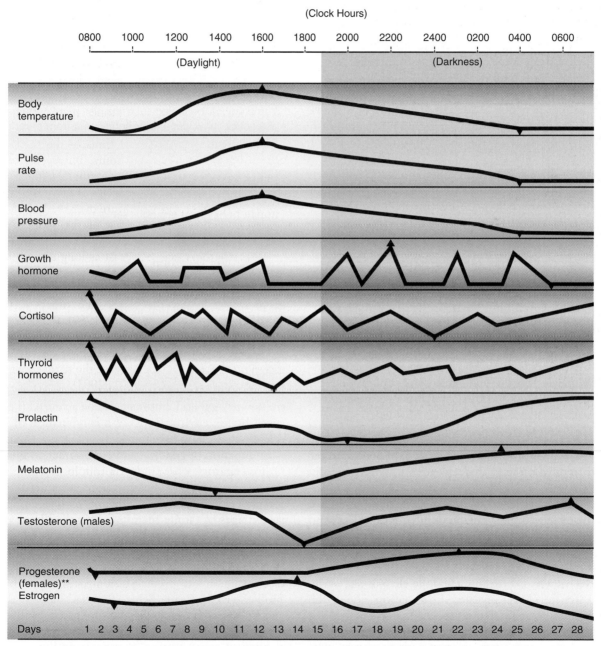

* ▼ indicates low point and ▲ indicates peak time of these biological factors within a 24-hour circadian rhythm.
** The female hormones are presented on a monthly rhythm because of their influence on the reproductive cycle.
  Daily rhythms of female gonadotropins are difficult to assay and are probably less significant than monthly.

FIGURE 4–10 Circadian biological rhythms.*

cycle generally develops about a 25-hour periodicity, which is close to the 24-hour normal circadian rhythm.

Sleep can be measured by the types of brain waves that occur during various stages of sleep activity. Dreaming episodes are characterized by rapid eye movement and are called REM sleep. Non-REM sleep is represented by six distinct stages.

1. **Stage 0—Alpha Rhythm**. This stage of the sleep–wake cycle is characterized by a relaxed, waking state with eyes closed. The alpha brain wave rhythm has a frequency of 8 to 12 cycles per second.
2. **Stage 1—Beta Rhythm**. Stage 1 characterizes the "transition" into sleep, or a period of dozing. Thoughts wander, and there is a drifting in and out of sleep. Beta brain wave rhythm has a frequency of 18 to 25 cycles per second.
3. **Stage 2—Theta Rhythm**. This stage characterizes the manner in which about half of sleep time is spent. Eye movement and muscular activity are minimal. Theta brain wave rhythm has a frequency of 4 to 7 cycles per second.
4. **Stage 3—Delta Rhythm**. This is a period of deep and restful sleep. Muscles are relaxed, heart rate and blood pressure fall, and breathing slows. No eye movement occurs. Delta brain wave rhythm has a frequency of 1.5 to 3 cycles per second.
5. **Stage 4—Delta Rhythm**. The stage of deepest sleep. Individuals who suffer from insomnia or other sleep disorders often do not experience this stage of sleep. Eye movement and muscular activity are minimal. Delta waves predominate.
6. **REM Sleep—Beta Rhythm**. The dream cycle. Eyes dart about beneath closed eyelids, moving more rapidly than when awake. The brain wave pattern is similar to that of stage 1 sleep. Heart and respiration rates increase and blood pressure may increase or decrease. Muscles are hypotonic during REM sleep.

Stages 2 through REM repeat themselves throughout the cycle of sleep. One is more likely to experience longer periods of stages 3 and 4 sleep early in the cycle and longer periods of REM sleep later in the sleep cycle. Most people experience REM sleep about four to five times during the night. The amount of REM sleep and deep sleep decreases with age, while the time spent in drowsy wakefulness and dozing increases.

Neurochemical Influences. A number of neurochemicals have been shown to influence the sleep–wake cycle. Several studies have revealed information about the sleep-inducing characteristics of serotonin. L-Tryptophan, the amino acid precursor to serotonin, has been used for many years as an effective sedative–hypnotic to induce sleep in individuals with sleep-onset disorder. Serotonin and norepinephrine both appear to be most active during non-REM sleep, whereas the neurotransmitter acetylcholine is activated during REM sleep

(Cardoso, 1997). The exact role of GABA in sleep facilitation is unclear, although the sedative effects of drugs that enhance GABA transmission, such as the benzodiazepines, suggest that this neurotransmitter plays an important role in regulation of sleep and arousal. Some studies have suggested that acetylcholine induces and prolongs REM sleep, whereas histamine appears to have an inhibitive effect. Neuroendocrine mechanisms seem to be more closely tied to circadian rhythms than to the sleep–wake cycle. One exception is growth hormone secretion, which exhibits increases during the early sleep period and may be associated with slow-wave sleep (Van Cauter et al., 1992).

> **Core Concept**
>
> **Genetics**
> The study of the biological transmission of certain characteristics (physical and/or behavioral) from parent to offspring.

GENETICS

Human behavioral genetics seeks to understand both the genetic and environmental contributions to individual variations in human behavior (McInerney, 2004). This type of study is complicated by the fact that behaviors, like all complex traits, involve *multiple genes*.

The term **genotype** refers to the total set of genes present in an individual at the time of conception, and coded in the DNA. The physical manifestations of a particular genotype are designated by characteristics that specify a specific **phenotype**. Examples of phenotypes include eye color, height, blood type, language, and hair type. As evident by the examples presented, phenotypes are not *only* genetic, but may also be acquired (i.e., influenced by the environment) or a combination of both. It is likely that many psychiatric disorders are the result of a combination of genetics and environmental influences.

Investigators who study the etiological implications for psychiatric illness may explore several risk factors. Studies to determine if an illness is *familial* compare the percentages of family members with the illness to those in the general population or within a control group of unrelated individuals. These studies estimate the prevalence of psychopathology among relatives, and make predictions about the predisposition to an illness based on familial risk factors. Schizophrenia, bipolar disorder, major depression, anorexia nervosa, panic disorder, somatization disorder, antisocial personality disorder, and alcoholism are examples of psychiatric illness in which familial tendencies have been indicated (Nurnberger, Goldin, & Gershon, 1994).

Studies that are purely genetic in nature search for a specific gene that is responsible for an individual having a particular illness. A number of disorders exist in which the mutation of a specific gene or change in the number or structure of a chromosome has been associated with the etiology. Examples include Huntington's disease, cystic fibrosis, phenylketonuria, Duchenne's muscular dystrophy, and Down's syndrome.

The search for genetic links to certain psychiatric disorders continues. Risk factors for early-onset Alzheimer's disease have been linked to mutations on chromosomes 21, 14, and 1 (National Institute on Aging, 2004). Other studies have linked a gene in the region of chromosome 19 that produces apolipoprotein E (ApoE) with late-onset Alzheimer's disease. Additional research is required before definitive confirmation can be made.

In addition to familial and purely genetic investigations, other types of studies have been conducted to estimate the existence and degree of genetic and environmental contributions to the etiology of certain psychiatric disorders. Twin studies and adoption studies have been successfully employed for this purpose.

Twin studies examine the frequency of a disorder in monozygotic (genetically identical) and dizygotic (fraternal; not genetically identical) twins. Twins are called *concordant* when both members suffer from the same disorder in question. Concordance in monozygotic twins is considered stronger evidence of genetic involvement than it is in dizygotic twins. Disorders in which twin studies have suggested a possible genetic link include alcoholism, schizophrenia, major depression, bipolar

disorder, anorexia nervosa, panic disorder, and obsessive–compulsive disorder (Kendler & Silverman, 1991; Nurnberger, Goldin, & Gershon, 1994).

Adoption studies allow comparisons to be made of the influences of genetics versus environment on the development of a psychiatric disorder. Knowles (2003) describes the following four types of adoption studies that have been conducted:

1. The study of adopted children whose biological parent(s) had a psychiatric disorder but whose adoptive parent(s) did not.
2. The study of adopted children whose adoptive parent(s) had a psychiatric disorder but whose biological parent(s) did not.
3. The study of adoptive and biological relatives of adopted children who developed a psychiatric disorder.
4. The study of monozygotic twins reared apart by different adoptive parents.

Disorders in which adoption studies have suggested a possible genetic link include alcoholism, schizophrenia, major depression, bipolar disorder, attention-deficit/hyperactivity disorder, and antisocial personality disorder (Knowles, 2003).

A summary of various psychiatric disorders and the possible biological influences discussed in this chapter is presented in Table 4–4. Various diagnostic procedures used to detect alteration in biological functioning that may contribute to psychiatric disorders are presented in Table 4–5.

TABLE 4–4 Biological Implications of Psychiatric Disorders

ANATOMICAL BRAIN STRUCTURES INVOLVED	NEUROTRANSMITTER HYPOTHESIS	POSSIBLE ENDOCRINE CORRELATION	IMPLICATIONS OF CIRCADIAN RHYTHMS	POSSIBLE GENETIC LINK
Schizophrenia				
Frontal cortex, temporal lobes, limbic system	Dopamine hyperactivity	Decreased prolactin levels	May correlate antipsychotic medication administration to times of lowest level	Twin, familial, and adoption studies suggest genetic link
Depressive Disorders				
Frontal lobes, limbic system, temporal lobes	Decreased levels of norepinephrine, dopamine, and serotonin	Increased cortisol levels; thyroid hormone hyposecretion; increased melatonin	DST* used to predict effectiveness of antidepressants; melatonin linked to depression during periods of darkness	Twin, familial, and adoption studies suggest a genetic link
Bipolar Disorder				
Frontal lobes, limbic system, temporal lobes	Increased levels of norepinephrine, dopamine, and serotonin in acute mania	Some indication of elevated thyroid hormones in acute mania		Twin, familial, and adoption studies suggest a genetic link
Panic Disorder				
Limbic system, midbrain	Increased levels of norepinephrine; decreased GABA activity	Elevated levels of thyroid hormones	May have some application for times of medication administration	Twin and familial studies suggest a genetic link

(Continued on following page)

TABLE 4–4 Biological Implications of Psychiatric Disorders *(Continued)*

ANATOMICAL BRAIN STRUCTURES INVOLVED	NEUROTRANSMITTER HYPOTHESIS	POSSIBLE ENDOCRINE CORRELATION	IMPLICATIONS OF CIRCADIAN RHYTHMS	POSSIBLE GENETIC LINK
Anorexia nervosa				
Limbic system, particularly the hypothalamus	Decreased levels of norepinephrine, serotonin, and dopamine	Decreased levels of gonadotropins and growth hormone; increased cortisol levels	DST* often shows same results as in depression	Twin and familial studies suggest a genetic link
Obsessive–Compulsive Disorder				
Limbic system, basal ganglia (specifically caudate nucleus)	Decreased levels of serotonin	Increased cortisol levels	DST* often shows same results as in depression	Twin studies suggest a possible genetic link
Alzheimer's Disease				
Temporal, parietal, and occipital regions of cerebral cortex; hippocampus	Decreased levels of acetylcholine, norepinephrine, serotonin, and somatostatin	Decreased corticotropin-releasing hormone	Decreased levels of acetylcholine and serotonin may inhibit hypothalamic-pituitary axis and interfere with hormonal releasing factors	Familial studies suggest a genetic predisposition; late-onset disorder linked to marker on chromosome 19; early-onset to chromosomes 21, 14, and 1

*DST = dexamethasone suppression test. Dexamethasone is a synthetic glucocorticoid that suppresses cortisol secretion via the feedback mechanism. In this test, 1 mg of dexamethasone is administered at 11:30 P.M. and blood samples are drawn at 8:00 A.M., 4:00 P.M., and 11:00 P.M. on the following day. A plasma value greater than 5 μg/dl suggests that the individual is not suppressing cortisol in response to the dose of dexamethasone. This is a positive result for depression and may have implications for other disorders as well.

TABLE 4–5 Diagnostic Procedures Used to Detect Altered Brain Functioning

EXAM	TECHNIQUE USED	PURPOSE OF THE EXAM AND POSSIBLE FINDINGS
Electroencephalography (EEG)	Electrodes are placed on the scalp in a standardized position. Amplitude and frequency of beta, alpha, theta, and delta brain waves are graphically recorded on paper by ink markers for multiple areas of the brain surface.	Measures brain electrical activity; identifies dysrhythmias, asymmetries, or suppression of brain rhythms; used in the diagnosis of epilepsy, neoplasm, stroke, metabolic or degenerative disease.
Computerized EEG mapping	EEG tracings are summarized by computer-assisted systems in which various regions of the brain are identified and functioning is interpreted by color coding or gray shading.	Measures brain electrical activity; used largely in research to represent statistical relationships between individuals and groups or between two populations of subjects (e.g., patients with schizophrenia vs. control subjects).
Computed tomographic (CT) scan	CT scan may be used with or without contrast medium. X-rays are taken of various transverse planes of the brain while a computerized analysis produces a precise reconstructed image of each segment.	Measures accuracy of brain structure to detect possible lesions, abscesses, areas of infarction, or aneurysm. CT has also identified various anatomical differences in patients with schizophrenia, organic mental disorders, and bipolar disorder.
Magnetic resonance imaging (MRI)	Within a strong magnetic field, the nuclei of hydrogen atoms absorb and reemit electromagnetic energy that is computerized and transformed into image information. No radiation or contrast medium is used.	Measures anatomical and biochemical status of various segments of the brain; detects brain edema, ischemia, infection, neoplasm, trauma, and other changes such as demyelination. Morphological differences have been noted in brains of patients with schizophrenia as compared with control subjects.
Positron emission tomography (PET)	The patient receives an intravenous (IV) injection of a radioactive substance (type depends on brain activity to be visualized). The head is surrounded by detectors that relay data to a computer that interprets the signals and produces the image.	Measures specific brain functioning, such as glucose metabolism, oxygen utilization, blood flow, and, of particular interest in psychiatry, neurotransmitter-receptor interaction.
Single photon emission computed tomography (SPECT)	The technique is similar to PET, but longer-acting radioactive substance must be used to allow time for a gamma-camera to rotate about the head and gather the data, which are then computer assembled into a brain image.	Measures various aspects of brain functioning, as with PET; has also been used to image activity of cerebrospinal fluid circulation.

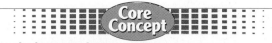

Core Concept

Psychoimmunology
The branch of medicine that studies the effects of psychological and social factors on the functioning of the immune system.

PSYCHOIMMUNOLOGY

Normal Immune Response

Cells responsible for *nonspecific* immune reactions include neutrophils, monocytes, and macrophages. They work to destroy the invasive organism and initiate and facilitate damaged tissue. If these cells are not effective in accomplishing a satisfactory healing response, *specific* immune mechanisms take over.

Specific immune mechanisms are divided into two major types: the cellular response and the humoral response. The controlling elements of the cellular response are the T lymphocytes (T cells); those of the humoral response are called B lymphocytes (B cells). When the body is invaded by a specific antigen, the T cells, and particularly the T4 lymphocytes (also called *T helper cells*), become sensitized to and specific for the foreign antigen. These antigen-specific T4 cells divide many times, producing antigen-specific T4 cells with other functions. One of these, the *T killer cell*, destroys viruses that reproduce inside other cells by puncturing the cell membrane of the host cell and allowing the contents of the cell, including viruses, to spill out into the bloodstream, where they can be engulfed by macrophages. Another cell produced through division of the T4 cells is the suppressor T cell, which serves to stop the immune response once the foreign antigen has been destroyed (Scanlon & Sanders, 2003).

The humoral response is activated when antigen-specific T4 cells communicate with the B cells in the spleen and lymph nodes. The B cells in turn produce the antibodies specific to the foreign antigen. Antibodies attach themselves to foreign antigens so that they are unable to invade body cells. These invader cells are then destroyed without being able to multiply.

Implications of the Immune System in Psychiatric Illness

In studies of the biological response to stress, it has been hypothesized that individuals become more susceptible to physical illness following exposure to a stressful stimulus or life event (see Chapter 1). This response is thought to be due to the effect of increased glucocorticoid release from the adrenal cortex following stimulation from the hypothalamic–pituitary–adrenal axis during stressful situations. The result is a suppression in lymphocyte proliferation and function.

Studies have shown that nerve endings exist in tissues of the immune system. The CNS has connections in both bone marrow and the thymus, where immune system cells are produced, and in the spleen and lymph nodes, where those cells are stored.

Growth hormone, which may be released in response to certain stressors, may enhance immune functioning, whereas testosterone is thought to inhibit immune functioning. Increased production of epinephrine and norepinephrine occurs in response to stress, and may decrease immunity. Serotonin has demonstrated both enhancing and inhibitory effects on immunity (Stein, Schleifer, & Keller, 1991).

Studies have correlated a decrease in lymphocyte functioning with periods of grief, bereavement, and depression, associating the degree of altered immunity with severity of the depression. A number of research studies have been conducted attempting to correlate the onset of schizophrenia to abnormalities of the immune system. These studies have considered autoimmune responses, viral infections, and immunogenetics (Sadock & Sadock, 2003). The role of these factors in the onset and course of schizophrenia remains unclear. Immunological abnormalities have also been investigated in a number of other psychiatric illnesses, including alcoholism, autism, and dementia.

Evidence exists to support a correlation between psychosocial stress and the onset of illness. Research is still required to determine the specific processes involved in stress-induced modulation of the immune system.

IMPLICATIONS FOR NURSING

The discipline of psychiatric/mental health nursing has always spoken of its role in holistic health care, but historical review reveals that emphasis has been placed on treatment approaches that focus on psychological and social factors. Psychiatric nurses must integrate knowledge of the biological sciences into their practices if they are to ensure safe and effective care to people with mental illness. In the Surgeon General's Report on Mental Health (U.S. Department of Health and Human Services, 1999), Dr. David Satcher wrote:

> The mental health field is far from a complete understanding of the biological, psychological, and sociocultural bases of development, but development clearly involves interplay among these influences. Understanding the process of development requires knowledge, ranging from the most fundamental level—that of gene expression and interactions between molecules and cells—all the way up to the highest

levels of cognition, memory, emotion, and language. The challenge requires integration of concepts from many different disciplines. A fuller understanding of development is not only important in its own right, but it is expected to pave the way for our ultimate understanding of mental health and mental illness and how different factors shape their expression at different stages of the life span.

To ensure a smooth transition from a psychosocial focus to one of biopsychosocial emphasis, nurses must have a clear understanding of the following:

Neuroanatomy and neurophysiology: the structure and functioning of the various parts of the brain and their correlation to human behavior and psychopathology.

Neuronal processes: the various functions of the nerve cells, including the role of neurotransmitters, receptors, synaptic activity, and informational pathways.

Neuroendocrinology: the interaction of the endocrine and nervous systems, and the role that the endocrine glands and their respective hormones play in behavioral functioning.

Circadian rhythms: regulation of biochemical functioning over periods of rhythmic cycles and their influence in predicting certain behaviors.

Genetic influences: hereditary factors that predispose individuals to certain psychiatric disorders.

Psychoimmunology: the influence of stress on the immune system and its role in the susceptibility to illness.

Psychopharmacology: the increasing use of psychotropics in the treatment of mental illness, demanding greater knowledge of psychopharmacological principles and nursing interventions necessary for safe and effective management.

Diagnostic technology: the importance of keeping informed about the latest in technological procedures for diagnosing alterations in brain structure and function.

Why are these concepts important to the practice of psychiatric/mental health nursing? The interrelationship between psychosocial adaptation and physical functioning has been established. Integrating biological and behavioral concepts into psychiatric nursing practice is essential for nurses to meet the complex needs of mentally ill clients. Psychobiological perspectives must be incorporated into nursing practice, education, and research to attain the evidence-based outcomes necessary for the delivery of competent care.

SUMMARY

A neurobiological transformation has occurred in psychiatry. Nurses must be cognizant of the interaction between biological and behavioral factors in the development and management of psychiatric illness. These current trends have made it essential for nurses to increase their knowledge about the structure and functioning of the brain. This includes the processes of neurotransmission and the function of various neurotransmitters. This is especially important in light of the increasing role of psychotropic medication in the treatment of psychiatric illness. Because the mechanism of action of many of these drugs occurs at synaptic transmission, nurses must understand this process so that they may predict outcomes and safely manage the administration of psychotropic medications.

The endocrine system plays an important role in human behavior through the hypothalamic–pituitary axis. Hormones and their circadian rhythm of regulation significantly influence a number of physiological and psychological life cycle phenomena, such as moods, sleep arousal, stress response, appetite, libido, and fertility.

Research continues to validate the role of genetics in psychiatric illness. Familial, twin, and adoption studies suggest that genetics may be implicated in the etiology of schizophrenia, bipolar disorder, depression, panic disorder, anorexia nervosa, alcoholism, and obsessive–compulsive disorder. Investigations to substantiate current data are ongoing and may reveal evidence of genetic influence in other psychiatric illnesses as well.

Psychoimmunology examines the impact of psychological factors on the immune system. Evidence exists to support a link between psychosocial stressors and suppression of the immune response. This is especially useful knowledge for nurses as they intervene to assist clients in the primary prevention of mental illness.

It is also important for nurses to keep abreast of the expanding diagnostic technologies available for detecting alterations in psychobiological functioning. Technologies such as magnetic resonance imagery (MRI) and positron emission tomography (PET) are facilitating the growth of knowledge linking mental illness to disorders of the brain.

The holistic concept of nursing has never been stronger than it is today. Integrating knowledge of the expanding biological focus into psychiatric nursing is essential if nurses are to meet the changing needs of today's psychiatric clients.

REVIEW QUESTIONS

SELF-EXAMINATION/LEARNING EXERCISE

Match the following parts of the brain to their functions described in the right-hand column:

_____ 1. Frontal lobe   a. Sometimes called the "emotional brain"; associated with multiple feelings and behaviors

_____ 2. Parietal lobe   b. Concerned with visual reception and interpretation

_____ 3. Temporal lobe   c. Voluntary body movement; thinking and judgment; expression of feeling

_____ 4. Occipital lobe   d. Integrates all sensory input (except smell) on way to cortex

_____ 5. Thalamus   e. Part of the cortex that deals with sensory perception and interpretation

_____ 6. Hypothalamus   f. Hearing, short-term memory, and sense of smell

_____ 7. Limbic system   g. Control over pituitary gland and autonomic nervous system; regulates appetite and temperature.

Select the answer that is most appropriate for each of the following questions.

8. At a synapse, the determination of further impulse transmission is accomplished by means of
   a. Potassium ions
   b. Interneurons
   c. Neurotransmitters
   d. The myelin sheath

9. A decrease in which of the following neurotransmitters has been implicated in depression?
   a. GABA, acetylcholine, and aspartate
   b. Norepinephrine, serotonin, and dopamine
   c. Somatostatin, substance P, and glycine
   d. Glutamate, histamine, and opioid peptides

10. Which of the following hormones has been implicated in the etiology of seasonal affective disorder (SAD)?
    a. Increased levels of melatonin
    b. Decreased levels of oxytocin
    c. Decreased levels of prolactin
    d. Increased levels of thyrotropin

11. In which of the following psychiatric disorders do genetic tendencies appear to exist?
    a. Schizophrenia
    b. Dissociative disorder
    c. Conversion disorder
    d. Narcissistic personality disorder

12. With which of the following diagnostic imaging technologies can neurotransmitter-receptor interaction be visualized?
    a. Magnetic resonance imaging (MRI)
    b. Positron emission tomography (PET)
    c. Electroencephalography (EEG)
    d. Computerized EEG mapping

13. During stressful situations, stimulation of the hypothalamic-pituitary-adrenal axis results in suppression of the immune system because of the effect of which of the following?
    a. Antidiuretic hormone from the posterior pituitary
    b. Increased secretion of gonadotropins from the gonads
    c. Decreased release of growth hormone from the anterior pituitary
    d. Increased glucocorticoid release from the adrenal cortex

REFERENCES

Cardoso, S.H. (1997). *Biochemical mechanisms of REM sleep.* Retrieved on June 11, 2002 from the World Wide Web at http://www.epub.org.br/cm/n02/mente/neuroestrut_i.htm

Dubovsky, S.L., Davies, R., & Dubovsky, A.N. (2003). Mood disorders. In R.E. Hales & S.C. Yudofsky (Eds.). *Textbook of clinical psychiatry* (4th ed.). Washington, DC: American Psychiatric Publishing.

Ho, B.C., Black, D.W., & Andreasen, N.C. (2003). Schizophrenia and other psychotic disorders. In R.E. Hales & S.C. Yudofsky (Eds.). *Textbook of clinical psychiatry* (4th ed.). Washington, DC: American Psychiatric Publishing.

Hughes, M. (1989). *Body clock: The effects of time on human health.* New York: Andromeda Oxford.

Sadock, B.J. & Sadock, V.A. (2003). *Synopsis of psychiatry: Behavioral sciences/clinical psychiatry* (9th ed.). Philadelphia: Lippincott Williams & Wilkins.

Kendler, K.S., & Silverman, J.M. (1991). Behavior genetics. In K. Davis, H. Klar, & J.T. Coyle (Eds.). *Foundations of psychiatry.* Philadelphia: W.B. Saunders.

Knowles, J.A. (2003). Genetics. In R.E. Hales, & S.C. Yudofsky (Eds.). *Textbook of psychiatry* (4th ed.). Washington, DC: American Psychiatric Publishing.

Lis, C.G., Grutsch, J.F., Wood, P., You, M., Rich, I., & Hrushesky, W.J. (2003). Circadian timing in cancer treatment: The biological foundation for an integrative approach. *Integrative Cancer Therapies,* 2(2), 105–111.

McInerney, J. (2004). Behavioral genetics. *The Human Genome Project.* Retrieved October 1, 2004 from http://www.ornl.gov/sci/techresources/Human Genome/elsi/behavior.shtml

Murphy, M., & Deutsch, S.I. (1991). Neurophysiological and neurochemical basis of behavior. In K. Davis, H. Klar, & J.T. Coyle (Eds.). *Foundations of psychiatry.* Philadelphia: W.B. Saunders.

National Institute on Aging. (2004). The Alzheimer's Disease Education and Referral Center. *Alzheimer's Disease Genetics.* Retrieved October 1, 2004 from http://www.nia.nih.gov/

Nurnberger, J.I., Goldin, L.R., & Gershon, E.S. (1994). Genetics of psychiatric disorders. In G. Winokur and P.J. Clayton (Eds.). *The medical basis of psychiatry* (2nd ed.). Philadelphia: W.B. Saunders.

Scanlon, V.C., & Sanders, T. (2003). *Essentials of anatomy and physiology* (4th ed.). Philadelphia: F.A. Davis.

Stein, M., Schleifer, S.J., & Keller, S.E. (1991). Stress and the immune system. In K. Davis, H. Klar, & J.T. Coyle (Eds.). *Foundations of psychiatry.* Philadelphia: W.B. Saunders.

U.S. Department of Health and Human Services. (1999). *Mental Health: A report of the Surgeon General—Executive Summary.* Rockville, MD: U.S. Department of Health and Human Services.

Van Cauter, E., Kerkhofs, M., Caufriez, A., Van Onderbergen, A., Thorner, M.O., & Copinschi, G. (1992). A quantitative estimation of growth hormone secretion in normal man: Reproducibility and relation to sleep and time of day. *Journal of Clinical Endocrinology and Metabolism, 74,* 1441–1450.

ETHICAL AND LEGAL ISSUES IN PSYCHIATRIC/ MENTAL HEALTH NURSING

CHAPTER OUTLINE

OBJECTIVES

ETHICAL CONSIDERATIONS

LEGAL CONSIDERATIONS

SUMMARY

REVIEW QUESTIONS

KEY TERMS

assault
autonomy
battery
beneficence
Christian ethics
civil law
common law
criminal law
defamation of
    character
ethical dilemma
ethical egoism
false imprisonment
informed consent

justice
Kantianism
libel
malpractice
natural law
negligence
nonmaleficence
privileged
    communication
slander
statutory law
tort
utilitarianism
veracity

CORE CONCEPTS

bioethics
ethics
moral behavior
right
values
values clarification

OBJECTIVES

After reading this chapter, the student will be able to:

1. Differentiate among *ethics, morals, values,* and *rights*.
2. Discuss ethical theories including utilitarianism, Kantianism, Christian ethics, natural law theories, and ethical egoism.
3. Define ethical dilemma.
4. Discuss the ethical principles of autonomy, beneficence, nonmaleficence, justice, and veracity.
5. Use an ethical decision-making model to make an ethical decision.

6. Describe ethical issues relevant to psychiatric/mental health nursing.
7. Define *statutory law* and *common law*.
8. Differentiate between civil and criminal law.
9. Discuss legal issues relevant to psychiatric/ mental health nursing.
10. Differentiate between *malpractice* and *negligence*.
11. Identify behaviors relevant to the psychiatric/mental health setting for which specific malpractice action could be taken.

urses are constantly faced with the challenge of making difficult decisions regarding good and evil or life and death. This chapter provides a reference for the student and practicing nurse of the basic ethical and legal concepts and their relationship to psychiatric/mental health nursing. A discussion of ethical theory is presented as a foundation upon which ethical decisions may be made. The American Nurses' Association (ANA) (2001) has established a code of ethics for nurses to use as a framework within which to make ethical choices and decisions (Table 5–1).

Because legislation determines what is *right* or *good* within a society, legal issues pertaining to psychiatric/mental health nursing are also discussed in this chapter. Definitions are presented, along with rights of psychiatric clients of which nurses must be aware. Nursing competency and client care accountability are compromised when the nurse has inadequate knowledge about the laws that regulate the practice of nursing.

Knowledge of the legal and ethical concepts presented in this chapter will enhance the quality of care the nurse provides in his or her psychiatric/mental health nursing practice, while also protecting the nurse within the parameters of legal accountability. Indeed, the very right to practice nursing carries with it the responsibility to maintain a specific level of competency and to practice in accordance with certain ethical and legal standards of care.

ETHICAL CONSIDERATIONS

Theoretical Perspectives

An *ethical theory* is a moral principle or a set of moral principles that can be used in assessing what is morally right or morally wrong (Ellis & Hartley, 2004). These principles provide guidelines for ethical decision-making.

Utilitarianism

The basis of **utilitarianism** is "the greatest-happiness principle," which holds that actions are right to the degree that they tend to promote happiness and wrong as

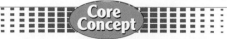

Ethics is the science that deals with the rightness and wrongness of actions (Aiken, 2004). **Bioethics** is the term applied to these principles when they refer to concepts within the scope of medicine, nursing, and allied health.

Moral behavior is defined as conduct that results from serious critical thinking about how individuals ought to treat others. Moral behavior reflects the way a person interprets basic respect for other persons, such as the respect for autonomy, freedom, justice, honesty, and confidentiality (Pappas, 2003).

Values are ideals or concepts that give meaning to the individual's life (Aiken, 2004). **Values clarification** is a process of self-exploration through which individuals identify and rank their own personal values. This process increases awareness about why individuals behave in certain ways. Values clarification is important in nursing to increase understanding about why certain choices and decisions are made over others and how values affect nursing outcomes.

A **right** is defined as "a valid, legally recognized claim or entitlement, encompassing both freedom from government interference or discriminatory treatment and an entitlement to a benefit or service" (Levy and Rubenstein, 1996). A right is *absolute* when there is no restriction whatsoever on the individual's entitlement. A *legal right* is one on which the society has agreed and formalized into law. Both the National League for Nursing (NLN) and the American Hospital Association (AHA) have established guidelines of patients' rights. Although these are not considered legal documents, nurses and hospitals are considered responsible for upholding these rights of patients.

■ TABLE 5–1	American Nurses' Association Code of Ethics for Nurses

1. The nurse, in all professional relationships, practices with compassion and respect for the inherent dignity, worth and uniqueness of every individual, unrestricted by consideration of social or economic status, personal attributes, or the nature of health problems.
2. The nurse's primary commitment is to the patient whether an individual, family, group or community.
3. The nurse promotes, advocates for and strives to protect the health, safety and rights of the patient.
4. The nurse is responsible and accountable for individual nursing practice and determines the appropriate delegation of tasks consistent with the nurse's obligation to provide optimum patient care.
5. The nurse owes the same duties to self as to others, including the responsibility to preserve integrity and safety, to maintain competence and to continue personal and professional growth.
6. The nurse participates in establishing, maintaining and improving healthcare environments and conditions of employment conducive to the provision of quality healthcare and consistent with the values of the profession through individual and collective action.
7. The nurse participates in the advancement of the profession through contributions to practice, education, administration, and knowledge development.
8. The nurse collaborates with other health professionals and the public in promoting community, national, and international efforts to meet health needs.
9. The profession of nursing, as represented by associations and their members, is responsible for articulating nursing values, for maintaining the integrity of the profession and its practice and for shaping social policy.

SOURCE: Reprinted with permission from American Nurses Association, Code of Ethics for Nurses with Interpretive Statements, © 2001 American Nurses Publishing, American Nurses Foundation/American Nurses Association, Washington, DC.

they tend to produce the reverse of happiness. Thus, the good is happiness and the right is that which promotes the good. Conversely, the wrongness of an action is determined by its tendency to bring about unhappiness. An ethical decision based on the utilitarian view looks at the end results of the decision. Action is taken based on the end results that produced the most good (happiness) for the most people.

Kantianism

Named for philosopher Immanuel Kant, **Kantianism** is directly opposed to utilitarianism. Kant argued that it is not the consequences or end results that make an action right or wrong; rather it is the principle or motivation on which the action is based that is the morally decisive factor. Kantianism suggests that our actions are bound by a sense of duty. This theory is often called *deontology* (from the Greek word *deon*, which means "that which is binding; duty"). Kantian-directed ethical decisions are made out of respect for moral law. For example, "I make this choice because it is morally right and my duty to do so" (not because of consideration for a possible outcome).

Christian Ethics

A basic principle that might be called a Christian philosophy is that which is known as the golden rule: "Do unto others as you would have them do unto you" and, alternatively, "Do not do unto others what you would not have them do unto you." The imperative demand of **Christian ethics** is to treat others as moral equals and to recognize the equality of other persons by permitting them to act as we do when they occupy a position similar to ours.

Natural Law Theories

The most general moral precept of the **natural law** theory is "do good and avoid evil." Based on the writings of St. Thomas Aquinas, natural-law theorists contend that ethics must be grounded in a concern for the human good. Although the nature of this "human good" is not expounded upon, Catholic theologians' view natural law as the law inscribed by God into the nature of things—as a species of divine law. According to this conception, the Creator endows all things with certain potentialities or tendencies that serve to define their natural end. The fulfillment of a thing's natural tendencies constitutes the specific good of that thing. For example, the natural tendency of an acorn is to become an oak. What then is the natural potential, or tendency, of human beings? Natural-law theorists focus on an attribute that is regarded as distinctively human, as separating human beings from the rest of worldly creatures; that is, the ability to live according to the dictates of reason. It is with this ability to reason that humans are able to choose "good" over "evil." In natural law, evil acts are never condoned, even if they are intended to advance the noblest of ends.

Ethical Egoism

Ethical egoism espouses that what is right and good is what is best for the individual making the decision. An individual's actions are determined by what is to his or her own advantage. The action may not be best for anyone else involved, but consideration is only for the individual making the decision.

Ethical Dilemmas

An **ethical dilemma** is a situation that requires an individual to make a choice between two equally unfavorable alternatives (Catalano, 2003). Evidence exists to support both moral "rightness" and moral "wrongness" related to a certain action. The individual who must make the choice experiences conscious conflict regarding the decision.

Ethical dilemmas arise when no explicit reasons exist that govern an action. Ethical dilemmas generally create a great deal of emotion. Often the reasons supporting each side of the argument for action are logical and appropriate. The actions associated with both sides are desirable in some respects and undesirable in others. In most situations, taking no action is considered an action taken.

Ethical Principles

Ethical principles are fundamental guidelines that influence decision-making. The ethical principles of autonomy, beneficence, nonmaleficence, veracity, and justice are helpful and used frequently by health care workers to assist with ethical decision-making.

Autonomy

The principle of **autonomy** arises from the Kantian duty of respect for persons as rational agents. This viewpoint emphasizes the status of persons as autonomous moral agents whose right to determine their destinies should always be respected. This presumes that individuals are always capable of making independent choices for themselves. Health care workers know this is not always the case. Children, comatose individuals, and persons who are seriously mentally ill are examples of clients who are incapable of making informed choices. In these instances, a representative of the individual is usually asked to intervene and give consent. However, health care workers must ensure that respect for an individual's autonomy is not disregarded in favor of what another person may view as best for the client.

Beneficence

Beneficence refers to one's duty to benefit or promote the good of others. Health care workers who act in their clients' interests are beneficent, provided their actions really do serve the client's best interest. In fact, some duties do seem to take preference over other duties. For example, the duty to respect the autonomy of an individual may be overridden when that individual has been deemed harmful to self or others. Aiken (2004) states, "The difficulty that sometimes arises in implementing the principle of beneficence lies in determining what exactly is good for another and who can best make that decision."

Nonmaleficence

Nonmaleficence is the requirement that health care providers do no harm to their clients, either intentionally or unintentionally (Aiken, 2004). Some philosophers suggest that this principle is more important than beneficence; that is, they support the notion that it is more important to avoid doing harm than it is to do good. In any event, ethical dilemmas often arise when a conflict exists between an individual's rights (the duty to promote good) and what is thought to best represent the welfare of the individual (the duty to do no harm). An example of this conflict might occur when administering chemotherapy to a cancer patient, knowing it will prolong his or her life, but create "harm" (side effects) in the short term.

Justice

The principle of **justice** has been referred to as the "justice as fairness" principle. It is sometimes referred to as *distributive justice*, and its basic premise lies with the right of individuals to be treated equally regardless of race, sex, marital status, medical diagnosis, social standing, economic level, or religious belief (Aiken, 2004). The concept of justice reflects a duty to treat all individuals equally and fairly. When applied to health care, this principle suggests that all resources within the society (including health care services) ought to be distributed evenly without respect to socioeconomic status. Thus, according to this principle, the vast disparity in the quality of care dispensed to the various classes within our society would be considered unjust. A more equitable distribution of care for all individuals would be favored.

Veracity

The principle of **veracity** refers to one's duty to always be truthful. Aiken (2004) states, "Veracity requires that the health care provider tell the truth and not intentionally deceive or mislead clients." There are times when limitations must be placed on this principle, such as when the truth would knowingly produce harm or interfere with

the recovery process. Being honest is not always easy, but rarely is lying justified. Clients have the right to know about their diagnosis, treatment, and prognosis.

A Model for Making Ethical Decisions

The following is a set of steps that may be used in making an ethical decision. These steps closely resemble the steps of the nursing process.

1. *Assessment.* Gather the subjective and objective data about a situation.
2. *Problem Identification.* Identify the conflict between two or more alternative actions.
3. *Plan:*
   a. Explore the benefits and consequences of each alternative.
   b. Consider principles of ethical theories.
   c. Select an alternative.
4. *Implementation.* Act on the decision made and communicate the decision to others.
5. *Evaluation.* Evaluate outcomes.

A schematic of this model is presented in Figure 5–1. A case study using this decision-making model is presented

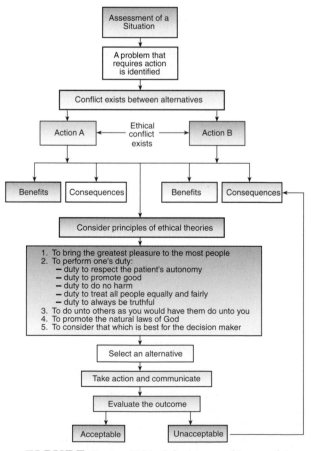

FIGURE 5–1 Ethical decision-making model.

TABLE 5–2	Ethical Decision Making—A Case Study

Step 1.   Assessment

Tonja is a 17-year-old girl who is currently on the psychiatric unit with a diagnosis of conduct disorder. Tonja reports that she has been sexually active since she was 14. She had an abortion when she was 15 and a second one just 6 weeks ago. She states that her mother told her she has "had her last abortion," and that she has to start taking birth control pills. She asks her nurse, Kimberly, to give her some information about the pills and to tell her how to go about getting some. Kimberly believes Tonja desperately needs information about birth control pills, as well as other types of contraceptives; however, the psychiatric unit is part of a Catholic hospital, and hospital policy prohibits distributing this type of information.

Step 2.   Problem Identification

A conflict exists between the client's need for information, the nurse's desire to provide that information, and the institution's policy prohibiting the provision of that information.

Step 3.   Alternatives—Benefits and Consequences

1. Alternative 1. Give the client information and risk losing job.
2. Alternative 2. Do not give client information and compromise own values of holistic nursing.
3. Alternative 3. Refer client to another source outside the hospital and risk reprimand from supervisor.

Step 4.   Consider Principles of Ethical Theories

1. Alternative 1. Giving the client information would certainly respect the client's autonomy and would benefit the client by decreasing her chances of becoming pregnant again. It would not be to the best advantage of Kimberly, in that she would likely lose her job. And according to the beliefs of the Catholic hospital, the natural laws of God would be violated.
2. Alternative 2. Withholding information restricts the client's autonomy. It has the potential for doing harm, in that without the use of contraceptives, the client may become pregnant again (and she implies that this is not what she wants). Kimberly's Christian ethic is violated in that this action is not what she would want "done unto her."
3. Alternative 3. A referral would respect the client's autonomy, would promote good, would do no harm (except perhaps to Kimberly's ego from the possible reprimand), and this decision would comply with Kimberly's Christian ethic.

Step 5.   Select an Alternative

Alternative 3 is selected based on the ethical theories of utilitarianism (does the most good for the greatest number), Christian ethics (Kimberly's belief of "Do unto others as you would have others do unto you"), and Kantianism (to perform one's duty), and the ethical principles of autonomy, beneficence, and nonmaleficence. The success of this decision depends on the client's follow-through with the referral and compliance with use of the contraceptives.

Step 6.   Take Action and Communicate

Taking action involves providing information in writing for Tonja, perhaps making a phone call and setting up an appointment for her with Planned Parenthood. Communicating suggests sharing the information with Tonja's mother. Communication also includes documentation of the referral in the client's chart.

Step 7.   Evaluate the Outcome

An acceptable outcome might indicate that Tonja did indeed keep her appointment at Planned Parenthood and is complying with the prescribed contraceptive regimen. It might also include Kimberly's input into the change process in her institution to implement these types of referrals to other clients who request them.

An unacceptable outcome might be indicated by Tonja's lack of follow-through with the appointment at Planned Parenthood or lack of compliance in using the contraceptives, resulting in another pregnancy. Kimberly may also view a reprimand from her supervisor as an unacceptable outcome, particularly if she is told that she must select other alternatives should this situation arise in the future. This may motivate Kimberly to make another decision—that of seeking employment in an institution that supports a philosophy more consistent with her own.

---

in Table 5–2. If the outcome is acceptable, action continues in the manner selected. If the outcome is unacceptable, benefits and consequences of the remaining alternatives are reexamined, and steps 3 through 7 in Table 5–2 are repeated.

Ethical Issues in Psychiatric/Mental Health Nursing

The Right to Refuse Medication

The AHA's (1992) Patient's Bill of Rights states: "The patient has the right to refuse treatment to the extent permitted by law, and to be informed of the medical consequences of his action" (Table 5–3). In psychiatry, refusal of treatment primarily concerns the administration of psychotropic medications. "To the extent permitted by law" may be defined within the U.S. Constitution and several of its amendments (e.g., the First Amendment, which addresses the rights of speech, thought, and expression; the Eighth Amendment, which grants the right to freedom from cruel and unusual punishment; and the Fifth and Fourteenth Amendments, which grant due process of law and equal protection for all). In psychiatry, "the medical consequences of his action" may include such steps as involuntary commitment, legal competency hearing, or client discharge from the hospital.

Although many courts are supporting a client's right to refuse medications in the psychiatric area, some limitations do exist. Weiss-Kaffie and Purtell (2001) state:

TABLE 5–3	American Hospital Association Patient's Bill of Rights

1. The patient has the right to considerate and respectful care.
2. The patient has the right to obtain from his physician complete current information concerning his diagnosis, treatment, and prognosis in terms the patient can be reasonably expected to understand. When it is not medically advisable to give such information to the patient, the information should be made available to an appropriate person in his behalf. He has the right to know by name the physician responsible for coordinating his care.
3. The patient has the right to receive from his physician information necessary to give informed consent prior to the start of any procedure and/or treatment. Except in emergencies, such information for informed consent should include but not necessarily be limited to the specific procedure and/or treatment, the medically significant risks involved, and the probable duration of incapacitation. Where medically significant alternatives for care or treatment exist, or when the patient requests information concerning medical alternatives, the patient has the right to such information. The patient also has the right to know the name of the person responsible for the procedures and/or treatment.
4. The patient has the right to refuse treatment to the extent permitted by law and to be informed of the medical consequences of his action.
5. The patient has the right to every consideration of his privacy concerning his own medical care program. Case discussion, consultation, examination, and treatment are confidential and should be conducted discreetly. Those not directly involved in his care must have the permission of the patient to be present.
6. The patient has the right to expect that all communications and records pertaining to his care should be treated as confidential.
7. The patient has the right to expect that within its capacity a hospital must make reasonable response to the request of a patient for services. The hospital must provide evaluation, service, and/or referral as indicated by the urgency of the case. When medically permissible, a patient may be transferred to another facility only after he has received complete information and explanation concerning the needs for and alternatives to such a transfer. The institution to which the patient is to be transferred must first have accepted the patient for transfer.
8. The patient has the right to obtain information as to any relationship of his hospital to other health care and educational institutions insofar as his care is concerned. The patient has the right to obtain information as to the existence of any professional relationships among individuals, by name, who are treating him.
9. The patient has the right to be advised if the hospital proposes to engage in or perform human experimentation affecting his care or treatment. The patient has the right to refuse to participate in such research projects.
10. The patient has the right to expect reasonable continuity of care. He has the right to know in advance what appointment times and physicians are available and where. The patient has the right to expect that the hospital will provide a mechanism whereby he is informed by his physician or a delegate of the physician of the patient's continuing health care requirements following discharge.
11. The patient has the right to examine and receive an explanation of his bill regardless of source of payment.
12. The patient has the right to know what hospital rules and regulations apply to his conduct as a patient.

SOURCE: AHA (1992), with permission.

The treatment team must determine that three criteria be met to force medication without client consent. The client must exhibit behavior that is dangerous to self or others; the medication ordered by the physician must have a reasonable chance of providing help to the client; and clients who refuse medication must be judged incompetent to evaluate the benefits of the treatment in question. (p. 361)

The Right to the Least-Restrictive Treatment Alternative

Health care personnel must attempt to provide treatment in a manner that least restricts the freedom of clients. The "restrictiveness" of psychiatric therapy can be described in the context of a continuum, based on severity of illness. Clients may be treated on an outpatient basis, in day hospitals, or in voluntary or involuntary hospitalization. Symptoms may be treated with verbal rehabilitative techniques and move successively to behavioral techniques, chemical interventions, mechanical restraints, or electroconvulsive therapy. The problem appears to arise in selecting the least restrictive means among involuntary chemical intervention, seclusion, and mechanical restraints. Sadock and Sadock (2003) state:

Distinguishing among these interventions on the basis of restrictiveness proves to be a purely subjective exercise

fraught with personal bias. Moreover, each of these three interventions is both more and less restrictive than each of the other two. Nevertheless, the effort should be made to think in terms of restrictiveness when deciding how to treat patients. (p. 1358)

LEGAL CONSIDERATIONS

In 1980, the 96th Congress of the United States passed the Mental Health Systems Act, which includes a Patient's Bill of Rights, for recommendation to the States. An adaptation of these rights is presented in Table 5-4.

Nurse Practice Acts

The legal parameters of professional and practical nursing are defined within each state by the state's nurse practice act. These documents are passed by the state legislature and in general are concerned with such provisions as the following:

● The definition of important terms, including the definition of nursing and the various types of nurses recognized
● A statement of the education and other training or requirements for licensure and reciprocity

TABLE 5-4	Bill of Rights for Psychiatric Patients

1. The right to appropriate treatment and related services in the setting that is most supportive and least restrictive to personal freedom.
2. The right to an individualized, written treatment or service plan; the right to treatment based on such plan; and the right to periodic review and revision of the plan based on treatment needs.
3. The right, consistent with one's capabilities, to participate in and receive a reasonable explanation of the care and treatment process.
4. The right to refuse treatment except in an emergency situation or as permitted by law.
5. The right not to participate in experimentation in the absence of informed, voluntary, written consent.
6. The right to freedom from restraint or seclusion except in an emergency situation.
7. The right to a humane treatment environment that affords reasonable protection from harm and appropriate privacy.
8. The right to confidentiality of medical records (also applicable following patient's discharge).
9. The right of access to medical records except information received from third parties under promise of confidentiality, and when access would be detrimental to the patient's health (also applicable following patient's discharge).
10. The right of access to use of the telephone, personal mail, and visitors, unless deemed inappropriate for treatment purposes.
11. The right to be informed of these rights in comprehensible language.
12. The right to assert grievances if rights are infringed.
13. The right to referral as appropriate to other providers of mental health services upon discharge.

SOURCE: Adapted from Mental Health Systems Act (1980).

- Broad statements that describe the scope of practice for various levels of nursing (APN, RN, LPN)
- Conditions under which a nurse's license may be suspended or revoked, and instructions for appeal
- The general authority and powers of the state board of nursing (Fedorka & Resnick, 2001)

Most nurse practice acts are general in their terminology, and do not provide specific guidelines for practice. Nurses must understand the scope of practice that is protected by their license, and should seek assistance from legal counsel if they are unsure about the proper interpretation of a nurse practice act.

Types of Law

There are two general categories or types of law that are of most concern to nurses: statutory law and common law. These laws are identified by their source or origin.

Statutory Law

A **statutory law** is a law that has been enacted by a legislative body, such as a county or city council, state legislature, or the Congress of the United States. An example of statutory law is the nurse practice acts.

Common Law

Common laws are derived from decisions made in previous cases. These laws apply to a body of principles that evolve from court decisions resolving various controversies. Because common law in the United States has been developed on a state basis, the law on specific subjects may differ from state to state. An example of a common law might be how different states deal with a nurse's refusal to provide care for a specific client.

Classifications Within Statutory and Common Law

Broadly speaking, there are two kinds of unlawful acts: civil and criminal. Both statutory law and common law have civil and criminal components.

Civil Law

Civil law protects the private and property rights of individuals and businesses. Private individuals or groups may bring a legal action to court for breach of civil law. These legal actions are of two basic types: torts and contracts.

Torts. A **tort** is a violation of a civil law in which an individual has been wronged. In a tort action, one party asserts that wrongful conduct on the part of the other has caused harm, and seeks compensation for harm suffered. A tort may be *intentional* or *unintentional*. Examples of unintentional torts are malpractice and negligence actions. An example of an intentional tort is the touching of another person without that person's consent. Intentional touching (e.g., a medical treatment) without the client's consent can result in a charge of battery, an intentional tort.

Contracts. In a contract action, one party asserts that the other party, in failing to fulfill an obligation, has breached the contract, and either compensation or performance of the obligation is sought as remedy. An example is an action by a mental health professional whose clinical privileges have been reduced or terminated in violation of an implied contract between the professional and a hospital.

Criminal Law

Criminal law provides protection from conduct deemed injurious to the public welfare. It provides for punishment of those found to have engaged in such conduct, which commonly includes imprisonment, parole conditions, a loss of privilege (such as a license), a fine, or any combination of these (Ellis & Hartley, 2004). An example of a violation of criminal law is the theft by a hospital employee of supplies or drugs.

Legal Issues in Psychiatric/Mental Health Nursing

Confidentiality and Right to Privacy

The Fourth, Fifth, and Fourteenth Amendments to the U.S. Constitution protect an individual's privacy. Most states have statutes protecting the confidentiality of client records and communications. The only individuals who have a right to observe a client or have access to medical information are those involved in his or her medical care.

Pertinent medical information may be released without consent in a life-threatening situation. If information is released in an emergency, the following information must be recorded in the client's record: date of disclosure, person to whom information was disclosed, reason for disclosure, reason written consent could not be obtained, and the specific information disclosed.

Most states have statutes that pertain to the doctrine of **privileged communication**. Although the codes differ markedly from state to state, most grant certain professionals privileges under which they may refuse to reveal information about, and communications with, clients. In most states, the doctrine of privileged communication applies to psychiatrists and attorneys; in some instances, psychologists, clergy, and nurses are also included.

In certain instances nurses may be called on to testify in cases in which the medical record is used as evidence. In most states, the right to privacy of these records is exempted in civil or criminal proceedings. Therefore, it is important that nurses document with these possibilities in mind. Strict record keeping using statements that are objective and nonjudgmental, having care plans that are specific in their prescriptive interventions, and keeping documentation that describes those interventions and their subsequent evaluation all serve the best interests of the client, the nurse, and the institution in case questions regarding care should arise. Documentation very often weighs heavily in malpractice case decisions.

The right to confidentiality is a basic one, especially so in psychiatry. Although societal attitudes are improving, individuals have experienced discrimination in the past for no other reason than for having a history of emotional illness. Nurses working in psychiatry must guard the privacy of their clients with great diligence.

Informed Consent

According to law, all individuals have the right to decide whether to accept or reject treatment (Guido, 2000). A health care provider can be charged with assault and battery for providing life-sustaining treatment to a client when the client has not agreed to it. The rationale for the doctrine of **informed consent** is the preservation and protection of individual autonomy in determining what will and will not happen to the person's body (Guido, 2000).

Informed consent is a client's permission granted to a physician to perform a therapeutic procedure, before which information about the procedure has been presented to the client with adequate time given for consideration about the pros and cons. The client should receive information such as what treatment alternatives are available; why the physician believes this treatment is most appropriate; the possible outcomes, risks, and adverse effects; the possible outcome should the client select another treatment alternative; and the possible outcome should the client choose to have no treatment. An example of a treatment in the psychiatric area that requires informed consent is electroconvulsive therapy.

There are some conditions under which treatment may be performed without obtaining informed consent. A client's refusal to accept treatment may be challenged under the following circumstances (Aiken, 2004; Guido, 2000; Cournos & Petrila, 1992; Levy & Rubenstein, 1996):

1. When a client is mentally incompetent to make a decision and treatment is necessary to preserve life or avoid serious harm
2. When refusing treatment endangers the life or health of another
3. During an emergency, in which a client is in no condition to exercise judgment
4. When the client is a child (consent is obtained from parent or surrogate)
5. In the case of therapeutic privilege. In therapeutic privilege, information about a treatment may be withheld if the physician can show that full disclosure would.
   a. Hinder or complicate necessary treatment
   b. Cause severe psychological harm
   c. Be so upsetting as to render a rational decision by the client impossible

Although most clients in psychiatric/mental health facilities are competent and capable of giving informed consent, those with severe psychiatric illness do not possess the cognitive ability to do so. If an individual has been legally determined to be mentally incompetent, consent is obtained from the legal guardian. Difficulty arises when no legal determination has been made, but the individual's current mental state prohibits informed decision making (e.g., the person who is psychotic, unconscious, or inebriated). In these instances, informed consent is usually obtained from the individual's nearest relative, or if none exists and time permits, the physician may ask the court to appoint a conservator or guardian. When time does not permit court intervention, permission may be sought from the hospital administrator.

A client or guardian always has the right to withdraw consent after it has been given. When this occurs, the physician should inform (or reinform) the client about the consequences of refusing treatment. If treatment has already been initiated, the physician should terminate treatment in a way least likely to cause injury to the client and inform the client or guardian of the risks associated with interrupted treatment (Guido, 2000).

The nurse's role in obtaining informed consent is usually defined by agency policy. A nurse may sign the consent form as witness for the client's signature. However, legal liability for informed consent lies with the physician. The nurse acts as client advocate to ensure that the following three major elements of informed consent have been addressed:

1. *Knowledge.* The client has received adequate information on which to base his or her decision.
2. *Competency.* The individual's cognition is not impaired to an extent that would interfere with decision making or, if so, that the individual has a legal representative.
3. *Free Will.* The individual has given consent voluntarily without pressure or coercion from others.

Restraints and Seclusion

An individual's privacy and personal security are protected by the U.S. Constitution and supported by the Mental Health Systems Act of 1980, out of which was conceived a Bill of Rights for psychiatric patients. These include "the right to freedom from restraint or seclusion except in an emergency situation."

In psychiatry, the term *restraints* generally refers to a set of leather straps that are used to restrain the extremities of an individual whose behavior is out of control and who poses an inherent risk to the physical safety and psychological well-being of the individual and staff (Joint Commission on Accreditation of Healthcare Organizations [JCAHO], 2000). Restraints are never to be used as punishment or for the convenience of staff. Other measures to decrease agitation, such as "talking down" (verbal intervention) and chemical restraints (tranquilizing medication) are usually tried first. If these interventions are ineffective, mechanical restraints may be instituted. *Seclusion* is another type of physical restraint in which the client is confined alone in a room from which he or she is unable to leave. The room is usually minimally furnished with items to promote the client's comfort and safety.

The Joint Commission on Accreditation of Healthcare Organizations (JCAHO) has released a set of revisions to its previous restraint and seclusion standards. The intent of these revisions is to reduce the use of this intervention

as well as to provide greater assurance of safety and protection to individuals placed in restraints or seclusion for reasons related to psychiatric disorders or substance abuse (Medscape, 2000). In addition to others, these provisions provide the following guidelines:

1. In the event of an emergency, restraints or seclusion may be initiated without a physician's order.
2. As soon as possible, but no longer than 1 hour after the initiation of restraints or seclusion, a qualified staff member must notify the physician about the individual's physical and psychological condition and obtain a verbal or written order for the restraints or seclusion.
3. Orders for restraints or seclusion must be reissued by a physician every 4 hours for adults age 18 and older, 2 hours for children and adolescents ages 9 to 17, and every hour for children younger than 9 years.
4. An in-person evaluation of the individual must be made by the physician within 4 hours of the initiation of restraints or seclusion of an adult age 18 or older and within 2 hours for children and adolescents ages 17 and younger.
5. Minimum time frames for an in-person re-evaluation by a physician include 8 hours for individuals ages 18 years and older, and 4 hours for individuals ages 17 and younger.
6. If an individual is no longer in restraints or seclusion when an original verbal order expires, the physician must conduct an in-person evaluation within 24 hours of initiation of the intervention.

Clients in restraints or seclusion must be observed and assessed every 10 to 15 minutes with regard to circulation, respiration, nutrition, hydration, and elimination. Such attention should be documented in the client's record.

False imprisonment is the deliberate and unauthorized confinement of a person within fixed limits by the use of verbal or physical means (Ellis & Hartley, 2004). Health care workers may be charged with false imprisonment for restraining or secluding—against the wishes of the client—anyone having been admitted to the hospital voluntarily. Should a voluntarily admitted client decompensate to a point that restraint or seclusion for protection of self or others is necessary, court intervention to determine competency and involuntary commitment is required to preserve the client's rights to privacy and freedom.

Commitment Issues
Voluntary Admissions

Each year, more than one million persons are admitted to health care facilities for psychiatric treatment, of which approximately two thirds are considered voluntary. To be admitted voluntarily, an individual makes direct application to the institution for services and may stay as long as treatment is deemed necessary. He or she may sign out of the hospital at any time, unless following a mental status examination the health care professional determines that the client may be harmful to self or others and recommends that the admission status be changed from voluntary to involuntary. Although these types of admissions are considered voluntary, it is important to ensure that the individual comprehends the meaning of his or her actions, has not been coerced in any manner, and is willing to proceed with admission.

Involuntary Commitment

Because involuntary hospitalization results in substantial restrictions of the rights of an individual, the admission process is subject to the guarantee of the Fourteenth Amendment to the U.S. Constitution that provides citizens protection against loss of liberty and ensures due process rights (Weiss-Kaffie & Purtell, 2001). Involuntary commitments are made for various reasons. Most states commonly cite the following criteria:

1. In an emergency situation (for the client who is dangerous to self or others)
2. For observation and treatment of mentally ill persons
3. When an individual is unable to take care of basic personal needs (the "gravely disabled")

Under the Fourth Amendment, individuals are protected from unlawful searches and seizures without probable cause. Therefore, the individual seeking the involuntary commitment must show probable cause why the client should be hospitalized against his or her wishes; that is, the person must show that there is cause to believe that the person would be dangerous to self or others, is mentally ill and in need of treatment, or is gravely disabled.

Emergency Commitments. Emergency commitments are sought when an individual manifests behavior that is clearly and imminently dangerous to self or others. These admissions are usually instigated by relatives or friends of the individual, police officers, the court, or health care professionals. Emergency commitments are time limited, and a court hearing for the individual is scheduled, usually within 72 hours. At that time the court may decide that the client may be discharged; or, if deemed necessary, and voluntary admission is refused by the client, an additional period of involuntary commitment may be ordered. In most instances, another hearing is scheduled for a specified time (usually in 7 to 21 days).

The Mentally Ill Person in Need of Treatment. A second type of involuntary commitment is for the observation and treatment of mentally ill persons in need of treatment. Most states have established definitions of what constitutes "mentally ill" for purposes of state involun-

tary admission statutes. Some examples include individuals who, because of severe mental illness, are:

● Unable to make informed decisions concerning treatment
● Likely to cause harm to self or others
● Unable to fulfill basic personal needs necessary for health and safety

In determining whether commitment is required, the court will look for substantial evidence of abnormal conduct—evidence that cannot be explained as the result of a physical cause. There must be "clear and convincing evidence" as well as "probable cause" to substantiate the need for involuntary commitment to ensure that an individual's rights under the Constitution are protected. The U.S. Supreme Court in *O'Connor v. Donaldson* held that the existence of mental illness alone does not justify involuntary hospitalization. State standards require a specific impact or consequence to flow from the mental illness that involves danger or an inability to care for one's own needs. These clients are entitled to court hearings with representation, at which time determination of commitment and length of stay are considered. Legislative statutes governing involuntary commitments vary from state to state.

Involuntary Outpatient Commitment. Involuntary outpatient commitment (IOC) is a court-ordered mechanism used to compel a person with mental illness to submit to treatment on an outpatient basis. A number of eligibility criteria for commitment to outpatient treatment have been cited (Appelbaum, 2001; Maloy, 1996; Torrey & Zdanowicz, 2001). Some of these include:

1. A history of repeated decompensation requiring involuntary hospitalization
2. Likelihood that without treatment the individual will deteriorate to the point of requiring inpatient commitment
3. Presence of severe and persistent mental illness (e.g., schizophrenia or bipolar disorder) and limited awareness of the illness or need for treatment
4. The presence of severe and persistent mental illness contributing to a risk of becoming homeless, incarcerated, or violent or of committing suicide
5. The existence of individualized treatment plan likely to be effective and a service provider who has agreed to provide the treatment

Most states have already enacted IOC legislation or currently have resolutions that speak to this topic on their agendas. Most commonly, clients who are committed into the IOC programs are those with severe and persistent mental illness, such as schizophrenia. The rationale behind the legislation is to reduce the numbers of readmissions and lengths of hospital stays of these clients. Concern lies in the possibility of violating the individual rights of psychiatric clients without significant improvement in treatment outcomes. One study at Bellevue hospital in New York found no difference in treatment outcomes between court-ordered outpatient treatment and voluntary outpatient treatment (Steadman et al., 2001). Other studies have shown positive outcomes, including a decrease in hospital readmissions, with IOC (Ridgely, Borum, & Petrila, 2001; Swartz et al., 2001). Continuing research is required to determine if IOC will improve treatment compliance and enhance quality of life in the community for individuals with severe and persistent mental illness.

The Gravely Disabled Client. A number of states have statutes that specifically define the "gravely disabled" client. For those that do not use this label, the description of the individual who, because of mental illness, is unable to take care of basic personal needs is very similar.

Gravely disabled is generally defined as a condition in which an individual, as a result of mental illness, is in danger of serious physical harm resulting from inability to provide for basic needs such as food, clothing, shelter, medical care, and personal safety. Inability to care for oneself cannot be established by showing that an individual lacks the resources to provide the necessities of life. Rather, it is the inability to make use of available resources.

Should it be determined that an individual is gravely disabled, a guardian, conservator, or committee will be appointed by the court to ensure the management of the person and his or her estate. To legally restore competency then requires another court hearing to reverse the previous ruling. The individual whose competency is being determined has the right to be represented by an attorney.

Nursing Liability

Mental health practitioners—psychiatrists, psychologists, psychiatric nurses, and social workers—have a duty to provide appropriate care based on the standards of their professions and the standards set by law. The standards of care for psychiatric/mental health nursing are presented in Chapter 9.

Malpractice and Negligence

The terms **malpractice** and **negligence** are often used interchangeably. Negligence has been defined as:

> The failure to exercise the standard of care that a reasonably prudent person would have exercised in a similar situation; any conduct that falls below the legal standard established to protect others against unreasonable risk of harm, except for conduct that is intentionally, wantonly, or willfully disregardful of others' rights. (Garner, 1999)

Any person may be negligent. In contrast, malpractice is a specialized form of negligence applicable only to professionals.

Black's Law Dictionary defines malpractice as:

> An instance of negligence or incompetence on the part of a professional. To succeed in a malpractice claim, a plaintiff must also prove proximate cause and damages. (Garner, 1999)

In the absence of any state statutes, common law is the basis of liability for injuries to clients caused by acts of malpractice and negligence of individual practitioners. In other words, most decisions of negligence in the professional setting are based on legal precedent (decisions that have previously been made about similar cases) rather than any specific action taken by the legislature.

To summarize, when the breach of duty is characterized as malpractice, the action is weighed against the professional standard. When it is brought forth as negligence, action is contrasted with what a reasonably prudent professional would have done in the same or similar circumstances.

Marchand (2001) cites the following basic elements of a nursing malpractice lawsuit:

1. The existence of a duty, owed by the nurse to a patient, to conform to a recognized standard of care
2. A failure to conform to the required nursing standard of care
3. Actual injury
4. A reasonably close causal connection between the nurse's conduct and the patient's injury

For the client to prevail in a malpractice claim, each of these elements must be proved. Juries' decisions are generally based on the testimony of expert witnesses, because members of the jury are laypeople and cannot be expected to know what nursing interventions should have been carried out. Without the testimony of expert witnesses, a favorable verdict usually goes to the defendant nurse.

Types of Lawsuits that Occur in Psychiatric Nursing

Most malpractice suits against nurses are civil actions; that is, they are considered breach of conduct actions on the part of the professional, for which compensation is being sought. The nurse in the psychiatric setting should be aware of the types of behaviors that may result in charges of malpractice.

Basic to the psychiatric client's hospitalization is his or her right to confidentiality and privacy. A nurse may be charged with *breach of confidentiality* for revealing aspects about a client's case, or even for revealing that an individual has been hospitalized, if that person can show that making this information known resulted in harm.

When shared information is detrimental to the client's reputation, the person sharing the information may be liable for **defamation of character**. When the information is in writing, the action is called **libel**. Oral defamation is called **slander**. Defamation of character involves communication that is malicious and false (Ellis & Hartley, 2004). Occasionally, libel arises out of critical, judgmental statements written in the client's medical record. Nurses need to be very objective in their charting, backing up all statements with factual evidence.

Invasion of privacy is a charge that may result when a client is searched without probable cause. Many institutions conduct body searches on mental clients as a routine intervention. In these cases, there should be a physician's order and written rationale showing probable cause for the intervention. Many institutions are reexamining their policies regarding this procedure.

Assault is an act that results in a person's genuine fear and apprehension that he or she will be touched without consent. **Battery** is the unconsented touching of another person. These charges can result when a treatment is administered to a client against his or her wishes and outside of an emergency situation. Harm or injury need not have occurred for these charges to be legitimate.

For confining a client against his or her wishes, and outside of an emergency situation, the nurse may be charged with false imprisonment. Examples of actions that may invoke these charges include locking an individual in a room; taking a client's clothes for purposes of detainment against his or her will; and retaining in mechanical restraints a competent voluntary client who demands to be released.

Avoiding Liability

Hall and Hall (2001) suggest the following proactive nursing actions in an effort to avoid nursing malpractice:

1. Responding to the patient
2. Educating the patient
3. Complying with the standard of care
4. Supervising care
5. Adhering to the nursing process
6. Documentation
7. Follow-up

In addition, it is a positive practice to develop and maintain a good interpersonal relationship with the client and his or her family. Some clients appear to be more "suit prone" than others. Suit-prone clients are often very critical, complaining, uncooperative, and even hostile. A natural response by the staff to these clients is to become defensive or withdrawn. Either of these behaviors increases the likelihood of a lawsuit should an unfavorable event occur (Ellis & Hartley, 2004). No matter how high the degree of technical competence and skill of the nurse, his or her insensitivity to a client's complaints and failure to meet the client's emotional needs often influence whether or not a lawsuit is generated. A great deal depends on the psychosocial skills of the health care professional.

SUMMARY

This chapter examined some of the ethical and legal issues relevant to psychiatric/mental health nursing in an effort to promote enhancement of quality of client care, as well as provide protection to the nurse within the parameters of legal accountability. Ethics is a branch of philosophy that deals with values related to human conduct, to the rightness and wrongness of certain actions, and to the goodness and badness of the motives and ends of such actions.

Clients have certain rights that are afforded them under the Constitution of the United States. Clients' rights have also been set forth by the AHA, the NLN, the American Civil Liberties Union, and the Mental Health Systems Act. Nurse practice acts and standards of professional practice guide the scope within which a nurse may legally practice. The ANA has established a Code for Nurses under which guidelines the professional nurse is expected to practice ethical nursing.

Ethical theories and principles are foundational guidelines that influence decision-making. Ethical theories include utilitarianism, Kantianism, Christian ethics, natural-law theories, and ethical egoism. Ethical principles include autonomy, beneficence, nonmaleficence, veracity, and justice. An individual's ethical philosophy affects his or her decision-making and ultimately the outcomes of those decisions.

Ethical issues in psychiatric/mental health nursing include the right to refuse medication and the right to the least-restrictive treatment alternative. An ethical decision-making model was presented along with a case study for application of the process.

Statutory laws are those that have been enacted by legislative bodies, and common laws are derived from decisions made in previous cases. Civil law protects the private and property rights of individuals and businesses, and criminal law provides protection from conduct deemed injurious to the public welfare. Both statutory law and common law have civil and criminal components.

Legal issues in psychiatric/mental health nursing center around confidentiality and the right to privacy, informed consent, restraints and seclusion, and commitment issues. Nurses are accountable for their own actions in relation to these issues, and violation can result in malpractice lawsuits against the physician, the hospital, and the nurse. Nurses must be aware of the kinds of behaviors that place them at risk for malpractice action. Developing and maintaining a good interpersonal relationship with the client and his or her family appears to be a positive factor when the question of malpractice is being considered.

REVIEW QUESTIONS

SELF-EXAMINATION/LEARNING EXERCISE

Match the following decision-making examples with the appropriate ethical theory:

_____ 1. Carol decides to go against family wishes and tell the client of his terminal status because that is what she would want if she were the client.

a. Utilitarianism

_____ 2. Carol decides to respect family wishes and not tell the client of his terminal status because that would bring the most happiness to the most people.

b. Kantianism

_____ 3. Carol decides not to tell the client about his terminal status because it would be too uncomfortable for her to do so.

c. Christian ethics

_____ 4. Carol decides to tell the client of his terminal status because her reasoning tells her that to do otherwise would be an evil act.

d. Natural law theories

_____ 5. Carol decides to tell the client of his terminal status because she believes it is her duty to do so.

e. Ethical egoism

Match the following nursing actions with the possible legal action with which the nurse may be charged:

_____ 6. The nurse assists the physician with electroconvulsive therapy on his client who has refused to give consent.

a. Breach of confidentiality

_____ 7. When the local newspaper calls to inquire why the mayor has been admitted to the hospital, the nurse replies, "He's here because he is an alcoholic."

b. Defamation of character

_____ 8. A competent, voluntary client has stated he wants to leave the hospital. The nurse hides his clothes in an effort to keep him from leaving.

c. Assault

_____ 9. Jack recently lost his wife and is very depressed. He is running for reelection to the Senate and asks the staff to keep his hospitalization confidential. The nurse is excited about having a Senator on the unit and tells her boyfriend about the admission, which soon becomes common knowledge. Jack loses the election.

d. Battery

_____ 10. Joe is very restless and is pacing a lot. The nurse says to Joe, "If you don't sit down in the chair and be still, I'm going to put you in restraints!"

e. False imprisonment

REFERENCES

Aiken, T.D. (2004). *Legal, ethical, and political issues in nursing* (2nd ed.). Philadelphia: F.A. Davis.

American Hospital Association (AHA). (1992). *A Patient's Bill of Rights*. Chicago: American Hospital Association.

American Nurses' Association (ANA). (2001). *Code of ethics for nurses with interpretive statements*. Washington, DC: ANA.

Appelbaum, P.S. (2001, March). Thinking carefully about outpatient commitment. *Psychiatric Services, 52*(3), 347–350.

Catalano, J.T. (2003). *Nursing now! Today's issues, tomorrow's trends* (3rd ed.). Philadelphia: F.A. Davis.

Cournos, F., & Petrila, J. (1992). Legal and ethical issues. In F.I. Kass, J.M. Oldham, & H. Pardes (Eds.). *The Columbia University College of Physicians and Surgeons complete guide to mental health*. New York: Henry Holt.

Ellis, J.R., & Hartley, C.L. (2004). *Nursing in today's world: Challenges, issues, and trends* (8th ed.). Philadelphia: Lippincott Williams & Wilkins

Fedorka, P., & Resnick, L.K. (2001). Defining nursing practice. In M.E. O'Keefe (Ed.). *Nursing practice and the law: Avoiding malpractice and other legal rights*. Philadelphia: F.A. Davis.

Garner, B.A. (Ed.). (1999). *Black's law dictionary*. St. Paul, MN: West Group.

Guido, G.W. (2000). *Legal and ethical issues in nursing* (3rd ed.). Upper Saddle River, NJ: Prentice-Hall.

Hall, J.K., & Hall, D. (2001). Negligence specific to nursing. In M.E. O'Keefe (Ed.). *Nursing practice and the law: Avoiding malpractice and other legal risks*. Philadelphia: F.A. Davis.

Joint Commission on Accreditation of Healthcare Organizations (JCAHO). (2000). *Restraint and Seclusion Standards for Behavioral Health*. Retrieved on May 16, 2000 from http://www.jcaho.org/standard/restraint_stds.html

Levy, R.M., & Rubenstein, L.S. (1996). *The rights of people with mental disabilities*. Carbondale, IL: Southern Illinois University Press.

Maloy, K.A. (1996). Does involuntary outpatient commitment work? In B.D. Sales & S.A. Shah (Eds.). *Mental health and law: Research, policy and services*. Durham, NC: Carolina Academic Press.

Marchand, L. (2001). Legal terminology. In M.E. O'Keefe (Ed.). *Nursing practice and the law: Avoiding malpractice and other legal risks*. Philadelphia: F.A. Davis.

Medscape Wire (2000). *Joint Commission Releases Revised Restraints Standards for Behavioral Healthcare*. Retrieved May 16, 2000 from http://psychiatry.medscape.com/MedscapeWire/2000/0500/medwire.0509.Joint.html.

Mental Health Systems Act. P.L. 96-398, Title V, Sect. 501.94 Stat. 1598, October 7, 1980.

Pappas, A. (2003). Ethical issues. In J. Zerwekh & J.C. Claborn (Eds.). *Nursing today: Transition and trends* (4th ed.). Philadelphia: W.B. Saunders.

Ridgely, M.S., Borum, R., & Petrila, J. (2001). *The effectiveness of involuntary outpatient treatment: Empirical evidence and the experience of eight states*. Santa Monica, CA: Rand Publications.

Schwarz, M., Swanson, J., Hiday, V., Wagner, H.R., Burns, B., & Borum, R. (2001). A randomized controlled trial of outpatient commitment in North Carolina. *Psychiatric Services, 52*(3), 325–329.

Steadman, H., Gounis, K., Dennis, D., Hopper, K., Roche, B., Swartz, M., & Robbins, P. (2001). Assessing the New York City involuntary outpatient commitment pilot program. *Psychiatric Services, 52*(3), 330–336.

Torrey, E.F. (2001). Outpatient commitment: What, Why, and for Whom. *Psychiatric Services 52*(3), 337–341.

Weiss-Kaffie, C.J., & Purtell, N.E. (2001). Psychiatric nursing. In M.E. O'Keefe (Ed.). *Nursing practice and the law: Avoiding malpractice and other legal risks*. Philadelphia: F.A. Davis.

6

C H A P T E R

CULTURAL CONCEPTS RELEVANT TO PSYCHIATRIC/MENTAL HEALTH NURSING

CHAPTER OUTLINE

OBJECTIVES

INTRODUCTION

HOW DO CULTURES DIFFER?

APPLICATION OF THE NURSING PROCESS

SUMMARY

REVIEW QUESTIONS

KEY TERMS

curandera
curandero
culture-bound
 syndromes
density
distance

folk medicine
shaman
stereotyping
territoriality
yin and yang

CORE CONCEPTS

culture
ethnicity

OBJECTIVES

After reading this chapter, the student will be able to:

1. Define and differentiate between *culture* and *ethnicity*.
2. Describe six phenomena on which to identify cultural differences.
3. Identify cultural variances, based on the six phenomena, for
   a. Northern European Americans.

   b. African Americans.
   c. Native Americans.
   d. Asian/Pacific Islander Americans.
   e. Latino Americans.
   f. Western European Americans.
4. Apply the nursing process in the care of individuals from various cultural groups.

INTRODUCTION

What is **culture**? How does it differ from **ethnicity**? Why are these questions important? The answers lie in the changing face of America. Immigration is not new in the United States. Indeed, most U.S. citizens are either immigrants or descendents of immigrants. This pattern continues because of the many individuals who

want to take advantage of the technological growth and upward mobility that exists in this country. Griffin (2002) states:

Most researchers agree that the United States, long a destination of immigrants, continues to grow more culturally diverse. According to the U.S. Census Bureau, the number of foreign-born residents in the country jumped from roughly 19.8 million to a little more than 28 million between

89

Culture describes a particular society's entire way of living, encompassing shared patterns of belief, feeling, and knowledge that guide people's conduct and are passed down from generation to generation. **Ethnicity** is a somewhat narrower term, and relates to people who identify with each other because of a shared heritage (Griffith, Gonzalez, & Blue, 2003).

1990 and 2000. What's more, experts predict that Caucasians, who now represent about 70 percent of the U.S. population, will account for barely more than 50 percent by the year 2050. (p. 14)

Why is this important? Cultural influences affect human behavior, the interpretation of human behavior, and the response to human behavior. It is therefore essential for nurses to understand the effects of these cultural influences if they are to work effectively with this diverse population. Caution must be taken, however, not to assume that all individuals who share a culture or ethnic group are clones. This constitutes **stereotyping**, and must be avoided. Many variations and subcultures are found within a culture. These differences may be related to status, ethnic background, residence, religion, education, or other factors (Purnell & Paulanka, 2003). Every individual must be appreciated for his or her uniqueness.

This chapter explores the ways in which various cultures differ. The nursing process is applied to the delivery of psychiatric/mental health nursing care for individuals from the following cultural groups: Northern European Americans, African Americans, Native Americans, Asian/Pacific Islander Americans, Latino Americans, and Western European Americans.

HOW DO CULTURES DIFFER?

It is difficult to generalize about any one specific group in a country that is known for its heterogeneity. Within our American "melting pot" any or all characteristics could apply to individuals within any or all of the cultural groups represented. As these differences continue to be integrated, one American culture will eventually emerge. This is already in evidence in certain regions of the country today. However, some differences still do exist, and it is important for nurses to be aware of certain cultural influences that may affect individuals' behaviors and beliefs, particularly as they apply to health care.

Giger and Davidhizar (2004) suggest six cultural phenomena that vary with application and use but yet are evidenced among all cultural groups: (1) communication, (2) space, (3) social organization, (4) time, (5) environmental control, and (6) biological variations.

Communication

All verbal and nonverbal behavior in the presence of another individual is communication. Therapeutic communication has always been considered an essential part of the nursing process and represents a critical element in the curricula of most schools of nursing. Communication has its roots in culture. Cultural mores, norms, ideas, and customs provide the basis for our way of thinking. Cultural values are learned and differ from society to society. Communication is expressed through language (the spoken vocabulary), paralanguage (the voice quality, intonation, rhythm, and speed of the spoken word), and gestures (touch, facial expression, eye movements, body posture, and physical appearance). The nurse who is planning care must have an understanding of the client's needs and expectations as they are being communicated. As a third party, an interpreter often complicates matters, but one may be necessary when the client does not speak the same language as the nurse. Interpreting is a very complex process, however, that requires a keen sensitivity to cultural nuances, and not just the translating of words into another language.

Space

Spatial determinants relate to the place where the communication occurs and encompass the concepts of **territoriality**, **density**, and **distance**. Territoriality refers to the innate tendency to own space. The need for territoriality is met only if the individual has control of a space, can establish rules for that space, and is able to defend the space against invasion or misuse by others (Giger & Davidhizar, 2004). Density refers to the number of people within a given environmental space and has been shown to influence interpersonal interaction. Distance is the means by which various cultures use space to communicate. Hall (1966) identified three primary dimensions of space in interpersonal interactions in the Western culture: the intimate zone (0 to 18 inches), the personal zone (18 inches to 3 feet), and the social zone (3 to 6 feet).

Social Organization

Cultural behavior is socially acquired through a process called *acculturation*, which involves acquiring knowledge and internalizing values (Giger & Davidhizar, 2004). Children are acculturated by observing adults within their social organizations. Social organizations include families, religious groups, and ethnic groups.

Time

An awareness of the concept of time is a gradual learning process. Some cultures place great importance on values that are measured by clock time. Punctuality and efficiency of time utilization are highly valued in the United States, whereas some cultures are actually scornful of clock time. Other cultural implications regarding time have to do with perception of time orientation. Whether individuals are present-oriented or future-oriented in their perception of time influences many aspects of their lives.

Environmental Control

The variable of environmental control has to do with the degree to which individuals perceive that they have control over their environment. Cultural beliefs and practices influence how an individual responds to their environment during periods of wellness and illness. To provide culturally appropriate care, the nurse should not only respect the individual's unique beliefs, but should also have an understanding of how these beliefs can be used to promote optimal health in the client's environment.

Biological Variations

Biological differences exist among people in various racial groups. Giger & Davidhizar (2004) state:

The strongest argument for including concepts on biological variations in nursing education and subsequently nursing practice is that scientific facts about biological variations can aid the nurse in giving culturally appropriate health care. (p. 136)

These differences include body structure (both size and shape), skin color, physiological responses to medication, electrocardiographic patterns, susceptibility to disease, and nutritional preferences and deficiencies.

APPLICATION OF THE NURSING PROCESS

Background Assessment Data

Table 6–1 presents a format for cultural assessment that may be used to gather information related to culture and ethnicity that is important for planning client care.

Northern European Americans

The language of the Northern European Americans has its roots in the language of the first English settlers to the United States, with the influence of immigrants from around the world. The descendants of these immigrants

TABLE 6–1	Cultural Assessment Tool

Client's name
Ethnic origin
Address
Birthdate
Name of significant other _____ Relationship
Primary language spoken _____ Second language spoken
How does client usually communicate with people who speak a different language?
Is an interpreter required? _____ Available?
Highest level of education achieved:
Occupation:
Presenting problem:
Has this problem ever occurred before?
If so, in what manner was it handled previously?
What is the client's usual manner of coping with stress?
Who is (are) the client's main support system(s)?
Describe the family living arrangements:
Who is the major decision maker in the family?
Describe client's/family members' roles within the family.

Describe religious beliefs and practices:
   Are there any religious requirements or restrictions that place limitations on the client's care?
   If so, describe:
Who in the family takes responsibility for health concerns?
Describe any special health beliefs and practices:

From whom does family usually seek medical assistance in time of need?
Describe client's usual emotional/behavioral response to:
   Anxiety:
   Anger:
   Loss/change/failure:
   Pain:
   Fear:

(Continued on following page)

TABLE 6-1	Cultural Assessment Tool *(Continued)*

Describe any topics that are particularly sensitive or that the client is unwilling to discuss (because of cultural taboos):_____

Describe any activities in which the client is unwilling to participate (because of cultural customs or taboos):_____

What are the client's personal feelings regarding touch?_____

What are the client's personal feelings regarding eye contact?_____

What is the client's personal orientation to time? (past, present, future)_____

Describe any particular illnesses to which the client may be bioculturally susceptible (e.g., hypertension and sickle cell anemia in African Americans):_____

Describe any nutritional deficiencies to which the client may be bioculturally susceptible (e.g., lactose intolerance in Native and Asian Americans)._____

Describe client's favorite foods:_____

Are there any foods the client requests or refuses because of cultural beliefs related to this illness (e.g., hot" and "cold" foods for Latino Americans and Asian Americans)? If so, please describe:_____
_____

Describe client's perception of the problem and expectations of health care:_____

now make up what is considered the dominant cultural group in the United States today. Specific dialects and rate of speech are common to various regions of the country. Northern European Americans value territory. Personal space is about 18 inches to 3 feet.

With the advent of technology and widespread mobility, less emphasis has been placed on the cohesiveness of the family. In 2003, the divorce rate was 3.8 divorces per 1000 population (National Center for Health Statistics, 2004). The value that was once placed on religion also seems to be diminishing in the American culture, with a reported decline in church attendance from 1991 to 2004 (Barna Research Online, 2004). Punctuality and efficiency are highly valued in the culture that promoted the work ethic, and most within this cultural group tend to be future oriented (Murray & Zentner, 2001).

Northern European Americans, particularly those who achieve middle-class socioeconomic status, value preventive medicine and primary health care. This value follows along with the socioeconomic group's educational level, successful achievement, and financial capability to maintain a healthy lifestyle. Most recognize the importance of regular physical exercise. Northern European Americans have medium body structure and fair skin, the latter of which is thought to be an evolutionary result of living in cold, cloudy Northern Europe (Giger & Davidhizar, 2004).

Beef and certain seafood, such as lobster, are regarded as high-status foods among many people in this culture (Giger & Davidhizar, 2004). Changing food habits may bring both good and bad news, however. The good news is that people are learning about eating healthier by decreasing the amount of fat and increasing the nutrients in their diets. The bad news is that Americans still enjoy fast food, and it conforms to their fast-paced lifestyles.

African Americans

The language dialect of many African Americans is different from what is considered standard English. The origin of the black dialect is not clearly understood but is thought to be a combination of various African languages and the languages of other cultural groups (e.g., Dutch, French, English, and Spanish) present in the United States at the time of its settlement. Personal space tends to be smaller than that of the dominant culture.

Patterns of discrimination date back to the days of slavery, and evidence of segregation still exists. This can be observed in some cities with the existence of predominantly black neighborhoods, churches, and schools. Some African Americans find it too difficult to try to assimilate into the mainstream culture and choose to remain within their own social organization.

In 2003, 44 percent of African American households were headed by a woman (U.S. Census Bureau, 2004a). Social support systems may be large and include sisters, brothers, aunts, uncles, cousins, boyfriends, girlfriends, neighbors, and friends. Many African Americans have a strong religious orientation, with the vast majority practicing some form of Protestantism (Harris, 2004).

African Americans who have assimilated into the dominant culture are likely to be well educated, professional, and future oriented. Some who have not become assimilated believe that planning for the future is hopeless, a belief based on their previous experiences and encounters with racism and discrimination (Cherry & Giger, 2004). They may be unemployed or have low-paying jobs, with little expectation for improvement. They are unlikely to value time or punctuality to the same degree as the dominant cultural group, which often causes them to be labeled as irresponsible.

Some African Americans, particularly those from the rural South, may reach adulthood never having encountered a physician. They receive their medical care from the local folk practitioner known as "granny," or "the old lady," or a "spiritualist." Incorporated into the system of **folk medicine** is the belief that health is a gift from God, whereas illness is a punishment from God or a retribution for sin and evil. Historically, African Americans have turned to folk medicine either because they could not afford the cost of medical treatment or because of the insensitive treatment by caregivers in the health care delivery system.

Height of African Americans varies little from their Northern European American counterparts. Skin color varies from white to very dark brown or black, which offered the ancestors of African Americans protection from the sun and tropical heat.

Hypertension occurs more frequently, and sickle cell anemia occurs predominantly in African Americans. Hypertension carries a strong hereditary risk factor, whereas sickle cell anemia is genetically derived. Alcoholism is a serious problem among members of the black community, leading to a high incidence of alcohol-related illness and death (Cherry & Giger, 2004).

The diet of most African Americans differs little from that of the mainstream culture. Some African Americans follow their heritage, however, and still enjoy what has come to be known as "soul" food. Some of these foods include poke salad, collard greens, beans, corn, fried chicken, black-eyed peas, grits, okra, and cornbread. These foods are now considered typical Southern fare and are regularly consumed and enjoyed by most individuals who inhabit the Southern region of the United States.

Native Americans

The Bureau of Indian Affairs (BIA) recognizes more than 554 Indian tribes and Alaska Native groups that speak more than 250 languages (BIA, 2001). Fewer than half of these still live on reservations, but most return home often to participate in family and tribal life and sometimes to retire. Touch is an aspect of communication that differs in Native Americans from the dominant American culture. Some Native Americans view the traditional handshake as somewhat aggressive. Instead, if a hand is offered to another, it may be accepted with a light touch or just a passing of hands (Still & Hodgins, 2003). Some Native Americans will not touch a dead person (Hanley, 2004).

Native Americans may appear silent and reserved. They may be uncomfortable expressing emotions because the culture encourages keeping private thoughts to oneself.

The concept of space is very concrete to Native Americans. Living space is often crowded, and includes members of both nuclear and extended families. A large network of kin is very important to Native Americans. A need for extended space exists, however, as demonstrated by a distance of many miles between individual homes or camps.

The primary social organizations of Native Americans are the family and the tribe. From infancy Native American children are taught the importance of these units. Traditions are passed down by the elderly, and children are taught to respect tradition and to honor wisdom.

Native Americans are very present-time oriented. The time sequences of importance for Native Americans are present, past, and future, with little emphasis on the future (Still & Hodgins, 2003). Not only are Native Americans not ruled by the clock, some do not even own clocks. The concept of time is very casual, and tasks are accomplished, not with the notion of a particular time in mind, but merely in a present-oriented time frame.

Religion and health practices are intertwined in the Native American culture. The medicine man (or woman) is called the **shaman**, and may use a variety of methods in his or her practice. Some depend on "crystal gazing" to diagnose illness, some sing and perform elaborate healing ceremonies, and some use herbs and other plants or roots to concoct remedies with healing properties. The Native American healers and U.S. Indian Health Service have worked together with mutual respect for many years. Hanley (2004) relates that a medicine man or medicine woman may confer with a physician regarding the care of a client in the hospital. Clients may sometimes receive hospital passes to participate in a healing ceremony held outside the hospital. Research studies have continued to show the importance of each of these health care systems in the overall wellness of Native American people.

Native Americans are typically of average height with reddish-tinted skin that may be light to medium brown. Their cheekbones are usually high and their noses have high bridges, probably an evolutionary result of living in very dry climates.

The risks of illness and premature death from alcoholism, diabetes, tuberculosis, heart disease, accidents, homicide, suicide, pneumonia, and influenza are greater for Native Americans than for the U.S. population as a whole (Indian Health Service [IHS], 2001). Alcoholism is a widespread problem among Native Americans (Shore, Manson, & Buchwald, 2002). It is thought to be a symptom of depression in many cases and to contribute to a number of other serious problems such as automobile accidents, homicides, spouse and child abuse, and suicides.

Nutritional deficiencies are not uncommon among tribal Native Americans. Fruits and green vegetables are often scarce in many of the federally defined Indian geographical regions. Meat and corn products are identified as preferred foods. Fiber intake is relatively low, while fat intake is often of the saturated variety. A large number of Native Americans living on or near reservations recognized by the federal or state government receive commodity foods supplied by the U.S. Department of Agriculture's food distribution program (U.S. Department of Agriculture, 2004).

Asian/Pacific Islander Americans

Asian Americans compose one of the largest ethnic groups in the United States today, totaling approximately

11 million people (U.S. Census Bureau, 2004b). The Asian American culture includes peoples (and their descendants) from Japan, China, Vietnam, the Philippines, Thailand, Cambodia, Korea, Laos, and the Pacific Islands. Although this discussion relates to these peoples as a single culture, it is important to keep in mind that a multiplicity of differences regarding attitudes, beliefs, values, religious practices, and language exist among these subcultures.

Many Asian Americans, particularly Japanese, are third- and even fourth-generation Americans. These individuals are likely to be acculturated to the U.S. culture. Ng (2001) describes three patterns common to Asian Americans in their attempt to adjust to the American culture:

1. The Traditionalists. These individuals tend to be the older generation Asians who hold on to the traditional values and practices of their native culture. They have strong internalized Asian values. Primary allegiance is to the biological family.
2. The Marginal People. These individuals reject the traditional values and totally embrace Western culture. Often they are members of the younger generations.
3. Asian Americans. These individuals incorporate traditional values and beliefs with Western values and beliefs. They become integrated into the American culture, while maintaining a connection with their ancestral culture.

The languages and dialects of Asian Americans are very diverse. In general, they do share a similar belief in harmonious interaction. To raise one's voice is likely to be interpreted as a sign of loss of control. The English language is very difficult to master, and even bilingual Asian Americans may encounter communication problems because of the differences in meaning assigned to nonverbal cues, such as facial gestures, verbal intonation and speed, and body movements. In Asian cultures, touching during communication has historically been considered unacceptable. However, with the advent of Western acculturation, younger generations of Asian Americans accept touching as more appropriate than did their ancestors. Eye contact is often avoided, as it connotes rudeness and lack of respect in some Asian cultures. Acceptable personal and social spaces are larger than in the dominant American culture. Some Asian Americans have a great deal of difficulty expressing emotions. Because of their reserved public demeanor, Asian Americans may be perceived as shy, cold, or uninterested.

The family is the ultimate social organization in the Asian American culture, and loyalty to family is emphasized above all else. Children are expected to obey and honor their parents. Misbehavior is perceived as bringing dishonor to the entire family. Filial piety (one's social obligation or duty to one's parents) is held in high regard.

Failure to fulfill these obligations can create a great deal of guilt and shame in an individual. A chronological hierarchy exists with the elderly maintaining positions of authority. Several generations, or even extended families, may share a single household.

Although education is highly valued among Asian Americans, many remain undereducated. Religious beliefs and practices are very diverse and exhibit influences of Taoism, Buddhism, Confucianism, Islam, and Christianity (Giger & Davidhizar, 2004).

Many Asian Americans are both past and present oriented. Emphasis is placed on the wishes of one's ancestors, while adjusting to demands of the present. Little value is given to prompt adherence to schedules or rigid standards of activities.

Restoring the balance of **yin and yang** is the fundamental concept of Asian health practices (Spector, 2004). Yin and yang represent opposite forces of energy, such as negative/positive, dark/light, cold/hot, hard/soft, and feminine/masculine. When there is a disruption in the balance of these forces of energy, illness can occur. In medicine, the opposites are expressed as "hot" and "cold," and health is the result of a balance between hot and cold elements (Wang, 2003). Food, medicines, and herbs are classified according to their hot and cold properties and are used to restore balance between yin and yang (cold and hot) thereby restoring health.

Asian Americans are generally small of frame and build. Obesity is very uncommon in this culture. Skin color ranges from white to medium brown, with yellow tones. Other physical characteristics include almond-shaped eyes with a slight droop to eyelids and sparse body hair, particularly in men, in whom chest hair is often absent. Hair on the head is commonly coarse, thick, straight, and black in color.

Rice, vegetables, and fish are the main staple foods of Asian Americans. Milk is seldom consumed because a large majority of Asian Americans experience lactose intolerance. With Western acculturation, their diet is changing, and unfortunately, with more meat being consumed, the percentage of fat in the diet is increasing.

Many Asian Americans believe that psychiatric illness is merely behavior that is out of control. They view this as a great shame to the individual and the family. They often attempt to manage the ill person on their own until they can no longer handle the situation. It is not uncommon for Asian Americans to somaticize. Expressing mental distress through various physical ailments may be viewed as more acceptable than expressing true emotions (Ishida & Inouye, 2004).

The incidence of alcohol dependence is low among Asians. This may be a result of a possible genetic intolerance of the substance. Some Asians develop unpleasant symptoms, such as flushing, headaches, and palpitations, on drinking alcoholic beverages. Research indicates that this is attributable to an isoenzyme variant that quickly converts alcohol to acetaldehyde and the absence of an isoenzyme that is needed to oxidize acetaldehyde. This results in a rapid accumulation of acetaldehyde that produces the unpleasant symptoms (Wall et al., 1997).

Latino Americans

Latino Americans are the fastest growing group of people in the United States comprising approximately 12 percent of the population (U.S. Census, 2004b). Only African Americans represent a larger ethnic minority group.

Latino Americans trace their ancestry to countries such as Mexico, Spain, Puerto Rico, Cuba, and other countries of Central and South America. The common language is Spanish, spoken with a number of dialects by the various peoples. Touch is a common form of communication among Latinos; however, they are very modest and are likely to withdraw from any infringement on their modesty (Murray & Zentner, 2001). Latinos tend to be very tactful and diplomatic and will often appear agreeable on the surface out of courtesy for the person with whom they are communicating. It is only after the fact when agreements remain unfulfilled that the true context of the interaction becomes clear.

Latino Americans are very group oriented. It is important for them to interact with large groups of relatives, during which a great deal of touching and embracing occurs. The family is the primary social organization and includes nuclear family members as well as numerous extended family members. The nuclear family is male dominated, and the father possesses ultimate authority.

Latino Americans tend to be present oriented. The concept of being punctual and giving attention to activities that relate to concern about the future are perceived as less important than present-oriented activities that cannot again be retrieved beyond the present time.

Roman Catholicism is the predominant religion among Latino Americans. Most Latinos identify with the Roman Catholic Church, even if they do not attend services. Religious beliefs and practices are likely to be strong influences in their lives. Especially in times of crisis, such as in cases of illness and hospitalization, Latino-Americans rely on priest and family to carry out important religious rituals, such as promise making, offering candles, visiting shrines, and offering prayers (Spector, 2004).

Folk beliefs regarding health are a combination of elements incorporating views of Roman Catholicism and Indian and Spanish ancestries. The folk healer is called a **curandero** (male) or **curandera** (female). Among traditional Latino Americans, the curandero is believed to have a gift from God for healing the sick and is often the first contact made when illness is encountered. Treatments used include massage, diet, rest, suggestions,

practical advice, indigenous herbs, prayers, magic, and supernatural rituals (Gonzalez & Kuipers, 2004). Many Latino Americans still subscribe to the "hot and cold theory" of disease. This concept is similar to the Asian perception of yin and yang discussed earlier in this chapter. Diseases and the foods and medicines used to treat them are classified as "hot" or "cold," and the intention is to restore the body to a balanced state.

Latino Americans are usually shorter than the average member of the dominant American culture. Skin color can vary from light tan to dark brown. Research indicates that there is less mental illness among Latino Americans than the general population. This may have to do with the strong cohesiveness of the family and the support that is given during times of stress. Because Latino Americans have clearly defined rules of conduct, fewer role conflicts occur within the family.

Western European Americans

Western European Americans have their origin in France, Italy, and Greece. Each of these cultures possesses its own unique language with a number of dialects noticeable within each language. Western Europeans are known to be very warm and affectionate people. They tend to be physically expressive, using a lot of body language, including hugging and kissing.

Like Latino Americans, Western European Americans are very family oriented. They interact in large groups, and it is not uncommon for several generations to live together or in close proximity of each other. A strong allegiance to the cultural heritage exists, and it is not uncommon, particularly among Italians, to find settlements of immigrants clustering together.

Roles within the family are clearly defined, with the man as the head of the household. Western European women view their role as mother and homemaker, and children are prized and cherished. The elderly are held in positions of respect and often are cared for in the home rather than placed in nursing homes.

Roman Catholicism is the predominant religion for the French and Italians; Greek Orthodox for the Greeks. A number of religious traditions are observed surrounding rites of passage. Masses and rituals are observed for births, first communions, marriages, anniversaries, and deaths.

Western Europeans tend to be present oriented with a somewhat fatalistic view of the future. A priority is placed on the here and now, and whatever happens in the future is perceived as God's will.

Most Western European Americans follow health beliefs and practices of the dominant American culture, but some folk beliefs and superstitions still endure. Spector (2004, p. 285) reports the following superstitions and practices of Italians as they relate to health and illness:

1. Congenital abnormalities can be attributed to the unsatisfied desire for food during pregnancy.
2. If a woman is not given food that she craves or smells, the fetus will move inside, and a miscarriage can result.
3. If a pregnant woman bends or turns or moves in a certain way, the fetus may not develop normally.
4. A woman must not reach during pregnancy because reaching can harm the fetus.
5. Sitting in a draft can cause a cold that can lead to pneumonia.

This author recalls her own Italian immigrant grandmother warming large collard greens in oil and placing them on swollen parotid glands during a bout with the mumps. The greens undoubtedly did nothing for the mumps, but they (along with the tender loving care) felt wonderful!

Western Europeans are typically of average stature. Skin color ranges from fair to medium brown. Hair and eyes are commonly dark, but some Italians have blue eyes and blond hair. Food is very important in the Western European American culture. Italian, Greek, and French cuisine is world famous, and food is used in a social manner, as well as for nutritional purposes. Wine is consumed by all (even the children) and is the beverage of choice with meals. However, among Greek Americans, drunkenness engenders social disgrace on the individual and the family (Tripp-Reimer & Sorofman, 1998).

Table 6–2 presents a summary of information related to the six cultural phenomena as they apply to the cultural groups discussed here.

Culture-Bound Syndromes

The *Diagnostic and Statistical Manual of Mental Disorders*, 4th Edition, *Text Revision* (*DSM-IV-TR*) (American Psychiatric Association [APA], 2000) recognizes various symptoms that are associated with specific cultures and that may be expressed differently from those of the dominant American culture. Although presentations associated with the major *DSM-IV-TR* categories can be found throughout the world, many of the responses are influenced by local cultural factors (APA, 2000). The *DSM-IV-TR* defines *culture-bound syndromes* as follows:

> Recurrent, locality-specific patterns of aberrant behavior and troubling experience that may or may not be linked to a particular DSM-IV diagnostic category. Many of these patterns are indigenously considered to be "illnesses," or at least afflictions, and most have local names. (p. 898)

It is important for nurses to understand that individuals from diverse cultural groups may exhibit these physical and behavioral manifestations. The syndromes are viewed within these cultural groups as folk, diagnostic categories with specific sets of experiences and observa-

tions (APA, 2000). Examples of culture-bound syndromes are presented in Table 6–3.

Diagnosis/Outcome Identification

Nursing diagnoses are selected based on the information gathered during the assessment process. With background knowledge of cultural variables and information uniquely related to the individual, the following nursing diagnoses may be appropriate:

1. Impaired verbal communication related to cultural differences evidenced by inability to speak the dominant language.
2. Anxiety (moderate to severe) related to entry into an unfamiliar health care system and separation from support systems evidenced by apprehension and suspicion, restlessness, and trembling.
3. Imbalanced nutrition, less than body requirements, related to refusal to eat unfamiliar foods provided in the health care setting, evidenced by loss of weight.
4. Spiritual distress related to inability to participate in usual religious practices because of hospitalization, evidenced by alterations in mood (e.g., anger, crying, withdrawal, preoccupation, anxiety, hostility, apathy, and so forth)

Outcome criteria related to these nursing diagnoses may include the following:
The Client:

1. Has had all basic needs fulfilled.
2. Has communicated with staff through an interpreter.
3. Has maintained anxiety at a manageable level by having family members stay with him or her during hospitalization.
4. Has maintained weight by eating foods that he or she likes brought to the hospital by family members.
5. Has restored spiritual strength through use of cultural rituals and beliefs and visits from a spiritual leader.

Planning/Implementation

The following interventions have special cultural implications for nursing:

1. Use an interpreter if necessary to ensure that there are no barriers to communication. Be careful with nonverbal communication because it may be interpreted differently by different cultures (e.g., Asians and Native Americans may be uncomfortable with touch and direct eye contact, whereas Latinos and Western Europeans perceive touch as a sign of caring).
2. Make allowances for individuals from other cultures to have family members around them and even participate in their care. Large numbers of extended family members are very important to African Americans, Native Americans, Asian Americans,

TABLE 6–2 Summary of Six Cultural Phenomena in Comparison of Various Cultural Groups

CULTURAL GROUP AND COUNTRIES OF ORIGIN	COMMUNICATION	SPACE	SOCIAL ORGANIZATION	TIME	ENVIRONMENTAL CONTROL	BIOLOGICAL VARIATIONS
Northern European Americans (England, Ireland, Germany, others)	National languages (although many learn English very quickly) Dialects (often regional) English More verbal than non-verbal	Territory valued Personal space: 18 inches to 3 feet Uncomfortable with personal contact and touch	Families: nuclear and extended Religions: Jewish and Christian Organizations: social community	Future oriented	Most value preventive medicine and primary health care through traditional health care delivery system Alternative methods on the increase	Health concerns: Cardiovascular disease Cancer Diabetes mellitus
African Americans (Africa, West Indian islands, Dominican Republic, Haiti, Jamaica)	National languages Dialects (pidgin, Creole, Gullah, French, Spanish) Highly verbal and nonverbal	Close personal space Comfortable with touch	Large, extended families Many female-headed households Strong religious orientation, mostly Protestant Community social organizations	Present oriented	Traditional health care delivery system Some individuals prefer to use folk practitioner ("granny" or voodoo healer) Home remedies	Health concerns: Cardiovascular disease Hypertension Sickle cell disease Diabetes mellitus Lactose intolerance
Native Americans (North America, Alaska, Aleutian Islands)	250 tribal languages recognized Comfortable with silence Direct eye contact considered rude	Large, extended space important Uncomfortable with touch	Families: nuclear and extended Children taught importance of tradition Social organizations: tribe and family most important	Present oriented	Religion and health practices intertwined Medicine man or woman (shaman) uses folk practices to heal Shaman may work with modern medical practitioner	Health concerns: Alcoholism Tuberculosis Accidents Diabetes mellitus Heart disease
Asian/Pacific Islander Americans (Japan, China, Korea, Vietnam, Philippines, Thailand, Cambodia, Laos, Pacific Islands, others)	More than 30 different languages spoken Comfortable with silence Uncomfortable with eye-to-eye contact Nonverbal connotations may be misunderstood	Large personal space Uncomfortable with touch	Families: nuclear and extended Children taught importance of family loyalty and tradition Many religions: Taoism, Buddhism, Islam, Christianity Community social organizations	Present oriented Past important and valued	Traditional health care delivery system Some prefer to use folk practices (e.g., yin and yang; herbal medicine; and moxibustion)	Health concerns: Hypertension Cancer Diabetes mellitus Thalassemia Lactose intolerance
Latino Americans (Mexico, Spain, Cuba, Puerto Rico, other countries of Central and South America)	Spanish, with many dialects	Close personal space Lots of touching and embracing Very group oriented	Families: nuclear and large extended families Strong ties to Roman Catholicism Community social organizations	Present oriented	Traditional health care delivery system Some prefer to use folk practitioner, called *curandero or curandera* Folk practices include "hot and cold" herbal remedies	Health concerns: Heart disease Cancer Diabetes mellitus Accidents Lactose intolerance
Western European Americans (France, Italy, Greece)	National languages Dialects	Close personal space Lots of touching and embracing Very group oriented	Families: nuclear and large extended families France and Italy: Roman Catholic Greece: Greek Orthodox	Present oriented	Traditional health care delivery system Lots of home remedies and practices based on superstition	Health concerns: Heart disease Cancer Diabetes mellitus Thalassemia

SOURCES: Spector (2004); Purnell & Paulanka (2003); Murrary & Zentner (2001); Geissler (1994); and Giger & Davidhizar (2004).

TABLE 6–3 Culture-Bound Syndromes

SYNDROME	CULTURE	SYMPTOMS
Amok	Malaysia, Laos, Philippines, Polynesia, Papua New Guinea, Puerto Rico	A dissociative episode followed by an outburst of violent, aggressive, or homicidal behavior directed at people and objects. May be associated with psychotic episode.
Ataque de nervios	Latin American and Latin Mediterranean groups	Uncontrollable shouting, crying, trembling, verbal or physical aggression, sometimes accompanied by dissociative experiences, seizurelike or fainting episodes, and suicidal gestures. Often occurs in response to stressful family event.
Bilis and colera (*muina*)	Latin American	Acute nervous tension, headache, trembling, screaming, stomach disturbances, and sometimes loss of consciousness. Thought to occur in response to intense anger or rage.
Boufee delirante	West Africa and Haiti	Sudden outburst of agitated and aggressive behavior, confusion, and psychomotor excitement. May be accompanied by hallucinations or paranoia.
Brain fag	West Africa	Difficulty concentrating, remembering, and thinking. Pain and pressure around head and neck; blurred vision. Associated with challenges of schooling.
Dhat	India	Severe anxiety and hypochondriasis associated with the discharge of semen, whitish discoloration of the urine, and feelings of weakness and exhaustion.
Falling-out or blacking out	Southern U.S. and the Caribbean	Sudden collapse. May or may not be preceded by dizziness. Person can hear but cannot move. Eyes are open, but individual claims inability to see.
Ghost sickness	American Indian tribes	Preoccupation with death and the deceased. Bad dreams, weakness, feelings of danger, loss of appetite, fainting, dizziness, fear anxiety, hallucinations, loss of consciousness, confusion, feelings of futility, and a sense of suffocation.
Hwa-byung (anger syndrome)	Korea	Insomnia, fatigue, panic, fear of impending death, dysphoric affect, indigestion, anorexia, dyspnea, palpitations, and generalized aches and pains. Attributed to the suppression of anger.
Koro	Southern and Eastern Asia	Sudden and intense anxiety that the penis (in males) or the vulva and nipples (in females) will recede into the body and cause death.
Latah	Malaysia, Indonesia	Hypersensitivity to sudden fright, often with echopraxia, echolalia, and dissociative or trancelike behavior.
Locura	Latinos in the U.S. and Latin America	Incoherence, agitation, hallucinations, ineffective social interaction, unpredictability, and possible violence. Attributed to genetics or environmental stress, or a combination of both.
Mal de ojo (evil eye)	Mediterranean cultures	Occurs primarily in children. Fitful sleep, crying, diarrhea, vomiting, and fever.
Nervios	Latinos in the U.S. and Latin America	Headaches, irritability, stomach disturbances, sleep difficulties, nervousness, easy tearfulness, inability to concentrate, trembling, tingling sensations and dizziness. Occurs in response to stressful life experiences.
Pibloktoq	Eskimo cultures	Abrupt dissociative episode accompanied by extreme excitement and sometimes followed by convulsions and coma lasting up to 12 hours.
Qi-gong psychotic reaction	China	Dissociative, paranoid, or other psychotic or nonpsychotic symptoms that occur in individuals who become overly involved in the Chinese health-enhancing practice of qi-gong ("exercise of vital energy")
Rootwork	African Americans, European Americans, Caribbean cultures	Anxiety, gastrointestinal complaints, weakness, dizziness, fear of being poisoned or killed. Symptoms are ascribed to hexing, witchcraft, sorcery, or the evil influence of another person.
Sangue dormido ("sleeping blood")	Portuguese Cape Verde Islanders	Pain, numbness, tremor, paralysis, convulsions, stroke, blindness, heart attack, infection, and miscarriage.
Shenjing shuairuo ("neurasthenia")	China	Physical and mental fatigue, dizziness, headaches, other pains, concentration difficulties, sleep disturbance, memory loss, gastrointestinal problems, sexual dysfunction, irritability, excitability, and various signs suggesting disturbance of the autonomic nervous systems.
Shenkui (Shenkuei)	China (Taiwan)	Anxiety or panic, with dizziness, backache, fatigability, general weakness, insomnia, frequent dreams and sexual dysfunction. Attributed to excessive semen loss.
Shin-byung	Korea	Anxiety, weakness, dizziness, fear, anorexia, insomnia, and gastrointestinal problems, with subsequent dissociation and possession by ancestral spirits.
Spell	African Americans and European Americans in southern U.S.	A trance state in which individuals "communicate" with deceased relatives or spirits. Not considered to be a folk illness, but may be misconstrued by clinicians as a psychosis.
Susto ("fright" or "soul loss")	Latin America, Mexico, Central America, and South America	Appetite and sleep disturbances, sadness, pains, headache, stomachache, and diarrhea. Attributed to a frightening event that causes the soul to leave the body and results in unhappiness and sickness.
Taijin kyofusho	Japan	Fear that one's body, body parts, or its functions displease, embarrass, or are offensive to other people in appearance, odor, facial expressions, or movements.
Zar	North African and Middle Eastern societies	Dissociative episodes that include shouting, laughing, hitting head against a wall, singing, or weeping. Person may withdraw and refuse to eat. Symptoms are attributed to being possessed by a spirit.

SOURCE: *Diagnostic and Statistical Manual of Mental Disorders*, 4th Edition, *Text Revision.* © 2000, American Psychiatric Association. With permission.

Latino Americans, and Western European Americans. To deny access to these family support systems could interfere with the healing process.

3. Ensure that the individual's spiritual needs are being met. Religion is an important source of support for many individuals, and the nurse must be tolerant of various rituals that may be connected with different cultural beliefs about health and illness.

4. Be aware of the differences in concept of time among the various cultures. Most members of the dominant American culture are future oriented and place a high value on punctuality and efficiency. Other cultures such as African Americans, Native Americans, Asian Americans, Latino Americans, and Western European Americans are more present oriented. Nurses must be aware that such individuals may not share the value of punctuality. They may be late to appointments and appear to be indifferent to some aspects of their therapy. Nurses must be accepting of these differences and refrain from allowing existing attitudes to interfere with delivery of care.

5. Be aware of different beliefs about health care among the various cultures, and recognize the importance of these beliefs to the healing process. If an individual from another culture has been receiving health care from a spiritualist, medicine man, granny, or curandero, it is important for the nurse to listen to what has been done in the past and even to consult with these cultural healers about the care being given to the client.

6. Follow the health care practices that the client views as essential, provided they do no harm or interfere with the healing process of the client. For example, the concepts of yin and yang and the "hot and cold" theory of disease are very important to the well-being of some Asians and Latinos, respectively. Try to ensure that a balance of these foods are included in the diet as an important reinforcement for traditional medical care.

7. Be aware of favorite foods of individuals from different cultures. The health care setting may seem strange and somewhat isolated, and for some individuals it feels good to have anything around them that is familiar. They may even refuse to eat foods that are unfamiliar to them. If it does not interfere with his or her care, allow family members to provide favorite foods for the client.

8. The nurse working in psychiatry must realize that psychiatric illness is unacceptable in some cultures. Individuals who believe that expressing emotions is unacceptable (e.g., Asian Americans and Native Americans) will present unique problems when they are clients in a psychiatric setting. Nurses must have patience and work slowly to establish trust in order to provide these individuals with the assistance they require.

Evaluation

Evaluation of nursing actions is directed at achievement of the established outcomes. Part of the evaluation process is continuous reassessment to ensure that the selected actions are appropriate and the goals and outcomes are realistic. Including the family and extended support systems in the evaluation process is essential if cultural implications of nursing care are to be measured. Modifications to the plan of care are made as the need is determined.

SUMMARY

Culture encompasses shared patterns of belief, feeling, and knowledge that guide people's conduct and are passed down from generation to generation. Ethnic groups are tied together by shared heritage. Nurses must understand concepts as they relate to various cultural groups while using caution to avoid stereotyping. Each person, regardless of cultural ties, must be considered unique.

Cultural groups differ in terms of communication, space, social organization, time, environmental control, and biological variations. Northern European Americans are the descendants of the first immigrants to the United States and make up the current dominant cultural group. They value punctuality, work responsibility, and a healthy lifestyle. The divorce rate is high in this cultural group and the structure of the family is changing. Religious ties have loosened.

African Americans trace their roots in the United States to the days of slavery. Many African Americans have assimilated into the dominant culture, but some remain tied to their own social organization by choice or by necessity. Forty-four percent of all African American households are headed by women. The social support systems are large, and many African Americans have strong religious ties, particularly to the Protestant faith. Some African Americans, particularly in the rural South, may still use folk medicine as a means of health care. Hypertension, sickle cell anemia, and alcoholism are serious health problems.

Many Native Americans still live on reservations. They speak many different languages and dialects. Native Americans appear silent and reserved and many are uncomfortable with touch and expressing emotions. A large network of family is important to Native Americans. They are very present-oriented and not ruled by a clock. Religion and health practices are intertwined, and the *shaman* (medicine man or woman) is the provider of care. Health problems include tuberculosis, diabetes, and alcoholism. Nutritional deficiencies are not uncommon.

Asian American languages are very diverse. Touching during communication has historically been considered unacceptable. Asian Americans have difficulty expressing emotions and may appear cold and aloof. Family loyalty is emphasized above all else, and extended family is very important. Health practices are based on the restoration of balance of yin and yang. Many Asian Americans believe that psychiatric illness is merely behavior that is out of control and to behave in such a manner is to bring shame on the family.

The common language of Latino Americans is Spanish. Large family groups are important to Latinos, and touch is a common form of communication. The predominant religion is Roman Catholicism and the church is often a source of strength in times of crisis. Health care may be delivered by a folk healer called a *curandero*, who uses various forms of treatment to restore the body to a balanced state.

Western European Americans have their origin in Italy, France, and Greece. They are warm and expressive and use touch as a common form of communication. Western European Americans are very family oriented, and most have a strong allegiance to the cultural heritage. The dominant religion is Roman Catholicism for the Italians and French and Greek Orthodoxy for the Greeks. Most Western European Americans follow the health practices of the dominant culture, but some folk beliefs and superstitions endure.

In this chapter, the nursing process was presented as the vehicle for delivery of care. A cultural assessment tool was included to assist in gathering information needed to plan appropriate care for individuals from various cultural groups.

Culture-bound syndromes are clusters of physical and behavioral symptoms that are considered as illnesses or "afflictions" by specific cultures and recognized as such by the *DSM-IV-TR*. Examples of these syndromes were presented as background assessment data.

REVIEW QUESTIONS

SELF-EXAMINATION/LEARNING EXERCISE

Select the answer that is most appropriate for each of the following questions.

1. Miss Lee is an Asian American on the psychiatric unit. She tells the nurse, "I must have the hot ginger root for my headache. It is the only thing that will help." What meaning does the nurse attach to this statement by Miss Lee?
   a. She is being obstinate and wants control over her care.
   b. She believes that ginger root has magical qualities.
   c. She subscribes to the restoration of health through the balance of yin and yang.
   d. Asian Americans refuse to take traditional medicine for pain.

2. Miss Lee (the same client from previous question) says she is afraid that no one from her family will visit her. On what belief does Miss Lee base her statement?
   a. Many Asian Americans do not believe in hospitals.
   b. Many Asian Americans do not have close family support systems.
   c. Many Asian Americans believe the body will heal itself if left alone.
   d. Many Asian Americans view psychiatric problems as bringing shame to the family.

3. Joe, a Native American, appears at the community health clinic with an oozing stasis ulcer on his lower right leg. It is obviously infected, and he tells the nurse that the shaman has been treating it with herbs. The nurse determines that Joe needs emergency care, but Joe states he will not go to the emergency department (ED) unless the shaman is allowed to help treat him. How should the nurse handle this situation?
   a. Contact the shaman and have him meet them at the ED to consult with the attending physician.
   b. Tell Joe that the shaman is not allowed in the ED.
   c. Explain to Joe that the shaman is at fault for his leg being in the condition it is in now.
   d. Have the shaman try to talk Joe into going to the ED without him.

4. When the shaman arrives at the hospital, Joe's physician extends his hand for a handshake. The shaman lightly touches the physician's hand, then quickly moves away. How should the physician interpret this gesture?
   a. The shaman is snubbing the physician.
   b. The shaman is angry that he was called away from his supper.
   c. The shaman does not believe in traditional medicine.
   d. The shaman does not feel comfortable with touch.

5. Sarah is an African American woman who receives a visit from the psychiatric home health nurse. A referral for a mental health assessment was made by the public health nurse, who noticed that Sarah was becoming exceedingly withdrawn. When the psychiatric nurse arrives, Sarah says to her, "No one can help me. I was an evil person in my youth, and now I must pay." How might the nurse assess this statement?
   a. Sarah is having delusions of persecution.
   b. Some African Americans believe illness is God's punishment for their sins.
   c. Sarah is depressed and just wants to be left alone.
   d. African Americans do not believe in psychiatric help.

6. Sarah says to the nurse, "Granny told me to eat a lot of poke greens and I would feel better." How should the nurse interpret this statement?
   a. Sarah's grandmother believes in the healing power of poke greens.
   b. Sarah believes everything her grandmother tells her.
   c. Sarah has been receiving health care from a "folk practitioner."
   d. Sarah is trying to determine if the nurse agrees with her grandmother.

7. Frank is a Latino American who has an appointment at the community health center for 1:00 P.M. The nurse is angry when Frank shows up at 3:30 P.M. stating, "I was visiting with my brother." How must the nurse interpret this behavior?
   a. Frank is being passive–aggressive by showing up late.
   b. This is Frank's way of defying authority.
   c. Frank is a member of a cultural group that is present oriented.
   d. Frank is a member of a cultural group that rejects traditional medicine.

8. The nurse must give Frank (the client from the previous question) a physical examination. She tells him to remove his clothing and put on an examination gown. Frank refuses. How should the nurse interpret this behavior?
   a. Frank does not believe in taking orders from a woman.
   b. Frank is modest and embarrassed to remove his clothes.
   c. Frank doesn't understand why he must remove his clothes.
   d. Frank does not think he needs a physical examination.

9. Maria is an Italian American who is in the hospital after having suffered a miscarriage at 5 months' gestation. Her room is filled with relatives who have brought a variety of foods and gifts for Maria. They are all talking, seemingly at the same time, and some, including Maria, are crying. They repeatedly touch and hug Maria and each other. How should the nurse handle this situation?
   a. Explain to the family that Maria needs her rest and they must all leave.
   b. Allow the family to remain and continue their activity as described, as long as they do not disturb other clients.
   c. Explain that Maria will not get over her loss if they keep bringing it up and causing her to cry so much.
   d. Call the family priest to come and take charge of this family situation.

10. Maria's mother says to the nurse, "If only Maria had told me she wanted the biscotti. I would have made them for her." What is the meaning behind Maria's mother's statement?
    a. Some Italian Americans believe a miscarriage can occur if a woman does not eat a food she craves.
    b. Some Italian Americans think biscotti can prevent miscarriage.
    c. Maria's mother is taking the blame for Maria's miscarriage.
    d. Maria's mother believes the physician should have told Maria to eat biscotti.

REFERENCES

American Psychiatric Association (APA). (2000). *Diagnostic and statistical manual of mental disorders* (4th ed.). *Text revision.* Washington, DC: American Psychiatric Association.

Barna Research Online. (2004). Church attendance. Retrieved October 8, 2004 from the World Wide Web at http://www.barna.org/

Bureau of Indian Affairs (BIA). (2001). *American Indian today.* Retrieved November 1, 2001 from the World Wide Web at http://www.doi.gov/bia/aitoday/aitoday.html.

Cherry, B., & Giger, J.N. (2004). African-Americans. In J.N. Giger & R.E. Davidhizar (Eds.). *Transcultural nursing: Assessment and intervention* (4th ed.). St. Louis: C.V. Mosby.

Geissler, E.M. (1994). *Pocket guide to cultural assessment.* St. Louis: Mosby Year Book.

Giger, J.N., & Davidhizar, R.E. (2004). *Transcultural nursing: Assessment and intervention* (4th ed.). St. Louis: C.V. Mosby.

Gonzalez, T., & Kuipers, J. (2004). Mexican Americans. In J.N. Giger & R.E. Davidhizar (Eds.). *Transcultural nursing: Assessment and intervention* (4th ed.). St. Louis: C.V. Mosby.

Griffin, H.C. (2002, December 12). Embracing diversity. *NurseWeek* [Special Edition], 14–15.

Griffith, E.E.H., Gonzalez, C.A., & Blue, H.C. (2003). Introduction to cultural psychiatry. In R.E. Hales & S.C. Yudofsky (Eds.).

Textbook of clinical psychiatry (4th ed.). Washington, DC: American Psychiatric Publishing.

Hanley, C.E. (2004). Navajos. In J.N. Giger & R.E. Davidhizar (Eds.). *Transcultural nursing: Assessment and intervention* (4th ed.). St. Louis: C.V. Mosby.

Harris, L. M. (2004). *African Americans.* Microsoft Encarta Online Encyclopedia. Retrieved October 13, 2004 from the World Wide Web at http://encarta.msn.com

Indian Health Service (IHS). (2001). *Important strides in Indian health.* Retrieved November 1, 2001 from the World Wide Webb at http://www.ihs.gov/MedicalPrograms/Nursing/nursing-strides.asp.

Ishida, D., & Inouye, J. (2004). Japanese Americans. In J.N. Giger & R.E. Davidhizar (Eds.). *Transcultural nursing: Assessment and intervention* (4th ed.). St. Louis: C.V. Mosby.

Murray, R.B., & Zentner, J.P. (2001). *Health promotion strategies through the life span* (7th ed.). Upper Saddle River, NJ: Prentice Hall.

National Center for Health Statistics. (2004). *Marriage and divorce.* Retrieved October 11, 2004 from the World Wide Web at http://www.cdc.gov/nchs/fastats/divorce.htm.

Ng, M. (2001). *The Asian-American struggle for identity and battle with racism.* Retrieved November 2, 2001 from the World Wide Web at http://www.stern.nyu.edu/~myn1/racism.htm

Purnell, L.D., & Paulanka, B.J. (2003). *Transcultural health care: A culturally competent approach* (2nd ed.). Philadelphia: F.A. Davis.

Shore, J., Manson, S.M., & Buchwald, D. (2002). Screening for alcohol abuse among urban Native Americans in a primary care setting. *Psychiatric Services 53*(6), 757–760.

Spector, R.E. (2004). *Cultural diversity in health and illness* (6th ed.). Upper Saddle River, N.J.: Pearson Prentice-Hall.

Still, O., & Hodgins, D. (2003). Navajo Indians. In L.D. Purnell & B.J. Paulanka (Eds.). *Transcultural health care: A culturally competent approach* (2nd ed.). Philadelphia: F.A. Davis.

Tripp-Reimer, T., & Sorofman, B. (1998). Greek-Americans. In L.D. Purnell & B.J. Paulanka (Eds.). *Transcultural health care: A culturally competent approach*. Philadelphia: F.A. Davis.

U.S. Census Bureau. (2004a). *American Families and Living Arrangements: March 2003.* Retrieved October 13, 2004 from the World Wide Web at http://www.census.gov/population/www/socdemo/hh-fam.html

U.S. Census Bureau. (2004b). *Population by Age, Sex, and Race and Hispanic Origin: March 2000.* Retrieved October 26, 2004 from the World Wide Web at http://www.census.gov

U.S. Department of Agriculture. (2004). *Food, nutrition, and consumer services.* Retrieved October 24, 2004 from the World Wide Web at http://www.aphis.usda.gov/anawg/Bluebook/guidefive.html

Wall, T.L., Peterson, C.M., Peterson, K.P., Johnson, M.L., Thomasson, H.R., Cole, M., & Ehlers, C.L. (1997). Alcohol metabolism in Asian-American men with genetic polymorphisms of aldehyde dehydrogenase. *Annals of Internal Medicine 127,* 376–379.

Wang, Y. (2003). People of Chinese heritage. In L.D. Purnell & B.J. Paulanka (Eds.). *Transcultural health care: A culturally competent approach* (2nd ed.). Philadelphia: F.A. Davis.

CLASSICAL REFERENCE

Hall, E.T. (1966). *The hidden dimension.* Garden City, NY: Doubleday.

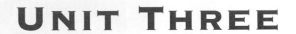

UNIT THREE

THERAPEUTIC APPROACHES IN PSYCHIATRIC NURSING CARE

RELATIONSHIP DEVELOPMENT

CHAPTER OUTLINE

OBJECTIVES
ROLE OF THE PSYCHIATRIC NURSE
DYNAMICS OF A THERAPEUTIC
NURSE–CLIENT RELATIONSHIP
CONDITIONS ESSENTIAL TO DEVELOPMENT
OF A THERAPEUTIC RELATIONSHIP

PHASES OF A THERAPEUTIC NURSE–
CLIENT RELATIONSHIP
SUMMARY
REVIEW QUESTIONS

KEY TERMS

attitude
belief
concrete thinking
confidentiality
countertransference
empathy
genuineness

rapport
sympathy
transference
unconditional positive
    regard
values

CORE CONCEPT

therapeutic
    relationship

OBJECTIVES

After reading this chapter, the student will be able to:

1. Describe the relevance of a therapeutic nurse–client relationship.
2. Discuss the dynamics of a therapeutic nurse–client relationship.
3. Discuss the importance of self-awareness in the nurse–client relationship.
4. Identify goals of the nurse–client relationship.
5. Identify and discuss essential conditions for a therapeutic relationship to occur.
6. Describe the phases of relationship development and the tasks associated with each phase.

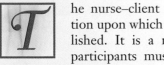

he nurse–client relationship is the foundation upon which psychiatric nursing is established. It is a relationship in which both participants must recognize each other as unique and important human beings. It is also a relationship in which mutual learning occurs. Peplau (1991) states:

Shall a nurse do things *for* a patient or can participant relationships be emphasized so that a nurse comes to do things *with* a patient as her share of an agenda of work to be ac-

complished in reaching a goal—health. It is likely that the nursing process is educative and therapeutic when nurse and patient can come to know and to respect each other, as persons who are alike, and yet, different, as persons who share in the solution of problems. (p. 9)

This chapter examines the role of the psychiatric nurse and the use of self as the therapeutic tool in the nursing of clients with emotional illness. Phases of the therapeutic relationship are explored and conditions essential to the development of a therapeutic relationship are

107

> ⬛ **Core Concept**
>
> **Therapeutic Relationship**
> An interaction between two people (usually a caregiver and a care receiver) in which input from both participants contributes to a climate of healing, growth promotion, and/or illness prevention.

discussed. The importance of values clarification in the development of self-awareness is emphasized.

ROLE OF THE PSYCHIATRIC NURSE

What is a nurse? Undoubtedly, this question would elicit as many different answers as the number of people to whom it was presented. Nursing as a *concept* has probably existed since the beginning of the civilized world, with the provision of "care" to the ill or infirm by anyone in the environment who took the time to administer to those in need. However, the emergence of nursing as a *profession* began only in the late 1800s with the graduation of Linda Richards from the New England Hospital for Women and Children in Boston upon achievement of the diploma in nursing. Since that time, the nurse's role has evolved from that of custodial caregiver and physician's handmaiden to recognition as a unique, independent member of the professional health care team.

Peplau (1991) identified several subroles within the role of the nurse:

1. **The Stranger.** A nurse is at first a stranger to the client. The client is also a stranger to the nurse. Peplau (1991) states:

   Respect and positive interest accorded a stranger is at first nonpersonal and includes the same ordinary courtesies that are accorded to a new guest who has been brought into any situation. This principle implies: (1) accepting the patient as he is; (2) treating the patient as an emotionally able stranger and relating to him on this basis until evidence shows him to be otherwise. (p. 44)

2. **The Resource Person.** According to Peplau, "a resource person provides specific answers to questions usually formulated with relation to a larger problem" (p. 47). In the role of resource person, the nurse explains, in language that the client can understand, information related to the client's health care.

3. **The Teacher.** In this subrole the nurse identifies learning needs and provides information required by the client or family to improve the health situation.

4. **The Leader.** According to Peplau, "democratic leadership in nursing situations implies that the patient will be permitted to be an active participant in designing nursing plans for him" (p. 49). Autocratic leadership promotes overvaluation of the nurse and clients'

substitution of the nurse's goals for their own. Laissez-faire leaders convey a lack of personal interest in the client.

5. **The Surrogate.** Outside of their awareness, clients often perceive nurses as symbols of other individuals. They may view the nurse as a mother figure, a sibling, a former teacher, or another nurse who has provided care in the past. This occurs when a client is placed in a situation that generates feelings similar to ones he or she has experienced previously. Peplau (1991) explains that the nurse-client relationship progresses along a continuum. When a client is acutely ill, he or she may incur the role of infant or child, while the nurse is perceived as the mother surrogate. Peplau (1991) states, "Each nurse has the responsibility for exercising her professional skill in aiding the relationship to move forward on the continuum, so that person to person relations compatible with chronological age levels can develop" (p. 55).

6. **The Counselor.** The nurse uses "interpersonal techniques" to assist clients to learn to adapt to difficulties or changes in life experiences. Peplau states, "Counseling in nursing has to do with helping the patient to remember and to understand fully what is happening to him in the present situation, so that the experience can be integrated with, rather than dissociated from, other experiences in life" (p. 64).

Peplau (1962) believed that the emphasis in psychiatric nursing is on the counseling subrole. How then does this emphasis influence the role of the nurse in the psychiatric setting? Many sources define the *nurse therapist* as having graduate preparation in psychiatric/mental health nursing. He or she has developed skills through intensive supervised educational experiences to provide helpful individual, group, or family therapy.

Peplau suggests that it is essential for the *staff nurse working in psychiatry* to have a general knowledge of basic counseling techniques. A therapeutic or "helping" relationship is established through use of these interpersonal techniques and is based on a knowledge of theories of personality development and human behavior.

Sullivan (1953) believed that emotional problems stem from difficulties with interpersonal relationships. Interpersonal theorists, such as Peplau and Sullivan, emphasize the importance of relationship development in the provision of emotional care. Through establishment of a satisfactory nurse–client relationship, individuals learn to generalize the ability to achieve satisfactory interpersonal relationships to other aspects of their lives.

DYNAMICS OF A THERAPEUTIC NURSE–CLIENT RELATIONSHIP

Travelbee (1971), who expanded on Peplau's theory of interpersonal relations in nursing, has stated that it is only when each individual in the interaction perceives the other as a unique human being that a relationship is possible. She refers not to a nurse–client relationship, but rather to a human-to-human relationship, which she describes as a "mutually significant experience." That is, both the nurse and the recipient of care have needs met when each views the other as a unique human being, not as "an illness," as "a room number," or as "all nurses" in general.

Therapeutic relationships are goal oriented. Ideally, the nurse and client decide together what the goal of the relationship will be. Most often the goal is directed at learning and growth promotion, in an effort to bring about some type of change in the client's life. In general, the goal of a therapeutic relationship may be based on a problem-solving model.

EXAMPLE:

Goal

The client will demonstrate more adaptive coping strategies for dealing with (specific life situation).

Interventions

1. Identify what is troubling the client at the present time.
2. Encourage the client to discuss changes he or she would like to make.
3. Discuss with the client which changes are possible and which are not possible.
4. Have the client explore feelings about aspects that cannot be changed and alternative ways of coping more adaptively.
5. Discuss alternative strategies for creating changes the client desires to make.
6. Weigh the benefits and consequences of each alternative.
7. Assist the client to select an alternative.
8. Encourage the client to implement the change.
9. Provide positive feedback for the client's attempts to create change.
10. Assist the client to evaluate outcomes of the change and make modifications as required.

Therapeutic Use of Self

Travelbee

Travelbee (1971) described the instrument for delivery of the process of interpersonal nursing as the *therapeutic use of self*, which she defined as "the ability to use one's personality consciously and in full awareness in an attempt to establish relatedness and to structure nursing interventions."

Use of the self in a therapeutic manner requires that the nurse have a great deal of self-awareness and self-understanding, that he or she has arrived at a philosophical belief about life, death, and the overall human condition. The nurse must understand that the ability

and extent to which one can effectively help others in time of need is strongly influenced by this internal value system—a combination of intellect and emotions.

Gaining Self-Awareness
Values Clarification

Knowing and understanding oneself enhances the ability to form satisfactory interpersonal relationships. Self-awareness requires that an individual recognize and accept what he or she values and learn to accept the uniqueness and differences in others. This concept is important in everyday life and in the nursing profession in general; but it is *essential* in psychiatric nursing.

An individual's value system is established very early in life and has its foundations in the value system held by the primary caregivers. It is culturally oriented; it may change many times over the course of a lifetime; and it consists of beliefs, attitudes, and values. Values clarification is one process by which an individual may gain self-awareness.

Beliefs. A **belief** is an idea that one holds to be true, and it can take any of several forms:

1. *Rational beliefs.* Ideas for which objective evidence exists to substantiate its truth.

EXAMPLE:

Alcoholism is a disease.

2. *Irrational beliefs.* Ideas that an individual holds as true despite the existence of objective contradictory evidence. Delusions can be a form of irrational beliefs.

EXAMPLE:

Once an alcoholic has been through detox and rehab, he or she can drink socially if desired. *if it is blind then it's not FAITH.*

3. *Faith* (sometimes called "blind beliefs"). An ideal that an individual holds as true for which no objective evidence exists. *FAITH is the substance of things hoped for, the evidence of things not seen. Heb 11:1*

EXAMPLE:

Belief in a higher power can help an alcoholic stop drinking. *WITHOUT FAITH IT is impossible to please him: for he that cometh to God must believe that he is*

4. *Stereotype.* A socially shared belief that describes a concept in an oversimplified or undifferentiated matter. *and that he is a rewarder of them that diligently seek him - Heb 11:6*

EXAMPLE:

All alcoholics are skid-row bums.

Attitudes. An **attitude** is a frame of reference around which an individual organizes knowledge about his or her world. An attitude also has an emotional component. It can be a prejudgment and may be selective and biased. Attitudes fulfill the need to find meaning in life and to

TABLE 7–1		The Process of Values Clarification	
LEVEL OF OPERATIONS	**CATEGORY**	**CRITERIA**	**EXPLANATION**
Cognitive	Choosing	1. Freely 2. From alternatives. 3. After careful consideration of the consequences	"This value is mine. No one forced me to choose it. I understand and accept the consequences of holding this value."
Emotional	Prizing	4. Satisfied; pleased with the choice 5. Making public affirmation of the choice, if necessary	"I am proud that I hold this value, and I am willing to tell others about it."
Behavioral	Acting	6. Taking action to demonstrate the value behaviorally 7. Demonstrating this pattern of behavior consistently and repeatedly	The value is reflected in the individual's behavior for as long as he or she holds it.

provide clarity and consistency for the individual. The prevailing stigma attached to mental illness is an example of a negative attitude. An associated belief might be that "all people with mental illness are dangerous."

Values. Values are abstract standards, positive or negative, that represent an individual's ideal mode of conduct and ideal goals. Some examples of ideal mode of conduct include seeking truth and beauty; being clean and orderly; and behaving with sincerity, justice, reason, compassion, humility, respect, honor, and loyalty. Examples of ideal goals are security, happiness, freedom, equality, ecstasy, fame, and power.

Values differ from attitudes and beliefs in that they are action oriented or action producing. One may hold many attitudes and beliefs without behaving in a way that shows they hold those attitudes and beliefs. For example, a nurse may believe that all clients have the right to be told the truth about their diagnosis; however, he or she may not always act on the belief and tell all clients the complete truth about their condition. Only when the belief is acted on does it become a value.

Attitudes and beliefs flow out of one's set of values. An individual may have thousands of beliefs and hundreds of attitudes, but his or her values probably number only in the dozens. Values may be viewed as a kind of core concept or basic standards that determine one's attitudes and beliefs, and ultimately, one's behavior. Raths, Merril, and Simon (1966) identified a seven-step process of valuing that can be used to help clarify personal values. This process is presented in Table 7–1. The process can be used by applying these seven steps to an attitude or belief that one holds. When an attitude or belief has met each of the seven criteria, it can be considered a value.

The Johari Window

The self arises out of self-appraisal and the appraisal of others and represents each individual's unique pattern of values, attitudes, beliefs, behaviors, emotions, and needs. Self-awareness is the recognition of these aspects and understanding about their impact on the self and others. The Johari Window is a representation of the self and a tool that can be used to increase self-awareness (Luft, 1970). The Johari Window is presented in Figure 7–1 and is divided into four quadrants.

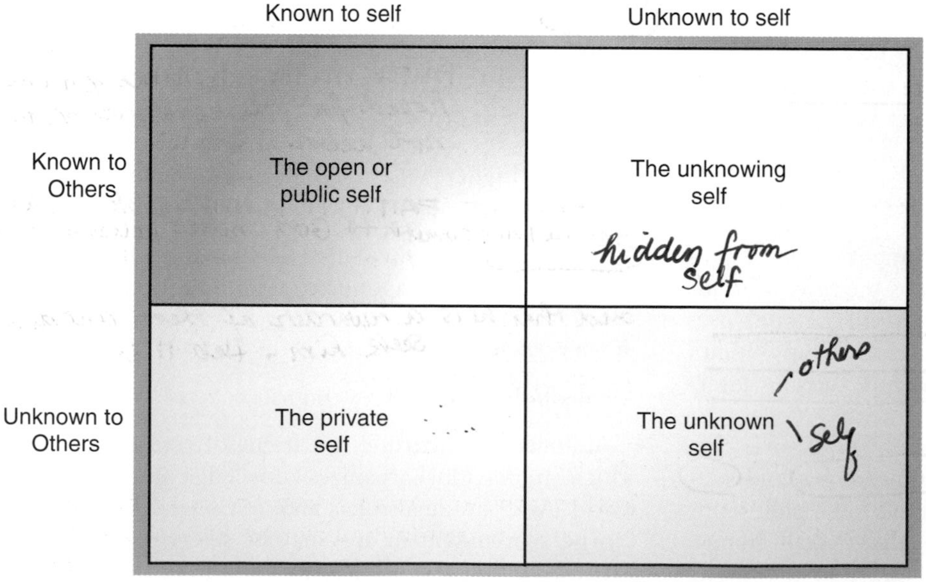

FIGURE 7–1 The Johari Window. (From Luft, J. *Group processes: An introduction to group dynamics.* National Press Books, Palo Alto, CA, 1970.

The Open or Public Self

The upper left quadrant of the window represents the part of the self that is public; that is, aspects of the self about which both the individual and others are aware.

EXAMPLE:

Susan, a nurse who is the adult child of an alcoholic, has strong feelings about helping alcoholics to achieve sobriety. She volunteers her time to be a support person on call to help recovering alcoholics. She is aware of her feelings and her desire to help others. Members of the Alcoholics Anonymous group in which she volunteers her time are also aware of Susan's feelings and they feel comfortable calling her when they need help refraining from drinking.

The Unknowing Self

The upper right (blind) quadrant of the window represents the part of the self that is known to others but remains hidden from the awareness of the individual.

EXAMPLE:

When Susan takes care of patients in detox, she does so without emotion, tending to the technical aspects of the task in a way that the clients perceive as cold and judgmental. She is unaware that she comes across to the clients in this way.

The Private Self

The lower left quadrant of the window represents the part of the self that is known to the individual, but which the individual deliberately and consciously conceals from others.

EXAMPLE:

Susan would prefer not to take care of the clients in detox because doing so provokes painful memories from her childhood. Because she does not want the other staff members to know about these feelings, however, she volunteers to take care of the detox clients whenever they are assigned to her unit.

The Unknown Self

The lower right quadrant of the window represents the part of the self that is unknown to both the individual and to others.

EXAMPLE:

Susan felt very powerless as a child growing up with an alcoholic father. She seldom knew in what condition she would find her father or what his behavior would be. She learned over the years to find small ways to maintain control over her life situation, and left home as soon as she graduated from high school. The need to stay in control has always been very important to Susan, and she is unaware that working with recovering alcoholics helps to fulfill this need in her. The people she is helping are also unaware that Susan is satisfying an unfulfilled personal need as she provides them with assistance.

The goal of increasing self-awareness by using the Johari Window is to increase the size of the quadrant that represents the open or public self. The individual who is open to self and others has the ability to be spontaneous and to share emotions and experiences with others. This individual also has a greater understanding of personal behavior and of others' responses to him or her. Increased self-awareness allows an individual to interact with others comfortably, to accept the differences in others, and to observe each person's right to respect and dignity.

CONDITIONS ESSENTIAL TO DEVELOPMENT OF A THERAPEUTIC RELATIONSHIP

Several characteristics that enhance the achievement of a therapeutic relationship have been identified. These concepts are highly significant to the use of self as the therapeutic tool in interpersonal relationship development.

Rapport

Getting acquainted and establishing **rapport** is the primary task in relationship development. Rapport implies special feelings on the part of both the client and the nurse based on acceptance, warmth, friendliness, common interest, a sense of trust, and a nonjudgmental attitude. Establishing rapport may be accomplished by discussing non-health–related topics. Travelbee (1971) states:

> [To establish rapport] is to create a sense of harmony based on knowledge and appreciation of each individual's uniqueness. It is the ability to be still and experience the other as a human being—to appreciate the unfolding of each personality one to the other. The ability to truly care for and about others is the core of rapport.

Trust *veracity*

To trust another, one must feel confidence in that person's presence, reliability, integrity, veracity, and sincere desire to provide assistance when requested. As previously discussed, trust is the initial developmental task described by Erikson. When this task has not been achieved, this component of relationship development becomes more difficult. That is not to say that trust cannot be established, but only that additional time and patience may be required on the part of the nurse.

It is imperative for the nurse to convey an aura of trustworthiness, which requires that he or she possess a sense of self-confidence. Confidence in the self is derived out of knowledge gained through achievement of personal and professional goals, as well as the ability to integrate these roles and to function as a unified whole.

Trust cannot be presumed; it must be earned. Trustworthiness is demonstrated through nursing interventions that convey a sense of warmth and caring to the client. These interventions are initiated simply and concretely and directed toward activities that address the client's basic needs for physiological and psychological safety and security. Many psychiatric clients experience **concrete thinking**, which focuses their thought processes on specifics rather than generalities, and immediate issues rather than eventual outcomes. Examples of nursing interventions that would promote trust in an individual who is thinking concretely include the following:

- Providing a blanket when the client is cold
- Providing food when the client is hungry
- Keeping promises
- Being honest (e.g., saying "I don't know the answer to your question, but I'll try to find out") and then following through
- Simply and clearly providing reasons for certain policies, procedures, and rules
- Providing a written, structured schedule of activities
- Attending activities with the client if he or she is reluctant to go alone
- Being consistent in adhering to unit guidelines
- Taking the client's preferences, requests, and opinions into consideration when possible in decisions concerning his or her care
- Ensuring **confidentiality**; providing reassurance that what is discussed will not be repeated outside the boundaries of the health care team

Trust is the basis of a therapeutic relationship. The nurse working in psychiatry must perfect the skills that foster the development of trust. Trust must be established for the nurse–client relationship to progress beyond the superficial level of tending to the client's immediate needs.

Respect

To show respect is to believe in the dignity and worth of an individual regardless of his or her unacceptable behavior. Rogers (1951) called this **unconditional positive regard**. The attitude is nonjudgmental, and the respect is unconditional in that it does not depend on the behavior of the client to meet certain standards. The nurse, in fact, may not approve of the client's lifestyle or pattern of behaving. With unconditional positive regard, however, the client is accepted and respected for no other reason than that he or she is considered to be a worthwhile and unique human being.

Many psychiatric clients have very little self-respect owing to the fact that, because of their behavior, they were frequently rejected by others in the past. Recognition that they are being accepted and respected as unique individuals on an unconditional basis can serve to elevate feelings of self-worth and self-respect. The nurse can convey an attitude of respect with the following interventions:

- Calling the client by name (and title, if the client prefers)
- Spending time with the client
- Allowing for sufficient time to answer the client's questions and concerns
- Promoting an atmosphere of privacy during therapeutic interactions with the client or when the client may be undergoing physical examination or therapy
- Always being open and honest with the client, even when the truth may be difficult to discuss
- Taking the client's ideas, preferences, and opinions into consideration when planning care
- Striving to understand the motivation behind the client's behavior, regardless of how unacceptable it may seem

Genuineness

The concept of **genuineness** refers to the nurse's ability to be open, honest, and "real" in interactions with the client. To be "real" is to be aware of what one is experiencing internally and to express this awareness in the therapeutic relationship. When one is genuine, there is *congruence* between what is felt and what is being expressed (Raskin & Rogers, 2005). The nurse who possesses the quality of genuineness responds to the client with truth and honesty, rather than with responses he or she may consider more "professional" or ones that merely reflect the "nursing role."

Genuineness may call for a degree of *self-disclosure* on the part of the nurse. This is not to say that the nurse must disclose to the client *everything* he or she is feeling or *all* personal experiences that may relate to what the client is going through. Indeed, care must be taken when using self-disclosure, to avoid transposing the roles of nurse and client.

When the nurse uses self-disclosure, a quality of "humanness" is revealed to the client, creating a role for the client to model in similar situations. The client may then feel more comfortable revealing personal information to the nurse.

Most individuals have an uncanny ability to detect other peoples' artificiality. When the nurse does not bring the quality of genuineness to the relationship, a reality base for trust cannot be established. These qualities are essential if the actualizing potential of the client is to be realized and for change and growth to occur (Raskin & Rogers, 2005).

Empathy

Empathy is the ability to see beyond outward behavior and to understand the situation from the client's point of view. With empathy, the nurse can accurately perceive and comprehend the meaning and relevance of the client's thoughts and feelings. The nurse must also be able to communicate this perception to the client by attempting to translate words and behaviors into feelings.

It is not uncommon for the concept of empathy to be confused with that of **sympathy**. The major difference is that with *empathy* the nurse "accurately perceives or understands" what the client is feeling and encourages the client to explore these feelings. With *sympathy* the nurse actually "shares" what the client is feeling, and experiences a need to alleviate distress. Schuster (2000) states:

> Empathy means that you remain emotionally separate from the other person, even though you can see the patient's viewpoint clearly. This is different from sympathy. Sympathy implies taking on the other's needs and problems as if they were your own and becoming emotionally involved to the point of losing your objectivity. To empathize rather then sympathize, you must show feelings but not get caught up in feelings or overly identify with the patient's and family's concerns. (p. 102)

Empathy is considered to be one of the most important characteristics of a therapeutic relationship. Accurate empathetic perceptions on the part of the nurse assist the client to identify feelings that may have been suppressed or denied. Positive emotions are generated as the client realizes that he or she is truly understood by another. As the feelings surface and are explored, the client learns aspects about self of which he or she may have been unaware. This contributes to the process of personal identification and the promotion of positive self-concept.

With empathy, while understanding the client's thoughts and feelings, the nurse is able to maintain sufficient objectivity to allow the client to achieve problem resolution with minimal assistance. With sympathy, the nurse actually feels what the client is feeling, objectivity is lost, and the nurse may become focused on relief of personal distress rather than on helping the client resolve the problem at hand. The following is an example of an empathetic and sympathetic response to the same situation.

Situation: B.J., age 29, is a client on the psychiatric unit with a diagnosis of dysthymic disorder. She is 5'5" tall and weights 295 lb. B.J. has been overweight all her life. She is single, has no close friends, and has never had an intimate relationship with another person. It is her first day on the unit, and she is refusing to come out of her room. When she appeared for lunch in the dining room following admission, she was embarrassed when several of the other clients laughed out loud and called her "fatso."

Sympathetic response: Nurse: "I can certainly identify with what you are feeling. I've been overweight most of my life, too. I just get so angry when people act like that. They are so insensitive! It's just so typical of skinny people to act that way. You have a right to want to stay away from them. We'll just see how loud they laugh when *you* get to choose what movie is shown on the unit after dinner tonight."

Empathetic response: Nurse: "You feel angry and embarrassed by what happened at lunch today." As tears fill B.J.'s eyes, the nurse encourages her to cry if she feels like it and to express her anger at the situation. She stays with B.J. but does not dwell on her *own* feelings about what happened. Instead she focuses on B.J. and what the client perceives are her most immediate needs at this time.

PHASES OF A THERAPEUTIC NURSE–CLIENT RELATIONSHIP

Psychiatric nurses use interpersonal relationship development as the primary intervention with clients in various psychiatric/mental health settings. This is congruent with Peplau's (1962) identification of *counseling* as the major subrole of nursing in psychiatry. If what Sullivan (1953) believed is true (i.e., that all emotional problems stem from difficulties with interpersonal relationships), then this role of the nurse in psychiatry becomes especially meaningful and purposeful. It becomes an integral part of the total therapeutic regimen.

The therapeutic interpersonal relationship is the means by which the nursing process is implemented. Through the relationship, problems are identified and resolution is sought. Tasks of the relationship have been categorized into four phases: the preinteraction phase, the orientation (introductory) phase, the working phase, and the termination phase. Although each phase is presented as specific and distinct from the others, there may be some overlapping of tasks, particularly when the interaction is limited. The major nursing goals during each phase of the nurse-client relationship are listed in Table 7–2.

Table 7–2	Phases of Relationship Development and Major Nursing Goals
Phase	**Goals**
1. Preinteraction	Explore self-perceptions.
2. Orientation (introductory)	Establish trust.
	Formulate contract for intervention.
3. Working	Promote client change.
4. Termination	Evaluate goal attainment.
	Ensure therapeutic closure.

The Preinteraction Phase

The preinteraction phase involves preparation for the first encounter with the client. Tasks include the following:

1. Obtaining available information about the client from his or her chart, significant others, or other health team members. From this information, the initial assessment is begun. This initial information may also allow the nurse to become aware of personal responses to knowledge about the client.
2. Examining one's feelings, fears, and anxieties about working with a particular client. For example, the nurse may have been reared in an alcoholic family and have ambivalent feelings about caring for a client who is alcohol dependent. All individuals bring attitudes and feelings from prior experiences to the clinical setting. The nurse needs to be aware of how these preconceptions may affect his or her ability to care for individual clients.

The Orientation (Introductory) Phase

During the orientation phase, the nurse and client become acquainted. Tasks include the following:

1. Creating an environment for the establishment of trust and rapport
2. Establishing a contract for intervention that details the expectations and responsibilities of both nurse and client
3. Gathering assessment information to build a strong client database
4. Identifying the client's strengths and limitations
5. Formulating nursing diagnoses
6. Setting goals that are mutually agreeable to the nurse and client
7. Developing a plan of action that is realistic for meeting the established goals
8. Exploring feelings of both the client and nurse in terms of the introductory phase. Introductions are often uncomfortable, and the participants may experience some anxiety until a degree of rapport has been established.

Interactions may remain on a superficial level until anxiety subsides. Several interactions may be required to fulfill the tasks associated with this phase.

The Working Phase

The therapeutic work of the relationship is accomplished during this phase. Tasks include the following:

1. Maintaining the trust and rapport that was established during the orientation phase
2. Promoting the client's insight and perception of reality
3. Problem solving using the model presented earlier in this chapter
4. Overcoming resistance behaviors on the part of the client as the level of anxiety rises in response to discussion of painful issues
5. Continuously evaluating progress toward goal attainment

Transference and Countertransference

Transference and countertransference are common phenomena that often arise during the course of a therapeutic relationship. **Transference** occurs when the client unconsciously displaces (or "transfers") to the nurse feelings formed toward a person from his or her past (Sadock & Sadock, 2003). These feelings toward the nurse may be triggered by something about the nurse's appearance or personality characteristics that remind the client of the person. Transference can interfere with the therapeutic interaction when the feelings being expressed include anger and hostility. Anger toward the nurse can be manifested by uncooperativeness and resistance to the therapy.

Transference can also take the form of overwhelming affection for the nurse or excessive dependency on the nurse. The nurse is overvalued and the client forms unrealistic expectations of the nurse. When the nurse is unable to fulfill those expectations or meet the excessive dependency needs, the client becomes angry and hostile.

Interventions for Transference. Hilz (2004) states,

In cases of transference, the relationship does not usually need to be terminated, except when the transference poses a serious barrier to therapy or safety. The nurse should work with the patient in sorting out the past from the present, and assist the patient into identifying the transference and reassign a new and more appropriate meaning to the current nurse-patient relationship. The goal is to guide the patient to independence by teaching them to assume responsibility for their own behaviors, feelings, and thoughts, and to assign the correct meanings to the relationships based on present circumstances instead of the past.

Countertransference refers to the nurse's behavioral and emotional response to the client. These responses may be related to unresolved feelings toward significant others from the nurse's past, or they may be generated in response to transference feelings on the part of the client. It is not easy to refrain from becoming angry when the client is consistently antagonistic, to feel flattered when showered with affection and attention by the client, or even to feel quite powerful when the client exhibits excessive dependency on the nurse. These feelings can interfere with the therapeutic relationship when they initiate the following types of behaviors:

● The nurse overidentifies with the client's feelings, as they remind him or her of problems from the nurse's past or present.
● The nurse and client develop a social or personal relationship.
● The nurse begins to give advice or attempts to "rescue" the client.
● The nurse encourages and promotes the client's dependence.
● The nurse's anger engenders feelings of disgust toward the client.
● The nurse feels anxious and uneasy in the presence of the client.
● The nurse is bored and apathetic in sessions with the client.
● The nurse has difficulty setting limits on the client's behavior.
● The nurse defends the client's behavior to other staff members.

The nurse may be completely unaware or only minimally aware of the countertransference as it is occurring (Hilz, 2004).

Interventions for Countertransference. Hilz (2004) states:

> The relationship usually should not be terminated in the presence of countertransference. Rather, the nurse or staff member experiencing the countertransference should be supportively assisted by other staff members to identify his or her feelings and behaviors and recognize the occurrence of the phenomenon. It may be helpful to have evaluative sessions with the nurse after his or her encounter with the patient, in which both the nurse and other staff members (who are observing the interactions) discuss and compare the exhibited behaviors in the relationship.

The Termination Phase

Termination of the relationship may occur for a variety of reasons: the mutually agreed-on goals may have been reached; the client may be discharged from the hospital; or in the case of a student nurse, it may be the end of a clinical rotation. Termination can be a difficult phase for both the client and nurse. Tasks include the following:

1. Bringing a therapeutic conclusion to the relationship. This occurs when:
   a. Progress has been made toward attainment of mutually set goals.
   b. A plan for continuing care or for assistance during stressful life experiences is mutually established by the nurse and client.
   c. Feelings about termination of the relationship are recognized and explored. Both the nurse and client may experience feelings of sadness and loss. The nurse should share his or her feelings with the client. Through these interactions, the client learns that it is acceptable to have these kinds of feelings at a time of separation. Through this knowledge, the client experiences growth during the process of termination.
   NOTE: When the client feels sadness and loss, behaviors to delay termination may become evident. If the nurse experiences the same feelings, he or she may allow the client's behaviors to delay termination. For therapeutic closure, the nurse must establish the reality of the separation and resist being manipulated into repeated delays by the client.

SUMMARY

Nurses who work in the psychiatric/mental health field use special skills, or "interpersonal techniques," to assist clients in adapting to difficulties or changes in life experiences. A therapeutic or "helping" relationship is established through use of these interpersonal techniques and is based on knowledge of theories of personality development and human behavior.

Therapeutic nurse–client relationships are goal oriented. Ideally, the goal is mutually agreed on by the nurse and client, and is directed at learning and growth promotion. The problem-solving model is used in an attempt to bring about some type of change in the client's life. The instrument for delivery of the process of interpersonal nursing is the therapeutic use of self, which requires that the nurse possess a strong sense of self-awareness and self-understanding.

A number of characteristics that enhance the achievement of a therapeutic relationship have been identified. They include rapport, trust, respect, genuineness, and empathy.

The tasks associated with the development of a therapeutic interpersonal relationship have been categorized into four phases: the preinteraction phase, the orientation (introductory) phase, the working phase, and the termination phase.

The concepts and tasks presented in this chapter can facilitate the promotion of a helping relationship and effective nursing care for clients requiring psychosocial intervention.

REVIEW QUESTIONS

SELF-EXAMINATION/LEARNING EXERCISE

Test your knowledge of therapeutic nurse–client relationships by answering the following questions:

1. Name the six subroles of nursing identified by Peplau.

2. Which subrole is emphasized in psychiatric nursing?

3. Why is relationship development so important in the provision of emotional care?

4. In general, what is the goal of a therapeutic relationship? What method is recommended for intervention?

5. What is the instrument for delivery of the process of interpersonal nursing?

6. Several characteristics that enhance the achievement of a therapeutic relationship have been identified. Match the therapeutic concept with the corresponding definition.

_____ 1. Rapport   a. The feeling of confidence in another person's presence, reliability, integrity, and desire to provide assistance

_____ 2. Trust   b. Congruence between what is felt and what is being expressed

_____ 3. Respect   c. The ability to see beyond outward behavior and to understand the situation from the client's point of view

_____ 4. Genuineness   d. Special feelings between two people based on acceptance, warmth, friendliness, and shared common interest

_____ 5. Empathy   e. Unconditional acceptance of an individual as a worthwhile and unique human being

7. Match the actions listed on the right to the appropriate phase of nurse–client relationship development on the left.

_____ 1. Preinteraction phase   a. Kim tells Nurse Jones she wants to learn more adaptive ways to handle her anger. Together, they set some goals.

_____ 2. Orientation (introductory) phase   b. The goals of therapy have been met, but Kim cries and says she has to keep coming to therapy in order to be able to handle her anger appropriately.

_____ 3. Working phase   c. Nurse Jones reads Kim's previous medical records. She explores her feelings about working with a woman who has abused her child.

_____ 4. Termination phase   d. Nurse Jones helps Kim practice various techniques to control her angry outbursts. She gives Kim positive feedback for attempting to improve maladaptive behaviors.

REFERENCES

Hilz, L.M. (2004). Transference and countertransference. *Kathi's mental health review*. Retrieved October 28, 2004 from the World Wide Web at http://www.toddlertime.com/terms/countertransference-transference-3.htm#Interventions

Peplau, H.E. (1991). *Interpersonal relations in nursing*. New York: Springer.

Raskin, N.J., & Rogers, C.R. (2005). Person-centered therapy.

In R.J. Corsini & D. Wedding (Eds.). *Current psychotherapies* (7th ed.). Belmont, CA: Wadsworth.

Sadock, B.J., & Sadock, V. A. (2003). *Synopsis of psychiatry: Behavioral sciences/clinical psychiatry* (9th ed.). Philadelphia: Lippincott Williams & Wilkins.

Schuster, P.M. (2000). *Communication: The key to the therapeutic relationship*. Philadelphia: F.A. Davis.

CLASSICAL REFERENCES

Luft, J. (1970). *Group processes: An introduction to group dynamics.* Palo Alto, CA: National Press Books.

Peplau, H.E. (1962). Interpersonal techniques: The crux of psychiatric nursing. *American Journal of Nursing, 62*(6), 50–54.

Raths, L., Merril, H., & Simon, S. (1966). *Values and teaching.* Columbus, OH: Merrill.

Rogers, C.R. (1951). *Client centered therapy.* Boston: Houghton Mifflin.

Sullivan, H.S. (1953). *The interpersonal theory of psychiatry.* New York: W.W. Norton.

Travelbee, J. (1971). *Interpersonal aspects of nursing* (2nd ed.). Philadelphia: F.A. Davis.

THERAPEUTIC COMMUNICATION

CHAPTER OUTLINE

OBJECTIVES

WHAT IS COMMUNICATION?

THE IMPACT OF PREEXISTING CONDITIONS

NONVERBAL COMMUNICATION

THERAPEUTIC COMMUNICATION TECHNIQUES

NONTHERAPEUTIC COMMUNICATION TECHNIQUES

ACTIVE LISTENING

PROCESS RECORDINGS

FEEDBACK

SUMMARY

REVIEW QUESTIONS

KEY TERMS

density
distance
intimate distance
paralanguage

personal distance
public distance
social distance
territoriality

CORE CONCEPTS

communication
therapeutic communication

OBJECTIVES

After reading this chapter, the student will be able to:

1. Discuss the transactional model of communication.
2. Identify types of preexisting conditions that influence the outcome of the communication process.
3. Define *territoriality*, *density*, and *distance* as components of the environment.

4. Identify components of nonverbal expression.
5. Describe therapeutic and nontherapeutic verbal communication techniques.
6. Describe active listening.
7. Discuss therapeutic feedback.

 evelopment of the *therapeutic interpersonal relationship* was described in Chapter 7 as the process by which nurses provide care for clients in need of psychosocial intervention. *Therapeutic use of self* was identified as the instrument for delivery of care. The focus of this chapter is on *techniques*—or, more specifically, *interpersonal communication techniques*—to facilitate the delivery of that care.

Hays and Larson (1963) have stated, "To relate therapeutically with a patient it is necessary for the nurse to understand his or her role and its relationship to the patient's illness." They describe the role of the nurse as providing the client with the opportunity to accomplish the following:

1. Identify and explore problems in relating to others.
2. Discover healthy ways of meeting emotional needs.
3. Experience a satisfying interpersonal relationship.

These goals are achieved through use of interpersonal communication techniques (both verbal and nonverbal).

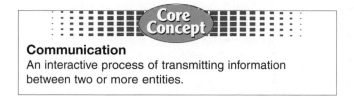

Communication

An interactive process of transmitting information between two or more entities.

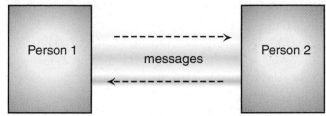

FIGURE 8–1 The Transactional Model of Communication.

The nurse must be aware of the therapeutic or nontherapeutic value of the communication techniques used with the client because they are the "tools" of psychosocial intervention.

WHAT IS COMMUNICATION?

It has been said that individuals "cannot not communicate." Every word that is spoken, every movement that is made, and every action that is taken or failed to be taken gives a message to someone. Interpersonal communication is a *transaction* between the sender and the receiver. In the transactional model of communication, both persons are participating simultaneously. They are mutually perceiving each other, simultaneously listening to each other, and simultaneously and mutually engaged in the process of creating meaning in a relationship (Yates, 2003). The transactional model is illustrated in Figure 8–1.

THE IMPACT OF PREEXISTING CONDITIONS

In all interpersonal transactions, both the sender and receiver bring certain preexisting conditions to the exchange that influences both the intended message and the way in which it is interpreted. Examples of these conditions include one's value system, internalized attitudes and beliefs, culture or religion, social status, gender,

background knowledge and experience, and age or developmental level. The type of environment in which the communication takes place may also influence the outcome of the transaction. Figure 8–2 shows how these influencing factors are positioned on the transactional model.

Values, Attitudes, and Beliefs

Values, attitudes, and beliefs are learned ways of thinking. Children generally adopt the value systems and internalize the attitudes and beliefs of their parents. Children may retain this way of thinking into adulthood or develop a different set of attitudes and values as they mature.

Values, attitudes, and beliefs can influence communication in numerous ways. For example, prejudice is expressed verbally through negative stereotyping.

One's value system may be communicated with behaviors that are more symbolic in nature. For example, an individual who values youth may dress and behave in a manner that is characteristic of one who is much younger. Persons who value freedom and the way of life in the United States may fly the U.S. flag in front of their homes each day. In each of these situations, a message is being communicated.

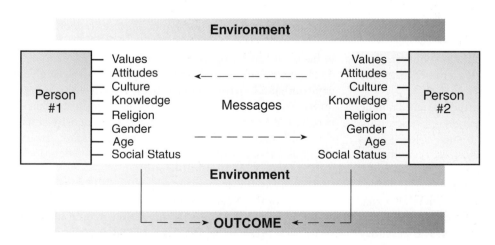

FIGURE 8–2 Factors influencing the Transactional Model of Communication.

Culture or Religion

Communication has its roots in culture. Cultural mores, norms, ideas, and customs provide the basis for our way of thinking. Cultural values are learned and differ from society to society. For example, in some European countries (e.g., Italy, Spain, and France), men may greet each other with hugs and kisses. These behaviors are appropriate in those cultures but would communicate a different message in the United States or Great Britain.

Religion can influence communication as well. Priests and ministers who wear clerical collars publicly communicate their mission in life. The collar may also influence the way in which others relate to them, either positively or negatively. Other symbolic gestures, such as wearing a cross around the neck or hanging a crucifix on the wall, also communicate an individual's religious beliefs.

Social Status

Studies of nonverbal indicators of social status or power have suggested that high-status persons are associated with gestures that communicate their higher-power position. For example, they use less eye contact, have a more relaxed posture, use louder voice pitch, place hands on hips more frequently, are "power dressers," have greater height, and maintain more distance when communicating with individuals considered to be of lower social status.

Gender

Gender influences the manner in which individuals communicate. Each culture has *gender signals* that are recognized as either masculine or feminine and provide a basis for distinguishing between members of each sex (Schuster, 2000). Examples include differences in posture, both standing and sitting, between many men and women in the United States. Men usually stand with thighs 10 to 15 degrees apart, the pelvis rolled back, and the arms slightly away from the body. Women often are seen with legs close together, the pelvis tipped forward, and the arms close to the body. When sitting, men may lean back in the chair with legs apart or may rest the ankle of one leg over the knee of the other. Women tend to sit more upright in the chair with legs together, perhaps crossed at the ankles, or one leg crossed over the other at thigh level.

Roles have historically been identified as either male or female. For example, in the United States masculinity typically was communicated through such roles as husband, father, breadwinner, doctor, lawyer, or engineer. Traditional female roles included those of wife, mother, homemaker, nurse, teacher, or secretary.

Gender signals are changing in U.S. society as sexual roles become less distinct. Behaviors that have been considered typically masculine or feminine in the past may now be generally acceptable in both sexes. Words such as "unisex" communicate a desire by some individuals to diminish the distinction between the sexes and minimize the discrimination of either. Gender roles are changing as both women and men enter professions that were once dominated by members of the opposite gender.

Age or Developmental Level

Age influences communication and it is never more evident than during adolescence. In their struggle to separate from parental confines and establish their own identity, adolescents generate a pattern of communication that is unique and changes from generation to generation. Words such as "dude," "awesome," "groovy," and "cool" have had special meaning for certain generations of adolescents.

Developmental influences on communication may relate to physiological alterations. One example is American Sign Language, the system of unique gestures used by many people who are deaf or hearing impaired. Individuals who are blind at birth never learn the subtle nonverbal gesticulations that accompany language and can totally change the meaning of the spoken word.

Environment in Which the Transaction Takes Place

The place where the communication occurs influences the outcome of the interaction. Some individuals who feel uncomfortable and refuse to speak during a group therapy session may be open and willing to discuss problems privately on a one-to-one basis with the nurse.

Territoriality, **density**, and **distance** are aspects of environment that communicate messages. *Territoriality* is the innate tendency to own space. Individuals lay claim to areas around them as their own. This influences communication when an interaction takes place in the territory "owned" by one or the other. Interpersonal communication can be more successful if the interaction takes place in a "neutral" area. For example, with the concept of territoriality in mind, the nurse may choose to conduct the psychosocial assessment in an interview room rather than in his or her office or in the client's room.

Density refers to the number of people within a given environmental space and has been shown to influence interpersonal interaction. Some studies indicate that a correlation exists between prolonged high-density situations and certain behaviors, such as aggression, stress, criminal activity, hostility toward others, and a deterioration of mental and physical health.

Distance is the means by which various cultures use space to communicate. Hall (1966) identified four kinds of spatial interaction, or distances, that people maintain from each other in their interpersonal interactions and the kinds of activities in which people engage at these various distances. **Intimate distance** is the closest distance that individuals will allow between themselves and others. In the United States, this distance, which is restricted to interactions of an intimate nature, is 0 to 18 inches. **Personal distance** is approximately 18 to 40 inches and reserved for interactions that are personal in nature, such as close conversations with friends or colleagues. Our **social distance** is about 4 to 12 feet away from the body. Interactions at this distance include conversations with strangers or acquaintances, such as at a cocktail party or in a public building. **Public distances** are those that exceed 12 feet. Examples include speaking in public or yelling to someone some distance away. This distance is considered public space, and communicants are free to move about in it during the interaction.

NONVERBAL COMMUNICATION   65-95% is nonVerbal

It has been estimated that 65 to 95 percent of all effective communication is nonverbal (Rankin, 2004). Some aspects of nonverbal expression have been discussed in the previous section on preexisting conditions that influence communication. Other components of nonverbal communication include physical appearance and dress, body movement and posture, touch, facial expressions, eye behavior, and vocal cues or paralanguage. These nonverbal messages vary from culture to culture.

Physical Appearance and Dress

Physical appearance and dress are part of the total nonverbal stimuli that influence interpersonal responses and, under some conditions, they are the primary determiners of such responses. Body coverings—both dress and hair—are manipulated by the wearer in a manner that conveys a distinct message to the receiver. Dress can be formal or casual, stylish or sloppy. Hair can be long or short, and even the presence or absence of hair conveys a message about the person. Other body adornments that are also considered potential communicative stimuli include tattoos, masks, cosmetics, badges, jewelry, and eyeglasses. Some jewelry worn in specific ways can give special messages (e.g., a gold band or diamond ring worn on the fourth finger of the left hand, a boy's class ring worn on a chain around a girl's neck, or a pin bearing Greek letters worn on the lapel). Some individuals convey a specific message with the total absence of any type of body adornment.

Body Movement and Posture

The way in which an individual positions his or her body communicates messages regarding self-esteem, gender

identity, status, and interpersonal warmth or coldness. The individual whose posture is slumped, with head and eyes pointed downward, conveys a message of low self-esteem. Specific ways of standing or sitting are considered to be either feminine or masculine within a defined culture. In the United States, to stand straight and tall with head high and hands on hips indicates a superior status over the person being addressed.

Reece and Whitman (1962) identified response behaviors that were used to designate individuals as either "warm" or "cold" persons. Individuals who were perceived as warm responded to others with a shift of posture toward the other person, a smile, direct eye contact, and hands that remained still. Individuals who responded to others with a slumped posture, by looking around the room, drumming fingers on the desk, and not smiling were perceived as cold.

Touch

Touch is a powerful communication tool. It can elicit both negative and positive reactions, depending on the people involved and the circumstances of the interaction. It is a very basic and primitive form of communication, and the appropriateness of its use is culturally determined.

Touch can be categorized according to the message communicated (Knapp, 1980):

1. **Functional-Professional**. This type of touch is impersonal and business-like. It is used to accomplish a task.

   > **EXAMPLE:**

   A tailor measuring a customer for a suit or a physician examining a client.

2. **Social-Polite**. This type of touch is still rather impersonal, but it conveys an affirmation or acceptance of the other person.

   > **EXAMPLE:**

   A handshake.

3. **Friendship–Warmth**. Touch at this level indicates a strong liking for the other person, a feeling that he or she is a friend.

   > **EXAMPLE:**

   Laying one's hand on the shoulder of another.

4. **Love–Intimacy**. This type of touch conveys an emotional attachment or attraction for another person.

   > **EXAMPLE:**

   Engaging in a strong, mutual embrace.

5. **Sexual–Arousal**. Touch at this level is an expression of physical attraction only.

EXAMPLE:

Touching another in the genital region.

Some cultures encourage more touching of various types than others. "Contact cultures" (e.g., France, Latin America, Italy) use a greater frequency of touch cues than do "noncontact cultures" (e.g., Germany, United States, Canada) (Givens, 2004a). The nurse should understand the cultural meaning of touch before using this method of communication in specific situations.

Facial Expressions

Next to human speech, facial expression is the primary source of communication. Facial expressions primarily reveal an individual's emotional states, such as happiness, sadness, anger, surprise, and fear. The face is a complex multimessage system. Facial expressions serve to complement and qualify other communication behaviors, and at times even take the place of verbal messages. A summary of feelings associated with various facial expressions is presented in Table 8–1.

TABLE 8–1	Summary of Facial Expressions
FACIAL EXPRESSION	ASSOCIATED FEELINGS
Nose	
Nostril flare	Anger; arousal
Wrinkling up	Dislike; disgust
Lips	
Grin; smile	Happiness; contentment
Grimace	Fear; pain
Compressed	Anger; frustration
Canine-type snarl	Disgust
Pouted; frown	Unhappiness; discontented; disapproval
Pursing	Disagreement
Sneer	Contempt; disdain
Brows	
Frown	Anger; unhappiness; concentration
Raised	Surprise; enthusiasm
Tongue	
Stick out	Dislike; disagree
Eyes	
Widened	Surprise; excitement
Narrowed; lids squeezed shut	Threat; fear
Stare	Threat
Stare/blink/look away	Dislike; disinterest
Eyes downcast; lack of eye contact	Submission; low self-esteem
Eye contact (generally intermittent, as opposed to a stare)	Self-confidence; interest

SOURCE: Adapted from Givens (2004b); Hughey (1990); and Archer (2004).

Eye Behavior

Eyes have been called the "windows of the soul." It is through eye contact that individuals view and are viewed by others in a revealing way. An interpersonal connectedness occurs through eye contact. In American culture, eye contact conveys a personal interest in the other person. Eye contact indicates that the communication channel is open, and it is often the initiating factor in verbal interaction between two people.

Eye behavior is regulated by social rules. These rules dictate where we can look, when we can look, for how long we can look, and at whom we can look. Staring is often used to register disapproval of the behavior of another. People are extremely sensitive to being looked at, and if the staring behavior violates social rules, they often assign meaning to it, such as the following statement implies: "He kept staring at me, and I began to wonder if I was dressed inappropriately or had mustard on my face!"

Gazing at another's eyes arouses strong emotions. Thus, eye contact rarely lasts longer than three seconds before one or both viewers experience a powerful urge to glance away. Breaking eye contact lowers stress levels (Givens, 2004c).

Vocal Cues, or Paralanguage

Paralanguage is the gestural component of the spoken word. It consists of pitch, tone, and loudness of spoken messages, the rate of speaking, expressively placed pauses, and emphasis assigned to certain words. These vocal cues greatly influence the way individuals interpret verbal messages. A normally soft-spoken individual whose pitch and rate of speaking increase may be perceived as being anxious or tense.

Different vocal emphases can alter interpretation of the message.

Three examples follow:

1. "I felt **SURE** you would notice the change."
   Interpretation: I was **SURE** you would, but you didn't.

2. "I felt sure **YOU** would notice the change."
   Interpretation: I thought **YOU** would, even if nobody else did.

3. "I felt sure you would notice the **CHANGE**."
   Interpretation: Even if you didn't notice anything else, I thought you would notice the **CHANGE**.

Verbal cues play a major role in determining responses in human communication situations. *How* a message is verbalized can be as important as *what* is verbalized.

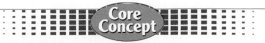

Core Concept

Therapeutic Communication
Caregiver verbal and nonverbal techniques that focus on the care receiver's needs and advance the promotion of healing and change. Therapeutic communication encourages exploration of feelings and fosters understanding of behavioral motivation. It is nonjudgmental, discourages defensiveness, and promotes trust.

THERAPEUTIC COMMUNICATION TECHNIQUES

Hays and Larson (1963) identified a number of techniques to assist the nurse in interacting more therapeutically with clients. These are the "technical procedures" carried out by the nurse working in psychiatry, and they should serve to enhance development of a therapeutic nurse–client relationship. Table 8–2 includes a list of

TABLE 8–2	Therapeutic Communication Techniques	
TECHNIQUE	**EXPLANATION/RATIONALE**	**EXAMPLES**
Using silence	Gives the client the opportunity to collect and organize thoughts, to think through a point, or to consider introducing a topic of greater concern than the one being discussed.	
Accepting	Conveys an attitude of reception and regard	"Yes, I understand what you said." Eye contact; nodding.
Giving recognition	Acknowledging and indicating awareness; better than complimenting, which reflects the nurse's judgment.	"Hello, Mr. J. I notice that you made a ceramic ash tray in OT." "I see you made your bed."
Offering self	Making oneself available on an unconditional basis, increasing client's feelings of self-worth	"I'll stay with you awhile." "We can eat our lunch together." "I'm interested in you."
Giving broad openings	Allows the client to take the initiative in introducing the topic; emphasizes the importance of the client's role in the interaction.	"What would you like to talk about today?" "Tell me what you are thinking."
Offering general leads	Offers the client encouragement to continue.	"Yes, I see." "Go on." "And after that?"
Placing the event in time or sequence	Clarifies the relationship of events in time so that the nurse and client can view them in perspective	"What seemed to lead up to...?" "Was this before or after...?" "When did this happen?"
Making observations	Verbalizing what is observed or perceived. This encourages the client to recognize specific behaviors and compare perceptions with the nurse.	"You seem tense." "I notice you are pacing a lot." "You seem uncomfortable when you..."
Encouraging description of perceptions	Asking the client to verbalize what is being perceived; often used with clients experiencing hallucinations	"Tell me what is happening now." "Are you hearing the voices again?" "What do the voices seem to be saying?"
Encouraging comparison	Asking the client to compare similarities and differences in ideas, experiences, or interpersonal relationships. This helps the client recognize life experiences that tend to recur as well as those aspects of life that are changeable.	"Was this something like...?" "How does this compare with the time when...?" "What was your response the last time this situation occurred?"
Restating	The main idea of what the client has said is repeated; lets the client know whether or not an expressed statement has been understood and gives him or her the chance to continue, or to clarify if necessary.	Cl: "I can't study. My mind keeps wandering." Ns: "You have difficulty concentrating." Cl: "I can't take that new job. What if I can't do it?" Ns: "You're afraid you will fail in this new position."
Reflecting	Questions and feelings are referred back to the client so that they may be recognized and accepted, and so that the client may recognize that his or her point of view has value—a good technique to use when the client asks the nurse for advice.	Cl: "What do you think I should do about my wife's drinking problem?" Ns: "What do *you* think you should do?" Cl: "My sister won't help a bit toward my mother's care. I have to do it all!" Ns: "You feel angry when she doesn't help."
Focusing	Taking notice of a single idea or even a single word; works especially well with a client who is moving rapidly from one thought to another. This technique is *not* therapeutic, however, with the client who is very anxious. Focusing should not be pursued until the anxiety level has subsided	"This point seems worth looking at more closely. Perhaps you and I can discuss it together."

(Continued on following page)

TABLE 8–2 Therapeutic Communication Techniques *(Continued)*

TECHNIQUE	EXPLANATION/RATIONALE	EXAMPLES
Exploring	Delving further into a subject, idea, experience, or relationship; especially helpful with clients who tend to remain on a superficial level of communication. However, if the client chooses not to disclose further information, the nurse should refrain from pushing or probing in an area that obviously creates discomfort.	"Please explain that situation in more detail." "Tell me more about that particular situation."
Seeking clarification and validation	Striving to explain that which is vague or incomprehensible and searching for mutual understanding. Clarifying the meaning of what has been said facilitates and increases understanding for both client and nurse.	"I'm not sure that I understand. Would you please explain?" "Tell me if my understanding agrees with yours." "Do I understand correctly that you said…?"
Presenting reality	When the client has a misperception of the environment, the nurse defines reality or indicates his or her perception of the situation for the client.	"I understand that the voices seem real to you, but I do not hear any voices." "There is no one else in the room but you and me."
Voicing doubt	Expressing uncertainty as to the reality of the client's perceptions; often used with clients experiencing delusional thinking.	"I find that hard to believe." "That seems rather doubtful to me."
Verbalizing the implied	Putting into words what the client has only implied or said indirectly; it can also be used with the client who is mute or is otherwise experiencing impaired verbal communication. This clarifies that which is *implicit* rather than *explicit*.	Cl: "It's a waste of time to be here. I can't talk to you or anyone." Ns: "Are you feeling that no one understands?" Cl: (Mute) Ns: "It must have been very difficult for you when your husband died in the fire."
Attempting to translate words into feelings	When feelings are expressed indirectly, the nurse tries to "desymbolize" what has been said and to find clues to the underlying true feelings.	Cl: "I'm way out in the ocean." Ns: "You must be feeling very lonely now."
Formulating a plan of action	When a client has a plan in mind for dealing with what is considered to be a stressful situation, it may serve to prevent anger or anxiety from escalating to an unmanageable level.	"What could you do to let your anger out harmlessly?" "Next time this comes up, what might you do to handle it more appropriately?"

SOURCE: Adapted from Hays & Larson (1963).

these techniques, a short explanation of their usefulness, and examples of each.

NONTHERAPEUTIC COMMUNICATION TECHNIQUES

Several approaches are considered to be barriers to open communication between the nurse and client. Hays and Larson (1963) identified a number of these techniques, which are presented in Table 8–3. Nurses should recognize and eliminate the use of these patterns in their relationships with clients. Avoiding these communication barriers maximizes the effectiveness of communication and enhances the nurse-client relationship.

ACTIVE LISTENING

To listen actively is to be attentive to what the client is saying, both verbally and nonverbally. Attentive listening creates a climate in which the client can communicate. With active listening the nurse communicates acceptance and respect for the client, and trust is enhanced. A climate is established within the relationship that promotes openness and honest expression.

Several nonverbal behaviors have been designated as facilitative skills for attentive listening. Those listed here can be identified by the acronym SOLER:

S—Sit squarely facing the client. This gives the message that the nurse is there to listen and is interested in what the client has to say.

O—Observe an open posture. Posture is considered "open" when arms and legs remain uncrossed. This suggests that the nurse is "open" to what the client has to say. With a "closed" position, the nurse can convey a somewhat defensive stance, possibly invoking a similar response in the client.

L—Lean forward toward the client. This conveys to the client that you are involved in the interaction, interested in what is being said, and making a sincere effort to be attentive.

E—Establish eye contact. Eye contact, intermittently directed, is another behavior that conveys the nurse's involvement and willingness to listen to what the client has to say. The absence of eye contact or the constant shifting of eye contact elsewhere in the environment

TABLE 8–3   Nontherapeutic Communication Techniques

TECHNIQUE	EXPLANATION/RATIONALE	EXAMPLES
Giving reassurance	Indicates to the client that there is no cause for anxiety, thereby devaluing the client's feelings; may discourage the client from further expression of feelings if he or she believes they will only be downplayed or ridiculed	"I wouldn't worry about that if I were you" "Everything will be all right." **Better to say:** "We will work on that together."
Rejecting	Refusing to consider or showing contempt for the client's ideas or behavior. This may cause the client to discontinue interaction with the nurse for fear of further rejection.	"Let's not discuss…" "I don't want to hear about…" **Better to say:** "Let's look at that a little closer."
Giving approval or disapproval	Sanctioning or denouncing the client's ideas or behavior; implies that the nurse has the right to pass judgment on whether the client's ideas or behaviors are "good" or "bad," and that the client is expected to please the nurse. The nurse's acceptance of the client is then seen as conditional depending on the client's behavior.	"That's good. I'm glad that you…" "That's bad. I'd rather you wouldn't…" **Better to say:** "Let's talk about how your behavior invoked anger in the other clients at dinner."
Agreeing/disagreeing	Indicating accord with or opposition to the client's ideas or opinions; implies that the nurse has the right to pass judgment on whether the client's ideas or opinions are "right" or "wrong." Agreement prevents the client from later modifying his or her point of view without admitting error. Disagreement implies inaccuracy, provoking the need for defensiveness on the part of the client.	"That's right. I agree." "That's wrong. I disagree." "I don't believe that." **Better to say:** "Let's discuss what you feel is unfair about the new community rules."
Giving advice	Telling the client what to do or how to behave implies that the nurse knows what is best, and that the client is incapable of any self-direction. It nurtures the client in the dependent role by discouraging independent thinking.	"I think you should…" "Why don't you…" **Better to say:** "What do *you* think you should do?"
Probing	Persistent questioning of the client; pushing for answers to issues the client does not wish to discuss. This causes the client to feel used and valued only for what is shared with the nurse and places the client on the defensive.	"Tell me how your mother abused you when you were a child." "Tell me how you feel toward your mother now that she is dead." "Now tell me about…" **Better technique:** The nurse should be aware of the client's response and discontinue the interaction at the first sign of discomfort.
Defending	Attempting to protect someone or something from verbal attack. To defend what the client has criticized is to imply that he or she has no right to express ideas, opinions, or feelings. Defending does not change the client's feelings and may cause the client to think the nurse is taking sides against the client.	"No one here would lie to you." "You have a very capable physician. I'm sure he only has your best interests in mind." **Better to say:** "I will try to answer your questions and clarify some issues regarding your treatment."
Requesting an explanation	Asking the client to provide the reasons for thoughts, feelings, behavior, and events. Asking "why" a client did something or feels a certain way can be very intimidating, and implies that the client must defend his or her behavior or feelings.	"Why do you think that?" "Why do you feel this way?" "Why did you do that?" **Better to say:** "Describe what you were feeling just before that happened."
Indicating the existence of an external source of power	Attributing the source of thoughts, feelings, and behavior to others or to outside influences. This encourages the client to project blame for his or her thoughts or behaviors on others rather than accepting the responsibility personally.	"What makes you say that?" "What made you do that?" "What made you so angry last night?" **Better to say:** "You became angry when your brother insulted your wife."
Belittling feelings expressed	When the nurse misjudges the degree of the client's discomfort, a lack of empathy and understanding may be conveyed. The nurse may tell the client to "perk up" or "snap out of it." This causes the client to feel insignificant or unimportant. When one is experiencing discomfort, it is no relief to hear that others are or have been in similar situations.	Cl: "I have nothing to live for. I wish I were dead." Ns: "Everybody gets down in the dumps at times. I feel that way myself sometimes." **Better to say:** "You must be very upset. Tell me what you are feeling right now."

(Continued on following page)

TABLE 8–3	Nontherapeutic Communication Techniques *(Continued)*	
TECHNIQUE	**EXPLANATION/RATIONALE**	**EXAMPLES**
Making stereotyped comments	Cliches and trite expressions are meaningless in a nurse-client relationship. When the nurse makes empty conversation, it encourages a like response from the client.	"I'm fine, and how are you?" "Hang in there. It's for your own good." "Keep your chin up." **Better to say:** "The therapy must be difficult for you at times. How do you feel about your progress at this point?"
Using denial	When the nurse denies that a problem exists, he or she blocks discussion with the client and avoids helping the client identify and explore areas of difficulty.	Cl: "I'm nothing." Ns: "Of course you're something. Everybody is somebody. **Better to say:** "You're feeling like no one cares about you right now."
Interpreting	With this technique the therapist seeks to make conscious that which is unconscious, to tell the client the meaning of his experience.	"What you really mean is…" "Unconsciously you're saying…" **Better technique:** The nurse must leave interpretation of the client's behavior to the psychiatrist. The nurse has not been prepared to perform this technique, and in attempting to do so, may endanger other nursing roles with the client."
Introducing an unrelated topic	Changing the subject causes the nurse to take over the direction of the discussion. This may occur in order to get to something that the nurse wants to discuss with the client or to get away from a topic that he or she would prefer not to discuss.	Cl: "I don't have anything to live for." Ns: "Did you have visitors this weekend?" **Better technique:** The nurse must remain open and free to hear the client, to take in all that is being conveyed, both verbally and nonverbally.

SOURCE: Adapted from Hays & Larson (1963).

gives the message that the nurse is not really interested in what is being said.

NOTE: Ensure that eye contact conveys warmth and is accompanied by smiling and intermittent nodding of the head, and does not come across as staring or glaring, which can create intense discomfort in the client.

R—Relax. Whether sitting or standing during the interaction, the nurse should communicate a sense of being relaxed and comfortable with the client. Restlessness and fidgetiness communicate a lack of interest and may convey a feeling of discomfort that is likely to be transferred to the client.

PROCESS RECORDINGS

Process recordings are written reports of verbal interactions with clients. They are verbatim (to the extent that this is possible) accounts, written by the nurse or student as a tool for improving interpersonal communication techniques. Although the process recording can take many forms, it usually includes the verbal and nonverbal communication of both nurse and client. It provides a means for the nurse to analyze both the content and the pattern of the interaction. The process recording, which is not considered documentation, should be used as a learning tool for professional development. An example of one type of process recording is presented in Table 8–4.

FEEDBACK

Feedback is a method of communication for helping the client consider a modification of behavior. Feedback gives information to clients about how they are being perceived by others. It should be presented in a manner that discourages defensiveness on the part of the client. Feedback can be useful to the client if presented with objectivity by a trusted individual.

Some criteria about useful feedback include the following:

1. Feedback is descriptive rather than evaluative and focuses on the behavior rather than on the client. Avoiding evaluative language reduces the need for the client to react defensively. Objective descriptions allow clients to take the information and use it in whatever way they choose. When the focus is on the client, the nurse makes judgments about the client.

EXAMPLE:

Descriptive and focused on behavior	"Jane was very upset in group today when you called her 'fatty' and laughed at her in front of the others."
Evaluative	"You were very rude and inconsiderate to Jane in group today."
Focus on client	"You are a very insensitive person."

TABLE 8–4	Sample Process Recording			
NURSE VERBAL (NONVERBAL)	**CLIENT VERBAL (NONVERBAL)**	**NURSE'S THOUGHTS AND FEELINGS CONCERNING THE INTERACTION**	**ANALYSIS OF THE INTERACTION**
Do you still have thoughts about harming yourself? (Sitting facing the client; looking directly at client)	Not really. I still feel sad, but I don't want to die. (Looking at hands in lap.)	Felt a little uncomfortable. Always a hard question to ask.	**Therapeutic.** Asking a direct question about suicidal intent.
Tell me what you were feeling before you took all the pills the other night. (Still using SOLER techniques of active listening.)	I was just so angry! To think that my husband wants a divorce now that he has a good job. I worked hard to put him through college. (Fists clenched. Face and neck reddened.)	Beginning to feel more comfortable. Client seems willing to talk and I think she trusts me.	**Therapeutic.** Exploring. Delving further into the experience.
You wanted to hurt him because you felt betrayed. (SOLER)	Yes! If I died, maybe he'd realize that he loved me more than that other woman. (Tears starting to well up in her eyes.)	Starting to feel sorry for her.	**Therapeutic.** Attempting to translate words into feelings.
Seems like a pretty drastic way to get your point across. (Small frown.)	I know. It was a stupid thing to do. (Wiping eyes.)	Trying hard to remain objective.	**Nontherapeutic.** Sounds disapproving. Better to have pursued her feelings.
How are you feeling about the situation now? (SOLER)	I don't know. I still love him. I want him to come home. I don't want him to marry her. (Starting to cry again.)	Wishing there was an easy way to help relieve some of her pain.	**Therapeutic.** Focusing on her feelings.
Yes, I can understand that you would like things to be the way they were before. (Offer client a tissue.)	(Silence. Continues to cry softly.)	I'm starting to feel some anger toward her husband. Sometimes it's so hard to remain objective!	**Therapeutic.** Conveying empathy.
What do you think are the chances of your getting back together? (SOLER)	None. He's refused marriage counseling. He's already moved in with her. He says it's over. (Wipes tears. Looks directly at nurse.)	Relieved to know that she isn't using denial about the reality of the situation.	**Therapeutic.** Reflecting. Seeking client's perception of the situation.
So how are you preparing to deal with this inevitable outcome? (SOLER)	I'm going to do the things we talked about: join a divorced women's support group; increase my job hours to full-time; do some volunteer work; and call the suicide hot line if I feel like taking pills again. (Looks directly at nurse. Smiles.)	Positive feeling to know that she remembers what we discussed earlier and plans to follow through.	**Therapeutic.** Formulating a plan of action.
It won't be easy. But you have come a long way, and I feel you have gained strength in your ability to cope. (Standing. Looking at client. Smiling.)	Yes, I know I will have hard times. But I also know I have support, and I want to go on with my life and be happy again. (Standing, smiling at nurse)	Feeling confident that the session has gone well; hopeful that the client will succeed in what she wants to do with her life.	**Therapeutic.** Presenting reality.

2. Feedback should be specific rather than general. Information that gives details about the client's behavior can be used more easily than a generalized description for modifying the behavior.

EXAMPLE:

General   "You just don't pay attention."

Specific   "You were talking to Joe when we were deciding on the issue. Now you want to argue about the outcome."

3. Feedback should be directed toward behavior that the client has the capacity to modify. To provide feedback about a characteristic or situation that the client cannot change only provokes frustration.

EXAMPLE:

Can modify   "I noticed that you did not want to hold your baby when the nurse brought her to you."

Cannot modify   "Your baby daughter is mentally retarded because you took drugs when you were pregnant."

4. Feedback should impart information rather than offer advice. Giving advice fosters dependence and may

convey the message to the client that he or she is not capable of making decisions and solving problems independently. It is the client's right and privilege to be as self-sufficient as possible.

EXAMPLE:

Imparting information	"There are various methods of assistance for people who want to lose weight, such as Overeaters Anonymous, Weight Watchers, regular visits to a dietitian, and the Physician's Weight Loss Program. You can decide what is best for you."
Giving advice	"You obviously need to lose a great deal of weight. I think the Physician's Weight Loss Program would be best for you."

5. Feedback should be well timed. Feedback is most useful when given at the earliest appropriate opportunity following the specific behavior.

EXAMPLE:

Prompt response	"I saw you hit the wall with your fist just now when you hung up the phone after talking to your mother."
Delayed response	"You need to learn some more appropriate ways of dealing with your anger. Last week after group I saw you pounding your fist against the wall."

SUMMARY

Interpersonal communication is a transaction between the sender and the receiver. In all interpersonal transactions, both the sender and receiver bring certain preexisting conditions to the exchange that influences both the intended message and the way in which it is interpreted.

Examples of these conditions include one's value system, internalized attitudes and beliefs, culture or religion, social status, gender, background knowledge and experience, age or developmental level, and the type of environment in which the communication takes place.

Nonverbal expression is a primary communication system in which meaning is assigned to various gestures and patterns of behavior. Some components of nonverbal communication include physical appearance and dress, body movement and posture, touch, facial expressions, eye behavior, and vocal cues or paralanguage. The meaning of each of these nonverbal components is culturally determined.

Hays and Larson (1963) have described various techniques of communication that can facilitate interaction between nurse and client. They have also identified a number of barriers in communication that can interfere with a satisfactory nurse–client interaction. Examples of both were presented in this chapter.

Active listening is described as being attentive to what the client is saying, through both verbal and nonverbal cues. Facilitative skills for attentive listening include sitting squarely facing the client, observing an open posture, leaning forward toward the client, establishing eye contact, and relaxing. They can be identified by the acronym SOLER.

Feedback is a method of communication for helping the client consider a modification of behavior. It is most useful when it is presented as follows:

1. Is descriptive rather than evaluative.
2. Focuses on behavior rather than on the person.
3. Is specific rather than general.
4. Is directed toward behavior that the client can change.
5. Imparts information rather than gives advice.
6. Is well timed.

The nurse must be aware of the therapeutic or nontherapeutic value of the communication techniques used with the client because they are the "tools" of psychosocial intervention.

REVIEW QUESTIONS

SELF-EXAMINATION/LEARNING EXERCISE

Test your knowledge about the concept of communication by answering the following questions:

1. Describe the transactional model of communication.

2. List eight types of preexisting conditions that can influence the outcome of the communication process.

3. Define *territoriality*. How does it affect communication?

4. Define *density*. How does it affect communication?

5. Identify four types of spatial distance and give an example of each.

6. Identify six components of nonverbal communication that convey special messages and give an example of each.

7. Describe five facilitative skills for active, or attentive, listening that can be identified by the acronym SOLER.

Identify the correct answer in each of the following questions. Provide explanation where requested. Identify the technique used (both therapeutic and nontherapeutic) in all choices given.

8. A client states: "I refuse to shower in this room. I must be very cautious. The FBI has placed a camera in here to monitor my every move." Which of the following is the therapeutic response? What is this technique called?
   a. "That's not true."
   b. "I have a hard time believing that is true."

9. Nancy, a depressed client who has been unkempt and untidy for weeks, today comes to group therapy wearing a clean dress, makeup, and having washed and combed her hair. Which of the following responses by the nurse is most appropriate? Give the rationale.
   a. "Nancy, I see you have put on a clean dress and combed your hair."
   b. "Nancy, you look wonderful today!"

10. Dorothy was involved in an automobile accident while under the influence of alcohol. She swerved her car into a tree and narrowly missed hitting a child on a bicycle. She is in the hospital with multiple abrasions and contusions. She is talking about the accident with the nurse. Which of the following statements by the nurse is most appropriate? Identify the therapeutic or nontherapeutic technique in each.
    a. "Now that you know what can happen when you drink and drive, I'm sure you won't let it happen again. I'm sure everything will be okay."
    b. "That was a terrible thing you did. You could have killed that child!"
    c. "Now I guess you'll have to buy a new car. Can you afford that?"
    d. "What made you do such a thing?"
    e. "Tell me how you are feeling about what happened."

11. Judy has been in the hospital for 3 weeks. She has used Valium "to settle my nerves" for the past 15 years. She was admitted by her psychiatrist for safe withdrawal from the drug. She has passed the physical symptoms of withdrawal at this time, but states to the nurse, "I don't know if I will make it without Valium after I go home. I'm already starting to feel nervous. I have so many personal problems." Which is the most appropriate response by the nurse? Identify the technique in each.

a. "Why do you think you have to have drugs to deal with your problems?"
b. "You'll just have to pull yourself together. Everybody has problems, and everybody doesn't use drugs to deal with them. They just do the best that they can."
c. "I don't want to talk about that now. Look at that sunshine. It's beautiful outside. You and I are going to take a walk!"
d. "Starting today you and I are going to think about some alternative ways for you to deal with those problems—things that you can do to decrease your anxiety without resorting to drugs."

12. Mrs. S. asks the nurse, "Do you think I should tell my husband about my affair with my boss?" Give one therapeutic response and one nontherapeutic response, give your rationale, and identify the technique used in each response.

13. Carol, an adolescent, just returned from group therapy and is crying. She says to the nurse, "All the other kids laughed at me! I try to fit in, but I always seem to say the wrong thing. I've never had a close friend. I guess I never will." Which is the most appropriate response by the nurse? Identify each technique used.
a. "You're feeling pretty down on yourself right now."
b. "Why do you feel this way about yourself?"
c. "What makes you think you will never have any friends?"
d. "The next time they laugh at you, you should just get up and leave the room!"
e. "I'm sure they didn't mean to hurt your feelings."
f. "Keep your chin up and hang in there. Your time will come."

REFERENCES

Archer, D. (2004). *Exploring nonverbal communication.* Retrieved October 31, 2004 at http://nonverbal.ucsc.edu/index.html

Givens, D.B. (2004a). *The nonverbal dictionary.* Center for Nonverbal Studies. Retrieved October 31, 2004 at http://members.aol.com/nonverbal2/diction1.htm

Givens, D.B. (2004b). *The nonverbal dictionary.* Center for Nonverbal Studies. Retrieved October 31, 2004 at http://members.aol.com/nonverbal3/facialx.htm

Givens, D.B. (2004c). *The nonverbal dictionary.* Center for Nonverbal Studies. Retrieved October 31, 2004 at http://members.aol.com/nonverbal3/eyecon.htm

Hughey, J.D. (1990). *Speech communication.* Stillwater, OK: Oklahoma State University.

Rankin, J. (2004). *Body language training.* Retrieved October 31, 2004 from the World Wide Web at http://www.jrbodylanguage.com/

Schuster, P.M. (2000). *Communication: The key to the therapeutic relationship.* Philadelphia: F.A. Davis.

Yates, D. (2003). *Communication models.* Seton Hall University. Department of Communication. Retrieved October 31, 2004 at http://pirate.shu.edu/~yatesdan/Tutorial.htm

CLASSICAL REFERENCES

Hall, E.T. (1966). *The hidden dimension.* Garden City, NY: Doubleday.

Hays, J.S., & Larson, K.H. (1963). *Interacting with patients.* New York: Macmillan.

Knapp, M.L. (1980). *Essentials of nonverbal communication.* New York: Holt, Rinehart & Winston.

Reece, M., & Whitman, R. (1962). Expressive movements, warmth, and verbal reinforcement. *Journal of Abnormal and Social Psychology, 64,* 234–236.

THE NURSING PROCESS IN PSYCHIATRIC/MENTAL HEALTH NURSING

CHAPTER OUTLINE

OBJECTIVES

THE NURSING PROCESS

WHY NURSING DIAGNOSIS?

NURSING CASE MANAGEMENT

APPLYING THE NURSING PROCESS IN THE PSYCHIATRIC SETTING

CONCEPT MAPPING

DOCUMENTATION OF THE NURSING PROCESS

SUMMARY

REVIEW QUESTIONS

KEY TERMS

case manager
case management
concept mapping
critical pathways of
    care
Focus Charting®
interdisciplinary
managed care

nursing interventions
    classification (NIC)
nursing outcomes
    classification (NOC)
nursing process
PIE charting
problem-oriented
    recording

CORE CONCEPTS

assessment
evaluation
nursing diagnosis
outcomes

OBJECTIVES

After reading this chapter, the student will be able to:

1. Define *nursing process.*
2. Identify six steps of the nursing process and describe nursing actions associated with each.
3. Describe the benefits of using nursing diagnosis.
4. Discuss the list of nursing diagnoses approved by NANDA International for clinical use and testing.

5. Define and discuss the use of case management and critical pathways of care in the clinical setting.
6. Apply the six steps of the nursing process in the care of a client within the psychiatric setting.
7. Document client care that validates use of the nursing process.

ANA

or many years the **nursing process** has provided a systematic framework for the delivery of nursing care. It is nursing's means of fulfilling the requirement for a *scientific methodology* in order to be considered a profession.

This chapter examines the steps of the nursing process as they are set forth by the American Nurses' Association (ANA) in *Nursing: Scope and Standards of Practice* (ANA, 2004). A list of the nursing diagnoses approved for clinical use and testing by NANDA International is presented. An explanation is provided for the implementation of case management and the tool used in the delivery of care with this methodology, critical pathways of care. A description of concept mapping is included, and documentation that validates the use of the nursing process is discussed.

THE NURSING PROCESS

Definition

The nursing process consists of six steps and uses a problem-solving approach that has come to be accepted as nursing's scientific methodology. It is goal directed, with the objective being delivery of quality client care.

Nursing process is dynamic, not static. It is an ongoing process that continues for as long as the nurse and client have interactions directed toward change in the client's physical or behavioral responses. Figure 9–1 presents a schematic of the ongoing nursing process.

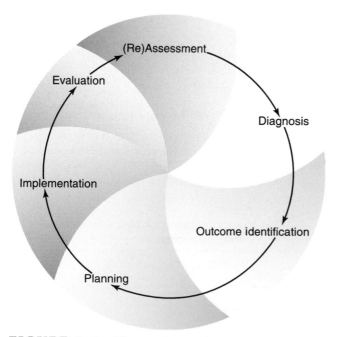

FIGURE 9–1 The ongoing nursing process.

Standards of Care

ANA
APNA
ISPMHN

The ANA, in collaboration with the American Psychiatric Nurses Association and the International Society of Psychiatric-Mental Health Nurses, has delineated a set of standards that psychiatric nurses are expected to follow as they provide care for their clients. The ANA (2000) states,

> Standards of care pertain to professional nursing activities that are demonstrated by the nurse through the nursing process. These involve assessment, diagnosis, outcome identification, planning, implementation, and evaluation. The nursing process is the foundation of clinical decision making and encompasses all significant action taken by nurses in providing psychiatric-mental health care to all clients. (p. 28)

Following are the standards with rationale as set forth by the ANA (2000).

Core Concept

Assessment
A systematic, dynamic process by which the nurse, through interaction with the client, significant others, and health care providers, collects and analyzes data about the client. Data may include the following dimensions: physical, psychological, sociocultural, spiritual, cognitive, functional abilities, developmental, economic, and lifestyle (ANA, 2004).

Standard I. Assessment

The Psychiatric/Mental Health Nurse Collects Patient Health Data.

Rationale. The assessment interview—which requires linguistically and culturally effective communication skills, interviewing, behavioral observation, record review, and comprehensive assessment of the patient and relevant systems—enables the psychiatric/mental health nurse to make sound clinical judgments and plan appropriate interventions with the client (ANA, 2000, p. 28).

In this first step, information is gathered from which to establish a database for determining the best possible care for the client. Information for this database is gathered from a variety of sources including interviewing the client or family, observing the client and his or her environment, consulting other health team members, reviewing the client's records, and conducting a nursing physical examination. A biopsychosocial assessment tool based on the stress-adaptation framework is included in Table 9–1.

TABLE 9–1 Nursing History and Assessment Tool

I. General Information

Client name: _____   Allergies: _____

Room number: _____   Diet: _____

Doctor: _____   Height/weight: _____

Age: _____   Vital signs: TPR/BP _____

Sex: _____   Name and phone no. of significant other: _____

Race: _____   City of residence: _____

Dominant language: _____   Diagnosis (admitting & current): _____

Marital status: _____

Chief complaint: _____

Conditions of admission.

Date: _____   Time: _____

Accompanied by: _____

Route of admission (wheelchair; ambulatory; cart): _____

Admitted from: _____

II. Predisposing Factors

A. *Genetic Influences*

1. Family configuration (use genograms):

   Family of origin: Present family:

   Family dynamics (describe significant relationships between family members): _____
   _____
   _____
   _____
   _____

2. Medical/psychiatric history:

   a. Client: _____
   _____

   b. Family members: _____
   _____

3. Other genetic influences affecting present adaptation. This might include effects specific to gender, race, appearance, such as genetic physical defects, or any other factor related to genetics that is affecting the client's adaptation that has not been mentioned elsewhere in this assessment.
   _____
   _____

B. *Past Experiences*

1. Cultural and social history:

   a. Environmental factors (family living arrangements, type of neighborhood, special working conditions): _____
   _____

   b. Health beliefs and practices (personal responsibility for health; special self-care practices): _____
   _____

   c. Religious beliefs and practices: _____
   _____

   d. Educational background: _____
   _____

   e. Significant losses/changes (include dates): _____
   _____

   f. Peer/friendship relationships: _____
   _____

   g. Occupational history: _____
   _____

   h. Previous pattern of coping with stress: _____
   _____

   i. Other lifestyle factors contributing to present adaptation: _____
   _____
   _____

(Continued on following page)

TABLE 9–1   **Nursing History and Assessment Tool** (*Continued*)

   C. *Existing Conditions*
      1. Stage of development (Erikson):
         a. Theoretically: _____
         b. Behaviorally: _____
         c. Rationale: _____
         _____
         _____

      2. Support systems: _____

      3. Economic security: _____
         _____

      4. Avenues of productivity/contribution:
         a. Current job status: _____
         _____
         b. Role contributions and responsibility for others: _____
         _____

III. Precipitating Event
    Describe the situation or events that precipitated this illness/hospitalization: _____
    _____
    _____

IV. Client's Perception of the Stressor
    Client's or family member's understanding or description of stressor/illness and expectations of hospitalization: _____
    _____
    _____
    _____

V. Adaptation Responses
   A. *Psychosocial*
      1. Anxiety level (circle level, and check the behaviors that apply): mild moderate severe panic
        calm _____ friendly _____ passive _____ alert _____ perceives environment correctly _____ cooperative _____
        impaired attention _____ "jittery" _____ unable to concentrate _____ hypervigilant _____ tremors _____ rapid speech _____
        withdrawn _____ confused _____ disoriented _____ fearful _____ hyperventilating _____ misinterpreting the environment
        (hallucinations or delusions) _____ depersonalization _____ obsessions _____ compulsions _____ somatic complaints _____
        excessive hyperactivity _____ other _____
      2. Mood/affect (circle as many as apply): happiness sadness dejection despair elation euphoria suspiciousness
        apathy (little emotional tone)   anger/hostility
      3. Ego defense mechanisms (describe how used by client):
        Projection _____
        Suppression _____
        Undoing _____
        Displacement _____
        Intellectualization _____
        Rationalization _____
        Denial _____
        Repression _____
        Isolation _____
        Regression _____
        Reaction Formation _____
        Splitting _____
        Religiosity _____
        Sublimation _____
        Compensation _____
      4. Level of self-esteem (circle one): low moderate high
        Things client likes about self:_____
        Things client would like to change about self:_____
        _____
        Objective assessment of self-esteem:
        Eye contact:_____
        General appearance:_____
        _____
        Personal hygiene:_____
        Participation in group activities and interactions with others: _____
        _____
      5. Stage and manifestations of grief (circle one): denial anger bargaining depression acceptance
        Describe the client's behaviors that are associated with this stage of grieving in response to loss or change: _____
        _____
        _____
        _____

(Continued on opposite page)

6. Thought processes (circle as many as apply): clear   logical   easy to follow   relevant   confused   blocking   delusional   rapid flow of thoughts   slowness in thought association   suspicious
   recent memory: loss   intact
   remote memory: loss   intact
   other: _____

7. Communication patterns (circle as many as apply): clear   coherent   slurred speech   incoherent   neologisms   loose associations   flight of ideas   aphasic   perseveration   rumination   tangential speech   loquaciousness   slow, impoverished speech
   speech impediment (describe):_____
   other:_____
   _____

8. Interaction patterns (describe client's pattern of interpersonal interactions with staff and peers on the unit, e.g., manipulative, withdrawn, isolated, verbally or physically hostile, argumentative, passive, assertive, aggressive, passive-aggressive, other): _____
   _____
   _____
   _____

9. Reality orientation (check those that apply):
   Oriented to: time _____   person _____
                    place _____   situation _____

10. Ideas of destruction to self/others?   Yes   No
    If yes, consider plan; available means:_____
    _____
    _____
    _____

B. *Physiological*
1. Psychosomatic manifestations (describe any somatic complaints that may be stress-related): _____
   _____

2. Drug history and assessment:
   Use of prescribed drugs:

NAME	DOSAGE	PRESCRIBED FOR	RESULTS

   Use of over-the-counter drugs:

NAME	DOSAGE	USED FOR	RESULTS

   Use of street drugs or alcohol:

NAME	AMOUNT USED	HOW OFTEN USED	WHEN LAST USED	EFFECTS PRODUCED

3. Pertinent physical assessments:
   a. Respirations: normal _____   labored _____
                Rate _____   Rhythm _____
   b. Skin: warm _____   dry _____   moist _____   cool _____
          clammy _____   pink _____   cyanotic _____
          poor turgor _____   edematous _____
          Evidence of: rash_____   bruising_____
            needle tracts _____   hirsutism _____   loss of hair _____
            other _____
   c. Musculoskeletal status: weakness _____   tremors _____
          Degree of range of motion (describe limitations) _____
          _____
          Pain (describe) _____
          _____
          Skeletal deformities (describe) _____
          Coordination (describe limitations) _____
   d. Neurological status:
          History of (check all that apply):   seizures _____
          (describe method of control) _____
          headaches (describe location and frequency)_____
          fainting spells _____   dizziness _____
          tingling/numbness (describe location)_____

(Continued on following page)

TABLE 9–1 **Nursing History and Assessment Tool** *(Continued)*

e. Cardiovascular: B/P _____ Pulse _____
   History of (check all that apply):
       hypertension _____ palpitations _____
       heart murmur _____ chest pain _____
       shortness of breath _____ pain in legs _____
       phlebitis _____ ankle/leg edema _____
       numbness/tingling in extremities _____
       varicose veins _____

f. Gastrointestinal:
   Usual diet pattern: _____
   Food allergies: _____
   Dentures? _____ Upper _____ Lower _____
   Any problems with chewing or swallowing? _____
   Any recent change in weight? _____
   Any problems with:
       indigestion/heartburn? _____
           relieved by _____
       nausea/vomiting? _____
           relieved by _____
   History of ulcers? _____
   Usual bowel pattern:_____
       Constipation? _____ Diarrhea? _____
   Type of self-care assistance provided for either of the above problems:_____

g. Genitourinary/Reproductive:
   Usual voiding pattern: _____
   Urinary hesitancy? _____ Frequency? _____
   Nocturia?_____ Pain/burning? _____
   Incontinence? _____
   Any genital lesions? _____
       Discharge? _____ Odor? _____
   History of sexually transmitted disease? _____
       If yes, please explain: _____

   Any concerns about sexuality/sexual activity? _____

   Method of birth control used:_____
   Females:
       Date of last menstrual cycle:_____
       Length of cycle:_____
       Problems associated with menstruation? _____

   Breasts: Pain/tenderness? _____
               Swelling? _____ Discharge? _____
               Lumps? _____ Dimpling? _____
   Practice breast self-examination? _____
       Frequency? _____
   Males:
       Penile discharge? _____
       Prostate problems? _____

h. Eyes: YES   NO   EXPLAIN
   Glasses?   ____   ____   _____
   Contacts?   ____   ____   _____
   Swelling?   ____   ____   _____
   Discharge?   ____   ____   _____
   Itching?   ____   ____   _____
   Blurring?   ____   ____   _____
   Double vision? ____   ____   _____

i. Ears   YES   NO   EXPLAIN
   Pain?   ____   ____   _____
   Drainage?   ____   ____   _____
   Difficulty hearing? ____ ____   _____
   Hearing aid?   ____   ____   _____
   Tinnitus?   ____   ____   _____

j. Medication side effects:
   What symptoms is the client experiencing that may be attributed to current medication usage? _____
   _____
   _____

k. Altered lab values and possible significance: _____
   _____
   _____

(Continued on opposite page)

l. Activity/rest patterns:
Exercise (amount, type, frequency):_____

Leisure time activities: _____

Patterns of sleep: Number of hours per night:_____
Use of sleep aids? _____
Pattern of awakening during the night? _____

Feel rested upon awakening? _____
m. Personal hygiene/activities of daily living:
Patterns of self-care: independent _____
Requires assistance with: mobility _____
hygiene _____
toileting _____
feeding _____
dressing _____
other _____
Statement describing personal hygiene and general appearance:_____

n. Other pertinent physical assessments: _____

VI. Summary of Initial Psychosocial/Physical Assessment:

Knowledge Deficits Identified:

Nursing Diagnoses Indicated:

Core Concept

Nursing Diagnosis
Nursing diagnoses are clinical judgments about individual, family, or community responses to actual or potential health problems/life processes. A nursing diagnosis provides the basis for selection of nursing interventions to achieve outcomes for which the nurse is accountable" (NANDA-I, 2005).

Standard II. Diagnosis

The Psychiatric/Mental Health Nurse Analyzes the Assessment Data in Determining Diagnoses.

Rationale. The basis for providing psychiatric/mental health nursing care is the recognition and identification of patterns of response to actual or potential psychiatric illnesses, mental health problems, and potential comorbid physical illnesses (ANA, 2000, p. 30).

In the second step, data gathered during the assessment are analyzed. Diagnoses and potential problem statements are formulated and prioritized. Diagnoses

conform to accepted classification systems, such as the NANDA International Nursing Diagnosis Classification (see Table 9–2); International Classification of Diseases (WHO, 1993); and *DSM-IV-TR* (APA, 2000) (see Appendix C).

Core Concept

Outcomes
Measurable, expected, patient-focused goals that translate into observable behaviors (ANA, 2004).

Standard III. Outcome Identification

The Psychiatric/Mental Health Nurse Identifies Expected Outcomes Individualized to the Patient.

Rationale. Within the context of providing nursing care, the ultimate goal is to influence health outcomes and improve the patient's health status (ANA, 2000, p. 31).

Expected outcomes are derived from the diagnosis. They must be measurable and estimate a time for attainment. They must be realistic for the client's capabilities,

Exchanging

- Imbalanced nutrition: More than body requirements
- Imbalanced nutrition: Less than body requirements
- Risk for imbalanced nutrition: More than body requirements
- Readiness for enhanced nutrition*
- Risk for infection
- Risk for imbalanced body temperature
- Hypothermia
- Hyperthermia
- Ineffective thermoregulation
- Autonomic dysreflexia
- Risk for autonomic dysreflexia
- Constipation
- Perceived constipation
- Diarrhea
- Bowel incontinence
- Risk for constipation
- Impaired urinary elimination
- Readiness for enhanced urinary elimination*
- Stress urinary incontinence
- Reflex urinary incontinence
- Urge urinary incontinence
- Functional urinary incontinence
- Total urinary incontinence
- Risk for urge urinary incontinence
- Urinary retention
- Ineffective tissue perfusion (specify type: renal, cerebral, cardiopulmonary, gastrointestinal, peripheral)
- Readiness for enhanced fluid balance*
- Risk for imbalanced fluid volume
- Excess fluid volume
- Deficient fluid volume
- Risk for deficient fluid volume
- Decreased cardiac output
- Impaired gas exchange
- Ineffective airway clearance
- Ineffective breathing pattern
- Impaired spontaneous ventilation
- Dysfunctional ventilatory weaning response
- Risk for injury
- Risk for suffocation
- Risk for poisoning
- Risk for trauma
- Risk for aspiration
- Risk for disuse syndrome
- Risk for sudden infant death syndrome*
- Latex allergy response
- Risk for latex allergy response
- Ineffective protection
- Impaired tissue integrity
- Impaired oral mucous membrane
- Impaired skin integrity
- Risk for impaired skin integrity
- Impaired dentition
- Decreased intracranial adaptive capacity
- Disturbed energy field

Communicating

- Impaired verbal communication
- Readiness for enhanced communication*

Relating

- Impaired social interaction
- Social isolation
- Risk for loneliness
- Ineffective role performance
- Impaired parenting
- Risk for impaired parenting
- Readiness for enhanced parenting*
- Risk for impaired parent/infant/child attachment
- Sexual dysfunction
- Interrupted family processes
- Readiness for enhanced family processes*

- Caregiver role strain
- Risk for caregiver role strain
- Dysfunctional family processes: Alcoholism
- Parental role conflict
- Ineffective sexuality patterns

Valuing

- Spiritual distress
- Risk for spiritual distress
- Readiness for enhanced spiritual well-being
- Impaired religiosity**
- Readiness for enhanced religiosity**
- Risk for impaired religiosity**

Choosing

- Ineffective coping
- Impaired adjustment
- Defensive coping
- Ineffective denial
- Disabled family coping
- Compromised family coping
- Readiness for enhanced family coping
- Readiness for enhanced community coping
- Ineffective community coping
- Readiness for enhanced coping*
- Ineffective therapeutic regimen management
- Noncompliance (specify)
- Ineffective family therapeutic regimen management
- Ineffective community therapeutic regimen management
- Effective therapeutic regimen management
- Readiness for enhanced management of therapeutic regimen*
- Decisional conflict (specify)
- Health-seeking behaviors (specify)

Moving

- Impaired physical mobility
- Risk for peripheral neurovascular dysfunction
- Risk for perioperative-positioning injury
- Impaired walking
- Risk for falls
- Wandering
- Impaired wheelchair mobility
- Impaired transfer ability
- Impaired bed mobility
- Activity intolerance
- Fatigue
- Risk for activity intolerance
- Disturbed sleep pattern
- Sleep deprivation
- Readiness for enhanced sleep*
- Deficient diversional activity
- Impaired home maintenance
- Ineffective health maintenance
- Delayed surgical recovery
- Adult failure to thrive
- Feeding self-care deficit
- Impaired swallowing
- Ineffective breastfeeding
- Interrupted breastfeeding
- Effective breastfeeding
- Ineffective infant feeding pattern
- Bathing/hygiene self-care deficit
- Dressing/grooming self-care deficit
- Toileting self-care deficit
- Delayed growth and development
- Risk for delayed development
- Risk for disproportionate growth
- Relocation stress syndrome
- Risk for relocation stress syndrome
- Risk for disorganized infant behavior

(Continued on opposite page)

Moving (*continued*)
- Disorganized infant behavior
- Readiness for enhanced organized infant behavior
- Sedentary lifestyle**

Perceiving
- Disturbed body image
- Readiness for enhanced self-concept
- Chronic low self-esteem
- Situational low self-esteem
- Risk for situational low self-esteem
- Disturbed personal identity
- Disturbed sensory perception (specify: visual, auditory, kinesthetic, gustatory, tactile, olfactory)
- Unilateral neglect
- Hopelessness
- Powerlessness
- Risk for powerlessness

Knowing
- Deficient knowledge (specify)
- Readiness for enhanced knowledge (specify)*
- Impaired environmental interpretation syndrome
- Acute confusion
- Chronic confusion

- Disturbed thought processes
- Impaired memory

Feeling
- Acute pain
- Chronic pain
- Nausea
- Dysfunctional grieving
- Anticipatory grieving
- Chronic sorrow
- Risk for other-directed violence
- Self-mutilation
- Risk for self-mutilation
- Risk for self-directed violence
- Risk for suicide
- Post-trauma syndrome
- Rape-trauma syndrome
- Rape-trauma syndrome: Compound reaction
- Rape-trauma syndrome: Silent reaction
- Risk for post-trauma syndrome
- Anxiety
- Death anxiety
- Fear
- Risk for dysfunctional grieving**

*New nursing diagnoses, 2003.
** New nursing diagnoses, 2005.
SOURCE: *NANDA Nursing Diagnoses: Definitions & Classification 2005–2006.* (2005). Philadelphia: North American Nursing Diagnosis Association. With permission.

and are most effective when formulated by the interdisciplinary members, the client, and significant others together.

Nursing Outcomes Classification (NOC). The **nursing outcomes classification (NOC)** is a comprehensive, standardized classification of patient/client outcomes developed to evaluate the effects of nursing interventions (Johnson, Maas, & Moorhead, 2004). The outcomes have been linked to NANDA diagnoses and to the **Nursing Interventions Classification (NIC).** NANDA, NIC, and NOC represent all domains of nursing and can be used together or separately (Johnson et al., 2001).

Each NOC outcome has a label name, a definition, a list of indicators to evaluate client status in relation to the outcome, and a five-point Likert scale to measure client status (Johnson et al., 2001). The 330 NOC outcomes include 311 individual level outcomes, 10 family and 9 community level outcomes (Johnson, Maas, & Moorhead, 2004).

Standard IV. Planning

The Psychiatric/Mental Health Nurse Develops a Plan of Care that Is Negotiated Among the Patient, Nurse, Family, and Health Care Team and Prescribes Evidence-Based Interventions to Attain Expected Outcomes.

Rationale. A plan of care is used to guide therapeutic intervention systematically, document progress, and achieve the expected patient outcomes (ANA, 2000, p. 32).

The care plan is individualized to the client's mental health problems, condition, or needs and is developed in collaboration with the client, significant others, and interdisciplinary team members, if possible. For each diagnosis identified, the most appropriate interventions, based on current psychiatric/mental health nursing practice and research, are selected. Client education and necessary referrals are included. Priorities for delivery of nursing care are determined.

Nursing Interventions Classification (NIC). The Nursing Interventions Classification (NIC) is a comprehensive, standardized language describing treatments that nurses perform in all settings and in all specialties. NIC includes both physiological and psychosocial interventions, as well as those for illness treatment, illness prevention, and health promotion (Dochterman & Bulechek, 2004). NIC interventions are comprehensive, based on research, and reflect current clinical practice. They were developed inductively based on existing practice.

NIC contains 514 interventions each with a definition and a detailed set of activities that describe what a nurse does to implement the intervention. The use of a standardized language is thought to enhance continuity of care and facilitate communication among nurses and between nurses and other providers.

Standard V. Implementation

The Psychiatric/Mental Health Nurse Implements the Interventions Identified in the Plan of Care.

Rationale. In implementing the plan of care, psychiatric/mental health nurses use a wide range of interventions designed to prevent mental and physical illness, and promote, maintain, and restore mental and physical health. Psychiatric/mental health nurses select interventions according to their level of practice. At the basic level, the nurse may select counseling, milieu therapy, self-care activities, psychobiological interventions, health teaching, case management, health promotion and health maintenance, crisis intervention, community-based care, psychiatric home health care, telehealth, and a variety of other approaches to meet the mental health needs of patients. In addition to the intervention options available to the basic-level psychiatric/mental health nurse, at the advanced level the certified specialist may provide consultation, engage in psychotherapy, and prescribe pharmacological agents in accordance with state statutes or regulations (ANA, 2000, p. 33).

Interventions selected during the planning stage are executed, taking into consideration the nurse's level of practice, education, and certification. The care plan serves as a blueprint for delivery of safe, ethical, and appropriate interventions. Documentation of interventions also occurs at this step in the nursing process.

Several specific interventions are included among the standards of psychiatric/mental health clinical nursing practice (ANA, 2000):

Standard Va. Counseling. The psychiatric/mental health nurse uses counseling interventions to assist clients in improving or regaining their previous coping abilities, fostering mental health, and preventing mental illness and disability.

Standard Vb. Milieu Therapy. The psychiatric/mental health nurse provides, structures, and maintains a therapeutic environment in collaboration with the client and other health care clinicians.

Standard Vc. Promotion of Self-Care Activities. The psychiatric/mental health nurse structures interventions around the client's activities of daily living to foster self-care and mental and physical well-being.

Standard Vd. Psychobiological Interventions. The psychiatric/mental health nurse uses knowledge of psychobiological interventions and applies clinical skills to restore the client's health and prevent further disability.

Standard Ve. Health Teaching. The psychiatric/mental health nurse, through health teaching, assists clients in achieving satisfying, productive, and healthy patterns of living.

Standard Vf. Case Management. The psychiatric/mental health nurse provides case management to coordinate comprehensive health services and ensure continuity of care.

Standard Vg. Health Promotion and Health Maintenance. The psychiatric/mental health nurse employs strategies and interventions to promote and maintain health and prevent mental illness.

Advanced Practice Interventions

Standard Vh. Psychotherapy. The certified specialist in psychiatric/mental health nursing uses individual, group, and family psychotherapy, and other therapeutic treatments to assist clients in preventing mental illness and disability, treating mental health disorders, and improving mental health status and functional abilities.

Standard Vi. Prescriptive Authority and Treatment. The certified specialist in psychiatric/mental health nursing uses prescriptive authority, procedures, and treatments in accordance with state and federal laws and regulations, to treat symptoms of psychiatric illness and improve functional health status.

Standard Vj. Consultation. The certified specialist in psychiatric/mental health nursing provides consultation to enhance the abilities of other clinicians to provide services for clients and effect change in the system.

> **Core Concept**
> **Evaluation**
> The process of determining both the client's progress toward the attainment of expected outcomes and the effectiveness of nursing care.

Standard VI. Evaluation

The Psychiatric/Mental Health Nurse Evaluates the Client's Progress in Attaining Expected Outcomes.

Rationale. Nursing care is a dynamic process involving change in the client's health status over time, giving rise to the need for data, different diagnoses, and modifications in the plan of care. Therefore, evaluation is a continuous process of appraising the effect of nursing and the treatment regimen on the client's health status and expected health outcomes (ANA, 2000, p. 40).

During the evaluation step, the nurse measures the success of the interventions in meeting the outcome criteria. The client's response to treatment is documented, validating use of the nursing process in the delivery of care. The diagnoses, outcomes, and plan of care are reviewed and revised as need is determined by the evaluation.

WHY NURSING DIAGNOSIS?

The concept of **nursing diagnosis** is not new. For centuries, nurses have identified specific client responses for which nursing interventions were used in an effort to improve quality of life. However, the autonomy of practice to which nurses were entitled by virtue of their licensure was historically lacking in the provision of nursing care. Nurses assisted physicians as required, and performed a group of specific tasks that were considered within their scope of responsibility.

The term *diagnosis* in relation to nursing first began to appear in the literature in the early 1950s. The formalized organization of the concept, however, was initiated only in 1973 with the convening of the First Task Force to Name and Classify Nursing Diagnoses. The Task Force of the National Conference Group on the Classification of Nursing Diagnoses was developed during this conference (NANDA International, 2004a). These individuals were charged with the task of identifying and classifying nursing diagnoses.

Also in the 1970s, the ANA began to write standards of practice around the steps of the nursing process, of which nursing diagnosis is an inherent part. This format encompassed both the general and specialty standards outlined by the ANA. The standards of psychiatric/mental health nursing practice are summarized in Table 9–3.

From this progression a statement of policy was published in 1980 and included a definition of nursing. The ANA defined nursing as "the diagnosis and treatment of human responses to actual or potential health problems" (ANA, 2003). This definition has been expanded to more appropriately describe nursing's commitment to society and to the profession itself. The ANA (2003) defines nursing as follows:

> Nursing is the protection, promotion, and optimization of health and abilities, prevention of illness and injury, alleviation of suffering through the diagnosis and treatment of human response, and advocacy in the care of individuals, families, communities, and populations. (p. 6)

Nursing diagnosis is an inherent component of both the original and expanded definitions.

TABLE 9–3 Standards of Psychiatric-Mental Health Clinical Nursing Practice

Standard I. Assessment

The psychiatric/mental health nurse collects client health data.

Standard II. Diagnosis

The psychiatric/mental health nurse analyzes the assessment data in determining diagnoses.

Standard III. Outcome Identification

The psychiatric/mental health nurse identifies expected outcomes individualized to the client.

Standard IV. Planning

The psychiatric/mental health nurse develops a plan of care that is negotiated among the client, nurse, family, and health care team and prescribes evidence based interventions to attain expected outcomes.

Standard V. Implementation

The psychiatric/mental health nurse implements the interventions identified in the plan of care.

Standard Va. Counseling

The psychiatric/mental health nurse uses counseling interventions to assist clients in improving or regaining their previous coping abilities, fostering mental health, and preventing mental illness and disability.

Standard Vb. Milieu Therapy

The psychiatric/mental health nurse provides, structures, and maintains a therapeutic environment in collaboration with the client and other health care clinicians.

Standard Vc. Promotion of Self-Care Activities

The psychiatric/mental health nurse structures interventions around the client's activities of daily living to foster self-care and mental and physical well-being.

Standard Vd. Psychobiological Interventions

The psychiatric/mental health nurse uses knowledge of psychobiological interventions and applies clinical skills to restore the client's health and prevent further disability.

Standard Ve. Health Teaching

The psychiatric/mental health nurse, through health teaching, assists clients in achieving satisfying, productive, and healthy patterns of living.

Standard Vf. Case Management

The psychiatric/mental health nurse provides case management to coordinate comprehensive health services and ensure continuity of care.

Standard Vg. Health Promotion and Health Maintenance

The psychiatric/mental health nurse employs strategies and interventions to promote and maintain health and prevent mental illness.

Advanced Practice Interventions (Vh, Vi, & Vj)

Standard Vh. Psychotherapy

The certified specialist in psychiatric/mental health nursing uses individual, group, and family psychotherapy, and other therapeutic treatments to assist clients in preventing mental illness and disability, treating mental health disorders, and improving mental health status and functional abilities.

Standard Vi. Prescriptive Authority and Treatment

The certified specialist in psychiatric/mental health nursing uses prescriptive authority, procedures, and treatments in accordance with state and federal laws and regulations, to treat symptoms of psychiatric illness and improve functional health status.

Standard Vj. Consultation

The certified specialist in psychiatric/mental health nursing provides consultation to enhance the abilities of other clinicians to provide services for clients and effect change in the system.

Standard VI. Evaluation

The psychiatric/mental health nurse evaluates the client's progress in attaining expected outcomes.

SOURCE: *Scope and Standards of Psychiatric-Mental Health Nursing Practice,* American Nurses Association (2000). With permission.

Decisions regarding professional negligence are made based on the standards of practice defined by the ANA and the individual state nursing practice acts. A number of states have incorporated the steps of the nursing process, including nursing diagnosis, into the scope of nursing practice described in their nursing practice acts. When this is the case, it is the legal duty of the nurse to show that nursing process and nursing diagnosis were accurately implemented in the delivery of nursing care.

NANDA International evolved from the original task force that was convened in 1973 to name and classify nursing diagnoses. The major purpose of NANDA International is to "increase the visibility of nursing's contribution to patient care by continuing to develop, refine, and classify phenomena of concern to nurses" (NANDA International, 2004b). A list of nursing diagnoses approved by NANDA-I for use and testing is presented in Table 9–2. This list is by no means exhaustive or all-inclusive. For purposes of this text, however, the existing list will be used in an effort to maintain a common language within nursing and to encourage clinical testing of what is available.

The use of nursing diagnosis affords a degree of autonomy that historically has been lacking in the practice of nursing. Nursing diagnosis describes the client's condition, facilitating the prescription of interventions and establishment of parameters for outcome criteria based on what is uniquely nursing. The ultimate benefit is to the client, who receives effective and consistent nursing care based on knowledge of the problems that he or she is experiencing and of the most beneficial nursing interventions to resolve them.

NURSING CASE MANAGEMENT

With the advent of diagnosis-related groups (DRGs) and shorter hospital stays, the concept of **case management** has evolved. Case management is an innovative model of care delivery that can result in improved client care. Within this model, clients are assigned a manager who negotiates with multiple providers to obtain diverse services. This type of health care delivery process serves to decrease fragmentation of care while striving to contain cost of services.

Case management in the acute care setting strives to organize client care through an episode of illness so that specific clinical and financial outcomes are achieved within an allotted time frame. Commonly, the allotted time frame is determined by the established protocols for length of stay as defined by the DRGs.

Case management has been shown to be an effective method of treatment for individuals with a chronic mental illness. This type of care strives to improve function-ing by assisting the individual to solve problems, improve work and socialization skills, promote leisure-time activities, and enhance overall independence.

Ideally, case management incorporates concepts of care at the primary, secondary, and tertiary levels of prevention. Various definitions have emerged and should be clarified, as follows.

Managed care refers to a strategy employed by purchasers of health services who make determinations about various types of services in order to maintain quality and control costs (Bower, 1992). In a managed care program, individuals receive health care based on need, as assessed by coordinators of the providership. Managed care exists in many settings, including (but not limited to) the following:

- Insurance-based programs
- Employer-based medical providerships
- Social service programs
- The public health sector

Managed care may exist in virtually any setting in which medical providership is a part of the service; that is, in any setting in which an organization (whether private or government-based) is responsible for payment of health care services for a group of people. Examples of managed care are the health maintenance organizations (HMOs) and preferred provider organizations (PPOs).

Case management is the method used to achieve managed care. It is the actual coordination of services required to meet the needs of the client. Goals of case management are to:

> facilitate access to needed services and coordinate care for clients within the fragmented health care delivery system, prevent avoidable episodes of illness among at-risk clients, and control or reduce the cost of care borne by the client or third-part payers. (Bower, 1992, p. 8)

Types of clients who benefit from case management include (but are not limited to) the following:

- The frail elderly
- The developmentally disabled
- The physically handicapped
- The mentally handicapped
- Individuals with long-term medically complex problems that require multifaceted, costly care (e.g., high-risk infants, those with human immunodeficiency virus [HIV] or acquired immunodeficiency syndrome [AIDS], and transplant clients)
- Individuals who are severely compromised by an acute episode of illness or an acute exacerbation of a chronic illness (e.g., schizophrenia)

The **case manager** is responsible for negotiating with multiple health care providers to obtain a variety of services for the client. Bower (1992) states, "Nurses are particularly suited to provide case management for clients with multiple health problems that have a health-related component." The very nature of nursing, which incorporates knowledge about the biological, psychological, and sociocultural aspects related to human functioning, makes nurses highly appropriate as case managers. The ANA recommends that the minimum preparation for a nurse case manager is a baccalaureate degree in nursing with 3 years of appropriate clinical experience (Bower, 1992). Some case management programs prefer master's-prepared clinical nurse specialists who have experience working with the specific populations for whom the case management service will be rendered.

Critical Pathways of Care

Critical pathways of care (CPCs) have emerged as the tools for provision of care in a case management system. A critical pathway is a type of abbreviated plan of care that provides outcome-based guidelines for goal achievement within a designated length of stay. CPCs have been included in this text for selected psychiatric diagnoses. A sample CPC is presented in Table 9–4. Only one nursing diagnosis is used in this sample. A CPC may have nursing diagnoses for several individual problems.

Critical pathways of care are meant to be used by the entire interdisciplinary team, which may include nurse case manager, clinical nurse specialist, social worker, psy-

---

TABLE 9–4   **Sample Critical Pathway of Care for Client in Alcohol Withdrawal**

Estimated Length of Stay: 7 Days—Variations from Designated Pathway Should Be Documented in Progress Notes

Nursing Diagnoses and Categories of Care	Time Dimension	Goals and/or Actions	Time Dimension	Goals and/or Actions	Time Dimension	Discharge Outcome
Risk for injury related to CNS agitation					Day 7	Client shows no evidence of injury obtained during ETOH withdrawal
Referrals	Day 1	Psychiatrist Assess need for: Neurologist Cardiologist Internist			Day 7	Discharge with follow-up appointments as required.
Diagnostic studies	Day 1	Blood alcohol level Drug screen Chemistry profile Urinalysis Chest X-ray ECG	Day 4	Repeat of selected diagnostic studies as necessary.		
Additional assessments	Day 1 Day 1–5 Ongoing Ongoing	VS q4h I&O Restraints p.r.n. Assess withdrawal symptoms: tremors, nausea/vomiting, tachycardia, sweating, high blood pressure, seizures, insomnia, hallucinations	Day 2–3 Day 6 Day 4	VS q8h if stable DC I&O Marked decrease in objective withdrawal symptoms	Day 4–7 Day 7	VS b.i.d.; remain stable Discharge; absence of objective withdrawal symptoms
Medications	Day 1 Day 2 Day 1–6 Day 1–7	*Librium 200 mg in divided doses Librium 160 mg in divided doses Librium p.r.n. Maalox ac & hs *Note: Some physicians may elect to use Serax or Tegretol in the detoxification process	Day 3 Day 4	Librium 120 mg in divided doses Librium 80 mg in divided doses	Day 5 Day 6 Day 7	Librium 40 mg DC Librium Discharge; no withdrawal symptoms
Client education			Day 5	Discuss goals of AA and need for outpatient therapy	Day 7	Discharge with information regarding AA attendance or outpatient treatment

chiatrist, psychologist, dietitian, occupational therapist, recreational therapist, chaplain, and others. The team decides what categories of care are to be performed, by what date, and by whom. Each member of the team is then expected to carry out his or her functions according to the time line designated on the CPC. The nurse, as case manager, is ultimately responsible for ensuring that each of the assignments is carried out. If variations occur at any time in any of the categories of care, rationale must be documented in the progress notes.

For example, with the sample CPC presented, the nurse case manager may admit the client into the detoxification center. The nurse contacts the psychiatrist to inform him or her of the admission. The psychiatrist performs additional assessments to determine if other consults are required. The psychiatrist also writes the orders for the initial diagnostic work-up and medication regimen. Within 24 hours, the interdisciplinary team meets to decide on other categories of care, to complete the CPC, and to make individual care assignments from the CPC. This particular sample CPC relies heavily on nursing care of the client through the critical withdrawal period. However, other problems for the same client, such as imbalanced nutrition, impaired physical mobility, or spiritual distress, may involve other members of the team to a greater degree. Each member of the team stays in contact with the nurse case manager regarding individual assignments. Ideally, team meetings are held daily or every other day to review progress and modify the plan as required.

CPCs can be standardized, as they are intended to be used with uncomplicated cases. A CPC can be viewed as protocol for various clients with problems for which a designated outcome can be predicted.

APPLYING THE NURSING PROCESS IN THE PSYCHIATRIC SETTING

Based on the definition of mental health set forth in Chapter 2, the role of the nurse in psychiatry focuses on helping the client successfully adapt to stressors within the environment. Goals are directed toward change in thoughts, feelings, and behaviors that are age appropriate and congruent with local and cultural norms.

Therapy within the psychiatric setting is very often team, or **interdisciplinary**, oriented. Therefore, it is important to delineate nursing's involvement in the treatment regimen. Nurses are indeed valuable members of the team. Having progressed beyond the role of custodial caregiver in the psychiatric setting, nurses now provide services that are defined within the scope of nursing practice. Nursing diagnosis is helping to define these nursing boundaries, providing the degree of autonomy and professionalism that has for so long been unrealized.

For example, a newly admitted client with the medical diagnosis of schizophrenia may be demonstrating the following behaviors:

● Inability to trust others
● Verbalizing hearing voices
● Refusing to interact with staff and peers
● Expressing a fear of failure
● Poor personal hygiene

From these assessments, the treatment team may determine that the client has the following problems:

● Paranoid delusions
● Auditory hallucinations
● Social withdrawal
● Developmental regression

Team goals would be directed toward the following:

● Reducing suspiciousness
● Terminating auditory hallucinations
● Increasing feelings of self-worth

From this team treatment plan, nursing may identify the following nursing diagnoses:

1. Disturbed sensory perception, auditory (evidenced by hearing voices)
2. Disturbed thought processes (evidenced by delusions)
3. Low self-esteem (evidenced by fear of failure and social withdrawal)
4. Self-care deficit (evidenced by poor personal hygiene)

Nursing diagnoses are prioritized according to life-threatening potential. Maslow's hierarchy of needs is a good model to follow in prioritizing nursing diagnoses. In this instance, disturbed sensory perception (auditory) is identified as the priority nursing diagnosis, because the client may be hearing voices that command him or her to harm self or others. Nursing in psychiatry, regardless of the setting—hospital (inpatient or outpatient), office, home, community—is goal-directed care. The goals (or expected outcomes) are client oriented, are measurable, and focus on resolution of the problem (if this is realistic) or on a more short-term outcome (if resolution is unrealistic). For example, in the previous situation, expected outcomes for the identified nursing diagnoses might be as follows:

1. The client will demonstrate trust in one staff member within 5 days.
2. The client will verbalize understanding that the voices are not real (not heard by others) within 10 days.
3. The client will complete one simple craft project within 7 days.
4. The client will take responsibility for own self-care and perform activities of daily living independently by time of discharge.

Nursing's contribution to the interdisciplinary treatment regimen will focus on establishing trust on a one-to-one basis (thus reducing the level of anxiety that is promoting hallucinations), giving positive feedback for small day-to-day accomplishments in an effort to build self-esteem, and assisting with and encouraging independent self-care. These interventions describe *independent nursing* actions and goals that are evaluated apart from, while also being directed toward achievement of, the *team's* treatment goals.

In this manner of collaboration with other team members, nursing provides a service that is unique and based on sound knowledge of psychopathology, scope of practice, and legal implications of the role. Although there is no dispute that "following doctor's orders" continues to be accepted as a priority of care, nursing intervention that enhances achievement of the overall goals of treatment is being recognized for its important contribution. The nurse who administers a medication prescribed by the physician to decrease anxiety may also choose to stay with the anxious client and offer reassurance of safety and security, thereby providing an independent nursing action that is distinct from, yet complementary to, the medical treatment.

CONCEPT MAPPING*

Concept mapping is a diagrammatic teaching and learning strategy that allows students and faculty to visualize interrelationships between medical diagnoses, nursing diagnoses, assessment data, and treatments. The concept map care plan is an innovative approach to planning and organizing nursing care. Basically, it is a diagram of client problems and interventions. Compared to the commonly used column format care plans, concept map care plans are more succinct. They are practical, realistic, and time saving, and they serve to enhance critical-thinking skills and clinical reasoning ability.

The nursing process is foundational to developing and using the concept map care plan, just as it is with all types of nursing care plans. Client data are collected and analyzed, nursing diagnoses are formulated, outcome criteria are identified, nursing actions are planned and implemented, and the success of the interventions in meeting the outcome criteria is evaluated.

The concept map care plan may be presented in its entirety on one page, or the assessment data and nursing diagnoses may appear in diagram format on one page, with outcomes, interventions, and evaluation written on a second page. In addition, the diagram may appear in circular format, with nursing diagnoses and interventions branching off the "client" in the center of the diagram. Or, it may begin with the "client" at the top of the diagram, with branches emanating in a linear fashion downward.

As stated previously, the concept map care plan is based on the components of the nursing process. Accordingly, the diagram is assembled in the nursing process stepwise fashion, beginning with the client and his or her reason for needing care, nursing diagnoses with subjective and objective clinical evidence for each, nursing interventions, and outcome criteria for evaluation.

Figure 9–2 presents one example of a concept map care plan. It is assembled for the hypothetical client with schizophrenia discussed in the previous section on "Applying the Nursing Process in the Psychiatric Setting." Various colors may be used in the diagram to designate various components of the care plan. Lines are drawn to connect the various components to indicate any relationships that exist. For example, there may be a relationship between two nursing diagnoses (e.g., between the nursing diagnoses of pain or anxiety and disturbed sleep pattern). A line between these nursing diagnoses should be drawn to show the relationship.

Concept map care plans allow for a great deal of creativity on the part of the user, and permits viewing the "whole picture" without generating a great deal of paperwork. Because they reflect the steps of the nursing process, concept map care plans also are valuable guides for documentation of client care. Doenges, Moorhouse, and Murr (2005) state,

> As students, you are asked to develop plans of care that often contain more detail than what you see in the hospital plans of care. This is to help you learn how to apply the nursing process and create individualized client care plans. However, even though much time and energy may be spent focusing on filling the columns of traditional clinical care plan forms, some students never develop a holistic view of their clients and fail to visualize how each client need interacts with other identified needs. A new technique or learning tool [concept mapping] has been developed to assist you in visualizing the linkages, enhance your critical thinking skills, and facilitate the creative process of planning client care. (p. 33)

DOCUMENTATION OF THE NURSING PROCESS

Equally important as using the nursing process in the delivery of care is the written documentation that it has been used. Some contemporary nursing leaders are advocating that with solid standards of practice and procedures in place within the institution, nurses need only chart when there has been a deviation in the care as outlined by that standard. However, many legal decisions are still based on the precept that "if it was not charted, it was not done."

Because nursing process and nursing diagnosis are mandated by nursing practice acts in some states, documentation of their use is being considered in those states as evidence in determining certain cases of negligence by

---

*Content in this section is adapted from Doenges, Moorhouse, & Murr (2005) and Schuster (2002).

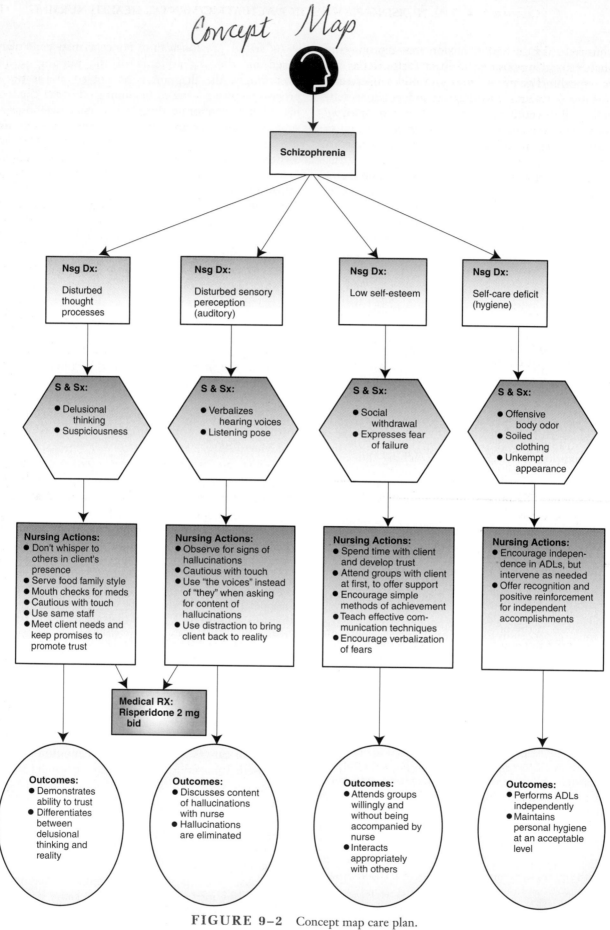

FIGURE 9–2 Concept map care plan.

nurses. Some health care organization accrediting agencies also require that nursing process be reflected in the delivery of care. Therefore, documentation must bear written testament to the use of the nursing process.

A variety of documentation methods can be used to reflect use of the nursing process in the delivery of nursing care. Three examples are presented here: problem-oriented recording (POR), Focus Charting®, and the problem, intervention, evaluation (PIE) system of documentation.

Problem-Oriented Recording

Problem-oriented recording follows the subjective, objective, assessment, plan, implementation, and evaluation (SOAPIE) format. It has as its basis a list of problems. When it is used in nursing, the problems (nursing diagnoses) are identified on a written plan of care with appropriate nursing interventions described for each. Documentation written in the SOAPIE format includes the following:

S = Subjective data: Information gathered from what the client, family, or other source has said or reported
O = Objective data: Information gathered by direct observation of the person performing the assessment; may include a physiological measurement such as blood pressure or a behavioral response such as affect
A = Assessment: The nurse's interpretation of the subjective and objective data
P = Plan: The actions or treatments to be carried out (may be omitted in daily charting if the plan is clearly explained in the written nursing care plan and no changes are expected)
I = Intervention: Those nursing actions that were actually carried out
E = Evaluation of the problem following nursing intervention (some nursing interventions cannot be evaluated immediately, so this section may be optional)

Table 9–5 shows how POR corresponds to the steps of the nursing process. Following is an example of a three-column documentation in the POR format.

DATE/TIME	PROBLEM	PROGRESS NOTES
6-22-04 1000	Social isolation	**S:** States he does not want to sit with or talk to others; "they frighten me" **O:** Stays in room alone unless strongly encouraged to come out; no group involvement; at times listens to group conversations from a distance but does not interact; some hypervigilance and scanning noted. **A:** Inability to trust; panic level of anxiety; delusional thinking **I:** Initiated trusting relationship by spending time alone with the client; discussed his feelings regarding interactions with others; accompanied client to group activities; provided positive feedback for voluntarily participating in assertiveness training

Focus Charting

Another type of documentation that reflects use of the nursing process is **Focus Charting**. Focus Charting differs from POR in that the main perspective has been changed from "problem" to "focus," and data, action, and response (DAR), has replaced SOAPIE.

Lampe (1985) suggests that a focus for documentation can be any of the following:

1. Nursing diagnosis
2. Current client concern or behavior
3. Significant change in the client status or behavior
4. Significant event in the client's therapy

The focus cannot be a medical diagnosis. The documentation is organized in the format of DAR. These categories are defined as follows:

D = Data: Information that supports the stated focus or describes pertinent observations about the client

---

TABLE 9–5	**Validation of the Nursing Process with Problem-Oriented Recording**	
PROBLEM-ORIENTED RECORDING	**WHAT IS RECORDED**	**NURSING PROCESS**
S and O (Subjective and Objective data)	Verbal reports to, and direct observation and examination by, the nurse	Assessment
A (Assessment)	Nurse's interpretation of S and O	Diagnosis and outcome identification
P (Plan) Omitted in charting if written plan describes care to be given	Description of appropriate nursing actions to resolve the identified problem	Planning
I (Intervention)	Description of nursing actions actually carried out	Implementation
E (Evaluation)	A reassessment of the situation to determine results of nursing actions implemented	Evaluation

TABLE 9–6	Validation of the Nursing Process with Focus Charting	
FOCUS CHARTING	WHAT IS RECORDED	NURSING PROCESS
D (Data)	Information that supports the stated focus or describes pertinent observations about the client.	Assessment
Focus	A nursing diagnosis; current client concern or behavior; significant change in client status; significant event in the client's therapy. **NOTE:** If outcome appears on written care plan, it need not be repeated in daily documentation unless a change occurs.	Diagnosis and outcome identification
A (Action)	Immediate or future nursing actions that address the focus; appraisal of the care plan along with any changes required.	Plan and implementation
R (Response)	Description of client responses to any part of the medical or nursing care.	Evaluation

A = Action: Immediate or future nursing actions that address the focus, and evaluation of the present care plan along with any changes required

R = Response: Description of client's responses to any part of the medical or nursing care.

Table 9–6 shows how Focus Charting corresponds to the steps of the nursing process. Following is an example of a three-column documentation in the DAR format.

DATE/TIME	FOCUS	PROGRESS NOTES
6-22-04 1000	Social isolation related to mistrust, panic anxiety, delusions	**D:** States he does not want to sit with or talk to others; they "frighten" him; stays in room alone unless strongly encouraged to come out; no group involvement; at times listens to group conversations from a distance, but does not interact; some hypervigilance and scanning noted **A:** Initiated trusting relationship by spending time alone with client; discussed his feelings regarding interactions with others; accompanied client to group activities; provided positive feedback for voluntarily participating in assertiveness training **R:** Cooperative with therapy; still acts uncomfortable in the presence of a group of people; accepted positive feedback from nurse

The PIE Method

PIE, or more specifically "APIE" (assessment, problem, intervention, evaluation), is a systematic method of documenting to nursing process and nursing diagnosis. A problem-oriented system, **PIE charting** uses accompanying flow sheets that are individualized by each institution. Criteria for documentation are organized in the following manner:

A = Assessment: A complete client assessment is conducted at the beginning of each shift. Results are documented under this section in the progress notes. Some institutions elect instead to use a daily client assessment sheet designed to meet specific needs of the unit. Explanation of any deviation from the norm is included in the progress notes.

P = Problem: A problem list, or list of nursing diagnoses, is an important part of the APIE method of charting. The name or number of the problem being addressed is documented in this section.

I = Intervention: Nursing actions are performed, directed at resolution of the problem.

E = Evaluation: Outcomes of the implemented interventions are documented, including an evaluation of client responses to determine the effectiveness of nursing interventions and the presence or absence of progress toward resolution of a problem.

Table 9–7 shows how APIE charting corresponds to the steps of the nursing process. Following is an example of a three-column documentation in the APIE format.

TABLE 9–7	Validation of the Nursing Process with APIE Method	
APIE CHARTING	WHAT IS RECORDED	NURSING PROCESS
A (Assessment)	Subjective and objective data about the client that are gathered at the beginning of each shift	Assessment
P (Problem)	Name (or number) of nursing diagnosis being addressed from written problem list, and identified outcome for that problem. **NOTE:** If outcome appears on written care plan, it need not be repeated in daily documentation unless a change occurs.	Diagnosis and outcome identification
I (Intervention)	Nursing actions performed, directed at problem resolution	Plan and implementation
E (Evaluation)	Appraisal of client responses to determine effectiveness of nursing interventions	Evaluation

DATE/TIME	PROBLEM	PROGRESS NOTES
6-22-04 1000	Social isolation	**A:** States he does not want to sit with or talk to others; they "frighten" him; stays in room alone unless strongly encouraged to come out; no group involvement; at times listens to group conversations from a distance but does not interact; some hypervigilance and scanning noted **P:** Social isolation related to inability to trust, panic level of anxiety, and delusional thinking **I:** Initiated trusting relationship by spending time alone with client; discussed his feelings regarding interactions with others; accompanied client to group activities; provided positive feedback for voluntarily participating in assertiveness training **E:** Cooperative with therapy; still uncomfortable in the presence of a group of people; accepted positive feedback from nurse.

SUMMARY

The nursing process provides a methodology by which nurses may deliver care using a systematic, scientific approach. The focus is goal directed and based on a decision-making or problem-solving model, consisting of six steps: assessment, diagnosis, outcome identification, planning, implementation, and evaluation.

Nursing diagnosis is inherent within the nursing process. The concept of nursing diagnosis is not new, but became formalized only with the organization of NANDA in the 1970s. Nursing diagnosis defines the scope and boundaries for nursing, thereby offering a degree of autonomy and independence so long restricted within the practice of nursing. Nursing diagnosis also provides a common language for nursing and assists nurses to provide consistent, quality care for their clients based on an increase in the body of nursing knowledge through research. A list of the nursing diagnoses approved by NANDA for use and testing was presented.

The psychiatric nurse uses the nursing process to assist clients to adapt successfully to stressors within the environment. Goals are directed toward change in thoughts, feelings, and behaviors that are age-appropriate and congruent with local and cultural norms. The nurse serves as a valuable member of the interdisciplinary treatment team, working both independently and cooperatively with other team members. Nursing diagnosis, in its ability to define the scope of nursing practice, is facilitating nursing's role in the psychiatric setting by differentiating that which is specifically nursing from interventions associated with other disciplines.

Nursing in psychiatry is goal-directed care. These goals are evaluated apart from, while also being directed toward achievement of, the team's treatment goals. The role of case management in psychiatric nursing is being expanded, and some institutions that employ this concept are using CPCs as the tool for treatment planning. The concept of case management was explored in this chapter and a sample CPC was included with an explanation for its use. Concept mapping, an innovative strategy for planning and organizing nursing care, was also presented.

Nurses must document that the nursing process has been used in the delivery of care. Its use is mandated in some states by their nurse practice act and also required by some health-care organization accrediting agencies. Three methods of documentation—POR, Focus Charting, and the PIE system—were presented with examples to demonstrate how they reflect use of the nursing process.

REVIEW QUESTIONS

SELF-EXAMINATION/LEARNING EXERCISE

Test your knowledge of nursing process by supplying the information requested.

1. Name the six steps of the nursing process.

2. Identify the step of the nursing process to which each of the following nursing actions applies:
   a. Obtains a short-term contract from the client to seek out staff if feeling suicidal
   b. Identifies nursing diagnosis: Risk for suicide
   c. Determines if nursing interventions have been appropriate to achieve desired results
   d. Client's family reports recent suicide attempt
   e. Prioritizes the necessity for maintaining a safe environment for the client
   f. Establishes goal of care: Client will not harm self during hospitalization.

3. S.T. is a 15-year-old girl who has just been admitted to the adolescent psychiatric unit with a diagnosis of anorexia nervosa. She is 5'5" tall and weighs 82 lb. She was elected to the cheerleading squad for the fall but states that she is not as good as the others on the squad. The treatment team has identified the following problems: refusal to eat, occasional purging, refusing to interact with staff and peers, and fear of failure.

   Formulate three nursing diagnoses and identify outcomes for each that nursing could use as a part of the treatment team to contribute both independently and cooperatively to the team treatment plan.

4. Review various methods of documentation that reflect delivery of nursing care via the nursing process. Practice making entries for the case described in question 3 using the various methods.

REFERENCES

American Nurses' Association (ANA). (2004). *Nursing: Scope and standards of practice*. Washington, DC: ANA.
American Nurses' Association. (2003). *Nursing's social policy statement* (2nd ed). Washington, DC: ANA.
American Nurses' Association. (2000). *Scope and standards of psychiatric-mental health nursing practice*. Washington, DC: American Nurses' Association.
American Psychiatric Association (APA). (2000). *Diagnosis and statistical manual of mental disorders* (4th ed.) *Text revision*. Washington, DC: American Psychiatric Association.
Bower, K.A. (1992). *Case management by nurses*. Washington, DC: American Nurses Publishing.
Doenges, M.E., Moorhouse, M.F., & Murr, A.C. (2005). *Nursing diagnosis manual: Planning, individualizing, and documenting client care*. Philadelphia: F.A. Davis.
Dochterman, J.M., & Bulechek, G. (2004). Nursing interventions classification overview. Retrieved November 1, 2004 from the World Wide Web at http://www.nursing.uiowa.edu/centers/cncce/nic/nicoverview.htm
Johnson, M., Bulechek, G., Dochterman, J.M., Maas, M., &

Moorhead, S. (2001). *Nursing diagnoses, outcomes, & interventions: NANDA, NOC, and NIC linkages*. St. Louis: C.V. Mosby.
Johnson, M., Maas, M., & Moorhead, S. (2004). Nursing outcomes classification overview. Retrieved November 1, 2004 from the World Wide Web at http://www.nursing.uiowa.edu/centers/cncce/noc/nocoverview.htm
Lampe, S.S. (1985). Focus charting: Streamlining documentation. *Nursing Management, 16*(7), 43–46.
NANDA International. (2005). *Nursing diagnoses: Definitions and classification, 2005–2006*. Philadelphia: NANDA International.
NANDA International. (2004a). *History and historical highlights 1973 through 1998*. Retrieved November 2, 2004 from the World Wide Web at http://www.nanda.org/html/history1.html
NANDA International. (2004b). *About NANDA International*. Retrieved November 2, 2004 from the World Wide Web at http://www.nanda.org/html/about.html
Schuster, P.M. (2002). *Concept mapping: A critical-thinking approach to care planning*. Philadelphia: F.A. Davis.
World Health Organization (WHO). (1993). *International classification of diseases* (10th ed.). Geneva: World Health Organization.

THERAPEUTIC GROUPS

CHAPTER OUTLINE

OBJECTIVES

FUNCTIONS OF A GROUP

TYPES OF GROUPS

PHYSICAL CONDITIONS THAT INFLUENCE
GROUP DYNAMICS

CURATIVE FACTORS

PHASES OF GROUP DEVELOPMENT

LEADERSHIP STYLES

MEMBER ROLES

PSYCHODRAMA

THE ROLE OF THE NURSE IN
GROUP THERAPY

SUMMARY

REVIEW QUESTIONS

KEY TERMS

altruism
autocratic
catharsis
democratic

laissez-faire
psychodrama
universality

CORE CONCEPTS

group
group therapy

OBJECTIVES

After reading this chapter, the student will be able to:

1. Define a group.
2. Discuss eight functions of a group.
3. Identify various types of groups.
4. Describe physical conditions that influence groups.
5. Discuss "curative factors" that occur in groups.
6. Describe the phases of group development.

7. Identify various leadership styles in groups.
8. Identify various roles that members assume within a group.
9. Discuss psychodrama as a specialized form of group therapy.
10. Describe the role of the nurse in group therapy.

 uman beings are complex creatures who share their activities of daily living with various *groups* of people. Sampson and Marthas (1990) state:

We are *biological* organisms possessing qualities shared with all living systems and with others of our species. We are *psychological* beings with distinctly human capabilities for thought, feeling, and action. We are also *social* beings, who function as part of the complex webs that link us with other people. (p. 3)

Health care professionals not only share their personal lives with groups of people but also encounter multiple group situations in their professional operations. Team conferences, committee meetings, grand rounds, and in-service sessions are but a few. In psychiatry, work with clients and families often takes the form of groups. With group work, not only does the nurse have the opportunity to reach out to a greater number of people at one time, but those individuals also assist each other by bringing to the group and sharing their feelings,

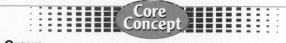

Group

A *group* is a collection of individuals whose association is founded on shared commonalities of interest, values, norms, or purpose. Membership in a group is generally by chance (born into the group), by choice (voluntary affiliation), or by circumstance (the result of life-cycle events over which an individual may or may not have control).

opinions, ideas, and behaviors. Clients learn from each other in a group setting.

This chapter explores various types and methods of therapeutic groups that can be used with psychiatric clients, and the role of the nurse in group intervention.

FUNCTIONS OF A GROUP

Sampson and Marthas (1990) have outlined eight functions that groups serve for their members. They contend that groups may serve more than one function and usually serve different functions for different members of the group. The eight functions are as follows:

1. **Socialization**. The cultural group into which we are born begins the process of teaching social norms. This is continued throughout our lives by members of other groups with which we become affiliated.
2. **Support**. One's fellow group members are available in time of need. Individuals derive a feeling of security from group involvement.
3. **Task Completion**. Group members provide assistance in endeavors that are beyond the capacity of one individual alone or when results can be achieved more effectively as a team.
4. **Camaraderie**. Members of a group provide the joy and pleasure that individuals seek from interactions with significant others.
5. **Informational**. Learning takes place within groups. Explanations regarding world events occur in groups. Knowledge is gained when individual members learn how others in the group have resolved situations similar to those with which they are currently struggling.
6. **Normative**. This function relates to the ways in which groups enforce the established norms.
7. **Empowerment**. Groups help to bring about improvement in existing conditions by providing support to individual members who seek to bring about change. Groups have power that individuals on their own do not.
8. **Governance**. An example of the governing function is that of rules being made by committees within a larger organization.

TYPES OF GROUPS

The functions of a group vary depending on the reason the group was formed. Clark (1994) identifies three types of groups in which nurses most often participate: task, teaching, and supportive/therapeutic groups.

Task Groups

The function of a task group is to accomplish a specific outcome or task. The focus is on solving problems and making decisions to achieve this outcome. Often a deadline is placed on completion of the task, and such importance is placed on a satisfactory outcome that conflict in the group may be smoothed over or ignored in order to focus on the priority at hand.

Teaching Groups

Teaching, or educational, groups exist to convey knowledge and information to a number of individuals. Nurses can be involved in teaching groups of many varieties, such as medication education, childbirth education, breast self-examination, and effective parenting classes. These groups usually have a set time frame or a set number of meetings. Members learn from each other as well as from the designated instructor. The objective of teaching groups is verbalization or demonstration by the learner of the material presented by the end of the designated period.

Supportive/Therapeutic Groups

The primary concern of support groups is to prevent future upsets by teaching participants effective ways of dealing with emotional stress arising from situational or developmental crises.

Group Therapy

A form of psychosocial treatment in which a number of clients meet together with a therapist for purposes of sharing, gaining personal insight, and improving interpersonal coping strategies.

For the purposes of this text, it is important to differentiate between "therapeutic groups" and "**group therapy**." Leaders of group therapy generally have advanced degrees in psychology, social work, nursing, or medicine. They often have additional training or experience under the supervision of an accomplished professional in conducting group psychotherapy based on various theoretical frameworks such as psychoanalytic, psychodynamic, interpersonal, or family dynamics. Approaches based on these theories are used by the group therapy leaders to encourage improvement in the ability of group members to function on an interpersonal level.

Therapeutic groups, on the other hand, are based to a lesser degree in theory. Focus is more on group relationships, interactions among group members, and the consideration of a selected issue. Like group therapists, individuals who lead therapeutic groups must be knowledgeable in *group process*; that is, the *way* in which group members interact with each other. Interruptions, silences, judgments, glares, and scapegoating are examples of group processes (Clark, 1994). They must also have thorough knowledge of *group content*, the topic or issue being discussed within the group, and the ability to present the topic in language that can be understood by all group members. Many nurses who work in psychiatry lead supportive/therapeutic groups.

Self-Help Groups

An additional type of group, in which nurses may or may not be involved, is the self-help group. Self-help groups have grown in numbers and in credibility in recent years. They allow clients to talk about their fears and relieve feelings of isolation, while receiving comfort and advice from others undergoing similar experiences (Harvard Medical School, 1998). Examples of self-help groups are Alzheimer's Disease and Related Disorders, Anorexia Nervosa and Associated Disorders, Weight Watchers, Alcoholics Anonymous, Reach to Recovery, Parents Without Partners, Overeaters Anonymous, Adult Children of Alcoholics, and many others related to specific needs or illnesses. These groups may or may not have a professional leader or consultant. They are run by the members, and leadership often rotates from member to member.

Nurses may become involved with self-help groups either voluntarily or because their advice or participation has been requested by the members. The nurse may function as a referral agent, resource person, member of an advisory board, or leader of the group. Self-help groups are a valuable source of referral for clients with specific problems. However, nurses must be knowledgeable about the purposes of the group, membership, leadership, benefits, and problems that might threaten the success of the group before making referrals to their clients for a specific self-help group. The nurse may find it necessary to attend several meetings of a particular group, if possible, to assess its effectiveness of purpose and appropriateness for client referral.

PHYSICAL CONDITIONS THAT INFLUENCE GROUP DYNAMICS

Seating

The physical conditions for the group should be set up so that there is no barrier between the members. For example, a circle of chairs is better than chairs set around a table. Members should be encouraged to sit in different chairs each meeting. This openness and change creates an uncomfortableness that encourages anxious and unsettled behaviors that can then be explored within the group.

Size

Various authors have suggested different ranges of size as ideal for group interaction: 4 to 7 (Huber, 1996), 2 to 15 (Sampson & Marthas, 1990), and 4 to 12 (Clark, 1994). Group size does make a difference in the interaction among members. The larger the group, the less time is available to devote to individual members. In fact, in larger groups, those more aggressive individuals are most likely to be heard, whereas quieter members may be left out of the discussions altogether. On the other hand, larger groups provide more opportunities for individuals to learn from other members. The wider range of life experiences and knowledge provides a greater potential for effective group problem solving. Studies have indicated that a composition of 7 or 8 members provides a favorable climate for optimal group interaction and relationship development.

Membership

Whether the group is open or closed ended is another condition that influences the dynamics of group process. Open-ended groups are those in which members leave and others join at any time while the group exists. The continuous movement of members in and out of the group creates the type of uncomfortableness described previously that encourages unsettled behaviors in individual members and fosters the exploration of feelings. These are the most common types of groups held on short-term inpatient units, although they are used in outpatient and long-term care facilities as well. Closed-ended groups usually have a predetermined, fixed time frame. All members join at the time the group is organized and terminate at the end of the designated time period. Closed-ended groups are often composed of individuals with common issues or problems they wish to address.

CURATIVE FACTORS

Why are therapeutic groups helpful? Yalom (1985) identified 11 curative factors that individuals can achieve

YALOM - CURATIVE FACTORS

through interpersonal interactions within the group. Some of the factors are present in most groups in varying degrees. These curative factors identified by Yalom include the following:

1. **The Instillation of Hope.** By observing the progress of others in the group with similar problems, a group member garners hope that his or her problems can also be resolved.

2. **Universality.** Individuals come to realize that they are not alone in the problems, thoughts, and feelings they are experiencing. Anxiety is relieved by the support and understanding of others in the group who share similar (universal) experiences.

3. **The Imparting of Information**. Knowledge is gained through formal instruction as well as the sharing of advice and suggestions among group members.

4. **Altruism. Altruism** is assimilated by group members through mutual sharing and concern for each other. Providing assistance and support to others creates a positive self-image and promotes self-growth.

5. **The Corrective Recapitulation of the Primary Family Group.** Group members are able to re-experience early family conflicts that remain unresolved. Attempts at resolution are promoted through feedback and exploration.

6. **The Development of Socializing Techniques**. Through interaction with and feedback from other members within the group, individuals are able to correct maladaptive social behaviors and learn and develop new social skills.

7. **Imitative Behavior.** In this setting, one who has mastered a particular psychosocial skill or developmental task can be a valuable role model for others. Individuals may imitate selected behaviors that they wish to develop in themselves.

8. **Interpersonal Learning.** The group offers many and varied opportunities for interacting with other people. Insight is gained regarding how one perceives and is being perceived by others.

9. **Group Cohesiveness.** Members develop a sense of belonging that separates the individual ("I am") from the group ("we are"). Out of this alliance emerges a common feeling that both individual members and the total group are of value to each other.

10. **Catharsis.** Within the group, members are able to express both positive and negative feelings—perhaps feelings that have never been expressed before—in a nonthreatening atmosphere. This **catharsis**, or open expression of feelings, is beneficial for the individual within the group.

11. **Existential Factors.** The group is able to help individual members take direction of their own lives and to accept responsibility for the quality of their existence.

It may be helpful for a group leader to explain these curative factors to members of the group. Positive responses are experienced by individuals who understand and are able to recognize curative factors as they occur within the group.

PHASES OF GROUP DEVELOPMENT

Groups, like individuals, move through phases of life-cycle development. Ideally, groups will progress from the phase of infancy to advanced maturity in an effort to fulfill the objectives set forth by the membership. Unfortunately, as with individuals, some groups become fixed in early developmental levels and never progress, or experience periods of regression in the developmental process. Three phases of group development are discussed here.

Phase I. Initial or Orientation Phase

Group Activities

The leader and members work together to establish the rules that will govern the group (e.g., when and where meetings will occur, the importance of confidentiality, how meetings will be structured). Goals of the group are established. Members are introduced to each other.

Leader Expectations

The leader is expected to orient members to specific group processes, encourage members to participate without disclosing too much too soon, promote an environment of trust, and ensure that rules established by the group do not interfere with fulfillment of the goals.

Member Behaviors

In phase I, members have not yet established trust and will respond to this lack of trust by being overly polite. There is a fear of not being accepted by the group. They may try to "get on the good side" of the leader with compliments and conforming behaviors. A power struggle may ensue as members compete for their positions in the "pecking order" of the group.

Phase II. Middle or Working Phase

Group Activities

Ideally, during the working phase, cohesiveness has been established within the group. This is when the productive work toward completion of the task is undertaken. Problem solving and decision making occur within the group. In the mature group, cooperation prevails, and differences and disagreements are confronted and resolved.

Leader Expectations

The role of leader diminishes and becomes more one of facilitator during the working phase. Some leadership functions are shared by certain members of the group as they progress toward resolution. The leader helps to resolve conflict and continues to foster cohesiveness among the members while ensuring that they do not deviate from the intended task or purpose for which the group was organized.

Member Behaviors

At this point trust has been established among the members. They turn more often to each other and less often to the leader for guidance. They accept criticism from each other, using it in a constructive manner to create change. Occasionally, subgroups will form in which two or more members conspire with each other to the exclusion of the rest of the group. To maintain group cohesion, these subgroups must be confronted and discussed by the entire membership. Conflict is managed by the group with minimal assistance from the leader.

Phase III. Final or Termination Phase

Group Activities

The longer a group has been in existence, the more difficult termination is likely to be for the members. Termination should be mentioned from the outset of group formation. It should be discussed in depth for several meetings prior to the final session. A sense of loss that precipitates the grief process may be evident, particularly in groups that have been successful in their stated purpose.

Leader Expectations

In the termination phase, the leader encourages the group members to reminisce about what has occurred within the group, to review the goals and discuss the actual outcomes, and to encourage members to provide feedback to each other about individual progress within the group. The leader encourages members to discuss feelings of loss associated with termination of the group.

Member Behaviors

Members may express surprise over the actual materialization of the end. This represents the grief response of denial, which may then progress to anger. Anger toward other group members or toward the leader may reflect feelings of abandonment (Sampson & Marthas, 1990). These feelings may lead to individual members' discussions of previous losses for which similar emotions were experienced. Successful termination of the group may help members develop the skills needed when losses occur in other dimensions of their lives.

LEADERSHIP STYLES

Three of the most common group leadership styles have been described by Lippitt and White (1958). They include autocratic, democratic, and laissez-faire.

Autocratic

Autocratic leaders have personal goals for the group. They withhold information from group members, particularly issues that may interfere with achievement of their own objectives. The message that is conveyed to the group is: "We will do it my way. My way is best." The focus in this style of leadership is on the leader. Members are dependent on the leader for problem solving, decision-making, and permission to perform. The approach of the autocratic leader is one of persuasion, striving to persuade others in the group that his or her ideas and methods are superior. Productivity is high with this type of leadership, but often morale within the group is low because of lack of member input and creativity.

Democratic

The **democratic** leadership style focuses on the members of the group. Information is shared with members in an effort to allow them to make decisions regarding achieving the goals for the group. Members are encouraged to participate fully in problem solving of issues that relate to the group, including taking action to effect change. The message that is conveyed to the group is: "Decide what must be done, consider the alternatives, make a selection, and proceed with the actions required to complete the task." The leader provides guidance and expertise as needed. Productivity is lower than it is with autocratic leadership, but morale is much higher because of the extent of input allowed all members of the group and the potential for individual creativity.

Laissez-Faire

This leadership style allows people to do as they please. There is no direction from the leader. In fact, the **laissez-faire** leader's approach is noninvolvement. Goals for the group are undefined. No decisions are made, no

TABLE 10–1	Leadership Styles—Similarities and Differences		
CHARACTERISTICS	AUTOCRATIC	DEMOCRATIC	LAISSEZ-FAIRE
1. Focus	Leader	Members	Undetermined
2. Task strategy	Members are persuaded to adopt leader ideas	Members engage in group problem solving	No defined strategy exists
3. Member participation	Limited	Unlimited	Inconsistent
4. Individual creativity	Stifled	Encouraged	Not addressed
5. Member enthusiasm and morale	Low	High	Low
6. Group cohesiveness	Low	High	Low
7. Productivity	High	High (may not be as high as autocratic)	Low
8. Individual motivation and commitment	Low (tend to work only when leader is present to urge them to do so)	High (satisfaction derived from personal input and participation)	Low (feelings of frustration from lack of direction or guidance)

problems are solved, and no action is taken. Members become frustrated and confused, and productivity and morale are low.

Table 10–1 outlines various similarities and differences among the three leadership styles.

MEMBER ROLES

Benne and Sheats (1948) identified three major types of roles that individuals play within the membership of the group. These are roles that serve to:

1. Complete the task of the group.
2. Maintain or enhance group processes.
3. Fulfill personal or individual needs.

Task roles and maintenance roles contribute to the success or effectiveness of the group. Personal roles satisfy needs of the individual members, sometimes to the extent of interfering with the effectiveness of the group.

Table 10–2 presents an outline of specific roles within these three major types and the behaviors associated with each.

PSYCHODRAMA

A specialized type of therapeutic group, called **psychodrama**, was introduced by J. L. Moreno, a Viennese psychiatrist. Moreno's method employs a dramatic approach in which clients become "actors" in life-situation scenarios.

The group leader is called the *director*, group members are the *audience*, and the *set*, or *stage*, may be specially designed or may just be any room or part of a room selected for this purpose. Actors are members from the audience who agree to take part in the "drama" by role-playing a situation about which they have been informed by the director. Usually the situation is an issue with which one individual client has been struggling. The

client plays the role of himself or herself and is called the *protagonist*. In this role, the client is able to express true feelings toward individuals (represented by group members) with whom he or she has unresolved conflicts.

In some instances, the group leader may ask for a client to volunteer to be the protagonist for that session. The client may choose a situation he or she wishes to enact and select the audience members to portray the roles of others in the life situation. The psychodrama setting provides the client with a safer and less threatening atmosphere than the real situation in which to express true feelings. Resolution of interpersonal conflicts is facilitated.

When the drama has been completed, group members from the audience discuss the situation they have observed, offer feedback, express their feelings, and relate their own similar experiences. In this way, all group members benefit from the session, either directly or indirectly.

Nurses often serve as actors, or role players, in psychodrama sessions. Leaders of psychodrama have graduate degrees in psychology, social work, nursing, or medicine with additional training in group therapy and specialty preparation to become a psychodramatist.

THE ROLE OF THE NURSE IN GROUP THERAPY

Nurses participate in group situations on a daily basis. In health care settings, nurses serve on or lead task groups that create policy, describe procedures, and plan client care. They are also involved in a variety of other groups aimed at the institutional effort of serving the consumer. Nurses are encouraged to use the steps of the nursing process as a framework for task group leadership.

In psychiatry, nurses may lead various types of therapeutic groups, such as client education, assertiveness training, support, parent, and transition to discharge groups, among others. To function effectively in the

ROLE	BEHAVIORS
TABLE 10–2	**Member Roles Within Groups**

Task Roles

Coordinator	Clarifies ideas and suggestions that have been made within the group; brings relationships together to pursue common goals.
Evaluator	Examines group plans and performance, measuring against group standards and goals.
Elaborator	Explains and expands upon group plans and ideas.
Energizer	Encourages and motivates group to perform at its maximum potential.
Initiator	Outlines the task at hand for the group and proposes methods for solution.
Orienter	Maintains direction within the group.

Maintenance Roles

Compromiser	Relieves conflict within the group by assisting members to reach a compromise agreeable to all.
Encourager	Offers recognition and acceptance of others' ideas and contributions.
Follower	Listens attentively to group interaction; is passive participant.
Gatekeeper	Encourages acceptance of and participation by all members of the group.
Harmonizer	Minimizes tension within the group by intervening when disagreements produce conflict.

Individual (Personal) Roles

Aggressor	Expresses negativism and hostility toward other members; may use sarcasm in effort to degrade the status of others.
Blocker	Resists group efforts; demonstrates rigid and sometimes irrational behaviors that impede group progress.
Dominator	Manipulates others to gain control; behaves in authoritarian manner.
Help-seeker	Uses the group to gain sympathy from others; seeks to increase self-confidence from group feedback; lacks concern for others or for the group as a whole.
Monopolizer	Maintains control of the group by dominating the conversation.
Mute or silent member	Does not participate verbally; remains silent for a variety of reasons—may feel uncomfortable with self-disclosure or may be seeking attention through silence.
Recognition seeker	Talks about personal accomplishments in an effort to gain attention for self.
Seducer	Shares intimate details about self with group; is the least reluctant of the group to do so; may frighten others in the group and inhibit group progress with excessive premature self-disclosure.

SOURCE: Adapted from Benne and Sheats (1948).

leadership capacity for these groups, nurses need to be able to recognize various processes that occur in groups (such as the phases of group development, the various roles that people play within group situations, and the motivation behind the behavior). They also need to be able to select the most appropriate leadership style for the type of group being led. Generalist nurses may develop these skills as part of their undergraduate education, or they may pursue additional study while serving and learning as the coleader of a group with a more experienced nurse leader.

Generalist nurses in psychiatry rarely serve as leaders of psychotherapy groups. American Nurses Association (ANA) guidelines specify that nurses who serve as group psychotherapists should have a minimum of a master's degree in psychiatric nursing. Other criteria that have been suggested are educational preparation in group theory, extended practice as a group coleader or leader under the supervision of an experienced psychotherapist, and participation in group therapy on an experiential level. Additional specialist training is required beyond the master's level to prepare nurses to become family therapists or psychodramatists.

Leading therapeutic groups is within the realm of nursing practice. Because group work is such a common therapeutic approach in the discipline of psychiatry, nurses working in this field must continually strive to

expand their knowledge and use of group process as a significant psychiatric nursing intervention.

SUMMARY

A *group* has been defined as a collection of individuals whose association is founded on shared commonalities of interest, values, norms, or purpose. Groups serve various functions for their members. Eight group functions were defined by Sampson and Marthas (1990). They include *socialization, support, task completion, camaraderie, informational, normative, empowerment,* and *governance.*

Three types of groups were identified: (1) task groups, whose function is to solve problems, make decisions, and achieve a specific outcome; (2) teaching groups, in which knowledge and information are conveyed to a number of individuals; and (3) supportive/therapeutic groups, whose function is to educate people to deal effectively with emotional stress in their lives. Self-help groups can be beneficial to clients with specific problems. In self-help groups, members share similar problems and help each other to prevent decompensation related to those problems. Professionals may or may not be a part of self-help groups.

Group therapy is differentiated from *therapeutic groups* by degree of educational preparation of the leader.

Group psychotherapists have advanced degrees in psychology, social work, medicine, or nursing. The focus of group psychotherapy is more theoretically based than it is in therapeutic groups.

Certain physical conditions, such as placement of the seating and size of the group, influence group interaction. Whether the group is open ended or closed ended can also affect group performance. In an *open-ended* group, members leave and others join at any time while the group exists. *Closed-ended* groups have a predetermined, fixed time frame. All members join the group at the same time and leave at the end of the designated time period.

Yalom (1985) identified a number of benefits that individuals derive from participation in therapeutic groups. He called these benefits *curative factors*. They include the instillation of hope, universality, the imparting of information, altruism, the corrective recapitulation of the primary family group, the development of socializing techniques, imitative behavior, interpersonal learning, group cohesiveness, catharsis, and existential factors.

Groups progress through three major phases of development. In the initial (orientation) phase, members are introduced to each other, rules and goals of the group are established, and a trusting relationship is initiated. In the second phase, called the middle or working phase, the actual work of the group takes place. As the group matures, trust is established and members cooperate in decision making and problem solving, with the leader at that time serving more as a facilitator. The final or termination phase can be difficult, particularly if the group has been together for a long time. A sense of loss can trigger the grief response, and it is essential that members confront these feelings and work through them before the final session.

Group leadership styles may vary. The *autocratic* leader concentrates on fulfillment of his or her own objectives for the group. This is achieved through persuasive selling of personal ideas to the group. Productivity is high with this type of leader, but morale and motivation are low. With a *democratic* leader, group members are encouraged to participate fully in the decision-making process. The leader provides guidance and expertise as needed. Productivity is lower than with autocratic leadership, but morale and motivation are much higher. In a group with *laissez-faire* leadership, the members essentially receive no direction at all. Goals are not established, decisions are not made, everyone does as he or she pleases, and confusion prevails. Productivity, morale, and motivation are low.

Members play various roles within groups. These roles are categorized according to *task roles*, *maintenance roles*, and *personal roles*. Task roles and maintenance roles contribute to the success or effectiveness of the group. Personal roles satisfy needs of the individual members, sometimes to the extent of interfering with the effectiveness of the group.

Psychodrama is a specialized type of group therapy that uses a dramatic approach in which clients become "actors" in life-situation scenarios. The psychodrama setting provides the client with a safer and less threatening atmosphere than the real situation in which to express and work through unresolved conflicts. Specialized training, in addition to a master's degree, is required for nurses to serve as psychodramatists.

Nurses lead various types of therapeutic groups in the psychiatric setting. Knowledge of human behavior in general and the group process in particular is essential to effective group leadership.

REVIEW QUESTIONS

SELF-EXAMINATION/LEARNING EXERCISE

Test your knowledge of group process by supplying the information requested.

1. Define a *group*.

2. Identify the type of group and leadership style in each of the following situations:
   a. N.J. is the nurse leader of a childbirth preparation group. Each week she shows various films and sets out various reading materials. She expects the participants to utilize their time on a topic of their choice or practice skills they have observed on the films. Two couples have dropped out of the group, stating, "This is a big waste of time."
   Type of group _____
   Style of leadership _____
   b. M.K. is a psychiatric nurse who has been selected to lead a group for women who desire to lose weight. The criterion for membership is that they must be at least 20 lb overweight. All have tried to lose weight on their own many times in the past without success. At their first meeting, M.K. provides suggestions as the members determine what their goals will be and how they plan to go about achieving those goals. They decided how often they wanted to meet, and what they planned to do at each meeting.
   Type of group _____
   Style of leadership _____
   c. J.J. is a staff nurse on a surgical unit. He has been selected as leader of a newly established group of staff nurses organized to determine ways to decrease the number of medication errors occurring on the unit. J.J. has definite ideas about how to bring this about. He has also applied for the position of Head Nurse on the unit and believes that if he is successful in leading the group toward achievement of its goals, he can also facilitate his chances for promotion. At each meeting he addresses the group in an effort to convince the members to adopt his ideas.
   Type of group _____
   Style of leadership _____

Match the situation on the right to the curative factor or benefit it describes on the left.

_____ 3. Instillation of hope

_____ 4. Universality

_____ 5. Imparting of information

_____ 6. Altruism

_____ 7. Corrective recapitulation of the primary family group

_____ 8. Development of socializing techniques

_____ 9. Imitative behavior

_____ 10. Interpersonal learning

a. Sam admires the way Jack stands up for what he believes. He decides to practice this himself.

b. Nancy sees that Jane has been a widow for 5 years now, and has adjusted well. She thinks maybe she can too.

c. Susan has come to realize that she has the power to shape the direction of her life.

d. John is able to have a discussion with another person for the first time in his life.

e. Linda now understands that her mother really did love her, although she was not able to show it.

f. Alice has come to feel as though the other group members are like a family to her. She looks forward to the meetings each week.

g. Tony talks in the group about the abuse he experienced as a child. He has never told anyone about this before.

h. Sandra felt so good about herself when she left group tonight. She had provided both physical and emotional support to Judy who shared for the first time about being raped.

_____ 11. Group cohesiveness

i. Judy appreciated Sandra's support as she expressed her feelings related to the rape. She had come to believe that no one else felt as she did.

_____ 12. Catharsis

j. Paul knew that people did not want to be his friend because of his violent temper. In the group he has learned to control his temper and form satisfactory inter-personal relationships with others.

_____ 13. Existential factors

k. Henry learned about the effects of alcohol on the body when a nurse from the chemical dependency unit spoke to the group.

Match the individual on the right to the role he or she is playing within the group.

_____ 14. Aggressor

a. Nancy talks incessantly in group. When someone else tries to make a comment, she refuses to allow him or her to speak.

_____ 15. Blocker

b. On the first day the group meets, Valerie shares the intimate details of her incestuous relationship with her father.

_____ 16. Dominator

c. Colleen listens with interest to everything the other members say, but she herself does not say anything in group.

_____ 17. Help seeker

d. Violet is obsessed with her physical appearance. Although she is beautiful, she has little self-confidence and needs continuous positive feedback. She states, "Maybe if I became a blond my boyfriend would love me more."

_____ 18. Monopolizer

e. Larry states to Violet, "Listen, dummy, you need more than blond hair to keep the guy around. A bit more in the brains department would help!"

_____ 19. Mute or silent member

f. At the beginning of the group meeting, Dan says, "All right now, I have a date tonight. I want this meeting over on time! I'll keep track of the time and let everyone know when their time is up. When I say you're done, you're done, understand?"

_____ 20. Recognition seeker

g. Joyce says, "I won my first beauty contest when I was 6 months old. Can you imagine? And I've been winning them ever since. I was prom queen when I was 16, Miss Rose Petal when I was 19, Miss Silver City at 21. Next I go to the state contest. It's just all so exciting!"

_____ 21. Seducer

h. Joe, an RN on the care-planning committee says, "What a stupid suggestion. Nursing Diagnosis!?!? I won't even discuss the matter. We have been doing our care plans this way for 20 years. I refuse to even consider changing."

REFERENCES

Clark, C.C. (1994). *The nurse as group leader* (3rd ed.). New York: Springer.

Harvard Medical School. (1998, March). Cancer in the Mind. *Harvard Mental Health Letter, 14*(9), 1–5.

Huber, D. (1996). *Leadership and nursing care management.* Philadelphia: W.B. Saunders.

Sampson, E.E., & Marthas, M. (1990). Group process for the health professions (3rd ed.). Albany, NY: Delmar.

CLASSICAL REFERENCES

Benne, K.B., & Sheats, P. (1948, Spring). Functional roles of group members. *Journal of Social Issues, 4*(2), 42–49.

Lippitt, R., & White, R.K. (1958). An experimental study of leadership and group life. In E.E. Maccoby, T.M. Newcomb, & E.L.

Hartley (Eds.). *Readings in social psychology* (3rd ed.). New York: Holt, Rinehart, & Winston

Yalom, I. (1985). *The theory and practice of group psychotherapy* (3rd ed.). New York: Basic Books.

INTERVENTION WITH FAMILIES

CHAPTER OUTLINE

OBJECTIVES

STAGES OF FAMILY DEVELOPMENT

MAJOR VARIATIONS

FAMILY FUNCTIONING

THERAPEUTIC MODALITIES WITH FAMILIES

THE NURSING PROCESS—A CASE STUDY

SUMMARY

REVIEW QUESTIONS

KEY TERMS

boundaries
disengagement
double-bind
   communication
enmeshment
family structure
family system
genogram
marital schism

marital skew
paradoxical
   intervention
pseudohostility
pseudomutuality
reframing
scapegoating
subsystems
triangles

CORE CONCEPTS

family
family therapy

OBJECTIVES

After reading this chapter, the student will be able to:

1. Define the term *family*.
2. Identify stages of family development.
3. Describe major variations to the American middle-class family life cycle.
4. Discuss characteristics of adaptive family functioning.
5. Describe behaviors that interfere with adaptive family functioning.
6. Discuss the essential components of family systems, structural, and strategic therapies.
7. Construct a family genogram.
8. Apply the steps of the nursing process in therapeutic intervention with families.

 hat is a family? Wright and Leahey (2000) propose the following definition: a family is who they say they are. Many family forms exist within society today, such as the biological family of procreation, the nuclear family that incorporates one or more members of the extended family (family of origin), the sole-parent family, the stepfamily, the communal family, and the homosexual couple or family. Labeling individuals as "families" based on their group composition may not be the best way, however. Instead, family consideration may be more appropriately determined based on attributes of affection, strong emotional ties, a sense of belonging, and durability of membership (Wright & Leahey, 2000).

Many nurses have interactions with family members on a daily basis. A client's illness or hospitalization affects all members of the family, and nurses must understand how to work with the family as a unit, knowing that family members can have a profound effect on the client's healing process.

Nurse generalists should be familiar with the tasks associated with adaptive family functioning. With this knowledge, they are able to assess family interaction and recognize problems when they arise. They can provide support to families with an ill member and make referrals to other professionals when assistance is required to restore adaptive functioning.

Nurse specialists usually possess an advanced degree in nursing. Some nurse specialists have education or experience that qualifies them to perform family therapy. Family therapy is broadly defined as "a form of intervention in which members of a family are assisted to identify and change problematic, maladaptive, self-defeating, repetitive relationship patterns" (Goldenberg & Goldenberg, 2005). Family therapy has a strong theoretical focus, and a number of conceptual approaches have been introduced and suggested as frameworks for this intervention.

This chapter explores the stages of family development and compares the "typical" family within various subcultures. Characteristics of adaptive family functioning and behaviors that interfere with this adaptation are discussed. Theoretical components of selected therapeutic approaches are described. Instructions for construction of a family genogram are included. Nursing process provides the framework for nursing intervention with families.

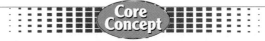

Family
A group of individuals who are bound by strong emotional ties, a sense of belonging, and a passion for being involved in one another's lives (Wright, Watson, & Bell, 1996).

STAGES OF FAMILY DEVELOPMENT

Carter and McGoldrick (1999) have identified six stages that describe the family life cycle. It is acknowledged that these tasks would vary greatly among diverse cultural groups, as well as the various forms of families previously described. These stages, however, provide a valuable framework from which the nurse may study families, emphasizing expansion (the addition of members), contraction (the loss of members), and realignment of relationships as members experience developmental changes. These stages of family development are summarized in Table 11–1.

TABLE 11–1	Stages of the Family Life Cycle	
FAMILY LIFE CYCLE STAGES	**EMOTIONAL PROCESS OF TRANSITION: KEY PRINCIPLES**	**CHANGES REQUIRED IN FAMILY STATUS TO PROCEED DEVELOPMENTALLY**
I. The Single Young Adult	Accepting separation from parents and emotional and financial responsibility for self	• Differentiation of self in relation to family of origin • Development of intimate peer relationships • Establishment of self in respect to work and financial independence
II. The Newly Married Couple	Commitment to new system	• Formation of marital system • Realignment of relationships with extended families and friends to include spouse
III. The Family with Young Children	Accepting new generation of members into the system	• Adjusting marital system to make space for child(ren) • Joining in child rearing, financial and household tasks • Realignment of relationships with extended family to include parenting and grandparenting roles
IV. The Family with Adolescents	Increasing flexibility of family boundaries to permit children's independence and grandparents' increasing dependence	• Shifting of parent/child relationships to permit adolescents to move in and out of system • Refocus on midlife marital and career issues • Beginning shift toward concerns for older generation
V. The Family Launching Grown Children	Accepting a multitude of exits from and entries into the family system	• Renegotiation of marital system as a dyad • Development of adult-to-adult relationships between grown children and their parents • Realignment of relationships to include in-laws and grandchildren • Dealing with disabilities and death of parents (grandparents)

(Continued on following page)

TABLE 11–1	Stages of the Family Life Cycle *(Continued)*	
FAMILY LIFE CYCLE STAGES	**EMOTIONAL PROCESS OF TRANSITION: KEY PRINCIPLES**	**CHANGES REQUIRED IN FAMILY STATUS TO PROCEED DEVELOPMENTALLY**
VI. The Family in Later Life	Accepting the shifting of generational roles	• Maintaining own and/or couple functioning and interests in face of physiological decline; exploration of new familial and social role options • Support for a more central role for middle generation • Making room in the system for the wisdom and experience of the elderly; supporting the older generation without overfunctioning for them • Dealing with loss of spouse, siblings, and other peers, and preparation for own death; life review and integration

SOURCE: From Carter, B & McGoldrick, M (eds). *The expanded family life cycle: Individual, family, and social perspectives* (3rd ed.) ©1999 by Allyn and Bacon. Reprinted by permission.

Stage I. The Single Young Adult

This model begins with the launching of the young adult from the family of origin. This is a difficult stage because young adults must decide what social standards from the family of origin will be preserved and what they will change for themselves to be incorporated into a new family. Tasks of this stage include forming an identity separate from the parents, establishing intimate peer relationships, and advancing toward financial independence. Problems can arise when either the young adults or the parents encounter difficulty terminating the interdependent relationship that has existed in the family of origin.

Stage II. The Newly Married Couple

Marriage is a difficult transition because renegotiation must include the integration of contrasting issues that each partner brings to the relationship and issues they may have redefined for themselves as a couple. In addition, the new couple must renegotiate relationships with parents, siblings, and other relatives in view of the new marriage. Tasks of this stage include establishing a new identity as a couple, realigning relationships with members of extended family, and making decisions about having children. Problems can arise if either partner remains too enmeshed with his or her family of origin or when the couple chooses to cut themselves off completely from extended family.

Stage III. The Family with Young Children

Adjustments in relationships must occur with the arrival of children. The entire family system is affected and role realignments are necessary for both new parents and new grandparents. Tasks of this stage include making adjustments within the marital system to meet the responsibilities associated with parenthood while maintaining the integrity of the couple relationship, sharing equally in the tasks of childrearing, and integrating the roles of extended family members into the newly expanded family organization. Problems can arise when parents lack knowledge about normal childhood development and adequate patience to allow children to express themselves through behavior.

Stage IV. The Family with Adolescents

This stage of family development is characterized by a great deal of turmoil and transition. Both parents who are approaching a midlife stage and adolescents are undergoing biological, emotional, and sociocultural changes that place demands on each individual and on the family unit. Grandparents, too, may require assistance with the tasks of later life. These developments can create a "sandwich" effect for the parents, who must deal with issues confronting three generations. Tasks of this stage include redefining the level of dependence so that adolescents are provided with greater autonomy while parents remain responsive to the teenager's dependency needs. Midlife issues related to marriage, career, and aging parents must also be resolved during this period. Problems can arise when parents are unable to relinquish control and allow the adolescent greater autonomy and freedom to make independent decisions or when parents are unable to agree and support each other in this effort.

Stage V. The Family Launching Grown Children

A great deal of realignment of family roles occurs during this stage. This stage is characterized by the intermittent exiting and entering of various family members. Children leave home for further education and careers; marriages occur, and new spouses, in-laws, and children enter the system; and new grandparent roles are established.

Adult-to-adult relationships among grown children and their parents are renegotiated. Tasks associated with this stage include reestablishing the bond of the dyadic marital relationship; realigning relationships to include grown children, in-laws, and new grandchildren; and accepting the additional caretaking responsibilities and eventual death of elderly parents. Problems can arise when feelings of loss and depression become overwhelming in response to the departure of children from the home, when parents are unable to accept their children as adults or cope with the disability or death of their own parents, and when the marital bond has deteriorated.

Stage VI. The Family in Later Life

This stage begins with retirement and lasts until the death of both spouses (Wright & Leahey, 2000). Most adults in their later years are still a prominent part of the family system, and many are able to offer support to their grown children in the middle generation. Tasks associated with this stage include exploring new social roles related to retirement and possible change in socioeconomic status; accepting some decline in physiological functioning; dealing with the deaths of spouse, siblings, and friends; and confronting and preparing for one's own death. Problems may arise when older adults have failed to fulfill the tasks associated with earlier levels of development and are dissatisfied with the way their lives have gone. They are unable to find happiness in retirement or emotional satisfaction with children and grandchildren and they are unable to accept the deaths of loved ones or to prepare for their own impending death.

MAJOR VARIATIONS

Divorce

Carter and McGoldrick (1999) also discuss stages and tasks of families experiencing divorce and remarriage. Currently, in the United States, about one half of all first marriages end in divorce (Kreider & Fields, 2002). Some statistics indicate that the divorce rate may be on the decline since the 1970s. In 2000, however, 16 percent of all families in the United States were headed by solo parents (Parents Without Partners, 2004). Stages in the family life cycle of divorce include deciding to divorce, planning the break-up of the system, separation, and divorce. Tasks include accepting one's own part in the failure of the marriage, working cooperatively on problems related to custody and visitation of children and finances, realigning relationships with extended family, and mourning the loss of the marriage relationship and the intact family.

After the divorce, the custodial parent must adjust to functioning as the single leader of an ongoing family while working to rebuild a new social network. The noncustodial parent must find ways to continue to be an effective parent while remaining outside the normal parenting role.

Remarriage *3/4 will remarry*

About three fourths of people who divorce will eventually remarry (Kreider & Fields, 2002). One fourth (4.5 million) of American families have at least one stepchild living in the household (Hanson, 2001). The challenges that face the joining of two established families are immense, and statistics reveal that the rate of divorce for remarried couples is even higher than the divorce rate following first marriages (Popenoe, 2002). Stages in the remarried family life cycle include entering the new relationship, planning the new marriage and family, and remarriage and reestablishment of family. Tasks include making a firm commitment to confronting the complexities of combining two families, maintaining open communication, facing fears, realigning relationships with extended family to include new spouse and children, and encouraging healthy relationships with biological (noncustodial) parents and grandparents.

Problems can arise when there is a blurring of boundaries between the custodial and noncustodial families. Children may contemplate, "Who is the boss now? Who is most important, the child or the new spouse? Mom loves her new husband more than she loves me. Dad lets me do more than my new step dad. I don't have to mind him; he's not my real dad." Confusion and distress for both the children and the parents can be avoided with the establishment of clear boundaries.

Goldenberg and Goldenberg (2004) state:

> Successful adaptation to stepfamily life calls for the ability to recognize and cope with a variety of problems: stepparents assuming a parental role, rule changes, jealousy and competition between stepsiblings as well as between birth parents and stepparents, loyalty conflicts in children between the absent parent and the stepparent, and financial obligations for child support while entering into a new marriage, to name but a few. Remarriage itself may resurrect old, unresolved feelings, such as anger and hurt left over from a previous marriage. (p. 372)

Cultural Variations

It is difficult to generalize about variations in family life cycle development according to culture. Most families have become acculturated to the U.S. society and conform to the life cycle stages previously described. Cultural diversity does exist, however, and nurses must be aware of possible differences in family expectations related to sociocultural beliefs. They must also be aware of a great deal of variation within ethnic groups as well as among them. Some variations that may be considered follow.

Marriage

A number of U.S. subcultures maintain traditional values in terms of marriage. Traditional views about family life and Roman Catholicism exert important influences on attitudes toward marriage in many Italian-American and Latino-American families. Although the tradition of arranged marriages is disappearing in Asian-American families, there is still frequently a much stronger influence by the family on mate selection than there is for other cultures in the United States (Earp, 2004). In these subcultures, the father is considered the authority figure and head of the household and the mother assumes the role of homemaker and caretaker. Family loyalty is intense and a breach of this loyalty brings considerable shame to the family.

Rabbi Bradley Bleifeld (2004) makes the following statement about Jewish families:

> The contemporary Jewish family is alive with a variety of faces, ages, and expressions—all vivid testimony to Jewish life in America today. No single snapshot could capture the infinite variety of what makes up today's Jewish family. We are so different; some single parents, some blended, some intermarried, some older, some younger. Diversity is both our challenge and our strength. And yet, we are so much the same. We still share our 3,000-year-old tradition. As one people, we strive to make this world a better place, to find some personal contentment through doing good deeds, and ultimately to contribute to the progress of our people and humanity by living good lives as Jews.

Children

In traditional Latino-American and Italian-American cultures, children are central to the family system. Many of these individuals have strong ties to Roman Catholicism, which historically has promoted marital relations for procreation only, and encouraged families to have large numbers of children. Regarding birth control, the Catechism of the Catholic Church (2000) states:

> Periodic continence, that is, the methods of birth regulation based on self-observation and the use of infertile periods, is in conformity with the objective criteria of morality. These methods respect the bodies of the spouses, encourage tenderness between them, and favor the education of an authentic freedom. In contrast, every action which, whether in anticipation of the conjugal act, or in its accomplishment, or in the development of its natural consequences, proposes, whether as an end or as a means, to render procreation impossible is intrinsically evil.

In the traditional Jewish community, having children is seen as a scriptural and social obligation. "You shall be fruitful and multiply" is a commandment of the Torah.

In traditional Asian-American cultures, sons are more highly valued than are daughters, and there is a strong preference for sons over daughters (Banister, 1999). Younger siblings are expected to follow the guidance of the oldest son throughout their lives, and when the father dies, the oldest son takes over the leadership of the family.

In all of these cultures, children are expected to be respectful of their parents and not bring shame to the family. Especially in the Asian culture, children learn a sense of obligation to their parents for bringing them into this world and caring for them when they were helpless. This is viewed as a debt that can never be truly repaid, and no matter what the parents may do, the child is still obligated to give respect and obedience.

Extended Family

The concept of extended family varies among societies (Purnell & Paulanka, 2003). The extended family is extremely important in the Western European, Latino, and Asian cultures, playing a central role in all aspects of life, including decision making.

In some U.S. subcultures, such as Asian, Latino, Italian, and Iranian, it is not uncommon to find several generations living together. Older family members are valued for their experience and wisdom. Because extended families often share living quarters, or at least live nearby, tasks of childrearing may be shared by several generations.

Divorce

In the Jewish community, divorce is often seen as a violation of family togetherness. Some Jewish parents take their child's divorce personally, with the response, "How could you possibly do this to me?"

Because Roman Catholicism has traditionally opposed divorce, those cultures that are largely Catholic have followed this dictate. Historically, a low divorce rate has existed among Italian Americans, Irish Americans, and Latino Americans. The number of divorces among these subcultures is on the rise, however, particularly in successive generations that have become more acculturated into a society where divorce is more acceptable.

FAMILY FUNCTIONING

Boyer and Jeffrey (1994) describe six elements on which families are assessed to be either functional or dysfunctional. Each can be viewed on a continuum, although families rarely fall at extreme ends of the continuum. Rather, they tend to be dynamic and fluctuate from one

TABLE 11–2	Family Functioning: Elements of Assessment	
	CONTINUUM	
ELEMENTS OF ASSESSMENT	FUNCTIONAL	DYSFUNCTIONAL
Communication	Clear, direct, open, and honest, with congruence between verbal and nonverbal	Indirect, vague, controlled, with many double-bind messages
Self-concept reinforcement	Supportive, loving, praising, approving, with behaviors that instill confidence	Unsupportive, blaming, "put-downs," refusing to allow self-responsibility
Family members' expectations	Flexible, realistic, individualized	Judgmental, rigid, controlling, ignoring individuality
Handling differences	Tolerant, dynamic, negotiating	Attacking, avoiding, surrendering
Family interactional patterns	Workable, constructive, flexible, and promoting the needs of all members	Contradictory, rigid, self-defeating, and destructive
Family climate	Trusting, growth-promoting, caring, general feeling of well-being	Distrusting, emotionally painful, with absence of hope for improvement

SOURCE: Adapted from Boyer & Jeffrey (1994).

point to another within the different areas. These six elements of assessment are described below and summarized in Table 11–2.

Communication

Functional communication patterns are those in which verbal and nonverbal messages are clear, direct, and congruent between sender and intended receiver. Family members are encouraged to express honest feelings and opinions, and all members participate in decisions that affect the family system. Each member is an active listener to the other members of the family.

Behaviors that interfere with functional communication include the following.

Making Assumptions

With this behavior, one assumes that others will know what is meant by an action or an expression (or sometimes even what one is thinking); or, on the other hand, assumes to know what another member is thinking or feeling without checking to make certain.

EXAMPLE:

A mother says to her teenage daughter, "You should have known that I expected you to clean up the kitchen while I was gone!"

Belittling Feelings

This action involves ignoring or minimizing another's feelings when they are expressed. This encourages the individual to withhold honest feelings to avoid being hurt by the negative response.

EXAMPLE:

When the young woman confides to her mother that she is angry because the grandfather has touched her breast, the mother responds, "Oh, don't be angry. He doesn't mean anything by that."

Failing to Listen

With this behavior, one does not hear what the other individual is saying. This can mean not hearing the words by "tuning out" what is being said, or it can be "selective" listening, in which a person hears only a selective part of the message or interprets it in a selective manner.

EXAMPLE:

The father explains to Johnny, "If the contract comes through and I get this new job, we'll have a little extra money and we will consider sending you to State U." Johnny relays the message to his friend, "Dad says I can go to State U!"

Communicating Indirectly

This usually means that an individual does not or cannot present a message to a receiver directly, so seeks to communicate through a third person.

EXAMPLE:

A father does not want his teenage daughter to see a certain boyfriend, but wants to avoid the angry response he expects from his daughter if he tells her so. He expresses his feelings to his wife, hoping she will share them with their daughter.

Presenting Double-Bind Messages

Double-bind communication conveys a "damned if I do and damned if I don't" message. A family member may respond to a direct request by another family member, only to be rebuked when the request is fulfilled.

EXAMPLE:

The father tells his son he is spending too much time playing football, and as a result, his grades are falling. He is expected to bring his grades up over the next 9 weeks or his car will be taken away. When the son tells the father he has quit the football team so he can study more, Dad responds angrily, "I won't allow any son of mine to be a quitter!"

Self-Concept Reinforcement

Functional families strive to reinforce and strengthen each member's self-concept, with the positive results being that family members feel loved and valued. Boyer and Jeffrey (1994) state:

> The manner in which children see and value themselves is influenced most significantly by the messages they receive concerning their value to other members of the family. Messages that convey praise, approval, appreciation, trust, and confidence in decisions and that allow family members to pursue individual needs and ultimately to become independent are the foundation blocks of a child's feelings of self-worth. Adults also need and depend heavily on this kind of reinforcement for their own emotional well-being. (p. 27)

Behaviors that interfere with self-concept reinforcement follow.

Expressing Denigrating Remarks

These remarks are commonly called "put downs." Individuals receive messages that they are worthless or unloved.

EXAMPLE:

A child spills a glass of milk at the table. The mother responds, "You are hopeless! How could anybody be so clumsy?!"

Withholding Supportive Messages

Some family members find it very difficult to provide others with reinforcing and supportive messages. This may be because they themselves have not been the recipients of reinforcement from significant others and have not learned how to provide support to others.

EXAMPLE:

A 10-year-old boy playing Little League baseball retrieves the ball and throws it to second base for an out. After the game he says to his Dad, "Did you see my play on second base?" Dad responds, "Yes, I did, son, but if you had been paying better attention, you could have caught the ball for a direct and immediate out."

Taking Over

This occurs when one family member fails to permit another member to develop a sense of responsibility and self-worth, by doing things for the individual instead of allowing him or her to manage the situation independently.

EXAMPLE:

Twelve-year-old Eric has a job delivering the evening paper, which he usually begins right after school. Today he must serve a 1-hour detention after school for being late to class yesterday. He tells his Mom, "Tommy said he would throw my papers for me today if I help him wash his Dad's car on Saturday." Mom responds, "Never mind. Tell Tommy to forget it. I'll take care of your paper route today."

Family Members' Expectations

All individuals have some expectations about the outcomes of the life situations they experience. These expectations are related to and significantly influenced by earlier life experiences. In functional families, expectations are realistic, thereby avoiding setting family members up for failure. In functional families, expectations are also flexible. Life situations are full of extraneous and unexpected interferences. Flexibility allows for changes and interruptions to occur without creating conflict. Finally, in functional families, expectations are individualized. Each family member is different, with different strengths and limitations. The outcome of a life situation for one family member may not be realistic for another. Each member must be valued independently, and comparison among members avoided.

Behaviors that interfere with adaptive functioning in terms of member expectations include the following.

Ignoring Individuality

This occurs when family members expect others to do things or behave in ways that do not fit with the latter's individuality or current life situation (Boyer & Jeffrey, 1994). This sometimes happens when parents expect their children to fulfill the hopes and dreams the parents have failed to achieve, yet the children have their own, different hopes and dreams.

EXAMPLE:

Bob, an only child, leaves for college next year. Bob's father, Robert, inherited a hardware store that was founded by Bob's great-grandfather and has been in the family for three generations. Robert expects Bob to major in business, work in the store after college, and take over the business when Robert retires. Bob, however, has a talent for writing, wants to major in journalism, and wants to work on a big-city newspaper when he graduates. Robert sees this as a betrayal of the family.

Demanding Proof of Love

Boyer and Jeffrey (1994) state:

> Family members place expectations on others' behavior that are used as standards by which the expecting member determines how much the other members care for him or her. The message attached to these expectations is: "If you will not be as I wish you to be, you don't love me." (p. 32)

EXAMPLE:

This is the message that Bob receives from his father in the example cited in the previous paragraph.

Handling Differences

It is difficult to conceive of two or more individuals living together who agree on everything all of the time. Serious problems in a family's functioning appear when differences become equated with "badness" or when disagreement is seen as "not caring" (Boyer & Jeffrey, 1994). Members of a functional family understand that it is acceptable to disagree and deal with differences in an open, nonattacking manner. Members are willing to hear the other person's position, respect the other person's right to hold an opposing position, and work to modify the expectations on both sides of the issue in order to negotiate a workable solution.

Behaviors that interfere with successful family negotiations follow.

Attacking

A difference of opinion can deteriorate into a direct personal attack and may be manifested by blaming another person, bringing up the past, making destructive comparisons, or lashing out with other expressions of anger and hurt (Boyer & Jeffrey, 1994).

EXAMPLE:

When Nancy's husband, John, buys an expensive set of golf clubs, Nancy responds, "How could you do such a thing? You know we can't afford those! No wonder we don't have a nice house like all our friends. You spend all our money before we can save for a down payment. You're so selfish! We'll never have anything nice and it's all your fault!"

Avoiding

With this tactic, differences are never acknowledged openly. The individual who disagrees avoids discussing it for fear that the other person will withdraw love or approval or become angry in response to the disagreement. Avoidance also occurs when an individual fears loss of control of his or her temper if the disagreement is brought out into the open.

EXAMPLE:

Vicki and Clint have been married 6 months. This is Vicki's second marriage and she has a 4-year-old son from her first marriage, Derek, who lives with her and Clint. Both Vicki and Clint work, and Derek goes to day care. Since the marriage 6 months ago, Derek cries every night continuously unless Vicki spends all her time with him, which she does in order to keep him quiet. Clint resents this but says nothing for fear he will come across as interfering; however, he has started going back to work in his office in the evenings to avoid the family situation.

Surrendering

The person who surrenders in the face of disagreement does so at the expense of denying his or her own needs or rights. The individual avoids expressing a difference of opinion for fear of angering another person or of losing approval and support.

EXAMPLE:

Elaine is the only child of wealthy parents. She attends an exclusive private college in a small New England town, where she met Andrew, the son of a farming couple from the area. Andrew attended the local community college for 2 years but chose to work on his parents' farm rather than continue college. Elaine and Andrew love each other and want to be married, but Elaine's parents say they will disown her if she marries Andrew, who they believe is below her social status. Elaine breaks off her relationship with Andrew rather than challenge her parents' wishes.

Family Interactional Patterns

Interactional patterns have to do with the ways in which families "behave." All families develop recurring, predictable patterns of interaction over time. These are often thought of as "family rules." The mentality conveys, "This is the way we have always done it" and provides a sense of security and stability for family members that comes from predictability. These interactions may have to do with communication, self-concept reinforcement, expressing expectations, and handling differences (all of the behaviors that were discussed previously), but because they are repetitive, and recur over time, they become the "rules" that govern patterns of interaction among family members.

Family rules are functional when they are workable, are constructive, and promote the needs of all family members. They are dysfunctional when they become contradictory, self-defeating, and destructive. Family therapists often find that individuals are unaware that dysfunctional family rules exist and may vehemently deny their existence even when confronted with a specific behavioral interaction. The development of dysfunctional interactional patterns occurs through a habituation process and out of fear of change or reprisal or a lack of knowledge as to how a given situation might be handled differently (Boyer & Jeffrey, 1994). Many are derived out of the parents' own growing-up experiences.

Patterns of interaction that interfere with adaptive family functioning include the following.

Patterns that Cause Emotional Discomfort

Interactions can promote hurt and anger in family members. This is particularly true of emotions that individuals feel uncomfortable expressing or are not permitted (according to "family rules") to express openly. These interactional patterns include behaviors such as never apologizing or never admitting that one has made a mistake, forbidding flexibility in life situations ("you must do it my way, or you will not do it at all"), making statements that devalue the worth of others, or withholding statements that promote increased self-worth.

EXAMPLE:

Priscilla and Bill had been discussing buying a new car but could not agree on the make or model to buy. One day, Bill appeared at Priscilla's office over the lunch hour and said, "Come outside and see our new car." In front of the building, Bill had parked a brand new sports car that he explained he had purchased with their combined savings. Priscilla was furious, but kept quiet and proceeded to finish her workday. At home she expressed her anger to Bill for making the purchase without consulting her. Bill refused to apologize or admit to making a mistake.

They both remained cool and hardly spoke to each other for weeks.

Patterns that Perpetuate or Intensify Problems Rather than Solve Them

When problems go unresolved over a long period of time, it sometimes appears to be easier just to ignore them. If problems of the same nature occur, the tendency to ignore them then becomes the safe and predictable pattern of interaction for dealing with this type of situation. This may occur until the problem intensifies to a point at which it can no longer be ignored.

EXAMPLE:

Dan works hard in the automobile factory and demands peace and quiet from his family when he comes home from work. His children have learned over the years not to share their problems with him because they fear his explosive temper. Their mother attempts to handle unpleasant situations alone as best she can. When son Ron was expelled from school for being caught smoking pot for the third time, Dan yelled, "Why wasn't I told about this before?"

Patterns that Are in Conflict with Each Other

Some family rules may appear to be functional—very workable and constructive—on the surface, but in practice may serve to destroy healthy interactional patterns. Boyer and Jeffrey (1994) describe the following scenario as an example.

EXAMPLE:

Dad insists that all members of the family eat dinner together every evening. No one may leave the table until everyone is finished because dinnertime is one of the few times left when the family can be together. Yet Dad frequently uses the time to reprimand Bobby about his poor grades in math, to scold Ann for her sloppy room, or to make not-so-subtle gibes at Mom for "spending all day on the telephone and never getting anything accomplished."

Family Climate

The atmosphere or climate of a family is composed of a blend of the feelings and experiences that are the result of family members' verbal and nonverbal sharing and interacting. Boyer and Jeffrey (1994) suggest that a positive family climate is founded on trust and is reflected in openness, appropriate humor and laughter, expressions of caring, mutual respect, a valuing of the quality of each individual, and a general feeling of well-being. A dysfunctional family climate is evidenced by tension, pain, physical disabilities, frustration, guilt, persistent anger, and feelings of hopelessness.

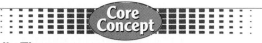

Family Therapy

A type of therapeutic modality in which the focus of treatment is on the family as a unit. It represents a form of intervention in which members of a family are assisted to identify and change problematic, maladaptive, self-defeating, repetitive relationship patterns (Goldenberg & Goldenberg, 2005).

THERAPEUTIC MODALITIES WITH FAMILIES

The Family as a System

General systems theory is a way of organizing thought according to the holistic perspective. A system is considered greater than the sum of its parts. A system is considered dynamic and ever changing. A change in one part of the system causes a change in the other parts of the system and in the system as a whole. When studying families, it is helpful to conceptualize a hierarchy of systems.

The family can be viewed as a system composed of various subsystems, such as the marital subsystem, parent–child subsystems, and sibling subsystems. Each of these subsystems is further divided into subsystems of individuals. The family system is also a subsystem of a larger suprasystem, such as the neighborhood or community. A schematic of a hierarchy of systems is presented in Figure 11–1.

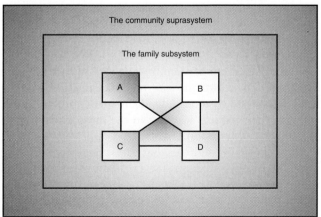

Key:
A = Father subsystem   CD = Sibling subsystem
B = Mother subsystem   AD = Parent-child subsystem
C = Child subsystem   BC = Parent-child subsystem
D = Child subsystem   AC = Parent-child subsystem
AB = Marital subsystem   BD = Parent-child subsystem

FIGURE 11–1   A hierarchy of systems.

Major Concepts

Bowen (1978) did a great deal of work with families using a systems approach. Bowen's theoretical approach to family therapy is composed of eight major concepts: (1) differentiation of self, (2) triangles, (3) nuclear family emotional process, (4) family projection process, (5) multigenerational transmission process, (6) sibling position profiles, (7) emotional cutoff, and (8) societal regression.

Differentiation of Self. Differentiation of self is the ability to define oneself as a separate being. The Bowen Theory suggests that "a person with a well-differentiated self recognizes his [or her] realistic dependence on others, but can stay calm and clear headed enough in the face of conflict, criticism, and rejection to distinguish thinking rooted in a careful assessment of the facts from thinking clouded by emotionality" (Georgetown Family Center, 2004a).

The degree of differentiation of self can be viewed on a continuum from high levels, in which an individual manifests a clearly defined sense of self, to low levels, or undifferentiated, in which emotional fusion exists and the individual is unable to function separately from a relationship system. Healthy families encourage differentiation, and the process of separation from the family ego mass is most pronounced during the ages of 2 to 5 and again between the ages of 13 and 15. Families that do not understand the child's need to be different during these times may perceive his or her behavior as objectionable.

Bowen (1971) used the term *stuck-togetherness* to describe the family with the fused ego mass. When family fusion occurs, none of the members has a true sense of self as an independent individual. Boundaries between members are blurred, and the family becomes enmeshed without individual distinguishing characteristics. In this situation, family members can neither gain true intimacy nor separate and become individuals.

Triangles. The concept of **triangle** refers to a three-person emotional configuration that is considered the basic building block of the family system. Bowen (1978) offers the following description of triangles:

> The basic building block of any emotional system is the triangle. When emotional tension in a two-person system exceeds a certain level, it triangles in a third person, permitting the tension to shift about within the triangle. Any two in the original triangle can add a new triangle. An emotional system is composed of a series of interlocking triangles. (p. 306)

Triangles are dysfunctional in that they offer relief from anxiety through diversion rather than through resolution of the issue. For example, when stress develops in a marital relationship, the couple may redirect their attention to a child, whose misbehavior gives them something on which to focus other than the tension in their relationship. When the dynamics within a triangle stabilize, a fourth person may be brought in to form additional triangles, in an effort to reduce tension. This triangulation can continue almost indefinitely as extended family and people outside the family, including the family therapist, can become entangled in the process. The therapist working with families must strive to remain "de-triangled" from this emotional system.

Nuclear Family Emotional Process. The nuclear family emotional process describes the patterns of emotional functioning in a single generation. The nuclear family begins with a relationship between two people who form a couple. The most open relationship usually occurs during courtship, when most individuals chose partners with similar levels of differentiation. The lower the level of differentiation, the greater the possibility of problems in the future. A degree of fusion occurs with permanent commitment. This fusion results in anxiety and must be dealt with by each partner in an effort to maintain a healthy degree of differentiation.

Family Projection Process. Spouses who are unable to work through the undifferentiation or fusion that occurs with permanent commitment may, when they become parents, project the resulting anxiety onto the children. This occurrence is manifested as a father-mother-child triangle. These triangles are common and exist in various gradations of intensity in most families with children.

The child who becomes the target of the projection may be selected for various reasons:

1. A particular child reminds one of the parents of an unresolved childhood issue.
2. The child is of a particular gender or position in the family.
3. The child is born with a deformity.
4. The parent has a negative attitude about the pregnancy.

This behavior is called **scapegoating**. It is harmful to both the child's emotional stability and ability to function outside the family. Goldenberg and Goldenberg (2005) state,

> Scapegoated family members assume the role assigned them, but they may become so entrenched in that role that they are unable to act otherwise. Particularly in dysfunctional families, individuals may be repeatedly labeled as the 'bad child'—incorrigible, destructive, unmanageable, troublesome—and they proceed to act accordingly. Scapegoated children are inducted into specific family roles, which over time become fixed and serve as the basis for chronic behavioral disturbance. (p. 386)

Multigenerational Transmission Process. Bowen (1978) describes the multigenerational transmission process as the manner in which interactional patterns are transferred from one generation to another. Attitudes, values, beliefs, behaviors, and patterns of interaction are passed along from parents to children over many lifetimes, so that it becomes possible to show in a family assessment that a certain behavior has existed within a family through multiple generations.

Genograms

A convenient way to plot a multigenerational assessment is with the use of **genograms**. Genograms offer the convenience of a great deal of information in a small amount of space. They can also be used as teaching tools with the family itself. An overall picture of the life of the family over several generations can be conveyed, including roles that various family members play as well as emotional distance between specific individuals. Areas for change can be easily identified. A sample genogram is presented in Figure 11–2.

Sibling Position Profiles. The thesis regarding sibling position profiles is that the position one holds in a family influences the development of predictable personality characteristics. For example, firstborn children are thought to be perfectionistic, reliable, and conscientious; middle children are described as independent, loyal, and intolerant of conflict; and youngest children tend to be charming, precocious, and gregarious (Leman & Leman, 1998). Bowen uses this to help determine level of differentiation within a family and the possible direction of the family projection process. For example, if an oldest child exhibits characteristics more representative of a youngest child, there is evidence that this child may be the product of triangulation. Sibling position profiles are also used when studying multigenerational transmission processes and verifiable data are missing for certain family members.

Emotional Cutoff. Emotional cutoff describes differentiation of self from the perception of the child. All individuals have some degree of unresolved emotional attachment to their parents and the lower the level of differentiation, the greater the degree of unresolved emotional attachment.

Emotional cutoff has very little to do with how far away one lives from the family of origin. Individuals who live great distances from their parents can still be undifferentiated, while some individuals are emotionally cut off from their parents who live in the same town or even the same neighborhood.

Bowen (1976) suggests that emotional cutoff is the result of dysfunction within the family of origin in which fusion has occurred and that emotional cutoff promotes the same type of dysfunction in the new nuclear family. He contends that maintaining some emotional contact with the family of origin promotes healthy differentiation.

Societal Regression. The Bowen theory views society as an emotional system. The concept of societal regres-

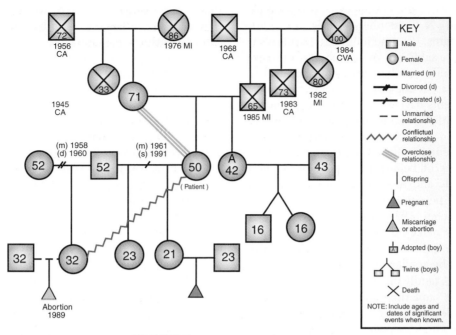

FIGURE 11–2   Sample genogram.

sion compares society's response to stress to the same type of response seen in individuals and families in response to emotional crisis: stress creates uncomfortable levels of anxiety, that leads to hasty solutions, which add to the problems, and the cycle continues. This concept of Bowen's theory is explained as follows (Georgetown Family Center, 2004b):

> Human societies undergo periods of regression and progression in their history. The current regression seems related to factors such as the population explosion, a sense of diminishing frontiers, and the depletion of natural resources. The 'symptoms' of societal regression include a growth of crime and violence, an increasing divorce rate, a more litigious attitude, a greater polarization between racial groups, less principled decision-making by leaders, the drug abuse epidemic, an increase in bankruptcy, and a focus on rights over responsibilities.

Goal and Techniques of Therapy

The goal of Bowen's systems approach to family therapy is to increase the level of differentiation of self, while remaining in touch with the family system. The premise is that intense emotional problems within the nuclear family can be resolved only by resolving undifferentiated relationships with the family of origin. Emphasis is given to the understanding of past relationships.

The therapeutic role is that of "coach" or supervisor, and emotional involvement with the family is minimized.

Therapist techniques include (Moriarty & Shepard, 2001):

1. Defining and clarifying the relationship between the family members.
2. Helping family members develop one-to-one relationships with each other and minimizing triangles within the system.
3. Teaching family members about the functioning of emotional systems.
4. Promoting differentiation by encouraging "I position" stands during the course of therapy.

The Structural Model

Structural family therapy is associated with a model developed by Minuchin (1974). In this model, the family is viewed as a social system within which the individual lives and to which the individual must adapt. The individual both contributes and responds to stresses within the family.

Major Concepts

Systems. The structural model views the family as a system. The structure of the **family system** is founded on a set of invisible principles that influence the interaction among family members. These principles concern how, when, and with whom to relate, and are established over time and through repeated transactions, until they become rules that govern the conduct of various family members (Goldenberg & Goldenberg, 2005).

Transactional Patterns. Transactional patterns are the rules that have been established over time that organize the ways in which family members relate to one another. A hierarchy of authority is one example of a transactional pattern. Usually, parents have a higher level of authority in a family than the children, so parental behavior reflects this role. A balance of authority may exist between husband and wife, or one may reflect a higher level than the other. These patterns of behavioral expectations differ from family to family and may trace their origin over generations of family negotiations.

Subsystems. Minuchin (1974) describes subsystems as smaller elements that make up the larger family system. Subsystems can be individuals or can consist of two or more persons united by gender, relationship, generation, interest, or purpose. A family member may belong to several subsystems at the same time, in which he or she may experience different levels of power and require different types of skills. For example, a young man has a different level of power and a different set of expectations in his father-son subsystem than in a subsystem with his younger brother.

Boundaries. **Boundaries** define the level of participation and interaction among subsystems. Boundaries are appropriate when they permit appropriate contact with others while preventing excessive interference. Clearly defined boundaries promote adaptive functioning. Maladaptive functioning can occur when boundaries are *rigid* or *diffuse*.

A rigid boundary is characterized by decreased communication and lack of support and responsiveness. Rigid boundaries prevent a subsystem (family member or subgroup) from achieving appropriate closeness or interaction with others in the system. Rigid boundaries promote **disengagement**, or extreme separateness, among family members.

A diffuse boundary is characterized by dependency and overinvolvement. Diffuse boundaries interfere with adaptive functioning because of the overinvestment, overinvolvement, and lack of differentiation between certain subsystems. Diffuse boundaries promote **enmeshment**, or exaggerated connectedness, among family members.

EXAMPLE:

Sally and Jim have been married for 12 years, during which time they have tried without success to have children. Six months ago they were thrilled to have the opportunity to adopt a 5-year-old girl, Annie. Since both Sally and Jim have full-time teaching jobs, Annie stays with her maternal grandmother, Krista, during the day after she gets home from half-day kindergarten.

At first, Annie was a polite and obedient child. However, in the last few months, she has become insolent and oppositional, and has temper tantrums when she cannot have her way. Sally and Krista agree that Annie should have whatever she desires and should not be punished for her behavior. Jim believes that discipline is necessary, but Sally and Krista refuse to enforce any guidelines he tries to establish. Annie is aware of this discordance and manipulates it to her full advantage.

In this situation, diffuse boundaries exist among the Sally-Krista-Annie subsystems. They have become enmeshed. They have also established a rigid boundary against Jim, disengaging him from the system.

Goal and Techniques of Therapy

The goal of structural family therapy is to facilitate change in the **family structure**. Family structure is changed with modification of the family "principles" or transactional patterns that are contributing to dysfunction within the family. The family is viewed as the unit of therapy, and all members are counseled together. Little, if any, time is spent exploring past experiences. The focus of structural therapy is on the present. Therapist techniques include the following:

1. **Joining the Family**. The therapist must become a part of the family if restructuring is to occur. The therapist joins the family but maintains a leadership position. He or she may at different times join various subsystems within the family, but ultimately includes the entire family system as the target of intervention.
2. **Evaluating the Family Structure**. Even though a family may come for therapy because of the behavior of one family member (the identified patient), the family as a unit is considered problematic. The family structure is evaluated by assessing transactional patterns, system flexibility and potential for change, boundaries, family developmental stage, and role of the identified patient within the system.
3. **Restructuring the Family**. An alliance or contract for therapy is established with the family. By becoming an actual part of the family, the therapist is able to manipulate the system and facilitate the circumstances and experiences that can lead to structural change.

The Strategic Model

The Strategic Model of family therapy uses the interactional or communications approach. Communication theory is viewed as the foundation for this model. Communication is the actual transmission of information among individuals. All behavior sends a message, so all behavior in the presence of two or more individuals is communication. In this model, families considered to be functional are open systems where clear and precise messages, congruent with the situation, are sent and received. Healthy communication patterns promote nurturance and individual self-worth. Dysfunctional families are viewed as partially closed systems in which communication is vague, and messages are often inconsistent and incongruent with the situation. Destructive patterns of communication tend to inhibit healthful nurturing and decrease individual feelings of self-worth.

Major Concepts

Double-Bind Communication. Double-bind communication occurs when a statement is made and succeeded by a contradictory statement. It also occurs when a statement is made accompanied by nonverbal expression that is inconsistent with the verbal communication. These incompatible communications can interfere with ego development in an individual and promote mistrust of all communications. Double-bind communication often results in a "damned if I do and damned if I don't" situation.

EXAMPLE:

A mother freely gives and receives hugs and kisses from her 6-year-old son some of the time, while at other times she pushes him away, saying, "Big boys don't act like that." The little boy receives a conflicting message and is presented with an impossible dilemma: "To please my mother I must not show her that I love her, but if I do not show her that I love her, I'm afraid I will lose her."

Pseudomutuality and Pseudohostility. A healthy functioning individual is able to relate to other people while still maintaining a sense of separate identity. In a dysfunctional family, patterns of interaction may be reflected in the remoteness or closeness of relationships. These relationships may reflect erratic interaction (i.e., sometimes remote and sometimes close), or inappropriate interaction (i.e., excessive closeness or remoteness).

Pseudomutuality and **pseudohostility** are seen as collective defenses against reality of the underlying meaning of the relationships in a dysfunctional family system. Pseudomutuality is characterized by a facade of mutual regard. Emotional investment is directed at maintaining outward representation of reciprocal fulfillment rather than in the relationship itself. The style of relating is fixed and rigid, and pseudomutuality allows family members to deny underlying fears of separation and hostility.

EXAMPLE:

Janet, age 16, is the only child of State Senator J. and his wife. Janet was recently involved in a joyriding experience with a group of teenagers her parents call "the wrong crowd." In family therapy, Mrs. J says, "We have always been a close family. I can't imagine why she is doing these things." Senator J. states, "I don't know another colleague who has a family that is as close as mine." Janet responds, "Yes, we are close. I just don't see my parents very much. Dad has been in politics since I was a baby, and Mom is always with him. I wish I could spend more time with them. But we are a close family."

Pseudohostility is also a fixed and rigid style of relating, but the facade being maintained is that of a state of chronic conflict and alienation among family members. This relationship pattern allows family members to deny underlying fears of tenderness and intimacy.

EXAMPLE:

Jack, 14, and his sister Jill, 15, will have nothing to do with each other. When they are together they can agree on nothing, and the barrage of "putdowns" is constant. This behavior reflects pseudohostility used by individuals who are afraid to reveal feelings of intimacy.

Schism and Skew. Lidz, Cornelison, Fleck, and Terry (1957) observed two patterns within families that relate to a dysfunctional marital dyad. A **marital schism** is defined as "a state of severe chronic disequilibrium and discord, with recurrent threats of separation." Each partner undermines the other, mutual trust is absent, and a competition exists for closeness with the children. Often a partner establishes an alliance with his or her parent against the spouse. Children lack appropriate role models.

Marital skew describes a relationship in which there is lack of equal partnership. One partner dominates the relationship and the other partner. The marriage remains intact as long as the passive partner allows the domination to continue. Children also lack role models when a marital skew exists.

Goal and Techniques of Therapy

The goal of strategic family therapy is to create change in destructive behavior and communication patterns among family members. The identified family *problem* is the unit of therapy, and all family members need not be counseled together. In fact, strategic therapists may prefer to see subgroups or individuals separately in an effort to achieve problem resolution. Therapy is oriented in the present and the therapist assumes full responsibility for devising an effective strategy for family change. Therapeutic techniques include the following:

1. **Paradoxical Intervention**. A paradox can be called a contradiction in therapy, or "prescribing the symptom." With **paradoxical intervention**, the therapist requests that the family continue to engage in the behavior that they are trying to change. Alternatively, specific directions may be given for continuing the defeating behavior. For example, a couple that regularly engages in insulting shouting matches is instructed to have one of these encounters on Tuesdays and Thursdays from 8:30 to 9:00 P.M. Boyer and Jeffrey (1994) explain:

   > A family using its maladaptive behavior to control or punish other people loses control of the situation when it finds itself continuing the behavior under a therapist's direction and being praised for following instructions. If the family disobeys the therapist's instruction, the price it pays is sacrificing the old behavior pattern and experiencing more satisfying ways of interacting with one another. A family that maintains it has no control over its behavior, or whose members contend that others must change before they can themselves, suddenly finds itself unable to defend such statements. (p. 125)

2. **Reframing**. Goldenberg and Goldenberg (2005) describe reframing as "relabeling problematic behavior by putting it into a new, more positive perspective that emphasizes its good intention." Therefore, with reframing, the *behavior* may not actually change, but the *consequences* of the behavior may change, owing to a change in the meaning attached to the behavior. This technique is sometimes referred to as positive reframing.

EXAMPLE:

Tom has a construction job and makes a comfortable living for his wife, Sue, and their two children. Tom and Sue have been arguing a lot and came to the therapist for counseling. Sue says Tom frequently drinks too much and is often late getting home from work. Tom counters, "I never used to drink on my way home from work, but Sue started complaining to me the minute I walked in the door about being so dirty and about tracking dirt and mud on 'her nice, clean floors.' It was the last straw when she made me undress before I came in the house and leave my dirty clothes and shoes in the garage. I thought a man's home was his castle. Well, I sure don't feel like a king. I need a few stiff drinks to face her nagging!"

The therapist used reframing to attempt change by helping Sue to view the situation in a more positive light. He suggested to Sue that she try to change her thinking by focusing on how much her husband must love her and her children to work as hard as he does. He asked her to

focus on the dirty clothes and shoes as symbols of his love for them and to respond to his "dirty" arrivals home with greater affection. This positive reframing set the tone for healing and for increased intimacy within the marital relationship.

The Evolution of Family Therapy

Goldenberg and Goldenberg (2004) describe Bowen's family theory and the structural and strategic models as "basic models of family therapy." They state:

> While noteworthy differences continue to exist in the theoretical assumptions each school of thought makes about the nature and origin of psychological dysfunction, in what precisely they look for in understanding family patterns, and in their strategies for therapeutic intervention, in practice the trend today is toward eclecticism and integration in family therapy. (p. 125)

Nichols and Schwartz (2004) suggest that contemporary family therapists "borrow from each other's arsenal of techniques." The basic models described here have provided a foundation for the progression and growth of the discipline of family therapy. Examples of newer models include the following:

● **Narrative therapy:** An approach to treatment that emphasizes the role of the stories people construct about their experience (Nichols & Schwartz, 2004, p. 442)
● **Feminist family therapy:** A form of collaborative, egalitarian, nonsexist intervention, applicable to both men and women, addressing family gender roles, patriarchal attitudes, and social and economic inequalities in male-female relationships (Goldenberg & Goldenberg, 2004, p. 508)
● **Social constructionist therapy:** Concerned with the assumptions or premises different family members hold about the problem. Efforts are focused on engaging families in conversations to solicit everyone's views, and not in imposing on families what is considered objectivity, truth, or "established knowledge" (Goldenberg & Goldenberg, 2004, p. 327)
● **Psychoeducational family therapy:** Therapy that emphasizes educating family members to help them understand and cope with a seriously disturbed family member (Nichols & Schwartz, 2004, p. 443)

The goal of most family therapy models is to provide the opportunity for change based on family members' perceptions of available options. The basic differences among models arise in how they go about achieving this goal. Goldenberg and Goldenberg (2004) state:

> Regardless of procedures, all attempt to create a therapeutic environment conducive to self-examination, to reduce dis-

comfort and conflict, to mobilize family resilience and empowerment, and to help the family members improve their overall functioning. (p. 463)

THE NURSING PROCESS

Assessment

Wright and Leahey (2000) have developed the Calgary Family Assessment Model (CFAM), a multidimensional model originally adapted from a framework developed by Tomm and Sanders (1983). The CFAM consists of three major categories: structural, developmental, and functional. Wright and Leahey (2000) state:

Each category contains several subcategories. It is important for each nurse to decide which subcategories are relevant and appropriate to explore and assess with each family at each point in time. That is, not all subcategories need to be assessed at a first meeting with a family, and some subcategories need never be assessed. If nurses use too many subcategories, they may become overwhelmed by all the data. If they and the family discuss too few subcategories, each may have a distorted view of the family situation. (p. 67)

A diagram of the CFAM is presented in Figure 11–3. The three major categories are listed, along with the subcategories for assessment under each. This diagram is used to assess the Marino family in the following case study.

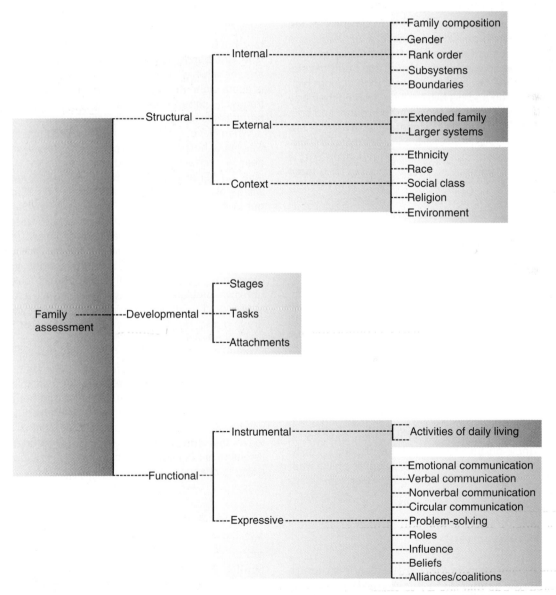

FIGURE 11–3   Branching diagram of the Calgary Family Assessment Model (CFAM). (From Wright, L.M., & Leahey, M. [2000]. *Nurses and families: A guide to family assessment and intervention* [3rd ed.]. Philadelphia: F.A. Davis.)

CASE STUDY

THE MARINO FAMILY

John and Nancy Marino have been married for 19 years. They have a 17-year-old son, Peter, and a 15-year-old daughter, Anna. Anna was recently hospitalized for taking an overdose of fluoxetine, her mother's prescription antidepressant. The family is attending family therapy sessions while Anna is in the hospital. Anna states, "I just couldn't take the fighting anymore! Our house is an awful place to be. Everyone hates each other, and everyone is unhappy. Dad drinks too much and Mom is always sick! Peter stays away as much as he can and I don't blame him. I would too if I had someplace to stay. I just thought I'd be better off dead."

John Marino, age 44, is the oldest of five children. His father, Paulo, age 66, is a first-generation Italian American whose parents immigrated from Italy in the early 1900s. Paulo retired last year after 32 years as a cutter in a meatpacking plant. His wife, Carla, age 64, has never worked outside the home. John and his siblings all worked at minimum-wage jobs during high school, and John and his two brothers worked their way through college. His two sisters married young, and both are housewives and mothers. John was able to go to law school with the help of loans, grants, and scholarships. He has held several positions since graduation and is currently employed as a corporate attorney for a large aircraft company.

Nancy, age 43, is the only child of Sam and Ethyl Jones. Sam, age 67, inherited a great deal of money from his family who had been in the shipping business. He is currently the Chief Executive Officer of this business. Ethyl, also 67, was an aspiring concert pianist when she met Sam. She chose to give up her career for marriage and family, although Nancy believes her mother always resented doing so. Nancy was reared in an affluent lifestyle. She attended private boarding schools as she was growing up and chose an exclusive college in the East to pursue her interest in art. She studied in Paris during her junior year. Nancy states that she was never emotionally close to her parents. They traveled a great deal, and she spent much of her time under the supervision of a nanny.

Nancy's parents were opposed to her marrying John. They perceived John's family to be below their social status. Nancy, on the other hand, loved John's family. She felt them to be very warm and loving, so unlike what she was used to in her own family. Her family are

Protestants and also disapproved of her marrying in the Roman Catholic church.

Family Dynamics

As their marriage progressed, Nancy's health became very fragile. She had continued her artistic pursuits but seemed to achieve little satisfaction from it. She tried to keep in touch with her parents but often felt spurned by them. They traveled a great deal and often did not even inform her of their whereabouts. They were not present at the birth of her children. She experiences many aches and pains and spends many days in bed. She sees several physicians, who have prescribed various pain medications, antianxiety agents, and antidepressants but can find nothing organically wrong. Five years ago she learned that John had been having an affair with his secretary. He promised to break it off and fired the secretary, but Nancy has had difficulty trusting him since that time. She brings up his infidelity whenever they have an argument, which is more and more often lately. When he is home, John drinks, usually until he falls asleep. Peter frequently comes home smelling of alcohol and a number of times has been clearly intoxicated.

When Nancy called her parents to tell them that Anna was in the hospital, Ethyl replied, "I'm sorry to hear that, dear. We certainly never had any of those kinds of problems on our side of the family. But I'm sure everything will be okay now that you are getting help. Please give our love to your family. Your father and I are leaving for Europe on Saturday and will be gone for 6 weeks."

Although more supportive, John's parents view this situation as somewhat shameful for the family. John's dad responded, "We had hard times when you were growing up, but never like this. We always took care of our own problems. We never had to tell a bunch of strangers about them. It's not right to air your dirty laundry in public. Bring Anna home. Give her your love and she will be okay."

In therapy, Nancy blames John's drinking and his admitted affair for all their problems. John states that he drinks because it is the only way he can tolerate his wife's complaining about his behavior and her many illnesses. Peter is very quiet most of the time but says he will be glad when he graduates in 4 months and can leave "this looney bunch of people." Anna cries as she listens to her family in therapy and says, "Nothing's ever going to change."

Structural Assessment

A graphic representation of the Marino family structure is presented in the genogram in Figure 11–4.

Internal Structure. This is a family that consists of a husband, wife, and their biological son and daughter who live together in the same home. They conform to the tra-

ditional gender roles. John is the eldest child from a rather large family, and Nancy has no siblings. In this family, their son, Peter, is the first-born and his sister, Anna, is 2 years younger. Neither spousal, sibling, nor spousal-sibling subsystems appear to be close in this family, and some are clearly conflictual. Problematic subsystems include John-Nancy, John-Nancy-children, and

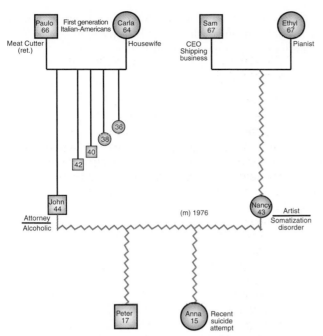

FIGURE 11–4 Genogram of the Marino family.

Nancy-Ethyl. The subsystem boundaries are quite rigid, and the family members appear to be emotionally disengaged from one another.

External Structure. This family has ties to extended family, although the availability of support is questionable. Nancy's parents offered little emotional support to her as a developing child. They never approved of her marriage to John and still remain distant and cold. John's family consists of a father, mother, two brothers, and two sisters. They are warm and supportive most of the time, but cultural influences interfere with their understanding of this current situation. At this time, the Marino family is probably receiving the most support from health care professionals who have intervened during Anna's hospitalization.

Context. John is a second-generation Italian American. His family of origin is large, warm, and supportive. However, John's parents believe that family problems should be dealt with in the family, and disapprove of bringing "strangers" in to hear what they consider to be private information. They believe that Anna's physical condition should be stabilized, and then she should be discharged to deal with family problems at home.

John and Nancy were reared in different social classes. In John's family, money was not available to seek out professional help for every problem that arose. Italian cultural beliefs promote the provision of help within the nuclear and extended family network. If outside counseling is sought, it is often with the family priest. John and Nancy did not seek this type of counseling because they no longer attend church regularly.

In Nancy's family, money was available to obtain the very best professional help at the first sign of trouble. However, Nancy's parents refused to acknowledge, both then and now, that any difficulty ever existed in their family situation.

The Marino family lives comfortably on John's salary as a corporate attorney. They have health insurance and access to any referrals that are deemed necessary. They are well educated but have been attempting to deny the dysfunctional dynamics that exist in their family.

Developmental Assessment

The Marino family is in stage IV of Carter and McGoldrick's family life cycle: the family with adolescents. In stage IV, parents are expected to respond to adolescents' requests for increasing independence, while being available to continue to fulfill dependency needs. They may also be required to provide additional support to aging grandparents. This is a time when parents may also begin to reexamine their own marital and career issues.

The Marino family is not fulfilling the dependency needs of its adolescents; in fact, they may be establishing premature independence. The parents are absorbed in their own personal problems to the exclusion of their children. Peter responds to this neglect by staying away as much as possible, drinking with his friends, and planning to leave home at the first opportunity. Anna's attempted suicide is a cry for help. She has needs that are unfulfilled by her parents, and this crisis situation may be required for them to recognize that a problem exists. This may be the time when they begin to reexamine their unresolved marital issues. Extended family are still self-supporting and do not require assistance from John and Nancy at this time.

Functional Assessment

Instrumental Functioning. This family has managed to adjust to the maladaptive functioning in an effort to meet physical activities of daily living. They subsist on fast food, or sometimes Nancy or Anna will prepare a meal. Seldom do they sit down at table to eat together. Nancy must take pain medication or sedatives to sleep. John usually drinks himself to sleep. Anna and Peter take care of their own needs independently. Often they do not even see their parents in the evenings. Each manages to do fairly well in school. Peter says, "I don't intend to ruin my chances of getting out of this hell hole as soon as I can!"

Expressive Functioning. John and Nancy Marino argue a great deal about many topics. This family seldom shows affection to one another. Nancy and Anna express sadness with tears, whereas John and Peter have a tendency to withdraw or turn to alcohol when experiencing unhappiness. Nancy somaticizes her internal pain, and numbs this pain with medication. Anna internalized her emotional pain until it became unbearable. A notable lack of constructive communication is evident.

This family is unable to solve its problems effectively. In fact, it is unlikely that it has even identified its problems, which undoubtedly have been in existence for a long while. These problems have only recently been revealed in light of Anna's suicide attempt.

Diagnosis

The following nursing diagnoses were identified for the Marino family:

1. **Interrupted family processes** related to unsuccessful achievement of family developmental tasks and dysfunctional coping strategies evidenced by inability of family members to relate to each other in an adaptive manner; adolescents' unmet dependency needs; and inability of family members to express a wide range of feelings and to send and receive clear messages.
2. **Disabled family coping** related to highly ambivalent family relationships and lack of support evidenced by inability to problem-solve; each member copes in response to dysfunctional family processes with destructive behavior (John drinks, Nancy somaticizes, Peter drinks and withdraws, and Anna attempts suicide).

Outcome Identification

The following criteria were identified as measurement of outcomes in counseling of the Marino family:

1. Family members will demonstrate effective communication patterns.
2. Family members will express feelings openly and honestly.
3. Family members will establish more adaptive coping strategies.
4. Family members will be able to identify destructive patterns of functioning and problem-solve them effectively.
5. Boundaries between spousal subsystems and spousal–children subsystems will become more clearly defined.
6. Family members will establish stronger bonds with extended family.

Planning/Implementation

The Marino family will undoubtedly require many months of outpatient therapy. It is even likely that each member will need individual psychotherapy in addition

to the family therapy. Once Anna has been stabilized physiologically and is discharged from the hospital, family/individual therapy will begin.

Several strategies for family therapy have been discussed in this chapter. As mentioned previously, family therapy has a strong theoretical framework and is performed by individuals with specialized education in family theory and process. Some clinical nurse specialists possess the credentials required to perform family therapy. It is important, however, for all nurses to have some knowledge about working with families, to be able to assess family interaction, and to recognize when problems exist.

Some interventions with the Marino family might include the following:

1. Create a therapeutic environment that fosters trust, and in which the family members can feel safe and comfortable. The nurse can promote this type of environment by being empathetic, listening actively (see Chapter 8), accepting feelings and attitudes, and being nonjudgmental.
2. Promote effective communication by
   a. Seeking clarification when vague and generalized statements are made (e.g., Anna states, "I just want my family to be like my friends' families." Nurse: "Anna, would you please explain to the group exactly what you mean by that?").
   b. Setting clear limits (e.g., "Peter, it is okay to state when you are angry about something that has been said. It is not okay to throw the chair against the wall.").
   c. Being consistent and fair (e.g., "I encourage each of you to contribute to the group process and to respect one another's opportunity to contribute equally.").
   d. Addressing each individual clearly and directly and encouraging family members to do the same (e.g., "Nancy, I think it would be more appropriate if you directed that statement to John instead of to me.").
3. Identify patterns of interaction that interfere with successful problem resolution. For example, John asks Nancy many "Why?" questions that keep her on the defensive. He criticizes her for "always being sick." Nancy responds by frequently reminding John of his infidelity. Peter and Anna interrupt each other and their parents when the level of conflict reaches a certain point. Provide examples of more appropriate ways to communicate that can improve interpersonal relationships and lead to more effective patterns of interaction.
4. Help the Marino family to identify problems that may necessitate change. Encourage each member to discuss a family process that he or she would like to change. As a group, promote discussion of what must take place for change to occur and allow each member

to explore whether he or she could realistically cooperate with the necessary requirements for change.

5. As the problem-solving process progresses, encourage all family members to express honest feelings. Address each one directly, "John (Nancy, Peter, Anna), how do you feel about what the others are suggesting?" Ensure that all participants understand that each member may express honest feelings (e.g., anger, sadness, fear, anxiety, guilt, disgust, helplessness) without criticism, judgment, or fear of personal reprisal.

6. Avoid becoming triangled in the family emotional system. Remain neutral and objective. Do not take sides in family disagreements; instead, provide alternative explanations and suggestions (e.g., "Perhaps we can look at that situation in a different light…").

7. Reframe vague problem descriptions into ones for which resolution is more realistic. For example, rather than defining the problem as "We don't love each other any more," the problem could be defined as, "We do not spend time together in family activities any more." This definition evolves from the family members' description of what they mean by the more general problem description.

8. Discuss present coping strategies. Encourage each family member to describe how he or she copes with stress and with the adversity within the family. Explore each member's possible contribution to the family's problems. Encourage family members to discuss possible solutions among themselves.

9. Identify community resources that may assist individual family members and provide support for establishing more adaptive coping mechanisms, for example, Alcoholics Anonymous for John, Al Anon for Nancy, and Al Ateen for Peter and Anna. Other groups that may be of assistance to this family include Emotions Anonymous, Parent's Support Group, Families Helping Families, Marriage Enrichment, Parents of Teenagers, and We Saved Our Marriage (WESOM). Local self-help networks often provide a directory of resources within specific communities.

10. Discuss with the family the possible need for psychotherapy for individual members. Provide names of therapists who would perform assessments to determine individual needs. Encourage follow-through with appointments.

11. Assist family members in planning leisure time activities together. This could include time to play together, exercise together, or engage in a shared project.

Evaluation

Evaluation is the final step in the nursing process. In this step, progress toward attainment of outcomes is measured.

1. Do family members demonstrate effective patterns of communication?
2. Can family members express feelings openly and honestly without fear of reprisal?
3. Can family members accept their own personal contribution to the family's problems?
4. Can individual members identify maladaptive coping methods and express a desire to improve?
5. Do family members work together to solve problems?
6. Can family members identify resources in the community from which they can seek assistance and support?
7. Do family members express a desire to form stronger bonds with the extended family?
8. Are family members willing to seek individual psychotherapy?
9. Are family members pursuing shared activities?

SUMMARY

Nurses interact with families daily. They must have sufficient knowledge of family functioning to assess family interaction and recognize when problems arise. Some nurse specialists perform therapy with families.

Carter and McGoldrick (1999) identified six stages that describe the family life cycle. They include the following:

1. The single young adult
2. The newly married couple
3. The family with young children
4. The family with adolescents
5. The family launching grown children
6. The family in later life

Carter and McGoldrick also discuss tasks of families experiencing divorce and remarriage, and those that vary according to cultural norms.

Families are assessed as functional or dysfunctional based on six elements (Boyer & Jeffrey, 1994). These elements include communication, self-concept reinforcement, family members' expectations, handling differences, family interactional patterns, and family climate.

Three models for family therapy were presented: the family as a system, the structural model, and the strategic model. Major concepts, goal, and techniques of therapy were presented for each. Several contemporary models were introduced. Explanation for use of the genogram in family assessment was included.

The nursing process, as the tool for delivery of nursing care, was presented in the form of a case study. Structure, development, and functioning were assessed; nursing diagnoses and outcome criteria were identified; and strategies for intervention and evaluation were discussed.

REVIEW QUESTIONS

SELF-EXAMINATION/LEARNING EXERCISE

Match the tasks in the column on the left to the family life cycle stages listed on the right.

_____ 1. Renegotiation of the marital system as a dyad

_____ 2. Differentiation of self in relation to family of origin.

_____ 3. Dealing with loss of spouse, siblings, and peers.

_____ 4. Adjusting marital system to make space for children

_____ 5. Formation of the marital system.

_____ 6. Refocus on midlife marital and career issues.

a. The Single Young Adult

b. The Newly Married Couple

c. The Family with Young Children

d. The Family with Adolescents

e. The Family Launching Grown Children

f. The Family in Later Life

Select the answer that is most appropriate in each of the following questions.

7. The nurse-therapist is counseling the Smith family: Mr. and Mrs. Smith, 10-year-old Rob, and 8-year-old Lisa. When Mr. and Mrs. Smith start to argue, Rob hits Lisa and Lisa starts to cry. The Smiths then turn their attention to comforting Lisa and scolding Rob, complaining that he is "out of control and we don't know what to do about his behavior." These dynamics are an example of
   a. Double-bind messages
   b. Triangulation
   c. Pseudohostility
   d. Multigenerational transmission

8. Using Bowen's systems approach to therapy with the Smith's, the therapist would:
   a. Try to change family principles that may be promoting dysfunctional behavior patterns.
   b. Strive to create change in destructive behavior through improvement in communication and interaction patterns.
   c. Encourage increase in the differentiation of individual family members.
   d. Promote change in dysfunctional behavior by encouraging the formation of more diffuse boundaries between family members.

9. Using the structural approach to therapy with the Smith's, the therapist would
   a. Try to change family principles that may be promoting dysfunctional behavior patterns.
   b. Strive to create change in destructive behavior through improvement in communications and interaction patterns.
   c. Encourage increase in the differentiation of individual family members
   d. Promote change in dysfunctional behavior by encouraging the formation of more diffuse boundaries between family members.

10. Using the strategic approach to therapy with the Smith's, the therapist would
   a. Try to change family principles that may be promoting dysfunctional behavior patterns.
   b. Strive to create change in destructive behavior through improvement in communication and interaction patterns.
   c. Encourage increase in the differentiation of individual family members
   d. Promote change in dysfunctional behavior by encouraging the formation of more diffuse boundaries between family members.

REFERENCES

Banister, J. (1999). *Son preference in Asia—Report of a symposium.* Washington, DC: U.S. Department of Commerce, Bureau of the Census.

Bleifeld, B. (2004). Jewish families. *Building a Jewish Home.* Retrieved November 17, 2004 from the World Wide Web at http://www.chsweb.org/mc/building02.html

Boyer, P.A., & Jeffrey, R.J. (1994). *A guide for the family therapist.* Northvale, NJ: Jason Aronson.

Carter, B., & McGoldrick, M. (1999). Overview: The expanded family life cycle: Individual, family, and social perspectives. In B. Carter & M. McGoldrick (Eds.). *The expanded family life cycle: Individual, family, and social perspectives* (3rd ed.). Boston: Allyn & Bacon.

Catechism of the Catholic Church (2nd ed.). (2000). Washington, DC: United States Conference of Catholic Bishops.

Earp, J.B.K. (2004). Korean Americans. In J.N. Giger and R.E. Davidhizar (Eds.). *Transcultural nursing: Assessment and Intervention* (4th ed.). St. Louis: C.V. Mosby.

Georgetown Family Center. (2004a). Bowen theory: Differentiation of self. Retrieved November 14, 2004 from the World Wide Web at http://www.georgetownfamilycenter.org/pages/conceptds.html

Georgetown Family Center. (2004b). Bowen theory: Societal emotional process. Retrieved November 14, 2004 from the World Wide Web at http://www.georgetownfamilycenter.org/pages/conceptsep.html

Goldenberg, I., & Goldenberg. H. (2004). *Family therapy: An overview* (6th ed.). Belmont, CA: Wadsworth.

Goldenberg, I., & Goldenberg, H. (2005). Family therapy. In R.J. Corsini & D. Wedding (Eds.). *Current Psychotherapies* (7th ed.). Belmont, CA: Wadsworth

Hanson, S.M.H. (2001). Family health care nursing: An introduction. In S.M.H. Hanson (Ed.). *Family health care nursing: Theory, practice, and research* (2nd ed.). Philadelphia: F.A. Davis.

Kreider, R.M., & Fields, J.M. (2002). Number, timing, and duration of marriages and divorces. *Current Population Reports, P70–80.* Washington, DC: U.S. Census Bureau.

Leman, K., & Leman, K. (1998). *The new birth order book: Why you are the way you are.* Grand Rapids, MI: Baker Books.

Moriarty, H.J., & Shepard, M.P. (2001). Family mental health nursing. In S.M.H. Hanson & S.T. Boyd (Eds.). *Family health care nursing: Theory, practice, and research.* (2nd ed.). Philadelphia: F.A. Davis.

Nichols, M.P., & Schwartz, R.C. (2004). *Family therapy: Concepts and methods* (6th ed.). Boston, MA: Allyn and Bacon.

Parents Without Partners. (2004). *Facts about single parent families.* Retrieved November 11, 2004 from the World Wide Web at http://www.parentswithoutpartners.org/Support1.htm

Popenoe, D. (2002). *The national marriage project at Rutgers University.* New Brunswick, NJ: Rutgers University.

Purnell, L.D., & Paulanka, B.J. (2003). Purnell's model for cultural competence. In L.D. Purnell & B.J. Paulanka (Eds.). *Transcultural health care: A culturally competent approach* (2nd ed.). Philadelphia: F.A. Davis.

Tomm, K., & Sanders, G. (1983). Family assessment in a problem oriented record. In J.C. Hansen, & B.F. Keeney (Eds.). *Diagnosis and assessment in family therapy.* London: Aspen Systems.

Wright, L.M., & Leahey, M. (2000). *Nurses and families: A guide to family assessment and intervention* (3rd ed.). Philadelphia: F.A. Davis.

Wright, L.M., Watson, W.L., & Bell, J.M. (1996). *Beliefs: The heart of healing in families and illness.* New York: Basic Books.

CLASSICAL REFERENCES

Bowen, M. (1971). The use of family theory in clinical practice. In J. Haley (Ed.). *Changing families.* New York: Grune & Stratton.

Bowen, M. (1976). Theory in the practice of psychotherapy. In P. Guerin (Ed.). *Family therapy: Theory and practice.* New York: Gardner Press.

Bowen, M. (1978). *Family therapy in clinical practice.* New York: Jason Aronson.

Lidz, T., Cornelison, A., Fleck, S., & Terry, D. (1957). The intrafamilial environment of schizophrenic patients: II. Marital schism and marital skew. *American Journal of Psychiatry, 114,* 241–248.

Minuchin, S. (1974). *Families and family therapy.* Cambridge, MA: Harvard University Press.

12
CHAPTER

MILIEU THERAPY—THE THERAPEUTIC COMMUNITY

CHAPTER OUTLINE

OBJECTIVES

MILIEU, DEFINED

CURRENT STATUS OF THE THERAPEUTIC COMMUNITY

BASIC ASSUMPTIONS

CONDITIONS THAT PROMOTE A THERAPEUTIC COMMUNITY

THE PROGRAM OF THERAPEUTIC COMMUNITY

THE ROLE OF THE NURSE

SUMMARY

REVIEW QUESTIONS

KEY TERMS

milieu

therapeutic community

CORE CONCEPT

milieu therapy

OBJECTIVES

After reading this chapter, the student will be able to:

1. Define *milieu therapy*.
2. Explain the goal of therapeutic community/ milieu therapy.
3. Identify seven basic assumptions of a therapeutic community.
4. Discuss conditions that characterize a therapeutic community.
5. Identify the various therapies that may be included within the program of the therapeutic community and the health care workers that make up the interdisciplinary treatment team.
6. Describe the role of the nurse on the interdisciplinary treatment team.

standard Vb of the Scope and Standards of Psychiatric-Mental Health Nursing Practice (ANA, 2000) states that, "The psychiatric-mental health nurse provides, structures, and maintains a therapeutic environment in collaboration with the client and other health care clinicians."

This chapter defines and explains the goal of milieu therapy. The conditions necessary for a therapeutic environment are discussed, and the roles of the various health care workers within the interdisciplinary team are delin-

eated. An interpretation of the nurse's role in milieu therapy is included.

MILIEU, DEFINED

The word *milieu* is French for "middle." The English translation of the word is "surroundings, or environment." In psychiatry, therapy involving the milieu, or environment, may be called milieu therapy, therapeutic community, or therapeutic environment. The goal of

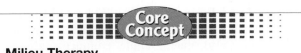

Milieu Therapy
A scientific structuring of the environment in order to effect behavioral changes and to improve the psychological health and functioning of the individual (Skinner, 1979).

milieu therapy is to manipulate the environment so that all aspects of the client's hospital experience are considered therapeutic. Within this therapeutic community setting the client is expected to learn adaptive coping, interaction, and relationship skills that can be generalized to other aspects of his or her life.

CURRENT STATUS OF THE THERAPEUTIC COMMUNITY

Milieu therapy came into its own during the 1960s through early 1980s. During this period, psychiatric inpatient treatment provided sufficient time to implement programs of therapy that were aimed at social rehabilitation. Nursing's focus of establishing interpersonal relationships with clients fit well within this concept of therapy. Patients were encouraged to be active participants in their therapy, and individual autonomy was emphasized.

The current focus of inpatient psychiatric care has changed. Hall (1995) states:

Care in inpatient psychiatric facilities can now be characterized as short and biologically based. By the time patients have stabilized enough to benefit from the socialization that would take place in a milieu as treatment program, they [often] have been discharged. (p. 51)

Although strategies for milieu therapy are still used, they have been modified to conform to the short-term approach to care or to outpatient treatment programs. Some programs (e.g., those for children and adolescents, clients with substance addictions, and geriatric clients) have successfully adapted the concepts of milieu treatment to their specialty needs (Bowler, 1991; DeSocio, Bowllan, & Staschak, 1997; Whall, 1991).

Many of the original concepts of milieu therapy are presented in this chapter. It is important to remember that a number of modifications to these concepts have been applied in practice for use in a variety of settings.

BASIC ASSUMPTIONS

Skinner (1979) outlined seven basic assumptions on which a therapeutic community is based:

1. **The Health in Each Individual Is to Be Realized and Encouraged to Grow**. All individuals are considered to have strengths as well as limitations. These healthy aspects of the individual are identified and serve as a foundation for growth in the personality and in the ability to function more adaptively and productively in all aspects of life.

2. **Every Interaction Is an Opportunity for Therapeutic Intervention**. Within this structured setting, it is virtually impossible to avoid interpersonal interaction. The ideal situation exists for clients to improve communication and relationship development skills. Learning occurs from immediate feedback of personal perceptions.

3. **The Client Owns His or Her Own Environment**. Clients make decisions and solve problems related to government of the unit. In this way, personal needs for autonomy as well as needs that pertain to the group as a whole are fulfilled.

4. **Each Client Owns His or Her Behavior**. Each individual within the therapeutic community is expected to take responsibility for his or her own behavior.

5. **Peer Pressure Is a Useful and a Powerful Tool**. Behavioral group norms are established through peer pressure. Feedback is direct and frequent, so that behaving in a manner acceptable to the other members of the community becomes essential.

6. **Inappropriate Behaviors Are Dealt with as They Occur**. Individuals examine the significance of their behavior, look at how it affects other people, and discuss more appropriate ways of behaving in certain situations.

7. **Restrictions and Punishment Are to Be Avoided**. Destructive behaviors can usually be controlled with group discussion. However, if an individual requires external controls, temporary isolation is preferred over lengthy restriction or other harsh punishment.

CONDITIONS THAT PROMOTE A THERAPEUTIC COMMUNITY

In a **therapeutic community** setting, everything that happens to the client, or within the client's environment, is considered to be part of the treatment program. The community setting is the foundation for the program of treatment. Community factors—such as social interactions, the physical structure of the treatment setting, and schedule of activities—may generate negative responses from some clients. These stressful experiences are used as examples to help the client learn how to manage stress more adaptively in real-life situations.

Under what conditions, then, is a hospital environment considered therapeutic? A number of criteria have been identified:

1. **Basic Physiological Needs Are Fulfilled**. As Maslow (1968) has suggested, individuals do not move to higher levels of functioning until the basic biological needs for food, water, air, sleep, exercise, elimination, shelter, and sexual expression have been met.

2. **The Physical Facilities Are Conducive to Achievement of the Goals of Therapy**. Space is provided so that each client has sufficient privacy, as well as physical space, for therapeutic interaction with others. Furnishings are arranged to present a homelike atmosphere—usually in spaces that accommodate communal living, dining, and activity areas—for facilitation of interpersonal interaction and communication.

3. **A Democratic Form of Self-Government Exists**. In the therapeutic community, clients participate in the decision making and problem solving that affect the management of the treatment setting. This is accomplished through regularly scheduled community meetings. These meetings are attended by staff and clients, and all individuals have equal input into the discussions. At these meetings, the norms and rules and behavioral limits of the treatment setting are set forth. This reinforces the democratic posture of the treatment setting, because these are expectations that affect all clients on an equal basis. An example might be the rule that no client may enter a room being occupied by a client of the opposite sex. Consequences of violating the rules are explained.

Other issues that may be discussed at the community meetings include those with which certain clients have some disagreements. A decision is then made by the entire group in a democratic manner. For example, several clients in an inpatient unit may disagree with the hours that have been designated for watching television on a weekend night. They may elect to bring up this issue at a community meeting and suggest an extension in television-viewing time. After discussion by the group, a vote will be taken, and clients and staff agree to abide by the expressed preference of the majority. Some therapeutic communities elect officers (usually a president and a secretary) who serve for a specified time. The president calls the meeting to order, conducts the business of discussing old and new issues, and asks for volunteers (or makes appointments, alternately, so that all clients have a turn) to accomplish the daily tasks associated with community living, for example, cleaning the tables after each meal and watering plants in the treatment facility. New assignments are made at each meeting. The secretary reads the minutes of the previous meeting and takes minutes of the current meeting. Minutes are important in the event that clients have a disagreement about issues that were discussed at various meetings. Minutes provide written evidence of decisions made by the group. In treatment settings where clients have short attention spans or disorganized thinking, meet-

ings are brief. Business is generally limited to introductions and expectations of the here and now. Discussions also may include comments about a recent occurrence in the group or something that has been bothering a member and about which he or she has some questions. These meetings are usually conducted by staff, although all clients have equal input into the discussions.

All clients are expected to attend the meetings. Exceptions are made for times when aspects of therapy interfere (e.g., scheduled testing, X-ray examinations, electroencephalograms). An explanation is made to clients present so that false perceptions of danger are not generated by another person's absence. All staff members are expected to attend the meetings, unless client care precludes their attendance.

4. **Responsibilities Are Assigned According to Client Capabilities**. Increasing self-esteem is an ultimate goal of the therapeutic community. Therefore, a client should not be set up for failure by being assigned a responsibility that is beyond his or her level of ability. By assigning clients responsibilities that promote achievement, self-esteem is enhanced. Consideration must also be given to times during which the client will show some regression in the treatment regimen. Adjustments in assignments should be made in a way that preserves self-esteem and provides for progression to greater degrees of responsibility as the client returns to previous level of functioning.

5. **A Structured Program of Social and Work-Related Activities Is Scheduled as Part of the Treatment Program**. Each client's therapeutic program consists of group activities in which interpersonal interaction and communication with other individuals are emphasized. Time is also devoted to personal problems. Various group activities may be selected for clients with specific needs (e.g., an exercise group for a person who expresses anger inappropriately, an assertiveness group for a person who is passive–aggressive, or a stress-management group for a person who is anxious). A structured schedule of activities is the major focus of a therapeutic community. Through these activities, change in the client's personality and behavior can be achieved. New coping strategies are learned and social skills are developed. In the group situation, the client is able to practice what he or she has learned to prepare for transition to the general community.

6. **Community and Family Are Included in the Program of Therapy in an Effort to Facilitate Discharge from Treatment**. An attempt is made to include family members, as well as certain aspects of the community that affect the client, in the treatment program. It is important to keep as many links to the client's life outside of therapy as possible. Family members are invited to participate in specific therapy groups and, in some instances, to share meals with the

client in the communal dining room. Connection with community life may be maintained through client group activities, such as shopping, picnicking, attending movies, bowling, and visiting the zoo. Inpatient clients may be awarded passes to visit family or may participate in work-related activities, the length of time being determined by the activity and the client's condition. These connections with family and community facilitate the discharge process and may help to prevent the client from becoming too dependent on the therapy.

THE PROGRAM OF THERAPEUTIC COMMUNITY

Care for clients in the therapeutic community is directed by an interdisciplinary treatment (IDT) team. An initial assessment is made by the admitting psychiatrist, nurse, or other designated admitting agent who establishes a priority of care. The IDT team determines a comprehensive treatment plan and goals of therapy and assigns intervention responsibilities. All members sign the treatment plan and meet regularly to update the plan as needed. Depending on the size of the treatment facility and scope of the therapy program, members representing a variety of disciplines may participate in the promotion of a therapeutic community. For example, an IDT team may include a psychiatrist, clinical psychologist, psychiatric clinical nurse specialist, psychiatric nurse, mental health technician, psychiatric social worker, occupational therapist, recreational therapist, art therapist, music therapist, psychodramatist, dietitian, and chaplain. Table 12–1 provides an explanation of responsibilities and educational preparation required for these members of the IDT team.

TABLE 12–1   The Interdisciplinary Treatment Team in Psychiatry

TEAM MEMBER	RESPONSIBILITIES	CREDENTIALS
Psychiatrist	Serves as the leader of the team. Responsible for diagnosis and treatment of mental disorders. Performs psychotherapy; prescribes medication and other somatic therapies.	Medical degree with residency in psychiatry and license to practice medicine
Clinical psychologist	Conducts individual, group, and family therapy. Administers, interprets, and evaluates psychological tests that assist in the diagnostic process.	Doctorate in clinical psychology with 2- to 3-year internship supervised by a licensed clinical psychologist. State license is required to practice.
Psychiatric clinical nurse specialist	Conducts individual, group, and family therapy. Presents educational programs for nursing staff. Provides consultation services to nurses who require assistance in the planning and implementation of care for individual clients.	Registered nurse with minimum of a master's degree in psychiatric nursing. Some institutions require certification by national credentialing association.
Psychiatric nurse	Provides ongoing assessment of client condition, both mentally and physically. Manages the therapeutic milieu on a 24-hour basis. Administers medications. Assists clients with all therapeutic activities as required. Focus is on one-to-one relationship development.	Registered nurse with hospital diploma, associate degree, or baccalaureate degree. Some psychiatric nurses have national certification.
Mental health technician (also called psychiatric aide or assistant or psychiatric technician)	Functions under the supervision of the psychiatric nurse. Provides assistance to clients in the fulfillment of their activities of daily living. Assists activity therapists as required in conducting their groups. May also participate in one-to-one relationship development.	Varies from state to state. Requirements include high school education, with additional vocational education or on-the-job training. Some hospitals hire individuals with baccalaureate degree in psychology in this capacity. Some states require a licensure examination to practice.
Psychiatric social worker	Conducts individual, group, and family therapy. Is concerned with client's social needs, such as placement, financial support, and community requirements. Conducts in-depth psychosocial history on which the needs assessment is based. Works with client and family to ensure that requirements for discharge are fulfilled and needs can be met by appropriate community resources.	Minimum of a master's degree in social work. Some states require additional supervision and subsequent licensure by examination.
Occupational therapist	Works with clients to help develop (or redevelop) independence in performance of activities of daily living. Focus is on rehabilitation and vocational training in which clients learn to be productive, thereby enhancing self-esteem. Creative activities and therapeutic relationship skills are used.	Baccalaureate or master's degree in occupational therapy

(Continued on following page)

TABLE 12-1	The Interdisciplinary Treatment Team in Psychiatry *(Continued)*	
TEAM MEMBER	**RESPONSIBILITIES**	**CREDENTIALS**
Recreational therapist	Uses recreational activities to promote clients to redirect their thinking or to rechannel destructive energy in an appropriate manner. Clients learn skills that can be used during leisure time and during times of stress following discharge from treatment. Examples include bowling, volleyball, exercises, and jogging. Some programs include activities such as picnics, swimming, and even group attendance at the state fair when it is in session.	Baccalaureate or master's degree in recreational therapy
Music therapist	Encourages clients in self-expression through music. Clients listen to music, play instruments, sing, dance, and compose songs that help them get in touch with feelings and emotions that they may not be able to experience in any other way.	Graduate degree with specialty in music therapy
Art therapist	Uses the client's creative abilities to encourage expression of emotions and feelings through artwork. Helps clients to analyze their own work in an effort to recognize and resolve underlying conflict.	Graduate degree with specialty in art therapy
Psychodramatist	Directs clients in the creation of a "drama" that portrays real-life situations. Individuals select problems they wish to enact, and other clients play the roles of significant others in the situations. Some clients are able to "act out" problems that they are unable to work through in a more traditional manner. All members benefit through intensive discussion that follows.	Graduate degree in psychology, social work, nursing, or medicine with additional training in group therapy and specialty preparation to become a psychodramatist
Dietitian	Plans nutritious meals for all clients. Works on consulting basis for clients with specific eating disorders, such as anorexia nervosa, bulimia nervosa, obesity, and pica.	Baccalaureate or master's degree with specialty in dietetics
Chaplain	Assesses, identifies, and attends to the spiritual needs of clients and their family members. Provides spiritual support and comfort as requested by client or family. May provide counseling if educational background includes this type of preparation.	College degree with advanced education in theology, seminary, or rabbinical studies

THE ROLE OF THE NURSE

Milieu therapy can take place in a variety of inpatient and outpatient settings. In the hospital, nurses are generally the only members of the IDT team who spend time with the clients on a 24-hour basis, and they assume responsibility for management of the therapeutic milieu. In all settings, the nursing process is used for the delivery of nursing care. Ongoing assessment, diagnosis, outcome identification, planning, implementation, and evaluation of the environment are necessary for the successful management of a therapeutic milieu. Nurses are involved in all day-to-day activities that pertain to client care. Suggestions and opinions of nursing staff are given serious consideration in the planning of care for individual clients. Information from the initial nursing assessment is used to create the IDT plan. Nurses have input into therapy goals and participate in the regular updates and modification of treatment plans.

In some treatment facilities, a separate nursing care plan is required in addition to the IDT plan. When this is the case, the nursing care plan must reflect diagnoses that are specific to nursing and include problems and interventions from the IDT plan that have been assigned specifically to the discipline of nursing.

In the therapeutic milieu, nurses are responsible for ensuring that clients' physiological needs are met. Clients must be encouraged to perform as independently as possible in fulfilling activities of daily living. However, the nurse must make ongoing assessments to provide assistance for those who require it. Assessing physical status is an important nursing responsibility that must not be overlooked in a psychiatric setting that emphasizes holistic care.

Reality orientation for clients who have disorganized thinking or who are disoriented or confused is important in the therapeutic milieu. Clocks with large hands and numbers, calendars that give the day and date in large print, and orientation boards that discuss daily activities and news happenings can help keep clients oriented to reality. Nurses should ensure that clients have written schedules of activities to which they are assigned and that they arrive at those activities on schedule. Some clients may require an identification sign on their door to remind them which room is theirs. All of these determinations are made from ongoing nursing assessments.

Nurses are responsible for the management of medication administration on inpatient psychiatric units. In some treatment programs, clients are expected to accept the responsibility and request their medication at the appropriate time. Although ultimate responsibility lies with the nurse, he or she must encourage clients to be self-reliant. Nurses must work with the clients to determine methods that result in achievement and provide positive feedback for successes.

A major focus of nursing in the therapeutic milieu is the one-to-one relationship, which grows out of a developing trust between client and nurse. Many clients with psychiatric disorders have never achieved the ability to trust. If this can be accomplished in a relationship with the nurse, the trust may be generalized to other relationships in the client's life. Developing trust means keeping promises that have been made. It means total acceptance of the individual as a person, separate from behavior that is unacceptable. It means responding to the client with concrete behaviors that are understandable to him or her (e.g., "If you are frightened, I will stay with you"; "If you are cold, I will bring you a blanket"; "If you are thirsty, I will bring you a drink of water"). Within an atmosphere of trust, the client is encouraged to express feelings and emotions and to discuss unresolved issues that are creating problems in his or her life.

The nurse is responsible for setting limits on unacceptable behavior in the therapeutic milieu. This requires stating to the client in understandable terminology what behaviors are not acceptable and what the consequences will be should the limits be violated. These limits must be established, written, and carried out by all staff. Consistency in carrying out the consequences of violation of the established limits is essential if the learning is to be reinforced.

The role of client teacher is important in the psychiatric area, as it is in all areas of nursing. Nurses must be able to assess learning readiness in individual clients. Do they want to learn? What is their level of anxiety? What is their level of ability to understand the information being presented? Topics for client education in psychiatry include information about medical diagnoses, side effects of medications, the importance of continuing to take medications, and stress management, among others. Some topics must be individualized for specific clients, whereas others may be taught in group situations. Table 12–2 outlines various topics of nursing concern for client education in psychiatry.

TABLE 12–2   The Therapeutic Milieu—Topics for Client Education

1. Ways to increase self-esteem
2. Ways to deal with anger appropriately
3. Stress-management techniques
4. How to recognize signs of increasing anxiety and intervene to stop progression
5. Normal stages of grieving and behaviors associated with each stage
6. Assertiveness techniques
7. Relaxation techniques
    a. Progressive relaxation
    b. Tense and relax
    c. Deep breathing
    d. Autogenics
8. Medications (specify)
    a. Reason for taking
    b. Harmless side effects
    c. Side effects to report to physician
    d. Importance of taking regularly
    e. Importance of not stopping abruptly
9. Effects of (substance) on the body
    a. Alcohol
    b. Other depressants
    c. Stimulants
    d. Hallucinogens
    e. Narcotics
    f. Cannabinols
10. Problem-solving skills
11. Thought-stopping/thought-switching technique
12. Sex education
    a. Structure and function of reproductive system
    b. Contraceptives
    c. Sexually transmitted diseases
13. The essentials of good nutrition
14. (For parents/guardians)
    a. Signs and symptoms of substance abuse
    b. Effective parenting techniques

Echternacht (2001) states:

Milieu therapy interventions are recognized as one of the basic-level functions of psychiatric-mental health nurses as addressed [in the American Nurses Association Scope and Standards of Psychiatric-Mental Health Nursing Practice, 2000]. Milieu therapy has been described as an excellent framework for operationalizing Peplau's interpretation and extension of Harry Stack Sullivan's Interpersonal Theory for use in nursing practice. (p. 39) Now is the time to rekindle interest in the therapeutic milieu concept and to reclaim nursing's traditional milieu intervention functions. Nurses need to identify the number of registered nurses necessary to carry out structured and unstructured milieu functions consistent with their Standards of Practice. (p. 43)

SUMMARY

In psychiatry, milieu therapy (or a therapeutic community) constitutes a manipulation of the environment in an effort to create behavioral changes and to improve the psychological health and functioning of the individual. The goal of therapeutic community is for the client to learn adaptive coping, interaction, and relationship skills that can be generalized to other aspects of his or her life. The community environment itself serves as the primary tool of therapy.

According to Skinner (1979), a therapeutic community is based on seven basic assumptions:

1. The health in each individual is to be realized and encouraged to grow.
2. Every interaction is an opportunity for therapeutic intervention.
3. The client owns his or her own environment.
4. Each client owns his or her behavior.
5. Peer pressure is a useful and a powerful tool.
6. Inappropriate behaviors are dealt with as they occur.
7. Restrictions and punishment are to be avoided.

Because the goals of milieu therapy relate to helping the client learn to generalize that which is learned to other aspects of his or her life, the conditions that promote a therapeutic community in the hospital setting are similar to the types of conditions that exist in real-life situations. They include the following:

1. The fulfillment of basic physiological needs.
2. Physical facilities that are conducive to achievement of the goals of therapy.
3. The existence of a democratic form of self-government.

4. The assignment of responsibilities according to client capabilities.
5. A structured program of social and work-related activities.
6. The inclusion of community and family in the program of therapy in an effort to facilitate discharge from treatment.

The program of therapy on the milieu unit is conducted by the IDT team. The team includes some, or all, of the following disciplines and may include others that are not specified here: psychiatrist, clinical psychologist, psychiatric clinical nurse specialist, psychiatric nurse, mental health technician, psychiatric social worker, occupational therapist, recreational therapist, art therapist, music therapist, psychodramatist, dietitian, and chaplain.

Nurses play a crucial role in the management of a therapeutic milieu. They are involved in the assessment, diagnosis, outcome identification, planning, implementation, and evaluation of all treatment programs. They have significant input into the IDT plans, which are developed for all clients. They are responsible for ensuring that clients' basic needs are fulfilled; assessing physical and psychosocial status; administering medication; helping the client develop trusting relationships; setting limits on unacceptable behaviors; educating clients; and ultimately, helping clients, within the limits of their capability, to become productive members of society.

REVIEW QUESTIONS

SELF-EXAMINATION/LEARNING EXERCISE

Test your knowledge of milieu therapy by supplying the information requested.

1. Define *milieu therapy*.

2. What is the goal of milieu therapy/therapeutic community?

Select the best response in each of the following questions:

3. In prioritizing care within the therapeutic environment, which of the following nursing interventions would receive the highest priority?
   a. Ensuring that the physical facilities are conducive to achievement of the goals of therapy.
   b. Scheduling a community meeting for 8:30 each morning.
   c. Attending to the nutritional and comfort needs of all clients.
   d. Establishing contacts with community resources.

4. In the community meeting, which of the following actions is most important for reinforcing the democratic posture of the therapy setting?
   a. Allowing each person a specific and equal amount of time to talk.
   b. Reviewing group rules and behavioral limits that apply to all clients.
   c. Reading the minutes from yesterday's meeting.
   d. Waiting until all clients are present before initiating the meeting.

5. One of the goals of therapeutic community is for clients to become more independent and accept self-responsibility. Which of the following approaches by staff best encourages fulfillment of this goal?
   a. Including client input and decisions into the treatment plan.
   b. Insisting that each client take a turn as "president" of the community meeting.
   c. Making decisions for the client regarding plans for treatment.
   d. Requiring that the client be bathed and dressed and attend breakfast on time each morning.

6. Client teaching is an important nursing function in milieu therapy. Which of the following statements by the client indicates the need for knowledge and a readiness to learn?
   a. "Get away from me with that medicine! I'm not sick!"
   b. "I don't need psychiatric treatment. It's my migraine headaches that I need help with."
   c. "I've taken Valium every day of my life for the last 20 years. I'll stop when I'm good and ready!"
   d. "The doctor says I have bipolar disorder. What does that really mean?"

Match the following activities with the responsible therapist from the IDT team.

_____ 7. Psychiatrist

_____ 8. Clinical psychologist

_____ 9. Psychiatric social worker

_____ 10. Psychiatric clinical nurse specialist

_____ 11. Psychiatric nurse

a. Helps clients plan, shop for, and cook a meal.

b. Locates halfway house and arranges living conditions for client being discharged from the hospital.

c. Helps clients get to know themselves better by having them describe what they feel when they hear a certain song.

d. Helps clients to recognize their own beliefs so that they may draw comfort from those beliefs in time of spiritual need.

e. Accompanies clients on community trip to the zoo.

——— 12. Mental health technician

——— 13. Occupational therapist

——— 14. Recreational therapist

——— 15. Music therapist

——— 16. Art therapist

——— 17. Psychodramatist

——— 18. Dietitian

——— 19. Chaplain

f. Diagnoses mental disorders, conducts psychotherapy, and prescribes somatic therapies.

g. Manages the therapeutic milieu on a 24-hour basis.

h. Conducts group and family therapies and administers and evaluates psychological tests that assist in the diagnostic process.

i. Conducts group therapies and provides consultation and education to staff nurses.

j. Assists staff nurses in the management of the milieu.

k. Encourages clients to express painful emotions by drawing pictures on paper.

l. Assesses needs, establishes, monitors, and evaluates a nutritional program for a client with anorexia nervosa.

m. Directs a group of clients in acting out a situation that is otherwise too painful for a client to discuss openly.

R E F E R E N C E S

American Nurses' Association (ANA). (2000). *Scope and standards of psychiatric-mental health nursing practice.* Washington DC: American Nurses' Association.

Bowler, J.B. (1991). Transformation into a healing healthcare environment: Recovering the possibilities of psychiatric/mental health nursing. *Perspectives in Psychiatric Care, 27*(2), 21–25.

DeSocio, J., Bowllan, N., & Staschak, S. (1997). Lessons learned in creating a safe and therapeutic milieu for children, adolescents, and families: Developmental considerations. *Journal of Child and Adolescent Psychiatric Nursing, 10*(4), 18–26.

Echternacht, M.R. (2001). Fluid group: Concept and clinical application in the therapeutic milieu. *Journal of the American Psychiatric Nurses Association, 7*(2), 39–44.

Hall, B.A. (1995). Use of milieu therapy: The context and environment as therapeutic practice for psychiatric-mental health nurses. In C.A. Anderson (Ed.). *Psychiatric nursing 1974 to 1994: A report on the state of the art.* St. Louis: Mosby-Year Book.

Whall, A.L. (1991). Using the environment to improve the mental health of the elderly. *Journal of Gerontological Nursing, 17*(7), 39.

C L A S S I C A L   R E F E R E N C E S

Maslow, A. (1968). *Towards a psychology of being* (2nd ed.). New York: D. Van Nostrand.

Skinner, K. (1979, August). The therapeutic milieu: Making it work. *Journal of Psychiatric Nursing and Mental Health Services, 17*, 38–44.

CRISIS INTERVENTION

CHAPTER OUTLINE

OBJECTIVES

CHARACTERISTICS OF A CRISIS

PHASES IN THE DEVELOPMENT
OF A CRISIS

TYPES OF CRISES

CRISIS INTERVENTION

PHASES OF CRISIS INTERVENTION:
THE ROLE OF THE NURSE

DISASTER NURSING

APPLICATION OF THE NURSING PROCESS

SUMMARY

REVIEW QUESTIONS

KEY TERMS

crisis intervention   disaster

CORE CONCEPT

crisis

OBJECTIVES

After reading this chapter, the student will be able to:

1. Define *crisis*.
2. Describe four phases in the development of a crisis.
3. Identify types of crises that occur in people's lives.
4. Discuss the goal of crisis intervention.

5. Describe the steps in crisis intervention.
6. Identify the role of the nurse in crisis intervention.
7. Apply the nursing process to care of victims of disasters.

S tressful situations are a part of everyday life. Any stressful situation can precipitate a crisis. Crises result in a disequilibrium from which many individuals require assistance to recover. Crisis intervention requires problem-solving skills that are often diminished by the level of anxiety accompanying disequilibrium. Assistance with problem solving during the crisis period preserves self-esteem and promotes growth with resolution.

In recent years, individuals in the United States have been faced with a number of catastrophic events, including natural disasters such as tornados, earthquakes, hurricanes, and floods. Also, manmade disasters, such as the Oklahoma City bombing and the attacks on the World Trade Center and the Pentagon, have created psychological stress of astronomical proportions in populations around the world.

This chapter examines the phases in the development

of a crisis and the types of crises that occur in people's lives. The methodology of crisis intervention, including the role of the nurse, is explored. A discussion of disaster nursing is also presented.

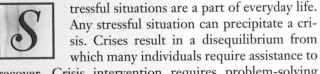

Crisis
A sudden event in one's life that disturbs homeostasis, during which usual coping mechanisms cannot resolve the problem (Lagerquist, 2001).

CHARACTERISTICS OF A CRISIS

A number of characteristics have been identified that can be viewed as assumptions upon which the concept of crisis is based (Aguilera, 1998; Caplan, 1964; Kaplan & Sadock, 1998). They include the following:

1. Crisis occurs in all individuals at one time or another and is not necessarily equated with psychopathology.
2. Crises are precipitated by specific identifiable events.
3. Crises are personal by nature. What may be considered a crisis situation by one individual may not be so for another.
4. Crises are acute, not chronic, and will be resolved in one way or another within a brief period.
5. A crisis situation contains the potential for psychological growth or deterioration.

Individuals who are in crisis feel helpless to change. They do not believe they have the resources to deal with the precipitating stressor. Levels of anxiety rise to the point that the individual becomes nonfunctional, thoughts become obsessional, and all behavior is aimed at relief of the anxiety being experienced. The feeling is overwhelming and may affect the individual physically as well as psychologically.

Bateman and Peternelj-Taylor (1998) state:

> Outside Western culture, a crisis is often viewed as a time for movement and growth. The Chinese symbol for crisis consists of the characters for *danger* and *opportunity* [Figure 13–1]. When a crisis is viewed as an opportunity for growth, those involved are much more capable of resolving related issues and more able to move toward positive changes. When the crisis experience is overwhelming because of its scope and nature or when there has not been adequate preparation for the necessary changes, the dangers seem paramount and overshadow any potential growth. The results are maladaptive coping and dysfunctional behavior. (pp. 144–145)

PHASES IN THE DEVELOPMENT OF A CRISIS

The development of a crisis situation follows a relatively predictable course. Caplan (1964) outlined four specific phases through which individuals progress in response to a precipitating stressor and that culminate in the state of acute crisis.

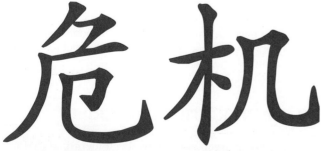

FIGURE 13-1 Chinese symbol for crisis.

Phase 1. *The individual is exposed to a precipitating stressor.* Anxiety increases; previous problem-solving techniques are employed.

Phase 2. *When previous problem-solving techniques do not relieve the stressor, anxiety increases further.* The individual begins to feel a great deal of discomfort at this point. Coping techniques that have worked in the past are attempted, only to create feelings of helplessness when they are not successful. Feelings of confusion and disorganization prevail.

Phase 3. *All possible resources, both internal and external, are called on to resolve the problem and relieve the discomfort.* The individual may try to view the problem from a different perspective, or even to overlook certain aspects of it. New problem-solving techniques may be used, and, if effectual, resolution may occur at this phase, with the individual returning to a higher, a lower, or the previous level of premorbid functioning.

Phase 4. *If resolution does not occur in previous phases, Caplan states that "the tension mounts beyond a further threshold or its burden increases over time to a breaking point. Major disorganization of the individual with drastic results often occurs."* Anxiety may reach panic levels. Cognitive functions are disordered, emotions are labile, and behavior may reflect the presence of psychotic thinking.

These phases are congruent with the transactional model of stress/adaptation outlined in Chapter 1. The relationship between the two perspectives is presented in Figure 13–2. Similarly, Aguilera (1998) spoke of "balancing factors" that affect the way in which an individual perceives and responds to a precipitating stressor. A schematic of these balancing factors is illustrated in Figure 13–3.

The paradigm set forth by Aguilera suggests that whether or not an individual experiences a crisis in response to a stressful situation depends upon the following three factors:

1. **The individual's perception of the event.** If the event is perceived realistically, the individual is more likely to draw upon adequate resources to restore equilibrium. If the perception of the event is distorted, attempts at problem solving are likely to be ineffective, and restoration of equilibrium goes unresolved.
2. **The availability of situational supports.** Aguilera states, "Situational supports are those persons who are available in the environment and who can be depended on to help solve the problem" (p. 37). Without adequate situational supports during a stressful situation, an individual is most likely to feel overwhelmed and alone.
3. **The availability of adequate coping mechanisms.** When a stressful situation occurs, individuals draw upon behavioral strategies that have been successful for them in the past. If these coping strategies work, a

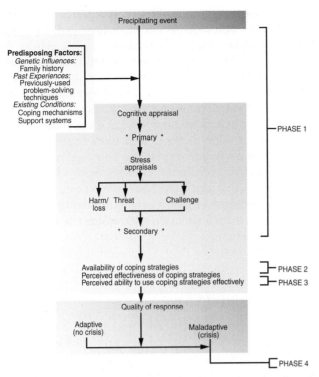

FIGURE 13–2 Relationship between transactional models of stress/adaptation and Caplan's phases in the development of a crisis.

crisis may be diverted. If not, disequilibrium may continue and tension and anxiety increase.

As previously set forth, it is assumed that crises are acute, not chronic, situations that will be resolved in one way or another within a brief period. Kaplan and Sadock (1998) state, "A crisis is self-limited and can last from a few hours to weeks. It is characterized by an initial phase in which anxiety and tension rise, followed by a phase in which problem-solving mechanisms are set in motion." Crises can become growth opportunities when individuals learn new methods of coping that can be preserved and used when similar stressors recur.

TYPES OF CRISES

Baldwin (1978) has identified six classes of emotional crises, which progress by degree of severity. As the measure of psychopathology increases, the source of the stressor changes from external to internal. The type of crisis determines the method of intervention selected.

Class 1: Dispositional Crises

Definition: An acute response to an external situational stessor.

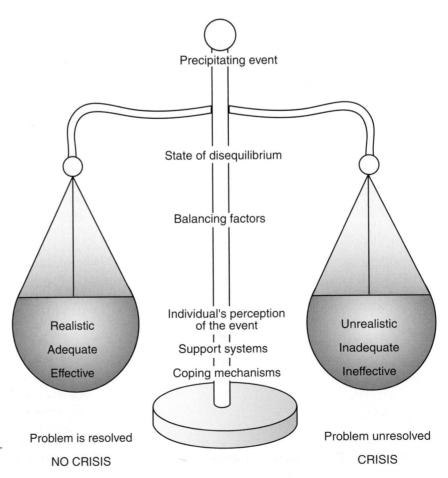

FIGURE 13–3 The effects of balancing factors in a stressful event.

EXAMPLE:

Nancy and Ted have been married for 3 years and have a 1-year-old daughter. Ted has been having difficulty with his boss at work. Twice during the past 6 months he has exploded in anger at home and become abusive with Nancy. Last night he became angry that dinner was not ready when he expected. He grabbed the baby from Nancy and tossed her, screaming, into her crib. He hit and punched Nancy until she feared for her life. This morning when he left for work, she took the baby and went to the emergency department of the city hospital, not having anywhere else to go.

Intervention: Nancy's physical wounds were cared for in the emergency department. The mental health counselor provided support and guidance in terms of presenting alternatives to her. Needs and issues were clarified, and referrals for agency assistance were made.

Class 2: Crises of Anticipated Life Transitions

Definition: Normal life-cycle transitions that may be anticipated but over which the individual may feel a lack of control.

EXAMPLE:

College student J.T. is placed on probationary status because of low grades this semester. His wife had a baby and had to quit her job. He increased his working hours from part time to full time to compensate, and therefore had little time for studies. He presents himself to the student-health nurse practitioner with numerous vague physical complaints.

Intervention: Physical examination should be performed (physical symptoms could be caused by depression) and ventilation of feelings encouraged. Reassurance and support should be provided as needed. The client should be referred to services that can provide financial and other types of needed assistance. Problematic areas should be identified and approaches to change discussed.

Class 3: Crises Resulting from Traumatic Stress

Definition: Crises precipitated by unexpected external stresses over which the individual has little or no control and from which he or she feels emotionally overwhelmed and defeated.

EXAMPLE:

Sally is a waitress whose shift ends at midnight. Two weeks ago, while walking to her car in the deserted parking lot, she was abducted by two men with guns, taken to an abandoned building, and raped and beaten. Since that time, her physical wounds have nearly healed. However, Sally cannot be alone, is constantly fearful, relives the experience in flashbacks and dreams, and is unable to eat, sleep, or work at her job in the restaurant. Her friend offers to accompany her to the mental health clinic.

Intervention: The nurse should encourage Sally to talk about the experience and to express her feelings associated with it. The nurse should offer reassurance and support; discuss stages of grief and how rape causes a loss of self-worth, triggering the grief response; identify support systems that can help Sally to resume her normal activities; and explore new methods of coping with emotions arising from a situation with which she has had no previous experience.

Class 4: Maturational/ Developmental Crises

Definition: Crises that occur in response to situations that trigger emotions related to unresolved conflicts in one's life. These crises are of internal origin and reflect underlying developmental issues that involve dependency, value conflicts, sexual identity, control, and capacity for emotional intimacy.

EXAMPLE:

Bob is 40 years old. He has just been passed over for a job promotion for the third time. He has moved many times within the large company for which he works, usually after angering and alienating himself from the supervisor. His father was domineering and became abusive when Bob did not comply with his every command. Over the years, Bob's behavioral response became one of passive-aggressiveness—first with his father, then with his supervisors. This third rejection has created feelings of depression and intense anxiety in Bob. At his wife's insistence, he has sought help at the mental health clinic.

Intervention: The primary intervention is to help the individual identify the unresolved developmental issue that is creating the conflict. Support and guidance are offered during the initial crisis period, then assistance is given to help the individual work through the underlying conflict in an effort to change response patterns that are creating problems in his current life situation.

Class 5: Crises Reflecting Psychopathology

Definition: Emotional crises in which preexisting psychopathology has been instrumental in precipitating the crisis or in which psychopathology significantly impairs or complicates adaptive resolution. Examples of psychopathology that may precipitate crises include borderline personality, severe neuroses, characterological disorders, or schizophrenia.

EXAMPLE:

Sonja, age 29, was diagnosed with borderline personality at age 18. She has been in therapy on a weekly basis for 10 years, with several hospitalizations for suicide attempts during that time. She has had the same therapist for the past 6 years. This therapist told Sonja today that she is to be married in 1 month and will be moving across the country with her new husband. Sonja is distraught and experiencing intense feelings of abandonment. She is found wandering in and out of traffic on a busy expressway, oblivious to her surroundings. Police bring her to the emergency department of the hospital.

Intervention: The initial intervention is to help bring down the level of anxiety in Sonja that has created feelings of unreality in her. She requires that someone stay with her and reassure her of her safety and security. After the feelings of panic anxiety have subsided, she should be encouraged to verbalize her feelings of abandonment. Regressive behaviors should be discouraged. Positive reinforcement should be given for independent activities and accomplishments. The primary therapist will need to pursue this issue of termination with Sonja at length. Referral to a long-term care facility may be required.

Class 6: Psychiatric Emergencies

Definition: Crisis situations in which general functioning has been severely impaired and the individual rendered incompetent or unable to assume personal responsibility. Examples include acutely suicidal individuals, drug overdoses, reactions to hallucinogenic drugs, acute psychoses, uncontrollable anger, and alcohol intoxication.

EXAMPLE:

Jennifer, age 16, had been dating Joe, the star high school football player, for 6 months. After the game on Friday night, Jennifer and Joe went to Jackie's house, where a number of high school students had gathered for an after-game party. No adults were present. About midnight, Joe told Jennifer that he did not want to date her anymore. Jennifer became hysterical, and Jackie was frightened by her behavior. She took Jennifer to her parent's bedroom and gave her a Valium from a bottle in her mother's medicine cabinet. She left Jennifer lying on her parent's bed and returned to the party downstairs. About an hour later, she returned to her parent's bedroom and found that Jennifer had removed the bottle of Valium from the cabinet and swallowed all of the tablets. Jennifer was unconscious and Jackie could not awaken her. An ambulance was called and Jennifer was transported to the local hospital.

Intervention: The crisis team monitored vital signs, ensured maintenance of adequate airway, initiated gastric lavage, and administered activated charcoal to minimize absorption. Jennifer's parents were notified and rushed to the hospital. The situation was explained to them, and they were encouraged to stay by her side. When the physical crisis was resolved, Jennifer was transferred to the psychiatric unit. In therapy, she was encouraged to ventilate her feelings regarding the rejection and subsequent overdose. Family therapy sessions were conducted in an effort to clarify interpersonal issues and to identify areas for change. On an individual level, Jennifer's therapist worked with her to establish more adaptive methods of coping with stressful situations.

CRISIS INTERVENTION

Individuals experiencing crises have an urgent need for assistance. In **crisis intervention** the therapist, or other intervener, becomes a part of the individual's life situation. Because of the individual's emotional state, he or she is unable to problem solve, so requires guidance and support from another to help mobilize the resources needed to resolve the crisis.

Lengthy psychological interpretations are obviously not appropriate for crisis intervention. It is a time for doing what is needed to help the individual get relief and for calling into action all the people and other resources required to do so.

Aguilera (1998) states:

> The goal of crisis intervention is the resolution of an immediate crisis. Its focus is on the supportive, with the restoration of the individual to his precrisis level of functioning or possibly to a higher level of functioning. The therapist's role is direct, supportive, and that of an active participant. (p. 24)

Crisis intervention takes place in both inpatient and outpatient settings. The basic methodology relies heavily on orderly problem-solving techniques and structured activities that are focused on change. Through adaptive change, crises are resolved and growth occurs. Because of the time limitation of crisis intervention, the individual must experience some degree of relief almost from the first interaction. Crisis intervention, then, is not aimed at major personality change or reconstruction (as may be the case in long-term psychotherapy), but rather at using a given crisis situation, at the very least, to restore functioning and, at most, to enhance personal growth.

PHASES OF CRISIS INTERVENTION: THE ROLE OF THE NURSE

Nurses respond to crisis situations on a daily basis. Crises can occur on every unit in the general hospital, in the home setting, the community health care setting, schools, offices, and in private practice. Indeed, nurses may be called on to function as crisis helpers in virtually any setting committed to the practice of nursing.

Aguilera (1998) describes four specific phases in the technique of crisis intervention. These phases are clearly comparable to the steps of the nursing process.

Phase 1. Assessment

In this phase, the crisis helper gathers information regarding the precipitating stressor and the resulting crisis that prompted the individual to seek professional help. A nurse in crisis intervention might perform some of the following assessments:

1. Ask the individual to describe the event that precipitated this crisis.
2. Determine when it occurred.
3. Assess the individual's physical and mental status.
4. Determine if the individual has experienced this stressor before. If so, what method of coping was used? Have these methods been tried this time?
5. If previous coping methods were tried, what was the result?
6. If new coping methods were tried, what was the result?
7. Assess suicide or homicide potential, plan, and means.
8. Assess the adequacy of support systems.
9. Determine level of precrisis functioning. Assess the usual coping methods, available support systems, and ability to problem solve.
10. Assess the individual's perception of personal strengths and limitations.
11. Assess the individual's use of substances.

Information from the comprehensive assessment is then analyzed, and appropriate nursing diagnoses reflecting the immediacy of the crisis situation are identified. Some nursing diagnoses that may be relevant include

1. Ineffective coping
2. Anxiety (severe to panic)
3. Disturbed thought processes
4. Risk for self- or other-directed violence
5. Rape-trauma syndrome
6. Post-trauma syndrome
7. Fear

Phase 2. Planning of Therapeutic Intervention

In the planning phase of the nursing process, the nurse selects the appropriate nursing actions for the identified nursing diagnoses. In planning the interventions, the type of crisis, as well as the individual's strengths and available resources for support, are taken into consideration. Goals are established for crisis resolution and a return to, or increase in, the precrisis level of functioning.

Phase 3. Intervention

During phase 3, the actions that were identified in phase 2 are implemented. The following interventions are the focus of nursing in crisis intervention:

1. Use a reality-oriented approach. The focus of the problem is on the here and now.
2. Remain with the individual who is experiencing panic anxiety.
3. Establish a rapid working relationship by showing unconditional acceptance, by active listening, and by attending to immediate needs.
4. Discourage lengthy explanations or rationalizations of the situation; promote an atmosphere for verbalization of true feelings.
5. Set firm limits on aggressive, destructive behaviors. At high levels of anxiety, behavior is likely to be impulsive and regressive. Establish at the outset what is acceptable and what is not, and maintain consistency.
6. Clarify the problem that the individual is facing. The nurse does this by describing his or her perception of the problem and comparing it with the individual's perception of the problem.
7. Help the individual determine what he or she believes precipitated the crisis.
8. Acknowledge feelings of anger, guilt, helplessness, and powerlessness, while taking care not to provide positive feedback for these feelings.
9. Guide the individual through a problem-solving process by which he or she may move in the direction of positive life change:
   a. Help the individual confront the source of the problem that is creating the crisis response.
   b. Encourage the individual to discuss changes he or she would like to make. Jointly determine whether or not desired changes are realistic.
   c. Encourage exploration of feelings about aspects that cannot be changed, and explore alternative ways of coping more adaptively in these situations.
   d. Discuss alternative strategies for creating changes that are realistically possible.
   e. Weigh benefits and consequences of each alternative.
   f. Assist the individual to select alternative coping strategies that will help alleviate future crisis situations.
10. Identify external support systems and new social networks from whom the individual may seek assistance in times of stress.

Phase 4. Evaluation of Crisis Resolution and Anticipatory Planning

To evaluate the outcome of crisis intervention, a reassessment is made to determine if the stated objective was achieved:

1. Have positive behavioral changes occurred?
2. Has the individual developed more adaptive coping strategies? Have they been effective?

3. Has the individual grown from the experience by gaining insight into his or her responses to crisis situations?
4. Does the individual believe that he or she could respond with healthy adaptation in future stressful situations to prevent crisis development?
5. Can the individual describe a plan of action for dealing with stressors similar to the one that precipitated this crisis?

During the evaluation period, the nurse and client summarize what has occurred during the intervention. They review what the individual has learned and "anticipate" how he or she will respond in the future. A determination is made regarding follow-up therapy; if needed, the nurse provides referral information.

DISASTER NURSING

Although there are many definitions of **disaster**, a common feature is that the event overwhelms local resources and threatens the function and safety of the community (Norwood, Ursano, & Fullerton, 2004). A violent disaster, whether natural or manmade, may leave devastation of property or life. Such tragedies also leave victims with a damaged sense of safety and well-being, and varying degrees of emotional trauma (Oklahoma State Department of Health [OSDH], 2001). Children, who lack life experiences and coping skills, are particularly vulnerable. Their sense of order and security has been seriously disrupted, and they are unable to understand that the disruption is time limited and that their world will eventually return to normal.

APPLICATION OF THE NURSING PROCESS

Background Assessment Data

Individuals respond to traumatic events in many ways. Grieving is a natural response following any loss, and it may be more extreme if the disaster is directly experienced or witnessed (OSDH, 2001). The emotional effects of loss and disruption may show up immediately or may appear weeks or months later.

Psychological and behavioral responses common in adults following trauma and disaster include anger; disbelief; sadness; anxiety; fear; irritability; arousal; numbing; sleep disturbance; and increases in alcohol, caffeine, and tobacco use (Norwood, Ursano, & Fullerton, 2004). Preschool children commonly experience separation anxiety, regressive behaviors, nightmares, and hyperactive or withdrawn behaviors. Older children may have difficulty concentrating, somatic complaints, sleep disturbances, and concerns about safety. Adolescents' responses are often similar to those of adults.

Norwood, Ursano, and Fullerton (2004) state:

Traumatic bereavement is recognized as posing special challenges to survivors. While the death of loved ones is always painful, an unexpected and violent death can be more difficult to assimilate. Family members may develop intrusive images of the death based on information gleaned from authorities or the media. Witnessing or learning of violence to a loved one also increases vulnerability to psychiatric disorders. The knowledge that one has been exposed to toxins is a potent traumatic stressor...and the focus of much concern in the medical community preparing for responses to terrorist attacks using biological, chemical, or nuclear agents. (p. 3)

Nursing Diagnoses/Outcome Identification

Information from the assessment is analyzed, and appropriate nursing diagnoses reflecting the immediacy of the situation are identified. Some nursing diagnoses that may be relevant include:

● Risk for injury (trauma, suffocation, poisoning)
● Risk for infection
● Anxiety (panic)
● Fear
● Spiritual distress
● Risk for post-trauma syndrome
● Ineffective community coping

The following criteria may be used for measurement of outcomes in the care of the client having experienced a traumatic event.
The client:

1. Experiences minimal/no injury to self.
2. Demonstrates behaviors necessary to protect self from further injury.
3. Identifies interventions to prevent/reduce risk of infection.
4. Is free of infection.
5. Maintains anxiety at manageable level.
6. Expresses beliefs and values about spiritual issues.
7. Demonstrates ability to deal with emotional reactions in an individually appropriate manner.
8. Demonstrates an increase in activities to improve community functioning.

Planning/Implementation

Table 13–1 provides a plan of care for the client who has experienced a traumatic event. Selected nursing diagnoses are presented, along with outcome criteria, appropriate nursing interventions, and rationales for each.

Evaluation

In the final step of the nursing process, a reassessment is conducted to determine if the nursing actions have been successful in achieving the objectives of care. Evaluation of the nursing actions for the client who has experienced

TABLE 13-1	Care Plan for the Client Who Has Experienced a Traumatic Event

NURSING DIAGNOSIS: ANXIETY (PANIC)/FEAR

RELATED TO: Real or perceived threat to physical well-being; threat of death; situational crisis; exposure to toxins; unmet needs

EVIDENCED BY: Persistent feelings of apprehension and uneasiness; sense of impending doom; impaired functioning; verbal expressions of having no control or influence over situation, outcome, or self-care; sympathetic stimulation; extraneous physical movements

OUTCOME CRITERIA	NURSING INTERVENTIONS	RATIONALE
Client will maintain anxiety at manageable level.	1. Determine degree of anxiety/fear present, associated behaviors (e.g., laughter, crying, calm or agitation, excited/hysterical behavior, expressions of disbelief and/or self-blame), and reality of perceived threat.	1. Clearly understanding client's perception is pivotal to providing appropriate assistance in overcoming the fear. Individual may be agitated or totally overwhelmed. Panic state increases risk for client's own safety as well as the safety of others in the environment.
	2. Note degree of disorganization.	2. Client may be unable to handle ADLs or work requirements and need more intensive intervention.
	3. Create as quiet an area as possible. Maintain a calm confident manner. Speak in even tone using short simple sentences.	3. Decreases sense of confusion or over-stimulation; enhances sense of safety. Helps client focus on what is said and reduces transmission of anxiety.
	4. Develop trusting relationship with the client.	4. Trust is the basis of a therapeutic nurse-client relationship and enables them to work effectively together.
	5. Identify whether incident has reactivated preexisting or coexisting situations (physical or psychological).	5. Concerns and psychological issues will be recycled every time trauma is re-experienced and affect how the client views the current situation.
	6. Determine presence of physical symptoms (e.g., numbness, headache, tightness in chest, nausea, and pounding heart)	6. Physical problems need to be differentiated from anxiety symptoms so appropriate treatment can be given.
	7. Identify psychological responses (e.g., anger, shock, acute anxiety, panic, confusion, denial). Record emotional changes.	7. Although these are normal responses at the time of the trauma, they will recycle again and again until they are dealt with adequately.
	8. Discuss with client the perception of what is causing the anxiety.	8. Increases the ability to connect symptoms to subjective feeling of anxiety, providing opportunity to gain insight/control and make desired changes.
	9. Assist client to correct any distortions being experienced. Share perceptions with client.	9. Perceptions based on reality will help to decrease fearfulness. How the nurse views the situation may help client to see it differently.
	10. Explore with client or significant other the manner in which client has previously coped with anxiety-producing events.	10. May help client regain sense of control and recognize significance of trauma.
	11. Engage client in learning new coping behaviors (e.g., progressive muscle relaxation, thought-stopping).	11. Replacing maladaptive behaviors can enhance ability to manage and deal with stress. Interrupting obsessive thinking allows client to use energy to address underlying anxiety, whereas continued rumination about the incident can retard recovery.
	12. Encourage use of techniques to manage stress and vent emotions such as anger and hostility.	12. Reduces the likelihood of eruptions that can result in abusive behavior.

(Continued on opposite page)

OUTCOME CRITERIA	NURSING INTERVENTIONS	RATIONALE
	13. Give positive feedback when client demonstrates better ways to manage anxiety and is able to calmly and realistically appraise the situation.	13. Provides acknowledgement and reinforcement, encouraging use of new coping strategies. Enhances ability to deal with fearful feelings and gain control over situation, promoting future successes.
	14. Administer medications as indicated: Antianxiety: diazepam, alprazolam, oxazepam; or Antidepressants: fluoxetine, paroxetine, bupropion	14. Provides temporary relief of anxiety symptoms, enhancing ability to cope with situation. To lift mood and help suppress intrusive thoughts and explosive anger.

NURSING DIAGNOSIS: SPIRITUAL DISTRESS

RELATED TO: Physical or psychological stress; energy-consuming anxiety; loss(es), intense suffering; separation from religious or cultural ties; challenged belief and value system

EVIDENCED BY: Expressions of concern about disaster and the meaning of life and death or belief systems; inner conflict about current loss of normality and effects of the disaster; anger directed at deity; engaging in self-blame; seeking spiritual assistance

OUTCOME CRITERIA	NURSING INTERVENTIONS	RATIONALE
Client expresses beliefs and values about spiritual issues.	1. Determine client's religious/spiritual orientation, current involvement, and presence of conflicts.	1. Provides baseline for planning care and accessing appropriate resources.
	2. Establish environment that promotes free expression of feelings and concerns. Provide calm, peaceful setting when possible.	2. Promotes awareness and identification of feelings so they can be dealt with.
	3. Listen to client's and significant others' expressions of anger, concern, alienation from God, belief that situation is a punishment for wrongdoing, etc.	3. It is helpful to understand the client's and significant others' points of view and how they are questioning their faith in the face of tragedy.
	4. Note sense of futility, feelings of hopelessness and helplessness, lack of motivation to help self.	4. These thoughts and feelings can result in the client feeling paralyzed and unable to move forward to resolve the situation.
	5. Listen to expressions of inability to find meaning in life and reason for living. Evaluate for suicidal ideation.	5. May indicate need for further intervention to prevent suicide attempt.
	6. Determine support systems available to client.	6. Presence or lack of support systems can affect client's recovery.
	7. Ask how you can be most helpful. Convey acceptance of client's spiritual beliefs and concerns.	7. Promotes trust and comfort, encouraging client to be open about sensitive matters.
	8. Make time for nonjudgmental discussion of philosophic issues and questions about spiritual impact of current situation.	8. Helps client to begin to look at basis for spiritual confusion. *Note:* There is a potential for care provider's belief system to interfere with client finding own way. Therefore, it is most beneficial to remain neutral and not espouse own beliefs.
	9. Discuss difference between grief and guilt and help client to identify and deal with each, assuming responsibility for own actions, expressing awareness of the consequences of acting out of false guilt.	9. Blaming self for what has happened impedes dealing with the grief process and needs to be discussed and dealt with.
	10. Use therapeutic communication skills of reflection and active-listening.	10. Helps client find own solutions to concerns.

(Continued on following page)

OUTCOME CRITERIA	NURSING INTERVENTIONS	RATIONALE
Client expresses beliefs and values about spiritual issues.	11. Encourage client to experience meditation, prayer, and forgiveness. Provide information that anger with God is a normal part of the grieving process.	11. This can help to heal past and present pain.
	12. Assist client to develop goals for dealing with life situation.	12. Enhances commitment to goal, optimizing outcomes and promoting sense of hope.
	13. Identify and refer to resources that can be helpful, e.g., pastoral/parish nurse or religious counselor, crisis counselor, psychotherapy, Alcoholics/Narcotics Anonymous.	13. Specific assistance may be helpful to recovery (e.g., relationship problems, substance abuse, suicidal ideation).
	14. Encourage participation in support groups.	14. Discussing concerns and questions with others can help client resolve feelings.

NURSING DIAGNOSIS: RISK FOR POST-TRAUMA SYNDROME

RELATED TO: Events outside the range of usual human experience; serious threat or injury to self or loved ones; witnessing horrors or tragic events; exaggerated sense of responsibility; survivor's guilt or role in the event; inadequate social support

OUTCOME CRITERIA	NURSING INTERVENTIONS	RATIONALE
Client demonstrates ability to deal with emotional reactions in an individually appropriate manner.	1. Determine involvement in event (e.g., survivor, significant other, rescue/aid worker, healthcare provider, family member).	1. All those concerned with a traumatic event are at risk for emotional trauma and have needs related to their involvement in the event. *Note:* Close involvement with victims affects individual responses and may prolong emotional suffering.
	2. Evaluate current factors associated with the event, such as displacement from home due to illness/injury, natural disaster, or terrorist attack. Identify how client's past experiences may affect current situation.	2. Affects client's reaction to current event and is basis for planning care and identifying appropriate support systems and resources.
	3. Listen for comments of taking on responsibility (e.g., "I should have been more careful or gone back to get her.")	3. Statements such as these are indicators of "survivor's guilt" and blaming self for actions.
	4. Identify client's current coping mechanisms.	4. Noting positive or negative coping skills provides direction for care.
	5. Determine availability and usefulness of client's support systems, family, social contacts, and community resources.	5. Family and others close to the client may also be at risk and require assistance to cope with the trauma.
	6. Provide information about signs and symptoms of post-trauma response, especially if individual is involved in a high-risk occupation.	6. Awareness of these factors helps individual identify need for assistance when signs and symptoms occur.
	7. Identify and discuss client's strengths as well as vulnerabilities.	7. Provides information to build on for coping with traumatic experience.
	8. Evaluate individual's perceptions of events and personal significance (e.g., rescue worker trained to provide life-saving assistance but recovering only dead bodies).	8. Events that trigger feelings of despair and hopelessness may be more difficult to deal with, and require long-term interventions.
	9. Provide emotional and physical presence by sitting with client/significant other and offering solace.	9. Strengthens coping abilities.
	10. Encourage expression of feelings. Note whether feelings expressed appear congruent with events experienced.	10. It is important to talk about the incident repeatedly. Incongruencies may indicate deeper conflict and can impede resolution.

(Continued on opposite page)

OUTCOME CRITERIA	NURSING INTERVENTIONS	RATIONALE
	11. Note presence of nightmares, reliving the incident, loss of appetite, irritability, numbness and crying, and family or relationship disruption.	11. These responses are normal in the early post-incident time frame. If prolonged and persistent, they may indicate need for more intensive therapy.
	12. Provide a calm, safe environment.	12. Helps client deal with the disruption in their life.
	13. Encourage and assist client in learning stress-management techniques.	13. Promotes relaxation and helps individual exercise control over self and what has happened.
	14. Recommend participation in debriefing sessions that may be provided following major disaster events.	14. Dealing with the stresses promptly may facilitate recovery from the event or prevent exacerbation.
	15. Identify employment, community resource groups.	15. Provides opportunity for ongoing support to deal with recurrent feelings related to the trauma.
	16. Administer medications as indicated, such as antipsychotics (e.g., chlorpromazine or haloperidol) or carbamazepine (Tegretol)	16. Low doses may be used for reduction of psychotic symptoms when loss of contact with reality occurs, usually for clients with especially disturbing flashbacks. Tegretol may be used to alleviate intrusive recollections/flashbacks, impulsivity, and violent behavior.

NURSING DIAGNOSIS: INEFFECTIVE COMMUNITY COPING

RELATED TO: Natural or man-made disasters (earthquakes, tornados, floods, reemerging infectious agents, terrorist activity); ineffective or nonexistent community systems (e.g., lack of or inadequate emergency medical system, transportation system, or disaster planning systems)

EVIDENCED BY: Deficits of community participation; community does not meet its own expectations; expressed vulnerability; community powerlessness; stressors perceived as excessive; excessive community conflicts; high illness rates

OUTCOME CRITERIA	NURSING INTERVENTIONS	RATIONALE
Client demonstrates an increase in activities to improve community functioning.	1. Evaluate community activities that are related to meeting collective needs within the community itself and between the community and the larger society. Note immediate needs, such as healthcare, food, shelter, funds.	1. Provides a baseline to determine community needs in relation to current concerns or threats.
	2. Note community reports of functioning including areas of weakness or conflict.	2. Provides a view of how the community itself sees these areas.
	3. Identify effects of related factors on community activities.	3. In the face of a current threat, local or national, community resources need to be evaluated, updated, and given priority to meet the identified need.
	4. Determine availability and use of resources. Identify unmet demands or needs of the community.	4. Information necessary to identify what else is needed to meet the current situation.
	5. Determine community strengths.	5. Promotes understanding of the ways in which the community is already meeting the identified needs.
	6. Encourage community members/groups to engage in problem-solving activities.	6. Promotes a sense of working together to meet the needs.
	7. Develop a plan jointly with the members of the community to address immediate needs.	7. Deals with deficits in support of identified goals.
	8. Create plans managing interactions within the community itself and between the community and the larger society.	8. Meets collective needs when the concerns/threats are shared beyond a local community.

(Continued on following page)

TABLE 13-1	Care Plan for the Client Who Has Experienced a Traumatic Event *(Continued)*	
OUTCOME CRITERIA	**NURSING INTERVENTIONS**	**RATIONALE**
	9. Make information accessible to the public. Provide channels for dissemination of information to the community as a whole (e.g., print media, radio/television reports and community bulletin boards, internet sites, speaker's bureau, reports to committees/councils/advisory boards).	9. Readily available accurate information can help citizens deal with the situation.
	10. Make information available in different modalities and geared to differing educational levels/cultures of the community.	10. Using languages other than English and making written materials accessible to all members of the community will promote understanding.
	11. Seek out and evaluate needs of underserved populations.	11. Homeless and those residing in lower income areas may have special requirements that need to be addressed with additional resources.

SOURCE: Doenges, Moorhouse, & Geissler (2002). With permission.

a traumatic event may be facilitated by gathering information utilizing the following types of questions.

1. Has the client escaped serious injury, or have injuries been resolved?
2. Have infections been prevented or resolved?
3. Is the client able to maintain anxiety at manageable level?
4. Does he or she demonstrate appropriate problem-solving skills?
5. Is the client able to discuss his or her beliefs about spiritual issues?
6. Does the client demonstrate the ability to deal with emotional reactions in an individually appropriate manner?
7. Does he or she verbalize a subsiding of the physical manifestations (e.g., pain, nightmares, flashbacks, fatigue) associated with the traumatic event?
8. Has there been recognition of factors affecting the community's ability to meet its own demands or needs?
9. Has there been a demonstration of increased activities to improve community functioning?
10. Has a plan been established and put in place to deal with future contingencies?

SUMMARY

A *crisis* is defined as "a sudden event in one's life that disturbs homeostasis, during which usual coping mechanisms cannot resolve the problem" (Lagerquist, 2001). All individuals experience crises at one time or another. This does not necessarily indicate psychopathology.

Crises are precipitated by specific identifiable events and are determined by an individual's personal perception of the situation. They are acute rather than chronic and generally last no more than a few hours to a few weeks.

Crises occur when an individual is exposed to a stressor and previous problem-solving techniques are ineffective. This causes the level of anxiety to rise. Panic may ensue when new techniques are tried and resolution fails to occur.

Baldwin (1978) identified six types of crises. They include dispositional crises, crises of anticipated life transitions, crises resulting from traumatic stress, maturation/developmental crises, crises reflecting psychopathology, and psychiatric emergencies. The type of crisis determines the method of intervention selected.

Crisis intervention is designed to provide rapid assistance for individuals who have an urgent need. Aguilera (1998) identifies the minimum therapeutic goal of crisis intervention as psychological resolution of the individual's immediate crisis and restoration to at least the level of functioning that existed before the crisis period. A maximum goal is improvement in functioning above the precrisis level.

Nurses regularly respond to individuals in crisis in all types of settings. Nursing process is the vehicle by which nurses assist individuals in crisis with a short-term problem-solving approach to change. A four-phase technique was outlined: assessment/analysis, planning of therapeutic intervention, intervention, and evaluation of crisis resolution and anticipatory planning. Through this structured method of assistance, nurses help individuals in crisis to develop more adaptive coping strategies for dealing with stressful situations in the future.

Nurses have many important skills that can assist individuals and communities in the wake of traumatic events. This chapter presented an example of disaster nursing as it is implemented through the six steps of the nursing process. A care plan for the client who has experienced a traumatic event was included.

REVIEW QUESTIONS

SELF-EXAMINATION/LEARNING EXERCISE

Select the best response to each of the following questions.

1. Which of the following is a correct assumption regarding the concept of crisis?
   a. Crises occur only in individuals with psychopathology.
   b. The stressful event that precipitates crisis is seldom identifiable.
   c. A crisis situation contains the potential for psychological growth or deterioration.
   d. Crises are chronic situations that recur many times during an individual's life.

2. Crises occur when an individual:
   a. Is exposed to a precipitating stressor.
   b. Perceives a stressor to be threatening.
   c. Has no support systems.
   d. Experiences a stressor and perceives coping strategies to be ineffective.

3. Amanda's mobile home was destroyed by a tornado. Amanda received only minor injuries, but is experiencing disabling anxiety in the aftermath of the event. This type of crisis is called:
   a. Crisis resulting from traumatic stress
   b. Maturational/developmental crisis
   c. Dispositional crisis
   d. Crisis of anticipated life transitions

4. The most appropriate crisis intervention with Amanda would be to:
   a. Encourage her to recognize how lucky she is to be alive.
   b. Discuss stages of grief and feelings associated with each.
   c. Identify community resources that can help Amanda.
   d. Suggest that she find a place to live that provides a storm shelter.

5. Jenny reported to the high school nurse that her mother drinks too much. She is drunk every afternoon when Jenny gets home from school. Jenny is afraid to invite friends over because of her mother's behavior. This type of crisis is called:
   a. Crisis resulting from traumatic stress
   b. Maturational/developmental crisis
   c. Dispositional crisis
   d. Crisis reflecting psychopathology

6. The most appropriate nursing intervention with Jenny would be to:
   a. Make arrangements for her to start attending Al-Ateen meetings.
   b. Help her identify the positive things in her life and recognize that her situation could be a lot worse than it is.
   c. Teach her about the effects of alcohol on the body and that it can be hereditary.
   d. Refer her to a psychiatrist for private therapy to learn to deal with her home situation.

7. Ginger, age 19 and an only child, left 3 months ago to attend a college of her choice 500 miles away from her parents. It is Ginger's first time away from home. She has difficulty making decisions and will not undertake anything new without first consulting her mother. They talk on the phone almost every day. Ginger has recently started having anxiety attacks. She consults the nurse practitioner in the student health center. This type of crisis is called:
   a. Crisis resulting from traumatic stress
   b. Dispositional crisis
   c. Psychiatric emergency
   d. Maturational/developmental crisis

8. The most appropriate nursing intervention with Ginger would be to:
   a. Suggest she move to a college closer to home.
   b. Work with Ginger on unresolved dependency issues.
   c. Help her find someone in the college town from whom she could seek assistance rather than calling her mother regularly.
   d. Recommend that the college physician prescribe an antianxiety medication for Ginger.

9. Marie, age 56, is the mother of five children. Her youngest child, who had been living at home and attending the local college, recently graduated and accepted a job in another state. Marie has never worked outside the home and has devoted her life to satisfying the needs of her husband and children. Since the departure of her last child from home, Marie has become more and more despondent. Her husband has become very concerned, and takes her to the local mental health center. This type of crisis is called:
   a. Dispositional crisis
   b. Crisis of anticipated life transitions
   c. Psychiatric emergency
   d. Crisis resulting from traumatic stress

10. The most appropriate nursing intervention with Marie would be to:
    a. Refer her to her family physician for a complete physical examination.
    b. Suggest she seek outside employment now that her children have left home.
    c. Identify convenient support systems for times when she is feeling particularly despondent.
    d. Begin grief work and assist her to recognize areas of self-worth separate and apart from her children.

11. The desired outcome of working with an individual who has witnessed a traumatic event and is now experiencing panic anxiety is:
    a. The individual will experience no anxiety.
    b. The individual will demonstrate hope for the future.
    c. The individual will maintain anxiety at a manageable level.
    d. The individual will verbalize acceptance of self as worthy.

REFERENCES

Aguilera, D.C. (1998). *Crisis intervention: Theory and methodology* (8th ed.). St. Louis: C.V. Mosby.
Bateman, A., & Peternelj-Taylor, C. (1998). Crisis intervention. In C.A. Glod (Ed.), *Contemporary psychiatric-mental health nursing: The brain-behavior connection*. Philadelphia: F.A. Davis.
Doenges, M.E., Moorhouse, M.F., & Geissler, A.C. (2002). *Nursing care plans: Guidelines for individualizing patient care* (6th ed.). Philadelphia: F.A. Davis.
Kaplan, H.I., & Sadock, B.J. (1998). *Synopsis of psychiatry: Behavioral sciences/clinical psychiatry* (8th ed.). Baltimore: Williams & Wilkins.
Lagerquist, S.L. (2001). *Davis's NCLEX-RN Success*. Philadelphia: F.A. Davis.
Norwood, A.E., Ursano, R.J., & Fullerton, C.S. (2004). *Disaster psychiatry: Principles and practice*. American Psychiatric Association. Retrieved November 22, 2004 from the World Wide Web at http://www.psych.org/disasterpsych/sl/principlespractice.cfm
Oklahoma State Department of Health [OSDH]. (2001). *After the storm: Helping families cope with disaster*. Oklahoma City, OK: State Department of Health.

CLASSICAL REFERENCES

Baldwin, B.A. (1978, July). A paradigm for the classification of emotional crises: Implications for crisis intervention. *American Journal of Orthopsychiatry, 48*(3), 538–551.
Caplan, G. (1964). *Principles of preventive psychiatry*. New York: Basic Books.

RELAXATION THERAPY

CHAPTER OUTLINE

OBJECTIVES

THE STRESS EPIDEMIC

PHYSIOLOGICAL, COGNITIVE, AND
BEHAVIORAL MANIFESTATIONS
OF RELAXATION

METHODS OF ACHIEVING RELAXATION

THE ROLE OF THE NURSE IN
RELAXATION THERAPY

SUMMARY

REVIEW QUESTIONS

KEY TERMS

biofeedback
meditation
mental imagery

progressive relaxation
stress management

CORE CONCEPTS

relaxation
stress

OBJECTIVES

After reading this chapter, the student will be able to:

1. Identify conditions for which relaxation is appropriate therapy.
2. Describe physiological and behavioral manifestations of relaxation.
3. Discuss various methods of achieving relaxation.
4. Describe the role of the nurse in relaxation therapy.

Researchers now know that stress has a definite effect on the body. They know that stress on the body can be caused by positive events as well as negative ones, and they know that prolonged stress can result in many physiological illnesses. Many times we hear "Relax, take it easy, don't work so hard, don't worry so much; you'll live longer that way." This is good advice no doubt, but it is easier to say than to do.

Nurses are in an ideal position to assist individuals in the management of stress in their lives. This chapter discusses the therapeutic benefits to the individual of regular participation in relaxation exercises. Various methods of achieving relaxation are described, and the nurse's role in helping individuals learn how to use relaxation techniques adaptively is explored.

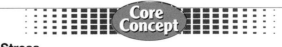

Stress
A biological, psychological, social, or chemical factor that causes physical or emotional tension and may be a factor in the etiology of certain illnesses.

THE STRESS EPIDEMIC

Individuals experience stress as a daily fact of life; it cannot be avoided. It is generated by both positive and negative experiences that require adjustment to various changes in one's current routine. Whether or not there is more stress today than in the past is unknown, but some experts have suggested that it has become more

207

pervasive. Perhaps this is due to the many uncertainties and salient risks that challenge our most basic value systems on a day-to-day basis.

In Chapter 1, a lengthy discussion was presented regarding the "fight or flight" response of the human body to stressful situations. This response served our ancestors well. The extra burst of adrenaline primed their muscles and focused their attention on the danger at hand. Indeed, the response provided early *Homo sapiens* with the essentials to deal with life-and-death situations, such as an imminent attack by a saber-toothed tiger or grizzly bear.

Today, with stress rapidly permeating our society, large segments of the population experience the "fight or flight" response on a regular basis. However, the physical reinforcements are not used in a manner by which the individual is returned to the homeostatic condition within a short period. The "fight or flight" emergency response is inappropriate to today's psychosocial stresses that persist over long periods. In fact, in today's society, rather than assisting with life-and-death situations, the response may actually be a contributing factor in some life-and-death situations. Dr. Joel Elkes, director of the behavioral medicine program at the University of Louisville, Kentucky, has said, "Our mode of life itself, the way we live, is emerging as today's principal cause of illness." Stress is now known to be a major contributor, either directly or indirectly, to coronary heart disease, cancer, lung ailments, accidental injuries, cirrhosis of the liver, and suicide—six of the leading causes of death in the United States (Karren, Hafen, Smith, & Frandsen, 2002).

Stress management has become a multimillion-dollar business in the United States. Corporation managers have realized increases in production by providing employees with stress-reduction programs. Hospitals and clinics have responded to the need for services that offer stress management information to individuals and groups.

When, then, is relaxation therapy required? The answer to this question depends largely on *predisposing factors*—the genetic influences, past experiences, and existing conditions that influence how an individual perceives and responds to stress. For example, temperament (i.e., behavioral characteristics that are present at birth) often plays a determining role in the individual's manner of responding to stressful situations. Some individuals, by temperament, naturally respond with a greater degree of anxiety than others.

Past experiences are occurrences that result in learned patterns that can influence an individual's adaptation response. They include previous exposure to the stressor or other stressors, learned coping responses, and degree of adaptation to previous stressors.

Existing conditions are the individual vulnerabilities that can influence the adequacy of the physical, psychological, and social resources for dealing with stressful situations. Examples include current health status, moti-

TABLE 14–1	**How Vulnerable Are You to Stress?**

Score each item from 1 (almost always) to 5 (never), according to how much of the time each statement applies to you.

_____ 1. I eat at least one hot, balanced meal a day.
_____ 2. I get 7 to 8 hours sleep at least four nights a week.
_____ 3. I give and receive affection regularly.
_____ 4. I have at least one relative within 50 miles on whom I can rely.
_____ 5. I exercise to the point of perspiration at least twice a week.
_____ 6. I smoke less than half a pack of cigarettes a day.
_____ 7. I take fewer than five alcoholic drinks a week.
_____ 8. I am the appropriate weight for my height.
_____ 9. I have an income adequate to meet basic expenses.
_____ 10. I get strength from my religious beliefs.
_____ 11. I regularly attend club or social activities.
_____ 12. I have a network of friends and acquaintances.
_____ 13. I have one or more friends to confide in about personal matters.
_____ 14. I am in good health (including eyesight, hearing, and teeth).
_____ 15. I am able to speak openly about my feelings when angry or worried.
_____ 16. I have regular conversations with the people I live with about domestic problems (e.g., chores, money, and daily living issues).
_____ 17. I do something for fun at least once a week.
_____ 18. I am able to organize my time effectively.
_____ 19. I drink fewer than three cups of coffee (or tea or colas) a day.
_____ 20. I take quiet time for myself during the day.
_____ TOTAL

To get your score, add up the figures and subtract 20. Any number over 30 indicates a vulnerability to stress. You are seriously vulnerable if your score is between 50 and 75, and extremely vulnerable if it is over 75.

SOURCE: From Miller and Smith (1983), Biobehavioral Institute of Boston, with permission.

vation, developmental maturity, severity and duration of the stressor, financial and educational resources, age, existing coping strategies, and a support system of caring others.

All individuals react to stress with predictable physiological and psychosocial responses. These predisposing factors determine the degree of severity of the response. Undoubtedly, there are very few people who would not benefit from some form of relaxation therapy. Miller and Rahe (1997) developed the Recent Life Changes Questionnaire, which correlated an individual's susceptibility to physical or psychological illness with his or her level of stress (see Chapter 1). The lay literature now provides various self-tests that individuals may perform to determine their vulnerability to stress. Two of these are presented in Tables 14–1 and 14–2.

PHYSIOLOGICAL, COGNITIVE, AND BEHAVIORAL MANIFESTATIONS OF RELAXATION

The physiological and behavioral manifestations of stress are well documented (see Chapters 1 and 2). A review of

TABLE 14-2	Are You "Stressed Out?"

Check yes or no for each of the following questions.

	Yes	No
1. Do you have recurrent headaches, neck tension, or back pain?	_____	_____
2. Do you often have indigestion, nausea, or diarrhea?	_____	_____
3. Have you unintentionally gained or lost 5–10 lb in the last month?	_____	_____
4. Do you have difficulty falling or staying asleep?	_____	_____
5. Do you often feel restless?	_____	_____
6. Do you have difficulty concentrating?	_____	_____
7. Do you drink alcohol, smoke, or take drugs to relax?	_____	_____
8. Have you had a major illness, surgery, or an accident in the past year?	_____	_____
9. Have you lost five or more days of work due to illness in the past 6 months?	_____	_____
10. Have you had a change in job status (been fired, laid off, promoted, demoted, and so on) in the past 6 months?	_____	_____
11. Do you work more than 48 hours a week?	_____	_____
12. Do you have serious financial problems?	_____	_____
13. Have you recently experienced family or marital problems?	_____	_____
14. Has a person of significance in your life died in the past year?	_____	_____
15. Have you been divorced or separated in the past year?	_____	_____
16. Do you find you've lost interest in hobbies, physical activity, and leisure time?	_____	_____
17. Have you lost interest in your relationship with your spouse, a relative, or a friend?	_____	_____
18. Do you find yourself watching more TV than you should?	_____	_____
19. Are you emotional or easily irritated lately?	_____	_____
20. Do you seem to experience more distress and discomfort than most people?	_____	_____

Scoring:
Each yes is worth 1 point; each no is worth 0.
Total your points:
  0–3 = mildly stressed
  4–6 = moderately stressed
  7 or more = extremely vulnerable. You may be at risk for stress-related illness.

SOURCE: From The Department of Psychiatry, St. Joseph Medical Center, Wichita, KS.

these symptoms is presented in Table 14–3. The persistence of these symptoms over long periods can contribute to the development of numerous stress-related illnesses.

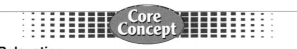

Relaxation
A decrease in tension or intensity, resulting in refreshment of body and mind. A state of refreshing tranquility.

The achievement of relaxation can counteract many of these symptoms. In a state of deep relaxation, the respiration rate may slow to as few as four to six breaths per minute and the heart rate to as low as 24 beats per minute (Pelletier, 1992). Blood pressure decreases and the meta-bolic rate slows down. Muscle tension diminishes, pupils constrict, and blood vessels in the periphery dilate leading to increased temperature and feeling of warmth in the extremities.

One's level of consciousness moves from beta activity, which occurs when one is mentally alert and actively thinking, to alpha activity, a state of altered consciousness (Davis, Eshelman, & McKay, 2000). Benefits associated with achievement of alpha consciousness include an increase in creativity, memory, and the ability to concentrate. Ultimately, an improvement in adaptive functioning may be realized.

When deeply relaxed, individuals are less attentive to distracting stimuli in the external environment. They will respond to questions directed at them but do not initiate verbal interaction. Physical demeanor is very composed.

TABLE 14-3	Physiological, Cognitive, and Behavioral Manifestations of Stress

PHYSIOLOGICAL	COGNITIVE	BEHAVIORAL
Epinephrine and norepinephrine are released into the bloodstream.	Anxiety increases.	Restlessness
Pupils dilate.	Confusion and disorientation may be evident.	Irritability
Respiration rate increases.	The person is unable to problem solve.	Use or misuse of defense mechanisms
Heart rate increases.	The person is unable to concentrate.	Disorganized routine functioning
Blood pressure increases.	Cognitive processes focus on achieving relief from anxiety.	Insomnia and anorexia
Digestion subsides.	Learning is inhibited.	Compulsive or bizarre behaviors (depending on level of anxiety being experienced)
Blood sugar increases.	Thoughts may reflect obsessions and ruminations.	
Metabolism increases.		
Serum free fatty acids, cholesterol, and triglycerides increase.		

TABLE 14–4	Physiological, Cognitive, and Behavioral Manifestations of Relaxation	
PHYSIOLOGICAL	**COGNITIVE**	**BEHAVIORAL**
Lower levels of epinephrine and norepinephrine in the blood	Change from beta consciousness to alpha consciousness	Distractibility to environmental stimuli is decreased.
Respiration rate decreases (sometimes as low as 4–6 breaths per minute).	Creativity and memory are enhanced.	Will respond to questions but does not initiate verbal interaction.
Heart rate decreases (sometimes as low as 24 beats per minute).	Increased ability to concentrate	Calm, tranquil demeanor; no evidence of restlessness
Blood pressure decreases.		Common mannerisms include eyes closed, jaws parted, palms open, fingers curled, and head slightly tilted to the side.
Metabolic rate slows down.		
Muscle tension diminishes.		
Pupils constrict.		
Vasodilation and increased temperature in the extremities.		

Virtually no muscle activity is observed. Eyes are closed, jaws may be slightly parted, and palms are open with fingers curled, but not clenched. Head may be slightly tilted to the side.

A summary of the physiological, cognitive, and behavioral manifestations of relaxation is presented in Table 14–4.

METHODS OF ACHIEVING RELAXATION

Deep Breathing Exercises

Deep breathing is a simple technique that is basic to most other relaxation skills. Tension is released when the lungs are allowed to breathe in as much oxygen as possible (Sobel & Ornstein, 1996). Breathing exercises have been found to be effective in reducing anxiety, depression, irritability, muscular tension, and fatigue (Davis, Eshelman, & McKay, 2000; Sobel & Ornstein, 1996). An advantage of this exercise is that it may be accomplished anywhere and at any time. A good guideline is to practice deep breathing for a few minutes three or four times a day or whenever a feeling of tenseness occurs.

Technique

1. Sit, stand, or lie in a comfortable position, ensuring that the spine is straight.
2. Place one hand on your abdomen and the other on your chest.
3. Inhale slowly and deeply through your nose. The abdomen should be expanding and pushing up on your hand. The chest should be moving only slightly.
4. When you have breathed in as much as possible, hold your breath for a few seconds before exhaling.
5. Begin exhaling slowly through the mouth, pursing your lips as if you were going to whistle. Pursing the lips helps to control how fast you exhale and keeps airways open as long as possible.
6. Feel the abdomen deflate as the lungs are emptied of air.
7. Begin the inhale–exhale cycle again. Focus on the sound and feeling of your breathing as you become more and more relaxed.
8. Continue the deep-breathing exercises for 5 to 10 minutes at a time. Once mastered, the technique may be used as often as required to relieve tension.

Progressive Relaxation

Progressive relaxation, a method of deep-muscle relaxation, was developed in 1929 by Chicago physician Edmond Jacobson. His technique is based on the premise that the body responds to anxiety-provoking thoughts and events with muscle tension. Excellent results have been observed with this method in the treatment of muscular tension, anxiety, insomnia, depression, fatigue, irritable bowel, muscle spasms, neck and back pain, high blood pressure, mild phobias, and stuttering (Davis, Eshelman, & McKay, 2000).

Technique

Each muscle group is tensed for 5 to 7 seconds and then relaxed for 20 to 30 seconds, during which time the individual concentrates on the difference in sensations between the two conditions. Soft, slow background music may facilitate relaxation.

1. Sit in a comfortable chair with your hands in your lap, your feet flat on the floor, and your eyes closed.
2. Begin by taking three deep, slow breaths, inhaling through the nose and releasing the air slowly through the mouth.
3. Now starting with the feet, pull the toes forward toward the knees, stiffen your calves, and hold for a count of five.
4. Now release the hold. Let go of the tension. Feel the sensation of relaxation and warmth as the tension flows out of the muscles.

5. Next, tense the muscles of the thighs and buttocks, and hold for a count of five.

6. Now release the hold. Feel the tension drain away, and be aware of the difference in sensation—perhaps a heaviness or feeling of warmth that you did not feel when the muscles were tensed. Concentrate on this feeling for a few seconds.

7. Next, tense the abdominal muscles. Hold for a count of five.

8. Now release the hold. Concentrate on the feeling of relaxation in the muscles. You may feel a warming sensation. Hold on to that feeling for 15 to 20 seconds.

9. Next, tense the muscles in the back and hold for a count of five.

10. Now release the hold. Feel the sensation of relaxation and warmth as the tension flows out of the muscles.

11. Next, tense the muscles of your hands, biceps, and forearms. Clench your hands into a tight fist. Hold for a count of five.

12. Now release the hold. Notice the sensations. You may feel tingling, warmth, or a light, airy feeling. Recognize these sensations as tension leaves the muscles.

13. Next, tense the muscles of the shoulders and neck. Shrug the shoulders tightly and hold for a count of five.

14. Now release the hold. Sense the tension as it leaves the muscles and experience the feeling of relaxation.

15. Next, tense the muscles of the face. Wrinkle the forehead, frown, squint the eyes, and purse the lips. Hold for a count of five.

16. Now release the hold. Recognize a light, warm feeling flowing into the muscles.

17. Now feel the relaxation in your whole body. As the tension leaves your entire being, you feel completely relaxed.

18. Open your eyes and enjoy renewed energy.

Modified (or Passive) Progressive Relaxation

Technique

In this version of total-body relaxation the muscles are not tensed. The individual learns to relax muscles by concentrating on the feeling of relaxation within the muscle. These instructions may be presented by one person for another or they may be self-administered. Relaxation may be facilitated by playing soft, slow background music during the activity.

1. Assume a comfortable position. Some suggestions include the following:
   a. Sitting straight up in a chair with hands in the lap or at sides and feet flat on the floor.
   b. Sitting in a reclining chair with hands in the lap or at sides and legs up on an elevated surface.
   c. Lying flat with head slightly elevated on pillow and arms at sides.

2. Close your eyes and take three deep breaths through your nose, slowly releasing the air through your mouth.

3. Allow a feeling of peacefulness to descend over you—a pleasant, enjoyable sensation of being comfortable and at ease.

4. Remain in this state for several minutes.

5. It is now time to turn your attention to various parts of your body.

6. We will begin with the muscles of the head, face, throat, and shoulders. Concentrate on these muscles, paying particular attention to those in the forehead and jaws. Feel the tension leave the area. The muscles start to feel relaxed, heavy, and warm. Concentrate on this feeling for a few minutes.

7. Now let the feeling of relaxation continue to spread downward to the muscles of your biceps, forearms, and hands. Concentrate on these muscles. Feel the tension dissolve, the muscles starting to feel relaxed and heavy. A feeling of warmth spreads through these muscles all the way to the fingertips. They are feeling very warm and very heavy. Concentrate on this feeling for a few minutes.

8. The tension is continuing to dissolve now, and you are feeling very relaxed. Turn your attention to the muscles in your chest, abdomen, and lower back. Feel the tension leave these areas. Allow these muscles to become very relaxed. They start to feel very warm and very heavy. Concentrate on this feeling for a few minutes.

9. The feeling of relaxation continues to move downward now as we move to the muscles of the thighs, buttocks, calves, and feet. Feel the tension moving down and out of your body. These muscles feel very relaxed now. Your legs are feeling very heavy and very limp. A feeling of warmth spreads over the area, all the way to the toes. You can feel that all the tension has been released.

10. Your whole body feels relaxed and warm. Listen to the music for a few moments and concentrate on this relaxed, warm feeling. Take several deep, slow breaths through your nose, releasing the air through your mouth. Continue to concentrate on how relaxed and warm you feel.

11. It is now time to refocus your concentration on the present and wake up your body to resume activity. Open your eyes and stretch or massage your muscles. Wiggle your fingers and toes. Take another deep breath, arise, and enjoy the feeling of renewed energy.

Meditation

Records and phenomenological accounts of meditative practices date back more than 2000 years, but only recently have empirical studies revealed the psychophysiological benefits of regular use (Pelletier, 1992). The goal of **meditation** is to gain "mastery over attention." It brings on a special state of consciousness, as attention is concentrated solely on one thought or object.

Historically, meditation has been associated with religious doctrines and disciplines by which individuals sought enlightenment with God or another higher power. However, meditation can be practiced independently from any religious philosophy and purely as a means of achieving inner harmony and increasing self-awareness.

During meditation, the respiration rate, heart rate, and blood pressure decrease. The overall metabolism declines, and the need for oxygen consumption is reduced. Alpha brain waves—those associated with brain activity during periods of relaxation—predominate (Pelletier, 1992).

Meditation has been used successfully in the prevention and treatment of various cardiovascular diseases. It has proved helpful in curtailing obsessive thinking, anxiety, depression, and hostility (Davis, Eshelman, & McKay, 2000). Meditation improves concentration and attention.

Technique

1. Select a quiet place and a comfortable position. Various sitting positions are appropriate for meditation. Examples include:
   a. Sitting in a chair with your feet flat on the floor approximately 6 inches apart, arms resting comfortably in your lap.
   b. Cross-legged on the floor or on a cushion.
   c. In the Japanese fashion with knees on floor, great toes together, pointed backward, and buttocks resting comfortably on bottom of feet.
   d. In the lotus yoga position, sitting on the floor with the legs flexed at the knees. The ankles are crossed and each foot rests on top of the opposite thigh.
2. Select an object, word, or thought on which to dwell. During meditation the individual becomes preoccupied with the selected focus. This total preoccupation serves to prevent distractions from interrupting attention. Examples of foci include:
   a. *Counting One's Breaths.* All attention is focused on breathing in and out.
   b. *Mantras.* A *mantra* is a syllable, word, or name that is repeated many times as you free your mind of thoughts. Any mantra is appropriate if it works to focus attention and prevent distracting thoughts.
   c. *Objects for Contemplation.* Select an object, such as a rock, a marble, or anything that does not hold a symbolic meaning that might cause distraction. Contemplate the object both visually and tactilely. Focus total attention on the object.
   d. *A Thought That Has Special Meaning to You.* With eyes closed, focus total attention on a specific thought or idea.
3. Practice directing attention on your selected focus for 10 to 15 minutes a day for several weeks. It is essential that the individual does not become upset if intrusive thoughts find their way into the meditation practice. They should merely be dealt with and dismissed as the individual returns to the selected focus of attention. Worrying about one's progress in the ability to meditate is a self-inhibiting behavior.

Mental Imagery

Mental imagery uses the imagination in an effort to reduce the body's response to stress. The frame of reference is very personal, based on what each individual considers to be a relaxing environment. Some might select a scene at the seashore, some might choose a mountain atmosphere, and some might choose floating through the air on a fluffy white cloud. The choices are as limitless as one's imagination. Following is an example of how one individual uses imagery for relaxation. The information is most useful when taped and played back at a time when the individual wishes to achieve relaxation.

Technique

Sit or lie down in a comfortable position. Close your eyes. Imagine that you and someone you love are walking along the seashore. No other people are in sight in any direction. The sun is shining, the sky is blue, and a gentle breeze is blowing. You select a spot to stop and rest. You lie on the sand and close your eyes. You hear the sound of the waves as they splash against the shore. The sun feels warm on your face and body. The sand feels soft and warm against your back. An occasional wave splashes you with a cool mist that dries rapidly in the warm sun. The coconut fragrance of your suntan lotion wafts gently and pleasantly in the air. You lie in this quiet place for what seems like a very long time, taking in the sounds of the waves, the warmth of the sun, and the cooling sensations of the mist and ocean breeze. It is very quiet. It is very warm. You feel very relaxed, very contented. This is your special place. You may come to this special place whenever you want to relax.

Biofeedback

Biofeedback is the use of instrumentation to become aware of processes in your body that you usually do not notice and to help bring them under voluntary control.

Biofeedback machines give immediate information about an individual's own biological conditions, such as muscle tension, skin surface temperature, brain-wave activity, skin conductivity, blood pressure, and heart rate (Sadock & Sadock, 2003). Some conditions that can be treated successfully with biofeedback include spastic colon, hypertension, tension and migraine headaches, muscle spasms/pain, anxiety, phobias, stuttering, and teeth grinding.

Technique

Biological conditions are monitored by the biofeedback equipment. Sensors relate muscle spasticity, body temperature, brain-wave activity, heart rate, and blood pressure. Each of these conditions will elicit a signal from the equipment, such as a blinking light, a measure on a meter, or an audible tone. The individual practices using relaxation and voluntary control to modify the signal, in turn indicating a modification of the autonomic function it represents.

Various types of biofeedback equipment have been developed for home use. Often they are less than effective, however, because they usually measure only one autonomic function. In fact, modification of several functions may be required to achieve the benefits of total relaxation.

Biofeedback can help monitor the progress an individual is making toward learning to relax. It is often used together with other relaxation techniques such as deep breathing, progressive relaxation, and mental imagery.

Special training is required to become a biofeedback practitioner. Nurses can support and encourage individuals learning to use this method of stress management. Nurses can also teach other techniques of relaxation that enhance the results of biofeedback training.

Physical Exercise

Regular exercise is viewed by many as one of the most effective methods for relieving stress. Physical exertion provides a natural outlet for the tension produced by the body in its state of arousal for "fight or flight." Following exercise, physiological equilibrium is restored, resulting in a feeling of relaxation and revitalization. Physical inactivity increases all causes of mortality and doubles the risk of cardiovascular disease, type 2 diabetes, and obesity. It also increases the risks of colon and breast cancer, high blood pressure, lipid disorders, osteoporosis, depression, and anxiety (World Health Organization [WHO], 2004).

Aerobic exercises strengthen the cardiovascular system and increase the body's ability to use oxygen more efficiently. Aerobic exercises include brisk walking, jogging, running, cycling, swimming, and dancing, among other activities. To achieve the benefits of aerobic exer-

cises, they must be performed regularly—for at least 30 minutes, three times per week.

Individuals can also benefit from low-intensity physical exercise. Although there is little benefit to the cardiovascular system, low-intensity exercise can help prevent obesity, relieve muscular tension, prevent muscle spasms, and increase flexibility. Examples of low-intensity exercise include slow walking, house cleaning, shopping, light gardening, calisthenics, and weight lifting.

Studies indicate that physical exercise can be effective in reducing general anxiety and depression. Vigorous exercise has been shown to increase levels of serotonin and beta-endorphins, both chemicals that have been implicated in mood regulation (Artal, 1998). Depressed people are often deficient in serotonin. Endorphins act as natural narcotics and mood elevators.

THE ROLE OF THE NURSE IN RELAXATION THERAPY

Nurses work with anxious clients in all departments of the hospital and in community and home health services. Individuals experience stress daily; it cannot be eliminated. Management of stress must be considered a lifelong function. Nurses can help individuals recognize the sources of stress in their lives and identify methods of adaptive coping.

Assessment

Stress management requires a holistic approach. Physical and psychosocial dimensions are considered in determining the individual's adaptation to stress. Following are some examples of assessment data for collection. Other assessments may need to be made, depending on specific circumstances of each individual.

1. Genetic influences
   a. Identify medical/psychiatric history of client and biological family members.
2. Past experiences
   a. Describe your living/working conditions.
   b. When did you last have a physical examination?
   c. Do you have a spiritual or religious position from which you derive support?
   d. Do you have a job? Have you experienced any recent employment changes or other difficulties on your job?
   e. What significant changes have occurred in your life in the last year?
   f. What is your usual way of coping with stress?
   g. Do you have someone to whom you can go for support when you feel stressed?
3. Client's perception of the stressor
   a. What do you feel is the major source of stress in your life right now?

4. Adaptation responses
   a. Do you ever feel anxious? Confused? Unable to concentrate? Fearful?
   b. Do you have tremors? Stutter or stammer? Sweat profusely?
   c. Do you often feel angry? Irritable? Moody?
   d. Do you ever feel depressed? Do you ever feel like harming yourself or others?
   e. Do you have difficulty communicating with others?
   f. Do you experience pain? What part of your body? When do you experience it? When does it worsen?
   g. Do you ever experience stomach upset? Constipation? Diarrhea? Nausea and vomiting?
   h. Do you ever feel your heart pounding in your chest?
   i. Do you take any drugs (prescription, over-the-counter, or street)?
   j. Do you drink alcohol? Smoke cigarettes? How much?
   k. Are you eating more/less than usual?
   l. Do you have difficulty sleeping?
   m. Do you have a significant other? Describe the relationship.
   n. Describe your relationship with other family members.
   o. Do you perceive any problems in your sexual lifestyle or behavior?

Diagnosis

Possible nursing diagnoses for individuals requiring assistance with stress management are listed here. Others may be appropriate for individuals with particular problems.

1. Adjustment, impaired
2. Anxiety (specify level)
3. Disturbed body image
4. Coping, defensive
5. Coping, ineffective
6. Decisional conflict (specify)
7. Denial, ineffective
8. Fear
9. Grieving, anticipatory
10. Grieving, dysfunctional
11. Hopelessness
12. Deficient knowledge (specify)
13. Pain (acute or chronic)
14. Parental role conflict
15. Post-trauma syndrome
16. Powerlessness
17. Rape-trauma syndrome
18. Role performance, ineffective
19. Low self-esteem
20. Sexual dysfunction
21. Sexuality patterns, ineffective
22. Sleep pattern, disturbed
23. Social interaction, impaired
24. Social isolation
25. Spiritual distress
26. Violence, risk for self-directed or other-directed

Outcome Identification/Implementation

The immediate goal for nurses working with individuals needing assistance with stress management is to help minimize current maladaptive symptoms. The long-term goal is to assist individuals toward achievement of their highest potential for wellness. Examples of outcome criteria may include:

1. Client will verbalize a reduction in pain following progressive relaxation techniques.
2. Client will be able to voluntarily control a decrease in blood pressure following 3 weeks of biofeedback training.
3. Client will be able to maintain stress at a manageable level by performing deep breathing exercises when feeling anxious.

Implementation of nursing actions has a strong focus on the role of client teacher. Relaxation therapy, as described in this chapter, is one way to help individuals manage stress. These techniques are well within the scope of nursing practice.

Evaluation

Evaluation requires that the nurse and client assess whether or not these techniques are achieving the desired outcomes. Various alternatives may be attempted and reevaluated.

Relaxation therapy provides alternatives to old, maladaptive methods of coping with stress. Lifestyle changes may be required and change does not come easily. Nurses must help individuals analyze the usefulness of these techniques in the management of stress in their daily lives.

SUMMARY

Stress is a part of our everyday lives. It can be positive or negative, but it cannot be eliminated. Keeping stress at a manageable level is a lifelong process.

Individuals under stress respond with a physiological arousal that can be dangerous over long periods. Indeed, the stress response has been shown to be a major contributor, either directly or indirectly, to coronary heart disease, cancer, lung ailments, accidental injuries, cirrhosis of the liver, and suicide—six of the leading causes of death in the United States.

Relaxation therapy is an effective means of reducing the stress response in some individuals. The degree of anxiety that an individual experiences in response to stress is related to certain predisposing factors, such as characteristics of temperament with which he or she was born, past experiences resulting in learned patterns of responding, and existing conditions, such as health status, coping strategies, and adequate support systems.

Deep relaxation can counteract the physiological and behavioral manifestations of stress. Various methods of relaxation therapy were presented: deep breathing exercises, progressive relaxation, passive progressive relaxation, meditation, mental imagery, biofeedback, and physical exercise.

Nurses use the nursing process to assist individuals in the management of stress. Assessment data are collected from which nursing diagnoses are derived. Outcome criteria that help individuals reduce current maladaptive symptoms and ultimately achieve their highest potential for wellness are identified. Implementation includes instructing clients and their families in the various techniques for achieving relaxation. Behavioral changes provide objective measurements for evaluation.

REVIEW QUESTIONS

SELF-EXAMINATION/LEARNING EXERCISE

1. **Learning exercise:** Practice some of the relaxation exercises presented in this chapter. It may be helpful to tape some of the exercises with soft music in the background. These tapes may be used with anxious clients or when you are feeling anxious yourself.

2. **Clinical activity:** Teach a relaxation exercise to a client. Practice it together. Evaluate the client's ability to achieve relaxation by performing the exercise.

3. **Case study:** Linda has just been admitted to the psychiatric unit. She was experiencing attacks of severe anxiety. Linda has worked in the typing pool of a large corporation for 10 years. She was recently promoted to private secretary for one of the executives. Some of her new duties include attending the board meetings and taking minutes, screening all calls and visitors for her boss, keeping track of his schedule, reminding him of important appointments, and making decisions for him in his absence. Linda felt comfortable in her old position, but has become increasingly fearful of making errors and incorrect decisions in her new job. Even though she is proud to have been selected for this position, she is constantly "nervous," has lost 10 pounds in 3 weeks, is having difficulty sleeping, and is having a recurrence of the severe migraine headaches she experienced as a teenager. She is often irritable with her husband and children for no apparent reason.
   a. Discuss some possible nursing diagnoses for Linda.
   b. Identify outcome criteria for Linda.
   c. Describe some relaxation techniques that may be helpful for her.

REFERENCES

Artal, M. (1998, October). Exercise against depression. *The physician and sportsmedicine, 26*(10). Retrieved December 19, 2004 from the World Wide Web at http://www.physsportsmed.com/issues/1998/10Oct/artal.htm

Davis, M.D., Eshelman, E.R., & McKay, M. (2000). *The relaxation and stress reduction workbook* (5th ed.). Oakland, CA: New Harbinger Publications.

Karren, K.J., Hafen, B.Q., Smith, N.L., & Frandsen, K.J. (2002). *Mind/Body Health: The effects of attitudes, emotions, and relationships* (2nd ed.). San Francisco: Benjamin Cummings.

Miller, L.H., & Smith, A.D. (1983, June 6). How vulnerable are you to stress? Brookline, MA: Biobehavioral Institute of Boston.

Miller, M.A., & Rahe, R.H. (1997). Life changes scaling for the 1990s. *Journal of Psychosomatic Research 43*(3), 279–292.

Pelletier, K.R. (1992). *Mind as healer, mind as slayer.* New York: Dell.

Sadock, B.J., & Sadock, V.A. (2003). *Synopsis of psychiatry: Behavioral sciences/clinical psychiatry* (9th ed.). Philadelphia: Lippincott Williams & Wilkins.

Sobel, D.S., & Ornstein, R. (1996). *The healthy mind, healthy body handbook.* Los Altos, CA: DR$_x$.

World Health Organization (WHO) (2004). *Sedentary lifestyle: A global public health problem.* Retrieved December 19, 2004 from the World Wide Web at http://www.who.int/hpr/physactiv/mfh.fs.sedentary.shtml

ASSERTIVENESS TRAINING

CHAPTER OUTLINE

OBJECTIVES

ASSERTIVE COMMUNICATION

BASIC HUMAN RIGHTS

RESPONSE PATTERNS

BEHAVIORAL COMPONENTS OF ASSERTIVE BEHAVIOR

TECHNIQUES THAT PROMOTE ASSERTIVE BEHAVIOR

THOUGHT-STOPPING TECHNIQUES

ROLE OF THE NURSE

SUMMARY

REVIEW QUESTIONS

KEY TERMS

aggressive
assertive
nonassertive
passive–aggressive
thought stopping

CORE CONCEPT

assertive behavior

OBJECTIVES

After reading this chapter, the student will be able to:

1. Define *assertive behavior*.
2. Discuss basic human rights.
3. Differentiate among nonassertive, assertive, aggressive, and passive–aggressive behaviors.
4. Describe techniques that promote assertive behavior.
5. Demonstrate thought stopping techniques.
6. Discuss the role of the nurse in assertiveness training.

lberti and Emmons (2001) ask:

> Are you able to express warm, positive feelings to another person? Are you comfortable starting a conversation with strangers at a party? Do you sometimes feel ineffective in making your desires clear to others? Do you have difficulty saying "no" to persuasive people? Are you often at the bottom of the "pecking order," pushed around by others? Or maybe you're the one who pushes others around to get your way? (pp. 4,5)

Assertive behavior promotes a feeling of personal power and self-confidence. These two components are commonly lacking in clients with emotional disorders. Becoming more assertive empowers individuals by promoting self-esteem, without diminishing the esteem of others.

This chapter describes a number of rights that are considered basic to human beings. Various kinds of behaviors are explored, including assertive, nonassertive, aggressive, and passive–aggressive. Techniques that pro-

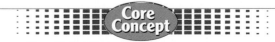

Assertive Behavior
Assertive behavior promotes equality in human relationships, enabling us to act in our own best interests, to stand up for ourselves without undue anxiety, to express honest feelings comfortably, to exercise personal rights without denying the rights of others (Alberti & Emmons, 2001).

mote assertive behavior and the nurse's role in assertiveness training are presented.

ASSERTIVE COMMUNICATION

Assertive behavior helps us feel good about ourselves and increases our self-esteem. It helps us feel good about other people and increases our ability to develop satisfying relationships with others. This is accomplished out of honesty, directness, appropriateness, and respecting one's own basic rights as well as the rights of others.

Honesty is basic to assertive behavior. Assertive honesty is not an outspoken declaration of everything that is on one's mind. It is instead an accurate representation of feelings, opinions, or preferences expressed in a manner that promotes self-respect and respect for others.

Direct communication is stating what one wants to convey with clarity and candor. Hinting and "beating around the bush" are indirect forms of communication.

Communication must occur in an appropriate context to be considered assertive. The location and timing, as well as the manner (tone of voice, nonverbal gestures) in which the communication is presented, must be correct for the situation.

BASIC HUMAN RIGHTS

A number of authors have identified a variety of "assertive rights" (Davis, McKay, & Eshelman, 2000; Lloyd, 2002; Powell & Enright, 1990; Schuster, 2000; Sobel & Ornstein, 1996). Many of these rights have been identified by participants in assertiveness training groups. Following is a composite of 10 basic assertive human rights adapted from the aggregation of sources.

1. The right to be treated with respect.
2. The right to express feelings, opinions, and beliefs.
3. The right to say "no" without feeling guilty.
4. The right to make mistakes and accept the responsibility for them.
5. The right to be listened to and taken seriously.
6. The right to change your mind.
7. The right to ask for what you want.
8. The right to put yourself first, sometimes.
9. The right to set your own priorities.
10. The right to refuse justification for your feelings or behavior.

In accepting these rights, an individual also accepts the responsibilities that accompany them. Rights and responsibilities are reciprocal entities. To experience one without the other is inherently destructive to an individual. Some responsibilities associated with basic assertive human rights are presented in Table 15–1.

RESPONSE PATTERNS

Individuals develop patterns of responding to others. Some of these patterns that have been identified include:

1. Watching other people (role modeling).
2. Being positively reinforced or punished for a certain response.
3. Inventing a response.
4. Not being able to think of a better way to respond.
5. Not developing the proper skills for a better response.
6. Consciously choosing a response style.

The nurse should be able to recognize his or her own pattern of responding, as well as that of others. Four response patterns are discussed here: nonassertive, assertive, aggressive, and passive–aggressive.

Nonassertive Behavior

Individuals who are **nonassertive** (sometimes called *passive*) seek to please others at the expense of denying their

---

■ TABLE 15–1	Assertive Rights and Responsibilities
RIGHTS ◄──────────────────────────────────► RESPONSIBILITIES	

RIGHTS	RESPONSIBILITIES
1. To be treated with respect ◄──────────►	To treat others in a way that recognizes their human dignity
2. To express feelings, opinions, and beliefs ◄──────►	To accept ownership of our feelings and show respect for those that differ from our own
3. To say "no" ◄──────────────►	To analyze each situation individually, recognizing all human rights as equal (others have the right to say "no," too)
4. To make mistakes ◄──────────►	To accept responsibility for own mistakes and to try to correct them
5. To be listened to ◄──────────►	To listen to others
6. To change your mind ◄──────────►	To accept the possible consequences that the change may incur; to accept the same flexibility in others
7. To ask for what you want ◄──────────►	To accept others' right to refuse your request
8. To put yourself first, sometimes ◄──────────►	To put others first, sometimes
9. To set your own priorities ◄──────────►	To consider one's limitations and strengths in directing independent activities; to be a dependable person
10. To refuse to justify feelings or behavior ◄──────────►	To accept ownership of own feelings/behavior; to accept others without requiring justification for their feelings/behavior

own basic human rights. They seldom let their true feelings show and often feel hurt and anxious because they allow others to choose for them. They seldom achieve their own desired goals (Alberti & Emmons, 2001). They come across as being very apologetic and tend to be self-deprecating. They use actions instead of words and hope someone will "guess" what they want. Their voices are hesitant, weak, and expressed in a monotone. Their eyes are usually downcast. They feel uncomfortable in interpersonal interactions. All they want is to please and to be liked by others. Their behavior helps them avoid unpleasant situations and confrontations with others; however, they often harbor anger and resentment.

Assertive Behavior

Assertive individuals stand up for their own rights while protecting the rights of others. Feelings are expressed openly and honestly. They assume responsibility for their own choices and allow others to choose for themselves. They maintain self-respect and respect for others by treating everyone equally and with human dignity. They communicate tactfully, using lots of "I" statements. Their voices are warm and expressive, and eye contact is intermittent but direct. These individuals desire to communicate effectively with, and be respected by, others. They are self-confident and experience satisfactory and pleasurable relationships with others.

Aggressive Behavior

Individuals who are **aggressive** defend their own basic rights by violating the basic rights of others. Feelings are often expressed dishonestly and inappropriately. They say what is on their mind, often at the expense of others. Aggressive behavior commonly results in a *putdown* of the receiver. Rights denied, the receiver feels hurt, defensive, and humiliated (Alberti & Emmons, 2001). Aggressive individuals devalue the self-worth of others on whom they impose their choices. They express an air of superiority, and their voices are often loud, demanding, angry, or cold, without emotion. Eye contact may be "to intimidate others by staring them down." They want to increase their feeling of power by dominating or humiliating others. Aggressive behavior hinders interpersonal relationships.

Passive–Aggressive Behavior

Passive–aggressive individuals defend their own rights by expressing resistance to social and occupational demands (APA, 2000). Sometimes called *indirect aggression*, this behavior takes the form of passive, nonconfrontive action (Alberti & Emmons, 2001). These individuals are devious, manipulative, and sly, and they undermine others with behavior that expresses the opposite of what they are feeling. They are highly critical and sarcastic. They allow others to make choices for them, then resist by using passive behaviors, such as procrastination, dawdling, stubbornness, and "forgetfulness." They use actions instead of words to convey their message, and the actions express covert aggression. They become sulky, irritable, or argumentative when asked to do something they do not want to do. They may protest to others about the demands but will not confront the person who is making the demands. Instead, they may deal with the demand by "forgetting" to do it. The goal is domination through retaliation. This behavior offers a feeling of control and power, although passive–aggressive individuals actually feel resentment and that they are being taken advantage of. They possess extremely low self-confidence. A comparison of these four behavior patterns is presented in Table 15–2.

TABLE 15–2	**Comparison of Behavioral Response Patterns**			
	NONASSERTIVE	**ASSERTIVE**	**AGGRESSIVE**	**PASSIVE-AGGRESSIVE**
Behavioral characteristics	Passive, does not express true feelings, self-deprecating, denies own rights	Stands up for own rights, protects rights of others, honest, direct, appropriate	Violates rights of others, expresses feelings dishonestly and inappropriately	Defends own rights with passive resistance, is critical and sarcastic; often expresses opposite of true feelings
Examples	"Uh, well, uh, sure, I'll be glad to stay and work an extra shift."	"I don't want to stay and work an extra shift today. I stayed over yesterday. It's someone else's turn today."	"You've got to be kidding!"	"Okay, I'll stay and work an extra shift." (Then to peer: "How dare she ask me to work over again! Well, we'll just see how much work she gets out of me!")
Goals	To please others; to be liked by others	To communicate effectively; to be respected by others	To dominate or humiliate others	To dominate through retaliation

(Continued on following page)

TABLE 15–2 Comparison of Behavioral Response Patterns *(Continued)*			
	NONASSERTIVE	**ASSERTIVE**	**AGGRESSIVE**	**PASSIVE-AGGRESSIVE**
Feelings	Anxious, hurt, disappointed with self, angry, resentful	Confident, successful, proud, self-respecting	Self-righteous, controlling, superior	Anger, resentment, manipulated, controlled
Compensation	Is able to avoid unpleasant situations and confrontations with others	Increased self-confidence, self-respect, respect for others, satisfying interpersonal relationships	Anger is released, increasing feeling of power and superiority	Feels self-righteous and in control
Outcomes	Goals not met; others meet *their* goals at nonassertive person's expense; anger and resentment grow; feels violated and manipulated	Goals met; desires most often fulfilled while defending own rights as well as rights of others	Goals may be met but at the expense of others; they feel hurt and vengeful	Goals not met, nor are the goals of others met due to retaliatory nature of the interaction

SOURCES: Alberti & Emmons (2001); Davis, Eshelman, & McKay, (2000); Lloyd, (2002); and Powell & Enright, 1990.

BEHAVIORAL COMPONENTS OF ASSERTIVE BEHAVIOR

Alberti and Emmons (2001) have identified several defining characteristics of assertive behavior:

1. **Eye contact**. Eye contact is considered appropriate when it is intermittent (i.e., looking directly at the person to whom one is speaking but looking away now and then). Individuals feel uncomfortable when someone stares at them continuously and intently. Intermittent eye contact conveys the message that one is interested in what is being said.

2. **Body posture**. Sitting and leaning slightly toward the other person in a conversation suggests an active interest in what is being said. Emphasis on an assertive stance can be achieved by standing with an erect posture, squarely facing the other person. A slumped posture conveys passivity or nonassertiveness.

3. **Distance/physical contact**. The distance between two individuals in an interaction or the physical contact between them has a strong cultural influence. For example, in the United States, intimate distance is considered approximately 18 inches from the body. We are very careful about whom we allow to enter this intimate space. Invasion of this space may be interpreted by some individuals as very aggressive.

4. **Gestures**. Nonverbal gestures may also be culturally related. Gesturing can add emphasis, warmth, depth, or power to the spoken word.

5. **Facial expression**. Various facial expressions convey different messages (e.g., frown, smile, surprise, anger, fear). It is difficult to "fake" these messages. In assertive communication, the facial expression is congruent with the verbal message.

6. **Voice**. The voice conveys a message by its loudness, softness, degree and placement of emphasis, and evidence of emotional tone.

7. **Fluency**. Being able to discuss a subject with ease and with obvious knowledge conveys assertiveness and self-confidence. This message is impeded by numerous pauses or filler words such as "and, uh …" or "you know …"

8. **Timing**. Assertive responses are most effective when they are spontaneous and immediate. However, most people have experienced times when it was not appropriate to respond (e.g., in front of a group of people) or times when an appropriate response is generated only after the fact ("If only I had said …"). Alberti and Emmons (2001) state that "… it is never too late to be assertive!" It is correct and worthwhile to seek out the individual at a later time and express the assertive response.

9. **Listening**. Assertive listening means giving the other individual full attention, by making eye contact, nodding to indicate acceptance of what is being said, and taking time to understand what is being said before giving a response.

10. **Thoughts**. Cognitive processes affect one's assertive behavior. Two such processes are (1) an individual's attitudes about the appropriateness of assertive behavior in general and (2) the appropriateness of assertive behavior for himself or herself specifically.

11. **Content**. Many times individuals do not respond to an unpleasant situation because "I just didn't know what to say." Perhaps *what* is being said is not as important as *how* it is said. Emotions should be expressed when they are experienced. It is also important to accept ownership of those emotions and not devalue the worth of another individual to assert oneself.

Assertive: "I'm really angry about what you said!"
Aggressive: "You're a real jerk for saying that!"

TECHNIQUES THAT PROMOTE ASSERTIVE BEHAVIOR

The following techniques have been shown to be effective in responding to criticism and avoiding manipulation by others.

1. **Standing up for one's basic human rights**

EXAMPLE:

"I have the right to express my opinion."

2. **Assuming responsibility for one's own statements**

EXAMPLE:

"I *don't want* to go out with you tonight," instead of "I *can't* go out with you tonight." The latter implies a lack of power or ability.

3. **Responding as a "broken record."** Persistently repeating in a calm voice what is wanted.

EXAMPLE:

Telephone salesperson: "I want to help you save money by changing long-distance services."
Assertive response: "I don't want to change my long-distance service."
Telephone salesperson: "I can't believe you don't want to save money!"
Assertive response: "I don't want to change my long-distance service."

4. **Agreeing assertively.** Assertively accepting negative aspects about oneself; admitting when an error has been made.

EXAMPLE:

Ms. Jones: "You sure let that meeting get out of hand. What a waste of time."
Ms. Smith: " Yes, I didn't do a very good job of conducting the meeting today."

5. **Inquiring assertively.** Seeking additional information about critical statements.

EXAMPLE:

Male board member: "You made a real fool of yourself at the board meeting last night."
Female board member: "Oh, really? Just what about my behavior offended you?"
Male board member: "You were so damned pushy!"
Female board member: "Were you offended that I spoke up for my beliefs, or was it because my beliefs are in direct opposition to yours?"

6. **Shifting from content to process.** Changing the focus of the communication from discussing the topic at hand to analyzing what is actually going on in the interaction.

EXAMPLE:

Wife: "Would you please call me if you will be late for dinner?"
Husband: "Why don't you just get off my back! I always have to account for every minute of my time with you!"
Wife: "Sounds to me like we need to discuss some other things here. What are you *really* angry about?"

7. **Clouding/fogging.** Concurring with the critic's argument without becoming defensive and without agreeing to change.

EXAMPLE:

Nurse 1: "You never come to the Nurses' Association meetings. I don't know why you even belong!"
Nurse 2: "You're right. I haven't attended very many of the meetings."

8. **Defusing.** Putting off further discussion with an angry individual until he or she is calmer.

EXAMPLE:

"You are very angry right now. I don't want to discuss this matter with you while you are so upset. I will discuss it with you in my office at 3 o'clock this afternoon."

9. **Delaying assertively.** Putting off further discussion with another individual until one is calmer.

EXAMPLE:

"That's a very challenging position you have taken, Mr. Brown. I'll need time to give it some thought. I'll call you later this afternoon."

10. **Responding assertively with irony.**

EXAMPLE:

Man: "I bet you're one of them so-called 'women's libbers,' aren't you?"
Woman: "Why, yes. Thank you for noticing."

THOUGHT-STOPPING TECHNIQUES

Assertive thinking is sometimes inhibited by repetitive, negative thoughts of which the mind refuses to let go. Individuals with low self-worth may be obsessed with thoughts such as, "I know he'd never want to go out with me. I'm too ugly (or plain, or fat, or dumb)" or "I just know I'll never be able to do this job well" or "I just can't seem to do anything right." This type of thinking fosters the belief that one's individual rights do not deserve the same consideration as those of others, and reflects nonassertive communication and behavioral response patterns.

Thought-stopping techniques, as described here, were developed by psychiatrist Joseph Wolpe (1990) and are intended to eliminate intrusive, unwanted thoughts.

Method

In a practice setting, with eyes closed, the individual concentrates on an unwanted recurring thought. Once the thought is clearly established in the mind, he or she shouts aloud: "STOP!" This action will interrupt the thought, and it is actually removed from one's awareness. The individual then immediately shifts his or her thoughts to one that is considered pleasant and desirable.

It is possible that the unwanted thought may soon recur, but with practice, the length of time between recurrences will increase until the unwanted thought is no longer intrusive.

Obviously, one cannot go about his or her daily life shouting, "STOP!" in public places. After a number of practice sessions, the technique is equally effective if the word "stop!" is used silently in the mind.

ROLE OF THE NURSE

It is important for nurses to become aware of and recognize their own behavioral responses. Are they mostly nonassertive? Assertive? Aggressive? Passive–aggressive? Do they consider their behavioral responses effective? Do they wish to change? Remember, all individuals have the right to choose whether or not they want to be assertive. A self-assessment of assertiveness is found in Table 15–3.

The ability to respond assertively is especially important to nurses who are committed to further development of the profession. Assertive skills facilitate the implementation of change—change that is required if the image of nursing is to be upgraded to the level of professionalism that most nurses desire. Assertive communication is useful in the political arena for nurses who choose to become involved at both state and national levels in striving to influence legislation and, ultimately, to improve the system of health care provision in our country.

Nurses who understand and use assertiveness skills themselves can in turn assist clients who wish to effect behavioral change in an effort to increase self-esteem and improve interpersonal relationships. The nursing process is a useful tool for nurses who are involved in helping clients increase their assertiveness.

Assessment

Nurses can help clients become more aware of their behavioral responses. Many tools for assessing the level of assertiveness have been attempted over the years. None have been very effective. Perhaps this is because it is so difficult to *generalize* when attempting to measure

---

■ TABLE 15–3   An Assertiveness Quiz

ASSIGN A NUMBER TO EACH ITEM USING THE FOLLOWING SCALE: 1 = NEVER; 3 = SOMETIMES; 5 = ALWAYS

_____ 1. I ask others to do things without feeling guilty or anxious.
_____ 2. When someone asks me to do something I don't want to do, I say no without feeling guilty or anxious.
_____ 3. I am comfortable when speaking to a large group of people.
_____ 4. I confidently express my honest opinions to authority figures (such as my boss).
_____ 5. When I experience powerful feelings (anger, frustration, disappointment, and so on), I verbalize them easily.
_____ 6. When I express anger, I do so without blaming others for "making me mad."
_____ 7. I am comfortable speaking up in a group situation.
_____ 8. If I disagree with the majority opinion in a meeting, I can "stick to my guns" without feeling uncomfortable or being abrasive.
_____ 9. When I make a mistake, I acknowledge it.
_____10. I tell others when their behavior creates a problem for me.
_____11. Meeting new people in social situations is something I do with ease and comfort.
_____12. When discussing my beliefs, I do so without labeling the opinions of others as "crazy," "stupid," "ridiculous," or "irrational."
_____13. I assume that most people are competent and trustworthy and do not have difficulty delegating tasks to others.
_____14. When considering doing something I have never done, I feel confident I can learn to do it.
_____15. I believe that my needs are as important as those of others, and I am entitled to have my needs satisfied.
_____ TOTAL SCORE

Scoring:
If your total score is 60 or higher, you have a consistently assertive philosophy and probably handle most situations well.
If your total score is 45–59, you have a fairly assertive outlook, but may benefit from some assertiveness training.
If your total score is 30–44, you may be assertive in some situations, but your natural response is either nonassertive or aggressive.
   Assertiveness training is suggested.
If your total score is 15–29, you have considerable difficulty being assertive. Assertiveness training is recommended.

SOURCE: Lloyd, S.R. (2002). *Developing positive assertiveness* (3rd ed.). With permission.

TABLE 15–4 Everyday Situations that May Require Assertiveness

At Work

How do you respond when:
1. You receive a compliment on your appearance or someone praises your work?
2. You are criticized unfairly?
3. You are criticized legitimately by a superior?
4. You have to confront a subordinate for continual lateness or sloppy work?
5. Your boss makes a sexual innuendo or makes a pass at you?

In Public

How do you respond when:
1. In a restaurant, the food you ordered arrives cold or over-cooked?
2. A fellow passenger in a no-smoking compartment lights a cigarette?
3. You are faced with an unhelpful shop assistant?
4. Somebody barges in front of you in a waiting line?
5. You take an inferior article back to a shop?

Among Friends

How do you respond when:
1. You feel angry with the way a friend has treated you?
2. A friend makes what you consider to be an unreasonable request?
3. You want to ask a friend for a favor?
4. You ask a friend for repayment of a loan of money?
5. You have to negotiate with a friend on which film to see or where to meet?

At Home

How do you respond when:
1. One of your parents criticizes you?
2. You are irritated by a persistent habit in someone you love?
3. Everybody leaves the cleaning-up chores to you?
4. You want to say "no" to a proposed visit to a relative?
5. Your partner feels amorous but you are not in the mood?

SOURCE: From Powell, T.J., & Enright, S J. (1990). *Anxiety and stress management*. London, Routledge. With permission.

assertive behaviors. Table 15-4 and Figure 15-1 represent examples of assertiveness inventories that could be personalized to describe life situations of individual clients more specifically. Obviously, "everyday situations that may require assertiveness" are not the same for all individuals.

Diagnosis

Possible nursing diagnoses for individuals needing assistance with assertiveness include:

1. Coping, defensive
2. Coping, ineffective
3. Decisional conflict
4. Denial, ineffective
5. Personal identity, disturbed
6. Powerlessness
7. Rape-trauma syndrome
8. Self-esteem, low
9. Social interaction, impaired
10. Social isolation

Outcome Identification/Implementation

The goal for nurses working with individuals needing assistance with assertiveness is to help them develop more satisfying interpersonal relationships. Individuals who do not feel good about themselves either allow others to violate their rights or cover up their low self-esteem by being overtly or covertly aggressive. Individuals should be given information regarding their individual human rights. They must know what these rights are before they can stand up for them.

Outcome criteria would be derived from specific nursing diagnoses. Some examples might include:

1. The client verbalizes and accepts responsibility for his or her own behavior.
2. The client is able to express opinions and disagree with the opinions of others in a socially acceptable manner and without feeling guilty.
3. The client is able to verbalize positive aspects about self.
4. The client verbalizes choices made in a plan to maintain control over his or her life situation.
5. The client approaches others in an appropriate manner for one-to-one interaction.

In a clinical setting, nurses can teach clients the techniques to use to increase their assertive responses. This can be done on a one-to-one basis or in group situations. Once these techniques have been discussed, nurses can assist clients to practice them through role-playing. Each client should compose a list of specific personal examples of situations that create difficulties for him or her. These situations will then be simulated in the therapy setting so that the client may practice assertive responses in a non-threatening environment. In a group situation, feedback from peers can provide valuable insight about the effectiveness of the response.

An important part of this type of intervention is to ensure that clients are aware of the differences among assertive, nonassertive, aggressive, and passive–aggressive behaviors in the same situation. When discussion is held about what the best (assertive) response would be, it is also important to discuss the other types of responses as well, so that clients can begin to recognize their pattern of response and make changes accordingly.

EXAMPLE:

Linda comes to day-hospital once a week to attend group therapy and assertiveness training. She has had problems with depression and low self-esteem. She is married to a man who is verbally abusive. He is highly critical, is seldom satisfied with anything Linda does, and blames her for negative consequences that occur in their lives, whether or not she is involved.

Since the group began, the nurse who leads the assertiveness training group has taught the participants

DIRECTIONS: Fill in each block with a rating of your assertiveness on a 5-point scale. A rating of 0 means you have no difficulty asserting yourself. A rating of 5 means that you are completely unable to assert yourself. Evaluation can be made by analyzing the scores:

1. totally by activity, including all of the different people categories
2. totally by people, including all of the different activity categories
3. on an individual basis, considering specific people and specific activities

PEOPLE\n\nACTIVITY	Friends of the same sex	Friends of the opposite sex	Intimate relations or spouse	Authority figures	Relatives/ family members	Colleagues and sub-ordinates	Strangers	Service workers; waiters; shop assistants, etc.
Giving and receiving compliments								
Asking for favors/help								
Initiating and maintaining conversation								
Refusing requests								
Expressing personal opinions								
Expressing anger/dis-pleasure								
Expressing liking, love, affection								
Stating your rights and needs								

FIGURE 15-1 Rating your assertiveness. (From Powell, T.J., & Enright, S.J. [1990]. *Anxiety and stress management.* London: Routledge, with permission.)

about basic human rights and the various types of response patterns. When the nurse asks for client situations to be presented in group, Linda volunteers to discuss an incident that occurred in her home this week. She related that she had just put some chicken on the stove to cook for supper when her 7-year-old son came running in the house yelling that he had been hurt. Linda went to him and observed that he had blood dripping down the side of his head from his forehead. He said he and some friends had been playing on the jungle gym in the school yard down the street, and he had fallen and hit his head. Linda went with him to the bathroom to clean the wound and apply some medication. Her husband, Raul, was reading the newspaper in the living room. By the time she got back to the chicken on the stove, it was burned and inedible. Her husband shouted, "You stupid woman! You can't do anything right!" Linda did not respond but burst into tears.

The nurse asked the other members in the group to present some ideas about how Linda could have responded to Raul's criticism. After some discussion, they agreed that Linda might have stated, "I made a mistake.

I am not stupid and I do lots of things right." They also discussed other types of responses and why they were less acceptable. They recognized that Linda's lack of verbal response and bursting into tears was a nonassertive response. They also agreed on other examples, such as:

1. An aggressive response might be, "Cook your own supper!" and toss the skillet out the back door.
2. A passive–aggressive response might be to fix sandwiches for supper and not speak to Raul for 3 days.

Practice on the assertive response began, with the nurse and various members of the group playing the role of Raul so that Linda could practice until she felt comfortable with the response. She participated in the group for 6 months, regularly submitting situations with which she needed help. She also learned from the situations presented by other members of the group. These weekly sessions gave Linda the self-confidence that she needed to stand up to Raul's criticism. She was aware of her basic human rights and, with practice, was able to stand up for them in an assertive manner. She was happy to report to the group after a few months that Raul seemed to be less critical and that their relationship was improving.

Evaluation

Evaluation requires that the nurse and client assess whether or not these techniques are achieving the desired outcomes. Reassessment might include the following questions:

Is the client able to accept criticism without becoming defensive?

Can the client express true feelings to (spouse, friend, boss, and so on) when his or her basic human rights are violated?

Is the client able to decline a request without feeling guilty?

Can the client verbalize positive qualities about himself or herself?

Does the client verbalize improvement in interpersonal relationships?

Assertiveness training serves to extend and create more flexibility in an individual's communication style so that he or she has a greater choice of responses in various situations. Although change does not come easily, assertiveness training can be an effective way of changing behavior. Nurses can assist individuals to become more assertive, thereby encouraging them to become what they want to be, promoting an improvement in self-esteem, and fostering a respect for their own rights and the rights of others.

SUMMARY

Assertive behavior helps individuals feel better about themselves by encouraging them to stand up for their own basic human rights. These rights have equal representation for all individuals. Along with rights comes an equal number of responsibilities. Part of being assertive includes living up to these responsibilities.

Assertive behavior increases self-esteem and the ability to develop satisfying interpersonal relationships. This is accomplished through honesty, directness, appropriateness, and respecting one's own rights, and the rights of others.

Individuals develop patterns of responding in various ways, such as role modeling, by receiving positive or negative reinforcement, or by conscious choice. These patterns can take the form of nonassertiveness, assertiveness, aggressiveness, or passive-aggressiveness.

Nonassertive individuals seek to please others at the expense of denying their own basic human rights. *Assertive* individuals stand up for their own rights while protecting the rights of others. Those who respond *aggressively* defend their own rights by violating the basic rights of others. Individuals who respond in a *passive–aggressive* manner defend their own rights by expressing resistance to social and occupational demands.

Some important behavioral considerations of assertive behavior include eye contact, body posture, distance/physical contact, gestures, facial expression, voice, fluency, timing, listening, thoughts, and content. Various techniques have been developed to assist individuals in the process of becoming more assertive.

Negative thinking can sometimes interfere with one's ability to respond assertively. Thought-stopping techniques help individuals remove negative, unwanted thoughts from awareness and promote the development of a more assertive attitude.

Nurses can assist individuals to learn and practice assertiveness techniques. The nursing process is an effective vehicle for providing the information and support to clients as they strive to create positive change in their lives.

REVIEW QUESTIONS

SELF-EXAMINATION/LEARNING EXERCISE

Identify each response in the space provided as nonassertive (NA), assertive (AS), aggressive (AG), or passive–aggressive (PA).

1. Your husband says, "You're crazy to think about going to college! You're not smart enough to handle the studies and the housework, too." You respond:
   _____ a. "I will do what I can, and the best that I can."
   _____ b. (Thinking to yourself): "We'll see how HE likes cooking dinner for a change."
   _____ c. "You're probably right. Maybe I should reconsider."
   _____ d. "I'm going to do what I want to do, when I want to do it, and you can't stop me!"

2. You are having company for dinner and they are due to arrive in 20 minutes. You are about to finish cooking and still have to shower and dress. The doorbell rings and it is a man selling a new product for cleaning windows. You respond:
   _____ a. "I don't do windows!" and slam the door in his face.
   _____ b. "I'll take a case," and write him a check.
   _____ c. "Sure, I'll take three bottles." Then to yourself you think: "I'm calling this company tomorrow and complaining to the manager about their salespeople coming around at dinnertime!"
   _____ d. "I'm very busy at the moment. I don't wish to purchase any of your product. Thank you."

3. You are in a movie theater that prohibits smoking. The person in the seat next to you just lit a cigarette and the smoke is very irritating. Your response is:
   _____ a. You say nothing.
   _____ b. "Please put your cigarette out. Smoking is prohibited."
   _____ c. You say nothing, but begin to frantically fan the air in front of you and cough loudly and convulsively.
   _____ d. "Put your cigarette out, you slob! Can't you read the 'no smoking' sign?"

4. You have been studying for a nursing exam all afternoon and lost track of time. Your husband expects dinner on the table when he gets home from work. You have not started cooking yet when he walks in the door and shouts, "Why the heck isn't dinner ready?" You respond:
   _____ a. "I'm sorry. I'll have it done in no time, honey." But then you move very slowly and take a long time to cook the meal.
   _____ b. "I'm tired from studying all afternoon. Make your own dinner, you bum! I'm tired of being your slave!"
   _____ c. "I haven't started dinner yet. I'd like some help from you."
   _____ d. "I'm so sorry. I know you're tired and hungry. It's all my fault. I'm such a terrible wife!"

5. You and your best friend, Jill, have had plans for 6 months to go on vacation together to Hawaii. You have saved your money and have plane tickets to leave in 3 weeks. She has just called you and reported that she is not going. She has a new boyfriend, they are moving in together, and she does not want to leave him. You are very angry with Jill for changing your plans. You respond:
   _____ a. "I'm very disappointed and very angry. I'd like to talk to you about this later. I'll call you."
   _____ b. "I'm very happy for you, Jill. I think it's wonderful that you and Jack are moving in together."
   _____ c. You tell Jill that you are very happy for her, but then say to another friend, "Well, that's the end of my friendship with Jill!"
   _____ d. "What? You can't do that to me! We've had plans! You're acting like a real slut!"

6. A typewritten report for your psychiatric nursing class is due tomorrow at 8:00 A.M. The assignment was made 4 weeks ago and, and yours is ready to turn in. Your roommate says, "I finally finished writing my report, but now I have to go to work, and I don't have time to type it. Please be a dear and type it for me; otherwise I'll fail!" You have a date with your boyfriend. You respond:

_____ a. "Okay, I'll call Ken and cancel our date."
_____ b. "I don't want to stay here and type your report. I'm going out with Ken."
_____ c. "You've got to be kidding! What kind of a fool do you take me for, anyway?"
_____ d. "Okay, I'll do it." However, when your roommate returns from work at midnight, you are asleep and the report has not been typed.

7. You are asked to serve on a committee on which you do not wish to serve. You respond:
_____ a. "Thank you, but I don't wish to be a member of that committee."
_____ b. "I'll be happy to serve." But then you don't show up for any of the meetings.
_____ c. "I'd rather have my teeth pulled!"
_____ d. "Okay, if I'm really needed, I'll serve."

8. You're on your way to the laundry room when you encounter a fellow dorm tenant who often asks you to "throw a few of my things in with yours." You view this as an imposition. He asks you where you're going. You respond:
_____ a. "I'm on my way to the Celtics game. Where do you think I'm going?"
_____ b. "I'm on my way to do some laundry. Do you have anything you want me to wash with mine?"
_____ c. "It's none of your damn business!"
_____ d. "I'm going to the laundry room. Please don't ask me to do some of yours. I resent being taken advantage of in that way."

9. At a hospital committee meeting, a fellow nurse who is the chairperson has interrupted you each time you have tried to make a statement. The next time it happens, you respond:
_____ a. "You make a lousy leader! You won't even let me finish what I'm trying to say!"
_____ b. By saying nothing.
_____ c. "Excuse me. I would like to finish my statement."
_____ d. By saying nothing, but you fail to complete your assignment and do not show up for the next meeting.

10. A fellow worker often borrows small amounts of money from you with the promise that she will pay you back "tomorrow." She currently owes you $15.00, and has not yet paid back any that she has borrowed. She asks if she can borrow a couple of dollars for lunch. You respond:
_____ a. "I've decided not to loan you any more money until you pay me back what you already borrowed."
_____ b. "I'm so sorry. I only have enough to pay for my own lunch today."
_____ c. "Get a life, will you? I'm tired of you sponging off me all the time!"
_____ d. "Sure, here's two dollars." Then to the other workers in the office: "Be sure you never lend Cindy any money. She never pays her debts. I'd be sure never to go to lunch with her if I were you!"

REFERENCES

Alberti, R.E., & Emmons, M.L. (2001). *Your perfect right* (8th ed.). Atascadero, CA: Impact Publishers.

American Psychiatric Association. (2000). *Diagnostic and statistical manual of mental Disorders* (4th ed.). *Text Revision*. Washington, DC: American Psychiatric Association.

Davis M., McKay, M., & Eshelman, E.R. (2000). *The relaxation and stress reduction workbook* (5th ed). Oakland, CA: New Harbinger Publications.

Lloyd, S.R. (2002). *Developing positive assertiveness* (3rd ed.). Menlo Park, CA: Crisp Publications.

Powell, T.J., & Enright, S.J. (1990). *Anxiety and stress management*. London: Routledge.

Schuster, P.M. (2000). *Communication: The key to the therapeutic relationship*. Philadelphia: F.A. Davis.

Sobel, D.S., & Ornstein, R. (1996). *The healthy mind/healthy body handbook*. New York: Patient Education Media.

Wolpe, J. (1990). *The practice of behavior therapy* (4th ed.). Elmsford, NY: Pergamon Press.

16
CHAPTER

PROMOTING SELF-ESTEEM

CHAPTER OUTLINE

OBJECTIVES

COMPONENTS OF SELF-CONCEPT

THE DEVELOPMENT OF SELF-ESTEEM

THE MANIFESTATIONS OF LOW
SELF-ESTEEM

BOUNDARIES

THE NURSING PROCESS

SUMMARY

REVIEW QUESTIONS

KEY TERMS

body image
boundaries
contextual stimuli
enmeshed boundaries
flexible boundaries
focal stimuli
moral–ethical self
personal identity

personal self
physical self
residual stimuli
rigid boundaries
self-consistency
self-expectancy
self-ideal

CORE CONCEPTS

self-concept
self-esteem

OBJECTIVES

After reading this chapter, the student will be able to:

1. Identify and define components of the self-concept.
2. Discuss influencing factors in the development of self-esteem and its progression through the life span.
3. Describe the verbal and nonverbal manifestations of low self-esteem.

4. Discuss the concept of boundaries and its relationship to self-esteem.
5. Apply the nursing process with clients who are experiencing disturbances in self-esteem.

 cKay and Fanning (2000) describe **self-esteem** as an emotional *sine qua non*, a component that is essential for psychological survival. They state, "Without some measure of self-worth, life can be enormously painful, with many basic needs going unmet."

The awareness of self (i.e., the ability to form an identity and then attach a value to it) is an important differentiating factor between humans and other animals. This

capacity for judgment, then, becomes a contributing factor in disturbances of self-esteem.

The promotion of self-esteem is about stopping self-judgments. It is about helping individuals change how they perceive and feel about themselves. This chapter describes the developmental progression and the verbal and behavioral manifestations of self-esteem. The concept of **boundaries** and its relationship to self-esteem is explored. Nursing care of clients with disturbances in

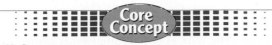

Self-Concept

Self-concept is the cognitive or thinking component of the self, and generally refers to the totality of a complex, organized, and dynamic system of learned beliefs, attitudes and opinions that each person holds to be true about his or her personal existence (Huitt, 2004).

self-esteem is described in the context of the nursing process.

COMPONENTS OF SELF-CONCEPT

Physical Self or Body Image

An individual's body image is a subjective perception of one's physical appearance based on self-evaluation and on reactions and feedback from others. Gorman, Raines, and Sultan (2002) state:

> Body image is the mental picture a person has of his or her own body. It significantly influences the way a person thinks and feels about his or her body as a whole, its functions, and the internal and external sensations associated with it. It also includes perceptions of the way others see the person's body and is central to self-concept and self-esteem. (p. 9)

An individual's body image may not necessarily coincide with his or her actual appearance. For example, individuals who have been overweight for many years and then lose weight often have difficulty perceiving of themselves as thin. They may even continue to choose clothing in the size they were before they lost weight.

A disturbance in one's body image may occur with changes in structure or function. Examples of changes in bodily structure include amputations, mastectomy, and facial disfigurements. Functional alterations are conditions such as colostomy, paralysis, and impotence. Alterations in body image are often experienced as losses.

Personal Identity

This component of the self-concept is composed of the moral–ethical self, the self-consistency, and the self-ideal/self-expectancy.

The **moral–ethical self** is that aspect of the personal identity that evaluates who the individual says he or she is. This component of the personal self observes, compares, sets standards, and makes judgments that influence an individual's self-evaluation.

Self-consistency is the component of the personal identity that strives to maintain a stable self-image. Even if the self-image is negative, because of this need for stability and self-consistency, the individual resists letting

go of the image from which he or she has achieved a measure of constancy.

Self-ideal/self-expectancy relates to an individual's perception of what he or she wants to be, to do, or to become. The concept of the ideal self arises out of the perception one has of the expectations of others. Disturbances in self-concept can occur when individuals are unable to achieve their ideals and expectancies.

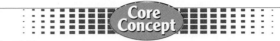

Self-Esteem

Self-esteem refers to the degree of regard or respect that individuals have for themselves and is a measure of worth that they place on their abilities and judgments.

Self-Esteem

Warren (1991) states:

> Self-esteem breaks down into two components: (1) the ability to say that "I am important," "I matter," and (2) the ability to say "I am competent," "I have something to offer to others and the world." (p. 1)

Maslow (1970) postulates that individuals must achieve a positive self-esteem before they can achieve self-actualization (see Chapter 2). On a day-to-day basis, one's self-value is challenged by changes within the environment. With a positive self-worth, individuals are able to adapt successfully to the demands associated with situational and maturational crises that occur. The ability to adapt to these environmental changes is impaired when individuals hold themselves in low esteem.

Self-esteem is very closely related to the other components of the self-concept. Just as with body image and personal identity, the development of self-esteem is largely influenced by the perceptions of how one is viewed by significant others. It begins in early childhood and vacillates throughout the life span.

THE DEVELOPMENT OF SELF-ESTEEM

How self-esteem is established has been the topic of investigation for a number of theorists and clinicians. From a review of personality theories, Coopersmith (1981) identified the following antecedent conditions of positive self-esteem.

1. **Power.** It is important for individuals to have a feeling of control over their own life situation and an ability to claim some measure of influence over the behaviors of others.
2. **Significance.** Self-esteem is enhanced when individuals feel loved, respected, and cared for by significant others.

3. **Virtue**. Individuals feel good about themselves when their actions reflect a set of personal, moral, and ethical values.
4. **Competence**. Positive self-esteem develops out of one's ability to perform successfully or achieve self-expectations and the expectations of others.
5. **Consistently set limits**. A structured lifestyle demonstrates acceptance and caring and provides a feeling of security.

Warren (1991) outlined the following focus areas to be emphasized by parents and others who work with children when encouraging the growth and development of positive self-esteem:

1. **A Sense of Competence**. Everyone needs to feel skilled at something. Warren (1991) states, "Children do not necessarily need to be THE best at a skill in order to have positive self-esteem; what they need to feel is that they have accomplished their PERSONAL best effort."
2. **Unconditional Love**. Children need to know that they are loved and accepted by family and friends regardless of success or failure. This is demonstrated by expressive touch, realistic praise, and separation of criticism of the person from criticism of the behavior.
3. **A Sense of Survival**. Everyone fails at something from time to time. Self-esteem is enhanced when individuals learn from failure and grow in the knowledge that they are stronger for having experienced it.
4. **Realistic Goals**. Low self-esteem can be the result of not being able to achieve established goals. Individuals may "set themselves up" for failure by setting goals that are unattainable. Goals can be unrealistic when they are beyond a child's capability to achieve, require an inordinate amount of effort to accomplish, and are based on exaggerated fantasy.
5. **A Sense of Responsibility**. Children gain positive self-worth when they are assigned areas of responsibility or are expected to complete tasks that they perceive are valued by others.
6. **Reality Orientation**. Personal limitations abound within our world, and it is important for children to recognize and achieve a healthy balance between what they can possess and achieve, and what is beyond their capability or control.

Other factors that have been found to be influential in the development of self-esteem include

1. **The Responses of Others**. The development of self-esteem can be positively or negatively influenced by the responses of others, particularly significant others, and by how individuals perceive those responses.
2. **Hereditary Factors**. Factors that are genetically determined, such as physical appearance, size, or inherited infirmity, can have an effect on the development of self-esteem.

3. **Environmental Conditions**. The development of self-esteem can be influenced by demands from the environment. For example, intellectual prowess may be incorporated into the self-worth of an individual who is reared in an academic environment.

Developmental Progression of the Self-Esteem Through the Life Span

The development of self-esteem progresses throughout the life span. Erikson's (1963) theory of personality development provides a useful framework for illustration (see Chapter 3). Erikson describes eight transitional or maturational crises, the resolution of which can have a profound influence on the self-esteem. If a crisis is successfully resolved at one stage, the individual develops healthy coping strategies that he or she can draw on to help fulfill tasks of subsequent stages. When an individual fails to achieve the tasks associated with a developmental stage, emotional growth is inhibited, and he or she is less able to cope with subsequent maturational or situational crises.

Trust Versus Mistrust

The development of trust results in a feeling of confidence in the predictability of the environment. Achievement of trust results in positive self-esteem through the instillation of self-confidence, optimism, and faith in the gratification of needs.

Unsuccessful resolution results in the individual experiencing emotional dissatisfaction with the self and suspiciousness of others, thereby promoting negative self-esteem.

Autonomy Versus Shame and Doubt

With motor and mental development come greater movement and independence within the environment. The child begins active exploration and experimentation. Achievement of the task results in a sense of self-control and the ability to delay gratification, as well as a feeling of self-confidence in one's ability to perform.

This task remains unresolved when the child's independent behaviors are restricted or when the child fails because of unrealistic expectations. Negative self-esteem is promoted by a lack of self-confidence, a lack of pride in the ability to perform, and a sense of being controlled by others.

Initiative Versus Guilt

Positive self-esteem is gained through initiative when creativity is encouraged and performance is recognized and positively reinforced. In this stage, children strive to develop a sense of purpose and the ability to initiate and direct their own activities.

This is the stage during which the child begins to develop a conscience. He or she becomes vulnerable to the labeling of behaviors as "good" or "bad." Guidance and discipline that rely heavily on shaming the child creates guilt and results in a decrease in self-esteem.

Industry Versus Inferiority

Self-confidence is gained at this stage through learning, competing, performing successfully, and receiving recognition from significant others, peers, and acquaintances. Negative self-esteem is the result of nonachievement, unrealistic expectations, or when accomplishments are consistently met with negative feedback. The child develops a sense of personal inadequacy.

Identity Versus Role Confusion

During adolescence, the individual is striving to redefine the sense of self. Positive self-esteem occurs when individuals are allowed to experience independence by making decisions that influence their lives.

Failure to develop a new self-definition results in a sense of self-consciousness, doubt, and confusion about one's role in life. This can occur when adolescents are encouraged to remain in the dependent position; when discipline in the home has been overly harsh, inconsistent, or absent; and when parental support has been lacking. These conditions are influential in the development of low self-esteem.

Intimacy Versus Isolation

Intimacy is achieved when one is able to form a lasting relationship or a commitment to another person, a cause, an institution, or a creative effort (Murray & Zentner, 2001). Positive self-esteem is promoted through this capacity for giving of oneself to another.

Failure to achieve intimacy results in behaviors such as withdrawal, social isolation, aloneness, and the inability to form lasting intimate relationships. Isolation occurs when love in the home has been deprived or distorted through the younger years, causing a severe impairment in self-esteem.

Generativity Versus Stagnation

Generativity promotes positive self-esteem through gratification from personal and professional achievements, and from meaningful contributions to others.

Failure to achieve generativity occurs when earlier developmental tasks are not fulfilled and the individual does not achieve the degree of maturity required to derive gratification out of a personal concern for the welfare of others. He or she lacks self-worth and becomes withdrawn and isolated.

Ego Integrity Versus Despair

Ego integrity results in a sense of self worth and self-acceptance as one reviews life goals, accepting that some were achieved and some were not. The individual has little desire to make major changes in how his or her life has progressed. Positive self-esteem is evident.

Individuals in despair possess a sense of self-contempt and disgust with how life has progressed. They feel worthless and helpless, and they would like to have a second chance at life. Earlier developmental tasks of self-confidence, self-identity, and concern for others remain unfulfilled. Negative self-esteem prevails.

THE MANIFESTATIONS OF LOW SELF-ESTEEM

Individuals with low self-esteem perceive themselves to be incompetent, unlovable, insecure, and unworthy. The number of manifestations exhibited is influenced by the degree to which an individual experiences low self-esteem. Roy (1976) categorized behaviors according to the type of stimuli that give rise to these behaviors and affirmed the importance of including this type of information in the nursing assessment. Stimulus categories are identified as *focal*, *contextual*, and *residual*. A summary of these types of influencing factors is presented in Table 16–1.

Focal Stimuli

A **focal stimulus** is the immediate concern that is causing the threat to self-esteem and the stimulus that is engendering the current behavior. Examples of focal stimuli include termination of a significant relationship, loss of employment, and failure to pass the nursing state board examination.

Contextual Stimuli

Contextual stimuli are all of the other stimuli present in the person's environment that *contribute* to the behavior being caused by the focal stimulus. Examples of contextual stimuli related to the previously mentioned focal stimuli might be a child of the relationship becoming emotionally disabled in response to the divorce, advanced age interfering with obtaining employment, or a significant other who states, "I knew you weren't smart enough to pass state boards."

TABLE 16–1	Factors that Influence Manifestations of Low Self-Esteem	
FOCAL	**CONTEXTUAL**	**RESIDUAL**
1. Any experience or situation causing the individual to question or decrease his or her value of self; experiences of loss are particularly significant.	1. Body changes experienced because of growth or illness. 2. Maturational crises associated with developmental stages. 3. Situational crises and the individual's ability to cope. 4. The individual's perceptions of feedback from significant others. 5. Ability to meet expectations of self and others. 6. The feeling of control one has over life situation. 7. One's self-definition and the use of it to measure self-worth. 8. How one copes with feelings of guilt, shame, and powerlessness. 9. How one copes with the required changes in self-perception. 10. Awareness of what affects self-concept and the manner with which these stimuli are dealt. 11. The number of failures experienced before judging self as worthless. 12. The degree of self-esteem one possesses. 13. How one copes with limits within the environment. 14. The type of support from significant others and how one responds to it. 15. One's awareness of and ability to express feelings. 16. One's current feeling of hope and comfort with the self.	1. Age and coping mechanisms one has developed. 2. Stressful situations previously experienced and how well one coped with them. 3. Previous feedback from significant others that contributed to self-worth. 4. Coping strategies developed through experiences with previous developmental crises. 5. Previous experiences with powerlessness and hopelessness and how one coped with them. 6. Coping with previous losses. 7. Coping with previous failures. 8. Previous experiences meeting expectations of self and others. 9. Previous experiences with control of self and the environment and quality of coping response. 10. Previous experience with decision making and subsequent consequences. 11. Previous experience with childhood limits, and whether or not those limits were clear, defined, and enforced.

SOURCE: From Driever (1976), with permission.

Residual Stimuli

Residual stimuli are factors that *may* influence one's maladaptive behavior in response to focal and contextual stimuli. An individual conducting a self-esteem assessment might *presume* from previous knowledge that certain beliefs, attitudes, experiences, or traits have an effect on client behavior, even though it cannot be clearly substantiated. For example, being reared in an atmosphere of ridicule and deprecation may be affecting current adaptation to failure on the state board examination.

Symptoms of Low Self-Esteem

Driever (1976) identified a number of behaviors manifested by the individual with low self-esteem. These behaviors are presented in Table 16–2.

TABLE 16–2	Manifestations of Low Self-Esteem

1. Loss of appetite/weight loss 2. Overeating 3. Constipation or diarrhea 4. Sleep disturbances (insomnia or difficulty falling or staying asleep) 5. Hypersomnia 6. Complaints of fatigue 7. Poor posture 8. Withdrawal from activities 9. Difficulty initiating new activities 10. Decreased libido 11. Decrease in spontaneous behavior 12. Expression of sadness, anxiety, or discouragement 13. Expression of feeling of isolation, being unlovable, unable to express or defend oneself, and too weak to confront or overcome difficulties 14. Fearful of angering others 15. Avoidance of situations of self-disclosure or public exposure 16. Tendency to stay in background; be a listener rather than a participant 17. Sensitivity to criticism; self-conscious 18. Expression of feelings of helplessness	19. Various complaints of aches and pains 20. Expression of being unable to do anything "good" or productive; expression of feelings of worthlessness and inadequacy 21. Expressions of self-deprecation, self-dislike, and unhappiness with self 22. Denial of past successes/accomplishments and of possibility for success with current activities 23. Feeling that anything one does will fail or be meaningless 24. Rumination about problems 25. Seeking reinforcement from others; making efforts to gain favors, but failing to reciprocate such behavior 26. Seeing self as a burden to others 27. Alienation from other by clinging and self-preoccupation 28. Self-accusatory 29. Demanding reassurance but not accepting it 30. Hostile behavior 31. Angry at self and others but unable to express these feelings directly 32. Decreased ability to meet responsibilities 33. Decreased interest, motivation, concentration 34. Decrease in self-care, hygiene

SOURCE: From Driever (1976), with permission.

BOUNDARIES

The word *boundary* is used to denote the personal space, both physical and psychological, that individuals identify as their own. Boundaries are sometimes referred to as limits: the limit or degree to which individuals feel comfortable in a relationship. Boundaries define and differentiate an individual's physical and psychological space from the physical and psychological space of others.

Boundaries help individuals define the self and are part of the individuation process. Individuals who are aware of their boundaries have a healthy self-esteem because they must know and accept their inner selves. The inner self includes beliefs, thoughts, feelings, decisions, choices, experiences, wants, needs, sensations, and intuitions.

Types of physical boundaries include physical closeness, touching, sexual behavior, eye contact, privacy (e.g., mail, diary, doors, nudity, bathroom, telephone), and pollution (e.g., noise and smoke), among others. Examples of invasions of physical boundaries are reading someone else's diary, smoking in a nonsmoking public area, and touching someone who does not wish to be touched.

Types of psychological boundaries include beliefs, feelings, choices, needs, time alone, interests, confidences, individual differences, and spirituality, among others. Examples of invasions of psychological boundaries are being criticized for doing something differently than others; having personal information shared in confidence told to others; and being told one "should" believe, feel, decide, choose, or think in a certain way.

Boundary Pliancy

Boundaries can be rigid, flexible, or enmeshed. The behavior of dogs and cats can be a good illustration of **rigid boundaries** and **flexible boundaries**. Most dogs want to be as close to people as possible. When "their people" walk into the room, the dog is likely to be all over them. They want to be where their people are and do what they are doing. Dogs have very flexible boundaries.

Cats, on the other hand, have very distinct boundaries. They do what they want, when they want. They decide how close they will be to their people, and when. Cats take notice when their people enter a room but may not even acknowledge their presence (until the cat decides the time is right). Their boundaries are less flexible than those of dogs.

Rigid Boundaries

Individuals who have rigid boundaries often have a hard time trusting others. They keep others at a distance, and are difficult to communicate with. They reject new ideas or experiences, and often withdraw, both emotionally and physically.

EXAMPLE:

Fred and Alice were seeing a marriage counselor because they were unable to agree on many aspects of raising their children and it was beginning to interfere with their relationship. Alice runs a day care service out of their home, and Fred is an accountant. Alice states, "He never once changed a diaper or got up at night with a child. Now that they are older, he refuses to discipline them in any way." Fred responds, "In my family, my Mom took care of the house and kids and my Dad kept us clothed and fed. That's the way it should be. It's Alice's job to raise the kids. It's my job to make the money." Fred's boundaries are considered rigid because he refuses to consider the ideas of others, or to experience alternative ways of doing things.

Flexible Boundaries

Healthy boundaries are flexible. That is, individuals must be able to let go of their boundaries and limits when appropriate. To have flexible boundaries, one must be aware of who is considered safe and when it is safe to let others invade our personal space.

EXAMPLE:

Nancy always takes the hour from 4 to 5 P.M. for her own. She takes no phone calls and tells the children that she is not to be disturbed during that hour. She reads or takes a long leisurely bath and relaxes before it is time to start dinner. Today her private time was interrupted when her 15-year-old daughter came home from school crying because she had not made the cheerleading squad. Nancy used her private time to comfort her daughter, who was experiencing a traumatic response to the failure.

Sometimes boundaries can be too flexible. Individuals with boundaries that are too loose are like chameleons. They take their "colors" from whomever they happen to be with at the time. That is, they allow others to make their choices and direct their behavior. For example, at a cocktail party Diane agreed with one person that the winter had been so unbearable she had hardly been out of the house. Later at the same party, she agreed with another person that the winter had seemed milder than usual.

Enmeshed Boundaries

Enmeshed boundaries occur when two people's boundaries are so blended together that neither can be sure where one stops and the other begins, or one individual's boundaries may be blurred with another's. The individual with the enmeshed boundaries may be unable to differentiate his or her feelings, wants, and needs from the other person's.

EXAMPLE:

1. Fran's parents are in town for a visit. They say to Fran, "Dear, we want to take you and Dave out to dinner tonight. What is your favorite restaurant?" Fran automatically responds, "Villa Roma," knowing that the Italian restaurant is Dave's favorite.
2. If a mother has difficulty allowing her daughter to individuate, the mother may perceive the daughter's experiences as happening to her. For example, Aileen got her hair cut without her mother's knowledge. It was styled with spikes across the top of her head. When her mother saw it, she said, "How dare you go around looking like that! What will people think of me?"

Establishing Boundaries

Boundaries are established in childhood. Unhealthy boundaries are the products of unhealthy, troubled, or dysfunctional families. The boundaries enclose painful feelings that have their origin in the dysfunctional family and that have not been dealt with. McKay and Fanning (2000) explain the correlation between unhealthy boundaries and self-esteem disturbances and how they can arise out of negative role models:

> Modeling self-esteem means valuing oneself enough to take care of one's own basic needs. When parents put themselves last, or chronically sacrifice for their kids, they teach them that a person is only worthy insofar as he or she is of service to others. When parents set consistent, supportive limits and protect themselves from overbearing demands, they send a message to their children that both are important and both have legitimate needs. (p. 312)

In addition to the lack of positive role models, unhealthy boundaries may also be the result of abuse or neglect. These circumstances can cause a delay in psychosocial development. The individual must then resume the grief process as an adult in order to continue the developmental progression. They learn to recognize feelings, work through core issues, and learn to tolerate emotional pain as their own. They complete the individuation process, go on to develop healthy boundaries, and learn to appreciate their self-worth.

THE NURSING PROCESS

Assessment

Clients with self-esteem problems may manifest any of the symptoms presented in Table 16–2. Some clients with disturbances in self-esteem will make direct statements that reflect guilt, shame, or negative self-appraisal, but often it is necessary for the nurse to ask specific questions to obtain this type of information. In particular, clients who have experienced abuse or other severe trauma often have kept feelings and fears buried for years, and behavioral manifestations of low self-esteem may not be readily evident.

Various tools for measuring self-esteem exist. One is presented in Table 16–3. This particular tool can be used as a self-inventory by the client, or it can be adapted and used by the nurse to format questions for assessing level of self-esteem in the client.

Diagnosis/Outcome Identification

NANDA International has accepted, for use and testing, three nursing diagnoses that relate to self-esteem. These diagnoses are chronic low self-esteem, situational low self-esteem, and risk for situational low self-esteem (NANDA International, 2003). Each is described here with its definitions and defining characteristics.

Chronic Low Self-Esteem

Definition: Long-standing negative self-evaluation/feelings about self or self-capabilities.

Defining Characteristics

Long-standing or chronic:

1. Self-negating verbalizations
2. Expressions of shame/guilt
3. Evaluations of self as unable to deal with events
4. Rationalizing away or rejection of positive feedback and exaggeration of negative feedback about self
5. Hesitation to try new things/situations

Other:

1. Frequent lack of success in work or other life events
2. Overly conforming, dependent on others' opinions
3. Lack of eye contact
4. Nonassertive/passive
5. Indecisive
6. Excessively seeks reassurance.

Situational Low Self-Esteem

Definition: Development of a negative perception of self-worth in response to a current situation (specify)

Defining Characteristics

1. Verbally reports current situational challenge to self-worth
2. Self-negating verbalizations
3. Indecisive, nonassertive behavior
4. Evaluation of self as unable to deal with situations or events
5. Expressions of helplessness and uselessness

TABLE 16–3	Self-Esteem Inventory

Place a check mark in the column that most closely describes your answer to each statement. Each check is worth the number of points listed above each column.

	3 OFTEN OR A GREAT DEAL	2 SOMETIMES	1 SELDOM OR OCCASIONALLY	0 NEVER OR NOT AT ALL
1. I become angry or hurt when criticized.				
2. I am afraid to try new things.				
3. I feel stupid when I make a mistake.				
4. I have difficulty looking people in the eye.				
5. I have difficulty making small talk.				
6. I feel uncomfortable in the presence of strangers.				
7. I am embarrassed when people compliment me.				
8. I am dissatisfied with the way I look.				
9. I am afraid to express my opinions in a group.				
10. I prefer staying home alone than participating in group social situations.				
11. I have trouble accepting teasing.				
12. I feel guilty when I say "no" to people.				
13. I am afraid to make a commitment to a relationship for fear of rejection.				
14. I believe that most people are more competent than I.				
15. I feel resentment toward people who are attractive and successful.				
16. I have trouble thinking of any positive aspects about my life.				
17. I feel inadequate in the presence of authority figures.				
18. I have trouble making decisions.				
19. I fear the disapproval of others.				
20. I feel tense, stressed out, or "uptight."				

Problems with low self-esteem are indicated by items scored with a "3" or by a total score higher than 46.

Risk for Situational Low Self-Esteem

Definition: At risk for developing negative perception of self worth in response to a current situation (specify)

Risk Factors

1. Developmental changes
2. Disturbed body image
3. Functional impairment (specify)
4. Loss (specify)
5. Social role changes (specify)
6. History of learned helplessness
7. History of abuse, neglect, or abandonment
8. Unrealistic self-expectations
9. Behavior inconsistent with values
10. Lack of recognition/rewards
11. Failures/rejections
12. Decreased power/control over environment
13. Physical illness (specify)

Outcome Criteria

The following criteria may be used for measurement of outcomes in the care of the client with disturbances of self-esteem.

The client:

1. Is able to express positive aspects about self and life situation.
2. Is able to accept positive feedback from others.
3. Is able to attempt new experiences.
4. Is able to accept personal responsibility for own problems.
5. Is able to accept constructive criticism without becoming defensive.
6. Is able to make independent decisions about life situation.
7. Uses good eye contact.
8. Is able to develop positive interpersonal relationships.
9. Is able to communicate needs and wants to others assertively.

Planning/Implementation

In Table 16–4, a plan of care using the three self-esteem diagnoses accepted by NANDA International is presented. Outcome criteria, appropriate nursing interventions, and rationales are included for each diagnosis.

Evaluation

Reassessment is conducted to determine if the nursing actions have been successful in achieving the objectives of

NURSING DIAGNOSIS: CHRONIC LOW SELF-ESTEEM

RELATED TO: Childhood neglect/abuse; numerous failures; negative feedback from others

EVIDENCED BY: Long-standing self-negating verbalizations and expressions of shame and guilt

OUTCOME CRITERIA	NURSING INTERVENTIONS	RATIONALE
Client will verbalize positive aspects of self and abandon judgmental self-perceptions.	1. Be supportive, accepting, and respectful without invading the client's personal space. 2. Discuss inaccuracies in self-perception with client. 3. Have client list success and strengths. Provide positive feedback. 4. Assess content of negative self-talk.	1. Individuals who have had longstanding feelings of low self-worth may be uncomfortable with personal attentiveness. 2. Client may not see positive aspects of self that others see, and bringing it to awareness may help change perception. 3. Helps client to develop internal self-worth and new coping behaviors. 4. Self-blame, shame, and guilt promote feelings of low self-worth. Depending on chronicity and severity of the problem, this is likely to be the focus of long-term psychotherapy with this client.

NURSING DIAGNOSIS: SITUATIONAL LOW SELF-ESTEEM

RELATED TO: Failure (either real or perceived) in a situation of importance to the individual or loss (either real or perceived) of a concept of value to the individual

EVIDENCED BY: Negative self-appraisal in a person with a previous positive self-evaluation

OUTCOME CRITERIA	NURSING INTERVENTIONS	RATIONALE
Client will identify source of threat to self-esteem and work through the stages of the grief process to resolve the loss or failure.	1. Convey an accepting attitude; encourage client to express self openly. 2. Encourage client to express anger. Do not become defensive if initial expression of anger is displaced on nurse/therapist. Assist client to explore angry feelings and direct them toward the intended object/person or other loss. 3. Assist client to avoid ruminating about past failures. Withdraw attention if client persists. 4. Client needs to focus on positive attributes if self-esteem is to be enhanced. Encourage discussion of past accomplishments and offer support in undertaking new tasks. Offer recognition of successful endeavors and positive reinforcement of attempts made.	1. An accepting attitude enhances trust and communicates to the client that you believe he or she is a worthwhile person, regardless of what is expressed. 2. Verbalization of feelings in a nonthreatening environment may help client come to terms with unresolved issues related to the loss. 3. Lack of attention to these undesirable behaviors may discourage their repetition. 4. Recognition and positive reinforcement enhance self-esteem and encourage repetition of desirable behaviors.

NURSING DIAGNOSIS: RISK FOR SITUATIONAL LOW SELF-ESTEEM

RISK FACTORS: Developmental or functional changes; disturbed body image; loss; history of abuse or neglect; unrealistic self-expectations; physical illness; failures/rejections.

OUTCOME CRITERIA	NURSING INTERVENTIONS	RATIONALE
Client's self-esteem will be preserved	1. Provide an open environment and trusting relationship. 2. Determine client's perception of the loss/failure and the meaning of it to him or her.	1. To facilitate client's ability to deal with current situation. 2. Assessment of the cause or contributing factor is necessary to provide assistance to the client.

(Continued on opposite page)

OUTCOME CRITERIA	NURSING INTERVENTIONS	RATIONALE
	3. Identify response of family or significant others to client's current situation.	3. This provides additional background assessment data with which to plan client's care.
	4. Permit appropriate expressions of anger.	4. Anger is a stage in the normal grieving process and must be dealt with for progression to occur.
	5. Provide information about normalcy of individual grief reaction.	5. Individuals who are unaware of normal feelings associated with grief may feel guilty and try to deny certain feelings.
	6. Discuss and assist with planning for the future. Provide hope, but avoid giving false reassurance.	6. In a state of anxiety and grief, individuals need assistance with decision-making and problem solving. They may find it difficult or impossible to envision any hope for the future.

care. Evaluation of the nursing actions for the client with self-esteem disturbances may be facilitated by gathering information using the following types of questions:

Is the client able to discuss past accomplishments and other positive aspects about his or her life?

Does the client accept praise and recognition from others in a gracious manner?

Is the client able to try new experiences without extreme fear of failure?

Can he or she accept constructive criticism now without becoming overly defensive and shifting the blame to others?

Does the client accept personal responsibility for problems, rather than attributing feelings and behaviors to others?

Does the client participate in decisions that affect his or her life?

Can the client make rational decisions independently?

Has he or she become more assertive in interpersonal relationships?

Is improvement observed in the physical presentation of self-esteem, such as eye contact, posture, changes in eating and sleeping, fatigue, libido, elimination patterns, self-care, and complaints of aches and pains?

SUMMARY

Emotional wellness requires that an individual have some degree of self-worth—a perception that he or she possesses a measure of value to self and others. Self-concept consists of body image, personal identity, and self-esteem. Body image encompasses one's appraisal of personal attributes, functioning, sexuality, wellness–illness state, and appearance.

The personal identity component is composed of the moral–ethical self, the self-consistency, and the self-ideal. The moral–ethical self functions as observer, standard setter, dreamer, comparer, and most of all evaluator of who the individual says he or she is. Self-consistency is the component of the personal identity that strives to maintain a stable self-image. Self-ideal relates to an individual's perception of what he or she wants to be, do, or become.

Self-esteem refers to the degree of regard or respect that individuals have for themselves and is a measure of worth that they place on their abilities and judgments. It is largely influenced by the perceptions of how one is viewed by significant others. Predisposing factors to the development of positive self-esteem include a sense of competence, unconditional love, a sense of survival, realistic goals, a sense of responsibility, and reality orientation. Genetics and environmental conditions may also be influencing factors.

The development of self-esteem progresses throughout the life span. Erikson's theory of personality development was used in this chapter as a framework for illustration of this progression.

The behaviors associated with low self-esteem are numerous. Stimuli that trigger these behaviors were presented according to focal, contextual, or residual types. Boundaries, or personal limits, help individuals define the self and are part of the individuation process. Boundaries are physical and psychological and may be rigid, flexible, or enmeshed. Unhealthy boundaries are often the result of dysfunctional family systems.

The nursing process was presented as the vehicle for delivery of care to clients needing assistance with self-esteem disturbances. An inventory for assessing self-esteem was included. The three nursing diagnoses relating to self-esteem that have been accepted by NANDA International were discussed, along with definitions and defining characteristics. Outcome criteria for clients with low self-esteem were presented. A plan of care for clients experiencing disturbances in self-esteem was included, along with reassessment questions for evaluation.

REVIEW QUESTIONS

SELF-EXAMINATION/LEARNING EXERCISE

Situation: Karen is 23 years old. She has always been a good student and liked by her peers. She made As and Bs in high school, was captain of the cheerleading squad, and was chosen best-liked girl by her senior classmates at graduation. She entered nursing school at a nearby university and graduated with a 3.2/4.0 grade point average in 4 years.

The summer after graduation, Karen took the state board examination and did not pass. She was disappointed but was allowed to continue working at her hospital job as a graduate nurse until she was able to take the examination again. After a few months, she retook the exam and again did not pass. She was not able to keep her job any longer and became despondent. She has sought counseling at the local mental health clinic.

Select the answers that are most appropriate for this situation.

1. Karen says to the psychiatric nurse, "I am a complete failure. I'm so dumb, I can't do anything right." What is the most appropriate nursing diagnosis for Karen?
   a. Chronic low self-esteem
   b. Situational low self-esteem
   c. Defensive coping
   d. Risk for situational low self-esteem.

2. Which of the following outcome criteria would be most appropriate for Karen?
   a. Karen is able to express positive aspects about herself and her life situation.
   b. Karen is able to accept constructive criticism without becoming defensive.
   c. Karen is able to develop positive interpersonal relationships.
   d. Karen is able to accept positive feedback from others.

3. Which of the following nursing interventions is best for Karen's specific problem?
   a. Encourage Karen to talk about her feeling of shame over the failure.
   b. Assist Karen to problem solve her reasons for failing the exam.
   c. Help Karen understand the importance of good self-care and personal hygiene in the maintenance of self-esteem.
   d. Explore with Karen her past successes and accomplishments.

4. The psychiatric nurse encourages Karen to express her anger. Why is this an appropriate nursing intervention?
   a. Anger is the basis for self-esteem problems.
   b. The nurse suspects that Karen was abused as a child.
   c. The nurse is attempting to guide Karen through the grief process.
   d. The nurse recognizes that Karen has long-standing repressed anger.

5. Karen is demonstrating a number of behaviors attributed to low self-esteem that were triggered by her failure of the examination. In Karen's case, failure of the exam can be considered a
   a. Focal stimulus
   b. Contextual stimulus
   c. Residual stimulus
   d. Spatial stimulus

Match the following words to the statements that follow:

_____ 6. "What do you want to do tonight?" "Whatever you want to do."   a. Rigid boundary

_____ 7. Twins Jan and Jean still dress alike even though they are grown and married.   b. Too flexible boundary

_____ 8. Karen's counselor asks her if she would like a hug.   c. Enmeshed boundary

_____ 9. Velma told Betty a secret that Mary had told her.

_____ 10. Tommy says to his friend, "I can't ever talk to my Daddy until after he has read his newspaper."

d. A boundary violation

e. Showing respect for the boundary of another

REFERENCES

Gorman, L.M., Raines, M.L., & Sultan, D.F. (2002). *Psychosocial nursing for general patient care* (2nd ed.). Philadelphia: F.A. Davis.

Huitt, W. (2004). *Self-concept and self-esteem*. Retrieved December 28, 2004 from the World Wide Web at http://chiron.valdosta.edu/whuitt/col/regsys/self.html

McKay, M., & Fanning, P. (2000). *Self-esteem: A proven program of cognitive techniques for assessing, improving, and maintaining your self-esteem* (3rd ed.). Oakland, CA: New Harbinger Publications.

Murray, R.B., & Zentner, J.P. (2001). *Health promotion strategies through the life span* (7th ed.). Upper Saddle River, NJ: Prentice-Hall.

NANDA International. (2005). *Nursing diagnoses: Definitions and classification 2005–2006*. Philadelphia: NANDA International.

Warren, J. (1991). Your child and self-esteem. *The Prairie View, 30*(2), 1.

CLASSICAL REFERENCES

Coopersmith, S. (1981). *The antecedents of self-esteem* (2nd ed.). Palo Alto, CA: Consulting Psychologists Press.

Driever, M.J. (1976). Problem of low self-esteem. In C. Roy (Ed.). *Introduction to nursing: An adaptation model*. Englewood Cliffs, NJ: Prentice-Hall.

Erikson, E.H. (1963). *Childhood and society* (2nd ed.). New York: W.W. Norton.

Maslow, A. (1970). *Motivation and personality* (2nd ed.). New York: Harper & Row.

Roy, C. (1976). *Introduction to nursing: An adaptation model*. Englewood Cliffs, N.J.: Prentice-Hall.

17
CHAPTER

ANGER/AGGRESSION
MANAGEMENT

CHAPTER OUTLINE

OBJECTIVES

ANGER AND AGGRESSION, DEFINED

PREDISPOSING FACTORS TO ANGER
AND AGGRESSION

THE NURSING PROCESS

SUMMARY

REVIEW QUESTIONS

KEY TERMS

modeling
operant conditioning

prodromal syndrome

CORE CONCEPTS

aggression
anger
anger management

OBJECTIVES

After reading this chapter, the student will be able to:

1. Define and differentiate between anger and aggression.
2. Identify when the expression of anger becomes a problem.
3. Discuss predisposing factors to the maladaptive expression of anger.
4. Apply the nursing process to clients expressing anger or aggression.
   a. **Assessment**: Describe physical and psychological responses to anger.
   b. **Diagnosis/outcome identification:**

Formulate nursing diagnoses and outcome criteria for clients expressing anger and aggression

   c. **Planning/intervention:** Describe nursing interventions for clients demonstrating maladaptive expressions of anger.
   d. **Evaluation**: Evaluate achievement of the projected outcomes in the intervention with clients demonstrating maladaptive expression of anger.

 nger need not be a negative expression. It is a normal human emotion that, when handled appropriately and expressed assertively, can provide an individual with a positive force to solve problems and make decisions concerning life situations. Anger becomes a problem when it is not expressed or when it is expressed aggressively. Violence occurs when individuals lose control of their anger. Violent acts are becoming commonplace in the United States. They are reported daily on the evening news, and health care workers see the results on a regular basis in the emergency departments of general hospitals.

This chapter addresses the concepts of anger and aggression. Predisposing factors to the maladaptative expression of anger are discussed, and the nursing process as a vehicle for delivery of care to assist clients in the management of anger and aggression is described.

ANGER AND AGGRESSION, DEFINED

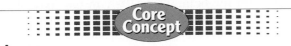

Anger
Anger is an emotional state that varies in intensity from mild irritation to intense fury and rage. It is accompanied by physiological and biological changes, such as increases in heart rate, blood pressure, and levels of the hormones epinephrine and norepinephrine (American Psychological Association, 2005a).

Anger is a normal, healthy emotion that serves as a warning signal and alerts us to potential threat or trauma. It triggers energy that sets us up for a good fight or quick flight, and can range from mild irritation to hot, fiery energy (Butterfield, 2000). Warren (1990) outlines some fundamental points about anger:

1. Anger is not a primary emotion, but it is typically experienced as an almost automatic inner response to hurt, frustration, or fear.
2. Anger is physiological arousal. It instills feelings of power and generates preparedness.
3. Anger and aggression are significantly different.
4. The expression of anger is learned.
5. The expression of anger can come under personal control.

Anger is a very powerful emotion. When it is denied or buried, it can precipitate a number of physical problems such as migraine headaches, ulcers, colitis, and even coronary heart disease. When turned inward on oneself, anger can result in depression and low self-esteem. When it is expressed inappropriately, it commonly interferes with relationships. When suppressed, anger may turn into resentment, which often manifests itself in negative, passive-aggressive behavior.

Anger creates a state of preparedness by arousing the sympathetic nervous system. The activation of this system results in increased heart rate and blood pressure, increased secretion of epinephrine (resulting in additional physiological arousal), and increased levels of serum glucose, among others. Anger prepares the body, physiologically, to fight. When anger goes unresolved, this physiological arousal can be the predisposing factor to a number of health problems. Even if the situation that created the anger is removed by miles or years, it can be replayed through the memory, reactivating the sympathetic arousal when this occurs.

Table 17-1 lists positive and negative functions of anger.

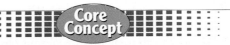

Aggression
Aggression is a behavior intended to threaten or injure the victim's security or self-esteem. It means "to go against," "to assault," or "to attack." It is a response that aims at inflicting pain or injury on objects or persons. Whether the damage is caused by words, fists, or weapons, the behavior is virtually always designed to punish. It is frequently accompanied by bitterness, meanness, and ridicule. An aggressive person is often vengeful (Warren, 1990, p. 81).

The term *anger* often takes on a negative connotation because of its link with aggression. Aggression is one way individuals express anger. It is sometimes used to try to force someone into compliance with the aggressor's wishes, but at other times the only objective seems to be the infliction of punishment and pain. In virtually all instances, aggression is a negative function or destructive use of anger.

TABLE 17–1	The Functions of Anger
POSITIVE FUNCTIONS OR CONSTRUCTIVE USES	**NEGATIVE FUNCTIONS OR DESTRUCTIVE USES**
Anger energizes and mobilizes the body for self-defense.	Without cognitive input, anger may result in impulsive behavior, disregarding possible negative consequences.
Communicated assertively, anger can promote conflict resolution.	Communicated passive-aggressively or aggressively, conflict escalates, and the problem that created the conflict goes unresolved.
Anger arousal is a personal signal of threat or injustice against the self. The signal elicits coping responses to deal with the distress.	Anger can lead to aggression when the coping response is displacement. Anger can be destructive if it is discharged against an object or person unrelated to the true target of the anger.
Anger is constructive when it provides a feeling of control over a situation and the individual is able to assertively take charge of a situation.	Anger can be destructive when the feeling of control is exaggerated and the individual uses the power to intimidate others.
Anger is constructive when it is expressed assertively, serves to increase self-esteem, and leads to mutual understanding and forgiveness.	Anger can be destructive when it masks honest feelings, weakens self-esteem, and leads to hostility and rage.

SOURCES: Adapted from Waughfield (2002) and Gorman, Raines, & Sultan (2002).

PREDISPOSING FACTORS TO ANGER AND AGGRESSION

A number of factors have been implicated in the way individuals express anger. Some theorists view aggression as purely biological, and some suggest that it results from individuals' interactions with their environments. It is likely a combination of both.

Modeling

Role **modeling** is one of the strongest forms of learning. Children model their behavior at a very early age after their primary caregivers, usually parents. How parents or significant others express anger becomes the child's method of anger expression.

Whether role modeling is positive or negative depends on the behavior of the models. Much has been written about the abused child becoming physically abusive as an adult.

Role models are not always in the home, however. Evidence supports the role of television violence as a predisposing factor to later aggressive behavior (American Psychological Association, 2005b). The American Psychiatric Association (2004) suggests that monitoring what children view and regulation of violence in the media are necessary to prevent this type of violent modeling.

Operant Conditioning

Operant conditioning occurs when a specific behavior is reinforced. A positive reinforcement is a response to the specific behavior that is pleasurable or produces the desired results. A negative reinforcement is a response to the specific behavior that prevents an undesirable result from occurring.

Anger responses can be learned through operant conditioning. For example, when a child wants something and has been told "no" by a parent, he or she might have a temper tantrum. If, when the temper tantrum begins, the parent lets the child have what is wanted, the anger has been positively reinforced (or rewarded).

An example of learning by negative reinforcement follows: A mother asks the child to pick up her toys and the child becomes angry and has a temper tantrum. If, when the temper tantrum begins, the mother thinks, "Oh, it's not worth all this!" and picks up the toys herself, the anger has been negatively reinforced (child was rewarded by not having to pick up her toys).

Neurophysiological Disorders

Some research has implicated epilepsy of temporal and frontal lobe origin in episodic aggression and violent behavior (Sadock & Sadock, 2003). Clients with episodic dyscontrol often respond to anticonvulsant medication.

Tumors in the brain, particularly in the areas of the limbic system and the temporal lobes; trauma to the brain, resulting in cerebral changes; and diseases, such as encephalitis (or medications that may effect this syndrome), have all been implicated in the predisposition to aggression and violent behavior. A study by Lee and associates (1998) showed that destruction of the amygdaloid body in patients with intractable aggression resulted in a reduction in autonomic arousal levels and in the number of aggressive outbursts.

Biochemical Factors

Violent behavior may be associated with hormonal dysfunction caused by Cushing's disease or hyperthyroidism (Tardiff, 2003). Studies have not supported a correlation between violence and increased levels of androgens or alterations in hormone levels associated with hypoglycemia or premenstrual syndrome.

Some research indicates that various neurotransmitters (e.g., epinephrine, norepinephrine, dopamine, acetylcholine, and serotonin) may play a role in the facilitation and inhibition of aggressive impulses (Sadock & Sadock, 2003).

Socioeconomic Factors

High rates of violence exist within the subculture of poverty in the United States. This has been attributed to lack of resources, breakup of families, alienation, discrimination, and frustration (Tardiff, 2003). An ongoing controversy exists as to whether economic inequality or absolute poverty is most responsible for violent behavior within this subculture. That is, does violence occur because individuals perceive themselves as disadvantaged relative to other persons, or does violence occur because of the deprivation itself? These concepts are not easily understood and are still under investigation.

Environmental Factors

Physical crowding may be related to violence through increased contact and decreased defensible space (Tardiff, 2003). A relationship between heat and aggression also has been indicated (Anderson, 2001). Moderately uncomfortable temperature appears to be associated with an increase in aggression, while extremely hot temperatures seem to decrease aggression.

A number of epidemiological studies have found a strong link between use of alcohol and violent behavior. Other substances, including cocaine, amphetamines, hallucinogens, and anabolic steroids, have also been associated with violent behavior (Tardiff, 2003).

Availability of firearms has been linked to commission of violent crimes (Violence Policy Center, 2002). Evidence exists to support the effectiveness of gun control legislation in decreasing the rate of homicides involving firearms.

THE NURSING PROCESS

Assessment

Nurses must be aware of the symptoms associated with anger and aggression in order to make an accurate assessment. The best intervention is prevention, so risk factors for assessing violence potential are also presented.

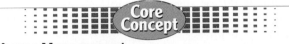

Anger Management
The use of various techniques and strategies to control responses to anger-provoking situations. The goal of anger management is to reduce both the emotional feelings and the physiological arousal that anger engenders.

Anger

Anger can be associated with a number of typical behaviors, including (but not limited to) the following:

Frowning facial expression
Clenched fists
Low-pitched verbalizations forced through clenched teeth
Yelling and shouting
Intense eye contact or avoidance of eye contact
Easily offended
Defensive response to criticism
Passive-aggressive behaviors
Emotional over control with flushing of the face
Intense discomfort; continuous state of tension

Anger has been identified as a stage in the grieving process. Individuals who become fixed in this stage may become depressed. In this instance, the anger is turned inward as a way for the individual to maintain control over the pent-up anger. Because of the negative connotation to the word *anger*, some clients will not acknowledge that what they are feeling is anger. These individuals need assistance to recognize their true feelings and to understand that anger is a perfectly acceptable emotion when it is expressed appropriately.

Aggression

Aggression can arise from a number of feeling states, including anger, anxiety, guilt, frustration, or suspicious-

ness. Aggressive behaviors can be classified as mild (e.g., sarcasm), moderate (e.g., slamming doors), severe (e.g., threats of physical violence against others), or extreme (e.g., physical acts of violence against others). Aggression may be associated with (but not limited to) the following defining characteristics:

Pacing, restlessness
Tense facial expression and body language
Verbal or physical threats
Loud voice, shouting, use of obscenities, argumentative
Threats of homicide or suicide
Increase in agitation, with overreaction to environmental stimuli
Panic anxiety, leading to misinterpretation of the environment
Disturbed thought processes; suspiciousness
Angry mood, often disproportionate to the situation

Kassinove and Tafrate (2002) state, "In contrast to anger, aggression is almost always goal directed and has the aim of harm to a specific person or object. Aggression is one of the negative outcomes that may emerge from general arousal and anger."

Intent is a requisite in the definition of aggression. It refers to behavior that is *intended* to inflict harm or destruction. Accidents that lead to *unintentional* harm or destruction are not considered aggression.

Assessing Risk Factors

Prevention is the key issue in the management of aggressive or violent behavior. The individual who becomes violent usually feels an underlying helplessness. Three factors that have been identified as important considerations in assessing for potential violence include the following:

1. Past history of violence
2. Client diagnosis
3. Current behavior

Past history of violence is widely recognized as a major risk factor for violence in a treatment setting. Also highly correlated with assaultive behavior is diagnosis. The diagnoses that have the strongest association with violent behavior are schizophrenia; organic brain disorders; mood disorders; antisocial, borderline, and intermittent explosive personality disorders; and substance use disorders (Sunderland, 1997).

Dubin (2003) states:

The successful management of aggression is predicated on the ability to predict which patients are most likely to become violent. Once such a prediction is made, rapid intervention can defuse the risk of violence. Violence usually does not occur without warning.

He describes a **"prodromal syndrome"** that is characterized by anxiety and tension, verbal abuse and profanity, and increasing hyperactivity. These escalating behaviors usually do not occur in stages but most often overlap and sometimes occur simultaneously. Behaviors associated with this prodromal stage include rigid posture; clenched fists and jaws; grim, defiant affect; talking in a rapid, raised voice; arguing and demanding; using profanity and threatening verbalizations; agitation and pacing; and pounding and slamming.

Most assaultive behavior is preceded by a period of increasing hyperactivity. Behaviors associated with the prodromal syndrome should be considered emergent and demand immediate attention. Keen observation skills and background knowledge for accurate assessment are critical factors in predicting potential for violent behavior.

Diagnosis/Outcome Identification

NANDA International does not include a separate nursing diagnosis for anger. The nursing diagnosis of dysfunctional grieving may be used when anger is expressed inappropriately and the etiology is related to a loss.

The following nursing diagnoses may be considered for clients demonstrating inappropriate expression of anger or aggression:

Ineffective coping related to negative role modeling and dysfunctional family system evidenced by yelling, name calling, hitting others, and temper tantrums as expressions of anger.

Risk for self-directed or other-directed violence related to having been nurtured in an atmosphere of violence.

Outcome Criteria

The following criteria may be used for measurement of outcomes in the care of the client needing assistance with management of anger and aggression.
The client:

1. Is able to recognize when he or she is angry, and seeks out staff/support person to talk about his or her feelings.
2. Is able to take responsibility for own feelings of anger.
3. Demonstrates the ability to exert internal control over feelings of anger.
4. Is able to diffuse anger before losing control.
5. Uses the tension generated by the anger in a constructive manner.
6. Does not cause harm to self or others.
7. Is able to use steps of the problem-solving process rather than becoming violent as a means of seeking solutions.

Planning/Implementation

In Table 17–2, a plan of care is presented for the client who expresses anger inappropriately. Outcome criteria, appropriate nursing interventions, and rationales are included for each diagnosis.

TABLE 17–2	Care Plan for the Individual Who Expresses Anger Inappropriately

NURSING DIAGNOSIS: INEFFECTIVE COPING
RELATED TO: Negative role modeling and dysfunctional family system
EVIDENCED BY: Yelling, name calling, hitting others, and temper tantrums as expressions of anger.

OUTCOME CRITERIA	NURSING INTERVENTIONS	RATIONALE
Client will be able to recognize anger in self and take responsibility before losing control.	1. Remain calm when dealing with an angry client	1. Anger expressed by the nurse will most likely incite increased anger in the client.
	2. Set verbal limits on behavior. Clearly delineate the consequences of inappropriate expression of anger and always follow through.	2. Consistency in enforcing the consequences is essential if positive outcomes are to be achieved. Inconsistency creates confusion and encourages testing of limits.
	3. Have the client keep a diary of angry feelings, what triggered them, and how they were handled.	3. This provides a more objective measure of the problem.
	4. Avoid touching the client when he or she becomes angry.	4. The client may view touch as threatening and could become violent.
	5. Help the client determine the true source of the anger.	5. Many times anger is being displaced onto a safer object or person. If resolution is to occur, the first step is to identify the source of the problem.
	6. It may be constructive to ignore initial derogatory remarks by the client.	6. Lack of feedback often extinguishes an undesirable behavior.

(Continued on opposite page)

7. Help the client find alternate ways of releasing tension, such as physical outlets, and more appropriate ways of expressing anger, such as seeking out staff when feelings emerge.

8. Role model appropriate ways of expressing anger assertively, such as, "I dislike being called names. I get angry when I hear you saying those things about me."

7. Client will likely need assistance to problem-solve more appropriate ways of behaving.

8. Role modeling is one of the strongest methods of learning.

NURSING DIAGNOSIS: RISK FOR SELF-DIRECTED OR OTHER-DIRECTED VIOLENCE

RISK FACTORS: Having been nurtured in an atmosphere of violence.

OUTCOME CRITERIA	NURSING INTERVENTIONS	RATIONALE

The client will not harm self or others.

The client will verbalize anger rather than hit others.

1. Observe client for escalation of anger (called the prodromal syndrome): increased motor activity, pounding, slamming, tense posture, defiant affect, clenched teeth and fists, arguing, demanding, and challenging or threatening staff.

2. When these behaviors are observed, first ensure that sufficient staff are available to help with a potentially violent situation. Attempt to defuse the anger beginning with the least restrictive means.

3. Techniques for dealing with aggression include:

   a. Talking down. Say, "John, you seem very angry. Let's go to your room and talk about it." (Ensure that client does not position self between door and nurse.)

   b. Physical outlets. "Maybe it would help if you punched your pillow or the punching bag for a while." "I'll stay here with you if you want."

   c. Medication. If agitation continues to escalate, offer client choice of taking medication voluntarily. If he or she refuses, reassess the situation to determine if harm to self or others is imminent.

   d. Call for assistance. Remove self and other clients from the immediate area. Call violence code, push "panic" button, call for assault team, or institute measures established by the institution. Sufficient staff to indicate a show of strength may be enough to deescalate the situation, and client may agree to take the medication.

   e. Restraints. If client is not calmed by "talking down" or by medication, use of mechanical restraints and/or seclusion may be necessary. Be sure to have sufficient staff available to assist. Figures 17–1, 17–2, and 17–3 illustrate ways in which staff can safely and appropriately deal with an out-of-control client. Follow protocol for restraints/seclusion established by the institution. JCAHO requires that the physician reissue a new order for restraints every 4 hours for adults and every 1-2 hours for children & adolescents. If the client has previously refused medication, administer after restraints have been applied. Most states consider this intervention appropriate in emergency situations or if a client would likely harm self or others.

1. Violence may be prevented if risks are identified in time.

2. The initial consideration must be having enough help to diffuse a potentially violent situation. Client rights must be honored, while preventing harm to client and others.

3. Aggression control techniques promote safety and reduce risk of harm to client and others:

   a. Promotes a trusting relationship and may prevent the client's anxiety from escalating.

   b. Provides effective way for client to release tension associated with high levels of anger.

   c. Provides the least restrictive method of controlling client behavior.

   d. Client and staff safety are of primary concern.

   e. Clients who do not have internal control over their own behavior may require external controls, such as mechanical restraints, in order to prevent harm to self or others.

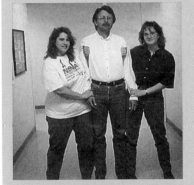

FIGURE 17–1 Walking a client to the seclusion room.

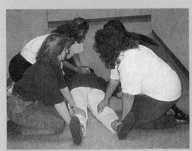

FIGURE 17–2 Staff restraint of a client in supine position. The client's head is controlled to prevent biting.

(Continued on following page)

TABLE 17–2	Care Plan for the Individual Who Expresses Anger Inappropriately *(Continued)*	
OUTCOME CRITERIA	**NURSING INTERVENTIONS**	**RATIONALE**

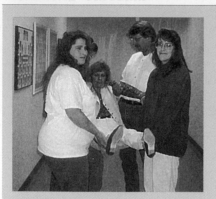

FIGURE 17–3 Transporting a client to the seclusion room.

f. Observation and documentation. Observe the client in restraints every 15 minutes (or according to institutional policy). Ensure that circulation to extremities is not compromised (check temperature, color, pulses). Assist client with needs related to nutrition, hydration, and elimination. Position client so that comfort is facilitated and aspiration can be prevented. Document all observations.

g. Ongoing assessment. As agitation decreases, assess client's readiness for restraint removal or reduction. With assistance from other staff members, remove one restraint at a time, while assessing client's response. This minimizes the risk of injury to client and staff.

h. Staff debriefing. It is important when a client loses control for staff to follow-up with a discussion about the situation. Tardiff (2003) states, "The violent episode should be discussed in terms of what happened, what would have prevented it, why seclusion or restraint was used (if it was), and how the patient or the staff felt in terms of using seclusion and restraint." It is also important to discuss the situation with other clients who witnessed the episode. It is important that they understand what happened. Some clients may fear that they could be secluded or restrained at some time for no apparent reason.

f. Client well being is a nursing priority.

g. Gradual removal of the restraints allows for testing of the client's self-control. Client and staff safety are of primary concern.

h. Debriefing diminishes the emotional impact of the intervention and provides an opportunity to clarify the need for the intervention, offer mutual feedback, and promote client's self-esteem (Norris & Kennedy, 1992).

Evaluation

Evaluation consists of reassessment to determine if the nursing interventions have been successful in achieving the objectives of care. The following type of information may be gathered to determine the success of working with a client exhibiting inappropriate expression of anger:

Is the client able to recognize when he or she is angry now?

Can the client take responsibility for these feelings and keep them in check without losing control?

Does the client seek out staff/support person to talk about feelings when they occur?

Is the client able to transfer tension generated by the anger into constructive activities?

Has harm to client and others been avoided?

Is the client able to solve problems adaptively without undue frustration and without becoming violent?

SUMMARY

Statistics show that violence is rampant in the United States. The precursor to violence is anger, which is a normal human emotion, and need not necessarily be a negative response. When used appropriately, anger can provide positive assistance with problem solving and decision-making in everyday life situations. Violence occurs when individuals lose control of their anger.

This chapter explores the concepts of anger and aggression. Anger is viewed as the emotional response to one's perception of a situation. It is a very powerful emotion and, when denied or buried, can precipitate a number of psychophysiological disorders. When it is turned inward on the self, it can result in depression. When expressed inappropriately, anger commonly interferes with interpersonal relationships. When it is suppressed, it often turns to resentment. Anger generates a physiological arousal comparable to the stress response discussed in Chapter 1.

Aggression is one way in which individuals express anger. It is behavior intended to threaten or injure the victim's security or self-esteem. It can be physical or verbal, but it is virtually always designed to punish. Aggression is a negative function or destructive use of anger.

Various predisposing factors to the way individuals express anger have been implicated. Some theorists suggest that the etiology is purely biological, whereas others believe it depends on psychological and environmental factors. Some possible predisposing factors include role modeling, operant conditioning, neurophysiological disorders (e.g., brain tumors, trauma, or diseases), biochem-

ical factors (e.g., increased levels of androgens or other alterations in hormone levels and neurotransmitter involvement), socioeconomic factors (e.g., living in poverty), and environmental factors (e.g., physical crowding, uncomfortable temperature, use of alcohol or drugs, and availability of firearms).

Nurses must be aware of the symptoms associated with anger and aggression in order to make an accurate assessment. Prevention is the key issue in the management of aggressive or violent behavior. Three elements have been identified as key risk factors in the potential for violence: (1) past history of violence, (2) client diagnosis, and (3) current behaviors. Nursing diagnoses and outcome criteria for working with clients expressing anger or aggression were discussed, and a care plan outlining appropriate interventions was presented.

REVIEW QUESTIONS

SELF-EXAMINATION/LEARNING EXERCISE

Situation: John, age 27, was brought to the emergency department by two police officers. He smelled strongly of alcohol, was loud, verbally abusive of staff, slurred his words, and had difficulty standing and walking without assistance. Blood alcohol level was measured at 293 mg/dL. John's girlfriend reported that they were at a party and he became violent, hitting her and threatening to kill others who tried to protect her. She reported that he gets drunk almost every day and has beaten her up a number of times. When told that he would be admitted to detox, he started cursing and hitting the staff who were trying to help him. He was admitted to the Detox Center of the Alcohol Treatment Unit with a diagnosis of Alcohol Intoxication. He was restrained for the protection of himself and others. His diagnosis was later changed to Alcohol Dependence, following conclusion of the withdrawal syndrome.

Please answer the following questions related to this situation.

1. The nurses on the unit wrote a priority nursing diagnosis of Risk for Other-Directed Violence for John. Using the assessment data provided, list the risk factors on which they based their diagnosis.

2. Which is the most appropriate *long-term* goal for the nursing diagnosis of Risk for Other-Directed Violence?
   a. The client will not verbalize anger or hit anyone.
   b. The client will verbalize anger rather than hit others.
   c. The client will not harm self or others.
   d. The client will be restrained if he becomes verbally or physically abusive.

3. Which is the most appropriate *short-term* goal for the nursing diagnosis of Risk for Other-Directed Violence?
   a. The client will not verbalize anger or hit anyone.
   b. The client will verbalize anger rather than hit others.
   c. The client will not harm self or others.
   d. The client will be restrained if he becomes verbally or physically abusive.

4. John is sitting in the dayroom watching TV with the other clients when the nurse approaches with his 5:00 P.M. dose of haloperidol. John says, "I feel in control now. I don't need any drugs." The nurse's best response is based on which of the following statements?
   a. John must have the medication, or he will become violent.
   b. John knows that if he will not take the medication orally, he will be restrained and given an intramuscular injection.
   c. John has the right to refuse the medication.
   d. John must take the medication at this time in order to maintain adequate blood levels.

5. Later that evening, the nurse hears John yelling in the dayroom. The nurse observes his increased agitation, clenched fists, and loud demanding voice. He is challenging and threatening staff and the other clients. The nurse's priority intervention would be:
   a. Call for assistance.
   b. Draw up a syringe of prn haloperidol.
   c. Ask John if he would like to talk about his anger.
   d. Tell John if he does not calm down he will have to be restrained.

6. John is placed in restraints in the seclusion room. Describe care of the client in restraints.

7. When John has been in restraints several hours, he tells the nurse he can maintain control and is ready to have the restraints removed. How does the nurse proceed?
   a. She removes the restraints.
   b. She calls for assistance to remove the restraints.
   c. She removes one restraint.
   d. She tells John he will have to wait until the doctor comes in.

8. Which of these procedures is important in following up an episode of violence on the unit? (More than one answer may apply.)
   a. Document all observations and occurrences.
   b. Conduct a debriefing with staff.
   c. Discuss what occurred with other clients who witnessed the incident.
   d. Warn the client that it could happen again if he becomes violent.

9. Later in the day when John is calm, he apologizes to the nurse. "I hope I didn't hurt anyone." The nurse's best response is:
   a. "This is our job. We know how to handle violent clients."
   b. "We understand you were out of control and didn't really mean to hurt anyone."
   c. "It is fortunate that no one was hurt. You will not be placed in restraints as long as you can control your behavior."
   d. "It is an unpleasant situation to have to restrain someone, but we have to think of the other clients. We can't have you causing injury to others. I just hope it won't happen again."

10. John and his girlfriend had an argument during her visit. Which behavior by John would indicate he is learning to adaptively problem solve his frustrations?
   a. John says to the nurse, "Give me some of that medication before I end up in restraints!"
   b. When his girlfriend leaves, John goes to the exercise room and punches on the punching bag.
   c. John says to the nurse, "I guess I'm going to have to dump that broad!"
   d. John says to his girlfriend, "You'd better leave before I do something I'm sorry for."

REFERENCES

American Psychiatric Association. (2004). *APA Position Statement on Violence*. Retrieved January 9, 2005 from the World Wide Web at http://www.psych.org/public_info/media_violence.cfm?

American Psychological Association. (2005a). *Controlling anger before it controls you*. Retrieved January 9, 2005 from the World Wide Web at http://www.apa.org/pubinfo/anger.html

American Psychological Association. (2005b). *Violence on television*. Retrieved January 9, 2005 from the World Wide Web at http://www.apa.org/pubinfo/violence.html

Anderson, C.A. (2001). Heat and violence. *Current Directions in Psychological Science 10*(1), 33–38.

Butterfield, P. (2000). *Understanding and managing anger: Diagnosis, treatment, and prevention*. Sunnyvale, CA: CorText Mind Matters Educational Seminars.

Dubin, W.R. (2003), Violent patients. In G. Bosker (Ed.). *The emergency medicine reports textbook of adult and pediatric emergency medicine*. Atlanta, GA: Thomson American Health Consultants.

Gorman, L.M., Raines, M.L., & Sultan, D.F. (2002). *Psychosocial nursing for general patient care* (2nd ed.). Philadelphia: F.A. Davis.

Lee, G.P., Bechara, A., Adolphs, R., Arena, J., Meador, K.J., Loring, D.W., & Smith, J.R. (1998). Clinical and physiological effects of stereotaxic bilateral amygdalotomy for intractable aggression. *Journal of Neuropsychiatry and Clinical Neurosciences 10*, 413–420.

Norris, M.K., & Kennedy, C.W. (1992). How patients perceive the seclusion process. *Journal of Psychosocial Nursing and Mental Health Services, 30*(3), 7–13.

Sadock, B.J. & Sadock, V.A. (2003). *Synopsis of psychiatry: Behavioral sciences/clinical psychiatry* (9th ed.). Philadelphia: Lippincott Williams & Wilkins.

Sunderland, T. (1997). Trends in violence and aggression. *Online coverage from the 150th annual meeting of the American Psychiatric Association, May 18 – 21, 1997*. Retrieved January 10, 2005 from the World Wide Web at http://www.dangerousbehaviour.com/Disturbing_News/Trends%20in%20Violence%20and%20Aggression.htm

Tardiff, K.J. (2003). Violence. In R.E. Hales, & S.C. Yudofsky (Eds.). *Textbook of clinical psychiatry* (4th ed.). Washington, DC: American Psychiatric Publishing.

Violence Policy Center. (2002). *Firearms and crime*. Retrieved on January 2, 2002 from the World Wide Web at http://www.vpc.org/studies/whercrim.htm

Warren, N.C. (1990). *Make anger your ally*. Colorado Springs, CO: Focus on the Family Publishing.

Waughfield, C.G. (2002). *Mental health concepts* (5th ed.). Clifton Park, NY: Thomson Delmar Learning.

THE SUICIDAL CLIENT

CHAPTER OUTLINE

OBJECTIVES

HISTORICAL PERSPECTIVES

EPIDEMIOLOGICAL FACTORS

RISK FACTORS

PREDISPOSING FACTORS: THEORIES
OF SUICIDE

APPLICATION OF THE NURSING
PROCESS WITH THE SUICIDAL CLIENT

SUMMARY

REVIEW QUESTIONS

KEY TERMS

altruistic suicide

anomic suicide

egoistic suicide

OBJECTIVES

After reading this chapter, the student will be able to:

1. Discuss epidemiological statistics and risk factors related to suicide.
2. Describe predisposing factors implicated in the etiology of suicide.
3. Differentiate between facts and fables regarding suicide.
4. Apply the nursing process to individuals exhibiting suicidal behavior.

 uicide is not a diagnosis or a disorder; it is a behavior. The Judeo-Christian belief has been that life is a gift from God and that taking it is strictly forbidden (Carroll-Ghosh, Victor, & Bourgeois, 2003). A recent, and more secular, view has influenced how some individuals view suicide in our society. Growing support for an individual's right to choose death over pain has been evidenced. Some individuals are striving to advance the cause of physician-assisted suicides for the terminally ill. Can suicide be a rational act? Most people in our society do not yet believe that it can.

Approximately 95 percent of all persons who commit or attempt suicide have a diagnosed mental disorder (Sadock & Sadock, 2003). This chapter explores suicide from an epidemiological and etiological perspective. Care of the suicidal client is presented in the context of the nursing process.

HISTORICAL PERSPECTIVES

In ancient Greece, suicide was an offense against the state and individuals who committed suicide were denied burial in community sites (Minois, 1999). In the culture of the imperial Roman army, individuals sometimes resorted to suicide to escape humiliation or abuse.

In the Middle Ages, suicide was viewed as a selfish or criminal act (Minois, 1999). Individuals who committed suicide were often denied cemetery burial and their property was confiscated and shared by the crown and the courts (MacDonald & Murphy, 1990). The issue of suicide changed during the period of the Renaissance. Although condemnation was still expected, the view became more philosophical, and intellectuals could discuss the issue more freely.

Most philosophers of the 17th and 18th centuries condemned suicide, but some writers recognized a connection between suicide and melancholy or other severe mental disturbances (Minois, 1999). Suicide was illegal in England until 1961, and only in 1993 was it decriminalized in Ireland.

Most religions consider suicide as a sin against God. Judaism, Christianity, Islam, Hinduism, and Buddhism all condemn suicide. In 1995, Pope John Paul II restated Church opposition to suicide, euthanasia, and abortion as crimes against life, not unlike homicide and genocide (Tondo & Baldessarini, 2001a).

EPIDEMIOLOGICAL FACTORS

Approximately 30,000 persons in the United States end their lives each year by suicide. These statistics have established suicide as the third leading cause of death (behind accidents and homicide) among young Americans ages 15 to 24 years, the fifth leading cause of death for ages 25 to 44, and the eighth leading cause of death for individuals age 45 to 64 (National Center for Health Statistics, 2004). Many more people attempt suicide than succeed, and countless others seriously contemplate the act without carrying it out. Suicide has become a major health care problem in the United States today.

Over the years confusion has existed over the reality of various notions regarding suicide. Some facts and fables relating to suicide are presented in Table 18–1.

RISK FACTORS

Marital Status

The suicide rate for single persons is twice that of married persons. Divorced, separated, or widowed persons have rates four to five times greater than those of the married (Tondo and Baldessarini, 2001b).

Gender

Women attempt suicide more, but men succeed more often. Successful suicides number about 70 percent for men and 30 percent for women. This has to do with the lethality of the means. Women tend to overdose; men use more lethal means such as firearms. In the United States, from 1970 to 2002, annual suicide rates per 100,000 rose from 16.8 to 17.9 in men, but decreased from 6.6 to 4.3 in women (National Center for Health Statistics, 2004). These differences between men and women may also reflect a tendency for women to seek and accept help

TABLE 18–1	Facts and Fables About Suicide
FABLES	**FACTS**
People who talk about suicide do not commit suicide. Suicide happens without warning.	Eight out of ten people who kill themselves have given definite clues and warnings about their suicidal intentions. Very subtle clues may be ignored or disregarded by others.
You cannot stop a suicidal person. He or she is fully intent on dying.	Most suicidal people are very ambivalent about their feelings regarding living or dying. Most are "gambling with death" and see it as a cry for someone to save them.
Once a person is suicidal, he or she is suicidal forever.	People who want to kill themselves are only suicidal for a limited time. If they are saved from feelings of self-destruction, they can go on to lead normal lives.
Improvement after severe depression means that the suicidal risk is over.	Most suicides occur within about 3 months after the beginning of "improvement," when the individual has the energy to carry out suicidal intentions.
Suicide is inherited, or "runs in families."	Suicide is not inherited. It is an individual matter and can be prevented. However, suicide by a close family member increases an individual's risk factor for suicide.
All suicidal individuals are mentally ill, and suicide is the act of a psychotic person.	Although suicidal persons are extremely unhappy, they are not necessarily psychotic or otherwise mentally ill. They are merely unable at that point in time to see an alternative solution to what they consider an unbearable problem.
Suicidal threats and gestures should be considered manipulative or attention-seeking behavior, and should not be taken seriously.	All suicidal behavior must be approached with the gravity of the potential act in mind. Attention should be given to the possibility that the individual is issuing a cry for help.
People usually commit suicide by taking an overdose of drugs.	Gunshot wounds are the leading cause of death among suicide victims.
If an individual has attempted suicide, he or she will not do it again.	Between 50% and 80% of all people who ultimately kill themselves have a history of a previous attempt.

SOURCES: From TWU (2005); USPHS (1999); and The Samaritans (2005).

from friends or professionals, whereas men often view help-seeking as a sign of weakness (Murphy, 1998).

Age

Suicide risk and age are positively correlated. This is particularly true with men. Although rates among women remain fairly constant throughout life, rates among men show a higher age correlation. The rates rise sharply during adolescence, peak between 40 and 50, and levels off until age 65, when it rises again for the remaining years (National Center for Health Statistics, 2004).

The suicide rate among young people ages 15 to 19 peaked in 1990 at 11.1 per 100,000 and declined to 7.4 per 100,000 in 2002 (National Center for Health Statistics, 2004). Several factors put adolescents at risk for suicide, including impulsive and high-risk behaviors, untreated mood disorders (e.g., major depression and bipolar disorder), access to lethal means (e.g., firearms), and substance abuse. The use of firearms, which accounts for about 49 percent of cases, is the most common method of completed suicide in children and adolescents (CDC, 2004).

The suicide rate for the elderly peaked in 1990 at 20.5 per 100,000 and declined to 15.6 per 100,000 in 2002 (National Center for Health Statistics, 2004). While the elderly make up less than 13 percent of the population, they account for 18 percent of all suicides (NIMH, 2003).

White men older than age 80 are at the greatest risk of all age/gender/race groups (see Figure 18–1). Eighty-one percent of elderly suicides are male, which is 13 times greater than for females, and firearms are the most common means of completing suicide (Hospice Association, 2002). The overall rate of suicide for women declines after age 65.

Religion

Historically, suicide rates among Roman Catholic populations have been lower than rates among Protestants and Jews (Sadock & Sadock, 2003). In a recent study published in the *American Journal of Psychiatry*, depressed men and women who consider themselves affiliated with a religion are less likely to attempt suicide than their non-religious counterparts (Dervic et al., 2004). The study showed no statistical significance for affiliation with any particular religious group, but only for the affiliation itself.

Socioeconomic Status

Individuals in the very highest and lowest social classes have higher suicide rates than those in the middle classes (Sadock & Sadock, 2003). With regard to occupation, suicide rates are higher among physicians, musicians,

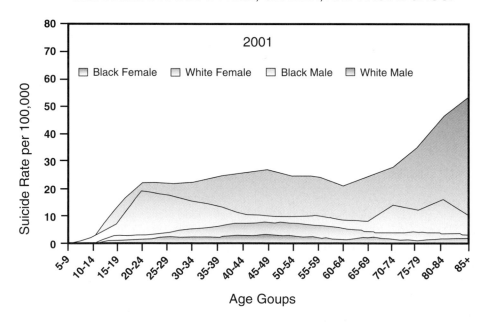

FIGURE 18–1   U.S. suicide rates by age, gender, and racial group. (From National Institute of Mental Health. Data from Center for Disease Control and Prevention, National Center for Health Statistics.)

dentists, law enforcement officers, lawyers, and insurance agents.

Ethnicity

With regard to ethnicity, most studies demonstrate that whites are at highest risk for suicide, followed by Native Americans, African Americans, Hispanic Americans, and Asian Americans (Carroll-Ghosh, Victor, & Burgeois, 2003).

Other Risk Factors

Individuals with mood disorders (major depression and bipolar disorder) are far more likely to commit suicide than those in any other psychiatric or medical risk group. Sadock and Sadock (2003) report, "Almost 95 percent of all people who commit or attempt suicide have a diagnosed mental disorder. Depressive disorders account for 80 percent of this figure." Suicide risk may increase early during treatment with antidepressants, as the return of energy brings about an increased ability to act out self-destructive wishes. Other psychiatric disorders that may account for suicidal behavior include psychoactive substance abuse disorders, schizophrenia, personality disorders, and anxiety disorders (Tondo & Baldessarini, 2001a).

Severe insomnia is associated with increased suicide risk, even in the absence of depression. Use of alcohol, and particularly a combination of alcohol and barbiturates, increases the risk of suicide. Psychosis, especially with command hallucinations, poses a higher than normal risk. Affliction with a chronic painful or disabling illness also increases the risk of suicide.

In 1994, the National Institute of Mental Health convened a workshop to study rates of suicide among gay men and lesbians. The committee stated that there was insufficient evidence to support a correlation between sexual orientation and suicidality. Responding to the statements made by this committee, Remafedi (1999) reported on a number of studies that have arrived at opposing conclusions. In a study of adult twins, it was found that men with same-sex partners were 6.5 times as likely as their twins to have attempted suicide (Herrell et al, 1999). Another study found that gay and lesbian subjects were at increased risk of psychiatric disorders and suicidal behaviors (Fergusson, Horwood, & Beautrais, 1999). Remafedi and associates (1998) found a higher degree of suicidality among homosexual adolescents than among their heterosexual counterparts.

Higher risk is also associated with a family history of suicide, especially in a same-sex parent. Persons who have made prior suicide attempts are at higher risk for suicide. About half of those who have who kill themselves have previously attempted suicide. Loss of a loved one through death or separation and lack of employment or increased financial burden also increase risk.

PREDISPOSING FACTORS: THEORIES OF SUICIDE

Psychological Theories

Anger Turned Inward. Freud (1957) believed that suicide was a response to the intense self-hatred that an individual possessed. The anger had originated toward a love object but was ultimately turned inward against the self. Freud believed that suicide occurred as a result of an earlier repressed desire to kill someone else. He interpreted suicide to be an aggressive act toward the self that often was really directed toward others.

Hopelessness. Carroll-Ghosh, Victor, and Bourgeois (2003) identify hopelessness as a central underlying factor in the predisposition to suicide. Beck and associates (1990) also found a high correlation between hopelessness and suicide.

Desperation and Guilt. Hendin (1991) identified desperation as another important factor in suicide. With desperation, an individual feels helpless to change, but he or she also feels that life is impossible without such change. Guilt and self-recrimination are other aspects of desperation. These affective components were found to be prominent in Vietnam veterans with posttraumatic stress disorder exhibiting suicidal behaviors (Carroll-Ghosh, Victor, & Bourgeois, 2003).

History of Aggression and Violence. Some studies have indicated that violent behavior often goes hand-in-hand with suicidal behavior (Carroll-Ghosh, Victor, & Bourgeois, 2003). These studies correlate the suicidal behavior in violent individuals to conscious rage, therefore citing rage as an important psychological factor underlying the suicidal behavior (Hendin, 1991).

Shame and Humiliation. Some individuals have viewed suicide as a "face-saving" mechanism—a way to prevent public humiliation following a social defeat such as a sudden loss of status or income. Often these individuals are too embarrassed to seek treatment or other support systems.

Developmental Stressors. Rich, Warsradt, and Nemiroff (1991) have associated developmental level with certain life stressors and their correlation to suicide. The stressors of conflict, separation, and rejection are associated with suicidal behavior in adolescence and early adulthood. The principal stressor associated with suicidal behavior in the 40- to 60-year-old group is economic problems. Medical illness plays an increasingly significant role after age 60 and becomes the leading predisposing factor to suicidal behavior in individuals older than age 80.

Sociological Theory

Durkheim (1951) studied the individual's interaction with the society in which he or she lived. He believed that the more cohesive the society, and the more that the individual felt an integrated part of the society, the less likely he or she was to commit suicide. Durkheim described three social categories of suicide:

Egoistic suicide is the response of the individual who feels separate and apart from the mainstream of society. Integration is lacking and the individual does not feel a part of any cohesive group (such as a family or a church).

Altruistic suicide is the opposite of egoistic suicide. The individual who is prone to altruistic suicide is excessively integrated into the group. The group is often governed by cultural, religious, or political ties, and allegiance is so strong that the individual will sacrifice his or her life for the group.

Anomic suicide occurs in response to changes that occur in an individual's life (e.g., divorce, loss of job) that disrupt feelings of relatedness to the group. An interruption in the customary norms of behavior instills feelings of "separateness," and fears of being without support from the formerly cohesive group.

Biological Theories

Genetics. Twin studies have shown a much higher concordance rate for monozygotic twins than for dizygotic twins. Recent studies with suicide attempters have focused on the genotypic variations in the gene for tryptophan hydroxylase, with results indicating significant association to suicidality (Abbar et al., 2001). These results suggest a possible existence of genetic predisposition toward suicidal behavior.

Neurochemical Factors. A number of studies have been conducted to determine if there is a correlation between neurochemical functioning in the central nervous system (CNS) and suicidal behavior. Some studies have revealed a deficiency of serotonin (measured as a decrease in the levels of 5-hydroxyindole acetic acid [5-HIAA] of the cerebrospinal fluid) in depressed clients who attempted suicide (Sadock & Sadock, 2003). Some changes in the noradrenergic system of suicide victims have also been reported.

APPLICATION OF THE NURSING PROCESS WITH THE SUICIDAL CLIENT

Assessment

The following items should be considered when conducting a suicidal assessment: demographics, presenting symptoms/medical-psychiatric diagnosis, suicidal ideas or acts, interpersonal support system, analysis of the suicidal crisis, psychiatric/medical/family history, and coping strategies. The Surgeon General, in his "Call to Action to Prevent Suicide," speaks of risk factors and protective factors (USPHS, 1999). Risk factors are associated with a greater potential for suicide and suicidal behavior, whereas protective factors are associated with reduced potential for suicide. These risk and protective factors are outlined in Table 18–2. Table 18–3 presents some additional guidelines for determining the degree of suicide potential.

TABLE 18–2 Suicide Risk Factors and Protective Factors	
RISK FACTORS	**PROTECTIVE FACTORS**
• Previous suicide attempt • Mental disorders—particularly mood disorders such as depression and bipolar disorder • Co-occurring mental and alcohol and substance abuse disorders • Family history of suicide • Hopelessness • Impulsive and/or aggressive tendencies • Barriers to accessing mental health treatment • Relational, social, work, or financial loss • Physical illness • Easy access to lethal methods, especially guns • Unwillingness to seek help because of stigma attached to mental and substance abuse disorders and/or suicidal thoughts • Influence of significant people—family members, celebrities, peers who have died by suicide—both through direct personal contact or inappropriate media representations • Cultural and religious beliefs—for instance, the belief that suicide is a noble resolution of a personal dilemma • Local epidemics of suicide that have a contagious influence • Isolation, a feeling of being cut off from other people	• Effective and appropriate clinical care for mental, physical, and substance abuse disorders • Easy access to a variety of clinical interventions and support for help seeking • Restricted access to highly lethal methods of suicide • Family and community support • Support from ongoing medical and mental health care relationships • Learned skills in problem solving, conflict resolution, and nonviolent handling of disputes • Cultural and religious beliefs that discourage suicide and support self-preservation instincts

SOURCE: U.S. Public Health Service, *The Surgeon General's Call To Action To Prevent Suicide.* Washington, DC: 1999.

TABLE 18–3	Assessing the Degree of Suicidal Risk		

| | INTENSITY OF RISK | | |
BEHAVIOR	LOW	MODERATE	HIGH
Anxiety	Mild	Moderate	High or panic
Depression	Mild	Moderate	Severe
Isolation; withdrawal	Some feelings of isolation; no withdrawal	Some feelings of helplessness, hopelessness, and withdrawal	Hopeless, helpless, withdrawn, and self-deprecating
Daily functioning	Fairly good in most activities	Moderately good in some activities	Not good in any activities
Resources	Several	Some	Few or none
Coping strategies being used	Generally constructive	Some that are constructive	Predominantly destructive
Significant others	Several who are available	Few or only one available	Only one or none available
Psychiatric help in past	None, or positive attitude toward	Yes, and moderately satisfied with results	Negative view of help received
Lifestyle	Stable	Moderately stable	Unstable
Alcohol or drug use	Infrequently to excess	Frequently to excess	Continual abuse
Previous suicide attempts	None, or of low lethality	One or more of moderate lethality	Multiple attempts of high lethality
Disorientation; disorganization	None	Some	Marked
Hostility	Little or none	Some	Marked
Suicidal plan	Vague, fleeting thoughts but no plan	Frequent thoughts, occasional ideas about a plan	Frequent or constant thought with a specific plan

SOURCE: From Hatten and Valente (1984), with permission.

Demographics

The following demographics are assessed:

Age. Suicide is highest in persons older than 50. Adolescents are also at high risk.

Gender. Males are at higher risk than females.

Ethnicity. Caucasians are at higher risk than are Native Americans, who are at higher risk than African Americans.

Martial Status. Single, divorced, and widowed are at higher risk than married.

Socioeconomic Status. Individuals in the highest and lowest socioeconomic classes are at higher risk than those in the middle classes.

Occupation. Professional health care personnel and business executives are at highest risk.

Method. Use of firearms presents a significantly higher risk than overdose of substances.

Religion. Individuals who are not affiliated with any religious group are at higher risk than those who have this type of affiliation.

Family History. Higher risk if individual has family history of suicide.

Presenting Symptoms/ Medical–Psychiatric Diagnosis

Assessment data must be gathered regarding any psychiatric or physical condition for which the client is being treated. Mood disorders (major depression and bipolar disorders) are the most common disorders that precede suicide. Individuals with substance use disorders are also at high risk. Other psychiatric disorders in which suicide may be a risk include anxiety disorders, schizophrenia, and borderline and antisocial personality disorders (Tondo & Baldessarini, 2001a). Other chronic and terminal physical illnesses have also precipitated suicidal acts.

Suicidal Ideas or Acts

How serious is the intent? Does the person have a plan? If so, does he or she have the means? How lethal are the means? Has the individual ever attempted suicide before? These are all questions that must be answered by the person conducting the suicidal assessment.

Individuals may leave both behavioral and verbal clues as to the intent of their act. Examples of behavioral clues include giving away prized possessions, getting financial affairs in order, writing suicide notes, or sudden lifts in mood (may indicate a decision to carry out the intent).

Verbal clues may be both direct and indirect. Examples of direct statements include "I want to die" or "I'm going to kill myself." Examples of indirect statements include "This is the last time you'll see me," "I won't be around much longer for the doctor to have to worry about," or "I don't have anything worth living for anymore."

Other assessments include determining whether the individual has a plan, and if so, whether he or she has the means to carry out that plan. If the person states the suicide will be carried out with a gun, does he or she have access to a gun? Bullets? If pills are planned, what kind of pills? Are they accessible?

Interpersonal Support System

Does the individual have support persons on whom he or she can rely during a crisis situation? Lack of a meaningful network of satisfactory relationships may implicate an individual at high risk for suicide during an emotional crisis.

Analysis of the Suicidal Crisis

The Precipitating Stressor. Adverse life events in combination with other risk factors such as depression may lead to suicide (NIMH, 2002). Life stresses accompanied by an increase in emotional disturbance include the loss of a loved person either by death or by divorce, problems in major relationships, changes in roles, or serious physical illness.

Relevant History. Has the individual experienced numerous failures or rejections that would increase his or her vulnerability for a dysfunctional response to the current situation?

Life-Stage Issues. The ability to tolerate losses and disappointments is often compromised if those losses and disappointments occur during various stages of life in which the individual struggles with developmental issues (e.g., adolescence, midlife).

Psychiatric/Medical/Family History

The individual should be assessed with regard to previous psychiatric treatment for depression, alcoholism, or for previous suicide attempts. Medical history should be obtained to determine presence of chronic, debilitating, or terminal illness. Is there a history of depressive disorder in the family, and has a close relative committed suicide in the past?

Coping Strategies

How has the individual handled previous crisis situations? How does this situation differ from previous ones?

Diagnosis/Outcome Identification

Nursing diagnoses for the suicidal client may include the following:

1. Risk for suicide related to feelings of hopelessness and desperation.
2. Hopelessness related to absence of support systems and perception of worthlessness.

The following criteria may be used for measurement of outcomes in the care of the suicidal client.
The client:

1. Has experienced no physical harm to self.
2. Sets realistic goals for self.
3. Expresses some optimism and hope for the future.

Planning/Implementation

Table 18–4 provides a plan of care for the hospitalized suicidal client. Nursing diagnoses are presented, along

TABLE 18–4	Care Plan for the Suicidal Client

NURSING DIAGNOSIS: RISK FOR SUICIDE
RELATED TO: Feelings of hopelessness and desperation

OUTCOME CRITERIA	NURSING INTERVENTIONS	RATIONALES
Client will not harm self.	1. Ask client directly: "Have you thought about harming yourself in any way? If so, what do you plan to do? Do you have the means to carry out this plan?"	1. The risk of suicide is greatly increased if the client has developed a plan and particularly if means exist for the client to execute the plan.
	2. Create a safe environment for the client. Remove all potentially harmful objects from client's access (sharp objects, straps, belts, ties, glass items, alcohol). Supervise closely during meals and medication administration. Perform room searches as deemed necessary.	2. Client safety is a nursing priority.
	3. Formulate a short-term verbal or written contract that the client will not harm self. When time is up, make another, and so forth. Secure a promise that the client will seek out staff when feeling suicidal.	3. A degree of the responsibility for his or her safety is given to the client. Increased feelings of self-worth may be experienced when client feels accepted unconditionally regardless of thoughts or behavior.

(Continued on opposite page)

OUTCOME CRITERIA	NURSING INTERVENTIONS	RATIONALES
	4. Maintain close observation of client. Depending on level of suicide precaution, provide one-to-one contact, constant visual observation, or every-15-minute checks. Place in room close to nurse's station; do not assign to private room. Accompany to off-unit activities if attendance is indicated. May need to accompany to bathroom.	4. Close observation is necessary to ensure that client does not harm self in any way. Being alert for suicidal and escape attempts facilitates being able to prevent or interrupt harmful behavior.
	5. Maintain special care in administration of medications.	5. Prevents saving up to overdose or discarding and not taking.
	6. Make rounds at frequent, *irregular* intervals (especially at night, toward early morning, at change of shift, or other predictably busy times for staff).	6. Prevents staff surveillance from becoming predictable. To be aware of client's location is important, especially when staff is busy and least available and observable.
	7. Encourage client to express honest feelings, including anger. Provide hostility release if needed.	7. Depression and suicidal behaviors may be viewed as anger turned inward on the self. If this anger can be verbalized in a nonthreatening environment, the client may be able to eventually resolve these feelings.

NURSING DIAGNOSIS: HOPELESSNESS

RELATED TO: Absence of support systems and perception of worthlessness

EVIDENCED BY: Verbal cues (despondent content, "I can't"); decreased affect; lack of initiative; suicidal ideas or attempts

OUTCOME CRITERIA	NURSING INTERVENTIONS	RATIONALES
Client will verbalize a measure of hope and acceptance of life and situations over which he or she has no control.	1. Identify stressors in client's life that precipitated current crisis.	1. Important to identify causative or contributing factors in order to plan appropriate assistance.
	2. Determine coping behaviors previously used and client's perception of effectiveness then and now.	2. It is important to identify client's strengths and encourage their use in current crisis situation.
	3. Encourage client to explore and verbalize feelings and perceptions.	3. Identification of feelings underlying behaviors helps client to begin process of taking control of own life.
	4. Provide expressions of hope to client in positive, low-key manner (e.g., "I know you feel you cannot go on, but I believe that things can get better for you. What you are feeling is temporary. It is okay if you don't see it just now." "You are very important to the people who care about you.")	4. Even though the client feels hopeless, it is helpful to hear positive expressions from others. The client's current state of mind may prevent him or her from identifying anything positive in life. It is important to accept the client's feelings nonjudgmentally and to affirm the individual's personal worth and value.
	5. Help client identify areas of life situation that are under own control.	5. The client's emotional condition may interfere with ability to problem solve. Assistance may be required to perceive the benefits and consequences of available alternatives accurately.
	6. Identify sources that client may use after discharge when crises occur or feelings of hopelessness and possible suicidal ideation prevail.	6. Client should be made aware of local suicide hotlines or other local support services from whom he or she may seek assistance following discharge from the hospital. A concrete plan provides hope in the face of a crisis situation.

with outcome criteria, appropriate nursing interventions, and rationales for each.

Intervention with the Suicidal Client Following Discharge (or Outpatient Suicidal Client)

In some instances, it may be determined that suicidal intent is low and that hospitalization is not required. Instead, the client with suicidal ideation may be treated in an outpatient setting. Guidelines for treatment of the suicidal client on an outpatient basis include the following:

1. The person should not be left alone. Arrangements must be made for the client to stay with family or friends. If this is not possible, hospitalization should be reconsidered.
2. Establish a no-suicide contract with the client. Formulate a written contract that the client will not harm himself or herself in a stated period of time. For example, the client writes, "I will not harm myself in any way between now and the time of our next counseling session," or "I will call the suicide hotline (or go to the emergency room) if I start to feel like harming myself." When the time period of this short-term contract has lapsed, a new contract is negotiated.
3. Enlist the help of family or friends to ensure that the home environment is safe from dangerous items, such as firearms or stockpiled drugs. Give support persons the telephone number of counselor or emergency contact person in the event that the counselor is not available.
4. Appointments may need to be scheduled daily or every other day at first until the immediate suicidal crisis has subsided.
5. Establish rapport and promote a trusting relationship. It is important for the suicide counselor to become a key person in the client's support system at this time.
6. Be direct. Talk openly and matter-of-factly about suicide. Listen actively and encourage expression of feelings, including anger. Accept the client's feelings in a nonjudgmental manner.
7. Discuss the current crisis situation in the client's life. Use the problem-solving approach (see Chapter 13). Offer alternatives to suicide. Macnab (1993) suggests the following statements:

   > You are incorrect in your belief that suicide is the only and the best solution to your problem. There are alternatives, and they are good. What is more, you will be alive to test them. (p. 265)

8. Help the client identify areas of life situation that are within his or her control and those that client does not have the ability to control. Discuss feelings associated with these control issues. It is important for the client to feel some control over his or her life situation in order to perceive a measure of self-worth.
9. The physician may prescribe antidepressants for an individual who is experiencing suicidal depression. It is wise to prescribe no more than a 3-day supply of the medication with no refills. The prescription can then be renewed at the client's next counseling session. **NOTE:** Sadock and Sadock (2003) state:

   > As the depression lifts, patients become energized and are thus able to put their suicidal plans into action. Sometimes, depressed patients, with or without treatment, suddenly appear to be at peace with themselves because they have reached a secret decision to commit suicide. Clinicians should be especially suspicious of such a dramatic clinical change, which may portend a suicidal attempt. (p. 921)

10. Macnab (1993) suggests the following steps in crisis counseling with the suicidal client:
    a. Focus on the current crisis and how it can be alleviated. Identify the client's appraisals of how things are, and how things will be. Note how these appraisals change in changing contexts.
    b. Note the client's reactivity to the crisis and how this can be changed. Discuss strategies and procedures for the management of anxiety, anger, and frustration.
    c. Work toward restoration of the client's self-worth, status, morale, and control. Introduce alternatives to suicide.
    d. Rehearse cognitive reconstruction—more positive ways of thinking about the self, events, the past, the present, and the future.
    e. Identify experiences and actions that affirm self-worth and self-efficacy.
    f. Encourage movement toward the new reality, with the coping skills required to manage adaptively.
    g. Be available for ongoing therapeutic support and growth.

Information for Family and Friends of the Suicidal Client

The following suggestions are made for family and friends of an individual who is suicidal:

1. Take any hint of suicide seriously. Anyone expressing suicidal feelings needs immediate attention.
2. Do not keep secrets. If a suicidal person says, "Promise you won't tell anyone," do not make that promise. Suicidal individuals are ambivalent about dying, and suicidal behavior is a cry for help. It is the part of the person that wants to stay alive that tells you about it. Get help for the person and for you. 1-800-

SUICIDE is a national hotline that is available 24 hours a day.

3. The Centers for Disease Control (CDC, 2002) offer the following suggestions for families and friends of suicidal persons:

    a. Be a good listener. If people express suicidal thoughts or feel depressed, hopeless, or worthless, be supportive. Let them know you are there for them and are willing to help them seek professional help.

    b. Many people find it awkward to put into words how another person's life is important for their own well-being, but it is important to stress that the person's life is important to you and to others. Emphasize in specific terms the ways in which the person's suicide would be devastating to you and to others.

    c. Express concern for individuals who express thoughts about committing suicide. The individual may be withdrawn and reluctant to discuss what he or she is thinking. Acknowledge the person's pain and feelings of hopelessness, and encourage the individual to talk to someone else if he or she does not feel comfortable talking with you.

    d. Familiarize yourself with suicide intervention sources, such as mental health centers and suicide hotlines.

    e. Ensure that access to firearms or other means of self-harm is restricted.

4. The Mental Health Sanctuary (2004) offers the following tips:

    a. Acknowledge and accept their feelings and be an active listener.

    b. Try to give them hope and remind them that what they are feeling is temporary.

    c. Stay with them. Do not leave them alone. Go to where they are, if necessary.

    d. Show love and encouragement. Hold them, hug them, touch them. Allow them to cry and express anger.

    e. Help them seek professional help.

    f. Remove any items from the home with which the person may harm himself or herself.

    g. If there are children present, try to remove them from the home. Perhaps another friend or relative can assist by taking them to their home. This type of situation can be extremely traumatic for children.

    h. DO NOT: judge suicidal people, show anger toward them, provoke guilt in them, discount their feelings, or tell them to "snap out of it." This is a very real and serious situation to suicidal individuals. They are in real pain. They feel the situation is hopeless and that there is no other way to resolve it aside from taking their own life.

Intervention with Families and Friends of Suicide Victims

Fraser (1994) states:

> For many people in a post-suicide situation there is a sudden and, for the most part, unexpected shattering of their lives. In addition to the grief and loss associated with the death of a close relative, there is an extra burden for the family members of a suicide victim. Part of that burden is the altered social world in which they suddenly find themselves. Their private sorrow has a public aspect and their grief and adjustment to it must be lived out within a social context which has little in the way of supporting structures of understanding of their plight. They must struggle as best they can with their own internal resources, resources which have been severely attenuated by this tragic event.

Suicide of a family member can induce a whole gamut of feelings in the survivors. Macnab (1993) identifies the following symptoms, which may be evident following the suicide of a loved one.

1. A sense of guilt and responsibility

2. Anger, resentment, and rage that can never find its "object"

3. A heightened sense of emotionality, helplessness, failure, and despair

4. A recurring self-searching: "If only I had done something," If only I had not done something," "If only...."

5. A sense of confusion and search for an explanation: "Why did this happen?" "What does it mean?" "What could have stopped it?" "What will people think?"

6. A sense of inner injury. The family feels wounded. They do not know how they will ever get over it and get on with life.

7. A severe strain is placed on relationships. A sense of impatience, irritability, and anger exists between family members.

8. A heightened vulnerability to illness and disease exists with this added burden of emotional stress.

Strategies for assisting survivors of suicide victims include:

1. Encourage the clients to talk about the suicide, each responding to the others' viewpoints, and reconstructing of events. Share memories.

2. Be aware of any blaming or scapegoating of specific family members. Discuss how each person fits into the family situation, both before and after the suicide.

3. Listen to feelings of guilt and self-persecution. Gently move the individuals toward the reality of the situation.

4. Encourage the family members to discuss individual relationships with the lost loved one. Focus on both

positive and negative aspects of the relationships. Gradually, point out the irrationality of any idealized concepts of the deceased person. The family must be able to recognize both positive and negative aspects about the person before grief can be resolved.

5. No two people grieve in the same way. It may appear that some family members are "getting over" the grief faster than others. All family members must be made to understand that if this occurs, it is not because they "care less," just that they "grieve differently." Variables that enter into this phenomenon include individual past experiences, personal relationship with the deceased person, and individual temperament and coping abilities.

6. Recognize how the suicide has caused disorganization in family coping. Reassess interpersonal relationships in the context of the event. Discuss coping strategies that have been successful in times of stress in the past, and work to reestablish these within the family. Identify new adaptive coping strategies that can be incorporated.

7. Identify resources that provide support: religious beliefs and spiritual counselors, close friends and relatives, survivors of suicide support groups. One on-line connection that puts individuals in contact with survivors groups specific to each state is http://www.afsp.org/survivor/groups.htm. A list of resources that provide information and help for issues regarding suicide is presented in Table 18–5.

Evaluation

Evaluation of the suicidal client is an ongoing process accomplished through continuous reassessment of the client, as well as determination of goal achievement. Once the immediate crisis has been resolved, extended psychotherapy may be indicated. The long-term goals of individual or group psychotherapy for the suicidal client would be for him or her to:

1. Develop and maintain a more positive self-concept.
2. Learn more effective ways to express feelings to others.
3. Achieve successful interpersonal relationships.
4. Feel accepted by others and achieve a sense of belonging.

A suicidal person feels worthless and hopeless. These goals serve to instill a sense of self-worth, while offering a measure of hope and a meaning for living.

TABLE 18–5	**Sources for Information Related to Issues of Suicide**
National Suicide Hotline 1-800-SUICIDE	**National Alliance for the Mentally Ill** http://www.nami.org 1-800-950-NAMI
American Association of Suicidology http://www.suicidology.org 1-202-237-2280	**National Depressive and Manic-Depressive Association (NDMDA)** http://www.dbsalliance.org/ 1-800-826-3632
American Foundation for Suicide Prevention http://www.afsp.org 1-888-333-AFSP	**National Institute of Mental Health** http://www.nimh.nih.gov 1-866-615-6464
American Psychiatric Association http://www.psych.org 1-703-907-7300	**National Mental Health Association** http://www.nmha.org 1-800-228-1114 1-800-969-NMHA
American Psychological Association http://www.apa.org 1-800-964-2000	**Screening for Mental Health** **Stop a Suicide Today!** http://www.stopasuicide.org 1-781-239-0071
Boys Town Cares for troubled boys and girls and families in crisis. Staff is trained to handle calls related to violence and suicide. http://www.girlsandboystown.org 1-800-448-3000 (crisis hotline) 1-402-498-1300	**Suicide Awareness—Voices of Education** http://www.save.org 1-612-946-7998
Centers for Disease Control and Prevention **National Center for Injury Prevention and Control** **Division of Violence Prevention** http://www.cdc.gov/ncipc 1-770-488-1506	**Centre for Suicide Prevention** http://www.suicideinfo.ca 1-403-245-3900
The Center for Mental Health Services http://www.mentalhealth.samhsa.gov/topics/explore/suicide/ 1-800-789-2647	**Suicide Prevention Advocacy Network** http://spanusa.org 1-202-449-3600

SUMMARY

Suicide is the eighth leading cause of death among adults ages 45 to 64, and the third leading cause of death among adolescents in the United States today. In assessing risk factors, it is important to consider marital status, gender, age, religion, socioeconomic status, ethnicity, occupation, family history, physical condition, support systems, precipitating stressors, coping strategies, seriousness of intent, and lethality and availability of method.

Predisposing factors include internalized anger, hopelessness, desperation and guilt, history of aggression and violence, shame and humiliation, developmental stressors, sociological influences, genetics, and neurochemical factors.

This chapter presented a plan for care of the suicidal client, both in the hospital and on an outpatient basis. Information for family and friends of a suicidal person and suggestions for counseling with families of suicide victims were also included.

Once the crisis intervention is complete, the individual may require long-term psychotherapy, during which he or she works to: (1) develop and maintain a more positive self-concept, (2) learn more effective ways to express feelings, (3) improve interpersonal relationships, and (4) achieve a sense of belonging and a measure of hope for living.

REVIEW QUESTIONS

SELF-EXAMINATION/LEARNING EXERCISE

Select the answer that is most appropriate for each of the following questions.

1. Which of the following individuals is at highest risk for suicide?
   a. Nancy, age 33, Asian American, Catholic, middle socioeconomic group, alcoholic
   b. John, age 72, white, Methodist, low socioeconomic group, diagnosis of metastatic cancer of the pancreas
   c. Carol, age 15, African American, Baptist, high socioeconomic group, no physical or mental health problems
   d. Mike, age 55, Jewish, middle socioeconomic group, suffered myocardial infarction a year ago

2. Some biological factors may be associated with the predisposition to suicide. Which of the following biological factors have been implicated?
   a. Genetics and decreased levels of serotonin
   b. Heredity and increased levels of norepinephrine
   c. Temporal lobe atrophy and decreased levels of acetylcholine
   d. Structural alterations of the brain and increased levels of dopamine

3. Theresa, age 27, was admitted to the psychiatric unit from the medical intensive care unit where she was treated for taking a deliberate overdose of her antidepressant medication, trazodone (Desyrel). She says to the nurse, "My boyfriend broke up with me. We had been together for 6 years. I love him so much. I know I'll never get over him." Which is the best response by the nurse?
   a. "You'll get over him in time, Theresa."
   b. "Forget him. There are other fish in the sea."
   c. "You must be feeling very sad about your loss."
   d. "Why do you think he broke up with you, Theresa?"

4. The nurse identifies the primary nursing diagnosis for Theresa as Risk for Suicide related to feelings of hopelessness from loss of relationship. Which is the outcome criterion that would most accurately measure achievement of this diagnosis?
   a. The client has experienced no physical harm to herself.
   b. The client sets realistic goals for herself.
   c. The client expresses some optimism and hope for the future.
   d. The client has reached a stage of acceptance in the loss of the relationship with her boyfriend.

5. Freudian psychoanalytic theory would explain Theresa's suicide attempt in which of the following ways?
   a. She feels hopeless about her future without her boyfriend.
   b. Without her boyfriend, she feels like an outsider with her peers.
   c. She is feeling intense guilt because her boyfriend broke up with her.
   d. She is angry at her boyfriend for breaking up with her and has turned the anger inward on herself.

6. Theresa says to the nurse, "When I get out of here, I'm going to try this again, and next time I'll choose a no-fail method." Which is the best response by the nurse?
   a. "You are safe here. We will make sure nothing happens to you."
   b. "You're just lucky your roommate came home when she did."
   c. "What exactly do you plan to do?"
   d. "I don't understand. You have so much to live for."

7. In determining degree of suicidal risk with Theresa, the nurse assesses the following behavioral manifestations: severely depressed, withdrawn, statements of worthlessness, difficulty accomplishing activities of daily living, no close support systems. The nurse identifies Theresa's risk for suicide as:

a. Low
b. Moderate
c. High
d. Unable to determine

8. Theresa is placed on suicide precautions on the psychiatric unit. Which of the following interventions is most appropriate in this instance?
   a. Obtain an order from the physician to place Theresa in restraints to prevent any attempts to harm herself.
   b. Check on Theresa every 15 minutes or assign a staff person to stay with her on a one-to-one basis.
   c. Obtain an order from the physician to give Theresa a sedative to calm her and reduce suicide ideas.
   d. Do not allow Theresa to participate in any unit activities while she is on suicide precautions.

9. All of the following interventions are appropriate for Theresa while she is on suicide precautions *except:*
   a. Remove all sharp objects, belts, and other potentially dangerous articles from Theresa's environment.
   b. Accompany Theresa to off-unit activities.
   c. Obtain a promise from Theresa that she will not do anything to harm herself for the next 12 hours.
   d. Put all of Theresa's possessions in storage and explain to her that she may have them back when she is off suicide precautions.

10. Success of long-term psychotherapy with Theresa could be measured by which of the following behaviors?
    a. Theresa has a new boyfriend.
    b. Theresa has an increased sense of self-worth.
    c. Theresa does not take antidepressants anymore.
    d. Theresa told her old boyfriend how angry she was with him for breaking up with her.

REFERENCES

Abbar, M., Courtet, P., Bellivier, F., Leboyer, M., Boulenger, J.P., Castelhau, D., Ferreira, M., Lambercy, C., Mouthon, D., Paoloni-Giacobino, A., Vessaz, M., Malafosse, A., & Buresi, C. (2001). Suicide attempters and the tryptophan hydroxylase gene. *Molecular Psychiatry, 6,* 268–273.

Beck, A.T., Brown, G., & Berchick, R.J. (1990). Relationship between hopelessness and ultimate suicide: A replication with psychiatric outpatients. *American Journal of Psychiatry, 147,* 190–195.

Carroll-Ghosh, T., Victor, B.S., & Bourgeois, J.A. (2003). Suicide. In R.E. Hales and S.C. Yudofsky (Eds.). *Textbook of clinical psychiatry* (4th ed.). Washington, DC: American Psychiatric Publishing.

Centers for Disease Control (CDC). (2002). *Preventing suicide.* Retrieved January 2, 2002 from the World Wide Web at http://www.cdc.gov/safeusa/suicide.htm

Centers for Disease Control (CDC). (2004). *Morbidity and Mortality Weekly Report, 53*(22), 471.

Dervic, K., Oquendo, M.A., Grunebaum, M.F., Ellis, S., Burke, A.K., & Mann, J.J. (2004). Religious affiliation and suicide attempt. *American Journal of Psychiatry, 161*(12), 2303–2308.

Fergusson, D.M., Horwood, L.J., & Beautrais, A.L. (1999). Is sexual orientation related to mental health problems and suicidality in young people? *Archives of General Psychiatry, 56*(10), 867–874.

Fraser, M. (1994). *What about us?: The legacy of suicide.* Retrieved January 6, 2002 from the World Wide Web at http://www.csu.edu.au/research/crsr/ruralsoc/v4n3p7.htm

Hatten, C.L., & Valente, S.M. (1984). *Suicide: Assessment and intervention* (2nd ed.). Norwalk, CT: Appleton-Century-Crofts.

Hendin, H. (1991). Psychodynamics of suicide, with particular reference to the young. *American Journal of Psychiatry, 148,* 1150–1158.

Herrell, R., Goldberg, J., True, W., Ramakrishnan, V., Lyons, M., Eisen, S., & Tsuang, M. (1999). Sexual orientation and suicidality: A co-twin control study in adult men. *Archives of General Psychiatry, 56*(10), 867–888.

Hospice Association, Inc. (2002). *Elderly suicide fact sheet.* Retrieved January 3, 2002 from the World Wide Web at http://hospice.hyper-mart.net/elderly.html

MacDonald, M., & Murphy, T.R. (1990). *Suicide in early modern England.* Oxford: Clarendon Press.

Macnab, F. (1993). *Brief psychotherapy: An integrative approach in clinical practice.* West Sussex, England: John Wiley & Sons.

Mental Health Sanctuary. (2004). *How to help a suicidal person.* Retrieved January 19, 2005 from the World Wide Web at http://www.mhsanctuary.com/suicide/sui2.htm

Minois, G. (1999). *History of suicide, voluntary death, in Western culture.* Baltimore: Johns Hopkins University Press.

Murphy, G.E. (1998). Why women are less likely than men to commit suicide. *Comprehensive Psychiatry, 39,* 165–175.

National Center for Health Statistics. (2004). *Health, United States, 2004.* Library of Congress Catalog Number 76-641496. Washington, DC: U.S. Government Printing Office.

National Institute of Mental Health (NIMH). (2002). *In harm's way: Suicide in America.* Retrieved January 5, 2002 from the World Wide Web at http://www.nimh.nih.gov/publicat/harmaway.cfm

National Institute of Mental Health (NIMH). (2003). *Older adults: Depression and suicide facts.* Retrieved January 18, 2005 from the World Wide Web at http://www.nimh.nih.gov/publicat/elderlydep suicide.cfm

Remafedi, G. (1999). Suicide and sexual orientation: Nearing the end of controversy? *Archives of General Psychiatry, 56*(10), 885–886.

Remafedi, G., French, S., Story, M., Resnick, M., & Blum, R. (1998). The relationship between suicide risk and sexual orientation: Results of a population-based study. *American Journal of Public Health, 88,* 57–60.

Rich, C.L., Warsradt, G.M., & Nemiroff, R.A. (1991). Suicide, stressors, and the life cycle. *American Journal of Psychiatry, 148,* 524–527.

Sadock, B.J., & Sadock, V.A. (2003). *Synopsis of psychiatry: Behavioral sciences/clinical psychiatry* (9th ed.). Philadelphia: Lippincott Williams & Wilkins.

Samaritans (The). (2005). *Suicide myths and misconceptions.* Retrieved January 17, 2005 from the World Wide Web at http://www.samaritansnyc.org/myths.html

Texas Women's University (TWU) Counseling Center. (2005). *Facts and fables about suicide.* Retrieved January 17, 2005 from the World Wide Web at http://www.twu.edu/o-sl/counseling/SH046.html

Tondo, L. & Baldessarini, R.J. (2001a). *Suicide: Historical, descriptive, and epidemiological considerations.* Retrieved March 6, 2003 from the World Wide Web at http://www.medscape.com/viewprogram/ 352

Tondo, L. & Baldessarini, R.J. (2001b). *Suicide: Causes and clinical management.* Retrieved March 6, 2003 from the World Wide Web at http://www.medscape.com/viewprogram/353

U.S. Public Health Service (USPHS). (1999). *The Surgeon General's call to action to prevent suicide.* Washington, DC: USPHS.

CLASSICAL REFERENCES

Durkheim, E. (1951). *Suicide: A study of sociology.* Glencoe, IL: Free Press.

Freud, S. (1957). *Mourning and melancholia,* Vol. 14 (standard ed.) London: Hogarth Press. (Original work published 1917.)

BEHAVIOR THERAPY

CHAPTER OUTLINE

OBJECTIVES

CLASSICAL CONDITIONING

OPERANT CONDITIONING

TECHNIQUES FOR MODIFYING CLIENT BEHAVIOR

ROLE OF THE NURSE IN BEHAVIOR THERAPY

SUMMARY

REVIEW QUESTIONS

KEY TERMS

aversive stimulus
classical conditioning
conditioned response
conditioned stimulus
contingency
  contracting
covert sensitization
discriminative
  stimulus
extinction
flooding
modeling
negative reinforcement
operant conditioning
overt sensitization

positive reinforcement
Premack principle
reciprocal inhibition
shaping
stimulus
  generalization
systematic
  desensitization
time out
token economy
unconditioned
  response
unconditioned
  stimulus

CORE CONCEPTS

behavior therapy
stimuli

OBJECTIVES

After reading this chapter, the student will be able to:

1. Discuss the principles of classical and operant conditioning as foundations for behavior therapy.
2. Identify various techniques used in the modification of client behavior.

3. Implement the principles of behavior therapy using the steps of the nursing process.

behavior is considered to be maladaptive when it is age inappropriate, when it interferes with adaptive functioning, or when others misunderstand it in terms of cultural inappropriateness. The behavioral approach to therapy is that people have become what they are through learning processes or, more correctly, through the interaction of the environment with their genetic endowment. The basic assumption is that problematic behaviors occur when there has been inadequate learning and therefore can be corrected through the provision of appropriate learning experiences. The principles of behavior therapy as we know it today are based on the early studies of **classical conditioning** by Pavlov (1927) and **operant conditioning** by Skinner (1938). Although in this text the concepts are presented separately for reasons of clarification, behavioral change procedures are often combined with cognitive procedures, and many behavior therapies are referred to as *cognitive–behavioral* therapies.

CLASSICAL CONDITIONING

Classical conditioning is a process of learning that was introduced by the Russian physiologist Pavlov. In his experiments with dogs, during which he hoped to learn more about the digestive process, he inadvertently discovered that organisms can learn to respond in specific ways if they are conditioned to do so.

In his trials he found that, as expected, the dogs salivated when they began to eat the food that was offered to them. This was a reflexive response that Pavlov called an **unconditioned response**. However, he also noticed that with time, the dogs began to salivate when the food came into their range of view, before it was even presented to them for consumption. Concluding that this response was not reflexive but had been learned, Pavlov called it a **conditioned response**. He carried the experiments even further by introducing an unrelated stimulus, one that had had no previous connection to the animal's food. He simultaneously presented the food with the sound of a bell. The animal responded with the expected reflexive salivation to the food. After a number of trials with the combined stimuli (food and bell), Pavlov found that the reflexive salivation began to occur when the dog was presented with the sound of the bell in the absence of food.

Core Concept

Stimulus
An environmental event that interacts with and influences an individual's behavior.

This was an important discovery in terms of how learning can occur. Pavlov found that unconditioned responses (salivation) occur in response to unconditioned stimuli (eating food). He also found that, over time, an unrelated stimulus (sound of the bell) introduced with the **unconditioned stimulus** could elicit the same response alone—that is, the conditioned response. The unrelated stimulus is called the **conditioned stimulus**. A graphic of Pavlov's classical conditioning model is presented in Figure 19–1. An example of the application of Pavlov's classical conditioning model to humans is shown in Figure 19–2. The process by which the fear response is elicited from similar stimuli (all individuals in white uniforms) is called **stimulus generalization**.

Sequence of Conditioning Operations:

1. UCS ---▶ UCR
   Unconditioned stimulus   Unconditioned response
   (eating food)   (salivation)

2. UCS ---▶ CR
   Unconditioned stimulus   Conditioned response
   (sight of food)   (salivation)

3. CS --▶ NR
   Conditioned stimulus   No response or
   (bell)   response unrelated to salivation

4. UCS + CS ------------------------------------▶ CR
   Unconditioned + Conditioned stimuli   Conditioned response
   (food)   (bell)   (salivation)

5. CS --▶ CR
   Conditioned stimulus   Conditioned response
   (bell)   (salivation)

FIGURE 19–1   Pavlov's model of classical conditioning.

OPERANT CONDITIONING

The focus of operant conditioning differs from that of classical conditioning. With classical conditioning, the focus is on behavioral responses that are elicited by specific objects or events. With operant conditioning, additional attention is given to the consequences of the behavioral response.

Operant conditioning was introduced by Skinner (1953), an American psychologist whose work was largely

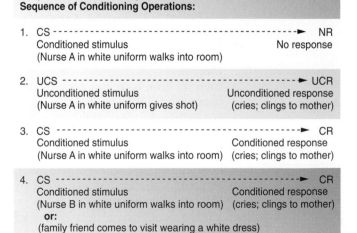

Classical Conditioning and Stimulus Generalization

Subject: 6-month-old baby
Sequence of Conditioning Operations:

1. CS --▶ NR
   Conditioned stimulus   No response
   (Nurse A in white uniform walks into room)

2. UCS ---▶ UCR
   Unconditioned stimulus   Unconditioned response
   (Nurse A in white uniform gives shot)   (cries; clings to mother)

3. CS --▶ CR
   Conditioned stimulus   Conditioned response
   (Nurse A in white uniform walks into room)   (cries; clings to mother)

4. CS --▶ CR
   Conditioned stimulus   Conditioned response
   (Nurse B in white uniform walks into room)   (cries; clings to mother)
   or:
   (family friend comes to visit wearing a white dress)

FIGURE 19–2   Example: classical conditioning and stimulus generalization.

influenced by Thorndike's (1911) law of effect—that is, that the connection between a stimulus and a response is strengthened or weakened by the consequences of the response. A number of terms need to be defined in order to understand the concept of operant conditioning.

As defined previously, stimuli are environmental events that interact with and influence an individual's behavior. Stimuli may precede or follow a behavior. A stimulus that follows a behavior (or response) is called a reinforcing stimulus or *reinforcer*. The function is called *reinforcement*. When the reinforcing stimulus increases the probability that the behavior will recur, it is called a *positive reinforcer*, and the function is called **positive reinforcement**. **Negative reinforcement**, on the other hand, is increasing the probability that a behavior will recur by removal of an undesirable reinforcing stimulus. A stimulus that follows a behavioral response and decreases the probability that the behavior will recur is called an **aversive stimulus** or *punisher*. Examples of these reinforcing stimuli are presented in Table 19–1.

Stimuli that precede a behavioral response and predict that a particular reinforcement will occur are called **discriminative stimuli**. Discriminative stimuli are under the control of the individual. The individual is said to be able to *discriminate* between stimuli and to *choose* according to the type of reinforcement he or she has come to associate with a specific stimulus. The following is an example of the concept of discrimination:

EXAMPLE:

Mrs. M. was admitted to the hospital from a nursing home 2 weeks ago. She has no family, and no one visits her. She is very lonely. Nurse A and Nurse B have taken care of Mrs. M. on a regular basis during her hospital stay. When she is feeling particularly lonely, Mrs. M. calls Nurse A to her room, for she has learned that Nurse A will stay and talk to her for a while, but Nurse B only takes care of her physical needs and leaves. She no longer seeks out Nurse B for emotional support and comfort.

After several attempts, Mrs. M. is able to discriminate between stimuli. She can predict with assurance that calling Nurse A (and not Nurse B) will result in the reinforcement she desires.

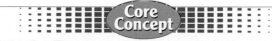

Core Concept

Behavior Therapy
A form of psychotherapy, the goal of which is to modify maladaptive behavior patterns by reinforcing more adaptive behaviors.

TECHNIQUES FOR MODIFYING CLIENT BEHAVIOR

Shaping

In **shaping** the behavior of another, reinforcements are given for increasingly closer approximations to the desired response. For example, in eliciting speech from an autistic child, the teacher may first reward the child for (a) watching the teacher's lips, then (b) for making any sound in imitation of the teacher, then (c) for forming sounds similar to the word uttered by the teacher. Shaping has been shown to be an effective way of modifying behavior for tasks that a child has not mastered on command or are not in the child's repertoire (Souders et al., 2002).

Modeling

Modeling refers to the learning of new behaviors by imitating the behavior in others. Role models are individuals who have qualities or skills that a person admires and wishes to imitate (Howard, 2000). Modeling occurs in various ways. Children imitate the behavior patterns of their parents, teachers, friends, and others. Adults and children alike model many of their behaviors after individuals observed on television and in movies. Unfortunately, modeling can result in maladaptive behaviors, as well as adaptive ones.

In the practice setting clients may imitate the behaviors of practitioners who are charged with their care. This can occur naturally in the therapeutic community environment. It can also occur in a therapy session in which the client watches a model demonstrate appropriate behaviors in a role-play of the client's problem. The client is then instructed to imitate the model's behaviors in a similar role-play and is positively reinforced for appropriate imitation.

TABLE 19–1	Examples of Reinforcing Stimuli		
TYPE	**STIMULUS**	**BEHAVIORAL RESPONSE**	**REINFORCING STIMULUS**
Positive	Messy room	Child cleans her messy room	Child gets allowance for cleaning room
Negative	Messy room	Child cleans her messy room	Child does not receive scolding from the mother.
Aversive	Messy room	Child does not clean her messy room	Child receives scolding from the mother.

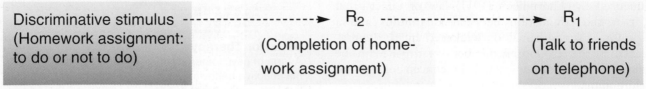

FIGURE 19–3   Example: Premack principle.

Premack Principle

This technique, named for its originator, states that a frequently occurring response (R_1) can serve as a positive reinforcement for a response (R_2) that occurs less frequently (Premack, 1959). This is accomplished by allowing R_1 to occur only after R_2 has been performed. For example, 13-year-old Jennie has been neglecting her homework for the past few weeks. She spends a great deal of time on the telephone talking to her friends. Applying the **Premack principle**, being allowed to talk on the telephone to her friends could serve as a positive reinforcement for completing her homework. A schematic of the Premack principle for this situation is presented in Figure 19–3.

Extinction

Extinction is the gradual decrease in frequency or disappearance of a response when the positive reinforcement is withheld. A classic example of this technique is its use with children who have temper tantrums. The tantrum behaviors continue as long as the parent gives attention to them but decrease and often disappear when the parent simply leaves the child alone in the room.

Contingency Contracting

In **contingency contracting**, a contract is drawn up among all parties involved. The behavior change that is desired is stated explicitly in writing. The contract specifies the behavior change desired and the reinforcers to be given for performing the desired behaviors. The negative consequences or punishers that will be rendered for not fulfilling the terms of the contract are also delineated. The contract is specific about how reinforcers and punishment will be presented; however, flexibility is important so that renegotiations can occur if necessary.

Token Economy

Token economy is a type of contingency contracting (although there may or may not be a written and signed contract involved) in which the reinforcers for desired behaviors are presented in the form of *tokens*. Essential to this type of technique is the prior determination of items and situations of significance to the client that can be employed as reinforcements. With this therapy, tokens are awarded when desired behaviors are performed and may be exchanged for designated privileges. For example, a client may be able to "buy" a snack or cigarettes for two tokens, a trip to the coffee shop or library for five tokens, or even a trip outside the hospital (if that is a realistic possibility) for another designated number of tokens. The tokens themselves provide immediate positive feedback, and clients should be allowed to make the decision of whether to spend the token as soon as it is presented or to accumulate tokens that may be exchanged later for a more desirable reward.

Time Out

Time out is an aversive stimulus or punishment during which the client is removed from the environment where the unacceptable behavior is being exhibited. The client is usually isolated so that reinforcement from the attention of others is absent.

Reciprocal Inhibition

Also called counter conditioning, **reciprocal inhibition** decreases or eliminates a behavior by introducing a more adaptive behavior, but one that is incompatible with the unacceptable behavior (Wolpe, 1958). An example is the introduction of relaxation exercises to an individual who is phobic. Relaxation is practiced in the presence of anxiety so that in time the individual is able to manage the anxiety in the presence of the phobic stimulus by engaging in relaxation exercises. Relaxation and anxiety are incompatible behaviors.

Overt Sensitization

Overt sensitization is a type of aversion therapy that produces unpleasant consequences for undesirable behavior.

For example, disulfiram (Antabuse) is a drug that is given to individuals who wish to stop drinking alcohol. If an individual consumes alcohol while on Antabuse therapy, symptoms of severe nausea and vomiting, dyspnea, palpitations, and headache will occur. Instead of the euphoric feeling normally experienced from the alcohol (the positive reinforcement for drinking), the individual receives a severe punishment that is intended to extinguish the unacceptable behavior (drinking alcohol).

Covert Sensitization

Covert sensitization relies on the individual's imagination to produce unpleasant symptoms rather than on medication. The technique is under the client's control and can be used whenever and wherever it is required. The individual learns, through mental imagery, to visualize nauseating scenes and even to induce a mild feeling of nausea. This mental image is visualized when the individual is about to succumb to an attractive but undesirable behavior. It is most effective when paired with relaxation exercises that are performed instead of the undesirable behavior. The primary advantage of covert sensitization is that the individual does not have to perform the undesired behaviors but simply imagines them.

Systematic Desensitization

Systematic desensitization is a technique for assisting individuals to overcome their fear of a phobic stimulus. It is "systematic" in that there is a hierarchy of anxiety-producing events through which the individual progresses during therapy. An example of a hierarchy of events associated with a fear of elevators may be as follows:

1. Discuss riding an elevator with the therapist.
2. Look at a picture of an elevator.
3. Walk into the lobby of a building and see the elevators.
4. Push the button for the elevator.
5. Walk into an elevator with a trusted person; disembark before the doors close.
6. Walk into an elevator with a trusted person; allow doors to close; then open the doors and walk out.
7. Ride one floor with a trusted person, and then walk back down the stairs.
8. Ride one floor with a trusted person and ride the elevator back down.
9. Ride the elevator alone.

As each of these steps is attempted, it is paired with relaxation exercises as an antagonistic behavior to anxiety. Generally, the desensitization procedures occur in the therapy setting by instructing the client to engage in relaxation exercises. When relaxation has been achieved, the client uses mental imagery to visualize the step in the hierarchy being described by the therapist. If the client becomes anxious, the therapist suggests relaxation exercises again, and presents a scene that is lower in the hierarchy. Therapy continues until the individual is able to progress through the entire hierarchy with manageable anxiety. The effects of relaxation in the presence of imagined anxiety-producing stimuli transfer to the real situation, once the client has achieved relaxation capable of suppressing or inhibiting anxiety responses (Ford-Martin, 2001). However, some clients are not successful in extinguishing phobic reactions through imagery. For these clients, *real-life desensitization* may be required. In these instances, the therapist may arrange for the client to be exposed to the hierarchy of steps in the desensitization process, but in real-life situations. Relaxation exercises may or may not be a part of real-life desensitization.

Flooding

This technique, sometimes called *implosive therapy*, is also used to desensitize individuals to phobic stimuli. It differs from systematic desensitization in that, instead of working up a hierarchy of anxiety-producing stimuli, the individual is "flooded" with a continuous presentation (through mental imagery) of the phobic stimulus until it no longer elicits anxiety. **Flooding** is believed to produce results faster than systematic desensitization; however, some therapists report more lasting behavioral changes with systematic desensitization. Some questions have also been raised in terms of the psychological discomfort that this therapy produces for the client. Flooding is contraindicated with clients for whom intense anxiety would be hazardous (e.g., individuals with heart disease or fragile psychological adaptation) (Sadock & Sadock, 2003).

ROLE OF THE NURSE IN BEHAVIOR THERAPY

The nursing process is the vehicle for delivery of nursing care with the client requiring assistance with behavior modification. The steps of the nursing process are illustrated in the following example case study.

CASE STUDY

(This example focuses on inpatient care, but these interventions can be modified and are applicable to various health care settings, including partial hospitalization, community outpatient clinic, home health, and private practice.)

ASSESSMENT

Sammy, age 8, has been admitted to the child psychiatric unit of a university medical center following evaluation by a child psychiatrist. His parents, Tom and Nancy, are at an impasse, and their marriage is suffering because of constant conflict over their son's behavior at home and at school. Tom complains bitterly that Nancy is overly permissive with their son. Tom reports that Sammy argues and has temper tantrums and insists on continuing games, books, and TV, whenever Nancy puts him to bed, so that an 8:30 P.M. bedtime regularly is delayed until 10:30 or later every night. Also, Nancy often cooks four or five different meals for her son's dinner if Sammy stubbornly insists that he will not eat what has been prepared. At school, several teachers have complained that the child is stubborn and argumentative, is often disruptive in the classroom, and refuses to follow established rules.

When asked by the psychiatric nurse about other maladaptive behaviors, such as destruction of property, stealing, lying, or setting fires, the parents denied that these had been a problem. During the interview, Sammy sat quietly without interrupting. He answered questions that were directed to him with brief responses and made light of the problems described by his parents and reported by his teachers.

During his first 3 days on the unit, the following assessments were made:

1. Sammy loses his temper when he cannot have his way. He screams, stomps his feet, and sometimes kicks the furniture.
2. Sammy refuses to follow directions given by staff. He merely responds, "No, I won't."
3. Sammy likes to engage in behaviors that annoy the staff and other children: belching loudly, scraping his fingernails across the blackboard, making loud noises when the other children are trying to watch television, opening his mouth when it is full of food.
4. Sammy blames others when he makes a mistake. He spilled his milk at lunchtime while racing to get to a specific seat he knew Tony wanted. He blamed the accident on Tony saying, "He made me do it! He tripped me!"

Upon completion of the initial assessments, the psychiatrist diagnosed Sammy with oppositional defiant disorder.

DIAGNOSIS/OUTCOME IDENTIFICATION

Nursing diagnoses and outcome criteria for Sammy include:

NURSING DIAGNOSES	OUTCOME CRITERIA
Noncompliance with therapy	Sammy participates in and cooperates during therapeutic activities.
Defensive coping	Sammy accepts responsibility for own behaviors and interacts with others without becoming defensive.
Impaired social interaction	Sammy interacts with staff and peers using age-appropriate, acceptable behaviors.

PLANNING/IMPLEMENTATION

A contract for Sammy's care was drawn up by the admitting nurse and others on the treatment team. Sammy's contract was based on a system of token economies. He discussed with the nurse the kinds of privileges he would like to earn. They included:

- Getting to wear his own clothes (5 tokens)
- Having a can of pop for a snack (2 tokens)
- Getting to watch 30 minutes of TV (5 tokens)
- Getting to stay up later on Friday nights with the other clients (7 tokens)
- Getting to play the video games (3 tokens)
- Getting to walk with the nurse to the gift shop to spend some of his money (8 tokens)
- Getting to talk to his parents/grandparents on the phone (5 tokens)
- Getting to go on the outside therapeutic recreation activities such as movies, the zoo, and picnics (10 tokens)

Tokens were awarded for appropriate behaviors:

- Gets out of bed when the nurse calls him (1 token)
- Gets dressed for breakfast (1 token)
- Presents himself for *all* meals in an appropriate manner, that is, no screaming, no belching, no opening his mouth when it is full of food, no throwing of food, staying in his chair during the meal, putting his tray away in the appropriate place when he is finished (2 tokens × 3 meals = 6 tokens)
- Completes hygiene activities (1 token)
- Accepts blame for own mistakes (1 token)
- Does not fight; uses no obscene language; does not "sass" staff (1 token)
- Remains quiet while others are watching TV (1 token)
- Participates and is not disruptive in unit meetings and group therapy sessions (2 tokens)
- Displays no temper tantrums (1 token)
- Follows unit rules (1 token)
- Goes to bed at designated hour without opposition (1 token)

Tokens are awarded at bedtime for absence of inappropriate behaviors during the day. For example, if Sammy has no temper tantrums during the day, he is awarded one token. Likewise, if Sammy has a temper tantrum (or exhibits other inappropriate behavior), he must pay back the token amount designated for that behavior. No other attention is given to inappropriate behaviors other than withholding and payback of tokens.

EXCEPTION: If Sammy is receiving reinforcement from peers for inappropriate behaviors, staff has the option of imposing time out or isolation until the behavior is extinguished.

The contract may be renegotiated at any time between Sammy and staff. Additional privileges or responsibilities may be added as they develop and are deemed appropriate.

All staff members are consistent with the terms of the contract and do not allow Sammy to manipulate. There are no exceptions without renegotiation of the contract.

NOTE: Parents meet regularly with the social worker from the treatment team. Effective parenting techniques are discussed, as are other problems identified within the marriage relationship. Parenting instruction coordinates with the pattern of behavior modification Sammy is receiving on the psychiatric unit. The importance of follow-through is emphasized, along with strong encouragement that the parents maintain a united front in disciplining Sammy. Oppositional behaviors are encouraged by divided management.

EVALUATION

Reassessment is conducted to determine if the nursing actions have been successful in achieving the objectives of Sammy's care. Evaluation can be facilitated by gathering information using the following questions:

- Does Sammy participate in and cooperate during therapeutic activities?
- Does he follow the rules of the unit (including mealtimes, hygiene, and bedtime) without opposition?
- Does Sammy accept responsibility for his own mistakes?
- Is he able to complete a task without becoming defensive?
- Does he refrain from interrupting when others are talking or making noise in situations where quiet is in order?
- Does he attempt to manipulate the staff?
- Is he able to express anger appropriately without tantrum behaviors?
- Does he demonstrate acceptable behavior in interactions with peers?

SUMMARY

The basic assumption of behavior therapy is that problematic behaviors occur when there has been inadequate learning and, therefore, can be corrected through the provision of appropriate learning experiences. The antecedents of today's principles of behavior therapy are largely the products of laboratory efforts by Pavlov and Skinner.

Pavlov introduced a process that came to be known as classical conditioning. He demonstrated in his trials with laboratory animals that a neutral stimulus could acquire the ability to elicit a conditioned response through pairing with an unconditioned stimulus. Previous responses had been reflexive in nature. Pavlov considered the conditioned response to be a new, learned response.

Skinner, in his model of operant conditioning, gave additional attention to the consequences of the response as an approach to learning new behaviors. His work was largely influenced by Thorndike's law of effect; that is, that the connection between a stimulus and a response is strengthened or weakened by the consequences of the response.

Various techniques for modifying client behavior have been applied. Those most widely used include shaping, modeling, the Premack principle, extinction, contingency contracting, token economy, time out, reciprocal inhibition, overt and covert sensitization, systematic desensitization, and flooding.

Nurses can implement behavior therapy techniques to help clients modify maladaptive behavior patterns. The nursing process is an systematic method of directing care for clients who require this type of assistance.

REVIEW QUESTIONS

SELF-EXAMINATION/LEARNING EXERCISE

Select the correct answer for each of the following questions:

1. A positive reinforcer:
   a. Increases the probability that a behavior will recur.
   b. Decreases the probability that a behavior will recur.
   c. Has nothing to do with modifying behavior.
   d. Always results in positive behavior.

2. A negative reinforcer:
   a. Increases the probability that a behavior will recur.
   b. Decreases the probability that a behavior will recur.
   c. Has nothing to do with modifying behavior.
   d. Always results in unacceptable behavior.

3. An aversive stimulus or punisher:
   a. Increases the probability that a behavior will recur.
   b. Decreases the probability that a behavior will recur.
   c. Has nothing to do with modifying behavior.
   d. Always results in unacceptable behavior.

Situation: B.J. has been out with his friends. He is late getting home. He knows his wife will be angry and will yell at him for being late. He stops at the florist's and buys a dozen red roses for her. Questions 4, 5, and 6 are related to this situation.

4. Which of the following behaviors represents positive reinforcement on the part of the wife?
   a. She meets him at the door, accepts the roses, and says nothing further about his being late.
   b. She meets him at the door, yelling that he is late, and makes him spend the night on the couch.
   c. She meets him at the door, expresses delight with the roses, and kisses him on the cheek.
   d. She meets him at the door and says, "How could you? You know I'm allergic to roses!"

5. Which of the following behaviors represents negative reinforcement on the part of the wife?
   a. She meets him at the door, accepts the roses, and says nothing further about his being late.
   b. She meets him at the door, yelling that he is late, and makes him spend the night on the couch.
   c. She meets him at the door, expresses delight with the roses, and kisses him on the cheek.
   d. She meets him at the door and says, "How could you? You know I'm allergic to roses!"

6. Which of the following behaviors represents an aversive stimulus on the part of the wife?
   a. She meets him at the door, accepts the roses, and says nothing further about his being late.
   b. She meets him at the door, yelling that he is late, and makes him spend the night on the couch.
   c. She meets him at the door, expresses delight with the roses, and kisses him on the cheek.
   d. She meets him at the door and says, "How could you? You know I'm allergic to roses!"

7. Fourteen-year-old Sally has been spending many hours after school watching TV. She has virtually stopped practicing her piano lessons. Her parents have told her that she may watch TV only after she has practiced the piano for 1 hour. This is an example of which behavior modification technique?
   a. Shaping
   b. Extinction
   c. Contingency contracting
   d. The Premack principle

8. Nancy has a fear of dogs. In helping her overcome this fear, the therapist is using systematic desensitization. List the following steps in the order in which the therapist would proceed. Having Nancy:
   a. Look at a real dog.
   b. Look at a stuffed toy dog.
   c. Pet a real dog.
   d. Pet the stuffed toy dog.
   e. Walk past a real dog.
   f. Look at a picture of a dog.

REFERENCES

Ford-Martin, P.A. (2001). *Behavioral therapy.* Retrieved January 22, 2005 from the World Wide Web at http://www.findarticles.com/cf_dls/g2603/0001/2603000194/p1/article.jhtml

Howard, D. (2000). *The effect of role modeling.* Retrieved January 20, 2005 from the World Wide Web at http://www.dianehoward.com/Effect_Role_Modeling.htm

Sadock, B.J., & Sadock, V.A. (2003). *Synopsis of psychiatry: Behavioral sciences/clinical psychiatry* (9th ed.). Philadelphia: Lippincott Williams & Wilkins.

Souders, M.C., DePaul, D., Freeman, K.G., & Levy, S.E. (2002). Caring for children and adolescents with autism who require challenging procedures. *Pediatric Nursing, 28*(6), 555–564.

CLASSICAL REFERENCES

Pavlov, I.P. (1927). *Conditioned reflexes.* London: Oxford University Press.

Premack, D. (1959). Toward empirical behavior laws: I. Positive reinforcement. *Psychological Review, 66,* 219–233.

Skinner, B.F. (1938) *The behavior of organisms.* New York: Appleton-Century-Crofts.

Skinner, B.F. (1953). *Science and human behavior.* New York: Macmillan.

Thorndike, E.L. (1911). *Animal intelligence.* New York: Macmillan.

Wolpe, J. (1958). *Psychotherapy by reciprocal inhibition.* Stanford, CA: Stanford University Press.

COGNITIVE THERAPY

KEY TERMS

arbitrary inference
automatic thoughts
catastrophic thinking
decatastrophizing
dichotomous thinking
distraction
magnification

minimization
overgeneralization
personalization
schemas
selective abstraction
Socratic questioning

CORE CONCEPTS

cognitive
cognitive therapy

OBJECTIVES

After reading this chapter, the student will be able to:

1. Discuss historical perspectives associated with cognitive therapy.
2. Identify various indications for cognitive therapy.
3. Describe goals, principles, and basic concepts of cognitive therapy.
4. Discuss a variety of cognitive therapy techniques.
5. Apply techniques of cognitive therapy within the context of the nursing process.

 right, Beck, and Thase (2003) state, "The writing of Epictetus in the *Enchiridion*, '*Men are disturbed not by things, but by the views which they take of them,*' captures the essence of the perspective that our ideas or thoughts are a controlling factor in our emotional lives." This concept provides a foundation on which the cognitive model is established. In cognitive therapy, the therapist's objective is to use a variety of methods to create change in the client's thinking and belief system in an effort to bring about lasting emotional and behavioral change (Beck, 1995).

This chapter examines the historical development of the cognitive model, defines the goals of therapy, and describes various techniques of the cognitive approach. A discussion of the role of the nurse in the implementation of cognitive behavioral techniques with clients is presented.

NOTE: Although in this text the concepts are presented separately for reasons of clarification, cognitive therapy procedures are often combined with behavioral modification techniques and may be referred to as *cognitive-behavioral* therapies.

panic disorder, GAD, social phobias, OCD, PTSD
EDO, SA PD Schizophrenia, Couples prob Bipolar DO
CHAPTER 20 • COGNITIVE THERAPY 275
hypochondriasis + somatoform - depression

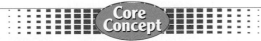

Core Concept

Cognitive
Relating to the mental processes of thinking and reasoning.

HISTORICAL BACKGROUND

Cognitive therapy has its roots in the early 1960s research on depression conducted by Aaron Beck (1963, 1964). Beck had been trained in the Freudian psychoanalytic view of depression as "anger turned inward." In his clinical research, he began to observe a common theme of negative cognitive processing in the thoughts and dreams of his depressed clients (Beck & Weishaar, 2005).

A number of theorists have both taken from and expanded upon Beck's original concept. The common theme is the rejection of the passive listening of the psychoanalytic method in favor of active, direct dialogues with clients (Beck & Weishaar, 2005). The work of contemporary behavioral therapists has also influenced the evolution of cognitive therapy. Behavioral techniques such as expectancy of reinforcement and modeling are used within the cognitive domain.

Lazarus and Folkman (1984), upon whose premise of *personal appraisal* and *coping* the conceptual format of this book is founded, have also contributed a great deal to the cognitive approach to therapy. The model for cognitive therapy is based on cognition, and more specifically, the personal cognitive appraisal by an individual of an event, and the emotions or behaviors that result from that appraisal. Personality—which undoubtedly influences our cognitive appraisal of an event—is viewed as having been shaped by the interaction between innate predisposition and environment (Beck, Freeman, & Davis, 2003). Whereas some therapies may be directed toward improvement in coping strategies or adaptiveness of behavioral response, cognitive therapy is aimed at modifying distorted cognitions about a situation.

INDICATIONS FOR COGNITIVE THERAPY

Cognitive therapy was originally developed for use in the treatment of depression. Today it is used for a broad range of emotional disorders. The proponents of cogni-

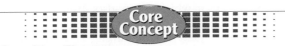

Core Concept

Cognitive Therapy
Cognitive therapy is a type of psychotherapy based on the concept of pathological mental processing. The focus of treatment is on the modification of distorted cognitions and maladaptive behaviors.

tive therapy suggest that the emphasis of therapy must be varied and individualized for clients according to their specific diagnosis, symptoms, and level of functioning. In addition to depression, cognitive therapy may be used with the following clinical conditions: panic disorder, generalized anxiety disorder, social phobias, obsessive–compulsive disorder, posttraumatic stress disorder, eating disorders, substance abuse, personality disorders, schizophrenia, couples' problems, bipolar disorder, hypochondriasis, and somatoform disorder (Beck, 1995; Sadock & Sadock, 2003; Wright, Beck, & Thase, 2003).

GOALS AND PRINCIPLES OF COGNITIVE THERAPY

Beck and associates (1987) define the goals of cognitive therapy in the following way:

The client will:

1. Monitor his or her negative, automatic thoughts.
2. Recognize the connections between cognition, affect, and behavior.
3. Examine the evidence for and against distorted automatic thoughts.
4. Substitute more realistic interpretations for these biased cognitions.
5. Learn to identify and alter the dysfunctional beliefs that predispose him or her to distort experiences.

Cognitive therapy is highly structured and short term, lasting from 12 to 16 weeks (Beck & Weishaar, 2005). Sadock and Sadock (2003) suggest that if a client does not improve within 25 weeks of therapy, a reevaluation of the diagnosis should be made. Although therapy must be tailored to the individual, the following principles underlie cognitive therapy for all clients (Beck, 1995).

Principle 1. Cognitive therapy is based on an ever-evolving formulation of the client and his or her problems in cognitive terms. The therapist identifies the event that precipitated the distorted cognition. Current thinking patterns that serve to maintain the problematic behaviors are reviewed. The therapist then hypothesizes about certain developmental events and enduring patterns of cognitive appraisal that may have predisposed the client to specific emotional and behavioral responses.

Principle 2. Cognitive therapy requires a sound therapeutic alliance. A trusting relationship between therapist and client must exist for cognitive therapy to succeed. The therapist must convey warmth, empathy, caring, and genuine positive regard. Development of a working relationship between therapist and client is an individual process, and clients with various disorders will require varying degrees of effort to achieve this therapeutic alliance.

Principle 3. Cognitive therapy emphasizes collaboration and active participation. Teamwork between therapist and client is emphasized. They decide together what to work on during each session, how often they should meet, and what homework assignments should be completed between sessions.

Principle 4. Cognitive therapy is goal oriented and problem focused. At the beginning of therapy, the client is encouraged to identify what he or she perceives to be the problem or problems. With guidance from the therapist, goals are established as outcomes of therapy. Assistance in problem solving is provided as required as the client comes to recognize and correct distortions in thinking.

Principle 5. Cognitive therapy initially emphasizes the present. Resolution of distressing situations that are based in the present usually lead to symptom reduction. It is therefore of more benefit to begin with current problems and delay shifting attention to the past until (1) the client expresses desire to do so, (2) the work on current problems produces little or no change; or (3) the therapist decides it is important to determine how dysfunctional ideas affecting the client's current thinking originated.

Principle 6. Cognitive therapy is educative, aims to teach the client to be his or her own therapist, and emphasizes relapse prevention. From the beginning of therapy, the client is taught about the nature and course of his or her disorder, about the cognitive model (i.e., how thoughts influence emotions and behavior), and about the process of cognitive therapy. The client is taught how to set goals, plan behavioral change, and intervene on his or her own behalf.

Principle 7. Cognitive therapy aims to be time limited. Clients often are seen weekly for a couple of months, followed by a number of biweekly sessions, then possibly a few monthly sessions. Some clients will want periodic "booster" sessions every few months.

Principle 8. Cognitive therapy sessions are structured. Each session has a set structure that includes (1) reviewing the client's week, (2) collaboratively setting the agenda for this session, (3) reviewing the previous week's session, (4) reviewing the previous week's homework, (5) discussing this week's agenda items, (6) establishing homework for next week, and (7) summarizing this week's session. This format focuses attention on what is important and maximizes the use of therapy time.

Principle 9. Cognitive therapy teaches clients to identify, evaluate, and respond to their dysfunctional thoughts and beliefs. Through gentle questioning and review of data, the therapist helps the client identify his or her dysfunctional thinking, evaluate the validity of the thoughts, and devise a plan of action. This is done by helping the client to examine evidence that supports or contradicts the accuracy of the thought, rather than directly challenging or confronting the belief.

Principle 10. Cognitive therapy uses a variety of techniques to change thinking, mood, and behavior. Techniques from various therapies may be used within the cognitive framework. Emphasis in treatment is guided by the client's particular disorder and directed toward modification of the client's dysfunctional cognitions that are contributing to the maladaptive behavior associated with their disorder. Examples of disorders and the dysfunctional thinking for which cognitive therapy may be of benefit are discussed later in this chapter.

BASIC CONCEPTS

Wright, Beck, and Thase (2003) state, "The general thrust of cognitive therapy is that emotional responses are largely dependent on cognitive appraisals of the significance of environmental cues." Basic concepts include **automatic thoughts** and **schemas** or core beliefs.

Automatic Thoughts

Automatic thoughts are those that occur rapidly in response to a situation and without rational analysis. These thoughts are often negative and based on erroneous logic. Beck and associates (1987) called these thoughts *cognitive errors*. Following are some examples of common cognitive errors.

Arbitrary Inference. In a type of thinking error known as **arbitrary inference**, the individual automatically comes to a conclusion about an incident without the facts to support it, or even sometimes despite contradictory evidence to support it.

> **EXAMPLE:**
>
> Two months ago, Mrs. B. sent a wedding gift to the daughter of an old friend. She has not yet received acknowledgment of the gift. Mrs. B. thinks, "They obviously think I have poor taste."

Overgeneralization (Absolutistic Thinking). Sweeping conclusions are **overgeneralizations** made based on one incident—a type of "all or nothing" kind of thinking.

> **EXAMPLE:**
>
> Frank submitted an article to a nursing journal and it was rejected. Frank thinks, "No journal will ever be interested in anything I write."

Dichotomous Thinking. An individual who is using **dichotomous thinking** views situations in terms of all-or-nothing, black-or-white, or good-or-bad.

> **EXAMPLE:**
>
> Frank submits an article to a nursing journal and the editor returns it and asks Frank to rewrite parts of it. Frank thinks, "I'm a bad writer," instead of recognizing that revision is a common part of the publication process.

mental filter

Selective Abstraction. A **selective abstraction** (sometimes referred to as *mental filter*) is a conclusion that is based on only a selected portion of the evidence. The selected portion is usually the negative evidence or what the individual views as a failure, rather than any successes that have occurred.

EXAMPLE:

Jackie just graduated from high school with a 3.98/4.00 grade point average. She won a scholarship to the large state university near her home. She was active in sports and activities in high school and well liked by all her peers. However, she is very depressed and dwells on the fact that she did not earn a scholarship to a prestigious Ivy League college to which she had applied.

Magnification. Exaggerating the negative significance of an event is known as **magnification**.

EXAMPLE:

Nancy hears that her colleague at work is having a cocktail party over the weekend and she is not invited. Nancy thinks, "She doesn't like me."

Minimization. Undervaluing the positive significance of an event is called **minimization**.

EXAMPLE:

Mrs. M. is feeling lonely. She calls her granddaughter Amy, who lives in a nearby town, and invites her to visit. Amy apologizes that she must go out of town on business and would not be able to visit at that time. While Amy is out of town, she calls Mrs. M. twice, but Mrs. M. still feels unloved by her granddaughter.

Catastrophic Thinking. Always thinking that the worst will occur without considering the possibility of more likely positive outcomes is considered **catastrophic thinking**.

EXAMPLE:

On Janet's first day in her secretarial job, her boss asked her to write a letter to another firm and put it on his desk

for his signature. She did so and left for lunch. When she returned, the letter was on her desk with a typographical error circled in red and a note from her boss to redo the letter. Janet thinks, "This is it! I will surely be fired now!"

Personalization. With **personalization**, the person takes complete responsibility for situations without considering that other circumstances may have contributed to the outcome.

EXAMPLE:

Jack, who sells vacuum cleaners door-to-door, has just given a two-hour demonstration to Mrs. W. At the end of the demonstration, Mrs. W tells Jack that she appreciates his demonstration, but she won't be purchasing a vacuum cleaner from him. Jack thinks, "I'm a lousy salesman" (when in fact, Mrs. W.'s husband lost his job last week and they have no extra money to buy a new vacuum cleaner at this time).

helplessness — unlovability

Schemas (Core Beliefs) — *deeper cognitive structures that serve to screen information from the environment*

Beck and Weishaar (2005) define cognitive schemas as:

> Structures that contain the individual's fundamental beliefs and assumptions. Schemas develop early in life from personal experience and identification with significant others. These concepts are reinforced by further learning experiences and, in turn, influence the formation of beliefs, values, and attitudes. (p. 245)

These schemas, or core beliefs, may be adaptive or maladaptive. They may be general or specific, and they may be latent, becoming evident only when triggered by a specific stressful stimulus. Schemas differ from automatic thoughts in that they are deeper cognitive structures that serve to screen information from the environment. For this reason they are often more difficult to modify than automatic thoughts. However, the same techniques are used at the schema level as at the level of automatic thoughts. Schemas can be positive or negative, and generally fall into two broad categories: those associated with *helplessness* and those associated with *unlovability* (Beck, 1995). Some examples of types of schemas are presented in Table 20–1.

TABLE 20–1	Examples of Schemas (or Core Beliefs)	
SCHEMA CATEGORY	**MALADAPTIVE/NEGATIVE**	**ADAPTIVE/POSITIVE**
Helplessness	No matter what I do, I will fail.	If I try and work very hard, I will succeed.
	I must be perfect. If I make one mistake, I will lose everything.	I am not afraid of a challenge. If I make a mistake, I will try again.
Unlovability	I'm stupid. No one would love me.	I'm a lovable person.
	I'm nobody without a man.	People respect me for myself.

TECHNIQUES OF COGNITIVE THERAPY

The three major components of cognitive therapy are didactic or educational aspects, cognitive techniques, and behavioral interventions (Sadock & Sadock, 2003; Wright, Beck, & Thase, 2003).

Didactic (Educational) Aspects

One of the basic principles of cognitive therapy is to prepare the client to eventually become his or her own cognitive therapist. The therapist provides information to the client about what cognitive therapy is, how it works, and the structure of the cognitive process. Explanation about expectations of both client and therapist is provided. Reading assignments are given in order to reinforce learning. Some therapists use audiotape or videotape sessions to teach clients about cognitive therapy. A full explanation about the relationship between depression (or anxiety, or whatever maladaptive response the client is experiencing) and distorted thinking patterns is an essential part of cognitive therapy.

Cognitive Techniques

Strategies used in cognitive therapy include recognizing and modifying automatic thoughts (cognitive errors) and recognizing and modifying schemas (core beliefs). Wright, Beck, and Thase (2003) identify the following techniques commonly used in cognitive therapy.

Recognizing Automatic Thoughts and Schemas

Socratic Questioning. In **Socratic questioning** (also called *guided discovery)*, the therapist questions the client about his or her situation. With Socratic questioning, the client is asked to describe feelings associated with specific situations. Questions are stated in a way that may stimulate in the client recognition of possible dysfunctional thinking and produce dissonance about the validity of the thoughts.

Imagery and Role-Play. When Socratic questioning does not produce the desired results, the therapist may choose to guide the client through imagery exercises or role-play in an effort to elicit automatic thoughts. Through guided imagery, the client is asked to "relive" the stressful situation by imagining the setting in which it occurred. Where did it occur? Who was there? What happened just prior to the stressful situation? What feelings did the client experience in association with the situation?

Role-play is not used as commonly as imagery. It is a technique that should be used only when the relationship between client and therapist is exceptionally strong and there is little likelihood of maladaptive transference occurring. With role-play, the therapist assumes the role of an individual within a situation that produces a maladaptive response in the client. The situation is played out in an effort to elicit recognition of automatic thinking on the part of the client.

Thought Recording. This technique, one of the most frequently used methods of recognizing automatic thoughts, is taught to and discussed with the client in the therapy session. Thought recording is assigned as homework for the client outside of therapy. In thought recording, the client is asked to keep a written record of situations that occur and the automatic thoughts that are elicited by the situation. This is called a "two-column" thought recording. Some therapists ask their clients to keep a "three-column" recording, which includes a description of the emotional response also associated with the situation, as illustrated in Table 20–2.

Modifying Automatic Thoughts and Schemas

Generating Alternatives. To help the client see a broader range of possibilities than had originally been considered, the therapist guides the client in generating alternatives.

Examining the Evidence. With this technique, the client and therapist set forth the automatic thought as the hypothesis, and they study the evidence both for and against the hypothesis.

Decatastrophizing. With the technique of **decatastrophizing**, the therapist assists the client to examine the validity of a negative automatic thought. Even if some validity exists, the client is then encouraged to review ways to cope adaptively, moving beyond the current crisis situation.

Reattribution. It is believed that depressed clients attribute life events in a negatively distorted manner; that is, they have a tendency "to blame themselves for adverse life events, and to believe that these negative situations will last indefinitely" (Wright, Beck, & Thase, 2003). Through Socratic questioning and testing of automatic

TABLE 20–2	Three-Column Thought Recording	
SITUATION	**AUTOMATIC THOUGHTS**	**EMOTIONAL RESPONSE**
Girlfriend broke up with me.	I'm a stupid person. No one would ever want to marry me.	Sadness; depression
I was turned down for a promotion.	Stupid boss!! He doesn't know how to manage people. It's not fair!	Anger

thoughts, this technique is aimed at reversing the negative attribution of depressed clients from internal and enduring to the more external and transient manner of nondepressed individuals.

Daily Record of Dysfunctional Thoughts (DRDT). DRDT is a tool commonly used in cognitive therapy to modify automatic thoughts. Two more columns are added to the three-column thought record presented earlier. Clients are then asked to rate the intensity of the thoughts and emotions on a 0- to-100 percent scale. The fourth column of the DRDT asks the client to describe a more rational cognition than the automatic thought identified in the second column and rate the intensity of the belief in the rational thought. In the fifth column, the client records any changes that have occurred as a result of modifying the automatic thought and the new rate of intensity associated with it. Table 20–3 presents an example of a DRDT as an extension to the three-column thought recording presented in Table 20–2.

Cognitive Rehearsal. This technique uses mental imagery to uncover potential automatic thoughts in advance of their occurrence in a stressful situation. A discussion is held to identify ways to modify these dysfunctional cognitions. The client is then given "homework" assignments to try these newly learned methods in real situations.

Behavioral Interventions

It is believed that in cognitive therapy, an interactive relationship exists between cognitions and behavior; that is, that cognitions affect behavior and behavior influences cognitions. With this concept in mind, a number of interventions are structured for the client to assist him or her to identify and modify maladaptive cognitions and behaviors. The following procedures, which are behavior-oriented, are directed toward helping clients learn more adaptive behavioral strategies that will in turn have a more positive effect on cognitions (Basco et al., 2004; Sadock & Sadock, 2003; Wright, Beck, & Thase, 2003):

1. **Activity Scheduling.** With this intervention, clients are asked to keep a daily log of their activities on an hourly basis and rate each activity, for mastery and pleasure, on a zero-to-ten scale. The schedule is then shared with the therapist and used to identify important areas needing concentration during therapy.
2. **Graded Task Assignments.** This intervention is used with clients who are facing a situation that they perceive as overwhelming. The task is broken down into subtasks that clients can complete one step at a time. Each subtask will have a goal and a time interval attached to it. Successful completion of each subtask helps to increase self-esteem and decrease feelings of helplessness.
3. **Behavioral Rehearsal.** Somewhat akin to, and often used in conjunction with, cognitive rehearsal, this technique uses role-play to "rehearse" a modification of maladaptive behaviors that may be contributing to dysfunctional cognitions.
4. **Distraction.** When dysfunctional cognitions have been recognized, activities are identified that can be used to **distract** clients and divert them from the intrusive thoughts or depressive ruminations that are contributing to the maladaptive responses.
5. **Miscellaneous Techniques.** Relaxation exercises, assertiveness training, role modeling, and social skills training are additional types of behavioral interventions that are used in cognitive therapy to assist clients to modify dysfunctional cognitions. Thought stopping techniques (described in Chapter 15) may also be used to restructure dysfunctional thinking patterns.

ROLE OF THE NURSE IN COGNITIVE THERAPY

Many of the techniques used in cognitive therapy are well within the scope of nursing practice, from generalist through specialist levels. Unfortunately, many nurses

| | | | | OUTCOME: |
SITUATION	**AUTOMATIC THOUGHT**	**EMOTIONAL RESPONSE**	**RATIONAL RESPONSE**	**EMOTIONAL RESPONSE**
Girlfriend broke up with me.	I'm a stupid person. No one would ever want to marry me. (95%)	Sadness; depression (90%)	I'm not stupid. Lots of people like me. Just because one person doesn't want to date me doesn't mean that no one would want to. (75%)	Sadness; depression (50%)
I was turned down for a promotion.	Stupid boss!! He doesn't know how to manage people. It's not fair! (90%)	Anger (95%)	I guess I have to admit the other guy's education and experience fit the position better than mine. The boss was being fair because he filled the position based on qualifications. I'll try for the next promotion that fits my qualifications better. (70%)	Anger (20%) Disappointment (80%) Hope (80%)

TABLE 20–3   Daily Record of Dysfunctional Thoughts (DRDT)

are not introduced to the major concepts of cognitive therapy during their nursing education. Cognitive therapy requires an understanding of educational principles and the ability to use problem-solving skills to guide clients' thinking through a reframing process. The scope of contemporary psychiatric nursing practice is expanding, and although psychiatric nurses have been using some of these techniques in various degrees within their

practices for years, it is important that knowledge and skills related to this type of therapy be promoted further. The value of cognitive therapy as a useful and cost-effective tool has been observed in a number of inpatient and community outpatient mental health settings.

The following case study is used to present the role of the nurse in cognitive therapy in the context of the nursing process.

CASE STUDY

ASSESSMENT

Sam is a 45-year-old white male admitted to the psychiatric unit of a general medical center by his family physician, Dr. Jones, who reported that Sam had become increasingly despondent over the last month. His wife reported that he had made statements such as, "Life is not worth living," and "I think I could just take all those pills Dr. Jones prescribed at one time, then it would all be over." He was admitted at 6:40 PM, via wheelchair from admissions, accompanied by his wife. He reports no known allergies. Vital signs upon admission were temperature, 97.9°F; P, 80; respirations, 16; and BP, 132/77. He is 5 feet 11 inches tall and weighs 160 pounds. He was referred to the psychiatrist on call, Dr. Smith. Orders include suicide precautions, level I; regular diet; chemistry profile and routine urinalysis in AM; Desyrel, 200 mg tid; Dalmane, 30 mg hs p.r.n. for sleep.

Family dynamics: Sam says he loves his wife and children and does not want to hurt them, but feels they no longer need him. He states, "They would probably be better off without me." His wife appears to be very concerned about his condition, though in his despondency, he seems oblivious to her feelings. His mother lives in a neighboring state, and he sees her infrequently. He admits that he is somewhat bitter toward her for allowing him and his siblings to "suffer from the physical and emotional brutality of their father." His siblings and their families live in distant states, and he sees them rarely, during holiday gatherings. He feels closest to the older of the two brothers.

Medical/psychiatric history: Sam's father died 5 years ago at age 65 of a myocardial infarction. Sam and both his brothers have a history of high cholesterol and triglyceride levels from approximately age 30. During his regular physical examination 1 month ago, Sam's family doctor recognized symptoms of depression and prescribed Elavil. Sam's mother has a history of depressive episodes. She was hospitalized once about 7 years ago for depression, and she has taken various antidepressant medications over the years. Her family physician has also prescribed Valium for her on numerous occasions for her "nerves." No other family members have a history of psychiatric problems.

Past experiences: Sam was the first child in a family of four. He is 2 years older than his sister and 4 years older than the third child, a brother. He was 6 years old

when his youngest sibling, also a boy, was born. Sam's father was a career Army man, who moved his family many times during their childhood years. Sam attended 15 schools from the time he entered kindergarten until he graduated from high school.

Sam reports that his father was very autocratic and had many rules that he expected his children to obey without question. Infraction resulted in harsh discipline. Because Sam was the oldest child, his father believed he should assume responsibility for the behavior of his siblings. Sam describes the severe physical punishment he received from his father when he or his siblings allegedly violated one of the rules. It was particularly intense when Sam's father had been drinking, which he did most evenings and weekends.

Sam's mother was very passive. Sam believes she was afraid of his father, particularly when he was drinking, so she quietly conformed to his lifestyle and offered no resistance, even though she did not agree with his disciplining of the children. Sam reports that he observed his father physically abusing his mother on a number of occasions, most often when he had been drinking.

Sam states that he had very few friends when he was growing up. With all the family moves, he gave up trying to make new friends because it became too painful to give them up when it was time to leave. He took a paper route when he was 13 years old and then worked in fast-food restaurants from age 15 on. He was a hard worker and never seemed to have difficulty finding work in any of the places where the family relocated. He states that he appreciated the independence and the opportunity of being away from home as much as his job would allow. "I guess I can honestly say I hated my father, and working was my way of getting away from all the stress that was going on in that house. I guess my dad hated me, too, because he never was satisfied with anything. I did. I never did well enough for him in school, on the job, or even at home. When I think of my dad now, the memories I have are of being criticized and beaten with a belt."

On graduation from high school, Sam joined the Navy, where he learned a skill that he used after discharge to obtain a job in a large aircraft plant. He also attended the local university at night, where he earned his accounting degree. When he completed his degree, he was reassigned to the administration department of the aircraft company, and he has been in the same position for 12 years without a promotion.

Precipitating event: Over the last 12 years, Sam has watched while a number of his peers were promoted to management positions. Sam has been considered for several of these positions but has never been selected. Last month a management position became available for which Sam felt he was qualified. He applied for this position, believing he had a good chance of being promoted. However, when the announcement was made, the position had been given to a younger man who had been with the company only 5 years. Sam seemed to accept the decision, but over the last few weeks he has become more and more withdrawn. He speaks to very few people at the office and is falling more and more behind in his work. At home, he eats very little, talks to family members only when they ask a direct question, withdraws to his bedroom very early in the evening, and does not come out until time to leave for work the next morning. Today, he refused to get out of bed or to go to work. His wife convinced him to talk to their family doctor, who admitted him to the hospital.

Client's perception of the stressor: Sam states that all his life he has "not been good enough at anything. I could never please my father. Now I can't seem to please my boss. What's the use of trying? I came to the hospital because my wife and my doctor are afraid I might try to kill myself. I must admit the thought has crossed my mind more than once. I seem to have very little motivation for living. I just don't care any more."

DIAGNOSES/OUTCOME IDENTIFICATION

The following nursing diagnoses were formulated for Sam:

1. Risk for suicide related to depressed mood and expressions of having nothing to live for.
2. Chronic low self-esteem related to lack of positive feedback and learned helplessness evidenced by a sense of worthlessness, lack of eye contact, social isolation, and negative/pessimistic outlook.

The following may be used as criteria for measurement of outcomes in the planning of care for Sam:

The client will:

1. Not harm self.
2. Acquire a feeling of hope for the future.
3. Demonstrate increased self-esteem and perception of self as a worthwhile person.

PLANNING/IMPLEMENTATION

Table 20–4 presents a nursing care plan for Sam employing some techniques associated with cognitive therapy that are within the scope of nursing practice. Rationales are presented for each intervention.

EVALUATION

Reassessment is conducted to determine if the nursing interventions have been successful in achieving the objectives of Sam's care. Evaluation can be facilitated by gathering information using the following questions:

1. Has self-harm to Sam been avoided?
2. Have Sam's suicidal ideations subsided?
3. Does Sam know where to seek help in a crisis situation?
4. Has Sam discussed the recent loss with staff and family?
5. Is Sam able to verbalize personal hope for the future?
6. Can Sam identify positive attributes about himself?
7. Does Sam demonstrate motivation to move on with his life without a fear of failure?

TABLE 20–4   Care Plan for "Sam" (An Example of Intervention with Cognitive Therapy)

NURSING DIAGNOSIS: RISK FOR SUICIDE
RELATED TO: Depressed mood

OUTCOME CRITERIA	NURSING INTERVENTIONS*	RATIONALE*
Sam will not harm himself.	1. Acknowledge Sam's feelings of despair.	1. Cognitive therapists actively pursue the client's point of view.
	2. Convey warmth, accurate empathy, and genuineness.	2. Cognitive therapists use these skills to understand the client's personal view of the world and to establish rapport.
	3. Through Socratic questioning, challenge irrational pessimism. Ask Sam to discuss what problems suicide would solve. Then try to get him to think of reasons for *not* attempting suicide.	3. Cognitive therapists use problem-solving techniques to help the suicidal client think beyond the immediate future.
	4. Begin a serious discussion of alternatives.	4. Cognitive therapists use this strategy to decrease feelings of hopelessness in suicidal clients.

(Continued on following page)

CASE STUDY (Continued)

TABLE 20–4	Care Plan for "Sam" (An Example of Intervention with Cognitive Therapy) (Continued)

NURSING DIAGNOSIS: CHRONIC LOW SELF-ESTEEM

RELATED TO: Lack of positive feedback and learned helplessness

EVIDENCED BY: A sense of worthlessness, lack of eye contact, social isolation, and negative/pessimistic outlook.

OUTCOME CRITERIA	NURSING INTERVENTIONS	RATIONALE
Sam will demonstrate increased self-esteem and perception of himself as a worthwhile person.	1. Ask Sam to keep a 3-column automatic thought recording. 2. Help Sam to recognize that his worth as a person is not tied to his promotion at work. The world will go on and he can survive this loss. 3. Help Sam to identify ways in which he could feel better about himself. For example, Sam states that he would like to update his computer skills, but he is afraid he is too old. Challenge his negative thinking about his age by using the cognitive therapy technique of "examining the evidence." 4. Ask Sam to expand on his 3-column automatic thought recording and make a daily record of dysfunctional thoughts (DRDT). 5. Discourage Sam's ruminating about his failures. May need to withdraw attention if he persists. Focus on past accomplishments and offer support in undertaking new tasks. Offer recognition of successful endeavors and positive reinforcement of attempts made.	1. Cognitive therapists use this tool to help clients identify automatic thoughts (cognitive errors). 2. Cognitive therapists use the technique of "decatastrophizing" to help clients get past a crisis situation. 3. Cognitive therapists use the technique of "generating alternatives" to help clients recognize that a broader range of possibilities may exist than may be evident at the moment. "Examining the evidence" may help Sam understand that self-improvement is worthwhile at any age. 4. Cognitive therapists use this tool to help clients examine their automatic thoughts and come up with more rational responses. 5. Cognitive therapy employs some techniques of behavior therapy. Lack of attention to undesirable behavior may discourage its repetition. Recognition and positive reinforcement enhance self-esteem and encourage repetition of desirable behaviors.

*Interventions and rationale for this diagnosis adapted from Harvard Medical School (2003) and Beck & Weishaar (2005).

SUMMARY

Cognitive therapy is founded on the premise that how people think significantly influences their feelings and behavior. Aaron Beck initiated the concept in the 1960s in his work with depressed clients. Since that time, it has been expanded for use with a number of emotional illnesses.

Cognitive therapy is short-term, highly structured, and goal-oriented therapy that consists of three major components: didactic, or educational, aspects; cognitive techniques; and behavioral interventions. The therapist teaches the client about the relationship between his or her illness and the distorted thinking patterns. Explanation about cognitive therapy and how it works is provided.

The therapist helps the client to recognize his or her negative automatic thoughts (sometimes called *cognitive errors*). Once these automatic thoughts have been identified, various cognitive and behavioral techniques are used to assist the client to modify the dysfunctional thinking patterns. Independent homework assignments are an important part of the cognitive therapist's strategy.

Many of the cognitive therapy techniques are within the scope of nursing practice. The role of the nurse was presented in this chapter in the context of the nursing process with a sample case study. As the role of the psychiatric nurse continues to expand, the knowledge and skills associated with a variety of therapies will need to be broadened. Cognitive therapy is likely to be one in which nurses will become more involved.

REVIEW QUESTIONS

SELF-EXAMINATION/LEARNING EXERCISE

Match the automatic thoughts on the left to the examples in the right-hand column:

_____ 1. Overgeneralization

_____ 2. Magnification

_____ 3. Catastrophic thinking

_____ 4. Personalization

a. Janet failed her first test in nursing school. She thinks, "Well, that's it! I'll never be a nurse."

b. When Jack is not accepted at the law school of his choice, he thinks, "I'm so stupid. No law school will ever accept me."

c. Nancy's new in-laws came to dinner for the first time. When Nancy's mother-in-law left some food on her plate, Nancy thought, "I must be a lousy cook."

d. Barbara burned the toast. She thinks, "I'm a totally incompetent person."

Situation: Opal is a 43-year-old woman who is suffering from depression and suicidal ideation. Answer the following questions about Opal related to cognitive therapy techniques:

5. Opal says, "I'm such a worthless person. I don't deserve to live." The therapist responds, "I would like for you to think about what problems committing suicide would solve." This therapist is using:
   a. Imagery
   b. Role-play
   c. Problem-solving
   d. Thought recording

6. The purpose of the thought recording technique is to help Opal:
   a. Identify automatic thoughts.
   b. Modify automatic thoughts.
   c. Identify rational alternatives.
   d. All of the above

7. The purpose of the Daily Record of Dysfunctional Thoughts is to help Opal:
   a. Identify automatic thoughts.
   b. Modify automatic thoughts.
   c. Identify rational alternatives.
   d. All of the above

8. Opal tells the therapist, "I thought I would just die when my husband told me he was leaving me. If I had been a better wife, he wouldn't have fallen in love with another woman. It's all my fault." The therapist asks Opal to think back to the day her husband told her he was leaving and to describe the situation and her feelings. This technique is called:
   a. Imagery
   b. Role-play
   c. Problem solving
   d. Thought recording

9. The therapist wants to use the technique of "examining the evidence." Which of the following statements reflects this technique:
   a. "How do you think you could have been a better wife?"
   b. "Okay, you say it's all your fault. Let's discuss why it might be your fault and then we will look at why it may not be."
   c. "Let's talk about what would make you a happier person."
   d. "Would you have wanted him to stay if he didn't really want to?"

10. The therapist teaches Opal that when the idea of herself as a worthless person starts to form in her mind, she should immediately start to whistle the tune of "Dixie." This is an example of the cognitive therapy technique of:
   a. Behavioral rehearsal
   b. Social skills training
   c. Distraction
   d. Generating alternatives

REFERENCES

Basco, M.R., McDonald, N., Merlock, M., & Rush, A.J. (2004). A cognitive-behavioral approach to treatment of bipolar I disorder. In J.H. Wright (Ed.). *Cognitive-behavioral therapy.* Washington, DC: American Psychiatric Publishing.

Beck, A.T., Freeman, A., & Davis, D.D. (2003). *Cognitive therapy of personality disorders* (2nd ed.). New York: The Guilford Press.

Beck, A.T., Rush, A.J., Shaw, B.F., & Emery, G. (1987). *Cognitive therapy of depression.* New York: The Guilford Press.

Beck, A.T., & Weishaar, M.E. (2005). Cognitive therapy. In R.J. Corsini and D. Wedding (Eds.). *Current psychotherapies* (7th ed.). Belmont, CA: Brooks/Cole.

Beck, J.S. (1995). *Cognitive therapy: Basics and beyond.* New York: The Guilford Press.

Harvard Medical School (2003). Confronting suicide—part II. *Harvard Mental Health Letter, 19*(12), 1–5.

Sadock, B.J., & Sadock, V.A. (2003). *Synopsis of psychiatry: Behavioral sciences/clinical psychiatry* (9th ed.). Philadelphia: Lippincott Williams & Wilkins.

Wright, J.H., Beck, A.T., & Thase, M.E. (2003). Cognitive therapy. In R.E. Hales & S.C. Yudofsky (Eds.). *Textbook of clinical psychiatry* (4th ed.). Washington, DC: American Psychiatric Publishing

CLASSICAL REFERENCES

Beck, A.T. (1963). Thinking and depression, I. Idiosyncratic content and cognitive distortions. *Archives of General Psychiatry, 9,* 324–333.

Beck, A.T. (1964). Thinking and depression, II. Theory and therapy. *Archives of General Psychiatry, 10,* 561–571.

Lazarus, R.S., & Folkman, S. (1984). *Stress, appraisal, and coping.* New York: Springer.

Psalm 56:13 For thou hast delivered my soul from death; wilt not thou deliver my feet from falling that I may walk before God in the light of the living?

PSYCHOPHARMACOLOGY

CHAPTER OUTLINE

OBJECTIVES
HISTORICAL PERSPECTIVES
HOW DO PSYCHOTROPICS WORK?

APPLYING THE NURSING PROCESS IN PSYCHOPHARMACOLOGICAL THERAPY
SUMMARY
REVIEW QUESTIONS

KEY TERMS

agranulocytosis
akathisia
akinesia
amenorrhea
dystonia
extrapyramidal
  symptoms
gynecomastia

hypertensive crisis
neuroleptic malignant
  syndrome
oculogyric crisis
priapism
retrograde ejaculation
serotonin syndrome
tardive dyskinesia

CORE CONCEPTS

neurotransmitter
psychotropic
  medication
receptor

OBJECTIVES

After reading this chapter, the student will be able to:

1. Discuss historical perspectives related to psychopharmacology.
2. Describe indications, actions, contraindications, precautions, side effects, and nursing implications for the following classifications of drugs:
   a. Antianxiety agents
   b. Antidepressants
   c. Mood-stabilizing agents
   d. Antipsychotics
   e. Antiparkinsonian agents
   f. Sedative-hypnotics
   g. Agents for attention-deficit/hyperactivity disorder
3. Apply the steps of the nursing process to the administration of psychotropic medications.

 he middle of the 20th century identifies a pivotal period in the treatment of the mentally ill. It was during this time that the phenothiazines were introduced into the United States. Before that time they had been used in France as preoperative medications. As Dr. Henri Laborit of the Hospital Boucicaut in Paris stated,

It was our aim to decrease the anxiety of the patients to prepare them in advance for their postoperative recovery. With these new drugs, the phenothiazines, we were seeing a profound psychic and physical relaxation... a real indifference to the environment and to the upcoming operation. It

seemed to me these drugs must have an application in psychiatry. (Sage, 1984)

Indeed they have had a significant application in psychiatry. Not only have they given many individuals a chance, without which they would have been unable to function, but also they have provided researchers and clinicians with information to study the origins and etiologies of mental illness. Knowledge gained from learning how these drugs work has promoted advancement in understanding how behavioral disorders develop. Dr. Arnold Scheibel, Director of the UCLA Brain Research Institute, stated,

[When these drugs came out] there was a sense of disbelief that we could actually do something substantive for the patients ... see them for the first time as sick individuals and not as something bizarre that we could literally not talk to. (Sage, 1984)

This chapter explores historical perspectives in the use of psychotropic medications in the treatment of mental illness. Seven classifications of medications are discussed, and their implications for psychiatric nursing are presented in the context of the steps of the nursing process.

Core Concept

Psychotropic Medication
Medication that affects psychic function, behavior, or experience.

HISTORICAL PERSPECTIVES

Historically, reaction to and treatment of the mentally ill ranged from benign involvement to intervention some would consider inhumane. Individuals with mental illness were feared because of common beliefs associating them with demons or the supernatural. They were looked upon as loathsome and often were mistreated.

Beginning in the late 18th century, a type of "moral reform" in the treatment of persons with mental illness began to occur. This resulted in the establishment of community and state hospitals concerned with the needs of persons with mental illness. Considered a breakthrough in the humanization of care, these institutions, however well intentioned, fostered the concept of custodial care. Clients were ensured the provision of food and shelter but received little or no hope of change for the future. As they became increasingly dependent upon the institution to fill their needs, the likelihood of their return to the family or community diminished.

The early part of the 20th century saw the advent of the somatic therapies in psychiatry. Individuals with mental illness were treated with insulin shock therapy, wet sheet packs, ice baths, electroconvulsive therapy, and psychosurgery. Prior to 1950, sedatives and amphetamines were the only significant psychotropic medications available. Even these had limited use because of their toxicity and addictive effects. Since the 1950s, the development of psychopharmacology has expanded to include widespread use of antipsychotic, antidepressant, and antianxiety medications. Research into how these drugs work has provided an understanding of the etiology of many psychiatric disorders.

Psychotropic medications are not intended to "cure" the mental illness. Most physicians who prescribe these medications for their clients use them as an adjunct to individual or group psychotherapy. Although their contribution to psychiatric care cannot be minimized, it must be emphasized that psychotropic medications relieve physical and behavioral symptoms. They do not resolve emotional problems.

Nurses must understand the legal implications associated with the administration of psychotropic medications. Laws differ from state to state, but most adhere to the client's right to refuse treatment. Exceptions exist in emergency situations when it has been determined that clients are likely to harm themselves or others.

Core Concept

Neurotransmitter
A chemical that is stored in the axon terminals of the presynaptic neuron. An electrical impulse through the neuron stimulates the release of the neurotransmitter into the synaptic cleft, which in turn determines whether another electrical impulse is generated.

Receptor
Molecules situated on the cell membrane that are binding sites for neurotransmitters

---

Reuptake – neurotransmitter inactivation/reabsorbed into the presynaptic neuron from which it was released

HOW DO PSYCHOTROPICS WORK?[*]

Most of the medications have their effects at the neuronal synapse, producing changes in neurotransmitter release and the receptors they bind to (see Figure 21–1). Researchers hypothesize that most antidepressants work by blocking the reuptake of neurotransmitters, specifically, serotonin and norepinephrine. *Reuptake* is the process of neurotransmitter inactivation by which the neurotransmitter is reabsorbed into the presynaptic neuron from which it had been released. Blocking the reuptake process allows more serotonin and norepinephrine to be available for neuronal transmission. Blockade of norepinephrine and serotonin may also result in undesirable side effects (see Table 21–1). Some antidepressants also block receptor sites that are unrelated to their mechanisms of action. These include α-adrenergic, histaminergic, and muscarinic cholinergic receptors. Blocking these receptors is also associated with the development of certain side effects.

Antipsychotic medications block dopamine receptors, and some affect muscarinic cholinergic, histaminergic, and α-adrenergic receptors. The "atypical" antipsychotics block a specific serotonin receptor. Benzodiazepines facilitate the transmission of the inhibitory neurotransmitter gamma-aminobutyric acid (GABA). The psychostimulants work by increasing norepinephrine, serotonin, and dopamine release.

Although each psychotropic medication affects neurotransmission, the specific drugs within each class have varying neuronal effects. Their exact mechanisms of action are unknown. Many of the neuronal effects occur acutely; however, the therapeutic effects may take weeks for some medications such as antidepressants and

---

[*]From Glod & Levy (1998), with permission.

EXACT Mechanisms of action are unknown
EFFECTS take weeks –

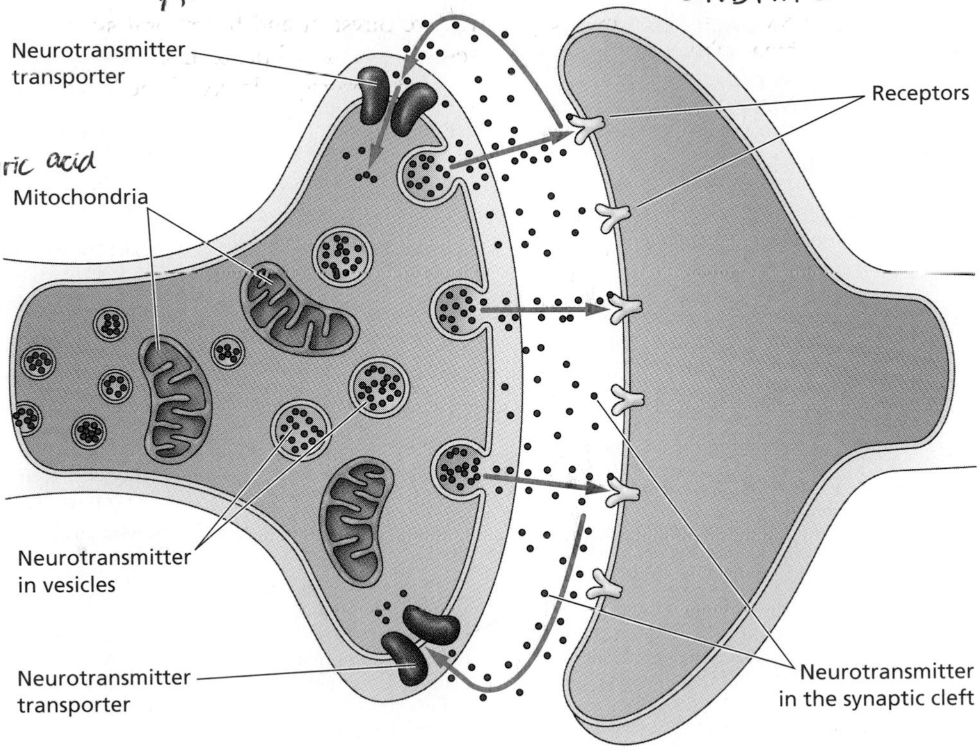

[handwritten top margin: antidepressants (block the reuptake) of neurotransmitters – serotonin + norepinephrine]

[handwritten left margin:
Neurotransmitters
Serotonin
norepinephrine
acetylcholine
glutamate
gamma-aminobutyric acid
dopamine
histamine]

AXON

DENDRITE

[handwritten right margin: Research shows that therapeutic effects are related to the nervous systems adaptation to increased levels of neurotransmitters these 'adaptive changes' result from a 'homeostatic mechanism' much like a thermostat' that that regulates the cell' and maintains equilibrium]

FIGURE 21–1 Area of synaptic transmission that is altered by drugs.

The transmission of electrical impulses from the axon terminal of one neuron to the dendrite of another is achieved by the controlled release of neurotransmitters into the synaptic cleft. Neurotransmitters include serotonin, norepinephrine, acetylcholine, dopamine, glutamate, gamma-aminobutyric acid (GABA), and histamine, among others. Prior to its release, the neurotransmitter is concentrated into specialized synaptic vesicles. Once fired, the neurotransmitter is released into the synaptic cleft where it encounters receptors on the postsynaptic membrane. Each neurotransmitter has receptors specific to it alone. Some neurotransmitters are considered to be *excitatory*, whereas others are *inhibitory*, a feature that determines whether another action potential will occur. In the synaptic cleft, the neurotransmitter rapidly diffuses, is catabolized by enzymatic action, or is taken up by the neurotransmitter transporters and returned to vesicles inside the axon terminal to await another action potential.

Psychotropic medications exert their effects in various ways in this area of synaptic transmission. Reuptake inhibitors block reuptake of the neurotransmitters by the transporter proteins, thus resulting in elevated levels of extracellular neurotransmitter. Drugs that inhibit catabolic enzymes promote excess buildup of the neurotransmitter at the synaptic site.

Some drugs cause receptor blockade, thereby resulting in a reduction in transmission and decreased neurotransmitter activity. These drugs are called *antagonists*. Drugs that increase neurotransmitter activity by direct stimulation of the specific receptors are called *agonists*.

[handwritten: receptor blockade – antagonists]
[handwritten: -↑ neurotransmitter activity by direct stimulation of the specific receptors – agonists]

antipsychotics. Acute alterations in neuronal function do not fully explain how these medications work. Long-term neuropharmacologic reactions to increased norepinephrine and serotonin levels relate more to their mechanisms of action. Recent research suggests that the therapeutic effects are related to the nervous system's adaptation to increased levels of neurotransmitters. These adaptive changes result from a homeostatic mechanism, much like a thermostat, that regulates the cell and maintains equilibrium.

[handwritten: Praise God! no one knows only God knows!!!]

APPLYING THE NURSING PROCESS IN PSYCHOPHARMACOLOGICAL THERAPY

An assessment tool for obtaining a drug history is provided in Table 21–2. This tool may be adapted for use by staff nurses admitting clients to the hospital, or by nurse practitioners who may wish to use it with prescriptive privileges. It may also be used when a client's signature of informed consent is required prior to pharmacological therapy.

Antianxiety Agents

Background Assessment Data

Indications. Antianxiety drugs are also called *anxiolytics* and *minor tranquilizers*. They are used in the treatment of anxiety disorders, anxiety symptoms, acute alcohol withdrawal, skeletal muscle spasms, convulsive disorders, status epilepticus, and preoperative sedation. Their use and efficacy for periods greater than 4 months have not been evaluated.

TABLE 21-1   Effects of Psychotropic Medications on Neurotransmitters

EXAMPLE OF MEDICATION	ACTION ON NEUROTRANSMITTER AND/OR RECEPTOR	PHYSIOLOGICAL EFFECTS	SIDE EFFECTS
SSRIs	Inhibit reuptake of serotonin (5-HT)	Reduce depression Control anxiety Control obsessions	Nausea, agitation, headache, sexual dysfunction
Tricyclic antidepressants	Inhibit reuptake of serotonin (5-HT) Inhibit reuptake of norepinephrine (NE) Block NE (α_1) receptor Block ACh receptor Block histamine (H_1) receptor	Reduce depression Relief of severe pain Prevent panic attacks	Sexual dysfunction (NE and 5-HT) Sedation, weight gain (H_1) Dry mouth, constipation, blurred vision, urinary retention (ACh) Postural hypotension and tachycardia (α_1)
MAO inhibitors	Increase NE and 5-HT by inhibiting the enzyme that degrades them (MAO-A)	Reduce depression Control anxiety	Sedation, dizziness Sexual dysfunction Hypertensive crisis (interaction with tyramine)
Trazodone and nefazodone	$5-HT_2$ receptor antagonism Adrenergic receptor blockade	Reduce depression Reduce anxiety	Nausea (5-HT) Sedation Orthostasis (α_1) Priapism (α_2)
SSNRIs: venlafaxine and duloxetine	Potent inhibitor of serotonin and norepinephrine reuptake Weak inhibitor of dopamine reuptake	Reduce depression Relieve pain of neuropathy (duloxetine) Relieve anxiety (venlafaxine)	Nausea (5-HT) $\uparrow$ sweating (5-HT) Insomnia (α) Tremors (α) Sexual dysfunction (5-HT)
Bupropion	Inhibits reuptake of 5-HT, NE, and dopamine (D)	Reduce depression Aid in smoking cessation $\downarrow$ symptoms of ADHD	Insomnia, dry mouth, tremor, seizures
Antipsychotics: phenothiazines and haloperidol	Strong D_2 receptor blockade Weaker blockade of ACh, H_1, α_1-adrenergic, and $5-HT_2$ receptors	Relief of psychosis Relief of anxiety (Some) provide relief from nausea and vomiting and intractable hiccoughs	Blurred vision, dry mouth, decreased sweating, constipation, urinary retention, tachycardia (ACh) EPS (D_2) $\uparrow$ plasma prolactin (D_2) Sedation; weight gain (H_1) Ejaculatory difficulty ($5-HT_2$) Orthostatic hypotension (α)
Antipsychotics (novel): clozapine, olanzapine, aripiprazole, quetiapine, risperidone, ziprasidone	Receptor antagonism of $5-HT_2$ $D_1 – D_5$ (varies with drug) H_1, α_1-adrenergic, muscarinic (ACh)	Relief of psychosis (with minimal or no EPS) Relief of anxiety Relief of acute mania	Potential with some of the drugs for mild EPS (D_2) Sedation, weight gain (H_1) Orthostasis and dizziness (α-adrenergic) Blurred vision, dry mouth, decreased sweating, constipation, urinary retention, tachycardia (ACh)
Antianxiety: benzodiazepines	Binds to BZ receptor sites on the $GABA_A$ receptor complex; increases receptor affinity for GABA	Relief of anxiety Sedation	Dependence (with long-term use) Confusion; memory impairment; motor incoordination
Antianxiety: buspirone ~BuSPAR~ *does not depress CNS* *Action unknown*	$5-HT_{1A}$ agonist D_2 agonist D_2 antagonist	Relief of anxiety	Nausea, headache, dizziness Restlessness

ACh, acetylcholine; BZ, benzodiazepine; EPS, extrapyramidal symptoms; GABA, gamma-aminobutyric acid; 5-HT, 5-hydroxytryptamine (serotonin); MAO, monoamine oxidase; NE, norepinephrine.

Examples of commonly used antianxiety agents are presented in Table 21–3.

Action. Antianxiety drugs depress subcortical levels of the central nervous system (CNS), particularly the limbic system and reticular formation. They may potentiate the effects of the powerful inhibitory neurotransmitter gamma-aminobutyric acid (GABA) in the brain, thereby producing a calming effect. All levels of CNS depression can be affected, from mild sedation to hypnosis to coma.

EXCEPTION: Buspirone (BuSpar) does not depress the CNS. Although its action is unknown, the drug is believed to produce the desired effects through interac-

TABLE 21-2	**Medication Assessment Tool**

Date _____ Client's Name _____ Age _____
Marital Status _____ Children _____ Occupation _____
Presenting Symptoms (subjective & objective) _____
_____

Diagnosis (DSM-IV-TR) _____
Current Vital Signs: Blood Pressure: Sitting _____/_____; Standing _____/_____; Pulse _____; Respirations _____

CURRENT/PAST USE OF PRESCRIPTION DRUGS (Indicate with "c" or "p" beside name of drug whether current or past use):

Name	Dosage	How Long Used	Why Prescribed	By Whom	Side Effects/Results

CURRENT/PAST USE OF OVER-THE-COUNTER DRUGS (Indicate with "c" or "p" beside name of drug whether current or past use):

Name	Dosage	How Long Used	Why Prescribed	By Whom	Side Effects/Results

CURRENT/PAST USE OF STREET DRUGS, ALCOHOL, NICOTINE, AND/OR CAFFEINE (Indicate with "c" or "p" beside name of drug):

Name	Amount Used	How Often Used	When Last Used	Effects Produced

Any allergies to food or drugs? _____
Any special diet considerations? _____
Do you have (or have you ever had) any of the following? If yes, provide explanation on the back of this sheet.

	Yes	No		Yes	No		Yes	No
1. Difficulty swallowing			12. Chest pain			23. Sexual dysfunction		
2. Delayed wound healing			13. Blood clots/pain in legs			24. Lumps in your breasts		
3. Constipation problems			14. Fainting spells			25. Blurred or double vision		
4. Urination problems			15. Swollen ankles/legs/hands			26. Ringing in the ears		
5. Recent change in elimination patterns			16. Asthma			27. Insomnia		
6. Weakness or tremors			17. Varicose veins			28. Skin Rashes		
7. Seizures			18. Numbness/tingling (location?)			29. Diabetes		
8. Headaches			19. Ulcers			30. Hepatitis (or other liver disease)		
9. Dizziness			20. Nausea/vomiting			31. Kidney disease		
10. High blood pressure			21. Problems with diarrhea			32. Glaucoma		
11. Palpitations			22. Shortness of breath					

Are you pregnant or breast feeding? _____ Date of last menses _____ Type of contraception used _____
Describe any restrictions/limitations that might interfere with your use of medication for your current problem. _____

Prescription orders: Patient teaching related to medications prescribed:

Lab work or referrals prescribed:

Nurse's signature _____   Client's signature _____

tions with serotonin, dopamine, and other neurotransmitter receptors.

Contraindications/Precautions. Antianxiety drugs are contraindicated in individuals with known hypersensitivity to any of the drugs within the classification (e.g., benzodiazepines). They should not be taken in combination with other CNS depressants and are contraindicated in pregnancy and lactation, narrow-angle glaucoma, shock, and coma.

Caution should be taken in administering these drugs to elderly or debilitated clients and clients with hepatic or renal dysfunction. (The dosage usually has to be decreased.) Caution is also required with individuals who have a history of drug abuse or addiction and with those

TABLE 21–3	Antianxiety Agents				
CHEMICAL CLASS	**GENERIC (TRADE) NAME**	**CONTROLLED CATEGORIES**	**HALF-LIFE (HR)**	**DAILY ADULT DOSAGE RANGE (MG)**	**AVAILABLE FORMS (MG)**
Antihistamines	Hydroxyzine (Atarax)		3	100–400	Tabs: 10, 25, 50, 100 Syrup: 10/5 ml
	(Vistaril)		3	100–400	Caps: 25, 50, 100 Oral Susp: 25/5 ml Inj: 25, 50
Benzodiazepines	Alprazolam (Xanax)	CIV	6–26	0.75–4	Tabs: 0.25, 0.5, 1.0, 2.0 ER: 0.5, 1, 2, 3 Oral Solu: 0.5/5 ml
	Chlordiazepoxide (Librium)	CIV	5–30	15–100	Caps: 5, 10, 25 Inj: 100
	Clonazepam (Klonopin)	CIV	18–50	1.5–20	Tabs: 0.5, 1.0, 2.0
	Clorazepate (Tranxene)	CIV	40–50	15–60	Tabs & Caps: 3.75, 7.5, 15 Single Dose: 11.25, 22.5
	Diazepam (Valium)	CIV	20–80	4–40	Tabs: 2, 5, 10 Oral Solu: 5/5 ml, 5/ml Inj: 5/ml
	Lorazepam (Ativan)	CIV	10–20	2–6	Tabs: 0.5, 1.0, 2.0 Oral Solu: 2/ml Inj: 2/ml, 4/ml
	Oxazepam (Serax)	CIV	5–20	30–120	Tabs: 15 Caps: 10, 15, 30
Propanediols	Meprobamate (Miltown)	CIV	6–17	400–2400	Tabs: 200, 400
Azaspirodecanediones	Buspirone (BuSpar)		2–11	15–60	Tabs: 5, 7.5, 10, 15, 30

who are depressed or suicidal. In depressed clients, CNS depressants can exacerbate symptoms.

Interactions. Increased effects of antianxiety agents can occur when taken concomitantly with alcohol, barbiturates, narcotics, antipsychotics, antidepressants, antihistamines, neuromuscular blocking agents, cimetidine, or disulfiram. Decreased effects can be noted with cigarette smoking and caffeine consumption.

Diagnosis

The following nursing diagnoses may be considered for clients receiving therapy with antianxiety agents:

1. Risk for injury related to seizures; panic anxiety; abrupt withdrawal after long-term use; effects of intoxication or overdose
2. Risk for activity intolerance related to side effects of sedation and lethargy
3. Risk for acute confusion related to action of the medication on the CNS

Planning/Implementation

The plan of care should include monitoring for the following side effects from antianxiety agents. Nursing implications related to each side effect are designated by an asterisk (*).

1. **Drowsiness, confusion, lethargy** (most common side effects)
   *Instruct the client not to drive or operate dangerous machinery while taking the medication.
2. **Tolerance; physical and psychological dependence** (does not apply to buspirone)
   *Instruct the client on long-term therapy not to quit taking the drug abruptly. Abrupt withdrawal can be life threatening. Symptoms include depression, insomnia, increased anxiety, abdominal and muscle cramps, tremors, vomiting, sweating, convulsions, and delirium.
3. **Ability to potentiate the effects of other CNS depressants**
   *Instruct the client not to drink alcohol or take other medications that depress the CNS while taking this medication.
4. **Possibility of aggravating symptoms in depressed persons**
   *Assess the client's mood daily.
   *Take necessary precautions for potential suicide.
5. **Orthostatic hypotension**
   *Monitor lying and standing blood pressure and pulse every shift.

CHAPTER 21 ● PSYCHOPHARMACOLOGY **291**

*Instruct the client to arise slowly from a lying or sitting position.

6. **Paradoxical excitement** (client develops symptoms opposite of the medication's desired effect)
*Withhold drug and notify the physician.

7. **Dry mouth**
*Have the client take frequent sips of water, suck on ice chips or hard candy, or chew sugarless gum.

8. **Nausea and vomiting**
*Have the client take the drug with food or milk.

9. **Blood dyscrasias**
*Symptoms of sore throat, fever, malaise, easy bruising, or unusual bleeding should be reported to the physician immediately.

10. **Delayed onset** (buspirone only)
*Ensure that the client understands there is a lag time of 10 days to 2 weeks between onset of therapy with buspirone and subsiding of anxiety symptoms. Client should continue to take the medication during this time.

NOTE: This medication is not recommended for p.r.n. administration because of this delayed therapeutic onset. There is no evidence that buspirone creates tolerance or physical dependence as do the CNS depressant anxiolytics.

Client/Family Education.

The client should:

● Not drive or operate dangerous machinery. Drowsiness and dizziness can occur.
● Not stop taking the drug abruptly, as this can produce serious withdrawal symptoms, such as depression, insomnia, anxiety, abdominal and muscle cramps, tremors, vomiting, sweating, convulsions, delirium.
● (With buspirone only): Be aware of lag time between start of therapy and subsiding of symptoms. Relief is usually evident within 10 to 14 days. The client must take the medication regularly, as ordered, so that it has sufficient time to take effect.
● Not consume other CNS depressants (including alcohol).
● Not take nonprescription medication without approval from physician.
● Rise slowly from sitting or lying position to prevent sudden drop in blood pressure.
● Report symptoms of sore throat, fever, malaise, easy bruising, unusual bleeding, or motor restlessness to physician immediately.
● Be aware of risks of taking this drug during pregnancy. (Congenital malformations have been associated with use during the first trimester.) The client should notify the physician of the desirability to discontinue the drug if pregnancy is suspected or planned.
● Be aware of possible side effects. The client should refer to written materials furnished by health care providers regarding the correct method of self-administration.
● Carry card or piece of paper at all times stating the names of medications being taken.

Outcome Criteria/Evaluation

The following criteria may be used for evaluating the effectiveness of therapy with antianxiety agents.
The client:

1. Demonstrates a reduction in anxiety, tension, and restless activity.
2. Experiences no seizure activity.
3. Experiences no physical injury.
4. Is able to tolerate usual activities without excessive sedation.
5. Exhibits no evidence of confusion.
6. Tolerates the medication without gastrointestinal distress.
7. Verbalizes understanding of the need for, side effects of, and regimen for self-administration.
8. Verbalizes possible consequences of abrupt withdrawal from the medication.

Antidepressants

Background Assessment Data

Indications. Antidepressant medications are used in the treatment of dysthymic disorder; major depression with melancholia or psychotic symptoms; depression associated with organic disease, alcoholism, schizophrenia, or mental retardation; depressive phase of bipolar disorder; and depression accompanied by anxiety. These drugs elevate mood and alleviate other symptoms associated with moderate-to-severe depression. Examples of commonly used antidepressant medications are presented in Table 21–4.

Action. These drugs ultimately work to increase the concentration of norepinephrine, serotonin, and/or dopamine in the body. This is accomplished in the brain by blocking the reuptake of these neurotransmitters by the neurons (tricyclics, selective serotonin reuptake inhibitors, and others). It also occurs when an enzyme, monoamine oxidase (MAO), that is known to inactivate norepinephrine, serotonin, and dopamine, is inhibited at various sites in the nervous system (MAO inhibitors [MAOIs]).

Contraindications/Precautions. Antidepressant drugs are contraindicated in individuals with hypersensitivity. They are also contraindicated in the acute recovery phase following myocardial infarction and in individuals with angle-closure glaucoma.

TABLE 21–4   Antidepressant Medications

CHEMICAL CLASS	GENERIC (TRADE) NAME	DAILY ADULT DOSAGE RANGE (MG)*	THERAPEUTIC PLASMA RANGES (NG/ML)	AVAILABLE FORMS (MG)
Tricyclics	Amitriptyline (Elavil; Endep)	50–300	110–250 (incl. metabolite)	Tabs: 10, 25, 50, 75, 100, 150 Inj: 10/ml
	Amoxapine (Asendin)	50–600	200–500	Tabs: 25, 50, 100, 150
	Clomipramine (Anafranil)	25–250	80–100	Caps: 25, 50, 75
	Desipramine (Norpramin)	25–300	125–300	Tabs: 10, 25, 50, 75, 100, 150
	Doxepin (Sinequan)	25–300	100–200 (incl. metabolite)	Caps: 10, 25, 50, 75, 100, 150 Oral Conc: 10/ml
	Imipramine (Tofranil)	30–300	200–350 (incl. metabolite)	Tabs: 10, 25, 50 Caps: 75, 100, 125, 150
	Nortriptyline (Aventyl; Pamelor)	30–100	50–150	Caps: 10, 25, 50, 75 Oral Solu: 10/5 ml
	Protriptyline (Vivactil)	15–60	100–200	Tabs: 5, 10
	Trimipramine (Surmontil)	50–300	180 (incl. metabolite)	Caps: 25, 50, 100
Selective serotonin reuptake inhibitors	Citalopram (Celexa)	20–60	Not well established	Tabs: 20, 40 Oral Solu: 10/5ml
	Fluoxetine (Prozac; Sarafem)	20–80	Not well established	Tabs: 10 Caps: 10, 20, 40 Caps (Delayed Release): 90 Oral Solu: 20/5 ml
	Fluvoxamine (Luvox)	50–300	Not well established	Tabs: 25, 50, 100
	Escitalopram (Lexapro)	10–20	Not well established	Tabs: 5, 10, 20 Oral Sol: 5/5 ml
	Paroxetine (Paxil)	10–50	Not well established	Tabs: 10, 20, 30, 40 Oral Susp: 10/5 ml
	Sertraline (Zoloft)	50–200	Not well established	Tabs: 25, 50, 100 Oral Conc: 20/ml
Monoamine oxidase inhibitors	Isocarboxazid (Marplan)	20–60	Not well established	Tabs: 10
	Phenelzine (Nardil)	45–90	Not well established	Tabs: 15
	Tranylcypromine (Parnate)	30–60	Not well established	Tabs: 10
Others	Bupropion (Zyban; Wellbutrin)	200–450	Not well established	Tabs: 75, 100 Tabs (SR): 100, 150, 200 Tabs (ER): 150, 300
	Maprotiline (Ludiomil)	50–225	200–300 (incl. metabolite)	Tabs: 25, 50, 75
	Mirtazapine (Remeron)	15–45	Not well established	Tabs: 15, 30, 45 Tabs (Sol): 15, 30, 45
	Trazodone (Desyrel)	150–600	800–1600	Tabs: 50, 100, 150, 300
	Nefazodone (Serzone)	200–600	Not well established	Tabs: 50, 100, 150, 200, 250
	Venlafaxine (Effexor)	75–375	Not well established	Tabs: 25, 37.5, 50, 75, 100 Caps (XR): 37.5, 75, 150
	Duloxetine (Cymbalta)	40–60	Not well established	Caps: 20, 30, 60

*Dosage requires slow titration; onset of therapeutic response may be 1 to 4 weeks.

Caution should be used in administering these drugs to elderly or debilitated clients and those with hepatic, renal, or cardiac insufficiency. (The dosage usually must be decreased.) Caution is also required with psychotic clients, with clients who have benign prostatic hypertrophy, and with individuals who have a history of seizures (may decrease seizure threshold).

NOTE: As these drugs take effect, and mood begins to lift, the individual may have increased energy with which to implement a suicide plan. Suicide potential often increases as level of depression decreases. The nurse should be particularly alert to sudden lifts in mood.

Interactions

Tricyclic Antidepressants. Hyperpyretic crisis, **hypertensive crisis**, severe seizures, and tachycardia may occur

guanethidine → *decreased therapeutic response*
Clonidine

when used with MAOIs. Use of these drugs may decrease therapeutic response to some antihypertensives (clonidine, guanethidine). Additive CNS depression occurs with concurrent use of CNS depressants. Additive sympathomimetic and anticholinergic effects occur with use of other drugs possessing these same properties. Increased effects of tricyclic antidepressants may occur with bupropion, cimetidine, haloperidol, selective serotonin reuptake inhibitors (SSRIs), and valproic acid.

MAO Inhibitors. Hypertensive crisis may occur with concurrent use of amphetamines, methyldopa, levodopa, dopamine, epinephrine, norepinephrine, reserpine, vasoconstrictors, or ingestion of tyramine-containing foods (Table 21–5). Hypertension or hypotension, coma, convulsions, and death may occur with meperidine or other narcotic analgesics when used with MAOIs. Additive hypotension may result with concurrent use of antihypertensives or spinal anesthesia and MAOIs. Additive hypoglycemia may result with concurrent use of insulin or oral hypoglycemic agents and MAOIs. Serious, potentially fatal adverse reactions may occur with concurrent use of other antidepressants, carbamazepine, cyclobenzaprine, maprotiline, furazolidone, procarbazine, or selegiline. Avoid using within 2 weeks of each other (5 weeks after therapy with fluoxetine).

Selective Serotonin Reuptake Inhibitors (SSRIs). Concurrent use with cimetidine may result in increased concentrations of SSRIs. Hypertensive crisis can occur if used within 14 days of MAOIs. Impairment of mental and motor skills may be potentiated with use of alcohol. **Serotonin syndrome** may occur with concurrent use of MAOIs, and other drugs that increase serotonin, such as tryptophan, amphetamines or other psychostimulants; other antidepressants that increase 5-HT levels; or buspirone, lithium, or dopamine agonists (e.g., amantadine, bromocriptine). Concomitant use of SSRIs may increase effects of hydantoins, tricyclic antidepressants, benzodiazepines, beta-blockers, carbamazepine, clozapine, haloperidol, phenothiazines, St. John's wort, sumatriptan, sympathomimetics, tacrine, theophylline, and warfarin.

Diagnosis

The following nursing diagnoses may be considered for clients receiving therapy with antidepressant medications:

1. Risk for suicide related to depressed mood
2. Risk for injury related to side effects of sedation, lowered seizure threshold, orthostatic hypotension, **priapism**, photosensitivity, arrhythmias, hypertensive crisis, or serotonin syndrome
3. Social isolation related to depressed mood
4. Constipation related to side effects of the medication

TABLE 21–5   Diet and Drug Restrictions for Clients on MAOI Therapy

FOODS CONTAINING TYRAMINE

HIGH TYRAMINE CONTENT (AVOID WHILE ON MAOI THERAPY)	MODERATE TYRAMINE CONTENT (MAY EAT OCCASIONALLY WHILE ON MAOI THERAPY)	LOW TYRAMINE CONTENT (LIMITED QUANTITIES PERMISSIBLE WHILE ON MAOI THERAPY)
Aged cheeses (cheddar, Swiss, Camembert, blue cheese, Parmesan, provolone, Romano, brie)	Gouda cheese, processed American cheese, mozzarella	Pasteurized cheeses (cream cheese, cottage cheese, ricotta)
Raisins, fava beans, flat Italian beans, Chinese pea pods	Yogurt, sour cream	Figs
Red wines (Chianti, burgundy, cabernet sauvignon)	Avocados, bananas	Distilled spirits (in moderation)
Smoked and processed meats (salami, bologna, pepperoni, summer sausage)	Beer, white wine, coffee, colas, tea, hot chocolate	
Caviar, pickled herring, corned beef, chicken or beef liver	Meat extracts, such as boullion	
Soy sauce, brewer's yeast, meat tenderizer (MSG)	Chocolate	

DRUG RESTRICTIONS

Ingestion of the following substances while on MAOI therapy could result in life-threatening hypertensive crisis. A 14-day interval is recommended between use of these drugs and an MAOI.

Other antidepressants (tricyclic; SSRIs)
Sympathomimetics: (epinephrine, dopamine, norepinephrine, ephedrine, pseudoephedrine, phenylephrine, phenylpropanolamine, over-the-counter cough and cold preparations)
Stimulants (amphetamines, cocaine, methyldopa, diet drugs)
Antihypertensives (methyldopa, guanethidine, reserpine)
Meperidine and (possibly) other opioid narcotics (morphine, codeine)
Antiparkinsonian agents (levodopa)

SOURCE: Adapted from Sadock & Sadock (2003) and Marangell et al. (2003).

Planning/Implementation

The plan of care should include monitoring for the following side effects from antidepressant medications. Nursing implications are designated by an asterisk (*). A general profile of the side effects of antidepressant medications is presented in Table 21–6.

1. **May occur with all chemical classes:**
   a. Dry mouth
      *Offer the client sugarless candy, ice, frequent sips of water.
      *Strict oral hygiene is very important.
   b. Sedation
      *Request an order from the physician for the drug to be given at bedtime.
      *Request that the physician decrease the dosage or perhaps order a less sedating drug.
      *Instruct the client not to drive or use dangerous equipment while experiencing sedation.
   c. Nausea
      *Medication may be taken with food to minimize GI distress.

   d. Discontinuation syndrome
      *All classes of antidepressants have varying potentials to cause discontinuation syndromes. Abrupt withdrawal following long-term therapy with SSRIs and venlafaxine may result in dizziness, lethargy, headache, and nausea. Fluoxetine is less likely to result in withdrawal symptoms because of its long half-life. Abrupt withdrawal from tricyclics may produce hypomania, akathisia, cardiac arrhythmias, and panic attacks. The discontinuation syndrome associated with MAOIs includes confusion, hypomania, and worsening of depressive symptoms. All antidepressant medication should be tapered gradually to prevent withdrawal symptoms (Haddad, 2001).
2. **Most commonly occur with tricyclics:**
   a. Blurred vision
      *Offer reassurance that this symptom should subside after a few weeks.
      *Instruct the client not to drive until vision is clear.
      *Clear small items from routine pathway to prevent falls.

TABLE 21–6 Side Effect Profiles of Antidepressant Medications

	CNS SIDE EFFECTS		CARDIOVASCULAR SIDE EFFECTS		OTHER SIDE EFFECTS		
	SEDATION	INSOMNIA/ AGITATION	ORTHOSTATIC HYPOTENSION	CARDIAC ARRHYTHMIA	GASTROINTES-TINAL DISTRESS	WEIGHT GAIN (>6 KG)	ANTICHO-LINERGIC*
Amitriptyline	4+	0	4+	3+	0	4+	4+
Desipramine	1+	1+	2+	2+	0	1+	1+
Doxepin	4+	0	2+	2+	0	3+	3+
Imipramine	3+	1+	4+	3+	1+	3+	3+
Nortriptyline	1+	0	2+	2+	0	1+	1+
Protriptyline	1+	1+	2+	2+	0	0	2+
Trimipramine	4+	0	2+	2+	0	3+	1+
Amoxapine	2+	2+	2+	3+	0	1+	2+
Maprotiline	4+	0	0	1+	0	2+	2+
Mirtazapine	4+	0	0	1+	0	2+	2+
Trazodone	4+	0	1+	0	1+	0	0
Nefazodone	3+	0	1+	0	1+	0	0
Bupropion	0	2+	0	1+	1+	0	0
Fluoxetine	0	2+	0	0	3+	0	0
Fluvoxamine	0	2+	0	0	3+	0	0
Paroxetine	0	2+	0	0	3+	0	0
Sertraline	0	2+	0	0	3+	0	0
Citalopram	1+	2+	0	0	3+	0	0
Escitalopram	0	2+	0	0	3+	0	0
Venlafaxine	0	2+	0	0	3+	0	0
Monoamine oxidase inhibitors (MAOIs)	1+	2+	2+	0	1+	2+	1+

KEY:
0 = Absent or rare.
1+ = Infrequent
2+, 3+ = Relatively common.
4+ = Frequent
*Dry mouth, blurred vision, urinary hesitancy, constipation.
SOURCE: Adapted from Depression Guideline Panel (1993); *Drug Facts & Comparisons* (2005); and Schatzberg, Cole, & DeBattista (2005).

b. Constipation
*Order foods high in fiber; increase fluid intake if not contraindicated; and encourage the client to increase physical exercise, if possible.

c. Urinary retention
*Instruct the client to report hesitancy or inability to urinate.
*Monitor intake and output.
*Try various methods to stimulate urination, such as running water in the bathroom or pouring water over the perineal area.

d. Orthostatic hypotension
*Instruct the client to rise slowly from a lying or sitting position.
*Monitor blood pressure (lying and standing) frequently, and document and report significant changes.
*Avoid long hot showers or tub baths.

e. Reduction of seizure threshold
*Observe clients with history of seizures closely.
*Institute seizure precautions as specified in hospital procedure manual.
*Bupropion (Wellbutrin) should be administered in doses of no more than 150 mg and should be given at least 6 hours apart. Bupropion has been associated with a relatively high incidence of seizure activity in anorexic and cachectic clients.

f. Tachycardia; arrhythmias
*Carefully monitor blood pressure and pulse rate and rhythm, and report any significant change to the physician.

g. Photosensitivity
*Ensure that client wears protective sunscreens, clothing, and sunglasses while outdoors.

h. Weight gain
*Provide instructions for reduced-calorie diet.
*Encourage increased level of activity, if appropriate.

3. **Most commonly occur with SSRIs:**
a. Insomnia; agitation
*Administer or instruct client to take dose early in the day.
*Instruct client to avoid caffeinated food and drinks.
*Teach relaxation techniques to use before bedtime.

b. Headache
*Administer analgesics, as prescribed.
*Request that the physician order another SSRI or another class of antidepressants

c. Weight loss (may occur early in therapy)
*Ensure that client is provided with caloric intake sufficient to maintain desired weight.
*Caution should be taken in prescribing these drugs for anorectic clients.
*Weigh client daily or every other day, at the same time, and on the same scale, if possible.
*After prolonged use, some clients may gain weight on SSRIs

d. Sexual dysfunction
*Men may report abnormal ejaculation or impotence.
*Women may experience delay or loss of orgasm.
*If side effect becomes intolerable, a switch to another antidepressant may be necessary.

e. Serotonin syndrome (may occur when two drugs that potentiate serotonergic neurotransmission are used concurrently [see "Interactions"])
*Most frequent symptoms include changes in mental status, restlessness, myoclonus, hyperreflexia, tachycardia, labile blood pressure, diaphoresis, shivering, and tremors.
*Discontinue offending agent immediately.
*The physician will prescribe medications to block serotonin receptors, relieve hyperthermia and muscle rigidity, and prevent seizures. Artificial ventilation may be required.
*The condition will usually resolve on its own once the offending medication has been discontinued. However, if the medication is not discontinued, the condition can progress to a more serious state and become fatal (Schatzberg, Cole, & DeBattista, 2003).

4. **Most commonly occur with MAOIs:**
a. Hypertensive crisis
*Hypertensive crisis occurs if the individual consumes foods containing tyramine while receiving MAOI therapy (see Table 21–5).
*Symptoms of hypertensive crisis include severe occipital headache, palpitations, nausea/vomiting, nuchal rigidity, fever, sweating, marked increase in blood pressure, chest pain, and coma.
*Treatment of hypertensive crisis: discontinue drug immediately; monitor vital signs; administer short-acting antihypertensive medication, as ordered by physician; use external cooling measures to control hyperpyrexia.

5. **Miscellaneous side effects:**
a. Priapism (with trazodone [Desyrel])
*Priapism is a rare side effect, but it has occurred in some men taking trazodone.
*If the client complains of prolonged or inappropriate penile erection, withhold medication dosage and notify the physician immediately.
*Priapism can become very problematic, requiring surgical intervention, and, if not treated successfully, can result in impotence.

b. Hepatic failure (with nefazodone [Serzone])
*Cases of life-threatening hepatic failure have been reported in clients treated with nefazodone.
*Advise clients to be alert for signs or symptoms suggestive of liver dysfunction (e.g., jaundice,

anorexia, GI complaints, or malaise) and to report them to physician immediately.

Client/Family Education.

The client should:

● Continue to take the medication even though the symptoms have not subsided. The therapeutic effect may not be seen for as long as 4 weeks. If after this length of time no improvement is noted, the physician may prescribe a different medication.

● Use caution when driving or operating dangerous machinery. Drowsiness and dizziness can occur. If these side effects become persistent or interfere with activities of daily living, the client should report them to the physician. Dosage adjustment may be necessary.

● Not stop taking the drug abruptly. To do so might produce withdrawal symptoms, such as nausea, vertigo, insomnia, headache, malaise, and nightmares.

● If taking a tricyclic, use sunscreens and wear protective clothing when spending time outdoors. The skin may be sensitive to sunburn.

● Report occurrence of any of the following symptoms to the physician immediately: sore throat, fever, malaise, yellowish skin, unusual bleeding, easy bruising, persistent nausea/vomiting, severe headache, rapid heart rate, difficulty urinating, anorexia/weight loss, seizure activity, stiff or sore neck, and chest pain.

● Rise slowly from a sitting or lying position to prevent a sudden drop in blood pressure.

● Take frequent sips of water, chew sugarless gum, or suck on hard candy if dry mouth is a problem. Good oral care (frequent brushing, flossing) is very important.

● Not consume the following foods or medications while taking MAOIs: aged cheese, wine (especially Chianti), beer, chocolate, colas, coffee, tea, sour cream, beef/chicken livers, canned figs, soy sauce, overripe and fermented foods, pickled herring, preserved sausages, yogurt, yeast products, broad beans, cold remedies, diet pills. To do so could cause a life-threatening hypertensive crisis.

● Avoid smoking while receiving tricyclic therapy. Smoking increases the metabolism of tricyclics, requiring an adjustment in dosage to achieve the therapeutic effect.

● Not drink alcohol while taking antidepressant therapy. These drugs potentiate the effects of each other.

● Not consume other medications (including over-the-counter medications) without the physician's approval while receiving antidepressant therapy. Many medications contain substances that, in combination with antidepressant medication, could precipitate a life-threatening hypertensive crisis.

● Notify physician immediately if inappropriate or prolonged penile erections occur while taking trazodone (Desyrel). If the erection persists longer than 1 hour, seek emergency room treatment. This condition is rare, but has occurred in some men who have taken trazodone. If measures are not instituted immediately, impotence can result.

● Not "double up" on medication if a dose of bupropion (Wellbutrin) is missed, unless advised to do so by the physician. Taking bupropion in divided doses will decrease the risk of seizures and other adverse effects.

● Be aware of possible risks of taking antidepressants during pregnancy. Safe use during pregnancy and lactation has not been fully established. These drugs are believed to readily cross the placental barrier; if so, the fetus could experience adverse effects of the drug. Inform the physician immediately if pregnancy occurs, is suspected, or is planned.

● Be aware of the side effects of antidepressants. Refer to written materials furnished by health care providers for safe self-administration.

● Carry a card or other identification at all times describing the medications being taken.

Outcome Criteria/Evaluation

The following criteria may be used for evaluating the effectiveness of therapy with antidepressant medications:
The client:

1. Has not harmed self.
2. Has not experienced injury caused by side effects such as priapism, hypertensive crisis, or photosensitivity.
3. Exhibits vital signs within normal limits.
4. Manifests symptoms of improvement in mood (brighter affect, interaction with others, improvement in hygiene, clear thought and communication patterns).
5. Willingly participates in activities and interacts appropriately with others.

Mood-stabilizing Agents

Background Assessment Data

For many years, the drug of choice for treatment and management of bipolar mania was lithium carbonate. However, in recent years, a number of investigators and clinicians in practice have achieved satisfactory results with several other medications, either alone or in combination with lithium. Table 21–7 provides information about the indications, actions, and contraindications and precautions of various medications being used as mood stabilizers.

TABLE 21–7 Mood-Stabilizing Agents

CLASSIFICATION: GENERIC (TRADE)	INDICATIONS	MECHANISM OF ACTION	CONTRAINDICATIONS/ PRECAUTIONS	DAILY ADULT DOSAGE RANGE (MG)	THERAPEUTIC PLASMA RANGE
Antimanic					
Lithium carbonate (Eskalith, Lithane; Lithobid)	Prevention and treatment of manic episodes of bipolar disorder. Also used for bipolar depression. Unlabeled uses: Major depression Neutropenia Cluster or migraine headache prophylaxis Alcohol dependence	Not fully understood, but may enhance reuptake of norepinephrine and serotonin, decreasing the levels in the body, resulting in decreased hyperactivity (may take 1–3 weeks for symptoms to subside).	Hypersensitivity. Cardiac or renal disease, dehydration; sodium depletion; brain damage; pregnancy and lactation. Caution with thyroid disorders, diabetes, urinary retention, history of seizures, and with the elderly.	Acute mania 1800–2400 Maintenance: 900–1200	Acute mania: 1.0–1.5 mEq/L Maintenance: 0.6–1.2 mEq/L
Anticonvulsants					
Clonazepam (Klonopin)	Absence, akinetic, and myoclonic seizures. Unlabeled use: bipolar mania.	Action in the treatment of bipolar disorder is unclear.	Hypersensitivity. Glaucoma, liver disease, lactation. Caution in elderly, liver/renal disease, pregnancy.	0.75–16	20–80 ng/ml
Carbamazepine (Tegretol)	Grand mal and psychomotor seizures. Unlabeled uses: bipolar mania, rage reactions, resistant schizophrenia	Action in the treatment of bipolar disorder is unclear.	Hypersensitivity. With MAOIs, lactation. Caution with elderly, liver/ renal/cardiac disease, pregnancy.	200–1200	4–12 µg/ml
Valproic acid (Depakene; Depakote)	Absence seizures; Unlabeled use: bipolar mania, migraine prophylaxis.	Action in the treatment of bipolar disorder is unclear.	Hypersensitivity; liver disease. Caution in elderly, renal/ cardiac diseases, pregnancy and lactation.	500–1500	50–100 µg/ml
Lamotrigine (Lamictal)	Generalized tonic-clonic seizures; absence and myoclonic seizures; Unlabeled use: bipolar disorder.	Action in the treatment of bipolar disorder is unclear.	Hypersensitivity. Caution in renal and hepatic insufficiency, pregnancy, lactation, and children < 16 years old.	100–200	No value established
Gabapentin (Neurontin)	Partial seizures with and without generalization in adults with epilepsy. Unlabeled use: bipolar disorder.	Action in the treatment of bipolar disorder is unclear.	Hypersensitivity. Caution in renal insufficiency, pregnancy, lactation, children, and the elderly.	900–1800	No value established
Topiramate (Topamax)	Partial onset seizures. Unlabeled use: Bipolar disorder.	Action in the treatment of bipolar disorder is unclear.	Hypersensitivity. Caution in renal and hepatic impairment, pregnancy, lactation, children, and the elderly.	50–400	No value established
Calcium Channel Blocker					
Verapamil (Calan; Isoptin)	Angina, arrhythmias, hypertension. Unlabeled use: bipolar mania, migraine headache prophylaxis.	Action in the treatment of bipolar disorder is unclear.	Hypersensitivity; heart block, hypotension, cardiogenic shock, congestive heart failure, pregnancy, lactation. Caution in liver or renal disease, cardiomyopathy, intracranial pressure, the elderly.	80–320	80–300 ng/ml

(Continued on following page)

TABLE 21–7	**Mood-Stabilizing Agents** (*Continued*)				
CLASSIFICATION: GENERIC (TRADE)	**INDICATIONS**	**MECHANISM OF ACTION**	**CONTRAINDICATIONS/ PRECAUTIONS**	**DAILY ADULT DOSAGE RANGE (MG)**	**THERAPEUTIC PLASMA RANGE**
Antipsychotics Olanzapine (Zyprexa) Aripiprazole (Abilify) Chlorpromazine (Thorazine) Quetiapine (Seroquel) Risperidone (Risperdal) Ziprasidone (Geodon)	Schizophrenia Bipolar mania	Action in the treatment of bipolar disorder is unclear	Hypersensitivity, children, lactation. Caution with hepatic or cardiovascular disease, history of seizures, comatose or other CNS-depression, prostatic hypertrophy, narrow-angle glaucoma, pregnancy, elderly and debilitated patients.	Olanzapine 5–20 Aripiprazole 10–30 Chlorpromazine 75–400 Quetiapine 400–800 Risperidone 1–6 Ziprasidone 40–160	Not established

Interactions

Lithium Carbonate. Increased renal excretion of lithium may occur with acetazolamide, osmotic diuretics, and theophylline. Decreased renal excretion of lithium may occur with nonsteroidal anti-inflammatory drugs and thiazide diuretics. There is an increased risk of neurotoxicity with concurrent use of lithium and carbamazepine, haloperidol, or methyldopa. Concurrent use with fluoxetine or loop diuretics may result in increased serum lithium levels. Increased effects of neuromuscular blocking agents or tricyclic antidepressants, and decreased pressor sensitivity of sympathomimetics can occur with concomitant use of lithium. Use of lithium with phenothiazines may result in neurotoxicity, decreased phenothiazine concentrations, or increased lithium concentration. Concurrent use with verapamil may result in decreased lithium levels or lithium toxicity.

Clonazepam. The effects of clonazepam may be increased with concomitant use of CNS depressants, cimetidine, hormonal contraceptives, disulfiram, fluoxetine, isoniazid, ketoconazole, metoprolol, propoxyphene, propranolol, or valproic acid. The effects of clonazepam are decreased by rifampin, barbiturates, theophylline, or phenytoin. Concomitant use may result in increased phenytoin levels and decreased efficacy of levodopa.

Carbamazepine. The effects of carbamazepine may be increased by verapamil, diltiazem, propoxyphene, erythromycin, clarithromycin, SSRIs, antidepressants, cimetidine, barbiturates, isoniazid, or danazol. The effects of carbamazepine may be decreased by felbamate, hydantoins, or phenobarbital. Concurrent use with carbamazepine may decrease levels of corticosteroids, doxycycline, felbamate, quinidine, warfarin, estrogen-containing contraceptives barbiturates, cyclosporine, benzodiazepines, theophylline, lamotrigine, valproic acid, bupropion, and haloperidol.

Valproic Acid. The effects of valproic acid may be increased by chlorpromazine, cimetidine, erythromycin, felbamate, or salicylates. The effects of valproic acid may be decreased by rifampin, carbamazepine, cholestyramine, lamotrigine, phenobarbital, or phenytoin. Concomitant use with valproic acid may increase the effects of tricyclic antidepressants, carbamazepine, CNS depressants, ethosuximide, lamotrigine, phenobarbital, phenytoin, warfarin and other antiplatelet agents, or zidovudine.

Lamotrigine. The effects of lamotrigine are increased by folate inhibitors or valproic acid. The effects of lamotrigine are decreased by primidone, phenobarbital, phenytoin, rifamycin, succinimides, or carbamazepine. Concomitant use with lamotrigine may decrease levels of valproic acid.

Gabapentin. Antacids reduce the bioavailability of gabapentin. Co-administration of gabapentin with cimetidine results in a small decrease in renal excretion of gabapentin.

Topiramate. The effects of topiramate may be decreased with phenytoin, carbamazepine, or valproic acid. Concomitant use of topiramate with alcohol or other CNS depressants can potentiate CNS depression or other cognitive or neuropsychiatric adverse events. A risk of renal stone formation exists with co-administration of topiramate with carbonic anhydrase inhibitors (e.g., acetazolamide or dichlorphenamide). Efficacy of oral contraceptives may be compromised when taken with topiramate. Serum digoxin level is decreased with concomitant topiramate administration.

Verapamil. Additive hypotension can occur with fentanyl, other antihypertensives, nitrates, alcohol, or quinidine. Antihypertensive effects of verapamil may be decreased with nonsteroidal anti-inflammatory drugs. Concurrent use with verapamil may increase serum levels of digoxin. Concomitant use of verapamil with beta-blockers, digoxin, disopyramide, or phenytoin may result in bradycardia, conduction defects, or congestive heart failure. Concurrent use may decrease the metabolism of and increase the risk of toxicity from cyclosporine, prazosin, quinidine, or carbamazepine. Verapamil may decrease the effectiveness of rifampin. Verapamil may increase the muscle-paralyzing effects of nondepolarizing neuromuscular-blocking agents. Verapamil effectiveness may be decreased by coadministration with vitamin D compounds and calcium. Verapamil may alter serum lithium levels.

Antipsychotics. Concomitant use may produce additive CNS depression with alcohol and other CNS depressants. Concomitant use of chlorpromazine and beta-blockers produces increased effects of both. Plasma concentrations of aripiprazole, olanzapine, risperidone, and ziprasidone are decreased with carbamazepine. Plasma concentrations of aripiprazole, risperidone, and ziprasidone are increased with ketoconazole and erythromycin. Effects of quetiapine are increased with concomitant use of cimetidine. Effects of olanzapine are increased with fluvoxamine or fluoxetine, and effects of risperidone are increased with fluoxetine and paroxetine. Effects of dopamine agonists are decreased with olanzapine, quetiapine, risperidone, and ziprasidone. Effects of aripiprazole are increased with concomitant use of quinidine. Effects of quetiapine are decreased with phenytoin or thioridazine, and effects of aripiprazole are decreased with valproate.

Diagnosis

The following nursing diagnoses may be considered for clients receiving therapy with mood-stabilizing agents:

1. Risk for injury related to manic hyperactivity
2. Risk for self-directed or other-directed violence related to unresolved anger turned inward on the self or outward on the environment
3. Risk for injury related to lithium toxicity
4. Risk for activity intolerance related to side effects of drowsiness and dizziness

Planning/Implementation

The plan of care should include monitoring for side effects of therapy with mood-stabilizing agents and intervening when required to prevent the occurrence of adverse events related to medication administration. Side effects and nursing implications for mood-stabilizing agents are presented in Table 21–8.

Lithium Toxicity. The margin between the therapeutic and toxic levels of lithium carbonate is very narrow. The usual ranges of therapeutic serum concentrations are:

TABLE 21–8   Side Effects and Nursing Implications of Mood-Stabilizing Agents

MEDICATION	SIDE EFFECTS	NURSING IMPLICATIONS
Antimanic		
Lithium carbonate (Eskalith, Lithane)	1. Drowsiness, dizziness, headache	1. Ensure that client does not participate in activities that require alertness, or operate dangerous machinery.
	2. Dry mouth; thirst	2. Provide sugarless candy, ice, frequent sips of water Ensure that strict oral hygiene is maintained.
	3. GI upset; nausea/vomiting	3. Administer medications with meals to minimize GI upset.
	4. Fine hand tremors	4. Report to physician, who may decrease dosage. Some physicians prescribe a small dose of beta-blocker propranolol to counteract this effect.
	5. Hypotension; arrhythmias; pulse irregularities	5. Monitor vital signs two or three times a day. Physician may decrease dose of medication.
	6. Polyuria; dehydration	6. May subside after initial week or two. Monitor daily intake and output and weight. Monitor skin turgor daily.
	7. Weight gain	7. Provide instructions for reduced calorie diet. Emphasize importance of maintaining adequate intake of sodium
Anticonvulsants		
Clonazepam (Klonopin) Carbamazepine (Tegretol) Valproic acid (Depakene; Depakote) Gabapentin (Neurontin) Lamotrigine (Lamictal) Topiramate (Topamax)	1. Nausea/vomiting	1. May give with food or milk to minimize GI upset.
	2. Drowsiness; dizziness	2. Ensure that client does not operate dangerous machinery or participate in activities that require alertness.
	3. Blood dyscrasias	3. Ensure that client understands the importance of regular blood tests while receiving anti-convulsant therapy.
	4. Prolonged bleeding time (with valproic acid)	4. Ensure that platelet counts and bleeding time are determined before initiation of therapy with valproic acid. Monitor for spontaneous bleeding or bruising
	5. Risk of severe rash (with lamotrigine)	5. Ensure that client is informed that he or she must report evidence of skin rash to physician immediately
	6. Decreased efficacy with oral contraceptives (with topiramate)	6. Ensure that client is aware of decreased efficacy of oral contraceptives with concomitant use.

(Continued on following page)

TABLE 21-8	Side Effects and Nursing Implications of Mood-Stabilizing Agents *(Continued)*	
MEDICATION	**SIDE EFFECTS**	**NURSING IMPLICATIONS**
Calcium Channel Blocker Verapamil (Calan; Isoptin)	1. Drowsiness; dizziness	1. Ensure that client does not operate dangerous machinery or participate in activities that require alertness.
	2. Hypotension; bradycardia	2. Take vital signs just before initiation of therapy and before daily administration of the medication. Physician will provide acceptable parameters for administration. Report marked changes immediately.
	3. Nausea	3. May give with food to minimize GI upset.
	4. Constipation	4. Encourage increased fluid (if not contraindicated) and fiber in the diet.
Antipsychotics Olanzapine (Zyprexa) Aripiprazole (Abilify) Chlorpromazine (Thorazine) Quetiapine (Seroquel) Risperidone (Risperdal) Ziprasidone (Geodon)	1. Drowsiness; dizziness	1. Ensure that client does not operate dangerous machinery or participate in activities that require alertness.
	2. Dry mouth; constipation	2. Provide sugarless candy or gum, ice, and frequent sips of water. Provide foods high in fiber; encourage physical activity and fluid if not contraindicated.
	3. Increased appetite; weight gain	3. Provide calorie-controlled diet; provide opportunity for physical exercise; provide diet and exercise instruction.
	4. ECG changes	4. Monitor vital signs. Observe for symptoms of dizziness, palpitations, syncope, or weakness.
	5. Extrapyramidal symptoms	5. Monitor for symptoms. Administer p.r.n. medication at first sign.
	6. Hyperglycemia and diabetes	6. Monitor blood glucose regularly. Observe for the appearance of symptoms of polydipsia, polyuria, polyphagia, and weakness at any time during therapy.

- For acute mania: 1.0 to 1.5 mEq/L
- For maintenance: 0.6 to 1.2 mEq/L

Serum lithium levels should be monitored once or twice a week after initial treatment until dosage and serum levels are stable, then monthly during maintenance therapy. Blood samples should be drawn 12 hours after the last dose.

Symptoms of lithium toxicity begin to appear at blood levels greater than 1.5 mEq/L and are dosage determinate. Symptoms include:

- **At serum levels of 1.5 to 2.0 mEq/L:** blurred vision, ataxia, tinnitus, persistent nausea and vomiting, severe diarrhea.
- **At serum levels of 2.0 to 3.5 mEq/L:** excessive output of dilute urine, increasing tremors, muscular irritability, psychomotor retardation, mental confusion, giddiness.
- **At serum levels above 3.5 mEq/L:** impaired consciousness, nystagmus, seizures, coma, oliguria/anuria, arrhythmias, myocardial infarction, cardiovascular collapse.

Lithium levels should be monitored prior to medication administration. The dosage should be withheld and the physician notified if the level reaches 1.5 mEq/L or at the earliest observation or report by the client of even the mildest symptom. If left untreated, lithium toxicity can be life threatening.

Lithium is similar in chemical structure to sodium, behaving in the body in much the same manner and competing with sodium at various sites in the body. If sodium intake is reduced or the body is depleted of its normal sodium (e.g., due to excessive sweating, fever, or diuresis), lithium is reabsorbed by the kidneys, increasing the possibility of toxicity. Therefore, the client must consume a diet adequate in sodium as well as 2500 to 3000 ml of fluid per day. Accurate records of intake, output, and client's weight should be kept on a daily basis.

Client/Family Education (for Lithium)

The client should:

- Take medication on a regular basis, even when feeling well. Discontinuation can result in return of symptoms.
- Not drive or operate dangerous machinery until lithium levels are stabilized. Drowsiness and dizziness can occur.
- Not skimp on dietary sodium intake. He or she should choose foods from the food pyramid and avoid "junk" foods. The client should drink six to eight large glasses of water each day and avoid excessive use of beverages

containing caffeine (coffee, tea, colas), which promote increased urine output.

- Notify the physician if vomiting or diarrhea occurs. These symptoms can result in sodium loss and an increased risk of toxicity.
- Carry card or other identification noting that he or she is taking lithium.
- Be aware of appropriate diet should weight gain become a problem. Include adequate sodium and other nutrients while decreasing number of calories.
- Be aware of risks of becoming pregnant while receiving lithium therapy. Use information furnished by health care providers regarding methods of contraception. Notify the physician as soon as possible if pregnancy is suspected or planned.
- Be aware of side effects and symptoms associated with toxicity. Notify the physician if any of the following symptoms occur: persistent nausea and vomiting, severe diarrhea, ataxia, blurred vision, tinnitus, excessive output of urine, increasing tremors, or mental confusion.
- Refer to written materials furnished by health care providers while receiving self-administered maintenance therapy. Keep appointments for outpatient follow-up; have serum lithium level checked every 1 to 2 months, or as advised by physician.

Client/Family Education (for Anticonvulsants)

The client should:

- Not stop taking drug abruptly. Physician will administer orders for tapering the drug when therapy is to be discontinued.
- Report the following symptoms to the physician immediately: unusual bleeding, spontaneous bruising, sore throat, fever, malaise, dark urine, and yellow skin or eyes.
- Not drive or operate dangerous machinery until reaction to the medication has been established.
- Avoid consuming alcoholic beverages and nonprescription medications without approval from physician.
- Carry card at all times identifying the name of medications being taken.

Client/Family Education (for Calcium Channel Blocker)

The client should:

- Take medication with meals if gastrointestinal (GI) upset occurs.
- Use caution when driving or when operating dangerous machinery. Dizziness, drowsiness, and blurred vision can occur.
- Not abruptly discontinue taking drug. To do so may precipitate cardiovascular problems.
- Report occurrence of any of the following symptoms to physician immediately: irregular heart beat, shortness of breath, swelling of the hands and feet, pronounced dizziness, chest pain, profound mood swings, severe and persistent headache.
- Rise slowly from a sitting or lying position to prevent a sudden drop in blood pressure.
- Not consume other medications (including over-the-counter medications) without the physician's approval.
- Carry card at all times describing medications being taken.

Client/Family Education for Antipsychotics

This information is included in the next section on "Antipsychotic Agents."

Outcome Criteria/Evaluation

The following criteria may be used for evaluating the effectiveness of therapy with mood-stabilizing agents.

The client:

1. Is maintaining stability of mood.
2. Has not harmed self or others.
3. Has experienced no injury from hyperactivity.
4. Is able to participate in activities without excessive sedation or dizziness.
5. Is maintaining appropriate weight.
6. Exhibits no signs of lithium toxicity.
7. Verbalizes importance of taking medication regularly and reporting for regular laboratory blood tests.

Antipsychotic Agents
Background Assessment Data

Indications. Antipsychotic drugs are also called *major tranquilizers* and *neuroleptics*. They are used in the treatment of acute and chronic psychoses, particularly when accompanied by increased psychomotor activity. Selected agents are used as antiemetics (chlorpromazine, perphenazine, prochlorperazine), in the treatment of intractable hiccoughs (chlorpromazine, perphenazine), and for the control of tics and vocal utterances in Tourette's disorder (haloperidol, pimozide). Examples of commonly used antipsychotic agents are presented in Table 21–9.

Action. The exact mechanism of action is not known. These drugs are thought to work by blocking

TABLE 21–9 Antipsychotic Agents

CHEMICAL CLASS	GENERIC (TRADE NAME)	DAILY DOSAGE RANGE (MG)	AVAILABLE FORMS (MG)
Phenothiazines	Chlorpromazine (Thorazine)	75–400	Tabs: 10, 25, 50, 100, 200 Oral conc: 100/ml Suppositories: 100 Inj: 25/ml
	Fluphenazine (Prolixin)	2.5–10	Tabs: 1, 2.5, 5, 10 Elixir: 2.5/5ml Inj: 2.5/ml Inj (long-acting): 25/ml
	Perphenazine (Trilafon)	12–64	Tabs: 2, 4, 8, 16 Oral conc: 16/5 ml Inj: 5/ml
	Prochlorperazine (Compazine)	15–150	Tabs: 5, 10 Caps (SR): 10, 15 Supp: 2.5, 5, 25 Syrup: 5/5ml Inj: 5/ml
	Thioridazine (Mellaril)	150–800	Tabs: 10, 15, 25, 50, 100, 150, 200 Conc: 30/ml, 100/ml
	Trifluoperazine (Stelazine)	4–40	Tabs: 1, 2, 5, 10
Thioxanthene	Thiothixene (Navane)	6–30	Caps: 1, 2, 5, 10, 20 Conc: 5/ml
Benzisoxazole	Risperidone (Risperdal)	1–6	Tabs: 0.25, 0.5, 1, 2, 3, 4 Oral solu: 1/ml Powder for inj: 25, 37.5, 50
Butyrophenone	Haloperidol (Haldol)	1–100	Tabs: 0.5, 1, 2, 5, 10, 20 Conc: 2/ml Inj: 5/ml Inj (long-acting): 50/ml, 100/ml
Dibenzoxazepine	Loxapine (Loxitane)	20–250	Caps: 5, 10, 25, 50
Dihydroindolone	Molindone (Moban)	15–225	Tabs: 5, 10, 25, 50
Dibenzodiazepine	Clozapine (Clozaril)	300–900	Tabs: 12.5, 25, 100
Diphenylbutylpiperidine	Pimozide (Orap)	2–10	Tabs: 1, 2
Thienobenzodiazepine	Olanzapine (Zyprexa)	5–20	Tabs: 2.5, 5, 7.5, 10, 15, 20 Powder for inj: 10
Dibenzothiazepine	Quetiapine (Seroquel)	150–750	Tabs: 25, 100, 200, 300
Benzothiazolylpiperazine	Ziprasidone (Geodon)	40–160	Caps: 20, 40, 60, 80 Powder for inj: 20
Dihydrocarbostyril	Aripiprazole (Abilify)	10–30	Tabs: 5, 10, 15, 20, 30

postsynaptic dopamine receptors in the basal ganglia, hypothalamus, limbic system, brain stem, and medulla. Newer medications may exert antipsychotic properties by blocking action on receptors specific to dopamine, serotonin, and other neurotransmitters. Antipsychotic effects may also be related to inhibition of dopamine-mediated transmission of neural impulses at the synapses (see Chapter 4).

Contraindications/Precautions. These drugs are contraindicated in clients with known hypersensitivity (cross-sensitivity may exist among phenothiazines). They should not be used when CNS depression is evident; when blood dyscrasias exist; in clients with Parkinson's disease; or in clients with liver, renal, or cardiac insufficiency.

Caution should be taken in administering these drugs to clients who are elderly, severely ill or debilitated, and to diabetic clients or clients with respiratory insufficiency, prostatic hypertrophy, or intestinal obstruction. Antipsychotics may lower seizure threshold. Individuals should avoid exposure to extremes in temperature while taking antipsychotic medication. Safety in pregnancy and lactation has not been established.

Interactions. Additive anticholinergic effects are observed when antipsychotics are taken concurrently with other drugs that produce these properties (e.g., antihistamines, antidepressants, antiparkinsonian agents). Additive hypotensive effects may occur with beta-adrenergic blocking agents (e.g., propranolol, metoprolol). Antacids and antidiarrheals may decrease absorption of antipsychotics. Barbiturates may increase metabolism and decrease effectiveness of antipsychotics. Additive CNS depression can occur with alcohol, antihistamines, antidepressants, sedative-hypnotics, and anxiolytics.

Diagnosis

The following nursing diagnoses may be considered for clients receiving antipsychotic therapy:

1. Risk for other-directed violence related to panic anxiety and mistrust of others
2. Risk for injury related to medication side effects of sedation, photosensitivity, reduction of seizure threshold, **agranulocytosis**, **extrapyramidal symptoms**, **tardive dyskinesia**, and **neuroleptic malignant syndrome**
3. Risk for activity intolerance related to medication side effects of sedation, blurred vision, and weakness
4. Noncompliance with medication regimen related to suspiciousness and mistrust of others

Planning/Implementation

The plan of care should include monitoring for the following side effects from antipsychotic medications. Nursing implications related to each side effect are designated by an asterisk (*). A profile of side effects comparing various antipsychotic medications is presented in Table 21–10.

TABLE 21–10   Comparison of Side Effects Among Antipsychotic Agents

CHEMICAL CLASS	GENERIC (TRADE) NAME	EXTRAPYRAMIDAL SYMPTOMS	SEDATION	ANTICHOLINERGIC	ORTHOSTATIC HYPOTENSION	SEIZURES
Phenothiazines	Chlorpromazine (Thorazine)	3	4	3	4	4
	Fluphenazine (Prolixin)	5	2	2	2	2
	Perphenazine (Trilafon)	4	2	2	2	3
	Prochlorperazine (Compazine)	4	3	2	2	4
	Thioridazine (Mellaril)	2	4	4	4	1
	Trifluoperazine (Stelazine)	4	2	2	2	2
Thioxanthenes	Thiothixene (Navane)	4	2	2	2	2
Benzisoxazole	Risperidone (Risperdal)	1	1	1	3	1
Butyrophenone	Haloperidol (Haldol)	5	1	1	1	1
Dibenzoxazepine	Loxapine (Loxitane)	4	3	2	3	4
Dihydroindolone	Molindone (Moban)	4	1	2	2	2
Dibenzodiazepine	Clozapine (Clozaril)	1	5	5	4	4
Thienobenzodiazepine	Olanzapine (Zyprexa)	1	3	2	1	1
Diphenylbutylpiperidine	Pimozide (Orap)	4	3	2	2	2
Dibenzothiazepine	Quetiapine (Seroquel)	1	3	2	1	1
Benzothiazolylpiperazine	Ziprasidone (Geodon)	1	2	1	1	1
Dihydrocarbostyril	Aripiprazole (Abilify)	2	2	1	3	2

KEY:
1 = Very low
2 = Low
3 = Moderate
4 = High
5 = Very high

SOURCE: Adapted from Schatzberg, Cole, & DeBattista (2005); *Drug Facts and Comparisons* (2005); and Tandon & Jibson (2003).

1. **Anticholinergic effects**
   a. Dry mouth
      *Provide the client with sugarless candy or gum, ice, and frequent sips of water.
      *Ensure that client practices strict oral hygiene.
   b. Blurred vision
      *Explain that this symptom will most likely subside after a few weeks.
      *Advise client not to drive a car until vision clears.
      *Clear small items from pathway to prevent falls.
   c. Constipation
      *Order foods high in fiber; encourage increase in physical activity and fluid intake if not contraindicated.
   d. Urinary retention
      *Instruct client to report any difficulty urinating; monitor intake and output.

2. **Nausea; GI upset**
   *Tablets or capsules may be administered with food to minimize GI upset.
   *Concentrates may be diluted and administered with fruit juice or other liquid; they should be mixed immediately before administration.

3. **Skin rash**
   *Report appearance of any rash on skin to physician.
   *Avoid spilling any of the liquid concentrate on skin; contact dermatitis can occur with some medications.

4. **Sedation**
   *Discuss with physician the possibility of administering the drug at bedtime.
   *Discuss with physician a possible decrease in dosage or an order for a less sedating drug.
   *Instruct client not to drive or operate dangerous equipment while experiencing sedation.

5. **Orthostatic hypotension**
   *Instruct client to rise slowly from a lying or sitting position
   *Monitor blood pressure (lying and standing) each shift; document and report significant changes.

6. **Photosensitivity**
   *Ensure that the client wears protective sunscreens, clothing, and sunglasses while spending time outdoors.

7. **Hormonal effects**
   a. Decreased libido, **retrograde ejaculation**, **gynecomastia** (men)
      *Provide explanation of the effects and reassurance of reversibility. If necessary, discuss with physician possibility of ordering alternate medication.
   b. Amenorrhea (women)
      *Offer reassurance of reversibility; instruct client to continue use of contraception, because **amenorrhea** does not indicate cessation of ovulation.
   c. Weight gain

      *Weigh client every other day; order calorie-controlled diet; provide opportunity for physical exercise; provide diet and exercise instruction.

8. **ECG changes**. ECG changes, including prolongation of the QT interval, are possible with most of the antipsychotics. This is particularly true with ziprasidone (Geodon). Caution is advised in prescribing this medication to individuals with history of arrhythmias. Conditions that produce hypokalemia and/or hypomagnesemia, such as diuretic therapy or diarrhea, should be taken into consideration when prescribing. Routine ECG should be taken before initiation of therapy and periodically during therapy.
   *Monitor vital signs every shift.
   *Observe for symptoms of dizziness, palpitations, syncope, or weakness.

9. **Reduction of seizure threshold**
   *Closely observe clients with history of seizures.
   ***NOTE:** This is particularly important with clients taking clozapine (Clozaril). Reportedly, seizures affect up to 5 percent of individuals who take this drug, depending on the dosage (Schatzberg, Cole, & DeBattista, 2005).

10. **Agranulocytosis**
    *Relatively rare with most of the antipsychotic drugs. It usually occurs within the first 3 months of treatment. Observe for symptoms of sore throat, fever, malaise. A complete blood count should be monitored if these symptoms appear.
    ***EXCEPTION:** There is a significant risk of agranulocytosis with clozapine (Clozaril). Agranulocytosis is a potentially fatal blood disorder in which the client's white blood cell (WBC) count can drop to extremely low levels. Individuals receiving clozapine therapy are required to have blood levels drawn weekly for the first 6 months of therapy. They are given a 1-week supply of medication at a time. If the WBC count falls below 3000 mm^3 or the granulocyte count falls below 1500 mm^3, clozapine therapy is discontinued. If the WBC remains within acceptable limits during the first 6 months of therapy, counts may be monitored every other week thereafter. The disorder is reversible if discovered in the early stages. However, this additional required technology of weekly blood tests has made this drug cost prohibitive for some people.

11. **Hypersalivation (with clozapine)**
    *A significant number of clients receiving clozapine (Clozaril) therapy experience extreme salivation. Offer support to the client because this may be an embarrassing situation. It may even be a safety issue (e.g., risk of aspiration) if the problem is very severe.

12. **Extrapyramidal symptoms (EPS)**
    *Observe for symptoms and report; administer antiparkinsonian drugs, as ordered (Table 21–11).

TABLE 21–11	Antiparkinsonian Agents Used to Treat Extrapyramidal Side Effects of Antipsychotic Drugs

Indication	Used to treat parkinsonism of various causes and drug-induced extrapyramidal reactions.
Action	Restores the natural balance of acetylcholine and dopamine in the CNS. The imbalance is a deficiency in dopamine that results in excessive cholinergic activity.
Contraindications/precautions	Antiparkinsonian agents are contraindicated in individuals with hypersensitivity. Anticholinergics should be avoided by individuals with angle-closure glaucoma; pyloric, duodenal, or bladder neck obstructions; prostatic hypertrophy; or myasthenia gravis.
	Caution should be used in administering these drugs to clients with hepatic, renal or cardiac insufficiency; elderly and debilitated clients; those with a tendency toward urinary retention; or those exposed to high environmental temperatures.
Common side effects	Anticholinergic effects (dry mouth, blurred vision, constipation, paralytic ileus, urinary retention, tachycardia, elevated temperature, decreased sweating), nausea/GI upset, sedation, dizziness, orthostatic hypotension, exacerbation of psychoses.

CHEMICAL CLASS	GENERIC (TRADE) NAME	DAILY DOSAGE RANGE (MG)	AVAILABLE FORMS (MG)
Anticholinergics	Benztropine (Cogentin)	1–8	Tabs: 0.5, 1, 2 Inj: 1/ml
	Biperiden (Akineton)	2–6	Tabs: 2
	Procyclidine (Kemadrin)	10–20	Tabs: 5
	Trihexyphenidyl (Artane)	1–15	Tabs: 2, 5
Antihistamines	Diphenhydramine (Benadryl)	25–300	Tabs/caps: 25, 50 Tabs (chewable): 12.5 Elixir/syrup: 12.5/5 ml Liquid/solu: 12.5/5ml Inj: 50/ml
Dopaminergic agonists	Amantadine (Symmetrel)	200–300	Caps: 100 Syrup: 50/5 ml

a. **Pseudoparkinsonism** (tremor, shuffling gait, drooling, rigidity)
   *Symptoms may appear 1 to 5 days following initiation of antipsychotic medication; occurs most often in women, the elderly, and dehydrated clients.

b. **Akinesia** (muscular weakness)
   *Same as for pseudoparkinsonism.

c. **Akathisia** (continuous restlessness and fidgeting)
   *This occurs most frequently in women; symptoms may occur 50 to 60 days following initiation of therapy.

d. **Dystonia** (involuntary muscular movements [spasms] of face, arms, legs, and neck)
   *This occurs most often in men and in people younger than 25 years of age.

e. **Oculogyric crisis** (uncontrolled rolling back of the eyes)
   *This may appear as part of the syndrome described as dystonia. It may be mistaken for seizure activity. Dystonia and oculogyric crisis should be treated as an emergency situation. The physician should be contacted, and intravenous benztropine mesylate (Cogentin) is commonly administered. Stay with the client and offer reassurance and support during this frightening time.

13. **Tardive dyskinesia** (bizarre facial and tongue movements, stiff neck, and difficulty swallowing)

*All clients receiving long-term (months or years) antipsychotic therapy are at risk.
*The symptoms are potentially irreversible.
*The drug should be withdrawn at the first sign, which is usually vermiform movements of the tongue; prompt action may prevent irreversibility.

14. **Neuroleptic malignant syndrome (NMS)**
    *This is a rare, but potentially fatal, complication of treatment with neuroleptic drugs. Routine assessments should include temperature and observation for parkinsonian symptoms.
    *Onset can occur within hours or even years after drug initiation, and progression is rapid over the following 24 to 72 hours.
    *Symptoms include severe parkinsonian muscle rigidity, hyperpyrexia up to 107°F, tachycardia, tachypnea, fluctuations in blood pressure, diaphoresis, and rapid deterioration of mental status to stupor and coma.
    *Discontinue neuroleptic medication immediately.
    *Monitor vital signs, degree of muscle rigidity, intake and output, level of consciousness.
    *The physician may order bromocriptine (Parlodel) or dantrolene (Dantrium) to counteract the effects of neuroleptic malignant syndrome.

15. **Hyperglycemia and diabetes.** Studies have suggested an increased risk of treatment-emergent hyperglycemia-related adverse events in clients using atypical antipsychotics (e.g., risperidone, clozapine,

olanzapine, quetiapine, ziprasidone, and aripiprazole). The FDA recommends that clients with diabetes starting on atypical antipsychotic drugs be monitored regularly for worsening of glucose control. Clients with risk factors for diabetes should undergo fasting blood glucose testing at the beginning of treatment and periodically thereafter. All clients taking these medications should be monitored for symptoms of hyperglycemia (polydipsia, polyuria, polyphagia, and weakness). If these symptoms appear during treatment, the client should undergo fasting blood glucose testing.

Client/Family Education

The client should:

- Use caution when driving or operating dangerous machinery. Drowsiness and dizziness can occur.
- Not stop taking the drug abruptly after long-term use. To do so might produce withdrawal symptoms, such as nausea, vomiting, dizziness, gastritis, headache, tachycardia, insomnia, and tremulousness.
- Use sunscreens and wear protective clothing when spending time outdoors. Skin is more susceptible to sunburn, which can occur in as little as 30 minutes.
- Report weekly (if receiving clozapine therapy) to have blood levels drawn and to obtain a weekly supply of the drug.
- Report the occurrence of any of the following symptoms to the physician immediately: sore throat, fever, malaise, unusual bleeding, easy bruising, persistent nausea and vomiting, severe headache, rapid heart rate, difficulty urinating, muscle twitching, tremors, darkly colored urine, excessive urination, excessive thirst, excessive hunger, weakness, pale stools, yellow skin or eyes, muscular incoordination, or skin rash.
- Rise slowly from a sitting or lying position to prevent a sudden drop in blood pressure.
- Take frequent sips of water, chew sugarless gum, or suck on hard candy, if dry mouth is a problem. Good oral care (frequent brushing, flossing) is very important.
- Consult the physician regarding smoking while on neuroleptic therapy. Smoking increases the metabolism of neuroleptics, requiring an adjustment in dosage to achieve a therapeutic effect.
- Dress warmly in cold weather, and avoid extended exposure to very high or low temperatures. Body temperature is harder to maintain with this medication.
- Not drink alcohol while on neuroleptic therapy. These drugs potentiate each other's effects.
- Not consume other medications (including over-the-counter products) without the physician's approval. Many medications contain substances that interact with neuroleptics in a way that may be harmful.
- Be aware of possible risks of taking neuroleptics during pregnancy. Safe use during pregnancy and lactation has not been established. Neuroleptics are thought to readily cross the placental barrier; if so, a fetus could experience adverse effects of the drug. Inform the physician immediately if pregnancy occurs, is suspected, or is planned.
- Be aware of side effects of neuroleptic drugs. Refer to written materials furnished by health care providers for safe self-administration.
- Continue to take the medication, even if feeling well and as though it is not needed. Symptoms may return if medication is discontinued.
- Carry a card or other identification at all times describing medications being taken.

Outcome Criteria/Evaluation

The following criteria may be used for evaluating the effectiveness of therapy with antipsychotic medications.
The client:

1. Has not harmed others.
2. Has not experienced injury caused by side effects of lowered seizure threshold or photosensitivity.
3. Maintains a WBC within normal limits.
4. Exhibits no symptoms of extrapyramidal side effects, tardive dyskinesia, neuroleptic malignant syndrome, or hyperglycemia.
5. Maintains weight within normal limits.
6. Tolerates activity unaltered by the effects of sedation or weakness.
7. Takes medication willingly.
8. Verbalizes understanding of medication regimen and the importance of regular administration.

Sedative-Hypnotics

Background Assessment Data

Indications. Sedative-hypnotics are used in the short-term management of various anxiety states and to treat insomnia. Selected agents are used as anticonvulsants and preoperative sedatives (phenobarbital, pentobarbital, secobarbital) and to reduce anxiety associated with drug withdrawal (chloral hydrate). Examples of commonly used sedative-hypnotics are presented in Table 21–12.

Action. Sedative-hypnotics cause generalized CNS depression. They may produce tolerance with chronic

TABLE 21–12	Sedative-Hypnotic Agents				
CHEMICAL CLASS	**GENERIC (TRADE) NAME**	**DAILY DOSAGE RANGE (MG)**	**CONTROLLED CATEGORIES**	**HALF-LIFE (HR)**	**AVAILABLE FORMS (MG)**
Barbiturates	Amobarbital (Amytal)	60–200	CII	16–40	Inj: powder, 250/vial, 500/vial
	Butabarbital (Butisol)	45–120	CIII	66–140	Tabs: 15, 30, 50, 100 Elixir: 30/5ml
	Mephobarbital (Mebaral)	32–200	CIV	11–67	Tabs: 32, 50, 100
	Pentobarbital (Ncmbutal)	60–100	CII	15–50	Caps: 100 Elixir: 20/5ml Inj: 50/ml
	Phenobarbital (Luminal)	30–200	CIV	53–118	Tabs: 15, 16, 30, 60, 90, 100 Caps: 16 Elixir: 15/5ml, 20/5ml Inj: 30/ml, 60/ml, 65/ml, 130/ml
	Secobarbital (Seconal)	100–200	CII	15–40	Caps: 100
Benzodiazepines	Estazolam (ProSom)	1–2	CIV	8–28	Tabs: 1, 2
	Flurazepam (Dalmane)	15–30	CIV	2–3 (active metabolite: 47–100)	Caps: 15, 30
	Quazepam (Doral)	7.5–15	CIV	41 (active metabolite: 47–100)	Tabs: 7.5, 15
	Temazepam (Restoril)	15–30	CIV	9–15	Caps: 7.5, 15, 30
	Triazolam (Halcion)	0.125–0.5	CIV	1.5–5.5	Tabs: 0.125, 0.25
Miscellaneous	Chloral hydrate (Noctec)	500–1000	CIV	8–10	Caps: 500 Syrup: 250/5ml, 500/5ml Supp: 324, 648
	Eszopiclone (Lunesta)	1–3	CIV	6	Tabs: 1, 2, 3
	Zaleplon (Sonata)	5–20	CIV	0.5–1.5	Caps: 5, 10
	Zolpidem (Ambien)	5–10	CIV	1.4–4	Tabs: 5, 10

use and have the potential for psychological or physical dependence.

Contraindications/Precautions. Sedative-hypnotics are contraindicated in individuals with hypersensitivity to the drug or to any drug within the chemical class.

Caution should be used in administering these drugs to clients with hepatic dysfunction or severe renal impairment. They should be used with caution in clients who may be suicidal or who may have been addicted to drugs previously. Hypnotic use should be short term. Elderly clients may be more sensitive to CNS depressant effects, and dosage reduction may be required.

Interactions. Additive CNS depression can occur when sedative-hypnotics are taken concomitantly with alcohol, antihistamines, antidepressants, phenothiazines, or any other CNS depressants. Barbiturates induce hepatic drug-metabolizing enzymes and can decrease the effectiveness of drugs metabolized by the liver. Sedative-hypnotics should not be used with MAOIs.

Diagnosis

The following nursing diagnoses may be considered for clients receiving therapy with sedative hypnotics:

1. Risk for injury related to abrupt withdrawal from long-term use or decreased mental alertness caused by residual sedation
2. Disturbed sleep pattern related to situational crises, physical condition, or severe level of anxiety
3. Risk for activity intolerance related to side effects of lethargy, drowsiness, and dizziness
4. Risk for acute confusion related to action of the medication on the CNS

Planning/Implementation

Refer to this section in the discussion of antianxiety medications.

Outcome Criteria/Evaluation

The following criteria may be used for evaluating the effectiveness of therapy with sedative-hypnotic medications:

The client:

1. Demonstrates a reduction in anxiety, tension, and restless activity.

TABLE 21–13	Agents for Attention-Deficit/Hyperactivity Disorder			
CHEMICAL CLASS	GENERIC (TRADE) NAME	DAILY DOSAGE RANGE (MG)	CONTROLLED CATEGORIES	AVAILABLE FORMS (MG)
Amphetamines	Dextroamphetamine sulfate (Dexedrine)	5–60	CII	Tabs: 5, 10 Caps (SR): 5, 10, 15
	Methamphetamine (Desoxyn)	5–25	CII	Tabs: 5
Amphetamine mixtures	Dextroamphetamine/amphetamine (Adderall)	5–60	CII	Tabs: 5, 7.5, 10, 12.5, 15, 20, 30 Caps (XR): 5, 10, 15, 20, 25, 30
Miscellaneous	Methylphenidate (Ritalin; Methylin; Concerta; Metadate)	10–60	CII	Tabs: 5, 10, 20 Tabs (chewable): 2.5, 5, 10 Tabs (ER): 10, 18, 20, 27, 36, 54 Caps (ER): 10, 20, 30, 40
	Dexmethylphenidate (Focalin)	5–20	CII	Tabs: 2.5, 5, 10
	Pemoline (Cylert)	37.5–112.5	CIV	Tabs: 18.75, 37.5, 75 Tabs (chewable): 37.5
	Atomoxetine (Strattera)	>70 kg: 40–100 ≤ 70 kg: 0.5–1.4 mg/kg	—	Caps: 10, 18, 25, 40, 60
	Bupropion (Wellbutrin)	3 mg/kg	—	Tabs: 75, 100 Tabs (SR): 100, 150, 200 Tabs (ER): 150, 300

2. Falls asleep within 30 minutes of taking the medication and remains asleep for 6 to 8 hours without interruption.
3. Is able to participate in usual activities without residual sedation.
4. Experiences no physical injury.
5. Exhibits no evidence of confusion.
6. Verbalizes understanding of taking the medication on a short-term basis.
7. Verbalizes understanding of potential for development of tolerance and dependence with long-term use.

Agents for Attention-Deficit/ Hyperactivity Disorder (ADHD)

Background Assessment Data

Indications. The medications in this section are used for ADHD in children and adults. Examples of commonly used agents for ADHD are presented in Table 21–13.

Action. CNS stimulants increase levels of neurotransmitters (probably norepinephrine, dopamine, and serotonin) in the CNS. They produce CNS and respiratory stimulation, dilated pupils, increased motor activity and mental alertness, diminished sense of fatigue, and brighter spirits. The CNS stimulants discussed in this section include dextroamphetamine sulfate, methamphetamine, amphetamine mixtures, methylphenidate, dexmethylphenidate, and pemoline.

Atomoxetine inhibits the reuptake of norepinephrine, and bupropion blocks the neuronal uptake of serotonin, norepinephrine, and dopamine. The exact mechanism by which these drugs produce the therapeutic effect in ADHD is unknown. They are not CNS stimulants.

Contraindications/Precautions. CNS stimulants are contraindicated in individuals with hypersensitivity to sympathomimetic amines. They should not be used in advanced arteriosclerosis, symptomatic cardiovascular disease, hypertension, hyperthyroidism, glaucoma, agitated or hyperexcitability states, in clients with a history of drug abuse, during or within 14 days of receiving therapy with MAOIs, in children younger than 3 years of age, and in pregnancy. Atomoxetine and bupropion are contraindicated in clients with hypersensitivity to the drugs or their components, and in concomitant use with, or within 2 weeks of using MAO inhibitors. Atomoxetine is contraindicated in clients with narrow-angle glaucoma. Bupropion is contraindicated in individuals with known or suspected seizure disorder, acute phase of myocardial infarction, and in clients with bulimia or anorexia nervosa.

Caution is advised in using CNS stimulants during lactation; with psychotic children; in Tourette disorder; in clients with anorexia or insomnia; in elderly, debilitated, or asthenic clients; and in clients with a history of suicidal or homicidal tendencies. Prolonged use may result in tolerance and physical or psychological dependence. Use atomoxetine and bupropion cautiously in clients with urinary retention; hepatic, renal, or cardiovascular disease; suicidal clients; pregnancy and lactation; and elderly and debilitated clients.

Interactions. Use of CNS stimulants within 14 days following administration of MAOIs may result in hypertensive crisis, headache, hyperpyrexia, intracranial hemorrhage, and bradycardia. Insulin requirements may be altered with CNS stimulants. Urine alkalinizers decrease excretion, enhancing the effects of amphetamines; urine acidifiers increase excretion, decreasing the effects. Decreased effects of both drugs can occur when administered concurrently with phenothiazines. With atomoxetine: increased cardiovascular effects with albuterol; increased risk of neuroleptic malignant syndrome when used within 14 days of MAO inhibitors; increased effects of atomoxetine with concomitant use of CYP 2D6 inhibitors (paroxetine, fluoxetine, quinidine). With bupropion: increased risk of seizures with other drugs that lower seizure threshold; acute toxicity of bupropion with concurrent use of MAOIs; hypertension, seizures, and death can occur when used within 14 days of MAOIs.

Diagnosis

The following nursing diagnoses may be considered for clients receiving therapy with agents for ADHD:

1. Risk for injury related to overstimulation and hyperactivity (CNS stimulants) or seizures (possible side effect of bupropion)
2. Risk for suicide secondary to major depression related to abrupt withdrawal after extended use (CNS stimulants)
3. Imbalanced nutrition, less than body requirements, related to side effects of anorexia and weight loss (CNS stimulants)
4. Disturbed sleep pattern related to overstimulation resulting from use of the medication (CNS stimulants) or side effect of insomnia with atomoxetine
5. Nausea related to side effects of atomoxetine or bupropion
6. Pain related to side effect of headache with atomoxetine or bupropion
7. Risk for activity intolerance related to side effects of sedation and dizziness with atomoxetine or bupropion

Planning/Implementation

The plan of care should include monitoring for the following side effects from agents for ADHD. Nursing implications related to each side effect are designated by an asterisk (*).

1. **Overstimulation, restlessness, insomnia** (CNS stimulants)
   *Assess mental status for changes in mood, level of activity, degree of stimulation, and aggressiveness.
   *Ensure that the client is protected from injury.
   *Keep stimuli low and environment as quiet as possible to discourage overstimulation.
   *To prevent insomnia, administer the last dose at least 6 hours before bedtime. Administer sustained-release forms in the morning.

2. **Palpitations, tachycardia** (CNS stimulants; atomoxetine)
   *Monitor and record vital signs at regular intervals (two or three times a day) throughout therapy. Report significant changes to the physician immediately.

3. **Anorexia, weight loss** (CNS stimulants; atomoxetine; bupropion)
   *To reduce anorexia, the medication may be administered immediately after meals. The client should be weighed regularly (at least weekly) when receiving therapy with CNS stimulants, atomoxetine, or bupropion because of the potential for anorexia/weight loss and temporary interruption of growth and development.

4. **Tolerance, physical and psychological dependence** (CNS stimulants)
   *Tolerance develops rapidly.
   *In children with behavior disorders, a drug "holiday" should be attempted periodically under direction of the physician to determine the effectiveness of the medication and the need for continuation.
   *The drug should not be withdrawn abruptly. To do so could initiate the following syndrome of symptoms: nausea, vomiting, abdominal cramping, headache, fatigue, weakness, mental depression, suicidal ideation, increased dreaming, and psychotic behavior.

5. **Nausea and vomiting** (atomoxetine and bupropion)
   *May be taken with food to minimize GI upset.

6. **Constipation** (atomoxetine and bupropion)
   *Increase fiber and fluid in diet, if not contraindicated.

7. **Potential for seizures** (bupropion)
   *Protect client from injury if seizure should occur. Instruct family and significant others of clients on bupropion therapy how to protect client during a seizure if one should occur. Ensure that doses of the medication are administered at least 8 hours apart.

Client/Family Education

The client should:

- Use caution in driving or operating dangerous machinery. Drowsiness, dizziness, and blurred vision can occur.
- Not stop taking CNS stimulants abruptly. To do so could produce serious withdrawal symptoms.
- Avoid taking CNS stimulants late in the day to prevent insomnia. Take no later than 6 hours before bedtime.
- Not take other medications (including over-the-counter drugs) without physician's approval. Many medications contain substances that, in combination with agents for ADHD, can be harmful.
- Diabetic clients should monitor blood sugar two or three times a day or as instructed by the physician. Be

aware of need for possible alteration in insulin requirements because of changes in food intake, weight, and activity.

● Avoid consumption of large amounts of caffeinated products (coffee, tea, colas, chocolate), as they may enhance the CNS stimulant effect.

● Notify physician if restlessness, insomnia, anorexia, or dry mouth becomes severe or if rapid, pounding heartbeat becomes evident.

● Be aware of possible risks of taking agents for ADHD during pregnancy. Safe use during pregnancy and lactation has not been established. Inform the physician immediately if pregnancy is suspected or planned.

● Be aware of potential side effects of agents for ADHD. Refer to written materials furnished by health care providers for safe self-administration.

● Carry a card or other identification at all times describing medications being taken.

Outcome Criteria/Evaluation

The following criteria may be used for evaluating the effectiveness of therapy with agents for ADHD.

The client:
1. Does not exhibit excessive hyperactivity.
2. Has not experienced injury.
3. Is maintaining expected parameters of growth and development.
4. Verbalizes understanding of safe self-administration and the importance of not withdrawing medication abruptly.

SUMMARY

Psychotropic medications are intended to be used as adjunctive therapy to individual or group psychotherapy. *Antianxiety agents* are used in the treatment of anxiety disorders and to alleviate acute anxiety symptoms. The benzodiazepines are the most commonly used group. They are CNS depressants and have a potential for physical and psychological dependence. They should not be discontinued abruptly following long-term use because they can produce a life-threatening withdrawal syndrome. The most common side effects are drowsiness, confusion, and lethargy.

Antidepressants elevate mood and alleviate other symptoms associated with moderate-to-severe depression. These drugs work to increase the concentration of norepinephrine and serotonin in the body. The tricyclics and related drugs accomplish this by blocking the reuptake of these chemicals by the neurons. Another group of antidepressants inhibit MAO, an enzyme that is known to inactivate norepinephrine and serotonin. They are called

MAO inhibitors (MAOIs). A third category of drugs block neuronal reuptake of serotonin, and has minimal or no effect on reuptake of norepinephrine or dopamine. They are called selective serotonin reuptake inhibitors (SSRIs). Antidepressant medications may take up to 4 weeks to produce the desired effect. The most common side effects are anticholinergic effects, sedation, and orthostatic hypotension. They can also reduce the seizure threshold. MAOIs can cause hypertensive crisis if products containing tyramine are consumed while taking these medications.

Lithium carbonate is widely used as a *mood-stabilizing agent*. Its mechanism of action is not fully understood, but it is thought to enhance the reuptake of norepinephrine and serotonin in the brain, thereby lowering the levels in the body, resulting in decreased hyperactivity. The most common side effects are dry mouth, GI upset, polyuria, and weight gain. There is a very narrow margin between the therapeutic and toxic levels of lithium. Serum levels must be drawn regularly to monitor for toxicity. Symptoms of lithium toxicity begin to appear at serum levels of approximately 1.5 mEq/L. If left untreated, lithium toxicity can be life-threatening.

Several other medications are used as mood-stabilizing agents. Two groups, anticonvulsants (carbamazepine, clonazepam, valproic acid, gabapentin, lamotrigine, and topiramate) and the calcium channel blocker, verapamil, have been used with some effectiveness. Their action in the treatment of bipolar mania is unknown. Most recently, a number of atypical antipsychotic medications have been used with success in the treatment of bipolar mania. These include olanzapine, aripiprazole, quetiapine, risperidone, and ziprasidone. Their action in the treatment of bipolar mania is not understood.

Antipsychotic drugs are used in the treatment of acute and chronic psychoses. Their action is unknown but is thought to decrease the activity of dopamine in the brain. The phenothiazines are a widely used group. Their most common side effects include anticholinergic effects, sedation, weight gain, reduction in seizure threshold, photosensitivity, and extrapyramidal symptoms. A newer generation of antipsychotic medications, which includes clozapine, risperidone, olanzapine, quetiapine, aripiprazoole, and ziprasidone may have an effect on dopamine, serotonin, and other neurotransmitters. They show promise of greater efficacy with fewer side effects.

Antiparkinsonian agents are used to counteract the extrapyramidal symptoms associated with antipsychotic medications. Antiparkinsonian drugs work to restore the natural balance of acetylcholine and dopamine in the brain. The most common side effects of these drugs are the anticholinergic effects. They may also cause sedation and orthostatic hypotension.

Sedative-hypnotics are used in the management of anxiety states and to treat insomnia. These CNS depressants have the potential for physical and psychological dependence. They are indicated for short-term use only. Side effects and nursing implications are similar to those described for antianxiety medications.

Several medications have been designated as *agents for treatment of ADHD*. These include CNS stimulants, which have the potential for physical and psychological dependence. Tolerance develops quickly with CNS stimulants, and they should not be withdrawn abruptly because they can produce serious withdrawal symptoms. The most common side effects are restlessness, anorexia, and insomnia. Other medications that have shown to be effective with ADHD include atomoxetine and bupropion. Their action in the treatment of ADHD is unknown.

REVIEW QUESTIONS

SELF-EXAMINATION/LEARNING EXERCISE

Select the answer that is most appropriate for each of the following questions.

1. Antianxiety medications produce a calming effect by:
   a. Depressing the CNS.
   b. Decreasing levels of norepinephrine and serotonin in the brain.
   c. Decreasing levels of dopamine in the brain.
   d. Inhibiting production of the enzyme MAO.

2. Nancy has a new diagnosis of panic disorder. Dr. S has written a p.r.n. order for alprazolam (Xanax) for when Nancy is feeling anxious. She says to the nurse, "Dr. S prescribed Buspirone for my friend's anxiety. Why did he order something different for me?" The nurse's answer is based on which of the following?
   a. Buspirone is not an antianxiety medication.
   b. Alprazolam and buspirone are essentially the same medication, so either one is appropriate.
   c. Buspirone has delayed onset of action and cannot be used on a p.r.n. basis.
   d. Alprazolam is the only medication that really works for panic disorder.

3. Education for the client who is taking MAOIs should include which of the following?
   a. Fluid and sodium replacement when appropriate, frequent drug blood levels, signs and symptoms of toxicity
   b. Lifetime of continuous use, possible tardive dyskinesia, advantages of an injection every 2 to 4 weeks
   c. Short-term use, possible tolerance to beneficial effects, careful tapering of the drug at end of treatment
   d. Tyramine-restricted diet, prohibitive concurrent use of over-the-counter medications without physician notification

4. There is a very narrow margin between the therapeutic and toxic levels of lithium carbonate. Symptoms of toxicity are most likely to appear if the serum levels exceed
   a. 0.15 mEq/L
   b. 1.5 mEq/L
   c. 15.0 mEq/L
   d. 150 mEq/L

5. Initial symptoms of lithium toxicity include:
   a. Constipation, dry mouth, drowsiness, oliguria
   b. Dizziness, thirst, dysuria, arrhythmias
   c. Ataxia, tinnitus, blurred vision, diarrhea
   d. Fatigue, vertigo, anuria, weakness

6. Antipsychotic medications are thought to decrease psychotic symptoms by:
   a. Blocking reuptake of norepinephrine and serotonin.
   b. Blocking the action of dopamine in the brain.
   c. Inhibiting production of the enzyme MAO.
   d. Depressing the CNS.

7. Part of the nurse's continual assessment of the client taking antipsychotic medications is to observe for extrapyramidal symptoms. Examples include:
   a. Muscular weakness, rigidity, tremors, facial spasms
   b. Dry mouth, blurred vision, urinary retention, orthostatic hypotension
   c. Amenorrhea, gynecomastia, retrograde ejaculation
   d. Elevated blood pressure, severe occipital headache, stiff neck

8. If the foregoing extrapyramidal symptoms should occur, which of the following would be a priority nursing intervention?
   a. Notify the physician immediately.
   b. Administer p.r.n. trihexyphenidyl (Artane).
   c. Withhold the next dose of antipsychotic medication.
   d. Explain to the client that these symptoms are only temporary and will disappear shortly.

9. A concern with children on long-term therapy with CNS stimulants for ADHD is:
   a. Addiction
   b. Weight gain
   c. Substance abuse
   d. Growth suppression

10. Doses of bupropion should be administered at least 8 hours apart and never doubled when a dose is missed. The reason for this is:
    a. To prevent orthostatic hypotension.
    b. To prevent seizures.
    c. To prevent hypertensive crisis.
    d. To prevent extrapyramidal symptoms.

REFERENCES

Bernstein, J.G. (1995). *Handbook of drug therapy in psychiatry* (3rd ed.). St. Louis: C.V. Mosby.

Depression Guideline Panel. (1993). *Depression in primary care:* Volume 2. *Treatment of major depression. Clinical practice guideline,* No. 5. Rockville, MD: U.S. Department of Health and Human Services, Public Health Service, Agency for Health Care Policy and Research. AHCPR Pub. No. 93-0551.

Drug facts and comparison (59th ed.). (2005). St. Louis: Wolters Kluwer.

Glod, C.A., & Levy, S. (1998). Psychopharmacology. In C.A. Glod (Ed.). *Contemporary psychiatric-mental health nursing: The brain-behavior connection.* Philadelphia: F.A. Davis.

Haddad, P.M. (2001). Antidepressant discontinuation syndromes: Clinical relevance, prevention, and management. *Drug Safety,* 24(3), 183–197.

Marangell, L.B., Silver, J.M., Goff, D.C., & Yudofsky, S.C. (2003). Psychopharmacology and electroconvulsive therapy. In R.E. Hales & S.C. Yudofsky (Eds.). *Textbook of clinical psychiatry* (4th ed.). Washington, DC: American Psychiatric Publishing.

Sadock, B.J., & Sadock, V.A. (2003). *Synopsis of psychiatry: Behavioral sciences/clinical psychiatry* (9th ed.). Philadelphia: Lippincott Williams & Wilkins.

Sage, D.L. (Producer) (1984). *The Brain: Madness.* Washington, DC: Public Broadcasting Company.

Schatzberg, A.F., Cole, J.O., & DeBattista, C. (2005). *Manual of clinical psychopharmacology* (5th ed.). Washington, DC: American Psychiatric Publishing.

Tandon, R., & Jibson, M.D. (2003). Safety and tolerability: How do second-generation atypical antipsychotics compare? *Current Psychosis & Therapeutic Reports,* 1:15–21.

22
CHAPTER

ELECTROCONVULSIVE
THERAPY

CHAPTER OUTLINE

OBJECTIVES

ELECTROCONVULSIVE THERAPY,
DEFINED

HISTORICAL PERSPECTIVES

INDICATIONS

CONTRAINDICATIONS

MECHANISM OF ACTION

SIDE EFFECTS

RISKS ASSOCIATED WITH
ELECTROCONVULSIVE THERAPY

THE ROLE OF THE NURSE IN
ELECTROCONVULSIVE THERAPY

SUMMARY

REVIEW QUESTIONS

KEY TERMS

insulin coma therapy   pharmacoconvulsive
                            therapy

CORE CONCEPT

electroconvulsive
therapy

OBJECTIVES

After reading this chapter, the student will be able to:

1. Define *electroconvulsive therapy*.
2. Discuss historical perspectives related to electroconvulsive therapy.
3. Discuss indications, contraindications, mechanism of action, and side effects of electroconvulsive therapy.

4. Identify risks associated with electroconvulsive therapy.
5. Describe the role of the nurse in the administration of electroconvulsive therapy.

 lectroconvulsive therapy (ECT) has had very bad press. In the movie *One Flew Over the Cuckoo's Nest*, it is depicted as a physically and emotionally brutal procedure imposed on unwilling clients in order to calm them. Today, ECT remains one of the most controversial treatments for psychological disorders and continues to be the subject of impassioned debate among various factions of society, within both the professional and lay communities.

Despite its controversial image, ECT has been used continuously for more than 50 years, longer than any other physical treatment available for mental illness. It has achieved this longevity because when administered properly, for the right illness, it can help as much as or more than any other treatment (Popolos, 2005).

This chapter explores the historical perspectives, indications and contraindications, mechanism of action, side effects, and risks associated with ECT. The role of the nurse in the care of the client receiving ECT is presented in the context of the nursing process.

314

ELECTROCONVULSIVE THERAPY, DEFINED

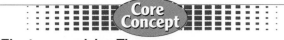

Electroconvulsive Therapy
The induction of a grand mal (generalized) seizure through the application of electrical current to the brain.

The stimulus is applied through electrodes that are placed either bilaterally in the front temporal region or unilaterally on the same side as the dominant hand (Marangell et al., 2003). Controversy exists over optimal placement of the electrodes in terms of possible greater efficacy with bilateral placement versus the potential in some clients for less confusion and acute amnesia with unilateral placement.

The amount of electrical stimulus applied is a point of controversy among clinicians. Dose of stimulation is based on the client's seizure threshold, which is highly variable among individuals. The duration of the seizure should be at least 25 seconds (Sadock & Sadock, 2003). Movements are very minimal because of the administration of a muscle relaxant before the treatment. The tonic phase of the seizure usually lasts 10 to 15 seconds and may be identified by a rigid plantar extension of the feet. The clonic phase follows and is usually characterized by rhythmic movements of the muscles that decrease in frequency and finally disappear. Because of the muscle relaxant, movements may be observed merely as a rhythmic twitching of the toes.

Most clients require an average of 6 to 12 treatments, but some may require up to 20 treatments (Sadock & Sadock, 2003). Treatments are usually administered every other day, three times per week. Treatments are performed on an inpatient basis for those who require close observation and care (e.g., clients who are suicidal, agitated, delusional, catatonic, or acutely manic). Those at less risk may have the option of receiving therapy at an outpatient treatment facility.

HISTORICAL PERSPECTIVES

The first electroconvulsive therapy treatment was performed in April 1938 by Italian psychiatrists Ugo Cerletti and Lucio Bini in Rome. Other somatic therapies had been tried before that time, in particular **insulin coma therapy** and **pharmacoconvulsive therapy**.

Insulin coma therapy was introduced by the German psychiatrist Manfred Sakel in 1933. His therapy was used for clients with schizophrenia. The insulin injection treatments would induce a hypoglycemic coma, which Sakel claimed was effective in alleviating schizophrenic symptoms. This therapy required vigorous medical and nursing intervention through the stages of induced coma. Some fatalities occurred when clients failed to respond to efforts directed at termination of the coma. The efficacy of insulin coma therapy has been questioned, and its use has been discontinued in the treatment of mental illness.

Pharmacoconvulsive therapy was introduced in Budapest in 1934 by Ladislas Meduna (Fink, 1999). He induced convulsions with intramuscular injections of camphor in oil in clients with schizophrenia. He based his treatment on clinical observation and on his theory that there was a biological antagonism between schizophrenia and epilepsy. Thus, by inducing seizures he hoped to reduce schizophrenic symptoms. Because he discovered that camphor was unreliable for inducing seizures, he began using pentylenetetrazol (Metrazol). Some successes were reported in terms of reduction of psychotic symptoms, and, until the advent of ECT in 1938, pentylenetetrazol was the most frequently used procedure for producing seizures in psychotic clients. There was a brief resurgence of pharmacoconvulsive therapy in the late 1950s, when flurothyl (Indoklon), a potent inhalant convulsant, was introduced as an alternative for individuals who were unwilling to consent to ECT for the treatment of depression and schizophrenia. Pharmacoconvulsive therapy is no longer used in psychiatry.

Periodic recognition of the important contribution of ECT in the treatment of mental illness has been evident in the United States. An initial acceptance was observed from 1940 to 1955, followed by a 20-year period in which ECT was considered objectionable by both the psychiatric profession and the lay public. A second wave of acceptance began around 1975 and has been increasing to the present. The period of nonacceptability coincided with the introduction of tricyclic and monoamine oxidase inhibitor antidepressant drugs and ended with the realization among many psychiatrists that the widely heralded replacement of ECT with these chemical agents had failed to materialize (Abrams, 2002). Some individuals showed improvement with ECT after failing to respond to other forms of therapy.

Currently, an estimated 100,000 people per year receive ECT treatments in the United States (Sadock & Sadock, 2003). The typical client is white, female, middle-aged and from a middle- to upper-income background, receiving treatment in a private or university hospital for major depression, usually after drug therapy has proved ineffective. Largely because of the expense involved, as well as the need for a team of highly skilled medical specialists, many public hospitals are not able to offer this service to their clients.

INDICATIONS

Major Depression

ECT has been shown to be effective in the treatment of severe depression. It appears to be particularly effective in depressed clients who are also experiencing psychotic symptoms and those with psychomotor retardation and neurovegetative changes, such as disturbances in sleep, appetite, and energy. These symptoms are associated with the diagnoses of major depressive disorder, major depressive disorder with psychotic or melancholic symptoms, and bipolar disorder depression (Sadock & Sadock, 2003). ECT is not often used as the treatment of choice for depressive disorders but is considered only after a trial of therapy with antidepressant medication has proved ineffective.

Mania

ECT is also indicated in the treatment of acute manic episodes of bipolar affective disorder (Marangell et al., 2003). At present it is rarely used for this purpose, having been superceded by the widespread use of antipsychotic drugs and/or lithium. However, it has been shown to be effective in the treatment of manic clients who do not tolerate or fail to respond to lithium or other drug treatment, or when life is threatened by dangerous behavior or exhaustion.

Schizophrenia

ECT can induce a remission in some clients who present with acute schizophrenia, particularly if it is accompanied by catatonic or affective (depression or mania) symptomatology (Sadock & Sadock, 2003). It does not appear to be of value to individuals with chronic schizophrenic illness.

Other Conditions

ECT has also been tried with clients experiencing a variety of neuroses, obsessive–compulsive disorders, and personality disorders. Little evidence exists to support the efficacy of ECT in the treatment of these conditions.

CONTRAINDICATIONS

The only absolute contraindication for ECT is increased intracranial pressure (from brain tumor, recent cardiovascular accident, or other cerebrovascular lesion). ECT is associated with a physiological rise in cerebrospinal fluid pressure during the treatment, resulting in increased intracranial pressure that could lead to brain stem herniation (Marangell et al., 2003).

Various other conditions, not considered absolute contraindications but rendering clients at high risk for the treatment, have been identified (Eisendrath & Lichtmacher, 2005; Marangell et al., 2003; Sadock & Sadock, 2003). These conditions are largely cardiovascular in nature and include myocardial infarction or cerebrovascular accident within the preceding 3 months, aortic or cerebral aneurysm, severe underlying hypertension, and congestive heart failure. Clients with cardiovascular problems are placed at risk because of the response of the body to the seizure itself. The initial vagal response results in a sinus bradycardia and drop in blood pressure. This is followed immediately by tachycardia and a hypertensive response. These changes can be life threatening to an individual with an already compromised cardiovascular system. Other factors that place clients at risk for ECT include severe osteoporosis, acute and chronic pulmonary disorders, and high-risk or complicated pregnancy.

MECHANISM OF ACTION

The exact mechanism by which ECT affects a therapeutic response is unknown. Several theories exist, but the one to which the most credibility has been given is the biochemical theory. A number of researchers have demonstrated that electric stimulation results in significant increases in the circulating levels of several neurotransmitters (Wahlund & von Rosen, 2003). These neurotransmitters include serotonin, norepinephrine, and dopamine, the same biogenic amines that are affected by antidepressant drugs. Additional evidence suggests that ECT may also result in increases in glutamate and gamma-aminobutyric acid (Ishihara & Sasa, 1999). The results of studies relating to the mechanism underlying the effectiveness of ECT are still ongoing and continue to be controversial.

SIDE EFFECTS

The most common side effects of ECT are temporary memory loss and confusion. Critics of the therapy argue that these changes represent irreversible brain damage. Proponents insist they are temporary and reversible. Marangell and associates (2003) state, "To date, no reliable data have shown permanent memory loss caused by modern ECT." Other researchers have suggested that varying degrees of memory loss may be evident in some clients up to 6 to 7 months following ECT (Popolos, 2002; Sadock & Sadock, 2003).

The controversy continues regarding the choice of unilateral versus bilateral ECT. Studies have shown that unilateral placement of the electrodes decreases the amount of memory disturbance. However, unilateral ECT often requires a higher stimulus dose or a greater number of treatments to match the efficacy of bilateral ECT in the relief of depression (Geddes, 2003).

RISKS ASSOCIATED WITH ELECTROCONVULSIVE THERAPY

Mortality

Studies indicate that the mortality rate from ECT is about 2 per 100,000 treatments (Marangell et al., 2003; Sadock & Sadock, 2003). Although the occurrence is rare, the major cause of death with ECT is from cardiovascular complications (e.g., acute myocardial infarction or cerebrovascular accident), usually in individuals with previously compromised cardiac status. Assessment and management of cardiovascular disease *prior to* treatment is vital in the reduction of morbidity and mortality rates associated with ECT.

Permanent Memory Loss

Marangell and associates (2003) state:

> The initial confusion and cognitive deficits associated with ECT treatment are usually temporary, lasting approximately 30 minutes. Whereas many patients report no problems with their memory, aside form the time immediately surrounding the ECT treatments, others report that their memory is not as good as it was before receiving ECT. To date, no reliable data have shown permanent memory loss caused by modern ECT. Prospective computed tomography and magnetic resonance imaging studies of the brain show no evidence of ECT-induced structural changes. (p. 1126)

Brain Damage

Brain damage from ECT remains a concern for those who continue to believe in its usefulness and efficacy as a treatment for depression. Critics of the procedure remain adamant in their belief that ECT always results in some degree of immediate brain damage (Frank, 2002). However, evidence is based largely on animal studies in which the subjects received excessive electrical dosages, and the seizures were unmodified by muscle paralysis and oxygenation (Abrams, 2003). Although this is an area for continuing study, there is no evidence to substantiate that ECT produces any permanent changes in brain structure or functioning (Sadock & Sadock, 2003).

THE ROLE OF THE NURSE IN ELECTROCONVULSIVE THERAPY

Nurses routinely assist with ECT, providing support before, during, and after the treatment to the client, family, and medical professionals who are conducting the therapy. The nursing process provides a systematic approach to the provision of care for the client receiving ECT.

Assessment

A complete physical examination must be completed by the appropriate medical professional prior to the initiation of ECT. This evaluation should include a thorough assessment of cardiovascular and pulmonary status as well as laboratory blood and urine studies. A skeletal history and X-ray assessment should also be considered.

The nurse may be responsible for ensuring that informed consent has been obtained from the client. If the depression is severe and the client is clearly unable to consent to the procedure, permission may be obtained from family or other legally responsible individual. Consent is secured only after the client or responsible individual acknowledges understanding of the procedure, including possible side effects and potential risks involved.

Nurses may also be required to assess:

- The client's mood and level of interaction with others
- Evidence of suicidal ideation, plan, and means
- Level of anxiety and fears associated with receiving ECT
- Thought and communication patterns
- Baseline memory for short- and long-term events
- Client and family knowledge of indications for, side effects of, and potential risks involved with ECT
- Current and past use of medications
- Baseline vital signs and history of allergies
- The client's ability to carry out activities of daily living

Diagnosis/Outcome Identification

Selection of appropriate nursing diagnoses for the client undergoing ECT is based on continual assessment before, during, and after treatment. Selected potential nursing diagnoses with outcome criteria for evaluation are presented in Table 22–1.

Planning/Implementation

ECT treatments are usually performed in the morning. The client is given nothing by mouth (NPO) for 4 to 8 hours before the treatment. Some institutional policies require that the client be placed on NPO status at midnight prior to the treatment day. The treatment team routinely consists of the psychiatrist, anesthesiologist, and two or more nurses.

Nursing interventions before the treatment include:

- Ensure that the physician has obtained informed consent and that a signed permission form is on the chart.

TABLE 22–1 Potential Nursing Diagnoses and Outcome Criteria for Client Receiving ECT	
NURSING DIAGNOSES	**OUTCOME CRITERIA**
Anxiety (moderate to severe) related to impending therapy	Client verbalizes a decrease in anxiety following explanation of procedure and expression of fears.
Deficient knowledge related to necessity for and side effects or risks of ECT	Client verbalizes understanding of need for and side effects/risks of ECT following explanation.
Risk for injury related to risks associated with ECT	Client undergoes treatment without sustaining injury
Risk for aspiration related to altered level of consciousness immediately following treatment	Client experiences no aspiration during ECT
Decreased cardiac output related to vagal stimulation occurring during the ECT	Client demonstrates adequate tissue perfusion during and after treatment (absence of cyanosis or severe change in mental status).
Disturbed thought processes related to side effects of temporary memory loss and confusion	Client maintains reality orientation following ECT treatment.
Self-care deficit related to incapacitation during postictal stage	Client's self-care needs are fulfilled at all times.
Risk for activity intolerance related to post-ECT confusion and memory loss	Client gradually increases participation in therapeutic activities to the highest level of personal capability.

● Ensure that the most recent laboratory reports (complete blood count, urinalysis) and results of electrocardiogram (ECG) and X-ray examination are available.

● Approximately 1 hour before treatment is scheduled, take vital signs and record them. Have the client void and remove dentures, eyeglasses or contact lenses, jewelry, and hairpins. Following institutional requirements, the client should change into hospital gown or, if permitted, into own loose clothing or pajamas. Client should remain in bed with side rails up.

● Approximately 30 minutes before treatment, administer the pretreatment medication as prescribed by the physician. The usual order is for atropine sulfate or glycopyrrolate (Robinul) given intramuscularly. Either of these medications may be ordered to decrease secretions and counteract the effects of vagal stimulation induced by the ECT.

● Stay with the client to help allay fears and anxiety. Maintain a positive attitude about the procedure, and encourage the client to verbalize feelings.

In the treatment room the client is placed on the treatment table in a supine position. The anesthesiologist administers intravenously a short-acting anesthetic, such as thiopental sodium (Pentothal) or methohexital sodium (Brevital). A muscle relaxant, usually succinylcholine chloride (Anectine), is given intravenously to prevent severe muscle contractions during the seizure, thereby reducing the possibility of fractured or dislocated bones. Because succinylcholine paralyzes respiratory muscles as well, the client is oxygenated with pure oxygen during and after the treatment, except for the brief interval of electrical stimulation, until spontaneous respirations return (Sadock & Sadock, 2003). A blood pressure cuff may be placed on the lower leg and inflated above systolic pressure prior to the injection of the succinyl-

choline. This is to ensure that the seizure activity can be observed in this one limb that is unaffected by the muscle relaxant.

An airway/bite block is placed in the client's mouth and he or she is positioned to facilitate airway patency. Electrodes are placed (either bilaterally or unilaterally) on the temples to deliver the electrical stimulation.

Nursing interventions during the treatment include:

● Ensure patency of airway. Provide suctioning if needed.
● Assist anesthesiologist with oxygenation as required.
● Observe readouts on machines monitoring vital signs and cardiac functioning.
● Provide support to the client's arms and legs during the seizure.
● Observe and record the type and amount of movement induced by the seizure.

After the treatment the anesthesiologist continues to oxygenate the client with pure oxygen until spontaneous respirations return. Most clients awaken within 10 or 15 minutes of the treatment and are confused and disoriented; however, some clients will sleep for 1 to 2 hours following the treatment. All clients require close observation in this immediate post treatment period.

Nursing interventions in the post treatment period include:

● Monitor pulse, respirations, and blood pressure every 15 minutes for the first hour, during which time the client should remain in bed.
● Position the client on side to prevent aspiration.
● Orient the client to time and place.
● Describe what has occurred.
● Provide reassurance that any memory loss the client may be experiencing is only temporary.

- Allow the client to verbalize fears and anxieties related to receiving ECT.
- Stay with the client until he or she is fully awake, oriented, and able to perform self-care activities without assistance.
- Provide the client with a highly structured schedule of routine activities in order to minimize confusion.

Evaluation

Evaluation of the effectiveness of nursing interventions is based on the achievement of the projected outcomes. Reassessment may be based on answers to the following questions:

- Was the client's anxiety maintained at a manageable level?
- Was the client/family teaching completed satisfactorily?
- Did the client/family verbalize understanding of the procedure, its side effects, and risks involved?
- Did the client undergo treatment without experiencing injury or aspiration?
- Has the client maintained adequate tissue perfusion during and following treatment? Have vital signs remained stable?
- With consideration to the individual client's condition and response to treatment, is the client reoriented to time, place, and situation?
- Have all of the client's self-care needs been fulfilled?
- Is the client participating in therapeutic activities to his or her maximum potential?
- What is the client's level of social interaction?

Careful documentation is an important part of the evaluation process. Some routine observations may be evaluated on flow sheets specifically identified for ECT. However, progress notes with detailed descriptions of client behavioral changes are essential to evaluate improvement and help determine the number of treatments that will be administered. Continual reassessment, planning, and evaluation will ensure that the client receives adequate and appropriate nursing care throughout the course of therapy.

SUMMARY

Electroconvulsive therapy is the induction of a grand mal seizure through the application of electrical current to the brain. It is a safe and effective treatment alternative for individuals with depression, mania, or schizoaffective disorder who do not respond to other forms of therapy.

Electroconvulsive therapy is contraindicated for individuals with increased intracranial pressure. Individuals with cardiovascular problems are at high risk for complications from ECT. Other factors that place clients at risk include severe osteoporosis, acute and chronic pulmonary disorders, and high-risk or complicated pregnancy.

The exact mechanism of action of ECT is unknown, but it is thought that the electrical stimulation results in significant increases in the circulating levels of the neurotransmitters serotonin, norepinephrine, and dopamine.

The most common side effects with ECT are temporary memory loss and confusion. Although it is rare, death must be considered a risk associated with ECT. When it does occur, the most common cause is cardiovascular complications. Other possible risks include permanent memory loss and brain damage, for which there is little substantiating evidence.

The nurse assists with ECT using the steps of the nursing process before, during, and after treatment. Important nursing interventions include ensuring client safety, managing client anxiety, and providing adequate client education. Nursing input into the ongoing evaluation of client behavior is an important factor in determining the therapeutic effectiveness of ECT.

REVIEW QUESTIONS

SELF-EXAMINATION/LEARNING EXERCISE

Select the answer that is most appropriate for each of the following questions.

1. Electroconvulsive therapy is most commonly prescribed for:
   a. Bipolar disorder, manic.
   b. Paranoid schizophrenia.
   c. Major depression.
   d. Obsessive–compulsive disorder.

2. Which of the following best describes the average number of ECT treatments given and the timing of administration?
   a. One treatment per month for 6 months
   b. One treatment every other day for a total of 6 to 10
   c. One treatment three times per week for a total of 20 to 30
   d. One treatment every day for a total of 10 to 15

3. Which of the following conditions is considered to be the only absolute contraindication for ECT?
   a. Increased intracranial pressure
   b. Recent myocardial infarction
   c. Severe underlying hypertension
   d. Congestive heart failure

4. Electroconvulsive therapy is thought to effect a therapeutic response by
   a. Stimulation of the CNS.
   b. Decreasing the levels of acetylcholine and monoamine oxidase.
   c. Increasing the levels of serotonin, norepinephrine, and dopamine.
   d. Altering sodium metabolism within nerve and muscle cells.

5. The most common side effects of ECT are:
   a. Permanent memory loss and brain damage.
   b. Fractured and dislocated bones.
   c. Myocardial infarction and cardiac arrest.
   d. Temporary memory loss and confusion.

Situation: Sam has just been admitted to the inpatient psychiatric unit with a diagnosis of major depression. Sam has been treated with antidepressant medication for 6 months without improvement. His psychiatrist has suggested a series of ECT treatments. Sam says to the nurse on admission, "I don't want to end up like McMurphy on *One Flew Over the Cuckoo's Nest*! I'm scared!" The following questions pertain to Sam.

6. Sam's priority nursing diagnosis at this time would be:
   a. Anxiety related to deficient knowledge about ECT.
   b. Risk for injury related to risks associated with ECT.
   c. Deficient knowledge related to negative media presentation of ECT.
   d. Disturbed thought processes related to side effects of ECT.

7. Which of the following statements would be most appropriate by the nurse in response to Sam's expression of concern?
   a. "I guarantee you won't end up like McMurphy, Sam."
   b. "The doctor knows what he is doing. There's nothing to worry about."
   c. "I know you are scared, Sam, and we're going to talk about what you can expect from the therapy."
   d. "I'm going to stay with you as long as you are scared."

8. The priority nursing intervention before starting Sam's therapy is to:
   a. Take vital signs and record.
   b. Have the patient void.
   c. Administer succinylcholine.
   d. Ensure that the consent form has been signed.

9. Atropine sulfate is administered to Sam for what purpose?
   a. To alleviate anxiety
   b. To decrease secretions
   c. To relax muscles
   d. As a short-acting anesthetic

10. Succinylcholine is administered to Sam for what purpose?
   a. To alleviate anxiety
   b. To decrease secretions
   c. To relax muscles
   d. As a short-acting anesthetic

REFERENCES

Abrams, R. (2002). *Electroconvulsive therapy* (4th ed). New York: Oxford University Press.

Eisendrath, S.J., & Lichtmacher, J.E. (2005). Psychiatric disorders. In L.M. Tierney, S.J. McPhee, & M.A. Papadakis (Eds.). *Current medical diagnosis & treatment*. New York: McGraw-Hill.

Fink, M. (1999). Images in psychiatry: Ladislas J. Meduna. *American Journal of Psychiatry, 156*(11), 1807.

Frank, L.R. (2002). Electroshock: A crime against the spirit. *Ethical Human Sciences & Services, 4*(1), 63–71.

Geddes, J.R. (2003). Efficacy and safety of electroconvulsive therapy in depressive disorders: A systematic review and meta-analysis. *The Lancet, 361*(9360), 799–808.

Ishihara, K., & Sasa, M. (1999). Mechanism underlying the therapeutic effects of electroconvulsive therapy (ECT) on depression. *Japanese Journal of Pharmacology, 80*(3), 185–189.

Marangell, L.B., Silver, J.M., Goff, D.C., & Yudofsky, S.C. (2003). Psychopharmacology and electroconvulsive therapy. In R.E. Hales & S.C. Yudofsky (Eds.). *Textbook of clinical psychiatry*. Washington, DC: American Psychiatric Publishing.

Popolos, D. (2005). All about ECT. Retrieved February 10, 2005 from the World Wide Web at http://www.schizophrenia.com/family/ect1.html

Sadock, B.J., & Sadock, V.A. (2003). *Synopsis of psychiatry: Behavioral sciences/clinical psychiatry* (9th ed.). Philadelphia: Lippincott Williams & Wilkins.

Wahlund, B., & von Rosen, D. (2003). ECT of major depressed patients in relation to biological and clinical variables: A brief overview. *Neuropsychopharmacology, 28*, S21–S26.

23
CHAPTER

COMPLEMENTARY
THERAPIES

CHAPTER OUTLINE

OBJECTIVES

COMMONALITIES AND CONTRASTS

TYPES OF COMPLEMENTARY THERAPIES

SUMMARY

REVIEW QUESTIONS

KEY TERMS

acupoints
acupressure
acupuncture
allopathic medicine
chiropractic medicine

meridians
qi
subluxation
yoga

CORE CONCEPTS

alternative medicine
complementary
  medicine

OBJECTIVES

After reading this chapter, the student will be able to:

1. Compare and contrast various types of conventional and alternative therapies.
2. Describe the philosophies behind various complementary therapies, including herbal medicine, acupressure and acupuncture, diet and nutrition, chiropractic medicine, thera-

peutic touch and massage, yoga, and pet therapy.
3. Discuss the historical background of various complementary therapies.
4. Describe the techniques used in various complementary therapies.

THE HISTORY OF MEDICINE

2000 BC—Here, eat this root.
1000 AD—That root is heathen. Here, say this prayer.
1850 AD—That prayer is superstition. Here, drink this potion.
1940 AD—That potion is snake oil. Here, swallow this pill.
1985 AD—That pill is ineffective. Here, take this antibiotic.
2000 AD—That antibiotic is ineffective and dangerous.
Here, eat this root.

Anonymous

*T*he connection between mind and body, and the influence of each on the other, is well recognized by all clinicians, and particularly by psychiatrists. Traditional medicine as it is currently practiced in the United States is based solely on scientific methodology. Traditional medicine, also known as **allopathic medicine**, is the type of medicine historically taught in U.S. medical schools.

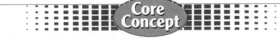

Alternative Medicine

Interventions that differ from the traditional or conventional biomedical treatment of disease. "Alternative" refers to an intervention that is used *instead* of conventional treatment.

A recent nationwide government survey found that 36 percent of U.S. adults aged 18 years and over use some form of alternative medicine. When prayer specifically for health reasons was included in the definition of alternative medicine, the number jumped to 62 percent (Center for Disease Control [CDC], 2004). More than $25 billion a year is spent on alternative medical therapies in the U.S. (Sadock & Sadock, 2003).

In 1991, an Office of Alternative Medicine (OAM) was established by the National Institutes of Health (NIH) to study nontraditional therapies and to evaluate their usefulness and their effectiveness. Since that time, the name has been changed to the National Center for Complementary Medicine and Alternative Medicine (NCCAM or CAM). The mission statement of the CAM states:

We are dedicated to exploring complementary and alternative healing practices in the context of rigorous science, educating and training CAM researchers, and disseminating authoritative information to the public and professionals. (NCCAM, 2002)

Although the CAM has not endorsed the methodologies, a list of alternative therapies has been established to be used in practice and for investigative purposes. This list is presented in Table 23–1.

Some health insurance companies and health maintenance organizations (HMOs) appear to be bowing to public pressure by including alternative providers in their networks of providers for treatments such as acupuncture and massage therapy. Chiropractic care has been covered by some third-party payers for many years. Individuals who seek alternative therapy, however, are often reimbursed at lower rates than those who choose traditional practitioners.

Complementary Medicine

A complementary therapy is an intervention that is different from, but used *in conjunction with,* traditional or conventional medical treatment.

Client education is an important part of complementary care. Positive lifestyle changes are encouraged, and practitioners serve as educators as well as treatment specialists. Complementary medicine is viewed as *holistic* health care, which deals not only with the physical perspective, but also the emotional and spiritual components of the individual. Dr. Tom Coniglione, former professor of medicine at the Oklahoma University Health Sciences Center has stated:

We must look at treating the "total person" in order to be more efficient and balanced within the medical community. Even finding doctors who are well-rounded and balanced has become a criteria in the admitting process for medical students. Medicine has changed from just looking at the "scientist perspective of organ and disease" to the total perspective of lifestyle and real impact/results to the patient. This evolution is a progressive and very positive shift in the right direction. (Coniglione, 1998)

Terms such as *harmony* and *balance* are often associated with complementary care. In fact, restoring harmony and balance between body and mind is often the goal of complementary health care approaches (Credit, Hartunian, & Nowak, 1998).

This chapter examines various complementary therapies by describing the therapeutic approach and identifying the conditions for which the therapy is intended.

TABLE 23–1	**Classification of Alternative Medicine Practices from the NIH Office of Alternative Medicine***

ALTERNATIVE SYSTEMS OF MEDICAL PRACTICE

Acupuncture
Anthroposophically extended medicine
Ayurveda
Community-based health care practices
Environmental medicine
Homeopathic medicine
Latin American rural practices
Native American practices
Natural products
Naturopathic medicine
Past life therapy
Shamanism
Tibetan medicine
Traditional Oriental medicine

BIOELECTROMAGNETIC APPLICATIONS

Blue light treatment and artificial lighting
Electroacupuncture
Electromagnetic fields
Electrostimulation and neuromagnetic stimulation devices
Magnetoresonance spectroscopy

DIET, NUTRITION, LIFESTYLE CHANGES

Changes in lifestyle
Diet
Gerson therapy
Macrobiotics
Megavitamins
Nutritional supplements

HERBAL MEDICINE

Echinacea (purple coneflower)
Ginger rhizome
Ginkgo biloba extract
Ginseng root
Wild chrysanthemum flower
Witch hazel
Yellowdock

MANUAL HEALING

Acupressure
Alexander technique
Biofield therapeutics
Chiropractic medicine
Feldenkrais method
Massage therapy
Osteopathy
Reflexology
Rolfing
Therapeutic touch
Trager method
Zone therapy

MIND/BODY CONTROL

Art therapy
Biofeedback
Counseling
Dance therapy
Guided imagery
Humor therapy
Hypnotherapy
Meditation
Music therapy
Prayer therapy
Psychotherapy
Relaxation techniques
Support groups
Yoga

PHARMACOLOGICAL & BIOLOGICAL TREATMENTS

Antioxidizing agents
Cell treatment
Chelation therapy
Metabolic therapy
Oxidizing agents (ozone, hydrogen peroxide)

*This list of complementary and alternative medical health care practices was developed by the ad hoc Advisory Panel to the Office of Alternative Medicine (OAM), National Institutes of Health (NIH). It was further refined at a workshop for alternative medicine researchers and practitioners. It was designed for the purposes of discussion and study, and is considered neither complete nor authoritative.

Although most are not founded in scientific principle, they have been shown to be effective in the treatment of certain disorders, and merit further examination as a viable component of holistic health care.

COMMONALITIES AND CONTRASTS

A number of commonalities and contrasts exist between complementary medicine and conventional health care. A summary of these characteristics is presented in Table 23–2.

TYPES OF COMPLEMENTARY THERAPIES

Herbal Medicine

The use of plants to heal is probably as old as humankind. Virtually every culture in the world has relied on herbs

and plants to treat illness. Clay tablets from about 4000 B.C. reveal that the Sumerians had apothecaries for dispensing medicinal herbs. At the root of Chinese medicine is the *Pen Tsao*, a Chinese text written around 3000 B.C., which contained hundreds of herbal remedies. When the Pilgrims came to America in the 1600s, they brought with them a variety of herbs to be established and used for medicinal purposes. The new settlers soon discovered that the Native Americans also had their own varieties of plants that they used for healing.

Many people are seeking a return to herbal remedies, because they perceive these remedies as being less potent than prescription drugs and as being free of adverse side effects. However, because the Food and Drug Administration (FDA) classifies herbal remedies as dietary supplements or food additives, their labels cannot indicate medicinal uses. They are not subject to FDA approval, and they lack uniform standards of quality control.

TABLE 23–2	**Commonalities and Contrasts Between Conventional and Complementary Therapies**
CONVENTIONAL	**COMPLEMENTARY**
Chemotherapy	Plants and other natural products
Curing/treating	Healing/ministering care
Individual viewed as disease category	Individual is viewed as a unique being
End-stage	Hope/hopefulness
Focus is on disease and illness	Focus is on health and wellness
Illness treatment	Health promotion and illness prevention
Nutrition is adjunct and supportive to treatment	Nutrition is the basis of health, wellness, and treatment
Objectivism: Person is separate from his/her disease	Subjectivism: person is integral to the illness
Patient	Person
Practitioner as authority	Practitioner as facilitator
Practitioner paternalism/patient dependency	Practitioner as partner/person empowerment
Positivism/materialism: data are physically measurable (through various types of energy systems for screening, diagnosis, and treatment)	Metaphysical: Entity is energy system or vital force that utilizes its own vital essences and energy forces to heal itself, prevent illness, and promote health
Reductionistic (emphasis placed on the cellular, organ, or system levels of the body)	Holistic (emphasis placed on treatment of the whole individual in his/her bio-psycho-social-cultural-and-spiritual context)
Specialist care	Self-care
Symptom relief	Alleviation of causative factors
Somatic (biological and physiological) model	Behavioral-psycho-social-spiritual model
Science is only source of knowledge and truth	Multiple sources of knowledge and truth
Technology/invasive	Natural/noninvasive

SOURCE: DeSantis, L. Alternative and complementary healing practices. In Catalano, J: *Nursing Now! Today's issues, Tomorrow's Trend* (3rd ed.). F.A. Davis Company, Philadelphia, 2003, p. 438. With permission.

Several organizations have been established to attempt regulation and control of the herbal industry. They include the Council for Responsible Nutrition, the American Herbal Association, and the American Botanical Council. The Commission E of the German Federal Health Agency is the group responsible for researching and regulating the safety and efficacy of herbs and plant medicines in Germany. All of the Commission E monographs of herbal medicines have been translated into English and compiled into one text (Blumenthal, 1998). This should prove to be an invaluable reference for practitioners of holistic medicine.

Until more extensive testing has been completed on humans and animals, the use of herbal medicines must be approached with caution and responsibility. *The notion that something being "natural" means it is therefore completely safe is a myth.* In fact, some of the plants from which even prescription drugs are derived are highly toxic in their natural state. Also, because of lack of regulation and standardization, ingredients may be adulterated. Their method of manufacture also may alter potency. For example, dried herbs lose potency rapidly because of exposure to air. In addition, it is often safer to use preparations that contain only one herb. There is a greater likelihood of unwanted side-effects with combined herbal preparations.

Table 23–3 lists information about common herbal remedies, with possible implications for psychiatric/men-

tal health nursing. Botanical names, medicinal uses, and safety profiles are included.

Acupressure and Acupuncture

Acupressure and **acupuncture** are healing techniques based on the ancient philosophies of traditional Chinese medicine dating back to 3000 B.C. The main concept behind Chinese medicine is that healing energy (**qi**) flows through the body along specific pathways called **meridians.** It is believed that these meridians of qi connect various parts of the body in a way similar to the way in which lines on a road map link various locations. The pathways link a conglomerate of points, called **acupoints.** Therefore, it is possible to treat a part of the body distant to another because they are linked by a meridian. Trivieri and Anderson (2002) state, "The proper flow of qi along energy channels (meridians) within the body is crucial to a person's health and vitality."

In acupressure, the fingers, thumbs, palms, or elbows are used to apply pressure to the acupoints. This pressure is thought to dissolve any obstructions in the flow of healing energy and to restore the body to a healthier functioning. In acupuncture, hair-thin, sterile, disposable, stainless-steel needles are inserted into acupoints to dissolve the obstructions along the meridians. The needles may be left in place for a specified length of time, they may be rotated, or a mild electric current may be

TABLE 23–3   Herbal Remedies

COMMON NAME (BOTANICAL NAME)	MEDICINAL USES/POSSIBLE ACTION	SAFETY PROFILE
Black cohosh (*Cimicifuga racemosa*)	May provide relief of menstrual cramps; improved mood; calming effect. Extracts from the roots are thought to have action similar to estrogen.	Generally considered safe in low doses. Occasionally causes GI discomfort. Toxic in large doses, causing dizziness, nausea, headaches, stiffness, and trembling. Should not take with heart problems, concurrently with antihypertensives, or during pregnancy.
Cascara sagrada (*Rhamnus purshiana*)	Relief of constipation	Generally recognized as safe; sold as over-the-counter drug in the United States. Should not be used during pregnancy. Contraindicated in bowel obstruction or inflammation.
Chamomile (*Matricaria chamomilla*)	As a tea, is effective as a mild sedative in the relief of insomnia. May also aid digestion, relieve menstrual cramps, and settle upset stomach.	Generally recognized as safe when consumed in reasonable amounts.
Echinacea (*Echinacea angustifolia* and *Echinacea purpurea*)	Stimulates the immune system; may have value in fighting infections and easing the symptoms of colds and flu.	Considered safe in reasonable doses. Observe for side effects of allergic reaction.
Fennel (*Foeniculum vulgare* or *Foeniculum officinale*)	Used to ease stomachaches and to aid digestion. Taken in a tea or in extracts to stimulate the appetites of people with anorexia (1–2 tsp. seeds steeped in boiling water for making tea)	Generally recognized as safe when consumed in reasonable amounts.
Feverfew (*Tanacetum parthenium*)	Prophylaxis and treatment of migraine headaches. Effective in either the fresh leaf or freeze-dried forms (2–3 fresh leaves [or equivalent] per day)	A small percentage of individuals may experience the adverse effect of temporary mouth ulcers. Considered safe in reasonable doses.
Ginger (*Zingiber officinale*)	Ginger tea to ease stomachaches and to aid digestion. Two powdered gingerroot capsules have shown to be effective in preventing motion sickness.	Generally recognized as safe in designated therapeutic doses.
Ginkgo (*Ginkgo biloba*)	Used to treat senility, short-term memory loss, and peripheral insufficiency. Has been shown to dilate blood vessels. Usual dosage is 120 mg/day.	Safety has been established with recommended dosages. Possible side effects include headache, GI problems, and dizziness. Contraindicated in pregnancy and lactation and in patients with bleeding disorder. Possible compound effect with concomitant use of aspirin or anticoagulants.
Ginseng (*Panax ginseng*)	The ancient Chinese saw this herb as one that increased wisdom and longevity. Current studies support a possible positive effect on the cardiovascular system. Action not known.	Generally considered safe. Side effects may include headache, insomnia, anxiety, skin rashes, diarrhea. Avoid concomitant use with anticoagulants.
Hops (*Humulus lupulus*)	Used in cases of nervousness, mild anxiety, and insomnia. Also may relieve the cramping associated with diarrhea. May be taken as a tea, in extracts, or capsules.	Generally recognized as safe when consumed in recommended dosages.
Kava-kava (*Piper methylsticum*)	Used to reduce anxiety while promoting mental acuity. Dosage: 150–300 mg bid.	Scaly skin rash may occur when taken at high dosage for long periods. Motor reflexes and judgment when driving may be reduced while taking the herb. Concurrent use with CNS depressants may produce additive tranquilizing effects. Recent reports of potential for liver damage. FDA is investigating. Should not be taken for longer than 3 months without a doctor's supervision.
Passion flower (*Passiflora incarnata*)	Used in tea, capsules, or extracts to treat nervousness and insomnia. Depresses the central nervous system to produce a mild sedative effect.	Generally recognized as safe in recommended doses.
Peppermint (*Mentha piperita*)	Used as a tea to relieve upset stomachs and headaches and as a mild sedative. Pour boiling water over 1 tbsp. dried leaves and steep to make a tea. Oil of peppermint is also used for inflammation of the mouth, pharynx, and bronchus.	Considered to be safe when consumed in designated therapeutic dosages.

(Continued on opposite page)

COMMON NAME (BOTANICAL NAME)	MEDICINAL USES/POSSIBLE ACTION	SAFETY PROFILE
Psyllium (*Plantago ovata*)	Psyllium seeds are a popular bulk laxative commonly used for chronic constipation. Also found to be useful in the treatment of hypercholesterolemia.	Approved as an over-the-counter drug in the United States.
Scullcap (*Scutellaria lateriflora*)	Used as a sedative for mild anxiety and nervousness.	Considered safe in reasonable amounts.
St. John's wort (*Hypericum perforatum*)	Used in the treatment of mild to moderate depression. May block reuptake of serotonin/norepinephrine and have a mild MAO inhibiting effect. Effective dose: 900 mg/day. May also have antiviral, antibacterial, and anti-inflammatory properties.	Generally recognized as safe when taken at recommended dosages. Side effects include mild GI irritation that is lessened with food; photosensitivity when taken in high dosages over long periods. Should not be taken with other psychoactive medications.
Valerian (*Valeriana officinals*)	Used to treat nervousness and insomnia. Produces restful sleep without morning "hangover." The root may be used to make a tea, or capsules are available in a variety of dosages. Mechanism of action is similar to benzodiazepines, but without addicting properties. Daily dosage range: 100–1000 mg.	Generally recognized as safe when taken at recommended dosages. Side effects may include mild headache or upset stomach. Taking doses higher than recommended may result in severe headache, nausea, morning grogginess, blurry vision. Should not be taken concurrently with CNS depressants.

SOURCES: Adapted from Sadock & Sadock (2003); Trivieri and Anderson (2002); Holt & Kouzi (2002); and PDR for Herbal Medicines (2000).

applied. An occasional tingling or numbness is experienced, but little to no pain is associated with the treatment (NCCAM, 2004).

The Western medical philosophy regarding acupressure and acupuncture is that they stimulate the body's own painkilling chemicals—the morphine-like substances known as *endorphins*. The treatment has been found to be effective in the treatment of asthma, headaches, dysmenorrhea, cervical pain, insomnia, anxiety, depression, substance abuse, stroke rehabilitation, nausea of pregnancy, postoperative and chemotherapy-induced nausea and vomiting, tennis elbow, fibromyalgia, low back pain, and carpal tunnel syndrome (NCCAM, 2004; Sadock & Sadock, 2003). A recent study suggests that acupuncture may aid in the treatment of cocaine dependence (Avants et al., 2000).

Acupuncture is gaining wide acceptance is the United States by both patients and physicians. This treatment can be administered at the same time other techniques are being used, such as conventional Western techniques, although it is essential that all health care providers have knowledge of all treatments being received. Acupuncture should be administered by a physician or an acupuncturist who is board certified by the National Commission for the Certification of Acupuncturists, which requires more than 1,000 hours of acupuncture training. Currently 34 states and the District of Columbia have set licensure standards for acupuncturists (Natural Healers, 2005).

Diet and Nutrition

The value of nutrition in the healing process has long been underrated. Lutz & Przytulski (2001) state:

Today many diseases are linked to lifestyle behaviors such as smoking, lack of adequate physical activity, and poor nutritional habits. Health care providers, in their role as educa-tors, emphasize the relationship between lifestyle and risk of disease. Many people, at least in industrialized countries, are increasingly managing their health problems and making personal commitments to lead healthier lives. Nutrition is, in part, a preventive science. Given sufficient resources, how and what one eats is a lifestyle choice. (p. 4)

Individuals select the foods they eat based on a number of factors, not the least of which is enjoyment. Eating must serve social and cultural, as well as nutritional, needs. The U.S. Departments of Agriculture (USDA) and Health and Human Services (USDHHS) have collaborated on a set of guidelines to help individuals understand what types of foods to eat and the healthy lifestyle they need to pursue in order to promote health and prevent disease. Following is a list of key recommendations from these guidelines (USDA/USDHHA, 2005):

Adequate Nutrients Within Calorie Needs

● Consume a variety of nutrient-dense foods and beverages within and among the basic food groups while choosing foods that limit the intakes of fat, cholesterol, added sugars, salt, and alcohol.

● Meet recommended intakes within energy needs by adopting a balanced eating pattern, such as the USDA Food Guide (Table 23–4). Table 23–5 provides a summary of information about essential vitamins and minerals.

Weight Management

● Maintain body weight in a healthy range, balance calories from foods and beverages with calories expended.

● To prevent gradual weight gain over time, make small decreases in food and beverage calories and increase physical activity.

TABLE 23-4   Sample USDA Food Guide at the 2000-Calorie Level

FOOD GROUPS AND SUBGROUPS	USDA FOOD GUIDE DAILY AMOUNT	EXAMPLES/EQUIVALENT AMOUNTS
Fruit Group	2 cups (4 servings)	$\frac{1}{2}$ cup equivalent is: • $\frac{1}{2}$ cup fresh, frozen, or canned fruit • 1 medium fruit • $\frac{1}{4}$ cup dried fruit • $\frac{1}{2}$ cup fruit juice
Vegetable Group	2.5 cups (5 servings) • Dark green vegetables: 3 cups/week • Orange vegetables: 2 cups/week • Legumes (dry beans/peas): 3 cups/week • Starchy vegetables: 3 cups/week • Other vegetables: 6.5 cups/week	$\frac{1}{2}$ cup equivalent is: • $\frac{1}{2}$ cup cut-up raw or cooked vegetable • 1 cup raw leafy vegetable • $\frac{1}{2}$ cup vegetable juice
Grain Group	6 ounce-equivalents • Whole grains: 3 ounce-equivalents • Other grains: 3 ounce-equivalents	1 ounce-equivalent is: • 1 slice bread • 1 cup dry cereal • $\frac{1}{2}$ cup cooked rice, pasta, cereal
Meat and Beans Group	5.5 ounce-equivalents	1 ounce-equivalent is: • 1 oz. cooked lean meat, poultry, or fish • 1 egg • $\frac{1}{4}$ cup cooked dry beans or tofu • 1 tbsp. peanut butter • $\frac{1}{2}$ oz. nuts or seeds
Milk Group	3 cups	1 cup equivalent is: • 1 cup low fat/fat-free milk • 1 cup low fat/fat-free yogurt • 1 $\frac{1}{2}$ oz. low-fat or fat-free natural cheese • 2 oz. low-fat or fat-free processed cheese
Oils	24 grams (6 tsp.)	1 tsp. equivalent is: • 1 tbsp. low-fat mayo • 2 tbsp. light salad dressing • 1 tsp. vegetable oil • 1 tsp. soft margarine with zero *trans* fat
Discretionary Calorie Allowance	267 calories Example of distribution: • Solid fats 18 grams (e.g., saturated & *trans* fats) • Added sugars 8 tsp. (e.g., sweetened cereals)	1 tbsp. added sugar equivalent is: • $\frac{1}{2}$ oz. jelly beans • 8 oz. lemonade Examples of solid fats: • Fat in whole milk/ice cream • Fatty meats Essential oils (above) are not considered part of the discretionary calories

SOURCE: *Dietary Guidelines for Americans 2005*. Washington, DC: USDA/USDHHS, 2005.

TABLE 23–5 Essential Vitamins and Minerals

VITAMIN/ MINERAL	FUNCTION	RDA*	NEW DRI (UL)**	FOOD SOURCES	COMMENTS
Vitamin A	Prevention of night blindness; calcification of growing bones; resistance to infection	Men: 1000 μg; Women: 800 μg	Men: 900 μg (3000 μg) Women: 700 μg (3000 μg)	Liver, butter, cheese, whole milk, egg yolk, fish, green leafy vegetables, carrots, pumpkin, sweet potatoes	May be of benefit in prevention of cancer, because of its antioxidant properties which are associated with control of free radicals that damage DNA and cell membranes.
Vitamin D	Promotes absorption of calcium and phosphorus in the small intestine; prevention of rickets	Men and women: 5 μg	Men and women: 5 μg (50 μg) (5–10 for ages 50–70 and 15 for >70)	Fortified milk and dairy products, egg yolk, fish liver oils, liver, oysters; formed in the skin by exposure to sunlight	Without vitamin D, very little dietary calcium can be absorbed.
Vitamin E	An antioxidant that prevents cell membrane destruction	Men: 10 mg; Women: 8 mg	Men and women: 15 mg (1000 mg)	Vegetable oils, wheat germ, whole grain or fortified cereals, green leafy vegetables, nuts	As an antioxidant, may have implications in the prevention of Alzheimer's disease, heart disease, breast cancer
Vitamin K	Synthesis of prothrombin and other clotting factors; normal blood coagulation	Men: 80 μg; Women: 65 μg	Men: 120 μg (ND)**** Women: 90 μg (ND)****	Green vegetables (collards, spinach, lettuce, kale, broccoli, brussel sprouts, cabbage), plant oils, and margarine	Individuals on anticoagulant therapy should monitor vitamin K intake.
Vitamin C	Formation of collagen in connective tissues; a powerful antioxidant; facilitates iron absorption; aids in the release of epinephrine from the adrenal glands during stress	Men and women: 60 mg	Men: 90 mg (2000 mg) Women: 75 mg (2000 mg)	Citrus fruits, tomatoes, potatoes, green leafy vegetables, strawberries	As an antioxidant, may have implications in the prevention of cancer, cataracts, heart disease. It may stimulate the immune system to fight various types of infection.
Vitamin B₁ (thiamine)	Essential for normal functioning of nervous tissue; coenzyme in carbohydrate metabolism	Men: 1.5 mg Women: 1.1 mg	Men: 1.2 mg (ND)**** Women: 1.1 mg (ND)****	Whole grains, legumes, nuts, egg yolk, meat, green leafy vegetables	Large doses may improve mental performance in people with Alzheimer's disease.
Vitamin B₂ (riboflavin)	Coenzyme in the metabolism of protein and carbohydrate for energy	Men: 1.7 mg Women: 1.3 mg	Men: 1.3 mg (ND)**** Women: 1.1 mg (ND)****	Meat, dairy products, whole or enriched grains, legumes, nuts	May help in the prevention of cataracts; high dose therapy may be effective in migraine prophylaxis (Schoenen et al., 1998).
Vitamin B₃ (niacin)	Coenzyme in the metabolism of protein and carbohydrates for energy	Men: 19 mg Women: 15 mg	Men: 16 mg (35 mg) Women: 14 mg (35 mg)	Milk, eggs, meats, legumes, whole grain and enriched cereals, nuts	High doses of niacin have been successful in decreasing levels of cholesterol in some individuals.
Vitamin B₆ (pyridoxine)	Coenzyme in the synthesis and catabolism of amino acids; essential for metabolism of tryptophan to niacin	Men: 2 mg Women: 1.6 mg	Men and women: 1.3 mg (100 mg) After age 50: Men: 1.7 mg Women: 1.5 mg	Meat, fish, grains, legumes, bananas, nuts, white and sweet potatoes	May decrease depression in some individuals by increasing levels of serotonin; deficiencies may contribute to memory problems; also used in the treatment of migraines and premenstrual discomfort.

(Continued on following page)

TABLE 23-5 **Essential Vitamins and Minerals** *(Continued)*

VITAMIN/ MINERAL	FUNCTION	RDA*	NEW DRI (UL)**	FOOD SOURCES	COMMENTS
Vitamin B$_{12}$	Necessary in the formation of DNA and the production of red blood cells; associated with folic acid metabolism	Men and women: 2 µg	Men and women: 2.4 µg (ND)****	Found in animal products (e.g., meats, eggs, dairy products)	Deficiency may contribute to memory problems. Vegetarians can get this vitamin from fortified foods. Intrinsic factor must be present in the stomach for absorption of vitamin B$_{12}$.
Folic acid (folate)	Necessary in the formation of DNA and the production of red blood cells	Men: 200 µg Women: 180 µg	Men and women: 400 µg (1000 µg)	Meat; green leafy vegetables; beans; peas; fortified cereals, breads, rice, and pasta	Important in women of childbearing age to prevent fetal neural tube defects; may contribute to prevention of heart disease and colon cancer
Calcium	Necessary in the formation of bones and teeth; neuron and muscle functioning; blood clotting	Men and women: 800 mg	Men and women: 1000 mg (2500 mg) After age 50: Men and women: 1200 mg	Dairy products, kale, broccoli, spinach, sardines, oysters, salmon	Calcium has been associated with preventing headaches, muscle cramps, osteoporosis, and premenstrual problems. Requires vitamin D for absorption.
Phosphorus	Necessary in the formation of bones and teeth; a component of DNA, RNA, ADP, and ATP; helps control acid–base balance in the blood	Men and women: 800 mg	Men and women: 700 mg (4000 mg)	Milk, cheese, fish, meat, yogurt, ice cream, peas, eggs	
Magnesium	Protein synthesis and carbohydrate metabolism; muscular relaxation following contraction; bone formation	Men: 350 mg Women: 280 mg	Men: 420 mg (350 mg)*** Women: 320 mg (350 mg)***	Green vegetables, legumes, seafood, milk, nuts, meat	May aid in prevention of asthmatic attacks and migraine headaches. Deficiencies may contribute to insomnia, premenstrual problems.
Iron	Synthesis of hemoglobin and myoglobin; cellular oxidation	Men and women: 10 mg (women who are breastfeeding and those of childbearing age: 15 mg)	Men: 8 mg (45 mg) Women: (45 mg) Childbearing age: 18 mg Over 50: 8 mg Pregnant: 27 mg Breastfeeding: 9 mg	Meat, fish, poultry, eggs, nuts, dark green leafy vegetables, dried fruit, enriched pasta and bread	Iron deficiencies can result in headaches and feeling chronically fatigued.
Iodine	Aids in the synthesis of T$_3$ and T$_4$	Men and women: 150 µg	Men and women: 150 µg (1100 µg)	Iodized salt, seafood	Exerts strong controlling influence on overall body metabolism.
Selenium	Works with vitamin E to protect cellular compounds from oxidation	Men: 70 µg Women: 55 µg	Men and women: 55 µg (400 µg)	Seafood, low-fat meats, dairy products, liver	As an antioxidant combined with vitamin E, may have some anti-cancer effect. Deficiency has also been associated with depressed mood.

(Continued on opposite page)

VITAMIN/ MINERAL	FUNCTION	RDA*	NEW DRI (UL)**	FOOD SOURCES	COMMENTS
Zinc	Involved in synthesis of DNA and RNA; energy metabolism and protein synthesis; wound healing; increased immune functioning; necessary for normal smell and taste sensation.	Men: 15 mg Women: 12 mg	Men: 11 mg (40 mg) Women: 8 mg (40 mg)	Meat, seafood, fortified cereals, poultry, eggs, milk	An important source for the prevention of infection and improvement in wound healing.

*Recommended Dietary Allowances, established by the Food and Nutrition Board of the Institute of Medicine, 1989.
**Dietary Reference Intakes (UL), the most recent set of dietary recommendations for adults established by the Food and Nutrition Board of the Institute of Medicine, © 2004. UL is the upper limit of intake considered to be safe for use by adults (includes total intake from food, water, and supplements).
***UL for magnesium applies only to intakes from dietary supplements, excluding intakes from food and water.
****ND = Not determined
SOURCES: Adapted from National Academy of Sciences (2004) and Council for Responsible Nutrition, Washington, D.C. (2001).

Physical Activity

● Engage in regular physical activity and reduce sedentary activities to promote health, psychological well-being, and a healthy body weight.
● To reduce the risk of chronic disease in adulthood, engage in at least 30 minutes of moderate-intensity physical activity, above usual activity, at work or home on most days of the week.
● To help manage body weight and prevent gradual, unhealthy body weight gain in adulthood, engage in approximately 60 minutes of moderate- to vigorous-intensity activity on most days of the week while not exceeding caloric intake requirements.
● To sustain weight loss in adulthood, participate in at least 60 to 90 minutes of daily moderate-intensity physical activity while not exceeding caloric intake requirements.
● Achieve physical fitness by including cardiovascular conditioning, stretching exercises for flexibility, and resistance exercises or calisthenics for muscle strength and endurance.

Food Groups to Encourage

Fruits and Vegetables. Choose a variety of fruits and vegetables each day. In particular, select from all five vegetable subgroups several times a week.

Whole Grains. Half the daily servings of grains should come from whole grains.

Milk and Milk Products. Daily choices of fat-free or low-fat milk or milk products are important. To help meet calcium needs, non-dairy calcium-containing alternatives may be selected by individuals with lactose intolerance or those who choose to avoid all milk products (e.g., vegans).

Food Groups to Moderate

Fats. Keep total fat intake between 20 and 35 percent of calories, with most fats coming from sources of polyunsaturated and monounsaturated fatty acids, such as fish, nuts, and vegetable oils. Consume less than 10 percent of calories from saturated fatty acids and less than 300 mg/day of cholesterol, and keep *trans* fatty acid consumption as low as possible.

Carbohydrates. Carbohydrate intake should comprise 45 to 64 percent of total calories, with the majority coming from fiber-rich foods. Important sources of nutrients from carbohydrates include fruits, vegetables, whole grains, and milk. Added sugars, caloric sweeteners, and refined starches should be used prudently.

Sodium Chloride. Consume less than 2300 mg (approximately 1 teaspoon of salt) of sodium per day. Choose and prepare foods with little salt. At the same time, consume potassium-rich foods, such as fruits and vegetables.

Alcoholic Beverages. Individuals who choose to drink alcoholic beverages should do so sensibly and in moderation—defined as the consumption of up to one drink per day for women and up to two drinks per day for men. One drink should count as:

● 12 ounces of regular beer (150 calories)
● 5 ounces of wine (100 calories)
● 1.5 ounces of 80-proof distilled spirits (100 calories)

Alcohol should be avoided by individuals who are unable to restrict their intake; women who are pregnant, may become pregnant, or are breastfeeding; and individuals who are taking medications that may interact with alcohol or who have specific medical conditions.

Chiropractic Medicine

Chiropractic medicine is probably the most widely used form of alternative healing in the United States. It was developed in the late 1800s by a self-taught healer named David Palmer. It was later reorganized and expanded by his son Joshua, a trained practitioner. Palmer's objective was to find a cure for disease and illness that did not use drugs, but instead relied on more natural methods of healing (Trivieri & Anderson, 2002). Palmer's theory behind chiropractic medicine was that energy flows from the brain to all parts of the body through the spinal cord and spinal nerves. When vertebrae of the spinal column become displaced, they may press on a nerve and interfere with the normal nerve transmission. Palmer named the displacement of these vertebrae **subluxation**, and he alleged that the way to restore normal function was to manipulate the vertebrae back into their normal positions. These manipulations are called *adjustments*.

Adjustments are usually performed by hand, although some chiropractors have special treatment tables equipped to facilitate these manipulations (Figure 23–1). Other processes used to facilitate the outcome of the spinal adjustment by providing muscle relaxation include massage tables, application of heat or cold, and ultrasound treatments.

The chiropractor takes a medical history and performs a clinical examination, which usually includes X-ray films of the spine. Today's chiropractors may practice "straight" therapy, that is, the only therapy provided is that of subluxation adjustments. *Mixer* is a term applied

to a chiropractor who combines adjustments with adjunct therapies, such as exercise, heat treatments, or massage.

Individuals seek treatment from chiropractors for many types of ailments and illnesses; the most common is back pain. In addition, chiropractors treat clients with headaches, neck injuries, scoliosis, carpal tunnel syndrome, respiratory and gastrointestinal disorders, menstrual difficulties, allergies, sinusitis, and certain sports injuries (Trivieri & Anderson, 2002). Some chiropractors are employed by professional sports teams as their team physicians.

Chiropractors are licensed to practice in all 50 states and treatment cost is covered by government and most private insurance plans. They treat over 20 million people in the United States annually (Sadock & Sadock, 2003).

Therapeutic Touch and Massage

Therapeutic Touch

Therapeutic touch was developed in the 1970s by Dolores Krieger, a nurse associated with the New York

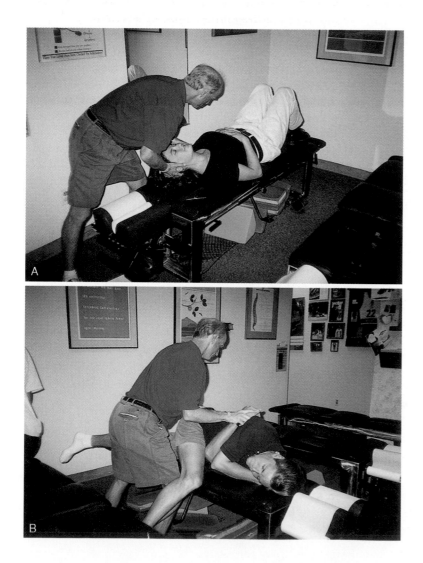

FIGURE 23–1 Chiropractic adjustments.

University School of Nursing. It is based on the philosophy that the human body projects a field of energy. When this field becomes blocked, pain or illness occurs. Practitioners of therapeutic touch use this method to correct the blockages, thereby relieving the discomfort and improving health.

Based on the premise that the energy field extends beyond the surface of the body, the practitioner need not actually touch the client's skin. The therapist's hands are passed over the client's body, remaining two to four inches from the skin. The goal is to repattern the energy field by performing slow, rhythmic, sweeping hand motions over the entire body (Credit et al., 1998). Heat should be felt where the energy is blocked. The therapist "massages" the energy field in that area, smoothing it out, and thus correcting the obstruction. Therapeutic touch is thought to reduce pain and anxiety and promote relaxation and health maintenance. It has proved to be useful in the treatment of chronic health conditions.

Massage

Massage is the technique of manipulating the muscles and soft tissues of the body. Chinese physicians prescribed massage for the treatment of disease more than 5000 years ago. The Eastern style focuses on balancing the body's vital energy (qi) as it flows through pathways (meridians), as described earlier in the discussion of acupressure and acupuncture. The Western style of massage affects muscles, connective tissues (e.g., tendons and ligaments), and the cardiovascular system. Swedish massage, which is probably the best known Western style, uses a variety of gliding and kneading strokes along with deep circular movements and vibrations to relax the muscles, improve circulation, and increase mobility (Trivieri & Anderson, 2002).

Massage has been shown to be beneficial in the following conditions: anxiety, chronic back and neck pain, arthritis, sciatica, migraine headaches, muscle spasms, insomnia, pain of labor and delivery, stress-related disorders, and whiplash. Massage is contraindicated in certain conditions, such as high blood pressure, acute infection, osteoporosis, phlebitis, skin conditions, and varicose veins. It also should not be performed over the site of a recent injury, bruise, or burn.

Massage therapists require specialized training in a program accredited by the American Massage Therapy Association and must pass the National Certification Examination for Therapeutic Massage and Bodywork.

Yoga

Yoga is thought to have developed in India some 5000 years ago and is attributed to an Indian physician and Sanskrit scholar named Patanjali. The objective of yoga is to integrate the physical, mental, and spiritual energies that enhance health and well-being (Trivieri & Anderson, 2002). Yoga has been found to be especially helpful in relieving stress and in improving overall physical and psychological wellness. Proper breathing is a major component of yoga. It is believed that yoga breathing—a deep, diaphramatic breathing—increases oxygen to brain and body tissues, thereby easing stress and fatigue, and boosting energy.

Another component of yoga is meditation. Individuals who practice the meditation and deep breathing associated with yoga find that they are able to achieve a profound feeling of relaxation (Figure 23–2).

The most familiar type of yoga practiced in Western countries is hatha yoga. Hatha yoga uses body postures, along with the meditation and breathing exercises, to achieve a balanced, disciplined workout that releases muscle tension, tones the internal organs, and energizes the mind, body, and spirit, to allow natural healing to occur (Credit et al., 1998). The complete routine of poses is designed to work all parts of the body—stretching and toning muscles, and keeping joints flexible. Studies have shown that yoga has provided beneficial effects to some individuals with back pain, stress, migraine, insomnia, high blood pressure, rapid heart rates, and limited mobility (Sadock & Sadock, 2003; Steinberg, 2002; Trivieri & Anderson, 2002).

Pet Therapy

The therapeutic value of pets is no longer just theory. Evidence has shown that animals can directly influence a person's mental and physical well-being. Many pet-therapy programs have been established across the country and the numbers are increasing regularly.

Several studies have provided information about the positive results of human interaction with pets. Some of these include:

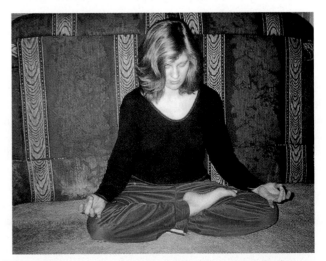

FIGURE 23–2 Achieving relaxation through the practice of yoga.

1. Petting a dog or cat has been shown to lower blood pressure. In one study, volunteers experienced a 7.1-mm Hg drop in systolic and an 8.1-mm Hg decrease in diastolic blood pressure when they talked to and petted their dogs, as opposed to reading aloud or resting quietly (Whitaker, 2000).

2. Bringing a pet into a nursing home or other institution for the elderly has been shown to enhance a client's mood and social interaction (Murray & Zentner, 2001).

3. One study of 96 patients who had been admitted to a coronary care unit for heart attack or angina revealed that in the year following hospitalization, the mortality rate among those who did not own pets was 22 percent higher than among pet owners (Whitaker, 2000).

4. Individuals with AIDS who have pets are less likely to suffer from depression than people with AIDS who don't own pets (Siegel et al., 1999).

Some researchers believe that animals actually may retard the aging process among those who live alone (Figure 23–3). Loneliness often results in premature death, and having a pet mitigates the effects of loneliness and isolation. Whitaker (2000) suggests:

> Though owning a pet doesn't make you immune to illness, pet owners are, on the whole, healthier than those who don't own pets. Study after study shows that people with pets have fewer minor health problems, require fewer visits to the doctor and less medication, and have fewer risk factors for heart disease, such as high blood pressure or cholesterol levels. (p. 7)

It may never be known precisely why animals affect humans they way they do, but for those who have pets to love, the therapeutic benefits come as no surprise. Pets provide unconditional, nonjudgmental love and affection, which can be the perfect antidote for a depressed mood or a stressful situation. The role of animals in the human healing process still requires more research, but its validity is now widely accepted in both the medical and lay communities.

SUMMARY

Alternative medicine includes those practices that differ from the usual traditional ones in the treatment of disease. *Complementary* therapies are those that work in partnership with traditional medical practice. This chapter has presented an overview of several complementary

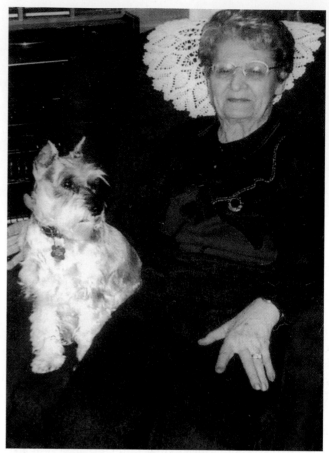

FIGURE 23–3 Healthy aging with pet.

therapies and provided information concerning the appropriateness of their use.

Complementary therapies help the practitioner view the client in a holistic manner. Most complementary therapies consider the mind and body connection and strive to enhance the body's own natural healing powers. The Office of Alternative Medicine of the National Institutes of Health has established a list of alternative therapies to be used in practice and for investigative purposes. More than $25 billion a year is spent on alternative medical therapies in the United States.

This chapter examined herbal medicine, acupressure, acupuncture, diet and nutrition, chiropractic medicine, therapeutic touch, massage, yoga, and pet therapy. Nurses must be familiar with these therapies, as more and more clients seek out the healing properties of these complementary care strategies.

REVIEW QUESTIONS

SELF-EXAMINATION/LEARNING EXERCISE

Match the following herbs with the uses for which they have been associated.

_____ 1. Chamomile

_____ 2. Echinacea

_____ 3. Feverfew

_____ 4. Ginkgo

_____ 5. Psyllium

_____ 6. St. John's wort

_____ 7. Valerian

a. For mild to moderate depression

b. To improve memory

c. To relieve upset stomach

d. For insomnia

e. To stimulate the immune system

f. For migraine headache

g. For constipation

8. Which of the following applies to Vitamin C?
   a. Coenzyme in protein metabolism; found in meat and dairy products.
   b. Necessary in formation of DNA; found in beans and other legumes.
   c. A powerful antioxidant; found in tomatoes and strawberries.
   d. Necessary for blood clotting; found in whole grains and bananas.

9. Which of the following applies to Calcium?
   a. Coenzyme in carbohydrate metabolism; found in whole grains and citrus fruits.
   b. Facilitates iron absorption; found in vegetable oils and liver.
   c. Prevents night blindness; found in egg yolk and cantaloupe.
   d. Important for nerve and muscle functioning; found in dairy products and oysters.

10. Subluxation is a term used by chiropractic medicine to describe
    a. Displacement of vertebrae in the spine.
    b. Adjustment of displaced vertebrae in the spine.
    c. Interference with the flow of energy from the brain.
    d. Pathways along which energy flows throughout the body.

REFERENCES

Avants, S.K., Margolin, A., Holford, T.R., & Kosten, T.R. (2000). A randomized controlled trial of auricular acupuncture for cocaine dependence. *Archives of Internal Medicine, 160*(15), 2305–2312.

Blumenthal, M. (Ed.). (1998). *The complete German Commission E monographs: Therapeutic guide to herbal medicines.* Austin, American Botanical Council.

Centers for Disease Control (CDC). (2004, May 27). Complementary and alternative medicine use among adults: United States, 2002. U.S. Department of Health and Human Services, National Center for Health Statistics. *Advance Data from Vital and Health Statistics, 343,* 1–20.

Coniglione, T. (1998, June). Our doctors must begin looking at the total person. *InBalance.* Oklahoma City, OK: The Balanced Healing Medical Center.

Council for Responsible Nutrition. (2001). Historical comparison of RDIs, RDAs, and DRIs, 1968 to present. Retrieved February 16, 2005 from the World Wide Web at http://www.crnusa.org/pdfs/CRNintakes.pdf

Credit, L.P., Hartunian, S.G., & Nowak, M.J. (1998). *Your guide to complementary medicine.* Garden City Park, NY: Avery Publishing Group.

DeSantis, L. (2003). Alternative and complementary healing practices. In J.T. Catalano (Ed.). *Nursing Now! Today's issues, tomorrow's trends* (3rd ed.). Philadelphia: F.A. Davis.

Friedmann, E., & Thomas, S.A. (1995). Pet ownership, social support, and one-year survival after acute myocardial infarction in the cardiac arrhythmia suppression trial. *American Journal of Cardiology, 76*(17), 1213.

Holt, G.A., & Kouzi, S. (2002). Herbs through the ages. In M.A. Bright (Ed.). *Holistic health and healing.* Philadelphia: F.A. Davis.

Lutz, C.A. & Przytulski, K.R. (2001). *Nutrition and diet therapy* (3rd ed.). Philadelphia: F.A. Davis.

Murray, R.B., & Zentner, J.P. (2001). *Health promotion strategies through the life span* (7th ed.). Upper Saddle River NJ: Prentice-Hall.

National Academy of Sciences. (2004). *Dietary Reference Intakes (DRIs) Tables.* Food and Nutrition Board, Institute of Medicine. Retrieved February 16, 2005 from the World Wide Web at http://www.iom.edu/file.asp?id=21372

National Center for Complementary and Alternative Medicine (NCCAM). (2004, December). *Get the facts: Acupuncture.* Bethesda, MD: National Institutes of Health.

National Center for Complementary and Alternative Medicine (NCCAM). (2002, May). *Office of special populations strategic plan to address racial and ethnic health disparities.* Bethesda, MD: National Institutes of Health.

Natural Healers. (2005). Acupuncture and Oriental Medicine Schools and Careers. Retrieved on February 15, 2005 from the World Wide Web at http://www.naturalhealers.com/

PDR for Herbal Medicines (2nd ed.). (2000). Montvale, NJ: Medical Economics Company.

Sadock, B.J., & Sadock, V.A. (2003). *Synopsis of psychiatry: Behavioral sciences/clinical psychiatry* (9th ed.). Philadelphia: Lippincott Williams & Wilkins.

Schoenen, J., Jacquy, J., & Lenaerts, M. (1998). Effectiveness of high-dose riboflavin in migraine prophylaxis: A randomized controlled trial. *Neurology, 50,* 466–469.

Siegel, J.M., Angulo, F.J., Detels, R., Wesch, J., & Mullen, A. (1999). AIDS diagnosis and depression in the Multicenter AIDS Cohort Study: The ameliorating impact of pet ownership. *AIDS Care, 11*(2), 157–170.

Steinberg, L. (2002). Yoga. In M.A. Bright (Ed.). *Holistic health and healing.* Philadelphia: F.A. Davis.

Trivieri, L., & Anderson, J.W. (2002). *Alternative medicine: The definitive guide.* Berkeley, CA: Celestial Arts.

U.S. Department of Agriculture & U.S. Department of Health and Human Services (2005). *Dietary guidelines for Americans 2005* (6th ed.). Washington, DC: USDA & USDHHS.

Whitaker, J. (2000). Pet owners are a healthy breed. *Health & Healing, 10*(10), 1–8.

CLIENT EDUCATION

KEY TERMS

affective domain
behavioral objective
cognitive domain
domains of learning
psychomotor domain

CORE CONCEPTS

client education
learning
teaching

OBJECTIVES

After reading this chapter, the student will be able to:

1. Identify three theories of teaching and learning: the behaviorist theory, the cognitive theory, and the humanistic theory.
2. Define and differentiate among the three domains of learning: affective, cognitive, and psychomotor.
3. Discuss teaching strategies appropriate for the adult learner, children and adolescents, and elderly individuals.
4. Assess clients' learning needs.
5. Formulate specific behavioral objectives for teaching plans of care.
6. Develop and implement teaching plans of care.
7. Evaluate and document teaching plans of care.

 eplau (1991) identified five sub-roles within the role of the nurse. These included stranger, resource person, teacher, leader, and surrogate (see Chapter 7). Peplau stated,

The role of teacher in nursing situations seems to be a combination of all of the roles [in nursing]. Teaching always proceeds from what the patient knows and it develops around his interest in wanting and being able to use additional medical information. Learning through experience, which is the kind that nurses wish to promote, requires development of novel plans and situations that can unfold and lead to open-ended outcomes (i.e., outcomes which are unique products within this situation) that are fruitful for nurse and patient. (p. 48)

Can nurses teach? Not only *can* they, but they *must*. Standard Ve of the *Standards of Psychiatric-Mental Health Nursing Practice* (ANA, 2000) pertains to "Health Teaching." It states, "The psychiatric-mental health nurse, through health teaching, assists patients in achieving satisfying, productive, and healthy patterns of living." On the state level, the nurse practice acts of all 50 states outlines health teaching, guidance, or counseling among the expectations of nursing practice. Since 1993, the Joint Commission on the Accreditation of Healthcare Organizations (JCAHO) has required that health care organizations show evidence that all patients receive health teaching (Rankin, Stallings, & London, 2005).

This chapter examines the nursing role of client educator. Theories of learning are discussed, and the nursing process is used as the tool to identify learning needs, formulate teaching plans, and evaluate teaching outcomes. Client teaching guides to accompany this chapter may be found in Appendix G.

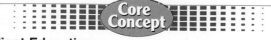

Client Education
The process of influencing behavior and producing the changes in knowledge, attitudes, and skills necessary to maintain or improve health. [It] is a holistic process with the goal of changing a patient's behavior to benefit his or her health status (Rankin, Stallings, & London, 2005).

HISTORICAL PERSPECTIVES

In the 19th century, client education by nurses focused on topics of sanitation, cleanliness, and care of the sick. However, in the early part of the 20th century, nurse educators were still expressing concern that nursing curricula dealing with health education were lacking in nursing schools. Public health work and primary prevention were coming to the forefront, and the importance of health teaching in these facets of nursing was being emphasized. In their 1937 *Curriculum Guide for Schools of Nursing*, the National League of Nursing Education, stated, "The nurse is essentially a teacher and an agent of health in whatever field she may be working" (National League of Nursing Education, 1937). A number of nursing conceptual models were developed that incorporated client education as an important component of nursing. Some of these nursing models and their client education focus are listed in Table 24–1.

The focus in the latter part of the 20th century moved from treatment of disease to prevention of illness and maintaining health. Hospital stays were shortened, and the need for health education increased to prepare clients for convalescence in their homes. As life span increases, so does the incidence of chronic illness and disability, with the subsequent need of the client and family for knowledge about the illness and its treatment.

In recent years there has been a movement on the part of consumers to take charge of their own health care. A client's right to take control of his or her own health care is a shift in position from earlier times when the physician controlled the medical situation, and clients were often left "in the dark" as far as knowledge of their condition was concerned. Consumers now demand that knowledge, and indeed, are entitled to it.

Nurses are in a dominant position to provide this knowledge on individual, family, small group, and community levels. It is their duty to do so.

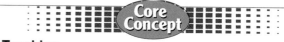

Teaching
The act of imparting knowledge or skill to another.

TABLE 24–1	Focus of Client Education Within Nursing Conceptual Models
CONCEPTUAL MODEL	**FOCUS OF CLIENT EDUCATION**
Peplau	Nursing is defined as an interpersonal process. Nursing is an educative instrument, a maturing force, that aims to promote forward movement of personality in the direction of creative, constructive, productive, personal, and community living.
Orem	The *supportive-educative nursing system* is a system in which the client is able to perform or can and should learn to perform required measures of therapeutic self-care but cannot do so without assistance. Helping techniques include support, guidance, provision of a developmental environment, and teaching.
Newman	Nursing is concerned with the total person. Nursing can intervene in the client's response to stress at three levels: primary, secondary, and tertiary prevention. Client education is a nursing intervention at all three levels, which are aimed at attaining, maintaining, or regaining optimum wellness.
Henderson	Nursing is an interpersonal process. The nurse assists the individual to learn, discover, or satisfy the curiosity that leads to normal development and health. Clients learn by the examples the nurse gives to them and by the answers the nurse offers to their questions.
Johnson	Nursing practice is directed toward restoring, maintaining, or attaining behavioral system balance at the highest possible level. Nurses intervene to change the behavioral elements through instruction or counseling and adding choices by teaching new skills.
Orlando	Nursing is an interpersonal process. Nursing activities include instructions, suggestions, directions, explanations, information, requests, and questions directed toward the client; making decisions for the client; handling the client's body; administering medications or treatments; and changing the client's immediate environment.

SOURCES: Peplau (1991); Orem (2001); George (2002); Furukawa & Howe (2002); Fawcett & Swoyer (1997).

THEORIES OF TEACHING AND LEARNING*

Theories of teaching and learning can be summarized according to three views: behaviorist, cognitive, and humanistic. In each of these views, the definition of learning, and consequently the definition of teaching, differ. The nurse can use concepts from each view to construct an effective teaching–learning situation in practice.

Behaviorist Theory

Behaviorist learning theory is based on the belief that there is a direct association between events or ideas (Bower & Hilgard, 1997). Behaviorists assume that people react to their environments and that behavior can be explained in mechanistic terms (Bigge & Shermis, 1998).

Learning is defined as a change in performance, including the development of habits or procedures in response to certain conditions, including need arousal, repeated practice, and reinforcement (Bower & Hilgard, 1997). Learning occurs when an unmet need produces sufficient motivation to satisfy that need. An unmet need causes tension, and the learner's desire to relieve the tension encourages action. The action is the response evoked by teacher-supplied stimuli. Through conditioning, or providing rewards for the desired response, the learner's needs are met and the tension is decreased. Need fulfillment accompanying the decrease in tension is also rewarding. If this pattern continues, habits develop through repeated practice.

Teaching is the arrangement of the contingencies of reinforcement (Skinner, 1968). The teacher controls the learning experience, and the learner is acted on by the teacher. The teacher specifies the desired response, and the learner, through trial and error, tries to produce the desired response. The teacher rewards the learner for correct or nearly correct responses.

To put it simply, Skinner (1968) noted that we learn by doing, by experience, and by trial and error. What is learned is that responses are emphasized, the situation where the responses occur is important, and consequences result from actions.

Cognitive Theory

Cognitive theory developed as researchers grew to believe that simple reflex arcs, or associations, could not adequately explain learning behavior. Cognitive learning theories are based on the assumption that learners interact with their environments. Learning occurs by focusing on the whole, rather than by studying the parts.

In cognitive theories, learning is considered an interaction between the learner and the environment, mediated by the teacher. Learning is internal; it occurs within the learner as new insights are formed or as cognitive structures are changed (Bigge & Shermis, 1998). Understanding is the focus of learning, and learners develop a coding system in their minds to store information. Thinking and conceptualizing are the learner's major activities, and the teacher evaluates cognitive development in the learners.

Teaching focuses on the relationships and organization of facts. Teaching involves creating situations that make meaningful learning experiences more likely for individual learners (Cantor, 1953). Teachers who understand the cognitive development of their learners and present organized subject matter appropriate to the learners produce learning.

Humanistic Theory

Humanistic theory is an approach to teaching and learning that involves being human in the process. Teachers and learners trust each other to be competent human beings who both learn through the process of self-discovery. Humanistic theory is a person-centered approach that involves specific values, which emphasize the individual and choice, responsibility, and creativity (Rogers, 1983).

Learning in humanistic theory has been called *significant*, or *experiential*, learning. Learning is the process of developing one's full potential. The elements of humanistic learning are (Rogers, 1983):

● The whole person, both feeling and cognition, is involved in learning.
● Learning is learner initiated.
● Learning is pervasive.
● Learning is learner evaluated.
● The essence of learning is meaning.

Learning may include practicing to make a new skill a habit or incorporating a new idea into one's own understanding, so long as the learner is actively involved in the process and not merely acted on by the teacher.

Teaching is the facilitation of learning (Rogers, 1983). The learner as a person, rather than as the subject matter, is the teacher's focus, and the learner is viewed as the one responsible for the learning. The teacher is available to assist the learner but is not necessarily the initiator of the process. Certain qualities of the humanistic teacher, including genuineness, appreciation of the learner, and empathic understanding, are essential to trusting the learner to develop and learn (Rogers, 1983).

---

*From Walsh, M., & Bernhard, L.A. (1998). Selected theories and models for advanced practice nursing. In C.M. Sheehy & M.C. McCarthy (Eds.). *Advanced practice nursing: Emphasizing common roles.* Philadelphia: F.A. Davis.

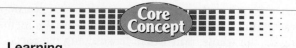

Learning
The act, process, or experience of becoming informed or of gaining knowledge or skill.

DOMAINS OF LEARNING[†]

Because learning is the acceptance and assimilation of information, it is incorporated into the learner's domains of knowledge and behavior. Note the difference reflected here between the knowledge and the demonstration of behaviors. We may "know" something, but either consciously or unconsciously decide not to demonstrate that behavior.

A *domain* is merely a category. There are three domains of learning or knowledge: affective, cognitive, and psychomotor.

Affective Domain

The **affective domain** includes attitudes, feelings, and values; for example, how the client feels about the importance of or the positive effect on his or her life of a needed dietary change will influence whether he or she will make the change. Often, the nursing goal is to incorporate the value of the diet into the person's belief system. However, cultural influence; cultural differences in the individual, family, or group; and the nurse's professional influences can all either positively or negatively affect whether the goal is achieved.

Cognitive Domain

The **cognitive domain** involves knowledge and thought processes within the individual's intellectual ability. Using the example of teaching a client about a low-fat diet, the cognitive domain involves understanding the information received about nutrition, diet, health conditions, and indications. The ability to conceptualize types of foods, gram counts, and dietary needs involves comprehension, application, and synthesis at an intellectual level before the actual behaviors are performed.

Psychomotor Domain

The **psychomotor domain** is the processing and demonstration of behaviors; the information has been intellectually processed, and the individual is displaying motor behaviors. To continue with the previous example, psychomotor skills are demonstrated by how the client

has performed on the changed diet, as seen in food diary reporting, preparing and ingesting appropriate foods, and even laboratory reports evaluating bodily functions.

It is important to consider these three domains in the teaching–learning process. Behavioral objectives, teaching content and methods, and evaluation of learning can be very different for the three domains and should be distinct. Remember, to achieve a lasting change in observed behavior (psychomotor domain), the value of that change (affective domain) and the intellectual capacity to understand and process the information for behavioral changes (cognitive domain) must first be present.

AGE AND DEVELOPMENTAL CONSIDERATIONS

The Adult Learner

Schuster (2000) outlines the following four adult learning principles—teaching strategies that are appropriate for client and family education.

1. **Build on Previous Experiences.** Adults learn by building on previous experiences. It is important to address any misconceptions or fears they may have related to previous experience with illness or injury. It is also important to know about clients' knowledge or understanding of the information you are wanting them to learn. In other words, how much do they know about the topic? Is what they know accurate? The answers to these questions become starting points for planning adult teaching. Nunnery (2005) states:

   > Adult learners are self-directing, have experiences that have shaped their identity, experience life events or a learning need that triggers their readiness to learn, have internal motivators, and demand an available, knowledgeable resource to assist them with practical problems and identified needs. (p. 216)

2. **Focus on Immediate Concerns First.** Adults want to learn what they need to know *now* (Schuster, 2000). They are generally concerned with solving an immediate problem. They want health professionals to tell them what they *need* to know versus what *is nice* to know (Rankin, Stallings, & London, 2005). They rarely want sophisticated, detailed explanations; instead, they want to know the basics of how to perform a prescribed regimen of health care and how to adapt it into their current lifestyle. Schuster (2000) states,

   > Always begin your teaching by finding the patient's immediate thoughts and needs. Adults must be involved in determining their own learning needs based on what they perceive to be the problem. You must know whether the patient sees his health problems the same way you do or whether he sees it differently before you suggest which behaviors he should change or how he should go about changing them. (p. 215)

[†]From Nunnery, R.K. (2005). Teaching-learning process. In R.K. Nunnery (Ed.). *Advancing your career: Concepts of professional nursing* (3rd ed.). Philadelphia: F.A. Davis.

3. **Adapt the Teaching to the Lifestyle.** Teaching must be tailored so that it is relevant to the client's present activities and responsibilities (Schuster, 2000). The client's current lifestyle must be taken into consideration when prescribing a particular health care regimen or proposing a specific behavioral change. Little good will it do to teach a client about a low-tyramine diet associated with the administration of an MAO inhibitor antidepressant if his wife is the sole purchaser and preparer of all his food. His wife must be included in the teaching. Also, if the client's lifestyle includes eating out often, it is important to help him learn which foods to avoid.

4. **Make the Client an Active Participant.** One key to successful teaching and learning in adults is active involvement throughout the process (Nunnery, 2005). Vella (2002) suggests that adult learners should be involved in identifying what needs to be learned, in planning the content of what is to be learned, and in evaluating what has been learned. Schuster (2000) states,

> Adults prefer to be independent and in control of the learning process and outcome. The patient must determine his own learning needs. In addition, this means the patient must actively participate. Teaching methods must be selected to facilitate active participation. Learning is faster and retention is better with the active involvement of the learner. (p. 215)

Teaching methods should include discussions and demonstrations that encourage the client to ask questions. The instructor should also ask questions, to validate what the client has learned. A lecture is not appropriate, except in large-group situations, because it discourages learner interaction.

Teaching Children and Adolescents[‡]

Although many of the same principles of adult learning also apply to children and adolescents, teaching young people demands more ingenuity and a somewhat different approach. Most importantly, it is essential to take the child's stage of cognitive development into consideration before embarking on pediatric client education (Piaget & Inhelder, 1969).

● **Birth to Age 2 Years—Sensorimotor Development.** During this stage, a child learns to differentiate the self from the environment. The child learns that his or her actions have effects on people and objects. Teaching should be aimed at the parents while making the child feel as secure and comfortable as possible, perhaps with familiar objects from the home environment.

● **Ages 2 to 7—Preoperational Development.** In the stage of preoperational development, children take

everything literally and cannot generalize. They often believe that illness is self-caused or punitive. They can manipulate equipment and be shown how to use equipment, such as stethoscopes and reflex hammers. They may practice on a doll. Encourage the child to express fears and be honest. Don't make false promises that a procedure won't hurt if indeed the child is likely to experience some pain.

● **Ages 7 to 12—Concrete Operational Thought Development.** During this stage, a child learns to understand cause-and-effect relationships and develops logical reasoning abilities. Simple drawings and the correct medical equipment should be used to facilitate learning. Explaining similar medical experiences of other children can be helpful at this stage, as they will be likely to relate the situations to their own. Redman (1993) states:

> Children of school age benefit from tours of hospital playrooms and wards and from discussion in which they can learn about their illness, its origins, and proposed plans of treatment. Because school-aged children have a more mature concept of causality, they have the capacity to understand that neither illness nor treatment is imposed on them because of their own misdeeds. (p. 91)

● **Ages 12 to 18—Formal Operations Development.** Children in this stage have well developed cognitive abilities. Increased amounts of technical information can be provided if the client wants to know more about what is happening to him or her. Children in this stage also are working to establish independence, and some resentment may be expressed toward healthcare professionals telling them what they should or should not do. Adolescents should be given the chance to discuss feelings and teaching should be performed without the parents present. Reassurance should be given that their confidentiality will be respected (as long as safety is not an issue).

In summary, Rankin, Stallings, and London (2005) state:

> Before teaching children, remember they have shorter attention spans, have greater need for support and nurturing, and learn more easily through active participation than do adults. Therefore, material must be presented in abbreviated format during a short time. Consistently and persistently show affection and offer praise to young patients during education sessions. By actively involving children in the learning process, we help them to more readily assimilate the information. (p. 125)

Teaching the Elderly

As the population ages, the need for teaching older clients increases. Teaching plans for middle-aged individuals must be modified for the elderly client. A mistake that is commonly made by health educators is to approach the older client as if he or she were a child

[‡]Adapted from Schuster, P.M. (2000). *Communication: The key to the therapeutic relationship*. Philadelphia: F.A. Davis.

(Rankin, Stallings, & London, 2005). This can be insulting to the client and demonstrates a lack of sensitivity on the part of the health care professional.

The ability to learn is not diminished by age. Studies, however, have shown that some aspects of learning do change with age. The ordinary slowing of reaction time with age for nearly all tasks or the overarousal of the central nervous system may account for lower performance levels on tests requiring rapid responses. Under conditions that allow for self-pacing by the participant, differences in accuracy of performance diminish. Ability to learn continues throughout life, although strongly influenced by interests, activity, motivation, health, and income (Williams, 1995). Adjustments do need to be made in teaching methodology and time allowed for learning.

There appears to be a high degree of regularity in intellectual functioning across the adult age span. Crystallized abilities, or knowledge acquired in the course of the socialization process, tend to remain stable over the adult life span. Fluid abilities, or abilities involved in solving novel problems, tend to decline gradually from young to old adulthood (Birren & Schaie, 2001). In other words, intellectual abilities of older people do not decline but do become obsolete. The age of their formal educational experiences is reflected in their intelligence scoring.

A number of biological changes occur with the aging process that require special adaptations in the teaching process when working with these individuals. Suggestions for teaching elderly clients, taking these biological changes into consideration, are presented in Table 24–2.

THE NURSING PROCESS IN CLIENT EDUCATION

Assessment

A comprehensive assessment tool is provided in Chapter 9. This tool includes information to assist the nurse in identifying knowledge deficits. Following are some spe-

TABLE 24–2   Biological Changes in the Elderly that May Affect the Learning Process

BIOLOGICAL CHANGES	SUGGESTIONS FOR MODIFICATION IN TEACHING
Vision Decreased visual acuity Presbyopia (blurred near vision) Cataract formation (cloudy vision) Decreased depth perception and peripheral vision	Use large-print materials with high contrast between black and white. Ensure minimal glare by using soft light positioned behind the client. Maintain low lighting in the room when using audiovisual materials.
Hearing Loss in sensitivity to discriminate sounds, particularly high-frequency sounds (presbycusis) General hearing loss related to (1) conduction problems (2) auditory nerve problems (3) disturbances in the brain	Speak clearly in a normal tone of voice. Speak to the person face-to-face. Avoid overarticulation. Encourage client to use hearing aid if he or she has one. May need to use a communication device, if appropriate (e.g., amplifier). Use visual aids to reinforce teaching. Ensure that extraneous, background noise is kept to a minimum.
Neurological System Decline in cognitive ability Impairment in short-term memory Increased distractibility Increased amount of time required to assimilate information	Present small amounts of information slowly. Repeat information frequently. Use audiovisual aids to reinforce teaching. Keep distracting stimuli to a minimum. Take frequent breaks. Allow increased amount of time for client discussion of the material.
Genitourinary (Women) Stress incontinence is common due to loss of muscle and sphincter control (Men) Prostatic hypertrophy may lead to urinary retention/frequency or incontinence	Frequent bathroom breaks will be necessary.
Musculoskeletal Osteoarthritis Osteoporosis Loss of muscle mass/tone Diminished storage of muscle glycogen, resulting in loss of energy reserve Impaired sense of balance	Take frequent rest breaks. Use comfortable chairs that provide support for arms and legs. Provide hand rails and available supports to prevent falls.
Cardiopulmonary Diminished cardiac output Decreased vital capacity Overall decline in energy reserves	Take frequent rest breaks. Teaching sessions must be brief.

SOURCES: Beers & Jones (2004); Birren & Schaie (2001); Rogers-Seidl (1996); and Boyd (1997).

cific topics of information that are especially important in assessing client learning needs.

Client's Understanding of the Current Health Problem

Ask the client what is his or her understanding of the current health condition. Ask what has been explained to him or her and what are some concerns. Redman (1993) suggests asking the following types of questions:

1. What do you know about your disease and treatment?
2. How do you cope with symptoms?
3. How do you manage stressful situations?
4. What concerns you the most right now?

Age and Developmental Level

It is important to assess whether the individual's age corresponds with current developmental level. Where should the client be in fulfilling developmental tasks according to his or her age? Where is he or she in actuality? If a client is developmentally delayed, this must be taken into consideration in formulating the teaching plan. Use of Erikson's stages (Chapter 3) is helpful in making this assessment.

Cultural Considerations

Does the client have cultural values that may interfere with his or her acceptance of certain health care recommendations? Does the client speak only a foreign language? Is an interpreter available? Does another member of the family take responsibility for the client's welfare? If so, can that individual be available for health teaching? Assess the value placed on certain health-care practices. Assess current health care practices specific to the culture (e.g., folk medicine practices). Are there certain religious beliefs that may prevent the client from seeking health care?

Learning Style and Reading Level

Pestonjee (2000) suggests the following types of questions to assess learning style:

1. What time of day do you learn best?
2. Do you like to read?
3. What do you like to read?
4. Would you prefer to read something first, or would you rather have me explain it to you?
5. Do you remember something better if you read it, hear it, or try it?

Winslow (2001) reports that the average adult in the United States cannot read above the eighth grade level. Some studies have shown that the number of years of school completed exceeds clients' actual reading abilities

by two to five years. Health care providers must prepare materials at the lowest possible reading level—preferably the sixth grade level or lower (Winslow, 2001).

Available Support Systems

What family and friends are available to the client? Are they supportive, both physically and emotionally? It is important to determine how family members perceive that the client's illness has affected the family. How willing are they to accept help from others? It is important to include the family or significant others in the client's health education. Rankin, Stallings, and London (2005) state, "Educating the patient without including the family frequently results in poor rehabilitation and poor cooperation with self-care measures, whether the patient is acutely ill or faces life with a long-term chronic illness" (p. 163).

Learning Readiness and Motivation

How do you know if your client is ready and motivated to learn? Has he or she accepted the diagnosis and decided to improve the current situation? What is his or her anxiety level? Learning cannot take place beyond the moderate level of anxiety (see Chapter 2). Is the current health state interfering with his or her ability to learn? Is the client motivated to improve the current health situation, or does he or she feel helpless in the face of this illness?

How is motivation assessed? That which serves as a motivator for one individual to change behavior or gain new information may be different for another individual. For example, one individual may decide to lose weight to feel more physically attractive, whereas another individual may do so because he or she fears the excess weight contributes to cardiac or other health problems. Some individuals may decide to quit smoking because they believe it is drying out their skin and contributing to wrinkles, while other persons may have fears of lung cancer. Nunnery (2005) states,

> The way the person views these future consequences of behavior becomes the motivation to behave or proceed in the present. This concept relates well to health teaching, in that the client can be motivated to learn with a realistic anticipation of the situation and consequences. Nurses can recognize client anticipation in the assessment phase, through interview data, diagnosis of the teaching and learning needs, and development of behavioral objectives. During this process, motivation can be assessed and stimulated by the client as well as by the professional nurse. (p. 219)

Financial Considerations

Does the client live on a small, fixed income? Does he or she have insurance? Will the health plan cover the cost of the client's health care needs (e.g., medication)? Will the client have to pay part of the costs? Schuster (2000) states,

> The reality for many patients is that they can't afford what nurses teach them to do. If that is the case, essentials will need to be separated from the alternatives. For example, perhaps a generic drug can be substituted for the more expensive brand name drug. (p. 230)

Nursing Diagnosis

Nursing diagnoses are statements of actual or potential health problems and are derived from the health assessment data. The nursing diagnosis of *deficient knowledge* is most frequently selected by nurses to use when a learning need has been identified. This is an appropriate choice, although learning needs also can be related to other nursing diagnoses and incorporated as a part of the total plan of care. For purposes of this chapter, the diagnosis of *deficient knowledge* will be detailed here (NANDA International, 2005).

Deficient Knowledge

Definition: Absence or deficiency of cognitive information related to a specific topic

Defining Characteristics

- Verbalization of the problem
- Inaccurate follow-through of instruction
- Inaccurate performance of test
- Inappropriate or exaggerated behaviors (e.g., hysterical, hostile, agitated, apathetic)

Related Factors

- Lack of exposure
- Lack of recall
- Information misinterpretation
- Cognitive limitation
- Lack of interest in learning
- Unfamiliarity with information resources

Outcome Identification

Developing Behavioral Objectives

Rankin, Stallings, and London (2005) state:

> Setting specific behavioral objectives for patient education ensures that learning interventions will be tailored to the client's unique situation and needs. Objectives describe the behaviors or actions the patient will perform to meet a goal. (p. 240)

Objectives let the learner know what is expected of him or her. They are a way of measuring learning outcomes, and are based on the three domains of learning described earlier in this chapter: cognitive, affective, and psychomotor.

A **behavioral** (or learning) **objective** has the following components:

Who:	The client
Will perform:	Action verb based on domains of learning
What:	Criteria (behavior to be measured)
How well:	Accurately (or with special conditions)
By when:	Time of evaluation

An example of a learning objective with these five components is as follows:

> Mr. T. *(who)* will list *(action verb)* five foods that should be avoided while taking MAO inhibitor *(what will be measured)* using handouts provided *(conditions)* by the end of the teaching session *(when)*.

Verbs must be of the action variety in order to be measurable. Words such as *understand* and *know* are not measurable, and therefore should be avoided in writing behavioral objectives. As previously stated, the action verbs should be based on the three domains of learning. The cognitive and psychomotor domains are relatively easy to measure. The affective domain is more difficult to measure because values and attitudes are more difficult to assess than knowledge, which can be measured with a paper-and-pencil test of information recalled (Nunnery, 2005). For example, in the case of a newly diagnosed diabetic, acceptance of the diagnosis is essential to developing long-range personal care skills. But to measure "acceptance" is a difficult task. Nunnery (2005) states:

> Although action verbs for the affective domain include *receiving, responding, valuing, organizing values,* and *characterizing,* this is a difficult domain of learning to evaluate. We must rely on the individual to communicate his or her attitudes, feelings, and values honestly through verbal and nonverbal behaviors. (p. 222)

Some examples of verbs that are appropriate for measuring these three domains are presented in Table 24–3.

Planning/Implementation

A teaching plan is a blueprint of what will be taught, how it will be taught, and how the results will be measured. Pestonjee (2000) states:

> The teaching plan should include clear, concise teaching actions, including *what* will be taught, *when* teaching will occur, *where* teaching will take place, *who* will teach and learn, and *how* teaching will occur. (p. 19)

TABLE 24–3	Action Verbs for Measuring Behaviors Within the Three Domains of Learning	
COGNITIVE	**AFFECTIVE**	**PSYCHOMOTOR**
Knowledge Level Identify List Define Recognize Repeat	**Receiving Level** Describe Identify Defend	**Imitation Level** Imitate Follow instructions Repeat Identify
Comprehension Level Describe Summarize Discuss Distinguish Explain	**Responding Level** Choose Compare Explain Express Relate	**Manipulation Level** Carry out Follow the procedure Practice Attempt
Application Level Apply Demonstrate Employ Use Implement	**Valuing Level** Help Join Initiate Propose	**Demonstration Level** Demonstrate skill in the procedure **Articulation Level** Use Apply
Analysis Level Assess Appraise Compare Contrast Critique Evaluate	**Organizing Values** Participate Perform Attempt State willingness	**Competence Level** Use Employ Adapt Modify Correct Rearrange Create Design
Synthesis Level Create Design Devise Generate	**Standing For** Accept Admit Heed Follow Influence Revise Serve	

SOURCES: Nunnery (2005); Rankin, Stallings, & London (2005); Redman (1993).

Plan What Will Be Taught

Once the behavioral objectives have been agreed upon by client and teacher, a specific content outline is developed to meet each objective. Teaching strategies and learning resources are listed on the plan as they relate to each objective.

Plan When the Teaching Will Take Place

Pestonjee (2000) suggests the following factors when planning teaching time:

● Consider the client's length of stay
● Offer options and allow the client to choose. For instance, what time of day does the client prefer to be taught? Some individuals prefer mornings, while others seem to have increased energy later in the day.
● Keep teaching sessions relatively short—generally no more than 30 minutes and possibly as short as 5 minutes. Watch for signs of inattention and fatigue on the part of the client.

Pestonjee (2000) states, "You can't plan for these, but always be ready to grab those 'golden teaching moments' when the patient is ready to learn—even when it means throwing your planned timetable out the window" (p. 19).

Plan Where the Teaching Will Take Place

Take comfort and privacy into consideration when deciding where to teach the client. Try to find a place with as few distractions as possible, away from the noise of the unit, the television, and the comings and goings of others. If family or significant others will be included in the teaching, ensure that there is enough room for everyone to sit comfortably. Be cognizant of external factors, such as temperature and lighting. It is important to consider the hierarchy of needs, and comfort measures must be fulfilled before the ability to learn can progress.

Plan How the Content Will Be Presented

It is important to determine, from the baseline assessment data, what is the most effective method of teaching the client. The client's preferred learning style and developmental learning level will have been assessed, and this information should be taken into consideration when selecting the most appropriate teaching methods. Pestonjee (2000) suggests the following teaching methods and materials:

TEACHING METHODS

- One-on-one sessions
- Small-group discussions and support groups
- Lectures
- Demonstration and return demonstrations
- Role-playing
- Games
- Programmed instruction

TEACHING MATERIALS

- Pamphlets
- Posters and flip charts
- Videos and closed-circuit television
- Computer-assisted instruction
- Audiocassettes
- Transparencies
- Chalk or dry-erase boards
- Models

A selected list of teaching strategies and advantages and disadvantages associated with each is presented in Table 24–4. Examples of teaching materials can be found in the electronic educational materials that accompany this text. These sample client teaching guides may be adapted and used by nurses and nursing students with clients who require this type of teaching.

Evaluation

Evaluation of the teaching–learning activity has a twofold purpose. First, were the behavioral objectives met? Has the client resolved an identified knowledge deficit? Second, evaluation can provide information about the teaching process itself. Were the teaching methods and materials appropriate for meeting the behavioral objectives? What problems or difficulties occurred during the teaching process? How will these problems be overcome in the future?

Care should be taken to select an evaluation method that accurately measures what the client has learned (i.e., to determine if the behavioral objectives have been met). Some ways of evaluating include:

- Return demonstrations
- Oral question and answer session
- Paper and pencil tests

TABLE 24–4 Teaching Strategies

STRATEGY	ADVANTAGES	DISADVANTAGES
Lecture	Easier to organize and transfer large amount of information Predictable, quicker, more efficient, and useful for a large group Allows teacher control over material being presented Easy to focus material	Lacks opportunity for feedback Risk of information overload Sustaining interest may be difficult Difficult to tailor material for the group
Discussion	Allows for continual feedback, attitude development and modification Flexible, able to be modified according to the motivation of the audience Able to identify confusion and resolve difficulties Serves as a vehicle for networking	Increases chance of getting off the focus Risk of discussion becoming pointless Allows participants to be dominant or passive Time-consuming
Demonstration	Activates many senses Clarifies the "whys" as a principle Commands interest Correlates theory with practice Allows for problem identification Helps learner receive well-directed practice	Time-consuming Does not cover all aspects of cognitive learning
Modeling	Facilitates active learning Bypasses defenses Effective with children	Ineffective without rapport Learning not always visible Risk for learner ambivalence
Programmed instruction	Allows learning at a self-directed pace Able to repeat sections at will Breaks down information into manageable increments Saves teacher time	Effectiveness depends on learner motivation Does not account for unplanned feedback, which can distance learner
Simulated environments, games, activities, and role playing	Greatest transfer of learning Facilitates learning of what is needed to cope with problem or environment Allows for practice that is most transferable	Facilitates unpredictable occurrences May be threatening to learner Time-consuming Achievement of outcomes is difficult
Team teaching	Uses competencies of more than one teacher Allows for learning among the teachers Accentuates divergent points of view	Lacks continuity and internal consistency Requires more planning Group processing slower Eliminates teacher autonomy

SOURCE: Babcock, D.E., & Miller, M.A. (1994). *Client education: Theory and practice* (1st ed.). St. Louis: C.V. Mosby. Reprinted with permission.

- Questionnaires or rating scales
- Pre- and post-tests
- Asking the client to problem solve in a hypothetical situation
- Direct observation of changes in behavior

These methods are appropriate for evaluating the cognitive and psychomotor domains of learning. Regarding evaluation of the affective domain, Nunnery (2005) states:

> Methods of evaluation in [the affective domain] include interviews, discussions, and observations that demonstrate certain beliefs and values. Another means of evaluating affective learning is a diary in which the client can record feelings and problems that arise between teaching sessions. Analyzing the content of the diaries can provide useful information on the affective domain, as well as knowledge gaps in cognitive processes. (p. 229)

DOCUMENTATION OF CLIENT EDUCATION

Documentation of client education should start with the initial learning assessment and continue through the final evaluation (Pestonjee, 2000). Documentation provides a permanent, legal record of teaching and learning. It serves as a communication medium among various health care professionals and helps maintain continuity of care. It is also required by some third-party payers and accrediting agencies, such as Medicare and the Joint Commission on Accreditation of Healthcare Organizations.

Documentation of teaching-learning may take the form of anecdotal notes, flowcharts, checklists, or even standardized teaching care plans (Boyd, 1997). Regardless of the form that the documentation takes, the following information should be included:

- Initial assessments and reassessments of client learning needs
- Nursing diagnoses
- Behavioral objectives identified by client and nurse
- Content presented and teaching strategies employed
- Objective report of learner(s) responses to teaching
- Evaluation of what the client learned, and how this was measured

The Problem-Oriented Recording (POR) format works particularly well for documenting client education. In the POR format, the subjective, objective, assessment, plan, intervention, and evaluation (SOAPIE) components are used for the entry. Following is an explanation of these components:

S = Subjective data: Information gathered from what the client, family, or other source has said or reported.

O = Objective data: Information gathered by direct observation of the person doing the assessment; may include a physiological measurement such as blood pressure or a behavioral response such as affect.

A = Assessment: The nurse's interpretation of the subjective and objective data.

P = Plan: The actions or treatments to be carried out.

I = Intervention: Those nursing actions that were actually carried out.

E = Evaluation of the problem following nursing intervention

An example of a client teaching documentation using this format is presented in Table 24–5.

TABLE 24–5   Documentation of Client Education Using SOAPIE Format

S:	Client stated, "The doctor told me I couldn't eat chocolate when I take this new medicine he prescribed. I don't understand why."
O:	Client approached nurse with this question. Expressed concern about having to follow a special diet while taking Nardil, a new prescription that he will be given on discharge.
A:	Deficient knowledge related to low-tyramine diet associated with the use of MAO Inhibitors
P:	1. Client will be able to name foods and over-the-counter medications to avoid while taking Nardil. 2. Client will be able to discuss reasons for avoiding these foods and medications while taking Nardil. 3. Client will carry a card in his wallet containing name of medication being taken.
I:	Presented client with handout naming foods and medications to avoid. Went over this handout with client and answered any questions he had. Presented client with handout describing hypertensive crisis. Discussed signs and symptoms with client and discussed reasons why these symptoms might occur. Stressed the importance of carrying a card in his wallet identifying the name of the medication he is taking. Followed up on this by making a small card with the name of the medication on it, which the client placed in his wallet. Answered questions that client presented. Allowed client to keep handouts, and told him that we would go over them again before his discharge.
E:	After going over the material, I asked the client to name some foods and medications that he would not be able to consume while he was taking Nardil. He was able to name these foods and medications, using the handout provided. I asked him to explain why avoiding these foods and medications was important, and he was able to state some of the symptoms that might occur if he did not comply. He stated that he would keep the card in his wallet in case anyone ever needed to know about his medication and he was unable to tell them. He also stated that he understood that hypertensive crisis could be a life-threatening situation if it should occur.

SUMMARY

Client education is defined as "the process of influencing behavior, producing changes in knowledge, attitudes, and skills required to maintain and improve health." Nurses must provide client education based on the standards of care, the nurse practice acts, and declarations from the Joint Commission on the Accreditation of Healthcare Organizations.

In the 19th century, client education by nurses focused on topics of sanitation, cleanliness, and care of the sick. The focus in the latter part of the 20th century moved from treatment of disease to prevention of illness and maintaining health. Hospital stays have been shortened, and with the increasing incidence of chronic illness and disability, the need of the client and family for knowledge about their illness and treatment is increasing.

This chapter presented an overview of the process of client education. A description of teaching and learning theories, including the behaviorist theory, the cognitive theory, and the humanistic theory was provided.

Domains of learning, including the affective, cognitive, and psychomotor domains, were described. An explanation of age and developmental considerations focused on strategies for teaching adults, children and adolescents, and the elderly.

The six steps of the nursing process were used to present the process of client education. Assessment should consider the client's understanding of the current health problem, age and developmental level, culture, learning style and reading level, available support systems, learning readiness and motivation, and financial situation. The nursing diagnosis of *deficient knowledge* is most frequently selected by nurses to use when a learning need has been identified. Definition, defining characteristics, and related factors, as described by NANDA International for the diagnosis of *deficient knowledge* were presented. Outcome identification included instructions for writing behavioral learning objectives. The final steps of the nursing process examined teaching strategies, methods of evaluation, and documentation of the teaching-learning process.

REVIEW QUESTIONS

SELF-EXAMINATION/LEARNING EXERCISE

Situation: Sarah is 13 years old. She was recently diagnosed with diabetes mellitus-type 1. She must learn how to manage her illness, including glucose monitoring, self-administration of insulin, urine ketone testing, nutrition, and exercise and activity. Sarah has been very withdrawn since being told about her condition. She became very depressed and has been seeing a counselor. She has finally agreed to allow the home health nurse, Ms. K., to begin diabetes education. Questions 1–5 apply to Sarah.

Select the answer that is most appropriate for the following questions.

1. Ms. K. has decided to try various approaches in her teaching to determine which method would be best with Sarah. She promises Sarah that when she has learned how to read the ketone tests correctly, they will go to the mall so that Sarah can buy the lip gloss she has been wanting. This is an example of
   a. The behaviorist learning theory
   b. The cognitive learning theory
   c. The humanistic learning theory
   d. The interpersonal learning theory.

2. Sarah says to Ms. K., "I'll be glad when I can give my own injections and don't have to rely on anyone else. I'll feel better then. Can we get started on that right away?" Ms. K. replies, "Sarah, you may decide what you want to learn next." This is an example of
   a. The behaviorist learning theory
   b. The cognitive learning theory
   c. The humanistic learning theory
   d. The interpersonal learning theory

3. After Ms. K. teaches Sarah about the effects of diabetes on the body, Sarah states, "I want to learn to do the right things so that I can stay healthy." This statement is an example of learning in the
   a. Cognitive domain
   b. Normative domain
   c. Psychomotor domain
   d. Affective domain

4. After explaining the procedure, Ms. K. demonstrated for Sarah how to draw up the medication from the vial into the syringe. Later she asked Sarah to perform this procedure while Ms. K. observed. This is an example of evaluation in the
   a. Cognitive domain
   b. Normative domain
   c. Psychomotor domain
   d. Affective domain

5. Ms. K. taught Sarah about which foods were most appropriate for her on her diabetic diet and how to coordinate diet, insulin, and exercise to maintain blood glucose levels. Following their lesson, Ms. K took Sarah to the grocery store and observed while Sarah purchased the appropriate foods to be used by Sarah and her mother in meal preparation. This is an example of evaluation in the
   a. Cognitive domain
   b. Normative domain
   c. Psychomotor domain
   d. Affective domain

6. Jim is recovering from a recent myocardial infarction (MI). His physician has left instructions that he is to receive teaching about a heart-healthy diet from the nurse. His first statement to the nurse when she arrives to begin the teaching is, "I have to eat lunch downtown 5 days a week. My co-workers and I have business lunches every day in a restaurant. How am I going to change the way I eat?" The nurse must teach Jim

a. That eating restaurant food every day is unhealthy
b. Which foods to choose when eating in a restaurant.
c. How to pack heart-healthy brown-bag lunches.
d. The importance of not doing business during lunch hours.

7. Sally is 8 years old. She is in the hospital to have her tonsils removed. She expresses her fear to the nurse. An appropriate response by the nurse would be:
   a. "Oh, there's nothing to be afraid of. Your doctor does this every day."
   b. "Don't be afraid. Just think! When it's over you can have all the ice cream you want!"
   c. "Let me tell you about my little girl. She just had her tonsils out last month."
   d. "You're throat will only hurt for a little while."

8. Edith is 72 years old. The nurse is teaching her about medication management. Edith states, "Oh, I don't know if I can learn this. I'm too old to learn anything new." Based on knowledge of the aging process, which of the following is a true statement?
   a. Ability to solve problems changes very little with advancing age.
   b. Intellectual functioning declines with advancing age.
   c. Cognitive functioning is rarely affected in aging individuals.
   d. Learning ability remains intact, but time required for learning increases with age.

9. The nurse is preparing a teaching plan to teach Sam about a low-tyramine diet. Which of the following is an appropriate behavioral learning objective for Sam?
   a. After a teaching session, Sam will list five foods high in tyramine.
   b. After a teaching session, Sam will have knowledge of foods high in tyramine.
   c. After a teaching session, Sam will verbalize understanding of foods high in tyramine.
   d. After a teaching session, Sam will know which foods to avoid while taking MAO inhibitor medication.

10. The nurse wants Sam to be able to synthesize the information learned about a low-tyramine diet. Which of the following behaviors on Sam's part demonstrates learning in the synthesis level of the cognitive domain?
   a. Sam describes the reason for following a low-tyramine diet.
   b. Sam creates a meal plan with the appropriate low-tyramine foods.
   c. Sam identifies which foods are high in tyramine from a list the nurse gives him.
   d. Sam is able to explain the consequences of eating foods high in tyramine while taking MAO inhibitor medication.

REFERENCES

American Nurses Association (ANA). (2000). *Scope and standards of psychiatric-mental health nursing practice.* Washington, DC: ANA.
Beers, M.H., & Jones, T.V. (Eds.). (2004). *Merck manual of health and aging.* Whitehouse Station, NJ: Merck.
Bigge, M.L., & Shermis, S.S. (1998). *Learning theories for teachers* (6th ed.). Boston: Addison Wesley Longman.
Birren, J.E., & Schaie, K.W. (Eds.). (2001). *Handbook of the psychology of aging.* New York: Elsevier Science.
Bower, G.H., & Hilgard, E.J. (1997). *Theories of learning* (5th ed.). Amarillo, TX: Paramount Communications Co.
Boyd, M.D. (1997). Health teaching in nursing practice. In M.H. Oermann (Ed.). *Professional nursing practice.* Stamford, CT: Appleton & Lange.
Fawcett, J., & Swoyer, B. (2005). Evolution and use of formal nursing knowledge. In R.K. Nunnery (Ed.). *Advancing your career: Concepts of professional nursing* (3rd ed.). Philadelphia: F.A. Davis.
Furukawa, C.Y., & Howe, J.K. (2002). Definition and components of nursing: Virginia Henderson. In J.B. George (Ed.). *Nursing theories: The base for professional nursing practice* (5th ed.). Upper Saddle River, NJ: Prentice-Hall.

George, J.B. (2002). The Newman systems model: Betty Newman. In J.B. George (Ed.). *Nursing theories: The base for professional nursing practice* (5th ed.). Upper Saddle River, NJ: Prentice-Hall.
NANDA International. (2005). *Nursing Diagnoses: Definitions & Classification 2005–2006.* Philadelphia: NANDA International.
Nunnery, R.K. (2005). Teaching-learning process. In R.K. Nunnery (Ed.). *Advancing your career: Concepts of professional nursing* (3rd ed.). Philadelphia: F.A. Davis.
Orem, D.E. (2001). *Nursing: Concepts of practice* (6th ed.). New York: Elsevier Science.
Peplau, H.E. (1991). *Interpersonal relations in nursing.* New York: Springer.
Pestonjee, S. F. (2000). *Nurse's handbook of patient education.* Springhouse, PA: Springhouse Corporation.
Rankin, S.H., Stallings, K.D., & London, F. (2005). *Patient education: Principles & practice* (5th ed.). Philadelphia: Lippincott Williams & Wilkins.
Redman, B.K. (1993). *The process of patient education.* St. Louis: Mosby Year Book.

Rogers-Seidl, F.F. (1996). *Geriatric nursing care plans* (2nd ed.). St. Louis: Mosby.

Schuster, P.M. (2000). *Communication: The key to the therapeutic relationship.* Philadelphia: F.A. Davis.

Vella, J. (2002). *Learning to listen, learning to teach: The power of dialogue in educating adults* (Revised). New York: John Wiley & Sons.

Williams, M.E. (1995). *The American Geriatrics Society's complete guide to aging and health.* New York: Harmony Books.

Winslow, E.H. (2001). Patient education materials: Can patients read them, or are they ending up in the trash? *American Journal of Nursing, 101*(10), 33–38.

CLASSICAL REFERENCES

Cantor, N. (1953). *The teaching-learning process.* New York: Dryden.

National League of Nursing Education. (1937). *A curriculum guide for schools of nursing.* New York: The League.

Piaget, J., & Inhelder, B. (1969). *The psychology of the child.* New York: Basic Books.

Rogers, C.R. (1983). *Freedom to learn for the 80s.* Columbus, OH: Merrill.

Skinner, B.F. (1968). *The technology of teaching.* New York: Appleton-Century-Crofts.

NURSING CARE OF CLIENTS WITH ALTERATIONS IN PSYCHOSOCIAL ADAPTATION

DISORDERS USUALLY FIRST DIAGNOSED IN INFANCY, CHILDHOOD, OR ADOLESCENCE

CHAPTER OUTLINE

KEY TERMS

aggression
autistic disorder
clinging
echolalia

impulsivity
negativism
palilalia

CORE CONCEPTS

disruptive behavior
  disorders
hyperactivity
impulsiveness

pervasive
  developmental
  disorders
temperament

OBJECTIVES

After reading this chapter, the student will be able to:

1. Identify psychiatric disorders usually first diagnosed in infancy, childhood, or adolescence.
2. Discuss predisposing factors implicated in the etiology of mental retardation, autistic disorder, attention-deficit/hyperactivity disorder, conduct disorder, oppositional defiant disorder, Tourette's disorder, and separation anxiety disorder.
3. Identify symptomatology and use the information in the assessment of clients with the aforementioned disorders.

4. Identify nursing diagnoses common to clients with these disorders and select appropriate nursing interventions for each.
5. Discuss relevant criteria for evaluating nursing care of clients with selected infant, childhood, and adolescent psychiatric disorders.
6. Describe treatment modalities relevant to selected disorders of infancy, childhood, and adolescence.

his chapter examines various disorders in which the symptoms usually first become evident during infancy, childhood, or adolescence. That is not to say that some of the disorders discussed in this chapter do not appear later in life or that symptoms associated with other disorders, such as major depression or schizophrenia, do not appear in childhood or adolescence. The basic concepts of care are applied to treatment in those instances, with consideration of the variances in age and developmental level.

Developmental theories were discussed in Chapter 3. Any nurse working with children or adolescents should be knowledgeable about "normal" stages of growth and development. At best, the developmental process is one that is fraught with frustrations and difficulties. Behavioral responses are individual and idiosyncratic. They are, indeed, *human* responses.

Whether or not a child's behavior indicates emotional problems is often difficult to determine. The *DSM-IV-TR* (American Psychiatric Association [APA], 2000) includes the following criteria among many of its diagnostic categories. An emotional problem exists if the behavioral manifestations:

● Are not age-appropriate.
● Deviate from cultural norms.
● Create deficits or impairments in adaptive functioning.

This chapter focuses on the nursing process in care of clients with mental retardation, autistic disorder, attention-deficit/hyperactivity disorder, conduct disorder, oppositional defiant disorder, Tourette's disorder, and separation anxiety disorder. Additional treatment modalities are included.

MENTAL RETARDATION

Mental retardation is defined by deficits in general intellectual functioning and adaptive functioning (APA, 2000). General intellectual functioning is measured by an individual's performance on intelligence quotient (IQ) tests. Adaptive functioning refers to the person's ability to adapt to the requirements of daily living and the expectations of his or her age and cultural group. The *DSM-IV-TR* diagnostic criteria for mental retardation are presented in Table 25–1.

Predisposing Factors

The *DSM-IV-TR* (APA, 2000) states that the etiology of mental retardation may be primarily biological or primarily psychosocial, or some combination of both. In approximately 30 to 40 percent of individuals seen in clinical settings, the etiology cannot be determined. Five major predisposing factors have been identified:

Hereditary Factors. Hereditary factors are implicated as the cause in approximately 5 percent of the cases. These factors include inborn errors of metabolism, such as Tay-Sachs disease, phenylketonuria, and hyperglycinemia. Also included are chromosomal disorders, such as Down syndrome and Klinefelter syndrome, and single-gene abnormalities, such as tuberous sclerosis and neurofibromatosis.

Early Alterations in Embryonic Development. Prenatal factors that result in early alterations in embryonic development account for approximately 30 percent of mental retardation cases. Damages may occur in response to toxicity associated with maternal ingestion of alcohol or other drugs. Maternal illnesses and infections during pregnancy (e.g., rubella, cytomegalovirus) and complications of pregnancy (e.g., toxemia, uncontrolled diabetes) also can result in congenital mental retardation (Sadock and Sadock, 2003).

Pregnancy and Perinatal Factors. Approximately 10 percent of cases of mental retardation are the result of factors that occur during pregnancy (e.g., fetal malnutrition, viral and other infections, and prematurity) or during the birth process. Examples of the latter include trauma to the head incurred during the process of birth, placenta previa or premature separation of the placenta, and prolapse of the umbilical cord.

General Medical Conditions Acquired in Infancy or Childhood. General medical conditions acquired during infancy or childhood account for approximately 5 percent of cases of mental retardation. They include infections, such as meningitis and encephalitis; poisonings, such as from insecticides, medications, and lead; and physical trauma, such as head injuries, asphyxiation, and hyperpyrexia (Sadock & Sadock, 2003).

Environmental Influences and Other Mental Disorders. Between 15 and 20 percent of cases of mental retardation are attributed to deprivation of nurturance and social, linguistic, and other stimulation, and to severe mental disorders, such as autistic disorder (APA, 2000).

Recognition of the cause and period of inception provides information regarding what to expect in terms of

---

TABLE 25–1
Diagnostic Criteria for Mental Retardation

A. Significantly subaverage general intellectual functioning: an IQ of approximately 70 or below on an individually administered IQ test (for infants, a clinical judgment of significantly subaverage intellectual functioning).
B. Concurrent deficits or impairments in adaptive functioning (i.e., the person's effectiveness in meeting the standards expected for his or her age by his or her cultural group) in at least two of the following areas: communication, self-care, home living, social/interpersonal skills, use of community resources, self-direction, functional academic skills, work, leisure, health, and safety.
C. The onset is before age 18 years.

SOURCE: From APA (2000), with permission.

behavior and potential. However, each child is different, and consideration must be given on an individual basis in every case.

Application of the Nursing Process

Background Assessment Data (Symptomatology)

The degree of severity of mental retardation is identified by the client's IQ level. Four levels have been delineated: mild, moderate, severe, and profound. The various behavioral manifestations and abilities associated with each of these levels of retardation are outlined in Table 25–2.

Nurses should assess and focus on each client's strengths and individual abilities. Knowledge regarding level of independence in the performance of self-care activities is essential to the development of an adequate plan for the provision of nursing care.

Diagnosis/Outcome Identification

Selection of appropriate nursing diagnoses for the mentally retarded client depends largely on the degree of severity of the condition and the client's capabilities. Possible nursing diagnoses include:

Risk for injury related to altered physical mobility or aggressive behavior.
Self-care deficit related to altered physical mobility or lack of maturity.
Impaired verbal communication related to developmental alteration.

Impaired social interaction related to speech deficiencies or difficulty adhering to conventional social behavior.
Delayed growth and development related to isolation from significant others; inadequate environmental stimulation; hereditary factors.
Anxiety (moderate to severe) related to hospitalization and absence of familiar surroundings.
Defensive coping related to feelings of powerlessness and threat to self-esteem.
Ineffective coping related to inadequate coping skills secondary to developmental delay.

The following criteria may be used for measurement of outcomes in the care of the client with mental retardation.

The client:

1. Has experienced no physical harm.
2. Has had self-care needs fulfilled.
3. Interacts with others in a socially appropriate manner.
4. Has maintained anxiety at a manageable level.
5. Is able to accept direction without becoming defensive.
6. Demonstrates adaptive coping skills in response to stressful situations.

Planning/Implementation

Table 25–3 provides a plan of care for the child with mental retardation using selected nursing diagnoses, outcome criteria, and appropriate nursing interventions and rationales.

Although this plan of care is directed toward the individual client, it is essential that family members or primary caregivers participate in the ongoing care of the

TABLE 25–2	Developmental Characteristics of Mental Retardation by Degree of Severity			
LEVEL (IQ)	**ABILITY TO PERFORM SELF-CARE ACTIVITIES**	**COGNITIVE/EDUCATIONAL CAPABILITIES**	**SOCIAL/COMMUNICATION CAPABILITIES**	**PSYCHOMOTOR CAPABILITIES**
Mild (50–70)	Capable of independent living, with assistance during times of stress.	Capable of academic skills to sixth-grade level. As adult can achieve vocational skills for minimum self-support.	Capable of developing social skills. Functions well in a structured, sheltered setting.	Psychomotor skills usually not affected, although may have some slight problems with coordination.
Moderate (35–49)	Can perform some activities independently. Requires supervision.	Capable of academic skill to second-grade level. As adult may be able to contribute to own support in sheltered workshop.	May experience some limitation in speech communication. Difficulty adhering to social convention may interfere with peer relationships.	Motor development is fair. Vocational capabilities may be limited to unskilled gross motor activities.
Severe (20–34)	May be trained in elementary hygiene skills. Requires complete supervision.	Unable to benefit from academic or vocational training. Profits from systematic habit training.	Minimal verbal skills. Wants and needs often communicated by acting-out behaviors.	Poor psychomotor development. Only able to perform simple tasks under close supervision.
Profound (below 20)	No capacity for independent functioning. Requires constant aid and supervision.	Unable to profit from academic or vocational training. May respond to minimal training in self-help if presented in the close context of a one-to-one relationship.	Little, if any, speech development. No capacity for socialization skills.	Lack of ability for both fine and gross motor movements. Requires constant supervision and care. May be associated with other physical disorders.

SOURCES: Adapted from APA (2000) and Sadock & Sadock (2003).

TABLE 25–3	Care Plan for the Child with Mental Retardation

NURSING DIAGNOSIS: RISK FOR INJURY
RELATED TO: Altered physical mobility or aggressive behavior

OUTCOME CRITERIA	NURSING INTERVENTIONS	RATIONALE
Client will not experience injury.	1. Create a safe environment for the client. 2. Ensure that small items are removed from area where client will be ambulating and that sharp items are out of reach. 3. Store items that client uses frequently within easy reach. 4. Pad siderails and headboard of client with history of seizures. 5. Prevent physical aggression and acting out behaviors by learning to recognize signs that client is becoming agitated.	1–5. Client safety is a nursing priority.

NURSING DIAGNOSIS: SELF-CARE DEFICIT
RELATED TO: Altered physical mobility or lack of maturity

OUTCOME CRITERIA	NURSING INTERVENTIONS	RATIONALE
Client will be able to participate in aspects of self-care.	1. Identify aspects of self-care that may be within the client's capabilities. Work on one aspect of self-care at a time. Provide simple, concrete explanations. Offer positive feedback for efforts. 2. When one aspect of self-care has been mastered to the best of the client's ability, move on to another. Encourage independence but intervene when client is unable to perform.	1. Positive reinforcement enhances self-esteem and encourages repetition of desirable behaviors. 2. Client comfort and safety are nursing priorities.

NURSING DIAGNOSIS: IMPAIRED VERBAL COMMUNICATION
RELATED TO: Developmental alteration

OUTCOME CRITERIA	NURSING INTERVENTIONS	RATIONALE
Client will be able to communicate needs and desires to staff.	1. Maintain consistency of staff assignment over time. 2. Anticipate and fulfill client's needs until satisfactory communication patterns are established. Learn (from family, if possible) special words client uses that are different from the norm. Identify nonverbal gestures or signals that client may use to convey needs if verbal communication is absent. Practice these communications skills repeatedly.	1. Consistency of staff assignments facilitates trust and the ability to understand client's actions and communications. 2. Some children with mental retardation, particularly at the severe level, can only learn by systematic habit training.

(Continued on opposite page)

NURSING DIAGNOSIS: IMPAIRED SOCIAL INTERACTION
RELATED TO: Speech deficiencies or difficulty adhering to conventional social behavior

OUTCOME CRITERIA	NURSING INTERVENTIONS	RATIONALE
Client will be able to interact with others using behaviors that are socially acceptable and appropriate to developmental level.	1. Remain with client during initial interactions with others on the unit. 2. Explain to other clients the meaning behind some of the client's nonverbal gestures and signals. Use simple language to explain to client which behaviors are acceptable and which are not. Establish a procedure for behavior modification with rewards for appropriate behaviors and aversive reinforcement for inappropriate behaviors.	1. Presence of a trusted individual provides a feeling of security. 2. Positive, negative, and aversive reinforcements can contribute to desired changes in behavior. These privileges and penalties are individually determined as staff learns the likes and dislikes of the client.

mentally retarded client. They need to receive information regarding the scope of the condition, realistic expectations and client potentials, methods for modifying behavior as required, and community resources from which they may seek assistance and support.

Evaluation

Evaluation of care given to the client with mental retardation should reflect positive behavioral changes. Evaluation is accomplished by determining if the goals of care have been met through implementation of the nursing actions selected. The nurse reassesses the plan and makes changes where required. Reassessment data may include information gathered by asking the following questions:

1. Have nursing actions providing for the client's safety been sufficient to prevent injury?
2. Have all of the client's self-care needs been fulfilled? Can he or she fulfill some of these needs independently?
3. Has the client been able to communicate needs and desires so that he or she can be understood?
4. Has the client learned to interact appropriately with others?
5. When regressive behaviors surface, can the client accept constructive feedback and discontinue the inappropriate behavior?
6. Has anxiety been maintained at a manageable level?
7. Has the client learned new coping skills through behavior modification? Does the client demonstrate evidence of increased self-esteem because of the accomplishment of these new skills and adaptive behaviors?
8. Have primary caregivers been taught realistic expectations of the client's behavior and methods for attempting to modify unacceptable behaviors?

> **Core Concept**
>
> **Pervasive Developmental Disorders**
> A group of disorders that are characterized by impairment in several areas of development, including social interaction skills and interpersonal communication. Included in this category are autistic disorder, Rett's disorder, childhood disintegrative disorder, and Asperger's disorder (APA, 2000).

9. Have primary caregivers been given information regarding various resources from which they can seek assistance and support within the community?

AUTISTIC DISORDER

Autistic disorder is characterized by a withdrawal of the child into the self and into a fantasy world of his or her own creation. The child has markedly abnormal or impaired development in social interaction and communication and a markedly restricted repertoire of activity and interests (APA, 2000). Activities and interests are restricted and may be considered somewhat bizarre.

The disorder is relatively rare and occurs four to five times more often in boys than in girls. Onset of the disorder occurs prior to age 3, and in most cases it runs a chronic course, with symptoms persisting into adulthood.

Predisposing Factors
Biological Factors

Neurological Implications. It is generally accepted that autism is caused by abnormalities in brain structures or functions (National Institute of Mental Health [NIMH], 2002). Abnormalities have been found in the area of the amygdala, which is known to help regulate aspects of social and emotional behavior. Elevated levels of serotonin have also been found in a number of people with autism. Magnetic resonance imagery (MRI) has been used to study brain activity of children with autistic disorder, revealing markedly less activity in the parietal areas and the corpus callosum than in their peers unaffected by the disorder (NIMH, 2002).

Popper and associates (2003) identify early developmental problems such as postnatal neurological infections, congenital rubella, phenylketonuria, and fragile X syndrome as possible implications in the predisposition to autistic disorder. Several studies have also implicated various structural and functional abnormalities in the brain. These include ventricular enlargement, left temporal lobe abnormalities, and increased glucose metabolism. Popper and associates (2003) state: "The neurobiological dysfunction appears to be quite diffuse, and no clear primary deficit is found in most autistic individuals."

Genetics

Recent research has revealed strong evidence that genetic factors may play a significant role in the etiology of autism (Popper et al., 2003). Studies have shown that parents who have one child with autism are at increased risk for having more than one child with autism (NIMH, 2002). Other studies with both monozygotic and dizygotic twins also have provided evidence of a genetic involvement. Research into how genetic factors influence the development of autistic disorder is now being conducted.

Perinatal Influences

Researchers at Kaiser Permanente in Oakland, California, recently found that women who suffered from asthma and/or allergies around the time of pregnancy were at increased risk of having a child affected by autism (Croen et al., 2005). Women with asthma and allergies recorded during the second trimester had a greater than twofold elevated risk of having a child affected by autism. The researchers have postulated that this may be due to maternal immune response during pregnancy, or that asthma and allergy may share environmental risk factors with autism spectrum disorders.

Application of the Nursing Process

Background Assessment Data (Symptomatology)

Impairment in Social Interaction. Children with autistic disorder do not form interpersonal relationships with others. They do not respond to or show interest in people. As infants they may have an aversion to affection and physical contact. As toddlers, the attachment to a significant adult may be either absent or manifested as exaggerated adherence behaviors. In childhood, there is failure to develop cooperative play, imaginative play, and friendships. Those children with minimal handicaps may eventually progress to the point of recognizing other children as part of their environment, if only in a passive manner.

Impairment in Communication and Imaginative Activity. Both verbal and nonverbal skills are affected. Language may be totally absent, or characterized by immature structure or idiosyncratic utterances whose meaning is clear only to those who are familiar with the child's past experiences. Nonverbal communication, such as facial expression or gestures, is often absent or socially inappropriate. The pattern of imaginative play is often restricted and stereotypical.

Restricted Activities and Interests. Even minor changes in the environment are often met with resistance, or sometimes with hysterical responses. Attachment to, or extreme fascination with, objects that move or spin (e.g., fans) is common. Routine may become an obsession, with minor alterations in routine leading to marked distress. Stereotyped body movements (hand-clapping, rocking, whole-body swaying) and verbalizations (repetition of words or phrases) are typical. Diet abnormalities may include eating only a few specific foods or consuming an excessive amount of fluids. Behaviors that are self-injurious, such as head banging or biting the hands or arms, may be evident.

The *DSM-IV-TR* (APA, 2000) diagnostic criteria for autistic disorder are presented in Table 25–4.

Diagnosis/Outcome Identification

Based on data collected during the nursing assessment, possible nursing diagnoses for the client with autistic disorder include:

Risk for self-mutilation related to neurological alterations.

Impaired social interaction related to inability to trust; neurological alterations.

Impaired verbal communication related to withdrawal into the self; inadequate sensory stimulation; neurological alterations.

Disturbed personal identity related to inadequate sensory stimulation; neurological alterations.

The following criteria may be used for measurement of outcomes in the care of the client with autistic disorder.

The client:

1. Exhibits no evidence of self-harm.
2. Interacts appropriately with at least one staff member.
3. Demonstrates trust in at least one staff member.
4. Is able to communicate so that he or she can be understood by at least one staff member.

TABLE 25–4	**Diagnostic Criteria for Autistic Disorder**

A. A total of six (or more) items from (1), (2), and (3), with at least two from (1), and one each from (2) and (3):
  1. Qualitative impairment in social interaction, as manifested by at least two of the following:
    (a) Marked impairment in the use of multiple nonverbal behaviors such as eye-to-eye gaze, facial expression, body postures, and gestures to regulate social interaction.
    (b) Failure to develop peer relationships appropriate to developmental level.
    (c) Lack of social or emotional reciprocity.
  2. Qualitative impairments in communication as manifested by at least one of the following:
    (a) Delay in, or total lack of, the development of spoken language (not accompanied by an attempt to compensate through alternative modes of communication such as gesture or mime).
    (b) In individuals with adequate speech, marked impairment in the ability to initiate or sustain a conversation with others.
    (c) Stereotyped and repetitive use of language or idiosyncratic language.
    (d) Lack of varied, spontaneous make-believe play or social imitative play appropriate to developmental level.
  3. Restricted repetitive and stereotyped patterns of behavior, interests, and activities, as manifested by at least one of the following:
    (a) Encompassing preoccupation with one or more stereotyped and restricted patterns of interest that is abnormal either in intensity or focus.
    (b) Apparently inflexible adherence to specific, nonfunctional routines or rituals.
    (c) Stereotyped and repetitive motor mannerisms (e.g., hand or finger flapping or twisting, or complex whole-body movements).
    (d) Persistent preoccupation with parts of objects.
B. Delays or abnormal functioning in at least one of the following areas, with onset prior to age 3 years:
  (1) social interaction, (2) language as used in social communication, or (3) symbolic or imaginative play.

SOURCE: From APA (2000), with permission.

5. Demonstrates behaviors that indicate he or she has begun the separation/individuation process.

Planning/Implementation

Table 25–5 provides a plan of care for the child with autistic disorder, including selected nursing diagnoses, outcome criteria, and appropriate nursing interventions and rationales.

Evaluation

Evaluation of care for the child with autistic disorder reflects whether the nursing actions have been effective in achieving the established goals. The nursing process calls for reassessment of the plan. Questions for gathering reassessment data may include:

1. Has the child been able to establish trust with at least *one* caregiver?
2. Have the nursing actions directed toward preventing mutilative behaviors been effective in protecting the client from self-harm?
3. Has the child attempted to interact with others? Has he or she received positive reinforcement for these efforts?
4. Has eye contact improved?
5. Has the child established a means of communicating

TABLE 25–5	**Care Plan for the Child with Autistic Disorder**

NURSING DIAGNOSIS: RISK FOR SELF-MUTILATION
RELATED TO: Neurological alterations

OUTCOME CRITERIA	NURSING INTERVENTIONS	RATIONALE
Client will not harm self.	1. Work with the child on a one-to-one basis.	1. One-to-one interaction facilitates trust.
	2. Try to determine if the self-mutilative behavior occurs in response to increasing anxiety, and if so, to what the anxiety may be attributed.	2. Mutilative behaviors may be averted if the cause can be determined and alleviated.
	3. Try to intervene with diversion or replacement activities and offer self to the child as anxiety level starts to rise.	3. Diversion and replacement activities may provide needed feelings of security and substitute for self-mutilative behaviors.
	4. Protect the child when self-mutilative behaviors occur. Devices such as a helmet, padded hand mitts, or arm covers may provide protection when the risk for self-harm exists.	4. Client safety is a priority nursing intervention.

(Continued on following page)

TABLE 25–5	Care Plan for the Child with Autistic Disorder *(Continued)*

NURSING DIAGNOSIS: IMPAIRED SOCIAL INTERACTION
RELATED TO: Inability to trust; neurological alterations

OUTCOME CRITERIA	NURSING INTERVENTIONS	RATIONALE
Client will initiate social interactions with caregiver.	1. Assign a limited number of caregivers to the child. Ensure that warmth, acceptance, and availability are conveyed. 2. Provide child with familiar objects, such as familiar toys or a blanket. Support child's attempts to interact with others. 3. Give positive reinforcement for eye contact with something acceptable to the child (e.g., food, familiar object). Gradually replace with social reinforcement (e.g., touch, smiling, hugging).	1. Warmth, acceptance, and availability, along with consistency of assignment, enhance the establishment and maintenance of a trusting relationship. 2. Familiar objects and presence of a trusted individual provide security during times of distress. 3. Being able to establish eye contact is essential to the child's ability to form satisfactory interpersonal relationships.

NURSING DIAGNOSIS: IMPAIRED VERBAL COMMUNICATION
RELATED TO: Withdrawal into the self; inadequate sensory stimulation; neurological alterations.

OUTCOME CRITERIA	NURSING INTERVENTIONS	RATIONALE
Client will establish a means of communicating needs and desires to others.	1. Maintain consistency in assignment of caregivers. 2. Anticipate and fulfill the child's needs until communication can be established. 3. Seek clarification and validation. 4. Give positive reinforcement when eye contact is used to convey nonverbal expressions.	1. Consistency facilitates trust and enhances the caregiver's ability to understand the child's attempts to communicate. 2. Anticipating needs helps to minimize frustration while the child is learning communication skills. 3. Validation ensures that the intended message has been conveyed. 4. Positive reinforcement increases self-esteem and encourages repetition.

NURSING DIAGNOSIS: DISTURBED PERSONAL IDENTITY
RELATED TO: Inadequate sensory stimulation; neurological alterations

OUTCOME CRITERIA	NURSING INTERVENTIONS	RATIONALE
Client will name own body parts as separate and individual from those of others.	1. Assist child to recognize separateness during self-care activities, such as dressing and feeding. 2. Assist the child in learning to name own body parts. This can be facilitated by the use of mirrors, drawings, and pictures of the child. Encourage appropriate touching of, and being touched by, others.	1. Recognition of body parts during dressing and feeding increases the child's awareness of self as separate from others. 2. All of these activities may help increase the child's awareness of self as separate from others.

his or her needs and desires to others? Have all self-care needs been met?

6. Does the child demonstrate an awareness of self as separate from others? Can he or she name own body parts and body parts of caregiver?

7. Can he or she accept touch from others? Does he or she willingly and appropriately touch others?

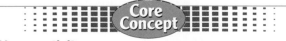

Hyperactivity

Excessive psychomotor activity that may be purposeful or aimless, accompanied by physical movements and verbal utterances that are usually more rapid than normal. Inattention and distractibility are common with hyperactive behavior.

ATTENTION-DEFICIT/ HYPERACTIVITY DISORDER

The essential feature of attention-deficit/hyperactivity disorder (ADHD) is a persistent pattern of inattention and/or hyperactivity-**impulsivity** that is more frequent and severe than is typically observed in individuals at a comparable level of development (APA, 2000). These children are highly distractible and unable to contain stimuli. Motor activity is excessive and movements are random and impulsive. Onset of the disorder is difficult to diagnose in children younger than age 4 years because their characteristic behavior is much more variable than that of older children. Frequently the disorder is not recognized until the child enters school. It is four to nine times more common in boys than in girls and may occur in as many as 3 to 7 percent of school-age children (APA, 2000). The *DSM-IV-TR* further categorizes the disorder into the following subtypes:

1. **Attention-Deficit/Hyperactivity Disorder, Combined Type.** This subtype is used if at least six symptoms of inattention and at least six symptoms of hyperactivity-impulsivity have persisted for at least 6 months. Most children and adolescents with the disorder have the combined type. It is not known whether the same is true of adults with the disorder.

2. **Attention Deficit/Hyperactivity Disorder, Predominantly Inattentive Type.** This subtype is used if at least six symptoms of inattention (but fewer than six symptoms of hyperactivity-impulsivity) have persisted for at least 6 months.

3. **Attention Deficit/Hyperactivity Disorder, Predominantly Hyperactive-Impulsive Type.** This subtype is used if at least six symptoms of hyperactivity-impulsivity (but fewer than six symptoms of inattention) have persisted for at least 6 months. In many cases, inattention still may be a significant clinical feature.

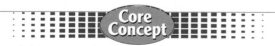

Core Concept

Impulsiveness
The trait of acting without reflection and without thought to the consequences of the behavior. An abrupt inclination to act (and the inability to resist acting) on certain behavioral urges.

Predisposing Factors

Biological Influences

Genetics. A number of studies have revealed supportive evidence of genetic influences in the etiology of ADHD. Results have indicated that a large number of parents of hyperactive children showed signs of hyperactivity during their own childhood; that hyperactive children are more likely than normal children to have siblings who are also hyperactive; and that when one twin of an identical twin pair has the disorder, the other is likely to have it too (National Institute of Mental Health [NIMH], 2000).

Biochemical Theory. Although it is believed that certain neurotransmitters—particularly dopamine, norepinephrine, and possibly serotonin—are involved in producing the symptoms associated with ADHD, their involvement is still under investigation. Abnormal levels of these neurotransmitters may be associated with the symptoms of hyperactivity, impulsivity, mood, and aggression often observed in individuals with the disorder.

Anatomical Influences. Recent studies have implicated alterations in specific areas of the brain in individuals with ADHD. These regions include the frontal lobes, basal ganglia, caudate nucleus, and cerebellum (Popper et al., 2003).

Prenatal, Perinatal, and Postnatal Factors. A recent study is consistent with an earlier finding that links maternal smoking during pregnancy and hyperkinetic-impulsive behavior in offspring (Linnet et al., 2005). Intrauterine exposure to toxic substances, including alcohol, can produce effects on behavior. Fetal alcohol syndrome includes hyperactivity, impulsivity, and inattention, as well as physical anomalies (Popper et al., 2003; Sadock & Sadock, 2003).

Perinatal influences that may contribute to ADHD are prematurity, signs of fetal distress, precipitated or prolonged labor, and perinatal asphyxia and low Apgar scores (Clunn, 1991). Postnatal factors that have been implicated include cerebral palsy, epilepsy, and other central nervous system (CNS) abnormalities resulting from trauma, infections, or other neurological disorders (Clunn, 1991; Popper et al., 2003).

Environmental Influences

Environmental Lead. Studies continue to provide evidence of the adverse effects on cognitive and behavioral development in children with elevated body levels of lead. Lead is pervasive in our environment, even though the government has placed tighter restrictions on the substance in recent years. A possible causal link between elevated lead levels and behavior associated with ADHD is still being investigated.

Diet Factors. The possible link between food dyes and additives, such as artificial flavorings and preservatives, was introduced in the mid-1970s. Studies on the effect of food and food-additive allergies remain controversial, largely because of the inconsistencies in the results. Striking improvement in behavior has been reported by some parents and teachers when hyperactive children are placed on a diet free of dyes and additives; however, results are inconclusive.

Another diet factor that has received much attention in its possible link to ADHD is sugar. A number of studies have been conducted in an effort to determine the effect of sugar on hyperactive behavior, and the results strongly suggest that sugar plays no role in hyperactivity. One study reported that ADHD children had fewer problems after a high-carbohydrate breakfast than after a high-protein one (Medscape Health, 2002).

What has been clear is that the etiological roles of both food additives and sugar have been greatly exaggerated. There are no reliable indications to date that either of these diet components plays a significant role in the development or exacerbation of hyperactivity.

Psychosocial Influences

Disorganized or chaotic environments or a disruption in family equilibrium may predispose some individuals to ADHD. A high degree of psychosocial stress, maternal mental disorder, paternal criminality, low socioeconomic status, and foster care have been implicated (Dopheide & Theesen, 1999).

Other psychosocial influences that have been implicated include family history of alcoholism, hysterical and sociopathic behaviors, and parental history of hyperactivity. Developmental learning disorders may also predispose to ADHD (Clunn, 1991).

Application of the Nursing Process

Background Assessment Data (Symptomatology)

A major portion of the hyperactive child's problems relate to difficulties in performing age-appropriate tasks. Hyperactive children are highly distractible and have extremely limited attention spans. They often shift from one uncompleted activity to another. Impulsivity, or deficit in inhibitory control, is also common.

Hyperactive children have difficulty forming satisfactory interpersonal relationships. They demonstrate behaviors that inhibit acceptable social interaction. They are disruptive and intrusive in group endeavors. They have difficulty complying with social norms. Some children with ADHD are very **aggressive** or oppositional, whereas others exhibit more regressive and immature behaviors. Low frustration tolerance and outbursts of temper are not uncommon.

Children with ADHD have boundless energy, exhibiting excessive levels of activity, restlessness, and fidgeting. They have been described as "perpetual motion machines," continuously running, jumping, wiggling, or squirming. They experience a greater than average number of accidents, from minor mishaps to more serious incidents that may lead to physical injury or the destruction of property.

The *DSM-IV-TR* diagnostic criteria for ADHD are presented in Table 25–6.

Diagnosis/Outcome Identification

Based on the data collected during the nursing assessment, possible nursing diagnoses for the child with ADHD include:

Risk for injury related to impulsive and accident-prone behavior and the inability to perceive self-harm.
Impaired social interaction related to intrusive and immature behavior.
Low self-esteem related to dysfunctional family system and negative feedback.
Noncompliance with task expectations related to low frustration tolerance and short attention span.

The following criteria may be used for measurement of outcomes in the care of the child with ADHD.

The client:

1. Has experienced no physical harm.
2. Interacts with others appropriately.
3. Verbalizes positive aspects about self.
4. Demonstrates fewer demanding behaviors.
5. Cooperatives with staff in an effort to complete assigned tasks.

Planning/Implementation

Table 25–7 provides a plan of care for the child with ADHD using nursing diagnoses common to the disorder, outcome criteria, and appropriate nursing interventions and rationales.

Evaluation

Evaluation of the care of a client with ADHD involves examining client behaviors following implementation of the nursing actions to determine if the goals of therapy have been achieved. Collecting data by using the following types of questions may provide appropriate information for evaluation.

1. Have the nursing actions directed at client safety been effective in protecting the child from injury?
2. Has the child been able to establish a trusting relationship with the primary caregiver?
3. Is the client responding to limits set on unacceptable behaviors?
4. Is the client able to interact appropriately with others?
5. Is the client able to verbalize positive statements about self?
6. Is the client able to complete tasks independently or with a minimum of assistance? Can he or she follow through after listening to simple instructions?
7. Is the client able to apply self-control to decrease motor activity?

TABLE 25-6   Diagnostic Criteria for Attention-Deficit/Hyperactivity Disorder

A. Either (1) or (2):
  1. Six (or more) of the following symptoms of inattention have persisted for at least 6 months to a degree that is maladaptive and inconsistent with developmental level:
    Inattention
    (a) Often fails to give close attention to details or makes careless mistakes in school work, work, or other activities.
    (b) Often has difficulty sustaining attention in tasks or play activities.
    (c) Often does not seem to listen when spoken to directly.
    (d) Often does not follow through on instructions and fails to finish schoolwork, chores, or duties in the workplace (not because of oppositional behavior or failure to understand instructions).
    (e) Often has difficulty organizing tasks and activities.
    (f) Often avoids, dislikes, or is reluctant to engage in tasks that require sustained mental effort (such as schoolwork or homework).
    (g) Often loses things necessary for tasks or activities (e.g., toys, school assignments, pencils, books, or tools)
    (h) Is often easily distracted by extraneous stimuli.
    (i) Is often forgetful in daily activities.

  2. Six (or more) of the following symptoms of hyperactivity-impulsivity have persisted for at least 6 months to a degree that is maladaptive and inconsistent with developmental level:
    Hyperactivity
    (a) Often fidgets with hands or feet or squirms in seat.
    (b) Often leaves seat in classroom or in other situations in which remaining seated is expected.
    (c) Often runs about or climbs excessively in situations in which it is inappropriate (in adolescents or adults, may be limited to subjective feelings of restlessness).
    (d) Often has difficulty playing or engaging in leisure activities quietly.
    (e) Is often "on the go" or often acts as if "driven by a motor."
    (f) Often talks excessively.
    Impulsivity
    (g) Often blurts out answers before questions have been completed.
    (h) Often has difficulty awaiting turn.
    (i) Often interrupts or intrudes on others (e.g., butts into conversations or games).

B. Some hyperactive-impulsive or inattentive symptoms that caused impairment were present before age 7 years.

C. Some impairment from the symptoms is present in two or more settings (e.g., at school or work and at home).

D. There is clear evidence of clinically significant impairment in social, academic, or occupational functioning.

E. The symptoms do not occur exclusively during the course of a pervasive developmental disorder, schizophrenia, or other psychotic disorder and are not better accounted for by another mental disorder (e.g., mood disorder, anxiety disorder, dissociative disorder, or a personality disorder).

Subtypes:
  1. **Attention-Deficit/Hyperactivity Disorder, Combined Type:** If both criteria A1 and A2 are met for the past 6 months.
  2. **Attention-Deficit/Hyperactivity Disorder, Predominantly Inattentive Type:** If criterion A1 is met but criterion A2 is not met for the past 6 months.
  3. **Attention-Deficit/Hyperactivity Disorder, Predominantly Hyperactive-Impulsive Type:** If criterion A2 is met but criterion A1 is not met for the past 6 months.

SOURCE: From APA (2000), with permission.

TABLE 25-7   Care Plan for the Child with Attention-Deficit/Hyperactivity Disorder

NURSING DIAGNOSIS: RISK FOR INJURY
RELATED TO: Impulsive and accident-prone behavior and the inability to perceive self-harm

OUTCOME CRITERIA	NURSING INTERVENTIONS	RATIONALE
Client will be free of injury.	1. Ensure that client has a safe environment. Remove objects from immediate area on which client could injure self as a result of random, hyperactive movements.	1. Objects that are appropriate to the normal living situation can be hazardous to the child whose motor activities are out of control.
	2. Identify deliberate behaviors that put the child at risk for injury. Institute consequences for repetition of this behavior.	2. Behavior can be modified with aversive reinforcement.
	3. If there is risk of injury associated with specific therapeutic activities, provide adequate supervision and assistance, or limit client's participation if adequate supervision is not possible.	3. Client safety is a nursing priority.

(Continued on following page)

NURSING DIAGNOSIS: IMPAIRED SOCIAL INTERACTION
RELATED TO: Intrusive and immature behavior

OUTCOME CRITERIA	NURSING INTERVENTIONS	RATIONALE
Client will observe limits set on intrusive behavior and will demonstrate ability to interact appropriately with others.	1. Develop a trusting relationship with the child. Convey acceptance of the child separate from the unacceptable behavior. 2. Discuss with client which behaviors are and are not acceptable. Describe in a matter-of-fact manner the consequences of unacceptable behavior. Follow through. 3. Provide group situations for client.	1. Unconditional acceptance increases feelings of self-worth. 2. Aversive reinforcement can alter undesirable behaviors. 3. Appropriate social behavior is often learned from the positive and negative feedback of peers.

NURSING DIAGNOSIS: LOW SELF-ESTEEM
RELATED TO: Dysfunctional family system and negative feedback

OUTCOME CRITERIA	NURSING INTERVENTIONS	RATIONALE
Client will demonstrate increased feelings of self-worth by verbalizing positive statements about self and exhibiting fewer demanding behaviors.	1. Ensure that goals are realistic. 2. Plan activities that provide opportunities for success. 3. Convey unconditional acceptance and positive regard. 4. Offer recognition of successful endeavors and positive reinforcement for attempts made. Give immediate positive feedback for acceptable behavior.	1. Unrealistic goals set client up for failure, which diminishes self-esteem. 2. Success enhances self-esteem. 3. Affirmation of client as worthwhile human being may increase self-esteem 4. Positive reinforcement enhances self-esteem and may increase the desired behaviors.

NURSING DIAGNOSIS: NONCOMPLIANCE (WITH TASK EXPECTATIONS)
RELATED TO: Low frustration tolerance and short attention span

OUTCOME CRITERIA	NURSING INTERVENTIONS	RATIONALE
Client will be able to complete assigned tasks independently or with a minimum of assistance.	1. Provide an environment for task efforts that is as free of distractions as possible. 2. Provide assistance on a one-to-one basis, beginning with simple, concrete instructions. 3. Ask client to repeat instructions to you. 4. Establish goals that allow client to complete a part of the task, rewarding each step-completion with a break for physical activity. 5. Gradually decrease the amount of assistance given, while assuring the client that assistance is still available if deemed necessary.	1. Client is highly distractible and is unable to perform in the presence of even minimal stimulation. 2. Client lacks the ability to assimilate information that is complicated or has abstract meaning. 3. Repetition of the instructions helps to determine client's level of comprehension. 4. Short-term goals are not so overwhelming to one with such a short attention span. The positive reinforcement (physical activity) increases self-esteem and provides incentive for client to pursue the task to completion. 5. This encourages the client to perform independently while providing a feeling of security with the presence of a trusted individual.

Psychopharmacological Intervention

Central nervous system stimulants are sometimes given to children with ADHD. Those commonly used include dextroamphetamine (Dexadrine), methylphenidate (Ritalin), pemoline (Cylert), and a dextroamphetamine/ amphetamine composite (Adderall). The actual mechanism by which these medications improve behavior associated with ADHD is not known. In most individuals, they produce stimulation, excitability, and restlessness. In children with ADHD, the effects include an increased attention span, control of hyperactive behavior, and improvement in learning ability.

Side effects include insomnia, anorexia, weight loss, tachycardia, and temporary decrease in rate of growth and development. Physical tolerance can occur (less with pemoline than with dextroamphetamine or methylphenidate).

In 2002, the U.S. Food and Drug Administration approved atomoxetine (Strattera), a medication specific for treating ADHD. Atomoxetine is a selective norepinephrine reuptake inhibitor. The exact mechanism by which it produces its therapeutic effect in ADHD is unknown. Side effects include headache, nausea and vomiting, upper abdominal pain, dry mouth, decreased appetite, weight loss, constipation, insomnia, increased blood pressure and heart rate, and sexual dysfunction.

Drugs in the antidepressant classification also have been used with some success in the treatment of ADHD. Commonly used medications in this category are bupropion (Wellbutrin), desipramine (Norpramin), nortriptyline (Pamelor), and imipramine (Tofranil).

Bupropion is distributed in a short- and long-lasting form. The side effects are similar to those of the stimulants: tachycardia, dizziness, shakiness, insomnia, nausea, anorexia, and weight loss. Individuals with a history of seizures or eating disorders should not take this medication.

The tricyclic antidepressants are useful for some ADHD symptoms, particularly attention and restlessness. The major side effects include sedation, dry mouth, increased appetite, changes in atrioventricular conduction of the heart, hypertension or hypotension, arrhythmias, and tachycardia. An electrocardiogram should be performed prior to initiation of therapy.

Route and Dosage Information

Dextroamphetamine (Dexedrine)
Dextroamphetamine/amphetamine composite (Adderall)

● PO (children age 3 to 5 years old): Initial dosage: 2.5 mg/day. This may be increased in increments of 2.5 mg/day at weekly intervals until the desired response is achieved.
● PO (children age 6 years or older): Initial dosage: 5 mg daily or twice a day. This may be increased in increments of 5 mg/day at weekly intervals until the desired response is achieved. Dosage rarely will exceed 40 mg/day. First dose of tablets or elixir forms may be given on awakening; additional doses at intervals of 4 to 6 hours. Sustained-release forms may be used for once-a-day dosage, given in the morning.

Methylphenidate (Ritalin)

● PO (children age 6 and older): Initial dosage 5 mg before breakfast and lunch. Dosage may be increased gradually in increments of 5 to 10 mg/day at weekly intervals. Maximum daily dosage: 60 mg. Sustained-release form may be used for once-a-day dosage, given in the morning.

Pemoline (Cylert)

● PO (children age 6 and older): Initial dosage: 37.5 mg/day, administered as a single dose each morning. Dosage may be gradually increased at 1-week intervals in increments of 18.75 mg/day until the desired effect is achieved. Effective dosage usually ranges from 56.25 to 75 mg/day. Maximum recommended dose: 112.5 mg/day. Clinical benefit may not be observed for 3 to 4 weeks.

Atomoxetine (Strattera)

● PO (Children and adults weighing more than 70 kg [154 lb]): Initial dose: 40 mg/day. Increase after a minimum of 3 days to a target total daily dose of 80 mg, as a single dose in the morning or 2 evenly divided doses in the morning and late afternoon or early evening. After 2 to 4 weeks, total dosage may be increased to a maximum of 100 mg, if needed.
● PO (Children and adults weighing 70 kg [154 lb] or less): Initial dose: 0.5 mg/kg per day. Increase after a minimum of 3 days to a target total daily dose of about 1.2 mg/kg taken either as a single dose in the morning or 2 evenly divided doses in the morning and late afternoon or early evening. Maximum daily dose: 1.4 mg/kg or 100 mg daily, whichever is less.

Bupropion (Wellbutrin)

● PO (children age 6 and older): 3 mg/kg per day.

Imipramine (Tofranil)

● PO (children age 6 and older): Initial dose: 1 mg/kg per day in divided doses, with increases every 2 to 3 weeks up to a maximum of 2.5 mg/kg per day.

Nursing Implications

● Assess the client's mental status for changes in mood, level of activity, degree of stimulation, and aggressiveness.

● Ensure that the client is protected from injury. Keep stimuli low and environment as quiet as possible to discourage overstimulation.

● To reduce anorexia, the medication may be administered immediately after meals. The client should be weighed regularly (at least weekly) while on therapy with CNS stimulants because of the potential for anorexia and weight loss and the temporary interruption of growth and development.

● To prevent insomnia, administer the last dose at least 6 hours before bedtime. Administer sustained-release forms in the morning.

● In children with behavior disorders, a drug "holiday" should be attempted periodically under direction of the physician to determine effectiveness of the medication and need for continuation.

● Ensure that the parents are aware of the delayed effects of pemoline. Therapeutic response may not be seen for 2 to 4 weeks. The drug should not be discontinued for lack of immediate results.

● Inform parents that over-the-counter (OTC) medications should be avoided while the child is receiving stimulant medication. Some OTC medications, particularly cold and hay fever preparations, contain sympathomimetic agents that could compound the effects of the stimulant and create a drug interaction that may be toxic to the child.

● Ensure that parents are aware that the drug should not be withdrawn abruptly. Withdrawal should be gradual and under the direction of the physician.

Core Concept

Disruptive Behavior Disorders
A disturbance of conduct severe enough to produce significant impairment in social, occupational, or academic functioning because of symptoms that range from oppositional defiant to moderate and severe conduct disturbances (Shahrokh & Hales, 2003).

CONDUCT DISORDER

With conduct disorder, there is a repetitive and persistent pattern of behavior in which the basic rights of others or major age-appropriate societal norms or rules are violated (APA, 2000). Physical aggression is common. The *DSM-IV-TR* divides this disorder into two subtypes based on the age at onset:

1. **Childhood-Onset Type.** This subtype is defined by the onset of at least one criterion characteristic of con-

duct disorder prior to age 10. Individuals with this subtype are usually boys, frequently display physical aggression, and have disturbed peer relationships. They may have had oppositional defiant disorder during early childhood, usually meet the full criteria for conduct disorder by puberty, and are likely to develop antisocial personality disorder in adulthood.

2. **Adolescent-Onset Type.** This subtype is defined by the absence of any criteria characteristic of conduct disorder prior to age 10. They are less likely to display aggressive behaviors and tend to have more normal peer relationships than those with childhood-onset type. They are also less likely to have persistent conduct disorder or develop antisocial personality disorder than those with childhood-onset type. The ratio of boys to girls is lower in adolescent-onset type than in childhood-onset type.

Core Concept

Temperament
Personality characteristics that define an individual's mood and behavioral tendencies. The sum of physical, emotional, and intellectual components that affect or determine a person's actions and reactions.

Predisposing Factors

Biological Influences

Genetics. Studies with monozygotic and dizygotic twins as well as with nontwin siblings have revealed a significantly higher number of conduct disorders among those who have family members with the disorder (APA, 2000). Although genetic factors appear to be involved in the etiology of conduct disorders, little is yet known about the actual mechanisms involved in genetic transmission. One recent study found that regions on chromosomes 19 and 2 may contain genes conferring risk to conduct disorder (Dick et al., 2004). In this study, the same region on chromosome 2 was also linked to alcohol dependence. These researchers report that childhood conduct disorder is known to be associated with the susceptibility for future alcohol problems. They have concluded that these findings suggest that some of the genes contributing to alcohol dependence in adulthood may also contribute to conduct disorder in childhood.

Temperament. The term **temperament** refers to personality traits that become evident very early in life and may be present at birth. Evidence suggests a genetic component in temperament and an association between temperament and behavioral problems later in life. Studies have shown that, without appropriate intervention, difficult temperament at age 3 has significant links to conduct disorder and movement into care or institutional life at age 17 (Bagley & Mallick, 2000).

Biochemical Factors. Studies have looked at various chemicals as biological markers. Alterations in the neurotransmitters norepinephrine and serotonin have been suggested by some studies (Comings et al., 2000; Searight et al., 2001). Some investigators have researched the possibility of testosterone association with violence. One study correlates higher levels of testosterone in pubertal boys with social dominance and association with deviant peers (Rowe et al., 2004).

Psychosocial Influences

Peer Relationships. Social groups have a significant impact on a child's development. Peers play an essential role in the socialization of interpersonal competence and skills acquired in this manner affect the child's long-term adjustment. Studies have shown that poor peer relationships during childhood were consistently implicated in the etiology of later deviance (Ladd, 1999). Aggression was found to be the principal cause of peer rejection, thus contributing to a cycle of maladaptive behavior.

Family Influences

The following factors related to family dynamics have been implicated as contributors in the predisposition to this disorder (Foley et al., 2004; Popper et al., 2003; Sadock & Sadock, 2003):

● Parental rejection
● Inconsistent management with harsh discipline
● Early institutional living
● Frequent shifting of parental figures
● Large family size
● Absent father
● Parents with antisocial personality disorder and/or alcohol dependence
● Association with a delinquent subgroup
● Marital conflict and divorce
● Inadequate communication patterns
● Parental permissiveness

Application of the Nursing Process

Background Assessment Data (Symptomatology)

The classic characteristic of conduct disorder is the use of physical aggression in the violation of the rights of others. The behavior pattern manifests itself it virtually all areas of the child's life (home, school, with peers, and in the community). Stealing, lying, and truancy are common problems. The child lacks feelings of guilt or remorse.

The use of tobacco, liquor, or nonprescribed drugs, as well as the participation in sexual activities, occurs earlier than the peer group's expected age. Projection is a common defense mechanism.

Low self-esteem is manifested by a "tough guy" image. Characteristics include poor frustration tolerance, irritability, and frequent temper outbursts. Symptoms of anxiety and depression are not uncommon.

Level of academic achievement may be low in relation to age and IQ.

Manifestations associated with ADHD (e.g., attention difficulties, impulsiveness, and hyperactivity) are very common in children with conduct disorder.

The *DSM-IV-TR* diagnostic criteria for conduct disorder are presented in Table 25–8.

Diagnosis/Outcome Identification

Based on the data collected during the nursing assessment, possible nursing diagnoses for the client with conduct disorder include:

Risk for other-directed violence related to characteristics of temperament, peer rejection, negative parental role models, dysfunctional family dynamics.
Impaired social interaction related to negative parental role models, impaired peer relations leading to inappropriate social behaviors.
Defensive coping related to low self-esteem and dysfunctional family system.
Low self-esteem related to lack of positive feedback and unsatisfactory parent–child relationship.

The following criteria may be used for measurement of outcomes in the care of the client with conduct disorder:

The client:

1. Has not harmed self or others.
2. Interacts with others in a socially appropriate manner.
3. Accepts direction without becoming defensive.
4. Demonstrates evidence of increased self-esteem by discontinuing exploitative and demanding behaviors toward others.

Planning/Implementation

Table 25–9 provides a plan of care for the child with conduct disorder using nursing diagnoses common to the disorder, outcome criteria, and appropriate nursing interventions and rationales.

Evaluation

Following the planning and implementation of care, evaluation is made of the behavioral changes in the child with conduct disorder. This is accomplished by deter-

TABLE 25–8   **Diagnostic Criteria for Conduct Disorder**

A. A repetitive and persistent pattern of behavior in which the basic rights of others or major age-appropriate societal norms or rules are violated, as manifested by the presence of three (or more) of the following criteria in the past 12 months, with at least one criterion present in the past 6 months:

1. **Aggression to people and animals**
   a. Often bullies, threatens, or intimidates others.
   b. Often initiates physical fights.
   c. Has used a weapon that can cause serious physical harm to others (e.g., a bat, brick, broken bottle, knife, gun)
   d. Has been physically cruel to people.
   e. Has been physically cruel to animals.
   f. Has stolen while confronting a victim (e.g., mugging, purse snatching, extortion, armed robbery).
   g. Has forced someone into sexual activity.

2. **Destruction of property**
   a. Has deliberately engaged in fire setting with the intention of causing serious damage.
   b. Has deliberately destroyed others' property (other than by fire setting).

3. **Deceitfulness or theft**
   a. Has broken into someone else's house, building, or car.
   b. Often lies to obtain goods or favors or to avoid obligations (i.e., "cons" others)
   c. Has stolen items of nontrivial value without confronting a victim (e.g., shoplifting, but without breaking and entering; forgery).

4. **Serious violations of rules**
   a. Often stays out at night despite parental prohibitions, beginning before age 13 years.
   b. Has run away from home overnight at least twice while living in parental or parental surrogate home (or once without returning for a lengthy period).
   c. Is often truant from school, beginning before age 13 years.

B. The disturbance in behavior causes clinically significant impairment in social, academic, or occupational functioning.

C. If the individual is age 18 years or older, criteria are not met for antisocial personality disorder.

Subtypes:
   1. **Childhood-Onset Type:** Onset of at least one criterion characteristic of conduct disorder prior to age 10 years.
   2. **Adolescent-Onset Type:** Absence of any criteria characteristic of conduct disorder prior to age 10 years.
   3. **Unspecified Onset:** Age at onset is not known.

SOURCE: From APA (2000), with permission.

TABLE 25–9   **Care Plan for Child/Adolescent with Conduct Disorder**

NURSING DIAGNOSIS: RISK FOR OTHER-DIRECTED VIOLENCE
RELATED TO: Characteristics of temperament, peer rejection, negative parental role models, dysfunctional family dynamics

OUTCOME CRITERIA	NURSING INTERVENTIONS	RATIONALE
Client will not harm others or others' property.	1. Observe client's behavior frequently through routine activities and interactions. Become aware of behaviors that indicate a rise in agitation.	1. Recognition of behaviors that precede the onset of aggression may provide the opportunity to intervene before violence occurs.
	2. Redirect violent behavior with physical outlets for suppressed anger and frustration.	2. Excess energy is released through physical activities inducing a feeling of relaxation.
	3. Encourage client to express anger and act as a role model for appropriate expression of anger.	3. Discussion of situations that create anger may lead to more effective ways of dealing with them.
	4. Ensure that a sufficient number of staff is available to indicate a show of strength if necessary.	4. This conveys an evidence of control over the situation and provides physical security for staff.
	5. Administer tranquilizing medication, if ordered, or use mechanical restraints or isolation room only if situation cannot be controlled with less restrictive means.	5. It is the client's right to expect the use of techniques that ensure safety of the client and others by the least restrictive means.

(Continued on opposite page)

NURSING DIAGNOSIS: IMPAIRED SOCIAL INTERACTION
RELATED TO: Negative parental role models; impaired peer relations leading to inappropriate social behavior

OUTCOME CRITERIA	NURSING INTERVENTIONS	RATIONALE
Client will be able to interact with staff and peers using age-appropriate, acceptable behaviors.	1. Develop a trusting relationship with the client. Convey acceptance of the person separate from the unacceptable behavior. 2. Discuss with client which behaviors are and are not acceptable. Describe in matter-of-fact manner the consequence of unacceptable behavior. Follow through. 3. Provide group situations for client.	1. Unconditional acceptance increases feeling of self-worth. 2. Aversive reinforcement can alter or extinguish undesirable behaviors. 3. Appropriate social behavior is often learned from the positive and negative feedback of peers.

NURSING DIAGNOSIS: DEFENSIVE COPING
RELATED TO: Low self-esteem and dysfunctional family system

OUTCOME CRITERIA	NURSING INTERVENTIONS	RATIONALE
Client will accept responsibility for own behaviors and interact with others without becoming defensive.	1. Explain to client the correlation between feelings of inadequacy and the need for acceptance from others and how these feelings provoke defensive behaviors, such as blaming others for own behaviors. 2. Provide immediate, matter-of-fact, non-threatening feedback for unacceptable behaviors. 3. Help identify situations that provoke defensiveness and practice through role-play more appropriate responses. 4. Provide immediate positive feedback for acceptable behaviors.	1. Recognition of the problem is the first step in the change process toward resolution. 2. Client may not realize how these behaviors are being perceived by others. 3. Role-playing provides confidence to deal with difficult situations when they actually occur. 4. Positive feedback encourages repetition, and immediacy is significant for these children who respond to immediate gratification.

NURSING DIAGNOSIS: LOW SELF-ESTEEM
RELATED TO: Lack of positive feedback and unsatisfactory parent/child relationship

OUTCOME CRITERIA	NURSING INTERVENTIONS	RATIONALE
Client will demonstrate increased feelings of self-worth by verbalizing positive statements about self and exhibiting fewer manipulative behaviors.	1. Ensure that goals are realistic. 2. Plan activities that provide opportunities for success. 3. Convey unconditional acceptance and positive regard. 4. Set limits on manipulative behavior. Take caution not to reinforce manipulative behaviors by providing desired attention. Identify the consequences of manipulation. Administer consequences matter-of-factly when manipulation occurs. 5. Help client understand that he or she uses this behavior in order to try to increase own self-esteem. Interventions should reflect other actions to accomplish this goal.	1. Unrealistic goals set client up for failure, which diminishes self-esteem. 2. Success enhances self-esteem. 3. Communicating that client is a worthwhile human being may increase self-esteem. 4. Aversive consequences may work to decrease unacceptable behaviors. 5. When the client feels better about self, the need to manipulate others will diminish.

mining if the goals of therapy have been achieved. Reassessment, the next step in the nursing process, may be initiated by gathering information using the following questions:

1. Have the nursing actions directed toward managing the client's aggressive behavior been effective?
2. Have interventions prevented harm to others or others' property?
3. Is the client able to express anger in an appropriate manner?
4. Has the client developed more adaptive coping strategies to deal with anger and feelings of aggression?
5. Does the client demonstrate the ability to trust others? Is he or she able to interact with staff and peers in an appropriate manner?
6. Is the client able to accept responsibility for his or her own behavior? Is there less blaming of others?
7. Is the client able to accept feedback from others without becoming defensive?
8. Is the client able to verbalize positive statements about self?
9. Is the client able to interact with others without engaging in manipulation?

OPPOSITIONAL DEFIANT DISORDER

Oppositional defiant disorder (ODD) is characterized by a pattern of negativistic, defiant, disobedient, and hostile behavior toward authority figures that occurs more frequently than is usually observed in individuals of comparable age and developmental level, and interferes with social, academic, or occupational functioning (APA, 2000). The disorder typically begins by 8 years of age, and usually not later than early adolescence. It is more prevalent in boys than in girls before puberty, but the rates are more closely equal after puberty. In a significant proportion of cases, ODD is a developmental antecedent to conduct disorder (APA, 2000).

Predisposing Factors

Biological Influences

Because the behaviors associated with ODD are very similar to those of conduct disorder, with the exception of violation of the rights of others, it is reasonable to speculate that they may share at least *some* of the same biological influences. What role, if any, genetics, temperament, or biochemical alterations play in the etiology of ODD is still being investigated. The study by Comings and associates (2000) suggests the genes for metabolism of dopamine, serotonin, and norepinephrine may be contributing factors in the development of ODD.

Family Influences

Opposition during various developmental stages is both normal and healthy. Children first exhibit oppositional behaviors at around 10 or 11 months of age, again as toddlers between 18 and 36 months of age, and finally during adolescence. Pathology is considered only when the developmental phase is prolonged, or when there is overreaction in the child's environment to his or her behavior.

Some children exhibit these behaviors in a more intense form than others. Sadock and Sadock (2003) report:

> Epidemiological studies of negativistic traits in nonclinical populations found such behavior in 16 to 22 percent of school-age children. (p. 1232)

Some parents interpret average or increased level of developmental oppositional behavior as hostility and a deliberate effort on the part of the child to be in control. If power and control are issues for parents, or if they exercise authority for their own needs, a power struggle can be established between the parents and the child that sets the stage for the development of ODD.

Popper and associates (2003) suggest that the following familial influences may play an etiological role in the development of ODD:

1. Parental problems in disciplining, structuring, and limit setting.
2. Identification by the child with an impulse-disordered parent who sets a role model for oppositional and defiant interactions with other people.
3. Parental unavailability (e.g., separation, evening work hours).

Application of the Nursing Process

Background Assessment Data (Symptomatology)

ODD is characterized by passive–aggressive behaviors such as stubbornness, procrastination, disobedience, carelessness, **negativism**, testing of limits, resistance to directions, deliberately ignoring the communication of others, and unwillingness to compromise. Other symptoms that may be evident are running away, school avoidance, school underachievement, temper tantrums, fighting, and argumentativeness. In severe cases, there may be elective mutism, enuresis, encopresis, or eating and sleeping problems (Harvard Medical School, 2002).

The oppositional attitude is directed toward adults, most particularly the parents. Symptoms of the disorder may or may not be evident in school or elsewhere in the community (APA, 2000).

Usually these children do not see themselves as being oppositional but view the problem as arising from others

TABLE 25–10	Diagnostic Criteria for Oppositional Defiant Disorder

A. A pattern of negativistic, hostile, and defiant behavior lasting at least 6 months, during which four (or more) of the following are present:
   1. Often loses temper.
   2. Often argues with adults
   3. Often actively defies or refuses to comply with adult requests or rules.
   4. Often deliberately annoys people.
   5. Often blames others for his or her mistakes or misbehavior.
   6. Is often touchy or easily annoyed by others.
   7. Is often angry and resentful.
   8. Is often spiteful or vindictive.

B. The disturbance in behavior causes clinically significant impairment in social, academic, or occupational functioning.

C. The behaviors do not occur exclusively during the course of a psychotic or mood disorder.

D. Criteria are not met for conduct disorder, and if the individual is age 18 years or older, criteria are not met for antisocial personality disorder.

SOURCE: From APA (2000), with permission.

whom they believe are making unreasonable demands on them. Interpersonal relationships are fraught with difficulty, including those with peers. These children are often friendless, perceiving human relationships as negative and unsatisfactory. School performance is usually poor because of their refusal to participate and their resistance to external demands.

The *DSM-IV-TR* (2000) diagnostic criteria for ODD is presented in Table 25–10.

Diagnosis/Outcome Identification

Based on the data collected during the nursing assessment, possible nursing diagnoses for the client with ODD include:

Noncompliance with therapy related to negative temperament, denial of problems, underlying hostility.

Defensive coping related to retarded ego development, low self-esteem, unsatisfactory parent–child relationship.

Low self-esteem related to lack of positive feedback, retarded ego development.

Impaired social interaction related to negative temperament, underlying hostility, manipulation of others.

The following criteria may be used for measurement of outcomes in the care of the client with ODD.

The client:

1. Complies with treatment by participating in therapies without negativism.
2. Accepts responsibility for his or her part in the problem.
3. Takes direction from staff without becoming defensive.
4. Does not manipulate other people.
5. Verbalizes positive aspects about self.
6. Interacts with others in an appropriate manner.

Planning/Implementation

Table 25–11 provides a plan of care for the child with ODD using nursing diagnoses common to the disorder, outcome criteria, and appropriate nursing interventions and rationales.

Evaluation

The evaluation step of the nursing process calls for reassessment of the plan of care to determine if the nursing actions have been effective in achieving the goals of therapy. The following questions can be used with the child or adolescent with ODD to gather information for the evaluation.

TABLE 25–11	Care Plan for the Child/Adolescent with Oppositional Defiant Disorder

NURSING DIAGNOSIS: NONCOMPLIANCE WITH THERAPY
RELATED TO: Negative temperament; denial of problems; underlying hostility

OUTCOME CRITERIA	NURSING INTERVENTIONS	RATIONALE
Client will participate in and cooperate during therapeutic activities.	1. Set forth a structured plan of therapeutic activities. Start with minimum expectations and increase as client begins to manifest evidence of compliance.	1. Structure provides security and one or two activities may not seem as overwhelming as the whole schedule of activities presented at one time.
	2. Establish a system of rewards for compliance with therapy and consequences for noncompliance. Ensure that the rewards and consequences are concepts of value to the client.	2. Positive, negative, and aversive reinforcements can contribute to desired changes in behavior.
	3. Convey acceptance of the client separate from the undesirable behaviors being exhibited. ("It is not *you*, but your *behavior*, that is unacceptable").	3. Unconditional acceptance enhances self-worth and may contribute to a decrease in the need for passive-aggression toward others.

(Continued on following page)

NURSING DIAGNOSIS: DEFENSIVE COPING
RELATED TO: Retarded ego development; low self-esteem; unsatisfactory parent/child relationship

OUTCOME CRITERIA	NURSING INTERVENTIONS	RATIONALE
Client will accept responsibility for own behaviors and interact with others without becoming defensive.	1. Help client recognize that feelings of inadequacy provoke defensive behaviors, such as blaming others for problems, and the need to "get even." 2. Provide immediate, nonthreatening feedback for passive-aggressive behavior. 3. Help identify situations that provoke defensiveness and practice through role-play more appropriate responses. 4. Provide immediate positive feedback for acceptable behaviors.	1. Recognition of the problem is the first step toward initiating change. 2. Because client denies responsibility for problems, he or she is denying the inappropriateness of behavior. 3. Role-playing provides confidence to deal with difficult situations when they actually occur. 4. Positive feedback encourages repetition, and immediacy is significant for these children who respond to immediate gratification.

NURSING DIAGNOSIS: LOW SELF-ESTEEM
RELATED TO: Lack of positive feedback; retarded ego development

OUTCOME CRITERIA	NURSING INTERVENTIONS	RATIONALE
Client will demonstrate increased feelings of self-worth by verbalizing positive statements about self and exhibiting fewer manipulative behaviors.	1. Ensure that goals are realistic. 2. Plan activities that provide opportunities for success. 3. Convey unconditional acceptance and positive regard. 4. Set limits on manipulative behavior. Take caution not to reinforce manipulative behaviors by providing desired attention. Identify the consequences of manipulation. Administer consequences matter-of-factly when manipulation occurs. 5. Help client understand that he or she uses this behavior in order to try to increase own self-esteem. Interventions should reflect other actions to accomplish this goal.	1. Unrealistic goals set client up for failure, which diminishes self-esteem. 2. Success enhances self-esteem. 3. Affirmation of client as worthwhile human being may increase self-esteem. 4. Aversive reinforcement may work to decrease unacceptable behaviors. 5. When client feels better about self, the need to manipulate others will diminish.

NURSING DIAGNOSIS: IMPAIRED SOCIAL INTERACTION
RELATED TO: Negative temperament; underlying hostility; manipulation of others

OUTCOME CRITERIA	NURSING INTERVENTIONS	RATIONALE
Client will be able to interact with staff and peers using age-appropriate, acceptable behaviors.	1. Develop a trusting relationship with the client. Convey acceptance of the person separate from the unacceptable behavior. 2. Explain to the client about passive-aggressive behavior. Explain how these behaviors are perceived by others. Describe which behaviors are not acceptable and role play more adaptive responses. Give positive feedback for acceptable behaviors. 3. Provide peer group situations for the client.	1. Unconditional acceptance increases feelings of self-worth and may serve to diminish feelings of rejection that have accumulated over a long period. 2. Role playing is a way to practice behaviors that do not come readily to the client, making it easier when the situation actually occurs. Positive feedback enhances repetition of desirable behaviors. 3. Appropriate social behavior is often learned from the positive and negative feedback of peers. Groups also provide an atmosphere for using the behaviors rehearsed in role-play.

1. Is the client cooperating with schedule of therapeutic activities? Is level of participation adequate?
2. Is the client's attitude toward therapy less negative?
3. Is the client accepting responsibility for problem behavior?
4. Is the client verbalizing the unacceptableness of his or her passive–aggressive behavior?
5. Is he or she able to identify which behaviors are unacceptable and substitute more adaptive behaviors?
6. Is the client able to interact with staff and peers without defending behavior in an angry manner?
7. Is the client able to verbalize positive statements about self?
8. Is increased self-worth evident with fewer manifestations of manipulation?
9. Is the client able to make compromises with others when issues of control emerge?
10. Is anger and hostility expressed in an appropriate manner? Can the client verbalize ways of releasing anger adaptively?
11. Is he or she able to verbalize true feelings instead of allowing them to emerge through use of passive-aggressive behaviors?

TOURETTE'S DISORDER

The essential feature of Tourette's disorder is the presence of multiple motor tics and one or more vocal tics (APA, 2000). They may appear simultaneously or at different periods during the illness. The disturbance causes marked distress and can interfere with social, occupational, or other important areas of functioning. The onset of the disorder is before age 18 years and is more common in boys than in girls. The duration of the disorder may be lifelong, although there may be periods of remission that last from weeks to years (APA, 2000). The symptoms usually diminish during adolescence and adulthood, and in some cases, disappear altogether by early adulthood.

Predisposing Factors
Biological Factors

Genetics. Tics are noted in two thirds of relatives of Tourette's disorder clients (Popper et al., 2003). Twin studies with both monozygotic and dizygotic twins suggest an inheritable component. Evidence suggests that Tourette's disorder may be transmitted in an autosomal pattern intermediate between dominant and recessive (Sadock & Sadock, 2003).

Biochemical Factors. Abnormalities in levels of dopamine, serotonin, dynorphin, gamma-aminobutyric acid (GABA), acetylcholine, and norepinephrine have been associated with Tourette's disorder (Popper et al., 2003). Neurotransmitter pathways through the basal ganglia, globus pallidus, and subthalamic regions appear to be involved.

Structural Factors. Neuroimaging brain studies have been consistent in finding dysfunction in the area of the basal ganglia. One recent study found a correlation between smaller size of corpus callosum and Tourette's disorder in children (Plessen et al., 2004).

Environmental Factors

Additional retrospective findings may be implicated in the etiology of Tourette's disorder. Complications of pregnancy (e.g., severe nausea and vomiting or excessive stress), low birth weight, head trauma, carbon monoxide poisoning, and encephalitis are thought to be associated with the onset of non-genetic Tourette's disorder. It is speculated that these environmental factors also may temper the genetic predisposition to the disorder.

Application of the Nursing Process
Background Assessment Data (Symptomatology)

The motor tics of Tourette's disorder may involve the head, torso, and upper and lower limbs. Initial symptoms may begin with a single motor tic, most commonly eye blinking, or with multiple symptoms. The *DSM-IV-TR* identifies simple motor tics as eye blinking, neck jerking, shoulder shrugging, facial grimacing, and coughing. Common complex motor tics include touching, squatting, hopping, skipping, deep knee bends, retracing steps, and twirling when walking.

Vocal tics include various words or sounds such as clicks, grunts, yelps, barks, sniffs, snorts, coughs and, in about 10 percent of cases, a complex vocal tic involving the uttering of obscenities (APA, 2000). Vocal tics may include repeating certain words or phrases out of context, repeating one's own sounds or words (**palilalia**), or repeating what others say (**echolalia**).

The movements and vocalizations are experienced as compulsive and irresistible, but they can be suppressed for varying lengths of time. They are exacerbated by stress and attenuated during periods in which the individual becomes totally absorbed by an activity. In most cases, tics are diminished during sleep (APA, 2000).

The age at onset of Tourette's disorder can be as early as age 2 years, but the disorder occurs most commonly during childhood (around age 6 to 7 years). Prevalence of the disorder is related to age, affecting many more children (5 to 30 per 10,000) than adults (1 to 2 per 10,000) (APA, 2000). The *DSM-IV-TR* diagnostic criteria for Tourette's disorder are presented in Table 25–12.

Diagnosis/Outcome Identification

Based on data collected during the nursing assessment, possible nursing diagnoses for the client with Tourette's disorder include:

TABLE 25–12	**Diagnostic Criteria for Tourette's Disorder**

A. Both multiple motor and one or more vocal tics have been present at some time during the illness, although not necessarily concurrently. (A *tic* is a sudden, rapid, recurrent, non-rhythmic, stereotyped motor movement or vocalization.)
B. The tics occur many times a day (usually in bouts) nearly every day or intermittently throughout a period of more than 1 year, and during this period there was never a tic-free period of more than 3 consecutive months.
C. The disturbance causes marked distress or significant impairment in social, occupational, or other important areas of functioning.
D. The onset is before age 18 years.
E. The disturbance is not due to the direct physiological effects of a substance (e.g., stimulants) or a general medical condition (e.g., Huntington's disease or postviral encephalitis).

SOURCE: From APA (2000), with permission.

Risk for self-directed or other-directed violence related to low tolerance for frustration.

Impaired social interaction related to impulsiveness, oppositional and aggressive behavior.

Low self-esteem related to shame associated with tic behaviors.

The following criteria may be used for measurement of outcomes in the care of the client with Tourette's disorder.

The client:

1. Has not harmed self or others.
2. Interacts with staff and peers in an appropriate manner.
3. Demonstrates self-control by managing tic behavior.
4. Follows rules of unit without becoming defensive.
5. Verbalizes positive aspects about self.

Planning/Implementation

Table 25–13 provides a plan of care for the child or adolescent with Tourette's disorder using selected nursing diagnoses, outcome criteria, and appropriate nursing interventions and rationales.

TABLE 25–13	**Care Plan for the Child or Adolescent with Tourette's Disorder**

NURSING DIAGNOSIS: RISK FOR SELF-DIRECTED OR OTHER-DIRECTED VIOLENCE
RELATED TO: Low tolerance for frustration

OUTCOME CRITERIA	NURSING INTERVENTIONS	RATIONALE
Client will not harm self or others.	1. Observe client's behavior frequently through routine activities and interactions. Become aware of behaviors that indicate a rise in agitation.	1. Stress commonly increases tic behaviors. Recognition of behaviors that precede the onset of aggression may provide the opportunity to intervene before violence occurs.
	2. Monitor for self-destructive behavior and impulses. A staff member may need to stay with the client to prevent self-mutilation.	2. Client safety is a nursing priority.
	3. Provide hand coverings and other restraints that prevent the client from self-mutilative behaviors.	3. Provide immediate external controls against self-aggressive behaviors.
	4. Redirect violent behavior with physical outlets for frustration.	4. Excess energy is released through physical activities and a feeling of relaxation is induced.

NURSING DIAGNOSIS: IMPAIRED SOCIAL INTERACTION
RELATED TO: Impulsiveness; oppositional and aggressive behavior

OUTCOME CRITERIA	NURSING INTERVENTIONS	RATIONALE
Client will be able to interact with staff and peers using age-appropriate, acceptable behaviors.	1. Develop a trusting relationship with the client. Convey acceptance of the person separate from the unacceptable behavior.	1. Unconditional acceptance increases feelings of self-worth.
	2. Discuss with client which behaviors are and are not acceptable. Describe in matter-of-fact manner the consequences of unacceptable behavior. Follow through.	2. Aversive reinforcement can alter undesirable behaviors.
	3. Provide group situations for client.	3. Appropriate social behavior is often learned from the positive and negative feedback of peers.

(Continued on opposite page)

NURSING DIAGNOSIS: LOW SELF-ESTEEM
RELATED TO: Shame associated with tic behaviors

OUTCOME CRITERIA	NURSING INTERVENTIONS	RATIONALE
Client will verbalize positive aspects about self not associated with tic behaviors.	1. Convey unconditional acceptance and positive regard.	1. Communication of client as a worthwhile human being may increase self-esteem.
	2. Set limits on manipulative behavior. Take caution not to reinforce manipulative behaviors by providing desired attention. Identify the consequences of manipulation. Administer consequences matter-of-factly when manipulation occurs.	2. Aversive consequences may work to decrease unacceptable behaviors.
	3. Help client understand that he or she uses manipulation to try to increase own self-esteem. Interventions should reflect other actions to accomplish this goal.	3. When client feels better about self, the need to manipulate others will diminish.
	4. If client chooses to suppress tics in the presence of others, provide a specified "tic time," during which he or she "vents" tics, feelings, and behaviors (alone or with staff).	4. Allows for release of tics and assists in sense of control and management of symptoms (Rosner & Pollice, 1991).
	5. Ensure that client has regular one-to-one time with nursing staff.	5. Provides opportunity for educating about illness and teaching management tactics. Assists in exploring feelings around illness and incorporating illness into a healthy sense of self (Rosner & Pollice, 1991).

Evaluation

Evaluation of care for the child with Tourette's disorder reflects whether or not the nursing actions have been effective in achieving the established goals. The nursing process calls for reassessment of the plan. Questions for gathering reassessment data may include:

1. Has the client refrained from causing harm to self or others during times of increased tension?
2. Has the client developed adaptive coping strategies for dealing with frustration to prevent resorting to self-destruction or aggression to others?
3. Is the client able to interact appropriately with staff and peers?
4. Is the client able to suppress tic behaviors when he or she chooses to do so?
5. Does the client set a time for "release" of the suppressed tic behaviors?
6. Does the client verbalize positive aspects about self, particularly as they relate to his or her ability to manage the illness?
7. Does the client comply with treatment in a nondefensive manner?

Psychopharmacological Intervention

Medications are used to reduce the severity of the tics in clients with Tourette's disorder. Pharmacotherapy is most effective when it is combined with psychosocial therapy, such as behavioral therapy, individual counseling or psychotherapy, and/or family therapy. Some cases of the disorder are mild and clients choose not to use medication until the symptoms become severe and more intense intervention is warranted. A number of medications have been used to treat Tourette's disorder. The most common ones are discussed here.

Haloperidol (Haldol). Haloperidol has been the drug of choice for Tourette's disorder. The dosage is 0.05 to 0.075 mg/kg per day in two to three divided doses. Children taking haloperidol can develop the same side effects associated with the neuroleptic as prescribed for psychotic disorders (see Chapter 21). Children should be monitored closely for efficacy and adverse effects of the medication. Because of the potential for adverse effects, it is advisable to reserve this medication for children with severe symptoms or with symptoms that interfere with their ability to function academically or socially.

Pimozide (Orap). Pimozide is a neuroleptic with a response rate and side effect profile similar to that of haloperidol. It is used in the management of severe motor or vocal tics that have failed to respond to more conventional treatment. Pimozide is not recommended for children younger than age 12 years. Dosage is initiated at 1 to 2 mg/day and increased weekly up to 3 to 5 mg/day.

Clonidine (Catapres). Clonidine is an alpha-adrenergic agonist that is approved for use as an antihypertensive agent. Results of studies on the efficacy of clonidine in the treatment of Tourette's disorder have been mixed. Some physicians use clonidine as a first choice because of the few side effects and relative safety associated with it. Common side effects include dry mouth, sedation, and dizziness or hypotension.

Atypical Antipsychotics. Atypical antipsychotics are less likely to cause extrapyramidal side effects than the older antipsychotics (e.g., haloperidol and pimozide). Risperidone, the most studied atypical antipsychotic in Tourette's disorder, has been shown to reduce symptoms by 21 to 61 percent when compared to placebo (results which are similar to that of pimozide and clonidine) (Dion et al., 2002). Both olanzapine and ziprasidone have demonstrated effectiveness in decreasing tic symptoms of Tourette's disorder. Weight gain and abnormal glucose tolerance associated with olanzapine may be troublesome side effects, and ziprasidone has been associated with increased risk of QTc interval prolongation (Stewart et al., 2003). Stewart and associates (2003) state:

> Further controlled trials of atypical antipsychotics in children and adolescents with tic disorders are needed. ECGs are recommended to monitor QTc intervals when using these medications.

SEPARATION ANXIETY DISORDER

The essential feature of separation anxiety disorder is excessive anxiety concerning separation from the home or from those to whom the person is attached (APA, 2000). The anxiety is beyond that which would be expected for the individual's developmental level and interferes with social, academic, occupational, or others areas of functioning. Onset may occur anytime before age 18 years and is more common in girls than in boys.

Predisposing Factors

Biological Influences

Genetics. Studies have been conducted in which the children of adult clients diagnosed as having separation anxiety disorder were studied. A second method, studying parents and other relatives of children diagnosed as having separation anxiety disorder, has also been used. The results have shown that a greater number of children with relatives who manifest anxiety problems develop anxiety disorders themselves than do children with no such family patterns. The results are significant enough to speculate that there is a hereditary influence in the development of separation anxiety disorder, but the mode of genetic transmission has not been determined.

Temperament. It is well established that children differ from birth, or shortly thereafter, on a number of temperamental characteristics. Sadock and Sadock (2003) state:

> The temperamental constellation of behavioral inhibition, excessive shyness, the tendency to withdraw from unfamiliar situations, and separation anxiety are all likely to have a genetic contribution. (p. 1260)

Individual differences in temperaments may be related to the acquisition of fear and anxiety disorders in childhood. This may be referred to as *anxiety proneness* or *vulnerability* and may denote an inherited "disposition" toward developing anxiety disorders.

Environmental Influences

Stressful Life Events. Studies have shown a relationship between life events and the development of anxiety disorders (Sadock & Sadock, 2003). It is thought that perhaps children who already are vulnerable or predisposed to developing anxiety disorders may be affected significantly by stressful life events. More research is needed before firm conclusions can be drawn.

Family Influences

Various theories expound on the idea that anxiety disorders in children are related to an overattachment to the mother. Sadock and Sadock (2003) attribute the major determinants of anxiety disorders to transactions relating to separation issues between mother (or mothering figure) and child. The *DSM-IV-TR* (APA, 2000) suggests that children with separation anxiety disorders come from close-knit families.

Some parents may instill anxiety in their children by overprotecting them from expectable dangers or by exaggerating the dangers of the present and the future (Sadock & Sadock, 2003). Some parents may also transfer their fears and anxieties to their children through role modeling. For example, a parent who becomes fearful in the presence of a small, harmless dog and retreats with dread and apprehension teaches the young child by example that this is an appropriate response.

Application of the Nursing Process

Background Assessment Data (Symptomatology)

Age at onset of this disorder may be as early as preschool age; it rarely begins as late as adolescence. In most cases, the child has difficulty separating from the mother.

Occasionally the separation reluctance is directed toward the father, siblings, or other significant individual to whom the child is attached. Anticipation of separation may result in tantrums, crying, screaming, complaints of physical problems, and **clinging** behaviors.

Reluctance or refusal to attend school is especially common in adolescence. Younger children may "shadow" or follow around the person from whom they are afraid to be separated. During middle childhood or adolescence they may refuse to sleep away from home (e.g., at a friend's house or at camp). Interpersonal peer relationships are usually not a problem with these children. They are generally well liked by their peers and are reasonably socially skilled.

Worrying is common, and relates to the possibility of harm coming to self or to the attachment figure. Younger children may even have nightmares to this effect.

Specific phobias are not uncommon (e.g., fear of the dark, ghosts, animals). Depressed mood is frequently present and often precedes the onset of the anxiety symptoms, which commonly occur following a major stressor. The *DSM-IV-TR* diagnostic criteria for separation anxiety disorder are presented in Table 25–14.

TABLE 25-14 Diagnostic Criteria for Separation Anxiety Disorder

A. Developmentally inappropriate and excessive anxiety concerning separation from home or from those to whom the individual is attached, as evidenced by three (or more) of the following:
   1. Recurrent excessive distress when separation from home or major attachment figures occurs or is anticipated.
   2. Persistent and excessive worry about losing, or about possible harm befalling, major attachment figures.
   3. Persistent and excessive worry that an untoward event will lead to separation from a major attachment figure (e.g., getting lost or being kidnapped).
   4. Persistent reluctance or refusal to go to school or elsewhere because of fear of separation.
   5. Persistently and excessively fearful or reluctant to be alone or without major attachment figures at home or without significant adults in other setting.
   6. Persistent reluctance or refusal to go to sleep without being near a major attachment figure or to sleep away from home.
   7. Repeated nightmares involving the theme of separation.
   8. Repeated complaints of physical symptoms (such as headaches, stomachaches, nausea, or vomiting) when separation from major attachment figures occurs or is anticipated.
B. The duration of the disturbance is at least 4 weeks.
C. The onset is before age 18 years.
D. The disturbance causes clinically significant distress or impairment in social, academic (occupational), or other important areas of functioning.
E. The disturbance does not occur exclusively during the course of a pervasive developmental disorder, schizophrenia, or other psychotic disorder and, in adolescents and adults, is not better accounted for by panic disorder with agoraphobia.

SOURCE: From APA (2000), with permission.

Diagnosis/Outcome Identification

Based on the data collected during the nursing assessment, possible nursing diagnoses for the client with separation anxiety disorder include:

Anxiety (severe) related to family history, temperament, overattachment to parent, negative role modeling.
Ineffective coping related to unresolved separation conflicts and inadequate coping skills evidenced by numerous somatic complaints.
Impaired social interaction related to reluctance to be away from attachment figure.

The following criteria may be used for measurement of outcomes in the care of the client with separation anxiety disorder.

The client:

1. Is able to maintain anxiety at manageable level.
2. Demonstrates adaptive coping strategies for dealing with anxiety when separation from attachment figure is anticipated.
3. Interacts appropriately with others and spends time away from attachment figure to do so.

Planning/Implementation

Table 25-15 provides a plan of care for the child or adolescent with separation anxiety, using nursing diagnoses common to this disorder, outcome criteria, and appropriate nursing interventions and rationales.

Evaluation

Evaluation of the child or adolescent with separation anxiety disorder requires reassessment of the behaviors for which the family sought treatment. Both the client and the family members will have to change their behavior. The following types of questions may provide assistance in gathering data required for evaluating whether the nursing interventions have been effective in achieving the goals of therapy.

1. Is the client able to maintain anxiety at a manageable level (i.e., without temper tantrums, screaming, "clinging")?
2. Have complaints of physical symptoms diminished?
3. Has the client demonstrated the ability to cope in more adaptive ways in the face of escalating anxiety?
4. Have the parents identified their role in the separation conflict? Are they able to discuss more adaptive coping strategies?
5. Does the client verbalize an intention to return to school?
6. Have nightmares and fears of the dark subsided?

TABLE 25–15   Care Plan for the Client with Separation Anxiety Disorder

NURSING DIAGNOSIS: ANXIETY (SEVERE)
RELATED TO: Family history; temperament; overattachment to parent; negative role modeling

OUTCOME CRITERIA	NURSING INTERVENTIONS	RATIONALE
Client will maintain anxiety at no higher than moderate level in the face of events that formerly have precipitated panic.	1. Establish an atmosphere of calmness, trust, and genuine positive regard. 2. Assure client of his or her safety and security. 3. Explore the child or adolescent's fears of separating from the parents. Explore with the parents possible fears they may have of separation from the child. 4. Help parents and child initiate realistic goals (e.g., child to stay with sitter for 2 hours with minimal anxiety; or, child to stay at friend's house without parents until 9 PM without experiencing panic anxiety). 5. Give, and encourage parents to give, positive reinforcement for desired behaviors.	1. Trust and unconditional acceptance are necessary for satisfactory nurse/client relationship. Calmness is important because anxiety is easily transmitted from one person to another. 2. Symptoms of panic anxiety are very frightening. 3. Some parents may have an underlying fear of separation from the child, of which they are unaware and which they are unconsciously transferring to the child. 4. Parents may be so frustrated with child's clinging and demanding behaviors that assistance with problem solving may be required. 5. Positive reinforcement encourages repetition of desirable behaviors.

NURSING DIAGNOSIS: INEFFECTIVE COPING
RELATED TO: Unresolved separation conflicts and inadequate coping skills
EVIDENCED BY: Numerous somatic complaints

OUTCOME CRITERIA	NURSING INTERVENTIONS	RATIONALE
Client will demonstrate use of more adaptive coping strategies (than physical symptoms) in response to stressful situations.	1. Encourage child or adolescent to discuss specific situations in life that produce the most distress and describe his or her response to these situations. Include parents in the discussion. 2. Help the child or adolescent who is perfectionistic to recognize that self-expectations may be unrealistic. Connect times of unmet self-expectations to the exacerbation of physical symptoms. 3. Encourage parents and child to identify more adaptive coping strategies that the child could use in the face of anxiety that feels overwhelming. Practice through role-play.	1. Client and family may be unaware of the correlation between stressful situations and the exacerbation of physical symptoms. 2. Recognition of maladaptive patterns is the first step in the change process. 3. Practice facilitates the use of the desired behavior when the individual is actually faced with the stressful situation.

NURSING DIAGNOSIS: IMPAIRED SOCIAL INTERACTION
RELATED TO: Reluctance to be away from attachment figure

OUTCOME CRITERIA	NURSING INTERVENTIONS	RATIONALE
Client will be able to spend time with staff and peers without excessive anxiety.	1. Develop a trusting relationship with client. 2. Attend groups with the child and support efforts to interact with others. Give positive feedback.	1. This is the first step in helping the client learn to interact with others. 2. Presence of a trusted individual provides security during times of distress. Positive feedback encourages repetition.

(Continued on opposite page)

OUTCOME CRITERIA	NURSING INTERVENTIONS	RATIONALE
	3. Convey to the child the acceptability of his or her not participating in group in the beginning. Gradually encourage small contributions until client is able to participate more fully.	3. Small successes will gradually increase self-confidence and decrease self-consciousness, so that client will feel less anxious in the group situation.
	4. Help client set small personal goals (e.g., "Today I will speak to one person I don't know").	4. Simple, realistic goals provide opportunities for success that increase self-confidence and may encourage the client to attempt more difficult objectives in the future.

7. Is the client able to interact with others away from the attachment figure?

8. Has the precipitating stressor been identified? Have strategies for coping more adaptively to similar stressors in the future been established?

GENERAL THERAPEUTIC APPROACHES

Behavior Therapy

Behavior therapy is based on the concepts of classical conditioning and operant conditioning (see Chapter 19). Behavior therapy is a common and effective treatment with disruptive behavior disorders. With this approach, rewards are given for appropriate behaviors and withheld when behaviors are disruptive or otherwise inappropriate. The principle behind behavior therapy is that positive reinforcements encourage repetition of desirable behaviors, and aversive reinforcements (punishments) discourage repetition of undesirable behaviors. Behavior modification techniques—the system of rewards and consequences—can be taught to parents to be used in the home environment. Consistency is an essential component.

In the treatment setting, individualized behavior modification programs are designed for each client. A case study example, based on a token economy, is presented in Chapter 19.

Family Therapy

Children cannot be separated from their families. Therapy for children and adolescents must involve the entire family if problems are to be resolved. Parents should be involved in designing and implementing the treatment plan for the child and should be involved in all aspects of the treatment process.

The genogram can be used to identify problem areas between family members (see Chapter 11). A genogram provides an overall picture of the life of the family over several generations, including roles that various family members play and emotional distance between specific individuals. Areas for change can be easily identified.

The impact of family dynamics on disruptive behavior disorders has been identified. The impact of disruptive behavior on family dynamics cannot be ignored. Family coping can become severely compromised with the chronic stress of dealing with a behavior-disordered child. It is therefore imperative that the treatment plan for the identified client be instituted within the context of family-centered care. Popper and associates (2003) state:

> Multimodal treatment of ADHD is currently the standard of care for children. There is a lot to be gained by supporting medication treatment with appropriate educational, psychosocial, and family interventions. (p. 854)

Group Therapy

Group therapy provides children and adolescents with the opportunity to interact within an association of their peers. This can be both gratifying and overwhelming, depending on the child.

Group therapy provides a number of benefits. Appropriate social behavior often is learned from the positive and negative feedback of peers. Opportunity is provided to learn to tolerate and accept differences in others, to learn that it is acceptable to disagree, to learn to offer and receive support from others, and to practice these new skills in a safe environment. It is a way to learn from the experiences of others.

Group therapy with children and adolescents can take several forms. Music therapy groups allow clients to express feelings through music, often when they are unable to express themselves in any other way. Art and activity/craft therapy groups allow individual expression through artistic means.

Group play therapy is the treatment of choice for many children between the ages of 3 and 9 years. Landreth and Bratton (2005) state:

Play therapy is to children what counseling or psychotherapy is to adults. Play provides children with a means of expressing their inner world. The use of toys enables children to transfer anxieties, fears, fantasies, and guilt to objects rather than people. In the process, children are safe from their own feelings and reactions because play enables children to distance themselves from traumatic events and experiences. For children, play therapy changes what may be unmanageable in reality into manageable situations through symbolic representation. This provides children with opportunities for learning to cope.

Psychoeducational groups are very beneficial for adolescents. The only drawback to this type of group is that it works best when the group is closed ended; that is, once the group has been formed, no one is allowed to join until the group has reached its preestablished closure. Members are allowed to propose topics for discussion. The leader serves as teacher much of the time and facilitates discussion of the proposed topic. Members may from time to time be presenters and serve as discussion leaders. Sometimes, psychoeducation groups evolve into traditional therapy discussion groups.

Psychopharmacology

Several of the disorders presented in this chapter are treated with medications. The appropriate pharmacology was presented following the section in which the disorder was discussed. Medication should never be the sole method of treatment. It is undeniable that medication can and does improve quality of life for families of children and adolescents with these disorders. However, research has indicated that medication alone is not as effective as a combination of medication and psychosocial therapy. It is important for families to understand that there is no way to "give him a pill and make him well." The importance of the psychosocial therapies cannot be overstressed. Some clinicians will not prescribe medications for a client unless he or she also participates in concomitant psychotherapy sessions. The beneficial effects of the medications promote improved coping ability, which in turn enhances the intent of the psychosocial therapy.

SUMMARY

Child and adolescent psychiatric nursing is a specialty that has been given too little attention. Most basic nursing curricula include minimal instruction in child psychiatric nursing. Even though nurses work in many areas that place them in ideal positions to identify emotionally disturbed children, many of them do not have sufficient knowledge of child psychopathology to recognize maladaptive behaviors.

This chapter has presented some of the most prevalent disorders identified by the *DSM-IV-TR* (APA, 2000) as first becoming evident in infancy, childhood, or adolescence. An explanation of various etiological factors was presented for each disorder to assist in the comprehension of underlying dynamics. These included biological, environmental, and family influences.

The nursing process was presented as the vehicle for delivery of care. Symptomatology for each of the disorders provided background assessment data. Nursing diagnoses identified specific behaviors that were targets for change. Both client and family were considered in the planning and implementation. Behavior modification is the focus of nursing intervention with children and adolescents. With families, attention is given to education and referrals to community resources from which they can derive support. Reassessment data provide information for evaluation of nursing interventions in achieving the desired outcomes.

Child psychiatry is an area in which nursing can make a valuable contribution. Nurses who choose this field have an excellent opportunity to serve in the promotion of emotional wellness for children and adolescents. A discussion of psychopharmacological intervention was included for the disorders in which this form of treatment is relevant.

IMPLICATIONS OF RESEARCH FOR EVIDENCE-BASED PRACTICE

Frame, K., Kelly, L., & Bayley, E. (2003). Increasing perceptions of self-worth in preadolescents diagnosed with ADHD. *Journal of Nursing Scholarship, 35(3), 225–229.*

Description of the Study: The theoretical framework for this study was based on the Roy adaptation model. The sample in this study consisted of 65 preadolescents diagnosed with ADD or ADHD in an upper-middle class community in the United States. Participants were randomly assigned to either the control group or the experimental group, and all completed the Harter's Self-Perception Profile for Children instrument at the beginning of the study and 4 weeks later. This tool was designed to measure perceptions of scholastic competence, social acceptance, athletic competence, physical appearance, behavioral conduct, and global self-worth. Children in the experimental group participated in a school-nurse facilitated support group that met twice weekly for 4 weeks. In the group, the participants were assisted to learn strategies for effective interactions with their peers, teachers, and families. Interventions served to promote adaptive self-evaluations and to address the unfavorable self-perceptions of many children with ADHD.

Results of the Study: On post-testing, participants in the support group scored significantly higher than controls on each of the six subscales, with significant increases on four of the subscales, including perceived social acceptance, perceived athletic competence, perceived physical appearance, and perceived global self-worth.

Implications for Nursing Practice: This study has implications for nurses who work with children, and particularly those who work with children diagnosed with ADHD. Because preadolescence is a time when children compare themselves, either positively or negatively, with their peers, group interaction is an especially significant intervention. The authors state, "The support group, with children helping children, enabled participants to engage in creative problem-solving and to develop solutions to their difficulties." This intervention was shown to promote positive perceptions and behaviors among children with ADD and ADHD. It is especially appropriate for the role of school nurse, but it is also consistent with the role of any nurse who interacts directly with children or adolescents who have similar problems.

TEST YOUR CRITICAL THINKING SKILLS

Jimmy, age 9, has been admitted to the child psychiatric unit with a diagnosis of attention-deficit/hyperactivity disorder. He has been unmanageable at school and at home, and was recently suspended from school for continuous disruption of his class. He refuses to sit in his chair or do his work. He yells out in class, interrupts the teacher and the other students, and lately has become physically aggressive when he cannot have his way. He was suspended after hitting his teacher when she asked him to return to his seat.

Jimmy's mother describes him as a restless and demanding baby, who grew into a restless and demanding toddler. He has never gotten along well with his peers. Even as a small child, he would take his friends' toys away from them or bite them if they tried to hold their own with him. His 5-year-old sister is afraid of him and refuses to be alone with him.

During the nurse's intake assessment, Jimmy paced the room or rocked in his chair. He talked incessantly on a superficial level and jumped from topic to topic. He told the nurse that he did not know why he was there. He acknowledged that he had some problems at school but said that was only because the other kids picked on him and the teacher did not like him. He said he got into trouble at home sometimes but that was because his parents liked his little sister better than they liked him.

The physician has ordered methylphenidate 5 mg twice a day for Jimmy. His response to this order is, "I'm not going to take drugs. I'm not sick!"

Answer the following questions related to Jimmy:

1. What are the pertinent assessment data to be noted by the nurse?
2. What is the primary nursing diagnosis for Jimmy?
3. Aside from client safety, to what problems would the nurse want to direct intervention with Jimmy?

REVIEW QUESTIONS

SELF-EXAMINATION/LEARNING EXERCISE

Select the answer that is most appropriate for each of the following questions.

1. In an effort to help the mild-to-moderately mentally retarded child develop satisfying relationships with others, which of the following nursing interventions is most appropriate?
   a. Interpret the child's behavior for others.
   b. Set limits on behavior that is socially inappropriate.
   c. Allow the child to behave spontaneously, for he or she has no concept of right or wrong.
   d. This child is not capable of forming social relationships.

2. The autistic child has difficulty with trust. With this in mind, which of the following nursing actions would be most appropriate?
   a. Encourage all staff to hold the child as often as possible, conveying trust through touch.
   b. Assign a different staff member each day so child will learn that everyone can be trusted.
   c. Assign same staff person as often as possible to promote feelings of security and trust.
   d. Avoid eye contact, as it is extremely uncomfortable for the child, and may even discourage trust.

3. Which of the following nursing diagnoses would be considered the *priority* in planning care for the autistic child?
   a. Risk for self-mutilation evidenced by banging head against wall
   b. Impaired social interaction evidenced by unresponsiveness to people
   c. Impaired verbal communication evidenced by absence of verbal expression
   d. Disturbed personal identity evidenced by inability to differentiate self from others

4. Which of the following activities would be most appropriate for the child with ADHD?
   a. Monopoly
   b. Volleyball
   c. Pool
   d. Checkers

5. Which of the following groups are most commonly used for drug management of the hyperactive child?
   a. CNS depressants (e.g., diazepam [Valium])
   b. CNS stimulants (e.g., methylphenidate [Ritalin])
   c. Anticonvulsants (e.g., phenytoin [Dilantin])
   d. Major tranquilizers (e.g., haloperidol [Haldol])

6. The child with ADHD has a nursing diagnosis of impaired social interaction. An appropriate nursing intervention for this child is:
   a. To socially isolate the child when interactions with others are inappropriate.
   b. To set limits with consequences on inappropriate behaviors.
   c. To provide rewards for appropriate behaviors.
   d. b and c
   e. a, b, and c

7. The nursing history and assessment of an adolescent with a conduct disorder might reveal all of the following behaviors *except*:
   a. Manipulation of others for fulfillment of own desires
   b. Chronic violation of rules
   c. Feelings of guilt associated with the exploitation of others
   d. Inability to form close peer relationships

8. Certain family dynamics often predispose adolescents to the development of conduct disorder. Which of the following patterns is thought to be a contributing factor?
   a. Parents who are overprotective
   b. Parents who have high expectations for their children
   c. Parents who consistently set limits on their children's behavior
   d. Parents who are alcohol dependent.

9. Which of the following is *least* likely to predispose a child to Tourette's disorder?
   a. Absence of parental bonding
   b. Family history of the disorder
   c. Abnormalities of brain neurotransmitters
   d. Structural abnormalities of the brain

10. Which of the following is the drug of choice for Tourette's disorder?
   a. Methylphenidate (Ritalin)
   b. Haloperidol (Haldol)
   c. Imipramine (Tofranil)
   d. Pemoline (Cylert)

REFERENCES

American Psychiatric Association. (2000). *Diagnostic and statistical manual of mental disorders* (4th ed.) *Text revision*. Washington, DC: American Psychiatric Association.

Bagley, C., & Mallick, K. (2000). Spiraling up and spiraling down: Implications of a long-term study of temperament and conduct disorder for social work with children. *Child & Family Social Work, 5*(4), 291–301.

Clunn, P. (1991). Child psychiatric nursing. St. Louis: Mosby-Year Book.

Comings, D.E., Gade-Andavolu, R., Gonzalez, N., Wu, S., Mahleman, D., Blake, H., Dietz, G., Saucier, G., & MacMurray, J.P. (2000). Comparison of the role of dopamine, serotonin, and noradrenaline genes in ADHD, ODD, and conduct disorder: Multivariate regression analysis of 20 genes. *Clinical Genetics, 57,* 178–196.

Croen, L.A., Grether, J.K., Yoshida, C.K., Odouli, R., & Van dewater, J. (2005). Maternal autoimmune diseases, asthma and allergies, and childhood autism spectrum disorders. *Archives of Pediatrics and Adolescent Medicine, 159,* 151–157.

Dick, D.M., Li, T-K, Edenberg, H.J., Hesselbrock, V, Kramer, J., Kuperman, S., Porjesz, B., Bucholz, K., Goate, A., Nurnberger, J., & Foroud, T. (2004). A genome-wide screen for genes influencing conduct disorder. *Molecular Psychiatry, 9*(1), 81–86.

Dion, Y., Annable, L., Sandor, P., & Chouinard, G. (2002). Risperidone in the treatment of Tourette syndrome: A double-blind, placebo-controlled trial. *Journal of Clinical Psychopharmacology, 22*(1), 31–39.

Dopheide, J.A., & Theesen, K.A. (1999). Disorders of childhood. In J.T. Dipiro, R.L. Talbert, & G.C. Yee (Eds.). *Pharmacotherapy: A pathophysiological approach* (4th ed.). New York: McGraw-Hill.

Foley, D.L., Eaves, L.J., Wormley, B., Silberg, J.L., Maes, H.H., Kuh, J., & Riley, B. (2004). Childhood adversity, monoamine oxidase A genotype, and risk for conduct disorder. *Archives of General Psychiatry, 61,* 738–744.

Harvard Medical School (2002). InteliHealth: Consumer health information. *Behavior disorders in children and teens.* Retrieved on February 4, 2002 from the World Wide Web at http://www.intelihealth.com/IH/ihtIH/EMIHC000/20722/8632/187947.html?d=dmtContent

Ladd, G.W. (1999). Peer relationships and social competence during early and middle childhood. *Annual Review of Psychology, 50,* 333–359.

Landreth, G., & Bratton, S. (2005). Play therapy. *ERIC Digests.* Retrieved March 4, 2005 from the World Wide Web at http://www.ericdigests.org/2000–1/play.html

Linnet, K.M., Wisborg, K., Obel, C., Secher, N.J., Thomsen, P.H., Agerbo, E., &, Henriksen, T.B. (2005). Smoking during pregnancy and the risk for hyperkinetic disorder in offspring. *Pediatrics, 116*(2), 462–467.

Medscape Health (2002). *What causes attention deficit hyperactivity disorder?* Retrieved February 3, 2002 from the World Wide Web at http://health.medscape.com/viewarticle/209223_6

National Institute of Mental Health (NIMH). (2002). *Autism.* NIH Publication No. 97-4023. Retrieved February 1, 2002 from the World Wide Web at http://www.nimh.nih.gov/publicat/autism.cfm#aut10

National Institute of Mental Health (NIMH). (2000). *Attention Deficit Hyperactivity Disorder (ADHD) – Questions and Answers.* Retrieved February 2, 2002 from the World Wide Web at http://www.nimh.nih.gov/publicat/adhdqa.cfm

Plessen, K.J., Wentzel-Larson, T., Hugdahl, K., Feineigle, P., Klein, J., Staib, L.H., Leckman, J.F., Bansal, R., & Peterson, B.S. (2004). Altered interhemispheric connectivity in individuals with Tourette's disorder. *American Journal of Psychiatry, 161,* 2028–2037.

Popper, C.W., Gammon, G.D., West, S.A., & Bailey, C.E. (2003). Disorders usually first diagnosed in infancy, childhood, or adolescence. In R.E. Hales & S.C. Yudofsky (Eds.). *Textbook of clinical psychiatry* (4th ed.). Washington, DC: The American Psychiatric Publishing.

Rosner, T.A., & Pollice, S.A. (1991). Tourette's syndrome. *Journal of Psychosocial Nursing, 29*(1), 4–9.

Rowe, R., Maughan, B., Worthman, C.M., Costello, E.J., & Angold, A. (2004). Testosterone, antisocial behavior, and social dominance in boys: Pubertal development and biosocial interaction. *Biological Psychiatry, 55*(5), 546–552.

Sadock, B.J., & Sadock, V.A. (2003). *Synopsis of psychiatry: Behavioral sciences/clinical psychiatry* (9th ed.). Philadelphia: Lippincott Williams & Wilkins.

Searight, H.R., Rottnek, F., & Abby, S.L. (2001). Conduct disorder: Diagnosis and treatment in primary care. *American Family Physician, 63*(8), 1579–1588.

Shahrokh, N.C. & Hales, R.E. (2003). *American psychiatric glossary* (8th ed.). Washington, DC: American Psychiatric Publishing.

Stewart, S.E., Geller, D., Spencer, T., & Gianini, L. (2003). Tics and Tourette's disorder: Which therapies, and when to use them. *Current Psychiatry Online.* Retrieved March 3, 2005 from the World Wide Web at http://www.currentpsychiatry.com/2003_10/1003_therapies.asp

@ INTERNET REFERENCES

- Additional information about Attention Deficit Hyperactivity Disorder may be located at the following Web sites:
  a. http://www.chadd.org
  b. http://www.nimh.nih.gov/healthinformation/adhdmenu.cfm

Additional information about Autism may be located at the following Web sites:

  a. http://www.autism-society.org
  b. http://www.nimh.nih.gov/healthinformation/autismmenu.cfm

- Additional information about medications to treat attention deficit hyperactivity disorder may be located at the following Web sites:
  a. http://www.fadavis.com/townsend
  b. http://www.laurus.com/library/healthguide/DrugGuide
  c. http://www.nimh.nih.gov/publicat/medicate.cfm

DELIRIUM, DEMENTIA, AND AMNESTIC DISORDERS

CHAPTER OUTLINE

OBJECTIVES

DELIRIUM

DEMENTIA

AMNESTIC DISORDERS

APPLICATION OF THE NURSING PROCESS

MEDICAL TREATMENT MODALITIES

SUMMARY

REVIEW QUESTIONS

KEY TERMS

aphasia

apraxia

ataxia

confabulation

primary dementia

pseudodementia

secondary dementia

sundowning

CORE CONCEPTS

amnesia

delirium

dementia

OBJECTIVES

After reading this chapter, the student will be able to:

1. Define and differentiate among *delirium, dementia,* and *amnestic disorder.*
2. Discuss predisposing factors implicated in the etiology of delirium, dementia, and amnestic disorders.
3. Identify symtomatology and use the information to assess clients with delirium, dementia, and amnestic disorders.
4. Identify nursing diagnoses common to clients with delirium, dementia, and

amnestic disorders, and select appropriate nursing interventions for each.
5. Identify topics for client and family teaching relevant to cognitive disorders.
6. Discuss criteria for evaluating nursing care of clients with delirium, dementia, and amnestic disorders.
7. Describe various treatment modalities relevant to care of clients with delirium, dementia, and amnestic disorders.

*T*his chapter discusses disorders in which a clinically significant deficit in cognition or memory exists, representing a significant change from a previous level of functioning. The *DSM-IV-TR* (APA, 2000) describes the etiology of these disorders as a general medical condition, a substance, or a combination of these factors.

These disorders were previously identified as *organic mental syndromes and disorders.* With the publication of the *DSM-IV* (APA, 1994), the name was changed to prevent the implication that *nonorganic* mental disorders do not have a biological basis.

These disorders constitute a large and growing public health problem. Scientists estimate that 4.5 million people currently have Alzheimer's disease (AD), the most common form of dementia, and the prevalence (the number of people with the disease at any one time) doubles for every 5-year age group beyond age 65 (National Institute on Aging [NIA], 2003). The disease affects one in ten people age 65 and older, one in five ages 75 to 85, and one in two age 85 and older (Laraia, 2004). Researchers estimate that by 2050, 13.2 million Americans will have AD if current population trends continue and no preventive treatments become available (Herbert et al., 2003). After heart disease and cancer, AD is the third most costly disease to society, accounting for $100 billion in yearly costs (NIA, 2003). This proliferation is not the result of an "epidemic." It has occurred because more people now survive into the high-risk period for dementia, which is middle age and beyond.

This chapter presents predisposing factors, clinical symptoms, and nursing interventions for care of clients with delirium, dementia, and amnestic disorders. The objective is to provide these individuals with the dignity and quality of life they deserve, while offering guidance and support to their families or primary caregivers.

Core Concept

Delirium

Delirium is a mental state characterized by a disturbance of cognition, which is manifested by confusion, excitement, disorientation, and a clouding of consciousness. Hallucinations and illusions are common.

DELIRIUM

A **delirium** is characterized by a disturbance of consciousness and a change in cognition that develop rapidly over a short period (APA, 2000). Symptoms of delirium include difficulty sustaining and shifting attention. The person is extremely distractible and must be repeatedly reminded to focus attention. Disorganized thinking prevails and is reflected by speech that is rambling, irrelevant, pressured, and incoherent, and that unpredictably switches from subject to subject. Reasoning ability and goal-directed behavior are impaired. Disorientation to time and place is common, and impairment of recent memory is invariably evident. Misperceptions of the environment, including illusions and hallucinations, prevail.

Level of consciousness is often affected, with a disturbance in the sleep–wake cycle. The state of awareness may range from that of hypervigilance to stupor or semicoma. Sleep may fluctuate between hypersomnolence and insomnia. Vivid dreams and nightmares are common.

Psychomotor activity may fluctuate between agitated, purposeless movements (e.g., restlessness, hyperactivity, striking out at nonexistent objects) and a vegetative state

resembling catatonic stupor. Various forms of tremor are frequently present.

Emotional instability may be manifested by fear, anxiety, depression, irritability, anger, euphoria, or apathy. These various emotions may be evidenced by crying, calls for help, cursing, muttering, moaning, acts of self-destruction, fearful attempts to flee, or attacks on others who are falsely viewed as threatening. Autonomic manifestations, such as tachycardia, sweating, flushed face, dilated pupils, and elevated blood pressure, are common.

The symptoms of delirium usually begin quite abruptly (e.g., following a head injury or seizure). At other times, they may be preceded by several hours or days of prodromal symptoms (e.g., restlessness, difficulty thinking clearly, insomnia or hypersomnolence, and nightmares). The slower onset is more common if the underlying cause is systemic illness or metabolic imbalance.

The duration of delirium is usually brief (e.g., 1 week; rarely more than 1 month) and, upon recovery from the underlying determinant, symptoms usually diminish over a 3- to 7-day period, but in some instances may take as long as 2 weeks (Sadock & Sadock, 2003). The age of the client and duration of the delirium influence rate of symptom resolution. Delirium may transition into a more permanent cognitive disorder (e.g., dementia) and also is associated with a high mortality rate (Bourgeois, Seaman, & Servis, 2003).

Predisposing Factors

The *DSM-IV-TR* (APA, 2000) differentiates between the disorders of delirium by their etiology, although they share a common symptom presentation. Categories of delirium include:

1. Delirium due to a general medical condition
2. Substance-induced delirium
3. Substance-intoxication delirium
4. Substance-withdrawal delirium
5. Delirium due to multiple etiologies

Delirium Due to a General Medical Condition

In this type of delirium, evidence must exist (from history, physical examination, or laboratory findings) to show that the symptoms of delirium are a direct result of the physiological consequences of a general medical condition (APA, 2000). Such conditions include systemic infections, metabolic disorders (e.g., hypoxia, hypercarbia, and hypoglycemia), fluid or electrolyte imbalances, hepatic or renal disease, thiamine deficiency, postoperative states, hypertensive encephalopathy, postictal states, and sequelae of head trauma (APA, 2000).

Substance-Induced Delirium

This disorder is characterized by the symptoms of delirium that are attributed to medication side effects or exposure to a toxin. The *DSM-IV-TR* (APA, 2000) lists the following examples of medications that have been reported to result in substance-induced delirium: anesthetics, analgesics, antiasthmatic agents, anticonvulsants, antihistamines, antihypertensive and cardiovascular medications, antimicrobials, antiparkinsonian drugs, corticosteroids, gastrointestinal medications, histamine H_2-receptor antagonists (e.g., cimetidine), immunosuppressive agents, lithium, muscle relaxants, and psychotropic medications with anticholinergic side effects. Toxins reported to cause delirium include organophosphate (anticholinesterase), insecticides, carbon monoxide, and volatile substances such as fuel or organic solvents.

Substance-Intoxication Delirium

With this disorder, the symptoms of delirium may arise within minutes to hours after taking relatively high doses of certain drugs such as cannabis, cocaine, and hallucinogens. It may take longer periods of sustained intoxication to produce delirium symptoms with alcohol, anxiolytics, or narcotics (APA, 2000).

Substance-Withdrawal Delirium

Withdrawal delirium symptoms develop after reduction or termination of sustained, usually high-dose use of certain substances, such as alcohol, sedatives, hypnotics, or anxiolytics (APA, 2000). The duration of the delirium is directly related to the half-life of the substance involved and may last from a few hours to 2 to 4 weeks.

Delirium Due to Multiple Etiologies

This diagnosis is used when the symptoms of delirium are brought on by more than one cause. For example, the delirium may be related to more than one general medical condition or it may be a result of the combined effects of a general medical condition and substance use (APA, 2000).

> **Core Concept**
>
> **Dementia**
> Dementia is defined by a loss of previous levels of cognitive, executive, and memory function in a state of full alertness (Bourgeois, Seaman, & Servis, 2003).

DEMENTIA

Dementia can be classified as either primary or secondary. **Primary dementias** are those, such as AD, in which the dementia itself is the major sign of some organic brain disease not directly related to any other organic illness. **Secondary dementias** are caused by or related to another disease or condition, such as human immunodeficiency virus (HIV) disease or a cerebral trauma.

In dementia, impairment is evident in abstract thinking, judgment, and impulse control. The conventional rules of social conduct are often disregarded. Behavior may be uninhibited and inappropriate. Personal appearance and hygiene are often neglected.

Language may or may not be affected. Some individuals may have difficulty naming objects, or the language may seem vague and imprecise. In severe forms of dementia, the individual may not speak at all (**aphasia**).

Personality change is common in dementia and may be manifested by either an alteration or accentuation of premorbid characteristics. For example, an individual who was previously very socially active may become apathetic and socially isolated. A previously neat person may become markedly untidy in his or her appearance. Conversely, an individual who may have had difficulty trusting others prior to the illness may exhibit extreme fear and paranoia as manifestations of the dementia.

The reversibility of a dementia is a function of the underlying pathology and of the availability and timely application of effective treatment (APA, 2000). Truly reversible dementia occurs in only a small percentage of cases and might be more appropriately termed *temporary* dementia. Reversible dementia can occur as a result of stroke, depression, side effects of certain medications, vitamin or nutritional deficiencies (especially B_{12} or folate), and metabolic disorders (Castiglioni, 2003). In most clients, dementia runs a progressive, irreversible course.

As the disease progresses, **apraxia**, which is the inability to carry out motor activities despite intact motor function, may develop. The individual may be irritable, moody, or exhibit sudden outbursts over trivial issues. The ability to work or care for personal needs independently will no longer be possible. These individuals can no longer be left alone because they do not comprehend their limitations and are therefore at serious risk for accidents. Wandering away from the home or care setting often becomes a problem.

Several causes have been described for the syndrome of dementia (see section on Predisposing Factors), but AD accounts for 60 to 80 percent of all cases (Castiglioni, 2003). The progressive nature of symptoms associated with AD has been described according to stages (Alzheimer's Association, 2005; Harvard Medical School, 1995a,b; Stanley, Blair, & Beare, 2005):

Stage 1. No Apparent Symptoms. In the first stage of the illness, there is no apparent decline in memory.

Stage 2. Forgetfulness. The individual begins to lose things or forget names of people. Losses in short-term memory are common. The individual is aware of the intellectual decline and may feel ashamed, becoming anxious and depressed, which in turn may worsen the symptom. Maintaining organization with lists and a structured routine provide some compensation. These symptoms often are not observed by others.

Stage 3. Mild Cognitive Decline. In this stage, there is interference with work performance, which becomes noticeable to coworkers. The individual may get lost when driving his or her car. Concentration may be interrupted. There is difficulty recalling names or words, which becomes noticeable to family and close associates. A decline occurs in the ability to plan or organize.

Stage 4. Mild-to-Moderate Cognitive Decline; Confusion. At this stage, the individual may forget major events in personal history, such as his or her own child's birthday; experience declining ability to perform tasks, such as shopping and managing personal finances; or be unable to understand current news events. He or she may deny that a problem exists by covering up memory loss with **confabulation** (creating imaginary events to fill in memory gaps). Depression and social withdrawal are common.

Stage 5. Moderate Cognitive Decline; Early Dementia. In the early stages of dementia, the individual loses the ability to perform some activities of daily living (ADLs) independently, such as hygiene, dressing, and grooming, and require some assistance to manage these on an ongoing basis. They may forget addresses, phone numbers, and names of close relatives. They may become disoriented about place and time, but they maintain knowledge about themselves. Frustration, withdrawal, and self-absorption are common.

Stage 6. Moderate-to-Severe Cognitive Decline; Middle Dementia. At this stage, the individual may be unable to recall recent major life events or even the name of his or her spouse. Disorientation to surroundings is common, and the person may be unable to recall the day, season, or year. The person is unable to manage ADLs without assistance. Urinary and fecal incontinence are common. Sleeping becomes a problem. Psychomotor symptoms include wandering, obsessiveness, agitation, and aggression. Symptoms seem to worsen in the late afternoon and evening—a phenomenon termed **sundowning**. Communication becomes more difficult, with increasing loss of language skills. Institutional care is usually required at this stage.

Stage 7. Severe Cognitive Decline; Late Dementia. In the end stages of AD, the individual is unable to recognize family members. He or she most commonly is bedfast and aphasic. Problems of immobility, such as decubiti and contractures, may occur.

Stanley, Blair, and Beare (2005) describe the late stages of dementia in the following manner:

During late-stage dementia, the person becomes more chairbound or bedbound. Muscles are rigid, contractures may develop, and primitive reflexes may be present. The person may have very active hands and repetitive movements, grunting, or other vocalizations. There is depressed immune system function, and this impairment coupled with immobility may lead to the development of pneumonia, urinary tract infections, sepsis, and pressure ulcers. Appetite decreases and dysphagia is present; aspiration is common. Weight loss generally occurs. Speech and language are severely impaired, with greatly decreased verbal communication. The person may no longer recognize any family members. Bowel and bladder incontinence are present and caregivers need to complete most ADLs for the person. The sleep-wake cycle is greatly altered, and the person spends a lot of time dozing and appears socially withdrawn and more unaware of the environment or surroundings. Death may be caused by infection, sepsis, or aspiration, although there are not many studies examining cause of death. (p. 358)

●

Predisposing Factors

The *DSM-IV-TR* (APA, 2000) differentiates between the disorders of dementia by their etiology, although they share a common symptom presentation. Categories of dementia include:

1. Dementia of the Alzheimer's type
2. Vascular dementia
3. Dementia due to HIV disease
4. Dementia due to head trauma
5. Dementia due to Parkinson's disease
6. Dementia due to Huntington's disease
7. Dementia due to Pick's disease
8. Dementia due to Creutzfeldt–Jakob disease
9. Dementia due to other general medical conditions
10. Substance-induced persisting dementia
11. Dementia due to multiple etiologies

Dementia of the Alzheimer's Type

This disorder is characterized by the syndrome of symptoms identified as dementia in the *DSM-IV-TR* and in the seven stages described previously. The onset of symptoms is slow and insidious, and the course of the disorder is generally progressive and deteriorating. The *DSM-IV-TR* further categorizes this disorder as *early onset* (first symptoms occurring at age 65 or younger) or *late onset* (first symptoms occurring after age 65) and by the clinical presentation of behavioral disturbance (such as wandering or agitation) superimposed on the dementia.

Refinement of diagnostic criteria now enables clinicians to use specific clinical features to identify the disease with considerable accuracy. Examination by computerized tomography (CT) scan or magnetic resonance imagery (MRI) reveals a degenerative pathology of the brain that includes atrophy, widened cortical sulci, and enlarged cerebral ventricles (Figures 26–1 and 26–2).

Microscopic examinations reveal numerous neurofibrillary tangles and senile plaques in the brains of clients with AD. These changes apparently occur as a part of the normal aging process. However, in clients with AD, they are found in dramatically increased numbers and their profusion is concentrated in the hippocampus and certain parts of the cerebral cortex.

Etiology. The exact cause of AD is unknown. Several hypotheses have been supported by varying amounts and quality of data. These hypotheses include:

1. **Acetylcholine Alterations**. Research has indicated that in the brains of Alzheimer's clients, the enzyme required to produce acetylcholine is dramatically reduced. The reduction seems to be greatest in the nucleus basalis of the inferior medial forebrain area (Cummings & Mega, 2003). This decrease in production of acetylcholine reduces the amount of the neurotransmitter that is released to cells in the cortex and hippocampus, resulting in a disruption of the cognitive processes. Other neurotransmitters implicated in the pathology and clinical symptoms of AD include norepinephrine, serotonin, dopamine, and the amino acid glutamate. It has been proposed that in dementia, excess glutamate leads to overstimulation of the N-methyl-D-aspartate (NMDA) receptors, leading to increased intracellular calcium, and subsequent neuronal degeneration and cell death.

2. **Plaques and Tangles.** As mentioned previously, an overabundance of structure called plaques and tangles appear in the brains of individuals with AD. The plaques are made of a protein called beta-amyloid, which are fragments of a larger protein called amyloid precursor protein (APP) (Alzheimer's Disease Education & Referral Center [ADEAR], 2005). Plaques are formed when these fragments clump together and mix with molecules and other cellular matter. Tangles are formed from a special kind of cellular protein called tau protein, whose function it is to provide stability to the neuron. In AD, the tau protein is chemically altered (ADEAR, 2005). Strands of the protein become tangled together, interfering with the neuronal transport system. It is not known whether the plaques and tangles cause AD or are a consequence of the AD process. It is thought that the plaques and tangles contribute to the destruction and death of neurons, leading to memory failure, personality changes, inability to carry out ADLs, and other features of the disease (ADEAR, 2005).

3. **Head Trauma.** The etiology of AD has been associated with serious head trauma (Munoz & Feldman, 2000). Studies have shown that some individuals who had experienced head trauma had subsequently (after years) developed AD. This hypothesis is being investigated as a possible cause. Munoz and Feldman (2000) report an increased risk for AD in individuals who are both genetically predisposed and who experience traumatic head injury.

plaques – protein called beta amyloid which are fragments of a larger protein Amyloid precursor protein

Tangles – formed from tau protein whose function is to provide stability to the neuron

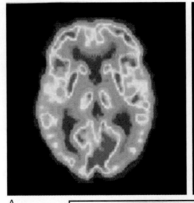
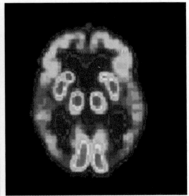
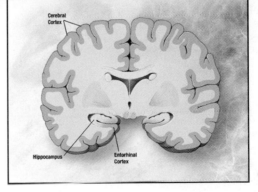

FIGURE 26–1 Changes in the Alzheimer's brain. *A.* PET scan showing metabolic activity in a normal brain. *B.* Diminished metabolic activity in the Alzheimer's diseased brain. *C.* Late stage Alzheimer's disease with generalized atrophy and enlargement of the ventricles and sulci. (SOURCE: Alzheimer's Disease Education & Referral Center, A Service of the National Institute on Aging. 2005. http://www.alzheimers.org/)

Brain Cross Sections

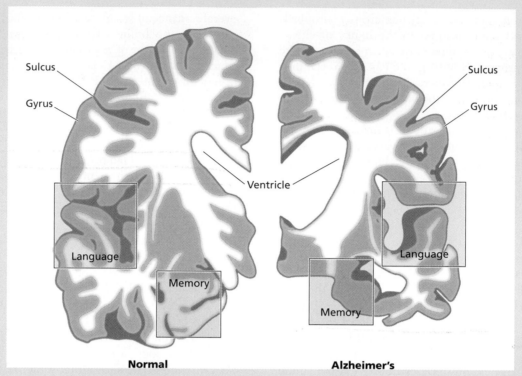

FIGURE 26–2 Neurobiology of Alzheimer's disease. (SOURCE: American Health Assistance Foundation, 2005, with permission. http://www.ahaf.org/alzdis/about/BrainAlzheimer.htm)

Neurotransmitters

A decrease in the neurotransmitter *acetylcholine* has been implicated in the etiology of Alzheimer's disease. Cholinergic sources arise from the brain stem and the basal forebrain to supply areas of the basal ganglia, thalamus, limbic structures, hippocampus, and cerebral cortex.

Cell bodies of origin for the *serotonin* pathways lie within the raphe nuclei located in the brain stem. Those for *norepinephrine* originate in the locus ceruleus. Projections for both neurotransmitters extend throughout the forebrain, prefrontal cortex, cerebellum, and limbic system. *Dopamine* pathways arise from areas in the midbrain and project to the frontal cortex, limbic system, basal ganglia, and thalamus. Dopamine neurons in the hypothalamus innervate the posterior pituitary.

Glutamate, an excitatory neurotransmitter, has largely descending pathways with highest concentrations in the cerebral cortex. It is also found in the hippocampus, thalamus, hypothalamus, cerebellum, and spinal cord.

Areas of the Brain Affected

Areas of the brain affected by Alzheimer's disease and associated symptoms include the following:

Frontal lobe:	Impaired reasoning ability. Unable to solve problems and perform familiar tasks. Poor judgment. Inability to evaluate the appropriateness of behavior. Aggressiveness.
Parietal lobe:	Impaired orientation ability. Impaired visuospatial skills (unable to remain oriented within own environment).
Occipital lobe:	Impaired language interpretation. Unable to recognize familiar objects.
Temporal lobe:	Inability to recall words. Inability to use words correctly (language comprehension). In late stages, some clients experience delusions, and hallucinations.
Hippocampus:	Impaired memory. Short-term memory is affected initially. Later, the individual is unable to form new memories.
Amygdala:	Impaired emotions: depression, anxiety, fear, personality changes, apathy, paranoia.
Neurotransmitters:	Alterations in acetylcholine, dopamine, norepinephrine, serotonin and others may play a role in behaviors such as restlessness, sleep impairment, mood, and agitation.

Medications and Their Effects on the Brain

1. Cholinesterase inhibitors (e.g., tacrine, donepezil, rivastigmine, and galantamine) act by inhibiting acetylcholinesterase, which slows the degradation of acetylcholine, thereby increasing concentrations of the neurotransmitter in the brain. Most common side effects include dizziness, GI upset, fatigue, and headache.

2. NMDA receptor antagonists (e.g., memantine) act by blocking NMDA receptors from excessive glutamate, preventing continuous influx of calcium into the cells, and ultimately slowing down neuronal degradation. Possible side effects include dizziness, headache, and constipation.

4. **Genetic Factors.** There is clearly a familial pattern with some forms of AD. Some families exhibit a pattern of inheritance that suggests possible autosomal-dominant gene transmission (Sadock & Sadock, 2003). Some studies indicate that early-onset cases are more likely to be familial than late-onset cases, and that from one third to one half of all cases may be of the genetic form. Some researchers believe that there is a link between AD and the alteration of a gene found on chromosome 21 (Munoz & Feldman, 2000; Saunders, 2001). People with Down syndrome, who carry an extra copy of chromosome 21, have been found to be unusually susceptible to AD (Lott & Head, 2005).

Some studies have linked the apolipoproteinE epsilon4 (*ApoE e4*) gene, found on chromosome 19, to an increased risk of late-onset AD (Poduslo & Yin, 2001). The presenilin 1 (*PS-1*) gene on chromosome 14 and the presenilin 2 (*PS-2*) gene on chromosome 1 have been associated with the onset of AD before age 65 years (Saunders, 2001).

Vascular Dementia *progression in "Steps"*

In this disorder, the clinical syndrome of dementia is due to significant cerebrovascular disease. The blood vessels of the brain are affected, and progressive intellectual deterioration occurs. Vascular dementia is the second most common form of dementia, ranking after AD (Black, 2005).

Vascular dementia differs from AD in that it has a more abrupt onset and runs a highly variable course. Progression of the symptoms occurs in "steps" rather than as a gradual deterioration; that is, at times the dementia seems to clear up and the individual exhibits fairly lucid thinking. Memory may seem better, and the client may become optimistic that improvement is occurring, only to experience further decline of functioning in a fluctuating pattern of progression. This irregular pattern of decline appears to be an intense source of anxiety for the client with this disorder.

In vascular dementia, clients suffer the equivalent of small strokes that destroy many areas of the brain. The pattern of deficits is variable, depending on which regions of the brain have been affected (APA, 2000). Certain focal neurological signs are commonly seen with vascular dementia, including weaknesses of the limbs, small-stepped gait, and difficulty with speech.

The disorder is more common in men than in women (APA, 2000). Arvanitakis (2000) states:

Prognosis for patients with vascular dementia is worse than that for Alzheimer's patients. The three-year mortality rate in cases over the age of 85 years old is quoted at 67 percent as compared to 42 percent in Alzheimer's disease, and 23 percent in non-demented individuals. However, outcome is ultimately dependent on the underlying risk factors and mechanism of disease, and further studies taking these distinctions into account are warranted.

The diagnosis can be subtyped when the dementia is superimposed with symptoms of delirium, delusions, or depressed mood.

Etiology. The cause of vascular dementia is directly related to an interruption of blood flow to the brain. Symptoms result from death of nerve cells in regions nourished by diseased vessels. Various diseases and conditions that interfere with blood circulation have been implicated.

High blood pressure is thought to be one of the most significant factors in the etiology of multiple small strokes or cerebral infarcts. Hypertension leads to damage to the lining of blood vessels. This can result in rupture of the blood vessel with subsequent hemorrhage or an accumulation of fibrin in the vessel with intravascular clotting and inhibited blood flow (DeMartinis, 2005). Dementia also can result from infarcts related to occlusion of blood vessels by particulate matter that travels through the bloodstream to the brain. These emboli may be solid (e.g., clots, cellular debris, platelet aggregates), gaseous (e.g., air, nitrogen), or liquid (e.g., fat, following soft tissue trauma or fracture of long bones).

Cognitive impairment can occur with multiple small infarcts (sometimes called "silent strokes") over time or with a single cerebrovascular insult that occurs in a strategic area of the brain. An individual may have both vascular dementia and AD simultaneously. This is referred to as *mixed dementia*, the prevalence of which is likely to increase as the population ages (Langa, Foster, & Larson, 2004).

Dementia Due to Human Immunodeficiency Virus

Infection with the human immunodeficiency virus-type 1 (HIV-1) produces a dementing illness called HIV-1–associated cognitive/motor complex. A less severe form, known as HIV-1–associated minor cognitive/motor disorder, also occurs. The severity of symptoms is correlated to the extent of brain pathology. The immune dysfunction associated with HIV disease can lead to brain infections by other organisms, and the HIV-1 also appears to cause dementia directly. In the early stages, neuropsychiatric symptoms may be manifested by barely perceptible changes in a person's normal psychological presentation. Severe cognitive changes, particularly confusion, changes in behavior, and sometimes psychoses, are not uncommon in the later stages.

With the advent of the highly active antiretroviral therapies (HAART), incidence rates of dementia associated with HIV disease have been on the decline.

However, it is possible that the prolonged life span of HIV-infected patients taking medications may actually increase the prevalence of this disorder in coming years (McArthur, 2004).

Dementia Due to Head Trauma

Serious head trauma can result in symptoms associated with the syndrome of dementia. Amnesia is the most common neurobehavioral symptoms following head trauma, and a degree of permanent disturbance may persist (Bourgeois, Seaman, & Servis, 2003). Repeated head trauma, such as the type experienced by boxers, can result in *dementia pugilistica*, a syndrome characterized by emotional lability, dysarthria, ataxia, and impulsivity (Sadock & Sadock, 2003).

Dementia Due to Parkinson's Disease

Dementia is observed in as many as 60 percent of clients with Parkinson's disease (Bourgeois, Seaman, & Servis, 2003). In this disease, there is a loss of nerve cells located in the substantia nigra, and dopamine activity is diminished, resulting in involuntary muscle movements, slowness, and rigidity. Tremor in the upper extremities is characteristic. In some instances, the cerebral changes that occur in dementia of Parkinson's disease closely resemble those of AD.

Dementia Due to Huntington's Disease

Huntington's disease is transmitted as a Mendelian dominant gene. Damage is seen in the areas of the basal ganglia and the cerebral cortex. The onset of symptoms (i.e., involuntary twitching of the limbs or facial muscles; mild cognitive changes; depression and apathy) is usually between age 30 and 50 years. The client usually declines into a profound state of dementia and **ataxia**. The average duration of the disease is based on age at onset. One study concluded that juvenile-onset and late-onset clients have the shortest duration (Foroud et al., 1999). In this study, the median duration of the disease was 21.4 years.

Dementia Due to Pick's Disease

The cause of Pick's disease is unknown, but a genetic factor appears to be involved. The clinical picture is strikingly similar to that of AD. One major difference is that the initial symptom in Pick's disease is usually personality change, whereas the initial symptom in AD is memory impairment. Studies reveal that pathology of Pick's disease results from atrophy in the frontal and temporal lobes of the brain, in contrast to AD, which is more widely distributed.

Dementia Due to Creutzfeldt–Jakob Disease

Creutzfeldt–Jakob disease is an uncommon neurodegenerative disease caused by a transmissible agent known as a "slow virus" or prion (APA, 2000). Five to 15 percent of cases have a genetic component. The clinical presentation is typical of the syndrome of dementia, along with involuntary movements, muscle rigidity, and ataxia. Symptoms may develop at any age in adults, but typically occur between ages 40 and 60 years. The clinical course is extremely rapid, with progressive deterioration and death within 1 year (Wise, Gray, & Seltzer, 1999).

Dementia Due to Other General Medical Conditions

A number of other general medical conditions can cause dementia. Some of these include endocrine conditions (e.g., hypoglycemia, hypothyroidism), pulmonary disease, hepatic or renal failure, cardiopulmonary insufficiency, fluid and electrolyte imbalances, nutritional deficiencies, frontal or temporal lobe lesions, central nervous system (CNS) or systemic infections, uncontrolled epilepsy, and other neurological conditions such as multiple sclerosis (APA, 2000).

Substance-Induced Persisting Dementia

The features associated with this type of dementia are those associated with dementias in general; however, evidence must exist from history, physical examination, or laboratory findings to show that the deficits are etiologically related to the persisting effects of substance use (APA, 2000). The term *persisting* is used to indicate that the dementia persists long after the effects of substance intoxication or substance withdrawal have subsided. The *DSM-IV-TR* identifies the following types of substances with which persisting dementia is associated:

1. Alcohol
2. Inhalants
3. Sedatives, hypnotics, and anxiolytics
4. Medications
   a. Anticonvulsants
   b. Intrathecal methotrexate
5. Toxins
   a. Lead
   b. Mercury
   c. Carbon monoxide
   d. Organophosphate insecticides
   e. Industrial solvents

TABLE 26–1	Etiological Factors Implicated in the Development of Delirium and/or Dementia	
BIOLOGICAL FACTORS		**EXOGENOUS FACTORS**
Hypoxia: any condition leading to a deficiency of oxygen to the brain		Birth trauma: prolonged labor, damage from use of forceps, other obstetric complications
Nutritional deficiencies: vitamins (particularly B and C); protein; fluid and electrolyte imbalances		Cranial trauma: concussion, contusions, hemorrhage, hematomas
Metabolic disturbances: porphyria; encephalopathies related to hepatic, renal, pancreatic, or pulmonary insufficiencies; hypoglycemia		Volatile inhalant compounds: gasoline, glue, paint, paint thinners, spray paints, cleaning fluids, typewriter correction fluid, varnishes, and lacquers
Endocrine dysfunction: thyroid, parathyroid, adrenal, pancreas, pituitary		Heavy metals: lead, mercury, manganese
Cardiovascular disease: stroke, cardiac insufficiency, atherosclerosis		Other metallic elements: aluminum
Primary brain disorders: epilepsy, Alzheimer's disease, Pick's disease, Huntington's disease, multiple sclerosis, Parkinson's disease		Organic phosphates: various insecticides
Infections: encephalitis, meningitis, pneumonia, septicemia, neurosyphilis (dementia paralytica), HIV disease, acute rheumatic fever, Creutzfeldt-Jakob disease		Substance abuse/dependence: alcohol, amphetamines, caffeine, cannabis, cocaine, hallucinogens, inhalants, nicotine, opioids, phencyclidine, sedatives, hypnotics, anxiolytics
Intracranial neoplasms		Other medications: anticholinergics, antihistamines, antidepressants, antipsychotics, antiparkinsonians, antihypertensives, steroids, digitalis
Congenital defects: prenatal infections, such as first-trimester maternal rubella		

The diagnosis is made according to the specific etiological substance involved. For example, if the substance known to cause the dementia is alcohol, the diagnosis is Alcohol-Induced Persisting Dementia. If the exact substance presumed to be causing the dementia were unknown, the diagnosis would be Unknown Substance-Induced Persisting Dementia.

Dementia Due to Multiple Etiologies

This diagnosis is used when the symptoms of dementia are attributed to more than one cause. For example, the dementia may be related to more than one medical condition or to the combined effects of a general medical condition and the long-term use of a substance (APA, 2000).

The etiological factors associated with delirium and dementia are summarized in Table 26–1.

Core Concept

Amnesia
The inability to retain or recall past experiences. The condition may be temporary or permanent, depending on etiology.

AMNESTIC DISORDERS

Amnestic disorders are characterized by an inability to learn new information (short-term memory deficit) despite normal attention, and an inability to recall previously learned information (long-term memory deficit). Events from the remote past often are recalled more easily than recently occurring ones. The

syndrome differs from dementia in that there is no impairment in abstract thinking or judgment, no other disturbances of higher cortical function, and no personality change.

Profound amnesia may result in disorientation to place and time, but rarely to self (APA, 2000). The individual may engage in confabulation—the creation of imaginary events to fill in memory gaps.

Some individuals will continue to deny that they have a problem despite evidence to the contrary. Others may acknowledge that a problem exists, but appear unconcerned. Apathy, lack of initiative, and emotional blandness are common. The person may appear friendly and agreeable, but the emotionality is superficial.

The onset of symptoms may be acute or insidious, depending on the pathological process causing the amnestic disorder. Duration and course of the illness may be quite variable and are also correlated with extent and severity of the cause.

Predisposing Factors

Amnestic disorders share a common symptom presentation of memory impairment but are differentiated in the *DSM-IV-TR* (APA, 2000) according to etiology:

1. Amnestic disorder due to a general medical condition
2. Substance-induced persisting amnestic disorder

Amnestic Disorder Due to a General Medical Condition

In this type of amnestic disorder, evidence must exist from the history, physical examination, or laboratory findings to show that the memory impairment is the direct physiological consequence of a general medical condition (APA, 2000). The diagnosis is specified further by indicating whether the symptoms are *transient* (present for no more than 1 month) or *chronic* (present for more than 1 month).

General medical conditions that may be associated with amnestic disorder include head trauma, cerebrovascular disease, cerebral neoplastic disease, cerebral anoxia, herpes simplex encephalitis, poorly controlled insulin-dependent diabetes, and surgical intervention to the brain (APA, 2000; Wise, Gray, & Seltzer, 1999).

Transient amnestic syndromes can occur from cerebrovascular disease, cardiac arrhythmias, migraine, thyroid disorders, and epilepsy (Bourgeois, Seaman, & Servis, 2003).

Substance-Induced Persisting Amnestic Disorder

In this disorder, evidence must exist from the history, physical examination, or laboratory findings that the memory impairment is related to the persisting effects of substance use (e.g., a drug of abuse, a medication, or toxin exposure) (APA, 2000). The term *persisting* is used to indicate that the symptoms exist long after the effects of substance intoxication or withdrawal have subsided. The *DSM-IV-TR* identifies the following substances with which amnestic disorder can be associated:

1. Alcohol
2. Sedatives, hypnotics, and anxiolytics
3. Medications
   a. Anticonvulsants
   b. Intrathecal methotrexate
4. Toxins
   a. Lead
   b. Mercury
   c. Carbon monoxide
   d. Organophosphate insecticides
   e. Industrial solvents

The diagnosis is made according to the specific etiological substance involved. For example, if the substance known to be the cause of the amnestic disorder is alcohol, the diagnosis would be Alcohol-Induced Persisting Amnestic Disorder.

APPLICATION OF THE NURSING PROCESS

Assessment

Nursing assessment of the client with delirium, dementia, or persisting amnesia is based on knowledge of the symptomatology associated with the various disorders described in the beginning of this chapter. Subjective and objective data are gathered by various members of the health care team. Clinicians report use of a variety of methods for obtaining assessment information.

The Client History

Nurses play a significant role in acquiring the client history, including the specific mental and physical changes that have occurred and the age at which the changes began. If the client is unable to relate information adequately, the data should be obtained from family members or others who would be aware of the client's physical and psychosocial history.

From the client history, nurses should assess the following areas of concern: (1) type, frequency, and severity of mood swings, personality and behavioral changes, and catastrophic emotional reactions; (2) cognitive changes, such as problems with attention span, thinking process, problem-solving, and memory (recent and remote); (3) language difficulties; (4) orientation to person, place, time, and situation; and (5) appropriateness of social behavior.

The nurse also should obtain information regarding current and past medication usage, history of other drug and alcohol use, and possible exposure to toxins. Knowledge regarding the history of related symptoms or specific illnesses (e.g., Huntington's disease, AD, Pick's disease, or Parkinson's disease) in other family members might be useful.

Physical Assessment

Assessment of physical systems by both the nurse and the physician has two main emphases: (1) signs of damage to the nervous system and (2) evidence of diseases of other organs that could affect mental function. Diseases of various organ systems can induce confusion, loss of memory, and behavioral changes. These causes must be considered in diagnosing cognitive disorders. In the neurological examination, the client is asked to perform maneuvers or answer questions that are designed to elicit information about the condition of specific parts of the brain or peripheral nerves. Testing will assess mental status and alertness, muscle strength, reflexes, sensory perception, language skills, and coordination. An example of a mental status examination for a client with dementia is presented in Table 26-2.

A battery of psychological tests may be ordered as part of the diagnostic examination. The results of these tests may be used to make a differential diagnosis between dementia and **pseudodementia** (depression). Depression is the most common mental illness in the elderly, but it is often misdiagnosed and treated inadequately. Cognitive symptoms of depression may mimic dementia, and because of the prevalence of dementia in the elderly, diag-

TABLE 26–2   Mental Status Examination for Dementia

Patient Name _____

Date _____

Age _____ **Sex** _____

Diagnosis _____

	Maximum	Client's Score
1. VERBAL FLUENCY		
Ask client to name as many animals as he/she can. (Time: 60 seconds) (Score 1 point/2 animals)	10 points	_____
2. COMPREHENSION		
a. Point to the ceiling	1 point	_____
b. Point to your nose and the window	1 point	_____
c. Point to your foot, the door, and ceiling	1 point	_____
d. Point to the window, your leg, the door, and your thumb	1 point	_____
3. NAMING AND WORD FINDING		
Ask the client to name the following as you point to them:		
a. Watch stem (winder)	1 point	_____
b. Teeth	1 point	_____
c. Sole of shoe	1 point	_____
d. Buckle of belt	1 point	_____
e. Knuckles	1 point	_____
4. ORIENTATION		
a. Date	2 points	_____
b. Day of week	2 points	_____
c. Month	1 point	_____
d. Year	1 point	_____

5. NEW LEARNING ABILITY

Tell the client: "I'm going to tell you four words, which I want you to remember." Have the client repeat the four words after they are initially presented, and then say that you will ask him/her to remember the words later. Continue with the examination, and at intervals of 5 and 10 minutes, ask the client to recall the words. Three different sets of words are provided here.

		5 min.	10 min.
a. Brown (Fun) (Grape)	2 points each:	_____	_____
b. Honesty (Loyalty) (Happiness)	2 points each:	_____	_____
c. Tulip (Carrot) (Stocking)	2 points each:	_____	_____
d. Eyedropper (Ankle) (Toothbrush)	2 points each:	_____	_____

6. VERBAL STORY FOR IMMEDIATE RECALL

Tell the client: "I'm going to read you a short story, which I want you to remember. Listen closely to what I read because I will ask you to tell me the story when I finish." Read the story slowly and carefully, but without pausing at the slash marks. After completing the paragraph, tell the client to retell the story as accurately as possible. Record the number of correct memories (information within the slashes) and describe confabulation if it is present. (1 point = 1 remembered item [13 maximum points])   **13 points   _____**

It was July / and the Rogers / had packed up / their four children / in the station wagon/ and were off / on vacation.
They were taking / their yearly trip / to the beach / at Gulf Shores.
This year / they were making / a special / 1-day stop / at The Aquarium / in New Orleans.
After a long day's drive / they arrived / at the motel / only to discover / that in their excitement / they had left / the twins / and their suitcases / in the front yard.

7. VISUAL MEMORY (HIDDEN OBJECTS)

Tell the client that you are going to hide some objects around the office (desk, bed) and that you want him/her to remember where they are. Hide four or five common objects (e.g., keys, pen, reflex hammer) in various places in the client's sight. After a delay of several minutes, ask the client to find the objects. (1 point per item found)

	Maximum	Client's Score
a. Coin	1 point	_____
b. Pen	1 point	_____
c. Comb	1 point	_____
d. Keys	1 point	_____
e. Fork	1 point	_____

(Continued on following page)

TABLE 26-2 **Mental Status Examination for Dementia** *(Continued)*

8. PAIRED ASSOCIATE LEARNING

Tell the client that you are going to read a list of words two at a time. The client will be expected to remember the words that go together (e.g., big—little). When he/she is clear on the directions, read the first list of words at the rate of one pair per second. After reading the first list, test for recall by presenting the first recall list. Give the first word of a pair and ask for the word that was paired with it. Correct incorrect responses and proceed to the next pair. After the first recall has been completed, allow a 10-second delay and continue with the second presentation and recall lists.

Presentation Lists

1	2
a. High—Low	a. Good—Bad
b. House—Income	b. Book—Page
c. Good—Bad	c. High—Low
d. Book—Page	d. House—Income

Recall Lists

1	2		
a. House _____	a. High _____	2 points	_____
b. Book _____	b. Good _____	2 points	_____
c. High _____	c. House _____	2 points	_____
d. Good _____	d. Book _____	2 points	_____

9. CONSTRUCTIONAL ABILITY

Ask client to reconstruct this drawing and to draw the other 2 items: 3 points   _____

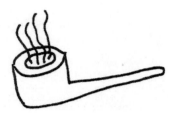

Draw a daisy in a flowerpot   3 points   _____

Draw a clock with all the numbers and set the clock at 2:30.   3 points   _____

10. WRITTEN COMPLEX CALCULATIONS

a. Addition	108 +79	1 point	_____
b. Subtraction	605 −86	1 point	_____
c. Multiplication	108 × 36	1 point	_____
d. Division	559÷43	1 point	_____

(Continued on opposite page)

11. PROVERB INTERPRETATION
Tell the client to explain the following sayings. Record the answers.

a. Don't cry over spilled milk.　　　　　　　　　　　　　　　　　　　　　　　　　2 points　　　_____

_____

b. Rome wasn't built in a day.　　　　　　　　　　　　　　　　　　　　　　　　　2 points　　　_____

_____

c. A drowning man will clutch at a straw.　　　　　　　　　　　　　　　　　　　2 points　　　_____

_____

d. A golden hammer can break down an iron door.　　　　　　　　　　　　　　2 points　　　_____

_____

e. The hot coal burns, the cold one blackens.　　　　　　　　　　　　　　　　　2 points　　　_____

_____

12. SIMILARITIES

a. Turnip _____ Cauliflower	2 points	_____
b. Car _____ Airplane	2 points	_____
c. Desk _____ Bookcase	2 points	_____
d. Poem _____ Novel	2 points	_____
e. Horse _____ Apple	2 points	_____

Maximum: 100 points　　　_____

Normal Individuals		Clients with Alzheimer's Disease	
Age Group	**Mean Score (standard deviation)**	**Stage**	**Mean Score (standard deviation)**
40–49	80.9 (9.7)	I	57.2 (9.1)
50–59	82.3 (8.6)	II	37.0 (7.8)
60–69	75.5 (10.5)	III	13.4 (8.1)
70–79	66.9 (9.1)		
80–89	67.9 (11.0)		

SOURCE: Adapted from Strub, R.L. & Black, F. W. (2000). *The Mental Status Examination in Neurology*, 4th ed., Philadelphia: F.A. Davis. With permission.

nosticians are often too eager to make this diagnosis. A comparison of symptoms of dementia and pseudodementia (depression) is presented in Table 26–3. Nurses can assist in this assessment by carefully observing and documenting these sometimes subtle differences.

Diagnostic Laboratory Evaluations

The nurse also may be required to help the client fulfill the physician's orders for special diagnostic laboratory evaluations. Many of these tests are routinely included with the physical examination and may include evaluation of blood and urine samples to test for various infections; hepatic and renal dysfunction; diabetes or hypoglycemia; electrolyte imbalances; metabolic and endocrine disorders; nutritional deficiencies; and presence of toxic substances, including alcohol and other drugs.

Other diagnostic evaluations may be made by electroencephalogram (EEG), which measures and records the brain's electrical activity. With CT scan, an image of the size and shape of the brain can be obtained. A technology called *positron emission tomography* (PET) reveals the metabolic activity of the brain, an evaluation some researchers believe will be important in the diagnosis of

TABLE 26–3	A Comparison of Dementia and Pseudodementia (Depression)	
SYMPTOM ELEMENT	**DEMENTIA**	**PSEUDODEMENTIA (DEPRESSION)**
Progression of symptoms	Slow	Rapid
Memory	Progressive deficits; recent memory loss greater than remote; may confabulate for memory "gaps"; no complaints of loss	More like forgetfulness; no evidence of progressive deficit; recent and remote loss equal; complaints of deficits; no confabulation (will more likely answer "I don't know")
Orientation	Disoriented to time and place; may wander in search of the familiar	Oriented to time and place; no wandering
Task performance	Consistently poor performance, but struggles to perform	Performance is variable; little effort is put forth
Symptom severity	Worse as the day progresses	Better as the day progresses
Affective distress	Appears unconcerned	Communicates severe distress
Appetite	Unchanged	Diminished
Attention and concentration	Impaired	Intact

AD. Magnetic resonance imaging (MRI) is used to obtain a computerized image of soft tissue in the body. It provides a sharp detailed picture of the tissues of the brain. A lumbar puncture may be performed to examine the cerebrospinal fluid for evidence of CNS infection or hemorrhage.

Diagnosis/Outcome Identification

Using information collected during the assessment, the nurse completes the client database, from which the selection of appropriate nursing diagnoses is determined. Possible nursing diagnoses for clients with cognitive disorders include:

Risk for trauma related to impairments in cognitive and psychomotor functioning.

Risk for suicide related to depressed mood secondary to awareness in decline of mental and/or physical capability.

Risk for other-directed violence related to impairment of impulse control; hallucinations.

Disturbed thought processes related to cerebral degeneration evidenced by disorientation, confusion, memory deficits, and inaccurate interpretation of the environment.

Low self-esteem related to loss of independent functioning evidenced by expressions of shame and self-degradation and progressive social isolation.

Self-care deficit related to disorientation, confusion, memory deficits evidenced by inability to fulfill ADLs.

The following criteria may be used for measurement of outcomes in the care of the client with cognitive disorders.

The client:

1. Has not experienced physical injury.
2. Has not harmed self or others.
3. Has maintained reality orientation to the best of his or her capability.
4. Discusses positive aspects about self and life.
5. Fulfills activities of daily living with assistance.

Planning/Implementation

Table 26–4 provides a plan of care for the client with a cognitive disorder (irrespective of etiology). Selected nursing diagnoses are presented, along with outcome criteria, appropriate nursing interventions, and rationales for each.

TABLE 26–4	Care Plan for the Client with a Cognitive Disorder

NURSING DIAGNOSIS: RISK FOR TRAUMA
RELATED TO: Impairments in cognitive and psychomotor functioning

OUTCOME CRITERIA	NURSING INTERVENTIONS	RATIONALE
Client will not experience injury.	The following measures may be instituted: a. Arrange furniture and other items in the room to accommodate client's disabilities. b. Store frequently used items within easy access. c. Do not keep bed in an elevated position. Pad siderails and headboard if client has history of seizures. Keep bedrails up when client is in bed (if regulations permit). d. Assign room near nurses' station; observe frequently. e. Assist client with ambulation. f. Keep a dim light on at night. g. If client is a smoker, cigarettes and lighter or matches should be kept at the nurses' station and dispensed only when someone is available to stay with client while he or she is smoking. h. Frequently orient client to place, time, and situation. i. If client is prone to wander, provide an area within which wandering can be carried out safely. j. Soft restraints may be required if client is very disoriented and hyperactive.	To ensure client safety.

(Continued on opposite page)

NURSING DIAGNOSIS: DISTURBED THOUGHT PROCESSES
RELATED TO: Cerebral degeneration
EVIDENCED BY: Disorientation, confusion, memory deficits, and inaccurate interpretation of the environment

OUTCOME CRITERIA	NURSING INTERVENTIONS	RATIONALE
Client will interpret the environment accurately and maintain reality orientation to the best of his or her cognitive ability.	1. Frequently orient client to reality. Use clocks and calendars with large numbers that are easy to read. Notes and large, bold signs may be useful as reminders. Allow client to have personal belongings. 2. Keep explanations simple. Use face-to-face interaction. Speak slowly and do not shout. 3. Discourage rumination of delusional thinking. Talk about real events and real people. 4. Monitor for medication side effects.	1. All of these items serve to help maintain orientation and aid in memory and recognition. 2. These interventions facilitate comprehension. Shouting may create discomfort, and in some instances, may provoke anger. 3. Rumination promotes disorientation. Reality orientation increases sense of self-worth and personal dignity. 4. Physiological changes in the elderly can alter the body's response to certain medications. Toxic effects may intensify altered thought processes.

NURSING DIAGNOSIS: SELF-CARE DEFICIT
RELATED TO: Disorientation, confusion, and memory deficits
EVIDENCED BY: Inability to fulfill ADLs

OUTCOME CRITERIA	NURSING INTERVENTIONS	RATIONALE
Client will accomplish ADLs to the best of his or her ability. Unfullfilled needs will be met by caregivers.	1. Provide a simple, structured environment: a. Identify self-care deficits and provide assistance as required. Promote independent actions as able. b. Allow plenty of time for client to perform tasks. c. Provide guidance and support for independent actions by talking the client through the task one step at a time. d. Provide a structured schedule of activities that does not change from day to day. e. ADLs should follow usual routine as closely as possible. f. Provide for consistency in assignment of daily caregivers. 2. Perform ongoing assessment of client's ability to fulfill nutritional needs, ensure personal safety, follow medication regimen, and communicate need for assistance with activities that he or she cannot accomplish independently. 3. Assess prospective caregivers' ability to anticipate and fulfill client's unmet needs. Provide information to assist caregivers with this responsibility. Ensure that caregivers are aware of available community support systems from which they may seek assistance when required. Examples include adult day care centers, housekeeping and homemaker services, respite care services, or the local chapter of a national support organization: a. For Parkinson's disease information: National Parkinson Foundation Inc. 1501 NW 9th Ave. Miami, FL 33136–1494 1-800-327-4545 b. For Alzheimer's disease information: Alzheimer's Association 225 N. Michigan Ave., Fl. 17 Chicago, IL 60601-7633 1-800-272-3900	1. To minimize confusion. 2. Client safety and security are nursing priorities. 3. To ensure provision and continuity of client care.

TABLE 26–5   Topics for Client/Family Education Related to Cognitive Disorders

1. Nature of the illness
   a. Possible causes
   b. What to expect
   c. Symptoms
2. Management of the illness
   a. Ways to ensure client safety
   b. How to maintain reality orientation
   c. Providing assistance with ADLs
   d. Nutritional information
   e. Difficult behaviors
   f. Medication administration
   g. Matters related to hygiene and toileting
3. Support services
   a. Financial assistance
   b. Legal assistance
   c. Caregiver support groups
   d. Respite care
   e. Home health care

Client/Family Education

The role of client teacher is important in the psychiatric area, as it is in all areas of nursing. A list of topics for client/family education relevant to cognitive disorders is presented in Table 26–5.

Evaluation

In the final step of the nursing process, reassessment occurs to determine if the nursing interventions have been effective in achieving the intended goals of care. Evaluation of the client with cognitive disorders is based on a series of short-term goals rather than on long-term goals. Resolution of identified problems is unrealistic for this client. Instead, outcomes must be measured in terms of slowing down the process rather than stopping or curing the problem. Evaluation questions may include the following:

1. Has the client experienced injury?
2. Does the client maintain orientation to time, person, place, and situation most of the time?
3. Is the client able to fulfill basic needs? Have those needs unmet by the client been fulfilled by caregivers?
4. Is confusion minimized by familiar objects and structured, routine schedule of activities?
5. Do the prospective caregivers have information regarding the progression of the client's illness?
6. Do caregivers have information regarding where to go for assistance and support in the care of their loved one?
7. Have the prospective caregivers received instruction in how to promote the client's safety, minimize confusion and disorientation, and cope with difficult client behaviors (e.g., hostility, anger, depression, agitation)?

MEDICAL TREATMENT MODALITIES

Delirium

The first step in the treatment of delirium should be the determination and correction of the underlying causes. Additional attention must be given to fluid and electrolyte status, hypoxia, anoxia, and diabetic problems. Staff members should remain with the client at all times to monitor behavior and provide reorientation and assurance. The room should maintain a low level of stimuli.

Some physicians prefer not to prescribe medications for the delirious client, reasoning that additional agents may only compound the syndrome of brain dysfunction. However, the agitation and aggression demonstrated by the delirious client may require chemical and/or mechanical restraint. Choice of specific therapy is made with consideration for the client's clinical condition and the underlying cause of the delirium. Low-dose neuroleptics are the pharmacological treatment of choice in most cases (Trzepacz et al., 2002). A benzodiazepine (e.g., lorazepam) is commonly used when the etiology is substance withdrawal (Eisendrath & Lichtmacher, 2005).

Dementia

Once a definitive diagnosis of dementia has been made, a primary consideration in the treatment of the disorder is the etiology. Focus must be directed to the identification and resolution of potentially reversible processes. Sadock and Sadock (2003) state:

> Once dementia is diagnosed, patients must undergo a complete medical and neurological workup, because 10 to 15 percent of all patients with dementia have a potentially reversible condition if treatment is initiated before permanent brain damage occurs. [Causes of potentially-reversible dementia include] hypothyroidism, normal pressure hydrocephalus, and brain tumors. (p. 339–340)

The need for general supportive care, with provisions for security, stimulation, patience, and nutrition, has been recognized and accepted. A number of pharmaceutical agents have been tried, with varying degrees of success, in the treatment of clients with dementia. Some of these drugs are described in the following section according to symptomatology for which they are indicated. (See Chapter 21 for side effects and nursing implications of the psychotropics.) A summary of medications for clients with dementia is provided in Table 26–6.

Cognitive Impairment

Antilirium physostigmine

The angiotensin-converting enzyme inhibitor physostigmine (Antilirium) has been shown to enhance cognitive functioning in individuals with mild-to-moderate AD (van Dyck et al., 2000).

TABLE 26–6	Selected Medications Used in the Treatment of Clients with Dementia			
MEDICATION	**CLASSIFICATION**	**FOR TREATMENT OF**	**DAILY DOSAGE RANGE**	**SIDE EFFECTS**
Tacrine (Cognex)	Cholinesterase inhibitor	Cognitive impairment	40–160 mg	Dizziness, headache, GI upset, elevated transaminase
Donepezil (Aricept)	Cholinesterase inhibitor	Cognitive impairment	5–10 mg	Insomnia, dizziness, GI upset, headache
Rivastigmine (Exelon)	Cholinesterase inhibitor	Cognitive impairment	6–12 mg	Dizziness, headache, GI upset, fatigue
Galantamine (Reminyl)	Cholinesterase inhibitor	Cognitive impairment	8–24 mg	Dizziness, headache, GI upset
Memantine (Namenda)	NMDA receptor antagonist	Cognitive impairment	5–20 mg	Dizziness, headache, constipation
Risperidone (Risperdal)	Antipsychotic	Agitation, aggression, hallucinations, thought disturbances, wandering	1–4 mg (Increase dosage cautiously)	Agitation, insomnia, headache, extrapyramidal symptoms
Olanzapine (Zyprexa)	Antipsychotic	Agitation, aggression, hallucinations, thought disturbances, wandering	5 mg (Increase dosage cautiously)	Hypotension, dizziness, sedation, constipation, weight gain
Quetiapine (Seroquel)	Antipsychotic	Agitation, aggression, hallucinations, thought disturbances, wandering	Initial dose 25 mg. Titrate slowly.	Hypotension, tachycardia, dizziness, drowsiness, headache
Haloperidol (Haldol)	Antipsychotic	Agitation, aggression, hallucinations, thought disturbances, wandering	1–4 mg (Increase dosage cautiously)	Dry mouth, blurred vision, orthostatic hypotension, extrapyramidal symptoms, sedation
Sertraline (Zoloft)	Antidepressant (SSRI)	Depression	50–100 mg	Fatigue, insomnia, sedation, GI upset, headache
Paroxetine (Paxil)	Antidepressant (SSRI)	Depression	10–40 mg	Dizziness, headache, insomnia, somnolence, GI upset
Nortriptyline (Pamelor)	Antidepressant (tricyclic)	Depression	30–50 mg	Anticholinergic, orthostatic hypotension, sedation, arrhythmia
Lorazepam (Ativan)	Antianxiety (benzodiazepine)	Anxiety	1–2 mg	Drowsiness, dizziness, GI upset, hypotension, tolerance, dependence
Oxazepam (Serax)	Antianxiety (benzodiazepine)	Anxiety	10–30 mg	Drowsiness, dizziness, GI upset, hypotension, tolerance, dependence
Temazepam (Restoril)	Sedative/hypnotic (benzodiazepine)	Insomnia	15 mg	Drowsiness, dizziness, GI upset, hypotension, tolerance, dependence
Zolpidem (Ambien)	Sedative/hypnotic (non-benzodiazepine)	Insomnia	5 mg	Headache, drowsiness, dizziness, GI upset
Zaleplon (Sonata)	Sedative/hypnotic (non-benzodiazepine)	Insomnia	5 mg	Headache, drowsiness, dizziness, GI upset
Trazodone (Desyrel)	Antidepressant (heterocyclic)	Depression and insomnia	50 mg	Dizziness, drowsiness, fatigue, dry mouth
Mirtazapine (Remeron)	Antidepressant (tetracyclic)	Depression and insomnia	7.5–15 mg	Somnolence, dry mouth, constipation, increased appetite

acetylcholine is (inactivated) by the enzyme acetylcholinesterase

Another classification of medications—cholinesterase inhibitors—is being used for treatment of mild to moderate cognitive impairment in AD. Some of the clinical manifestations of AD are thought to be the result of a deficiency of the neurotransmitter acetylcholine. In the brain, acetylcholine is inactivated by the enzyme acetylcholinesterase. Tacrine (Cognex), donepezil (Aricept), rivastigmine (Exelon), and galantamine (Reminyl) act by inhibiting acetylcholinesterase, which slows the degradation of acetylcholine, thereby increasing concentrations of the neurotransmitter in the cerebral cortex. Because their action relies on functionally intact cholinergic neurons, the effects of these medications may lessen as the disease process advances, and there is no evidence that these medications alter the course of the underlying dementing process.

Another medication, an *N*-methyl-D-aspartate (NMDA) receptor antagonist, was approved by the U.S. Food and Drug Administration (FDA) in 2003. The medication, memantine (Namenda), was approved for the treatment of moderate to severe AD. High levels of glutamate in the brains of Alzheimer's patients are thought to contribute to the symptomatology and decline in functionality. These high levels are caused by a dysfunction in glutamate transmission. In normal neurotransmission, glutamate plays an essential role in learning and memory by triggering NMDA receptors to allow a controlled amount of calcium to flow into a nerve cell (Alzheimer's Association, 2004). This creates the appropriate environment for information processing. In AD, there is a sustained release of glutamate, which results in a continuous influx of calcium into the nerve cells. This increased intracellular calcium concentration ultimately leads to disruption and death of the neurons. Memantine may protect cells against excess glutamate by partially blocking NMDA receptors. Memantine has shown in clinical trials to be effective in improving cognitive function and the ability to perform ADLs in clients with moderate to severe AD. Although it does not stop or reverse the effects of the disease, it has been shown to slow down the progression of the decline in functionality (Reisberg et al., 2003). Because the action of Memantine differs from that of the cholinesterase inhibitors, consideration is being given to possible co-administration of these medications. In one study, results showed statistically significant improvement in cognitive function, ADLs, behavior, and clinical global status in clients who took a combination of memantine and donepezil when compared to subjects who took a combination of donepezil and placebo (Tariot et al., 2004).

Agitation, Aggression, Hallucinations, Thought Disturbances, and Wandering

Antipsychotic medications are used to control agitation, aggression, hallucinations, thought disturbances, and wandering in clients with dementia. The newer antipsychotic medications—risperidone (Risperdal), olanzapine (Zyprexa), quetiapine (Seroquel), and ziprasidone (Geodon)—may be favored because of their lessened propensity to cause anticholinergic and extrapyramidal side effects, although additional research is still needed with geriatric clients and clients with dementia (Rabins et al., 2002). Haloperidol (Haldol) is still commonly used because of its proven efficacy in the behaviors associated with dementia, although it carries a higher potentiality of anticholinergic, extrapyramidal, and sedative side effects. The usual adult dosage of any medication must be decreased in the elderly.

Anticholinergic Effects. Many antipsychotic, antidepressant, and antihistaminic medications produce anticholinergic side effects, which include confusion, blurred

vision, constipation, dry mouth, dizziness, and difficulty urinating. Older people, and especially those with dementia, are particularly sensitive to these effects. Beers and Jones (2004) explain this phenomenon as follows:

> Older people are more likely to experience anticholinergic effects because as people age, the body produces less acetylcholine. Also, cells in many parts of the body (such as the digestive tract) have fewer sites where acetylcholine can attach to them. Thus, the acetylcholine produced is less likely to have an effect, and the effect of anticholinergic drugs is greater. (p. 48)

Depression [TCA - AVOIDED 2° Cardiac & anticholinergic Rxns]

Approximately 25 percent of people with AD also suffer from major depression (Lyketsos, 2003). Recognizing the symptoms of depression in these individuals is often a challenge. Depression—which affects thinking, memory, sleep, appetite, and interferes with daily life—is sometimes difficult to distinguish from dementia. Clearly, the existence of depression in the client with dementia complicates and worsens the individual's functioning.

Antidepressant medication is sometimes used in treatment of depression in dementia. The selective serotonin reuptake inhibitors (SSRIs) are considered by many to be the first line drug treatment for depression in the elderly because of their favorable side effect profile (Cummings et al., 2002). Although still used by some physicians, tricyclic antidepressants are often avoided because of cardiac and anticholinergic side effects. Trazodone may be a good choice, used at bedtime, for depression and insomnia. Dopaminergic agents (e.g., methylphenidate, amantadine, bromocriptine, and bupropion) may be helpful in the treatment of severe apathy (Rabins et al., 2002).

Anxiety

The progressive loss of mental functioning is a significant source of anxiety in the early stages of dementia. It is important that clients be encouraged to verbalize their feelings and fears associated with this loss. These interventions may be useful in reducing the anxiety of clients with dementia.

Antianxiety medications may be helpful but should not be used routinely or for prolonged periods. The least toxic and most effective of the antianxiety medications are the benzodiazepines. Examples include diazepam (Valium), chlordiazepoxide (Librium), alprazolam (Xanax), lorazepam (Ativan), and oxazepam (Serax). The drugs with shorter half-lives (e.g., lorazepam and oxazepam) are preferred to those longer-acting medications (e.g., diazepam), which promote a higher risk of oversedation and falls. Barbiturates are not appropriate as antianxiety agents because they frequently induce confusion and paradoxical excitement in elderly individuals.

Sleep Disturbances

Sleep problems are common in clients with dementia and often intensify as the disease progresses. Wakefulness and nighttime wandering create much distress and anguish in family members who are charged with protection of their loved one. Indeed, sleep disturbances are among the problems that most frequently initiate the need for placement of the client in a long-term care facility.

Some physicians treat sleep problems with sedative-hypnotic medications. The benzodiazepines may be useful for some clients but are indicated for relatively brief periods only. Examples include flurazepam (Dalmane), temazepam (Restoril), and triazolam (Halcion). Daytime sedation and cognitive impairment, in addition to paradoxical agitation in elderly clients, are of particular concern with these medications (Beers & Jones, 2004). The nonbenzodiazepine sedative-hypnotics zolpidem (Ambien) and zaleplon (Sonata) and the antidepressant trazodone (Desyrel) are also prescribed. Daytime sedation may also be a problem with these medications. As previously stated, barbiturates should not be used in elderly clients. Sleep problems are usually ongoing, and most clinicians prefer to use medications only to help an individual through a short-term stressful situation. Rising at the same time each morning; minimizing daytime sleep; participating in regular physical exercise (but no later than four hours before bedtime); getting proper nutrition; avoiding alcohol, caffeine, and nicotine; and retiring at the same time each night are behavioral approaches to sleep problems that may eliminate the need for sleep aids, particularly in the early stages of dementia. Because of the tremendous potential for adverse drug reactions in the elderly, many of whom are already taking multiple medications, pharmacological treatment of insomnia should be considered only after attempts at nonpharmacological strategies have failed.

SUMMARY

This chapter examined a group of disorders that constitute a large and growing public health concern. Cognitive disorders include delirium, dementia, and amnestic disorders.

A delirium is a disturbance of consciousness and a change in cognition that develop rapidly over a short period. Level of consciousness is often affected and psychomotor activity may fluctuate between agitated purposeless movements and a vegetative state resembling catatonic stupor. The symptoms of delirium usually begin quite abruptly and often are reversible and brief. Delirium may be caused by a general medical condition, substance intoxication or withdrawal, or ingestion of a medication or toxin.

Dementia is a syndrome of acquired, persistent intellectual impairment with compromised function in multiple spheres of mental activity, such as memory, language, visuospatial skills, emotion or personality, and cognition. Symptoms are insidious and develop slowly over time. In most clients, dementia runs a progressive, irreversible course. It may be caused by genetics, cardiovascular disease, infections, neurophysiological disorders, and other general medical conditions.

Amnestic disorders are characterized by an inability to learn new information despite normal attention and an inability to recall previously learned information. Remote past events are often more easily recalled than recent ones. The onset of symptoms may be acute or insidious, depending on the pathological process causing the amnestic disorder. Duration and course of the illness may be quite variable and are also correlated with extent and severity of the cause.

Nursing care of the client with a cognitive disorder is presented around the six steps of the nursing process. Objectives of care for the client experiencing an acute syndrome are aimed at eliminating the etiology, promoting client safety, and a return to highest possible functioning. Objectives of care for the client experiencing a chronic, progressive disorder are aimed at preserving the dignity of the individual, promoting deceleration of the symptoms, and maximizing functional capabilities.

Nursing interventions are also directed toward helping the client's family or primary caregivers learn about a chronic, progressive cognitive disorder. Education is provided about the disease process, expectations of client behavioral changes, methods for facilitating care, and sources of assistance and support as they struggle, both physically and emotionally, with the demands brought on by a disease process that is slowly taking their loved one away from them.

REVIEW QUESTIONS

SELF-EXAMINATION/LEARNING EXERCISE

Mrs. G. is 67 years old. Her husband brings her to the hospital. He explains that she has become increasingly confused and forgetful. Yesterday, she started a fire in the kitchen when she put some bacon on to fry and went off and forgot it on the stove. Her husband reports that sometimes she seems okay, and sometimes she is completely disoriented. The physician has made an admitting diagnosis of dementia, etiology unknown.

Select the answer that is most appropriate for each of the following questions.

1. Because the etiology of Mrs. G.'s symptoms is unknown, the physician will attempt to rule out the possibility that a reversible condition exists. An example of a treatable (reversible) form of dementia is one that is caused by:
   a. Multiple sclerosis
   b. Multiple small brain infarcts
   c. Electrolyte imbalances
   d. HIV disease

2. The physician rules out all reversible etiological factors and diagnoses Mrs. G. with Dementia of the Alzheimer's Type. The cause of this disorder is:
   a. Multiple small brain infarcts
   b. Chronic alcohol abuse
   c. Cerebral abscess
   d. Unknown

3. The *primary* nursing intervention in working with Mrs. G. would be:
   a. Ensuring that she receives food she likes, to prevent hunger.
   b. Ensuring that the environment is safe, to prevent injury.
   c. Ensuring that she meets the other patients, to prevent social isolation.
   d. Ensuring that she takes care of her own ADLs, to prevent dependence.

4. Some medications have been indicated to decrease the agitation, violence, and bizarre thoughts associated with dementia. A drug suggested for this use is:
   a. Risperidone (Risperdal)
   b. Tacrine (Cognex)
   c. Ergoloid (Hydergine)
   d. Diazepam (Valium)

5. Mrs. G. says to the nurse, "I have a date tonight. I always have a date on Christmas." The most appropriate response is:
   a. "Don't be silly. It's not Christmas, Mrs. G."
   b. "Today is Tuesday, Oct. 21, Mrs. G. We will have supper soon, and then your daughter will come to visit."
   c. "Who is your date with, Mrs. G.?"
   d. "I think you need some more medication, Mrs. G. I'll bring it to you now."

6. In addition to disturbances in her cognition and orientation, Mrs. G. may also show changes in her
   a. Hearing, speech, and vision.
   b. Energy, creativity, and coordination.
   c. Personality, speech, and mobility.
   d. Appetite, affect, and attitude.

7. Mrs. G. has trouble sleeping and wanders around at night. Which of the following nursing actions would be *best* to promote sleep in Mrs. G.?
   a. Ask the doctor to prescribe flurazepam (Dalmane).
   b. Ensure that Mrs. G. gets an afternoon nap so she will not be overtired at bedtime.

c. Make Mrs. G. a cup of tea with honey before bedtime.
d. Ensure that Mrs. G. gets regular physical exercise during the day.

8. Mrs. G.'s daughter says to the nurse, "I read an article about Alzheimer's and it said the disease is hereditary. Does that mean I'll get it when I'm old?" The nurse bases her response on the knowledge that which of the following factors is *not* associated with increased incidence of dementia of the Alzheimer's type?
   a. Multiple small strokes
   b. Family history of Alzheimer's disease
   c. Head trauma
   d. Advanced age

9. The physician determines that Mrs. G.'s dementia is related to cardiovascular disease and changes her diagnosis to vascular dementia. In explaining this disorder to Mrs. G.'s family, which of the following statements by the nurse is correct?
   a. "She will probably live longer than if her dementia was of the Alzheimer's type."
   b. "Vascular dementia shows step-wise progression. This is why she sometimes seems okay."
   c. "Vascular dementia is caused by plaques and tangles that form in the brain."
   d. "The cause of vascular dementia is unknown."

10. Which of the following interventions is most appropriate in helping Mrs. G with her ADLs?
    a. Perform ADLs for her while she is in the hospital.
    b. Provide her with a written list of activities she is expected to perform.
    c. Tell her that if her morning care is not completed by 9:00 A.M. it will be performed for her by the nurse's aide so that Mrs. G. can attend group therapy.
    d. Encourage her and give her plenty of time to perform as many of her ADLs as possible independently.

TEST YOUR CRITICAL THINKING SKILLS

Joe, a 62-year-old accountant, began having difficulty remembering details necessary to perform his job. He was also having trouble at home, failing to keep his finances straight, and forgetting to pay bills. It became increasingly difficult for him to function properly at work, and eventually he was forced to retire. Cognitive deterioration continued, and behavioral problems soon began. He became stubborn, verbally and physically abusive, and suspicious of most everyone in his environment. His wife and son convinced him to see a physician, who recommended hospitalization for testing.

At Joe's initial evaluation, he was fully alert and cooperative but obviously anxious and fidgety. He thought he was at his accounting office and he could not state what year it was. He could not say the names of his parents or siblings, nor did he know who was currently the president of the United States. He could not perform simple arithmetic calculations, write a proper sentence, or copy a drawing. He interpreted proverbs concretely and had difficulty stating similarities between related objects.

Laboratory serum studies revealed no abnormalities, but a CT scan showed marked cortical atrophy. The physician's diagnosis was Dementia of the Alzheimer's Type, Early Onset.

Answer the following questions related to Joe:

1. Identify the pertinent assessment data from which nursing care will be devised.
2. What is the primary nursing diagnosis for Joe?
3. How would outcomes be identified?

IMPLICATIONS OF RESEARCH FOR EVIDENCE-BASED PRACTICE

Yaffe, K., Barnes, D., Nevitt, M., Lui, L., & Covinsky, K. (2001). A prospective study of physical activity and cognitive decline in elderly women: Women who walk. *Archives of Internal Medicine, 161*(14), 1703–1708.

Description of the Study: Subjects included 5,925 predominantly white women, aged 65 and older, and who had completed a mean 13 years of education. They were all without baseline cognitive impairment or physical limitations. Cognitive performance was measured using a modified Mini-Mental State Examination at baseline and 6 to 8 years later. Physical activity was measured by self-reported blocks walked per week and by total kilocalories expended per week in recreation, blocks walked, and stairs climbed. Cognitive decline was defined as a 3-point decline or greater on repeated modified Mini-Mental State Examination.

Results of the Study: Participants were divided into quartiles according to physical activity (median number of blocks walked per week ranged from 7 to 175 per quartile). At follow-up, and after adjustment for age, education level, comorbid conditions, smoking status, estrogen use, and functional limitations, cognitive function had declined significantly less among women in the highest physical activity quartile compared with those in the lowest quartile. For every 1700 kcal/week expended on physical activity, there was a 14 percent decrease in the odds for cognitive decline.

Implications for Nursing Practice: Several studies have suggested that physical activity is positively associated with cognitive function in elderly persons. This study supports this hypothesis. These findings suggest the importance of exercise programs aimed at elderly persons. Nurses must educate their elderly clients about the importance of remaining active. Nurses may also participate in the planning and development of exercise, recreational, and leisure-time activities for the elderly.

REFERENCES

Alzheimer's Association. (2003). *Stages of Alzheimer's Disease.* Retrieved March 6, 2005 from the World Wide Web at http://www.alz.org

Alzheimer's Association (2004). *Fact sheet: About memantine.* Retrieved March 8, 2005 from the World Wide Web at http://www.alz.org

Alzheimer's Disease Education & Referral Center [ADEAR]. (2005). *Unraveling the Mystery.* Retrieved March 10, 2005 from the World Wide Web at http://www.alzheimers.org/unraveling/06.htm

American Psychiatric Association. (1994). *Diagnostic and statistical manual of mental disorders* (4th ed.). Washington, DC: American Psychiatric Association.

American Psychiatric Association. (2000). *Diagnostic and statistical manual of mental disorders* (4th ed.) *Text revision.* Washington, DC: American Psychiatric Association.

Arvanitakis, Z. (2000). *Dementia and vascular disease.* Duval County Medical Society. Retrieved March 7, 2005 from the World Wide Web at http://www.dcmsonline.org/jax-medicine/2000journals/February2000/vascdement.htm

Beers, M.H., & Jones, T.V. (Eds.). (2004). Drugs and aging. *The Merck manual of health and aging.* Whitehouse Station, NJ: Merck Research Laboratories.

Black, S.E. (2005). Vascular dementia: Stroke risk and sequelae define therapeutic approaches. *Postgraduate Medicine, 117*(1). Retrieved March 7, 2005 from http://www.postgradmed.com/issues/2005/01_05/black.htm

Bourgeois, J.A., Seaman, J.S., & Servis, M.E. (2003). Delirium, dementia, and amnestic disorders. In R.E. Hales & S.C. Yudofsky (Eds.). *Textbook of clinical psychiatry* (4th ed.). Washington, DC: American Psychiatric Publishing.

Castiglioni, A. (2003). Update: Memory loss and dementia. University of Alabama School of Medicine, Division of Continuing Medical Education. Retrieved March 6, 2005 from the World Wide Web at http://www-cme.erep.uab.edu/onlineCourses/dementia/ID0176.html

Cummings, J.L., Frank, J.C., Cherry, D., Kohatsu, N.D., Kemp, B., Hewett, L., & Mittman, B. (2002). Guidelines for managing Alzheimer's disease: Part II. Treatment. *American Family Physician, 65*(12), 2525–2534.

Cummings, J.L., & Mega, M.S. (2003). *Neuropsychiatry and behavioral neuroscience.* New York: Oxford University Press.

DeMartinis, J.E. (2005). Management of clients with hypertensive disorders. In J.M. Black & J.H. Hawks (Eds.). *Medical surgical nursing: Clinical management for positive outcomes* (7th ed.). St. Louis: W.B. Saunders.

Eisendrath, S.J., & Lichtmacher, J.E. (2005). Psychiatric disorders. In L.M. Tierney, S.J. McPhee, & M.A. Papadakis (Eds.). *Current medical diagnosis and treatment.* New York: McGraw-Hill.

Foroud, T., Gray, J., Ivashina, J., & Conneally, P.M. (1999). Differences in duration of Huntington's disease based on age at onset. *Journal of Neurology, Neurosurgery and Psychiatry, 66,* 52–56.

Harvard Medical School. (1995a, February). Update on Alzheimer's disease—Part I. *The Harvard Mental Health Letter.* Boston, MA: Harvard Medical School Publications Group.

Harvard Medical School. (1995b, March). Update on Alzheimer's disease—Part II. *The Harvard Mental Health Letter.* Boston, MA: Harvard Medical School Publications Group.

Herbert, L.E., Scherr, P.A., Bienias, J.L. Bennett, D.A., & Evans, D.A. (2003). Alzheimer's disease in the U.S. population: Prevalence estimates using the 2000 census. *Archives of Neurology, 60*(8), 1119–1122.

Langa, K.M., Foster, N.L., & Larson, E.B. (2004). Mixed dementia: Emerging concepts and therapeutic implications. *Journal of the American Medical Association, 292* (23), 2901–2908.

Laraia, M.T. (2004, January/February). Memantine: First NMDA receptor antagonist approved for the Treatment of Moderate to Severe Alzheimer's disease. *APNA News 16*(1), 12–13.

Lott, I.T., & Head, E. (2005). Alzheimer disease and Down syndrome: Factors in pathogenesis. *Neurobiology of Aging, 26*(3), 383–389.

Lyketsos, C.G., DelCampo, L., Steinberg, M., Miles, Q., Steele, C.D., Munro, C., Baker, A.S., Sheppard, J.E., Frangakis, C., Brandt, J., & Rabins, P.V. (2003). Treating depression in Alzheimer's disease. *Archives of General Psychiatry, 60*(7), 737–746.

McArthur, J. (2004). The Geneva Report. Update on neurology: HIV-associated dementia. Retrieved March 8, 2005 from the World Wide Web at http://www.hopkins-aids.edu/geneva/hilites_mcar_dem.html

Munoz, D.G., & Feldman, H. (2000). Causes of Alzheimer's disease. *Canadian Medical Association Journal, 162*(1), 65–72.

National Institute on Aging [NIA]. (2003). *2003 Progress Report on Alzheimer's Disease.* Washington, DC: National Institutes of Health, U.S. Department of Health and Human Services.

Newman, P.E. (2000). Alzheimer's disease revisited. *Medical Hypotheses, 54*(5), 774–776.

Poduslo, S.E., & Yin, X. (2001). A new locus on chromosome 19 linked with late-onset Alzheimer's disease. *Clinical Neuroscience and Neuropathology, 12*(17), 3759–3761.

Rabins, P., Bland, W., Bright-Long, L., Cohen, E., Katz, I., Rovner, B., Schneider, L., & Blacker, D. (2002). Practice guideline for the treatment of patients with Alzheimer's disease and other dementias of late life. *American Psychiatric Association Practice Guidelines for the Treatment of Psychiatric Disorders, Compendium 2002.* Washington, DC: American Psychiatric Association.

Reisberg, B., Doody, R., Stoffler, A., Schmitt, F., Ferris, S., & Mobius, H.J. (2003). Memantine in moderate-to-severe Alzheimer's disease. *New England Journal of Medicine, 348,* 1333–1341.

Sadock, B.J., & Sadock, V.A. (2003). *Synopsis of psychiatry: behavioral sciences/clinical psychiatry* (9th ed.). Philadelphia: Lippincott Williams & Wilkins.

Saunders, A.M. (2001). Gene identification in Alzheimer's disease. *Pharmacogenomics, 2*(3), 239–249.

Stanley, M., Blair, K.A., & Beare, P.G. (2005). *Gerontological nursing: Promoting successful aging with older adults* (3rd ed.). Philadelphia: F.A. Davis.

Tariot, P.N., Farlow, M.R., Grossberg, G.T., Graham, S.M., McDonald, S., & Gergel, I. (2004). Memantine treatment in patients with moderate to severe Alzheimer disease already receiving donepezil: A randomized controlled trial. *Journal of the American Medical Association, 291,* 317–324.

Trzepacz, P., Breitbart, W., Franklin, J., Levenson, J., Martini, D.R., & Wang, P. (2002). Practice guideline for the treatment of patients with delirium. *American Psychiatric Association Practice Guidelines for the Treatment of Psychiatric Disorders, Compendium 2002.* Washington, DC: American Psychiatric Association.

van Dyck, C.H., Newhouse, P., Falk, W.E., & Mattes, J.A. (2000). Extended-release physostigmine in Alzheimer's disease: A multicenter, double-blind, 12-week study with dose enrichment. *Archives of General Psychiatry, 57*(2), 157–164.

Wise, M.G., Gray, K.F., & Seltzer, B. (1999). Delirium, dementia, and amnestic disorders. In R.E. Hales & S.C. Yudofsky (Eds.). *Essentials of clinical psychiatry.* Washington, DC: American Psychiatric Press.

 INTERNET REFERENCES

Additional information about Alzheimer's disease may be located at the following Web sites:

- http://www.alz.org
- http://www.alzheimers.org/index.html
- http://www.ninds.nih.gov/disorders/alzheimersdisease/alzheimersdisease.htm
- http://www.ahcpr.gov/clinic/alzcons.htm

Information on caregiving can be located at the following Web site:

- http://www.aarp.org

Additional information about medications to treat Alzheimer's disease may be located at the following Web sites:

- http://www.fadavis.com/townsend
- http://www.laurus.com/library/healthguide/DrugGuide
- http://www.nimh.nih.gov/publicat/medicate.cfm

27
C H A P T E R

SUBSTANCE-RELATED DISORDERS

CHAPTER OUTLINE

OBJECTIVES

SUBSTANCE-USE DISORDERS

SUBSTANCE-INDUCED DISORDERS

CLASSES OF PSYCHOACTIVE SUBSTANCES

PREDISPOSING FACTORS

THE DYNAMICS OF SUBSTANCE-RELATED
DISORDERS

APPLICATION OF THE NURSING PROCESS

THE IMPAIRED NURSE

CODEPENDENCY

TREATMENT MODALITIES FOR SUBSTANCE-
RELATED DISORDERS

SUMMARY

REVIEW QUESTIONS

KEY TERMS

Alcoholics
   Anonymous
amphetamines
ascites
cannabis
codependence
detoxification
disulfiram
dual diagnosis
esophageal varices

hepatic
   encephalopathy
Korsakoff's
   psychosis
opioids
peer assistance
   programs
phencyclidine
substitution therapy
Wernicke's
   encephalopathy

CORE CONCEPTS

abuse
dependence
intoxication
withdrawal

OBJECTIVES

After reading this chapter, the student will be able to:

1. Define *abuse*, *dependence*, *intoxication*, and *withdrawal*.
2. Discuss predisposing factors implicated in the etiology of substance-related disorders.
3. Identify symptomatology and use the information in assessment of clients with various substance-use disorders and substance-induced disorders.
4. Identify nursing diagnoses common to clients with substance-use disorders and substance-induced disorders, and select appropriate nursing interventions for each.
5. Identify topics for client and family teaching

   relevant to substance-use disorders and substance-induced disorders.
6. Describe relevant outcome criteria for evaluating nursing care of clients with substance-use disorders and substance-induced disorders.
7. Discuss the issue of substance-related disorders within the profession of nursing.
8. Define codependency and identify behavioral characteristics associated with the disorder.
9. Discuss treatment of codependency.
10. Describe various modalities relevant to treatment of individuals with substance-use disorders and substance-induced disorders.

ubstance-related disorders are composed of two groups: the substance-use disorders (dependence and abuse) and the substance-induced disorders (intoxication, withdrawal, delirium, dementia, amnesia, psychosis, mood disorder, anxiety disorder, sexual dysfunction, and sleep disorders). This chapter discusses dependence, abuse, intoxication, and withdrawal. The remainder of the substance-induced disorders are included in the chapters with which they share symptomatology (e.g., substance-induced mood disorders are included in Chapter 29).

Drugs are a pervasive part of our society. Certain mood-altering substances are quite socially acceptable and are used moderately by many adult Americans. They include alcohol, caffeine, and nicotine. Society has even developed a relative indifference to an occasional abuse of these substances, despite documentation of their negative impact on health.

A wide variety of substances are produced for medicinal purposes. These include central nervous system (CNS) stimulants (e.g., **amphetamines**), CNS depressants (e.g., sedatives, tranquilizers), as well as numerous over-the-counter preparations designed to relieve nearly every kind of human ailment, real or imagined.

Some illegal substances have achieved a degree of social acceptance by various subcultural groups within our society. These drugs, such as marijuana and hashish, are by no means harmless, and the long-term effects are still being studied. On the other hand, the dangerous effects of other illegal substances (e.g., lysergic acid diethylamide [LSD], **phencyclidine**, cocaine, and heroin) have been well documented.

This chapter discusses the physical and behavioral manifestations and personal and social consequences related to the abuse of or dependency on alcohol, other CNS depressants, CNS stimulants, **opioids**, hallucinogens, and cannabinols. Wide cultural variations in attitudes exist regarding substance consumption and patterns of use. A high prevalence of substance use occurs between the ages of 18 and 24. Substance-related disorders are diagnosed more commonly in men than in women, but the gender ratios vary with the class of the substance (American Psychiatric Association [APA], 2000).

The concept of codependency is described in this chapter, as are aspects of treatment for the disorder. The issue of substance impairment within the profession of nursing is also explored. Nursing care for substance abuse, dependence, intoxication, and withdrawal is presented in the context of the six steps of the nursing process. Various medical and other treatment modalities are also discussed.

SUBSTANCE-USE DISORDERS

Substance Abuse

The *DSM-IV-TR* (APA, 2000) identifies substance abuse as a maladaptive pattern of substance use manifested by recurrent and significant adverse consequences related to repeated use of the substance. Substance abuse has also been referred to as any use of substances that poses significant hazards to health.

DSM-IV-TR Criteria for Substance Abuse

Substance abuse is described as a maladaptive pattern of substance use leading to clinically significant impairment or distress, as manifested by one (or more) of the following, occurring within a 12-month period:

1. Recurrent substance use resulting in a failure to fulfill major role obligations at work, school, or home (e.g., repeated absences or poor work performance related to substance use; substance-related absences, suspensions, or expulsions from school; neglect of children or household).
2. Recurrent substance use in situations in which it is physically hazardous (e.g., driving an automobile or operating a machine when impaired by substance use).
3. Recurrent substance-related legal problems (e.g., arrests for substance-related disorderly conduct).
4. Continued substance use despite having persistent or recurrent social or interpersonal problems caused or exacerbated by the effects of the substance (e.g., arguments with spouse about consequences of intoxication, physical fights).

> **Core Concept**
>
> **Dependence**
> A compulsive or chronic requirement. The need is so strong as to generate distress (either physical or psychological) if left unfulfilled.

Substance Dependence

Physical Dependence

Physical dependence on a substance is evidenced by a cluster of cognitive, behavioral, and physiological symptoms indicating that the individual continues use of the substance despite significant substance-related prob-

> **Core Concept**
>
> **Abuse**
> To use wrongfully or in a harmful way. Improper treatment or conduct that may result in injury.

lems (APA, 2000). As this condition develops, the repeated administration of the substance necessitates its continued use to prevent the appearance of unpleasant effects characteristic of the withdrawal syndrome associated with that particular drug. The development of physical dependence is promoted by the phenomenon of *tolerance*. Tolerance is defined as the need for increasingly larger or more frequent doses of a substance in order to obtain the desired effects originally produced by a lower dose.

Psychological Dependence

An individual is considered to be psychologically dependent on a substance when there is an overwhelming desire to repeat the use of a particular drug in order to produce pleasure or avoid discomfort. It can be extremely powerful, producing intense craving for a substance as well as its compulsive use.

DSM-IV-TR Criteria for Substance Dependence

At least three of the following characteristics must be present for a diagnosis of substance dependence:

1. Evidence of tolerance, as defined by either of the following:
   a. A need for markedly increased amounts of the substance to achieve intoxication or desired effects.
   b. Markedly diminished effect with continued use of the same amount of the substance.
2. Evidence of withdrawal symptoms, as manifested by either of the following:
   a. The characteristic withdrawal syndrome for the substance.
   b. The same (or a closely related) substance is taken to relieve or avoid withdrawal symptoms.
3. The substance is often taken in larger amounts or over a longer period than was intended.
4. There is a persistent desire or unsuccessful efforts to cut down or control substance use.
5. A great deal of time is spent in activities necessary to obtain the substance (e.g., visiting multiple doctors or driving long distances), use the substance (e.g., chain smoking), or recover from its effects.
6. Important social, occupational, or recreational activities are given up or reduced because of substance use.
7. The substance use is continued despite knowledge of having a persistent or recurrent physical or psychological problem that is likely to have been caused or exacerbated by the substance (e.g., current cocaine use despite recognition of cocaine-induced depression, or continued drinking despite recognition

that an ulcer was made worse by alcohol consumption).

SUBSTANCE-INDUCED DISORDERS

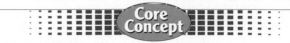

Intoxication
A physical and mental state of exhilaration and emotional frenzy or lethargy and stupor.

Substance Intoxication

Substance intoxication is defined as the development of a reversible substance-specific syndrome caused by the recent ingestion of (or exposure to) a substance (APA, 2000). The behavior changes can be attributed to the physiological effects of the substance on the CNS and develop during or shortly after use of the substance. This category does not apply to nicotine.

DSM-IV-TR Criteria for Substance Intoxication

1. The development of a reversible substance-specific syndrome caused by recent ingestion of (or exposure to) a substance.
   NOTE: Different substances may produce similar or identical syndromes.
2. Clinically significant maladaptive behavior or psychological changes that are due to the effect of the substance on the CNS (e.g., belligerence, mood lability, cognitive impairment, impaired judgment, impaired social or occupational functioning) and develop during or shortly after use of the substance.
3. The symptoms are not due to a general medical condition and are not better accounted for by another mental disorder.

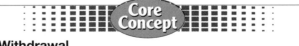

Withdrawal
The physiological and mental readjustment that accompanies the discontinuation of an addictive substance.

Substance Withdrawal

Substance withdrawal is the development of a substance-specific maladaptive behavioral change, with physiological and cognitive concomitants, that is due to the cessation of, or reduction in, heavy and prolonged substance use (APA, 2000). Withdrawal is usually, but not always, associated with substance dependence.

DSM-IV-TR Criteria for Substance Withdrawal

1. The development of a substance-specific syndrome caused by the cessation of (or reduction in) heavy and prolonged substance use.
2. The substance-specific syndrome causes clinically significant distress or impairment in social, occupational, or other important areas of functioning.
3. The symptoms are not due to a general medical condition and are not better accounted for by another mental disorder.

CLASSES OF PSYCHOACTIVE SUBSTANCES

The following 11 classes of psychoactive substances are associated with substance-use and substance-induced disorders. They include:

1. Alcohol
2. Amphetamines and related substances
3. Caffeine
4. **Cannabis**
5. Cocaine
6. Hallucinogens
7. Inhalants
8. Nicotine
9. Opioids
10. Phencyclidine (PCP) and related substances
11. Sedatives, hypnotics, or anxiolytics

PREDISPOSING FACTORS

A number of factors have been implicated in the predisposition to abuse of substances. At present, there is no single theory that can adequately explain the etiology of this problem. No doubt the interaction between various elements forms a complex collection of determinants that influence a person's susceptibility to abuse substances.

Biological Factors

Genetics

An apparent hereditary factor is involved in the development of substance-use disorders. This is especially evident with alcoholism, but less so with other substances. Children of alcoholics are three times more likely than other children to become alcoholics (Harvard Medical School, 2001). Studies with monozygotic and dizygotic twins have also supported the genetic hypothesis. Monozygotic (one egg, genetically identical) twins have a higher rate for concordance of alcoholism than dizygotic (two eggs, genetically nonidentical) twins (Sadock &

Sadock, 2003). Other studies have shown that biological offspring of alcoholic parents have a significantly greater incidence of alcoholism than offspring of nonalcoholic parents. This is true whether the child was reared by the biological parents or by nonalcoholic adoptive parents (Knowles, 2003).

Biochemical Factors

A second biological hypothesis relates to the possibility that alcohol may produce morphine-like substances in the brain that are responsible for alcohol addiction. These substances are formed by the reaction of biologically active amines (e.g., dopamine, serotonin) with products of alcohol metabolism, such as acetaldehyde (Jamal et al., 2003). Examples of these morphine-like substances include tetrahydropapaveroline and salsolinol. Some tests with animals have shown that injection of these compounds into the brain in small amounts results in patterns of alcohol addiction in animals that had previously avoided even the most dilute alcohol solutions (Behavioral Neuroscience Laboratory, 2002).

Psychological Factors

Developmental Influences

The psychodynamic approach to the etiology of substance abuse focuses on a punitive superego and fixation at the oral stage of psychosexual development (Sadock & Sadock, 2003). Individuals with punitive superegos turn to alcohol to diminish unconscious anxiety. Sadock and Sadock (2003) state, "Anxiety in people fixated at the oral stage may be reduced by taking substances, such as alcohol, by mouth." Alcohol may also serve to increase feelings of power and self worth in these individuals.

Personality Factors

Certain personality traits have been associated with a tendency toward addictive behavior. Some clinicians believe that low self-esteem, frequent depression, passivity, the inability to relax or to defer gratification, and the inability to communicate effectively are common in individuals who abuse substances. These personality characteristics cannot be called *predictive* of addictive behavior, yet for reasons not completely understood, they have been found to accompany addiction in many instances.

Substance abuse has also been associated with antisocial personality and depressive response styles. This may be explained by the inability of the individual with antisocial personality to anticipate the aversive consequences of his or her behavior. It is likely an effort on the part of the depressed person to treat the symptoms of discomfort associated with dysphoria. Achievement of relief then provides the positive reinforcement to continue abusing the substance.

Sociocultural Factors

Social Learning

The effects of modeling, imitation, and identification on behavior can be observed from early childhood onward. In relation to drug consumption, the family appears to be an important influence. Various studies have shown that children and adolescents are more likely to use substances if they have parents who provide a model for substance use. Peers often exert a great deal of influence in the life of the child or adolescent who is being encouraged to use substances for the first time. Modeling may continue to be a factor in the use of substances once the individual enters the work force. This is particularly true in a work setting that provides plenty of leisure time with coworkers and where drinking is valued and is used to express group cohesiveness.

Conditioning

Another important learning factor is the effect of the substance itself. Many substances create a pleasurable experience that encourages the user to repeat it. Thus, it is the intrinsically reinforcing properties of addictive drugs that "condition" the individual to seek out their use again and again. The environment in which the substance is taken also contributes to the reinforcement. If the environment is pleasurable, substance use is usually increased. Aversive stimuli within an environment are thought to be associated with a decrease in substance use within that environment.

Cultural and Ethnic Influences

Factors within an individual's culture help to establish patterns of substance use by molding attitudes, influencing patterns of consumption based on cultural acceptance, and determining the availability of the substance. For centuries, the French and Italians have considered wine an essential part of the family meal, even for the children. The incidence of alcohol dependency is low, and acute intoxication from alcohol is not common. However, the possibility of chronic physiological effects associated with lifelong alcohol consumption cannot be ignored.

Historically, a high incidence of alcohol dependency has existed within the Native American culture. Death rates from alcoholism among Native Americans are more than seven times the national average (Greer, 2004). Veterans Administration records show that 45 percent of the Indian veterans were alcohol dependent, or twice the rate for non-Indian veterans. A number of reasons have been postulated for alcohol abuse among Native Americans: a possible physical cause (difficulty metabolizing alcohol), children modeling their parents' drinking habits, unemployment and poverty, and loss of the traditional Native American religion that some believe has led to the increased use of alcohol to fill the spiritual gap (Newhouse, 1999).

The incidence of alcohol dependence is higher among northern Europeans than among southern Europeans. The Finns and the Irish use excessive alcohol consumption for the release of aggression, and the English "pub" is known for its attraction as a social meeting place.

Incidence of alcohol dependence among Asians is relatively low. This may be a result of a possible genetic intolerance of the substance. Some Asians develop unpleasant symptoms, such as flushing, headaches, nausea, and palpitations, when they drink alcohol. Research indicates that this is because of an isoenzyme variant that quickly converts alcohol to acetaldehyde, as well as the absence of an isoenzyme that is needed to oxidize acetaldehyde. This results in a rapid accumulation of acetaldehyde, which produces the unpleasant symptoms (Hanley, 2004).

THE DYNAMICS OF SUBSTANCE-RELATED DISORDERS

Alcohol Abuse and Dependence

A Profile of the Substance

Alcohol is a natural substance formed by the reaction of fermenting sugar with yeast spores. Although there are many alcohols, the kind in alcoholic beverages is known scientifically as ethyl alcohol and chemically as C_2H_5OH. Its abbreviation, ETOH, is sometimes seen in medical records and in various other documents and publications.

By strict definition, alcohol is classified as a food because it contains calories; however, it has no nutritional value. Different alcoholic beverages are produced by using different sources of sugar for the fermentation process. For example, beer is made from malted barley, wine from grapes or berries, whiskey from malted grains, and rum from molasses. Distilled beverages (e.g., whiskey, scotch, gin, vodka, and other "hard" liquors) derive their name from further concentration of the alcohol through a process called distillation.

The alcohol content varies by type of beverage. For example, most American beers contain 3 to 6 percent alcohol, wines average 10 to 20 percent, and distilled beverages range from 40 to 50 percent alcohol. The average-sized drink, regardless of beverage, contains a similar amount of alcohol. That is, 12 ounces of beer, 3 to 5 ounces of wine, and a cocktail with 1 ounce of whiskey all contain approximately 0.5 ounce of alcohol. If consumed at the same rate, they all would have an equal effect on the body.

Alcohol exerts a depressant effect on the CNS, resulting in behavioral and mood changes. The effects of alcohol on the CNS are proportional to the alcoholic concentration in the blood. Most states consider that an individual is legally intoxicated with a blood alcohol level of 0.08 to 0.10 percent.

The body burns alcohol at the rate of about 0.5 ounce per hour, so behavioral changes would not be expected to occur in an individual who slowly consumed only one averaged-sized drink per hour. Other factors do influence these effects, however, such as individual size and whether or not the stomach contains food at the time the alcohol is consumed. Alcohol is thought to have a more profound effect when an individual is emotionally stressed or fatigued (National Institute on Alcohol Abuse and Alcoholism [NIAAA], 2000).

Historical Aspects

The use of alcohol can be traced back to the Neolithic age. Beer and wine are known to have been used around 6400 B.C. With the introduction of distillation by the Arabs in the Middle Ages, alchemists believed that alcohol was the answer to all of their ailments. The word "whiskey," meaning "water of life," became widely known.

In America, Native Americans had been drinking beer and wine prior to the arrival of the first white visitors. Refinement of the distillation process made beverages with high alcohol content readily available. By the early 1800s, one renowned physician of the time, Benjamin Rush, had begun to identify the widespread excessive, chronic alcohol consumption as a disease and an addiction. The strong religious mores on which this country was founded soon led to a driving force aimed at prohibiting the sale of alcoholic beverages. By the middle of the 19th century, 13 states had passed prohibition laws. The most notable prohibition of major proportions was that in effect in the United States from 1920 to 1933. The mandatory restrictions on national social habits resulted in the creation of profitable underground markets that led to flourishing criminal enterprises. Furthermore, millions of dollars in federal, state, and local revenues from taxes and import duties on alcohol were lost. It is difficult to measure the value of this dollar loss against the human devastation and social costs that occur as a result of alcohol abuse in the United States today.

Patterns of Use/Abuse

About half of Americans aged 12 years and older report being current drinkers of alcohol (Substance Abuse and Mental Health Services Administration [SAMHSA],

2005). Of these about one fourth are binge drinkers or engage in heavy alcohol use.

Why do people drink? Drinking patterns in the United States show that people use alcoholic beverages to enhance the flavor of food with meals; at social gatherings to encourage relaxation and conviviality among the guests; and to promote a feeling of celebration at special occasions such as weddings, birthdays, and anniversaries. An alcoholic beverage (wine) is also used as part of the sacred ritual in some religious ceremonies. Therapeutically, alcohol is the major ingredient in many over-the-counter and prescription medicines that are prepared in concentrated form. Therefore, alcohol can be harmless and enjoyable—sometimes even beneficial—if it is used responsibly and in moderation. Like any other mind-altering drug, however, alcohol has the potential for abuse. Indeed, it is the most widely abused drug in the United States today. The National Council on Alcoholism and Drug Dependence (2005) reports:

> Alcoholism is the third leading cause of preventable death in the U.S. As the nation's number one health problem, addiction strains the health care system, the economy, harms family life and threatens public safety. One-quarter of all emergency room admissions, one-third of all suicides, and more than half of all homicides and incidents of domestic violence are alcohol-related. Heavy drinking contributes to illness in each of the top three causes of death: heart disease, cancer, and stroke. Almost half of all traffic fatalities are alcohol-related. Fetal alcohol syndrome is the leading known cause of mental retardation.

Jellinek (1952) outlined four phases through which the alcoholic's pattern of drinking progresses. Some variability among individuals is to be expected within this model of progression.

Phase I. The Prealcoholic Phase. This phase is characterized by the use of alcohol to relieve the everyday stress and tensions of life. As a child, the individual may have observed parents or other adults drinking alcohol and enjoying the effects. The child learns that use of alcohol is an acceptable method of coping with stress. Tolerance develops, and the amount required to achieve the desired effect increases steadily.

Phase II. The Early Alcoholic Phase. This phase begins with blackouts—brief periods of amnesia that occur during or immediately following a period of drinking. Now the alcohol is no longer a source of pleasure or relief for the individual but rather a drug that is *required* by the individual. Common behaviors include sneaking drinks or secret drinking, preoccupation with drinking and maintaining the supply of alcohol, rapid gulping of drinks, and further blackouts. The individual feels enormous guilt and becomes very defensive about his or her drinking. Excessive use of denial and rationalization is evident.

Phase III. The Crucial Phase. In this phase, the individual has lost control, and physiological dependence is clearly evident. This loss of control has been described as the inability to choose whether or not to drink. Binge drinking, lasting from a few hours to several weeks, is common. These episodes are characterized by sickness, loss of consciousness, squalor, and degradation. In this phase, the individual is extremely ill. Anger and aggression are common manifestations. Drinking is the total focus, and he or she is willing to risk losing everything that was once important in an effort to maintain the addiction. By this phase of the illness, it is not uncommon for the individual to have experienced the loss of job, marriage, family, friends, and most especially, self-respect.

Phase IV. The Chronic Phase. This phase is characterized by emotional and physical disintegration. The individual is usually intoxicated more than he or she is sober. Emotional disintegration is evidenced by profound helplessness and self-pity. Impairment in reality testing may result in psychosis. Life-threatening physical manifestations may be evident in virtually every system of the body. Abstention from alcohol results in a terrifying syndrome of symptoms that include hallucinations, tremors, convulsions, severe agitation, and panic. Depression and ideas of suicide are not uncommon.

Effects on the Body

Alcohol can induce a general, nonselective, reversible depression of the CNS. About 20 percent of a single dose of alcohol is absorbed directly and immediately into the bloodstream through the stomach wall. Unlike other "foods," it does not have to be digested. The blood carries it directly to the brain where the alcohol acts on the brain's central control areas, slowing down or depressing brain activity. The other 80 percent of the alcohol in one drink is processed only slightly more slowly through the upper intestinal tract and into the bloodstream. Only moments after alcohol is consumed, it can be found in all tissues, organs, and secretions of the body. Rapidity of absorption is influenced by various factors. For example, absorption is delayed when the drink is sipped, rather than gulped; when the stomach contains food, rather than being empty; and when the drink is wine or beer, rather than distilled beverages.

At low doses, alcohol produces relaxation, loss of inhibitions, lack of concentration, drowsiness, slurred speech, and sleep. Chronic abuse results in multisystem physiological impairments. These complications include (but are not limited to) those outlined in the following sections.

Peripheral Neuropathy. Peripheral neuropathy, characterized by peripheral nerve damage, results in pain, burning, tingling, or prickly sensations of the extremities. Researchers believe it is the direct result of deficiencies in the B vitamins, particularly thiamine. Nutritional deficiencies are common in chronic alcoholics because of insufficient intake of nutrients as well as the toxic effect of alcohol that results in malabsorption of nutrients. The process is reversible with abstinence from alcohol and restoration of nutritional deficiencies. Otherwise, permanent muscle wasting and paralysis can occur.

Alcoholic Myopathy. Alcoholic myopathy may occur as an acute or chronic condition. In the acute condition, the individual experiences a sudden onset of muscle pain, swelling, and weakness; a reddish tinge in the urine caused by myoglobin, a breakdown product of muscle excreted in the urine; and a rapid rise in muscle enzymes in the blood (Barclay, 2005). Muscle symptoms are usually generalized, but pain and swelling may selectively involve the calves or other muscle groups. Laboratory studies show elevations of the enzymes creatine phosphokinase (CPK), lactate dehydrogenase (LDH), aldolase, and aspartate aminotransferase (AST). The symptoms of chronic alcoholic myopathy include a gradual wasting and weakness in skeletal muscles. Neither the pain and tenderness nor the elevated muscle enzymes seen in acute myopathy are evident in the chronic condition.

Alcoholic myopathy is thought to be a result of the same B vitamin deficiency that contributes to peripheral neuropathy. Improvement is observed with abstinence from alcohol and the return to a nutritious diet with vitamin supplements.

Wernicke's Encephalopathy. **Wernicke's encephalopathy** represents the most serious form of thiamine deficiency in alcoholics. Symptoms include paralysis of the ocular muscles, diplopia, ataxia, somnolence, and stupor. If thiamine replacement therapy is not undertaken quickly, death will ensue.

Korsakoff's Psychosis. **Korsakoff's psychosis** is identified by a syndrome of confusion, loss of recent memory, and confabulation in alcoholics. It is frequently encountered in clients recovering from Wernicke's encephalopathy. In the United States, the two disorders are usually considered together and are called *Wernicke–Korsakoff syndrome*. Treatment is with parenteral or oral thiamine replacement.

Alcoholic Cardiomyopathy. The effect of alcohol on the heart is an accumulation of lipids in the myocardial cells, resulting in enlargement and a weakened condition. The clinical findings of alcoholic cardiomyopathy generally relate to congestive heart failure or arrhythmia. Symptoms include decreased exercise tolerance, tachycardia, dyspnea, edema, palpitations, and cough. Laboratory studies may show elevation of the enzymes creatine phosphokinase (CPK), aspartate aminotransferase (AST), alanine aminotransferase (ALT), and lactate dehydrogenase (LDH). Changes may be observed by electrocardiogram, and congestive heart failure may be evident on chest X-ray films (Tazbir & Keresztes, 2005).

The treatment is total permanent abstinence from alcohol. Treatment of the congestive heart failure may include rest, oxygen, digitalization, sodium restriction, and diuretics. Prognosis is encouraging if treated in the early stages. The death rate is high for individuals with advanced symptomatology.

Esophagitis. Esophagitis—inflammation and pain in the esophagus—occurs because of the toxic effects of alcohol on the esophageal mucosa. It also occurs because of frequent vomiting associated with alcohol abuse.

Gastritis. The effects of alcohol on the stomach include inflammation of the stomach lining characterized by epigastric distress, nausea, vomiting, and distention. Alcohol breaks down the stomach's protective mucosal barrier, allowing hydrochloric acid to erode the stomach wall. Damage to blood vessels may result in hemorrhage.

Pancreatitis. Pancreatitis may be categorized as *acute* or *chronic*. Acute pancreatitis usually occurs 1 or 2 days after a binge of excessive alcohol consumption. Symptoms include constant, severe epigastric pain, nausea and vomiting, and abdominal distention. The chronic condition leads to pancreatic insufficiency resulting in steatorrhea, malnutrition, weight loss, and diabetes mellitus.

Alcoholic Hepatitis. Alcoholic hepatitis is inflammation of the liver caused by long-term heavy alcohol use. Clinical manifestations include an enlarged and tender liver, nausea and vomiting, lethargy, anorexia, elevated white blood cell count, fever, and jaundice. **Ascites** and weight loss may be evident in more severe cases. With treatment—which includes strict abstinence from alcohol, proper nutrition, and rest—the individual can experience complete recovery. Severe cases can lead to cirrhosis or **hepatic encephalopathy**.

Cirrhosis of the Liver. In the United States, alcohol abuse is the leading cause of liver cirrhosis (Mayo Foundation for Medical Education and Research, 2005). Cirrhosis is the end-stage of alcoholic liver disease and results from long-term chronic alcohol abuse. There is widespread destruction of liver cells, which are replaced by fibrous (scar) tissue. Clinical manifestations include nausea and vomiting, anorexia, weight loss, abdominal pain, jaundice, edema, anemia, and blood coagulation abnormalities. Treatment includes abstention from alcohol, correction of malnutrition, and supportive care to prevent complications of the disease. Complications of cirrhosis include:

1. **Portal Hypertension.** Elevation of blood pressure through the portal circulation results from defective blood flow through the cirrhotic liver.
2. **Ascites.** Ascites, a condition in which an excessive amount of serous fluid accumulates in the abdominal cavity, occurs in response to portal hypertension. The increased pressure results in the seepage of fluid from the surface of the liver into the abdominal cavity.
3. **Esophageal Varices. Esophageal varices** are veins in the esophagus that become distended because of excessive pressure from defective blood flow through

the cirrhotic liver. As this pressure increases, these varicosities can rupture, resulting in hemorrhage and sometimes death.

4. **Hepatic Encephalopathy.** This serious complication occurs in response to the inability of the diseased liver to convert ammonia to urea for excretion. The continued rise in serum ammonia results in progressively impaired mental functioning, apathy, euphoria or depression, sleep disturbance, increasing confusion, and progression to coma and eventual death. Treatment requires complete abstention from alcohol, temporary elimination of protein from the diet, and reduction of intestinal ammonia using neomycin or lactulose (National Library of Medicine, 2002).

Leukopenia. The production, function, and movement of the white blood cells are impaired in chronic alcoholics. This condition, called leukopenia, places the individual at high risk for contracting infectious diseases as well as for complicated recovery.

Thrombocytopenia. Platelet production and survival is impaired as a result of the toxic effects of alcohol. This places the alcoholic at risk for hemorrhage. Abstinence from alcohol rapidly reverses this deficiency.

Sexual Dysfunction. Alcohol interferes with the normal production and maintenance of female and male hormones (National Institute on Alcohol Abuse and Alcoholism [NIAAA], 2005). For women, this can mean changes in the menstrual cycles and a decreased or loss of ability to become pregnant. For men, the decreased hormone levels result in a diminished libido, decreased sexual performance, and impaired fertility (NIAAA, 2005).

Alcohol Intoxication

Symptoms of alcohol intoxication include disinhibition of sexual or aggressive impulses, mood lability, impaired judgment, impaired social or occupational functioning, slurred speech, incoordination, unsteady gait, nystagmus, and flushed face. Intoxication usually occurs at blood alcohol levels between 100 and 200 mg/dl. Death has been reported at levels ranging from 400 to 700 mg/dl.

Alcohol Withdrawal

Within 4 to 12 hours of cessation of or reduction in heavy and prolonged (several days or longer) alcohol use, the following symptoms may appear: coarse tremor of hands, tongue, or eyelids; nausea or vomiting; malaise or weakness; tachycardia; sweating; elevated blood pressure; anxiety; depressed mood or irritability; transient hallucinations or illusions; headache; and insomnia. A complicated withdrawal syndrome may progress to *alcohol withdrawal delirium*. Onset of delirium is usually on the second or third day following cessation of or reduction in prolonged, heavy alcohol use. Symptoms include those described under the syndrome of delirium (Chapter 26).

Sedative, Hypnotic, or Anxiolytic Abuse and Dependence

A Profile of the Substance

The sedative-hypnotic compounds are drugs of diverse chemical structures that are all capable of inducing varying degrees of CNS depression, from tranquilizing relief of anxiety to anesthesia, coma, and even death. They are generally categorized as (1) barbiturates, (2) nonbarbiturate hypnotics, and (3) antianxiety agents. Effects produced by these substances depend on size of dose and potency of drug administered.

Table 27–1 presents a selected list of drugs included in these categories. Generic names are followed in parentheses by the trade names. Common street names for each category are also included.

Several principles have been identified that apply fairly uniformly to all CNS depressants:

1. **The effects of CNS depressants are additive with one another and with the behavioral state of the user.** For example, when these drugs are used in combination with each other or in combination with alcohol, the depressive effects are compounded. These intense depressive effects are often unpredictable and can even be fatal. Similarly, a person who is mentally depressed or physically fatigued may have an exaggerated response to a dose of the drug that would only slightly affect a person in a normal or excited state.
2. **CNS depressants are capable of producing physiological dependency.** If large doses of CNS depressants are repeatedly administered over a prolonged

duration, a period of CNS hyperexcitability occurs on withdrawal of the drug. The response can be quite severe, even leading to convulsions and death.
3. **CNS depressants are capable of producing psychological dependence.** CNS depressants have the potential to generate within the individual a psychic drive for periodic or continuous administration of the drug to achieve a maximum level of functioning or feeling of well-being.
4. **Cross-tolerance and cross-dependence may exist between various CNS depressants.** Cross-tolerance is exhibited when one drug results in a lessened response to another drug. Cross-dependence is a condition in which one drug can prevent withdrawal symptoms associated with physical dependence on a different drug (Julien, 2005).

Historical Aspects

Anxiety and insomnia, two of the most common human afflictions, were treated during the 19th century with opiates, bromide salts, chloral hydrate, paraldehyde, and alcohol (American Insomnia Association, 2005; Julien, 2005). Because the opiates were known to produce physical dependence, the bromides carried the risk of chronic bromide poisoning, and chloral hydrate and paraldehyde had an objectionable taste and smell, alcohol became the prescribed depressant drug of choice. Some people refused to use alcohol, however, either because they did not like the taste or for moral reasons, and others tended to take more than was prescribed. Therefore, a search for a better sedative drug continued.

Although barbituric acid was first synthesized in 1864, it was not until 1912 that phenobarbital was introduced into medicine as a sedative drug, the first of the struc-

---

TABLE 27–1   Sedative, Hypnotic, and Anxiolytic Drugs

CATEGORIES	GENERIC (TRADE) NAMES	COMMON STREET NAMES
Barbiturates	Pentobarbital (Nembutal)	Yellow jackets; yellow birds
	Secobarbital (Seconal)	GBs; red birds; red devils
	Amobarbital (Amytal)	Blue birds; blue angels
	Secobarbital/amobarbital (Tuinal)	Tooies; jelly beans
	Phenobarbital	
	Butabarbital	
Nonbarbiturate hypnotics	Chloral hydrate (Noctec)	Peter, Mickey
	Triazolam (Halcion)	Sleepers
	Flurazepam (Dalmane)	Sleepers
	Temazepam (Restoril)	Sleepers
	Quazepam (Doral)	Sleepers
Antianxiety agents	Diazepam (Valium)	Vs (color designates strength)
	Chlordiazepoxide (Librium)	Green and whites; roaches
	Meprobamate (Miltown)	Dolls; dollies
	Oxazepam (Serax)	Candy, downers (the benzodiazepines)
	Alprazolam (Xanax)	
	Lorazepam (Ativan)	
	Clorazepate (Tranxene)	
	Flunitrazepam (Rohypnol)	Date rape drug; roofies, R-2, rope, Mexican Valium

turally classified group of drugs called barbiturates (Julien, 2005). Since that time, more than 2500 barbiturate derivatives have been synthesized, but currently fewer than a dozen remain in medical use. Illicit use of the drugs for recreational purposes grew throughout the 1930s and 1940s.

Efforts to create depressant medications that were not barbiturate derivatives accelerated. By the mid-1950s the market for depressants had been expanded by the appearance of the nonbarbiturates glutethimide, ethchlorvynol, methyprylon, and meprobamate. Introduction of the benzodiazepines occurred around 1960 with the marketing of chlordiazepoxide (Librium), followed shortly by its derivative diazepam (Valium). The use of these drugs, and others within their group, has grown so rapidly that they have become some of the most widely prescribed medications in clinical use today. Their margin of safety is greater than that of barbiturates and the other nonbarbiturates. Prolonged use of even moderate doses is likely to result in physical and psychological dependence, however, with a characteristic syndrome of withdrawal that can be severe.

Patterns of Use/Abuse

Sadock and Sadock (2003) report that about 15 percent of all persons in the United States have had benzodiazepines prescribed by a physician. Of all the drugs used in clinical practice, the sedative-hypnotic-antianxiety drugs are among the most widely prescribed. The *DSM-IV-TR* states:

> In the United States, up to 90 percent of individuals hospitalized for medical care or surgery receive orders for sedative, hypnotic, or anxiolytic medications during their hospital stay, and more than 15 percent of American adults use these medications (usually by prescription) during any one year. (p. 291)

Two patterns of development of dependence and abuse are described. The first pattern is one of an individual whose physician originally prescribed the CNS depressant as treatment for anxiety or insomnia. Independently, the individual has increased the dosage or frequency from that which was prescribed. Use of the medication is justified on the basis of treating symptoms, but as tolerance grows, more and more of the medication is required

to produce the desired effect. Substance-seeking behavior is evident as the individual seeks prescriptions from several physicians in order to maintain sufficient supplies.

The second pattern, which the *DSM-IV-TR* reports is more frequent than the first, involves young people in their teens or early 20s who, in the company of their peers, use substances that were obtained illegally. The initial objective is to achieve a feeling of euphoria. The drug is usually used intermittently during recreational gatherings. This pattern of intermittent use leads to regular use and extreme levels of tolerance. Combining use with other substances is not uncommon. Physical and psychological dependence leads to intense substance-seeking behaviors, most often through illegal channels.

Effects on the Body

The sedative-hypnotic compounds induce a general depressant effect; that is, they depress the activity of the brain, nerves, muscles, and heart tissue. They reduce the rate of metabolism in a variety of tissues throughout the body, and in general, they depress any system that uses energy (Julien, 2005). Large doses are required to produce these effects. In lower doses these drugs appear to be more selective in their depressant actions. Specifically, in lower doses these drugs appear to exert their action on the centers within the brain that are concerned with arousal (e.g., the ascending reticular activating system, in the reticular formation, and the diffuse thalamic projection system).

As stated previously, the sedative-hypnotics are capable of producing all levels of CNS depression—from mild sedation to death. The level is determined by dosage and potency of the drug used. In Figure 27–1, a continuum of the CNS depressant effects is presented to demonstrate how increasing doses of sedative-hypnotic drugs affect behavioral depression.

The primary action of sedative-hypnotics is on nervous tissue. However, large doses may have an effect on other organ systems. Following is a discussion of the physiological effects of sedative-hypnotic/anxiolytic agents.

Effects on Sleep and Dreaming. Barbiturate use decreases the amount of sleep time spent in dreaming. During drug withdrawal, dreaming becomes vivid and excessive. Rebound insomnia and increased dreaming

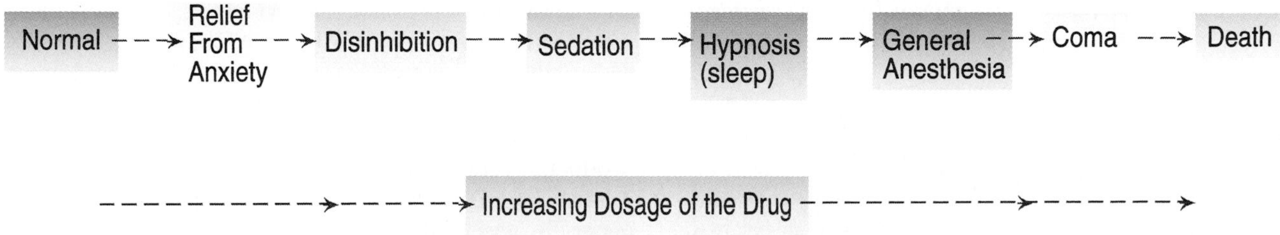

Normal - -→ Relief From Anxiety - -→ Disinhibition - -→ Sedation - -→ Hypnosis (sleep) - -→ General Anesthesia - -→ Coma - -→ Death

- - - - - - →- - - -→ Increasing Dosage of the Drug - - - - - - -→- - - -→

FIGURE 27–1 Continuum of behavioral depression.

(termed *REM rebound*) are not uncommon with abrupt withdrawal from long-term use of these drugs as sleeping aids (Julien, 2005).

Respiratory Depression. Barbiturates are capable of inhibiting the reticular activating system, resulting in respiratory depression (Sadock & Sadock, 2003). Additive effects can occur with the concurrent use of other CNS depressants, effecting a life-threatening situation.

Cardiovascular Effects. Hypotension may be a problem with large doses. Only a slight decrease in blood pressure is noted with normal oral dosage. High dosages of barbiturates may result in decreased cardiac output, decreased cerebral blood flow, and direct impairment of myocardial contractility (Habal, 2004).

Renal Function. In doses high enough to produce anesthesia, barbiturates may suppress urine function. At the usual sedative-hypnotic dosage, however, there is no evidence that they have any direct action on the kidneys.

Hepatic Effects. The barbiturates may produce jaundice with doses large enough to produce acute intoxication. Barbiturates stimulate the production of liver enzymes, resulting in a decrease in the plasma levels of both the barbiturates and other drugs metabolized in the liver (Habal, 2004). Preexisting liver disease may predispose an individual to additional liver damage with excessive barbiturate use.

Body Temperature. High doses of barbiturates can greatly decrease body temperature. It is not significantly altered with normal dosage levels.

Sexual Functioning. CNS depressants have a tendency to produce a biphasic response. There is an initial increase in libido, presumably from the primary disinhibitory effects of the drug. This initial response is then followed by a decrease in the ability to maintain an erection.

Sedative, Hypnotic, or Anxiolytic Intoxication

The *DSM-IV-TR* (APA, 2000) describes sedative, hypnotic, or anxiolytic intoxication as the presence of clinically significant maladaptive behavioral or psychological changes that develop during, or shortly after, use of one of these substances. These maladaptive changes may include inappropriate sexual or aggressive behavior, mood lability, impaired judgment, or impaired social or occupational functioning. Other symptoms that may develop with excessive use of sedatives, hypnotics, or anxiolytics include slurred speech, incoordination, unsteady gait, nystagmus, impairment in attention or memory, and stupor or coma.

Sedative, Hypnotic, or Anxiolytic Withdrawal

Withdrawal from sedatives, hypnotics, or anxiolytics produces a characteristic syndrome of symptoms that devel-

ops after a marked decrease in or cessation of intake after several weeks or more of regular use (APA, 2000). Onset of the symptoms depends on the drug from which the individual is withdrawing. A short-acting anxiolytic (e.g., lorazepam or oxazepam) may produce symptoms within 6 to 8 hours of decreasing blood levels, whereas withdrawal symptoms from substances with longer half-lives (e.g., diazepam) may not develop for more than a week, peak in intensity during the second week, and decrease markedly during the third or fourth week (APA, 2000).

Severe withdrawal is most likely to occur when a substance has been used at high dosages for prolonged periods. However, withdrawal symptoms also have been reported with moderate dosages taken over a relatively short duration. Withdrawal symptoms associated with sedatives, hypnotics, or anxiolytics include autonomic hyperactivity (e.g., sweating or pulse rate greater than 100), increased hand tremor, insomnia, nausea or vomiting, hallucinations, illusions, psychomotor agitation, anxiety, or grand mal seizures.

CNS Stimulant Abuse and Dependence

A Profile of the Substance

The CNS stimulants are identified by the behavioral stimulation and psychomotor agitation that they induce. They differ widely in their molecular structures and in their mechanisms of action. The amount of CNS stimulation caused by a certain drug depends on both the area in the brain or spinal cord that is affected by the drug and the cellular mechanism fundamental to the increased excitability (Kuhn, 1998).

Groups within this category are classified according to similarities in mechanism of action. The *psychomotor stimulants* induce stimulation by augmentation or potentiation of the neurotransmitters norepinephrine, epinephrine, or dopamine. The *general cellular stimulants* (caffeine and nicotine) exert their actions directly on cellular activity. Caffeine inhibits the enzyme phosphodiesterase, allowing increased levels of adenosine 3′, 5′-cyclic phosphate (cAMP), a chemical substance that promotes increased rates of cellular metabolism. Nicotine stimulates ganglionic synapses. This results in increased acetylcholine, which stimulates nerve impulse transmission to the entire autonomic nervous system. A selected list of drugs included in these categories is presented in Table 27–2.

The two most prevalent and widely used stimulants are caffeine and nicotine. Caffeine is readily available in every supermarket and grocery store as a common ingredient in coffee, tea, colas, and chocolate. Nicotine is the primary psychoactive substance found in tobacco products. When used in moderation, these stimulants tend to relieve fatigue and increase alertness. They are a generally accepted part of our culture; however, with increased social awareness regarding the health risks asso-

TABLE 27–2	CNS Stimulants	
CATEGORIES	**GENERIC (TRADE) NAMES**	**COMMON STREET NAMES**
Amphetamines	Dextroamphetamine (Dexedrine)	Dexies, uppers, truck drivers
	Methamphetamine (Desoxyn)	Meth, speed, crystal, ice
	3,4-Methylenedioxyamphetamine (MDMA)*	Adam, Ecstasy, Eve, XTC
	Amphetamine + dextroamphetamine (Adderall)	
Nonamphetamine stimulants	Phendimetrazine (Prelu-2)	Diet pills
	Benzphetamine (Didrex)	
	Diethylpropion (Tenuate)	
	Phentermine (Adipex-P; Ionamin)	
	Sibutramine (Meridia)	
	Methylphenidate (Ritalin)	Speed, uppers
	Dexmethylphenidate (Focalin)	
	Pemoline (Cylert)	
	Modafinil (Provigil)	
Cocaine	Cocaine hydrochloride	Coke, blow, toot, snow, lady, flake, crack
Caffeine	Coffee, tea, colas, chocolate	Java, mud, brew, cocoa
Nicotine	Cigarettes, cigars, pipe tobacco, snuff	Weeds, fags, butts, chaw, cancer sticks

*Cross-listed with the hallucinogens.

ciated with nicotine, its use has become stigmatized in some circles.

The more potent stimulants, because of their potential for physiological dependency, are under regulation by the Controlled Substances Act. These controlled stimulants are available for therapeutic purposes by prescription only; however, they are also clandestinely manufactured and widely distributed on the illicit market.

Historical Aspects

Cocaine is the most potent stimulant derived from nature. It is extracted from the leaves of the coca plant, which has been cultivated in the Andean highlands of South America since prehistoric times. Natives of the region chew the leaves of the plant for refreshment and relief from fatigue.

The coca leaves must be mixed with lime to release the cocaine alkaloid. The chemical formula for the pure form of the drug was obtained in 1960. Physicians began using the drug as an anesthetic in eye, nose, and throat surgeries. It has also been used therapeutically in the United States in a morphine–cocaine elixir designed to relieve the suffering associated with terminal illness. These therapeutic uses are now obsolete.

Cocaine has achieved a degree of acceptability within some social circles. It is illicitly distributed as a white crystalline powder, often mixed with other ingredients to increase its volume and, therefore, create more profits. The drug is most commonly "snorted," and chronic users may manifest symptoms that resemble the congested nose of a common cold. The intensely pleasurable effects of the drug create the potential for extraordinary psychological dependency.

Another form of cocaine commonly used in the United States, called "crack," is a cocaine alkaloid that is extracted from its powdered hydrochloride salt by mixing it with sodium bicarbonate and allowing it to dry into small "rocks" (APA, 2000). Because this type of cocaine can be easily vaporized and inhaled, its effects have an extremely rapid onset.

Amphetamine was first prepared in 1887. Various derivatives of the drug soon followed, and clinical use of the drug began in 1927. Amphetamines were used quite extensively for medical purposes through the 1960s, but recognition of their abuse potential has sharply decreased clinical use. Today, they are prescribed only to treat narcolepsy (a rare disorder resulting in an uncontrollable desire for sleep), hyperactivity disorders in children, and in certain cases of obesity. Clandestine production of amphetamines for distribution on the illicit market has become a thriving business.

The earliest history of caffeine is unknown and is shrouded by legend and myth. Caffeine was first discovered in coffee in 1820 and 7 years later in tea. Both beverages have been widely accepted and enjoyed as a "pick-me-up" by many cultures.

Tobacco was used by the aborigines from remote times. Introduced in Europe in the mid-16th century, its use grew rapidly and soon became prevalent in the Orient. Tobacco came to America with the settlement of the earliest colonies. Today, it is grown in many countries of the world, and although smoking is decreasing in most industrialized nations, it is increasing in the developing areas (APA, 2000).

Patterns of Use/Abuse

Because of their pleasurable effects, CNS stimulants have a high abuse potential. In 2003, about 2.3 million Americans were current cocaine users (SAMHSA, 2005). Use was highest among Americans ages 19 to 25.

Many individuals who abuse or are dependent on CNS stimulants began using the substance for the appetite-suppressant effect in an attempt at weight control (APA, 2000). Higher and higher doses are consumed in an effort to maintain the pleasurable effects. With continued use, the pleasurable effects diminish, and there is a corresponding increase in dysphoric effects. There is a persistent craving for the substance, however, even in the face of unpleasant adverse effects from the continued drug taking.

CNS stimulant abuse and dependence are usually characterized by either episodic or chronic daily, or almost daily, use. Individuals who use the substances on an episodic basis often "binge" on the drug with very high dosages followed by a day or two of recuperation. This recuperation period is characterized by extremely intense and unpleasant symptoms (called a "crash").

The daily user may take large or small doses and may use the drug several times a day or only at a specific time during the day. The amount consumed usually increases over time as tolerance occurs. Chronic users tend to rely on CNS stimulants to feel more powerful, more confident, and more decisive. They often fall into a pattern of taking "uppers" in the morning and "downers," such as alcohol or sleeping pills, at night.

The average American consumes two cups of coffee (about 200 mg of caffeine) per day. Caffeine is consumed in various amounts by 90 percent of the population. At a level of 500 to 600 mg of daily caffeine consumption, symptoms of anxiety, insomnia, and depression are not uncommon. It is also at this level that caffeine dependence and withdrawal can occur. Caffeine consumption is prevalent among children as well as adults. Table 27–3 lists some common sources of caffeine.

Next to caffeine, nicotine, an active ingredient in tobacco, is the most widely used psychoactive substance in U.S. society. Of the U.S. population, approximately 30 percent reported using a tobacco product in 2003 (SAMHSA, 2005). Since 1964, when the results of the first public health report on smoking were issued, the percentage of total smokers has been on the decline. The percentage of women and teenage smokers has declined more slowly than that of adult men, however. Approximately 400,000 people die annually because of tobacco use, and an estimated 60 percent of the direct health care costs in the United States go to treat tobacco-related illnesses (Sadock & Sadock, 2003).

Effects on the Body

The CNS stimulants are a group of pharmacological agents that are capable of exciting the entire nervous system. This is accomplished by increasing the activity or augmenting the capability of the neurotransmitter agents known to be directly involved in bodily activation and behavioral stimulation. Physiological responses vary markedly according to the potency and dosage of the drug.

CNS Effects. Stimulation of the CNS results in tremor, restlessness, anorexia, insomnia, agitation, and increased motor activity. Amphetamines, nonamphetamine stimulants, and cocaine produce increased alertness, decrease in fatigue, elation and euphoria, and subjective feelings of greater mental agility and muscular power. Chronic use of these drugs may result in compulsive behavior, paranoia, hallucinations, and aggressive behavior (*Street Drugs*, 2005).

Cardiovascular/Pulmonary Effects. Amphetamines can induce increased systolic and diastolic blood pressure, increased heart rate, and cardiac arrhythmias (*Street Drugs*, 2005). These drugs also relax bronchial smooth muscle.

Cocaine intoxication typically produces a rise in myocardial demand for oxygen and an increase in heart rate. Severe vasoconstriction may occur and can result in myocardial infarction, ventricular fibrillation, and sudden death. Inhaled cocaine can cause pulmonary hemorrhage, chronic bronchiolitis, and pneumonia. Nasal rhinitis is a result of chronic cocaine snorting.

Caffeine ingestion can result in increased heart rate, palpitations, extrasystoles, and cardiac arrhythmias. Caffeine induces dilation of pulmonary and general systemic blood vessels and constriction of cerebral blood vessels.

Nicotine stimulates the sympathetic nervous system, resulting in an increase in heart rate, blood pressure, and

TABLE 27–3	Common Sources of Caffeine
SOURCE	**CAFFEINE CONTENT (MG)**
Food and Beverages	
5–6 oz. brewed coffee	90–125
5–6 oz. instant coffee	60–90
5–6 oz. decaffeinated coffee	3
5–6 oz. brewed tea	70
5–6 oz. instant tea	45
8–12 oz. cola drinks	60
5–6 oz. cocoa	20
8 oz. chocolate milk	2–7
1 oz. chocolate bar	22
Prescription Medications	
APCs (aspirin, phenacetin, caffeine)	32
Cafergot	100
Darvon compound	32
Fiorinal	40
Migralam	100
Over-the-Counter Analgesics	
Anacin, Empirin, Midol, Vanquish	32
Excedrin Migraine (aspirin, acetaminophen, caffeine)	65
Over-the-Counter Stimulants	
No Doz Tablets	100
Vivarin	200
Caffedrine	250

cardiac contractility, thereby increasing myocardial oxygen consumption and demand for blood flow (Royal College of Physicians, 2000). Contractions of gastric smooth muscle associated with hunger are inhibited, thereby producing a mild anorectic effect.

Gastrointestinal and Renal Effects. Gastrointestinal (GI) effects of amphetamines are somewhat unpredictable; however, a decrease in GI tract motility commonly results in constipation. Contraction of the bladder sphincter makes urination difficult. Caffeine exerts a diuretic effect on the kidneys. Nicotine stimulates the hypothalamus to release antidiuretic hormone, reducing the excretion of urine. Because nicotine increases the tone and activity of the bowel, it may occasionally cause diarrhea.

Most CNS stimulants induce a small rise in metabolic rate and various degrees of anorexia. Amphetamines and cocaine can cause a rise in body temperature.

Sexual Functioning. CNS stimulants apparently promote the coital urge in both men and women. Women, more than men, report that stimulants make them feel sexier and have more orgasms. In fact, some men may experience sexual dysfunction with the use of stimulants. For the majority of individuals, however, these drugs exert a powerful aphrodisiac effect.

CNS Stimulant Intoxication

CNS stimulant intoxication produces maladaptive behavioral and psychological changes that develop during, or shortly after, use of these drugs. Amphetamine and cocaine intoxication typically produces euphoria or affective blunting; changes in sociability; hypervigilance; interpersonal sensitivity; anxiety, tension, or anger; stereotyped behaviors; or impaired judgment. Physical effects include tachycardia or bradycardia, pupillary dilation, elevated or lowered blood pressure, perspiration or chills, nausea or vomiting, weight loss, psychomotor agitation or retardation, muscular weakness, respiratory depression, chest pain, cardiac arrhythmias, confusion, seizures, dyskinesias, dystonias, or coma (APA, 2000).

Intoxication from caffeine usually occurs following consumption in excess of 250 mg. Symptoms include restlessness, nervousness, excitement, insomnia, flushed face, diuresis, GI disturbance, muscle twitching, rambling flow of thought and speech, tachycardia or cardiac arrhythmia, periods of inexhaustibility, and psychomotor agitation (APA, 2000).

CNS Stimulant Withdrawal

CNS stimulant withdrawal is the presence of a characteristic withdrawal syndrome that develops within a few hours to several days after cessation of, or reduction in, heavy and prolonged use (APA, 2000). Withdrawal from amphetamines and cocaine cause dysphoria, fatigue, vivid unpleasant dreams, insomnia or hypersomnia, increased appetite, and psychomotor retardation or agitation (APA, 2000). The *DSM-IV-TR* states:

> Marked withdrawal symptoms ('crashing') often follow an episode of intense, high-dose use (a "speed run"). This "crash" is characterized by intense and unpleasant feelings of lassitude and depression, generally requiring several days of rest and recuperation. Weight loss commonly occurs during heavy stimulant use, whereas a marked increase in appetite with rapid weight gain is often observed during withdrawal. Depressive symptoms may last several days to weeks and may be accompanied by suicidal ideation. (p. 227)

The *DSM-IV-TR* does not include a diagnosis of caffeine withdrawal. Sadock and Sadock (2003) state that a number of well controlled research studies indicate that caffeine withdrawal exists, however. They cite the following symptoms as typical: headache, fatigue, anxiety, irritability, depression, impaired psychomotor performance, nausea, vomiting, craving for caffeine, and muscle pain and stiffness.

Withdrawal from nicotine results in dysphoric or depressed mood; insomnia; irritability, frustration, or anger; anxiety; difficulty concentrating; restlessness; decreased heart rate; and increased appetite or weight gain (APA, 2000). A mild syndrome of nicotine withdrawal can appear when a smoker switches from regular cigarettes to low-nicotine cigarettes (Sadock & Sadock, 2003).

Inhalant Abuse and Dependence

A Profile of the Substance

Inhalant disorders are induced by inhaling the aliphatic and aromatic hydrocarbons found in substances such as fuels, solvents, adhesives, aerosol propellants, and paint thinners. Specific examples of these substances include gasoline, varnish remover, lighter fluid, airplane glue, rubber cement, cleaning fluid, spray paint, shoe conditioner, and typewriter correction fluid (Sadock & Sadock, 2003).

Patterns of Use/Abuse

Inhalant substances are readily available, legal, and inexpensive. These three factors make inhalants the drug of choice among poor people and among children and young adults. Use may begin by ages 9 to 12 and peak in the adolescent years; it is less common after age 35 (APA, 2000). A national government survey of drug use indicated that 9.7 percent of people in the United States acknowledged ever having used inhalants (SAMHSA, 2003). The highest use was seen in the 12- to 25-year-old age group.

Methods of use include "huffing"—a procedure in which a rag soaked with the substance is applied to the mouth and nose and the vapors breathed in. Another common method is called "bagging" in which the substance is placed in a paper or plastic bag and inhaled from the bag by the user. They may also be inhaled directly from the container or sprayed in the mouth or nose.

Sadock and Sadock (2003) report that:

> Inhalant use among adolescents may be most common in those whose parents or older siblings use illegal substances. Inhalant use among adolescents is also associated with an increased likelihood of conduct disorder or antisocial personality disorder. (p. 441)

Tolerance to inhalants has been reported with heavy use. A mild withdrawal syndrome has been documented but does not appear to be clinically significant (APA, 2000).

Children with inhalant disorder may use inhalants several times a week, often on weekends and after school (APA, 2000). Adults with inhalant dependence may use the substance at varying times during each day, or they may binge on the substance during a period of several days.

Effects on the Body

Inhalants are absorbed through the lungs and reach the CNS very rapidly. Inhalants generally act as a CNS depressant (Sadock & Sadock, 2003). The effects are relatively brief, lasting from several minutes to a few hours, depending on the specific substance and amount consumed.

Central Nervous System. Inhalants can cause both central and peripheral nervous system damage, which may be permanent (APA, 2000). Neurological deficits, such as generalized weakness and peripheral neuropathies, may be evident. Other CNS effects that have been reported with heavy inhalant use include cerebral atrophy, cerebellar degeneration, and white matter lesions resulting in cranial nerve or pyramidal tract signs.

Respiratory Effects. The *DSM-IV-TR* reports the following respiratory effects with inhalant use: upper- or lower-airway irritation, including increased airway resistance; pulmonary hypertension; acute respiratory distress; coughing; sinus discharge; dyspnea; rales; or rhonchi. Rarely, cyanosis may result from pneumonitis or asphyxia. Death may occur from respiratory or cardiovascular depression.

Gastrointestinal Effects. Abdominal pain, nausea, and vomiting may occur. A rash may be present around the individual's nose and mouth. Unusual breath odors are common.

Renal System Effects. Chronic renal failure, hepatorenal syndrome, and proximal renal tubular acidosis have been reported (APA, 2000).

Inhalant Intoxication

The *DSM-IV-TR* defines inhalant intoxication as "clinically significant maladaptive behavioral or psychological changes (e.g., belligerence, assaultiveness, apathy, impaired judgment, impaired social or occupational functioning) that developed during or shortly after, use of or exposure to volatile inhalants." Two or more of the following signs are present:

1. Dizziness
2. Nystagmus
3. Incoordination
4. Slurred speech
5. Unsteady gait
6. Lethargy
7. Depressed reflexes
8. Psychomotor retardation
9. Tremor
10. Generalized muscle weakness
11. Blurred vision or diplopia
12. Stupor or coma
13. Euphoria

The symptoms are not due to a general medical condition and are not better accounted for by another mental disorder.

Opioid Abuse and Dependence

A Profile of the Substance

The term *opioid* refers to a group of compounds that includes opium, opium derivatives, and synthetic substitutes. Opioids exert both a sedative and an analgesic effect, and their major medical uses are for the relief of pain, the treatment of diarrhea, and the relief of coughing. These drugs have addictive qualities; that is, they are capable of inducing tolerance and physiological and psychological dependence.

Opioids are popular drugs of abuse in that they desensitize an individual to both psychological and physiological pain and induce a sense of euphoria. Lethargy and indifference to the environment are common manifestations.

Opioid abusers usually spend much of their time nourishing their habit. Individuals who are opioid dependent are seldom able to hold a steady job that will support their need. They must therefore secure funds from friends, relatives, or whomever they have not yet alienated with their dependency-related behavior. It is not uncommon for individuals who are opioid-dependent to resort to illegal means of obtaining funds, such as burglary, robbery, prostitution, or selling drugs.

Methods of administration of opioid drugs include oral, snorting, or smoking, and by subcutaneous, intramuscular, and intravenous injection. A selected list of opioid substances is presented in Table 27–4.

Under close supervision, opioids are indispensable in the practice of medicine. They are the most effective agents known for the relief of intense pain. They also induce a pleasurable effect on the CNS, however, that promotes their abuse. The physiological and psychological dependence that occurs with opioids, as well as the development of profound tolerance, contribute to the addict's ongoing quest for more of the substance, regardless of the means.

TABLE 27–4	Opioids and Related Substances	
CATEGORIES	**GENERIC (TRADE) NAMES**	**COMMON STREET NAMES**
Opioids of natural origin	Opium (ingredient in various antidiarrheal agents)	Black stuff, poppy, tar, big O
	Morphine (Astramorph)	M, white stuff, Miss Emma
	Codeine (ingredient in various analgesics and cough suppressants)	Terp, schoolboy, syrup, cody
Opioid derivatives	Heroin	H, horse, junk, brown sugar, smack, skag, TNT, Harry
	Hydromorphone (Dilaudid)	DLs, 4s, lords, little D
	Oxycodone (Percodan; OxyContin)	Perks, perkies, Oxy, O.C.
	Hydrocodone (Vicodin)	Vike
Synthetic opiate-like drugs	Meperidine (Demerol)	Doctors
	Methadone (Dolophine)	Dollies, done
	Propoxyphene (Darvon)	Pinks and grays
	Pentazocine (Talwin)	Ts
	Fentanyl (Actiq; Duragesic)	Apache, China girl, China town, dance fever, goodfella, jackpot

Historical Aspects

Opium is the Greek word for "juice." In its crude form, opium is a brownish black, gummy substance obtained from the ripened pods of the opium poppy. References to the use of opiates have been found in the Egyptian, Greek, and Arabian cultures as early as 3000 B.C. The drug became widely used both medicinally and recreationally throughout Europe during the 16th and 17th centuries. Most of the opium supply came from China, where the drug was introduced by Arabic traders in the late 17th century. Morphine, the primary active ingredient of opium, was isolated in 1803 by the European chemist Frederich Serturner. Since that time, morphine, rather than crude opium, has been used throughout the world for the medical treatment of pain and diarrhea (Julien, 2005). This process was facilitated in 1853 by the development of the hypodermic syringe, which made it possible to deliver the undiluted morphine quickly into the body for rapid relief from pain.

This development also created a new variety of opiate user in the United States: one who was able to self-administer the drug by injection. During this time, there was also a large influx of Chinese immigrants into the United States, who introduced opium smoking to this country. By the early part of the 20th century, opium addiction was widespread.

In response to the concerns over widespread addiction, in 1914 the U.S. government passed the Harrison Narcotic Act, which created strict controls on the accessibility of opiates. Until that time, these substances had been freely available to the public without a prescription. The Harrison Act banned the use of opiates for other than medicinal purposes and drove the use of heroin underground. To this day, the beneficial uses of these substances are widely acclaimed within the medical profession, but the illicit trafficking of the drugs for recreational purposes continues to resist most efforts aimed at control.

Patterns of Use/Abuse

The development of opioid abuse and dependence may follow one of two typical behavior patterns. The first occurs in the individual who has obtained the drug by prescription from a physician for the relief of a medical problem. Abuse and dependency occur when the individual increases the amount and frequency of use, justifying the behavior as symptom treatment. He or she becomes obsessed with obtaining increasing amounts of the substance, seeking out several physicians in order to replenish and maintain supplies.

The second pattern of behavior associated with abuse and dependency of opioids occurs among individuals who use the drugs for recreational purposes and obtain them from illegal sources. Opioids may be used alone to induce the euphoric effects or in combination with stimulants or other drugs to enhance the euphoria or to counteract the depressant effects of the opioid. Tolerance develops and dependency occurs, leading the individual to procure the substance by whatever means is required to support the habit. SAMHSA (2003) reports:

Since the mid-1990s, the prevalence of lifetime heroin use increased for both youths and young adults. From 1995 to 2002, the rate among youths aged 12 to 17 increased from 0.1 to 0.4 percent; among young adults aged 18 to 25, the rate rose from 0.8 to 1.6 percent. During the latter half of the 1990s, the annual number of heroin initiates rose to a level not reached since the late 1970s. In 1974, there were an estimated 246,000 heroin initiates. Between 1988 and 1994, the annual number of new users ranged from 28,000 to 80,000. Between 1995 and 2001, the number of new heroin users was consistently greater than 100,000. Data suggest that there has been a rise in heroin use in recent years and that this rise has occurred among younger persons who are smoking or sniffing heroin rather than injecting. Some indicators exhibit an overall rise in heroin use, some display a rise in heroin use among youth, college students, and adolescents in small metropolitan areas, and others suggest that new users tend to smoke or sniff rather than inject. In addition, there is some evidence that the time between first use of marijuana and first use of heroin is decreasing.

Effects on the Body

Opiates are sometimes classified as *narcotic analgesics*. They exert their major effects primarily on the CNS, the eyes, and the GI tract. Chronic morphine use or acute morphine toxicity is manifested by a syndrome of sedation, chronic constipation, decreased respiratory rate, and pinpoint pupils. Intensity of symptoms is largely dose dependent. The following physiological effects are common with opioid use.

Central Nervous System. All opioids, opioid derivatives, and synthetic opioid-like drugs affect the CNS. Common manifestations include euphoria, mood changes, and mental clouding. Other common CNS effects include drowsiness and pain reduction. Pupillary constriction occurs in response to stimulation of the oculomotor nerve. CNS depression of the respiratory centers within the medulla results in respiratory depression. The antitussive response is due to suppression of the cough center within the medulla. The nausea and vomiting commonly associated with opiate ingestion is related to the stimulation of the centers within the medulla that trigger this response.

Gastrointestinal Effects. These drugs exert a profound effect on the GI tract. Both stomach and intestinal tone are increased, whereas peristaltic activity of the intestines is diminished. These effects lead to a marked decrease in the movement of food through the GI tract. This is a notable therapeutic effect in the treatment of severe diarrhea. In fact, no drugs have yet been developed that are more effective than the opioids for this purpose. However, constipation, and even fecal impaction, may be a serious problem for the chronic opioid user.

Cardiovascular Effects. In therapeutic doses, opioids have minimal effect on the action of the heart. Morphine is used extensively to relieve pulmonary edema and the pain of myocardial infarction in cardiac clients. At high doses, opioids induce hypotension, which may be caused by direct action on the heart or by opioid-induced histamine release.

Sexual Functioning. With opioids, there is decreased sexual function and diminished libido (Bruckenthal, 2001). Retarded ejaculation, impotence, and orgasm failure (in both men and women) may occur. Sexual side effects from opioids appear to be largely influenced by dosage.

Opioid Intoxication

Opioid intoxication constitutes clinically significant maladaptive behavioral or psychological changes that develop during, or shortly after, opioid use (APA, 2000).

Symptoms include initial euphoria followed by apathy, dysphoria, psychomotor agitation or retardation, and impaired judgment. Physical symptoms include pupillary constriction (or dilation due to anoxia from severe overdose), drowsiness, slurred speech, and impairment in attention or memory (APA, 2000). Symptoms are consistent with the half-life of most opioid drugs, and usually last for several hours. Severe opioid intoxication can lead to respiratory depression, coma, and even death.

Opioid Withdrawal

Opioid withdrawal produces a syndrome of symptoms that develops after cessation of, or reduction in, heavy and prolonged use of an opiate or related substance. Symptoms include dysphoric mood, nausea or vomiting, muscle aches, lacrimation or rhinorrhea, pupillary dilation, piloerection, sweating, abdominal cramping, diarrhea, yawning, fever, and insomnia. With short-acting drugs such as heroin, withdrawal symptoms occur within 6 to 12 hours after the last dose, peak within 1 to 3 days, and gradually subside over a period of 5 to 7 days (APA, 2000). With longer-acting drugs such as methadone, withdrawal symptoms begin within 1 to 3 days after the last dose and are complete in 10 to 14 days (Sadock & Sadock, 2003). Withdrawal from the ultra-short-acting meperidine begins quickly, reaches a peak in 8 to 12 hours, and is complete in 4 to 5 days (Sadock & Sadock, 2003).

Hallucinogen Abuse and Dependence

A Profile of the Substance

Hallucinogenic substances are capable of distorting an individual's perception of reality. They have the ability to alter sensory perception and induce hallucinations. For this reason they have sometimes been referred to as "mind expanding." Some of the manifestations have been likened to a psychotic break. The hallucinations experienced by an individual with schizophrenia, however, are most often auditory, whereas substance-induced hallucinations are usually visual (Mack, Franklin, & Frances, 2003). Perceptual distortions have been reported by some users as spiritual, as giving a sense of depersonalization (observing oneself having the experience), or as being at peace with self and the universe. Others, who describe their experiences as "bad trips," report feelings of panic and a fear of dying or going insane. A common danger reported with hallucinogenic drugs is that of "flashbacks," or a spontaneous recurrence of the hallucinogenic state without ingestion of the drug. These can occur months after the drug was last taken.

Recurrent use can produce tolerance, encouraging users to resort to higher and higher dosages. No evidence of physical dependence is detectable when the drug is withdrawn; however, recurrent use appears to induce

TABLE 27-5	Hallucinogens	
CATEGORIES	GENERIC (TRADE) NAMES	COMMON STREET NAMES
Naturally occurring hallucinogens	Mescaline (the primary active ingredient of the peyote cactus)	Cactus, mesc, mescal, half moon, big chief, bad seed, peyote
	Psilocybin and psilocin (active ingredients of *Psilocybe* mushrooms)	Magic mushroom, God's flesh, shrooms
	Ololiuqui (morning glory seeds)	Heavenly blue, pearly gates, flying saucers
Synthetic compounds	Lysergic acid diethylamide [LSD] (synthetically produced from a fungal substance found on rye or a chemical substance found in morning glory seeds)	Acid, cube, big D, California sunshine, microdots, blue dots, sugar, orange wedges, peace tablets, purple haze, cupcakes
	Dimethyltryptamine [DMT] and diethyltryptamine [DET] (chemical analogues of tryptamine)	Businessman's trip
	2,5-Dimethoxy-4-methylamphetamine [STP, DOM]	STP (serenity, tranquility, peace)
	Phencyclidine [PCP]	Angel dust, hog, peace pill, rocket fuel
	3,4-Methylene-dioxyamphetamine [MDMA]	XTC, Ecstasy, Adam, Eve
	Methoxy-amphetamine [MDA]	Love drug

a psychological dependence to the insight-inducing experiences that a user may associate with episodes of hallucinogen use (Sadock & Sadock, 2003). This psychological dependence varies according to the drug, the dose, and the individual user. Hallucinogens are highly unpredictable in the effects they may induce each time they are used.

Many of the hallucinogenic substances have structural similarities. Some are produced synthetically; others are natural products of plants and fungi. A selected list of hallucinogens is presented in Table 27-5.

Historical Aspects

Archeological data obtained with carbon-14 dating suggest that hallucinogens have been used as part of religious ceremonies and at social gatherings by Native Americans for as long as 7000 years (Goldstein, 2002). Use of the peyote cactus as part of religious ceremonies in the southwestern part of the United States still occurs today, although this ritual use has greatly diminished.

LSD was first synthesized in 1943 by Dr. Albert Hoffman (Goldstein, 2002). It was used as a clinical research tool to investigate the biochemical etiology of schizophrenia. It soon reached the illicit market, however, and its abuse began to overshadow the research effort.

The abuse of hallucinogens reached a peak in the late 1960s, waned during the 1970s, and returned to favor in the 1980s with the so-called designer drugs (e.g., 3,4-methylene-dioxyamphetamine [MDMA] and methoxy-amphetamine [MDA]). One of the most commonly abused hallucinogens today is PCP, even though many of its effects are perceived as undesirable. A number of deaths have been directly attributed to the use of PCP, and numerous accidental deaths have occurred as a result of overdose and of the behavioral changes the drug precipitates.

Several therapeutic uses of LSD have been proposed, including the treatment of chronic alcoholism and the

reduction of intractable pain such as occurs in malignant disease. A great deal more research is required regarding the therapeutic uses of LSD. At this time, there is no real evidence of the safety and efficacy of the drug in humans.

Patterns of Use/Abuse

Use of hallucinogens is usually episodic. Because cognitive and perceptual abilities are so markedly affected by these substances, the user must set aside time from normal daily activities for indulging in the consequences. The SAMHSA (2003) reports:

> The prevalence of lifetime hallucinogen use among youths aged 12 to 17 was at its highest level in 2001 (6.1 percent) but declined to 5.7 percent in 2002. Among young adults aged 18 to 25, use increased from 14.3 percent in 1992 to 24.2 percent in 2002. The increase in hallucinogen use in the 1990s appears to have been driven by the use of Ecstasy (i.e., MDMA).

The use of LSD does not lead to the development of physical dependence or withdrawal symptoms (Sadock & Sadock, 2003). However, tolerance does develop quickly and to a high degree. In fact, an individual who uses LSD repeatedly for a period of 3 to 4 days may develop complete tolerance to the drug. Recovery from the tolerance also occurs very rapidly (in 4 to 7 days), so that the individual is able to achieve the desired effect from the drug repeatedly and often.

PCP is usually taken episodically, in binges that can last for several days. Some chronic users take the substance daily, however. Physical dependence does not occur with PCP; however, psychological dependence characterized by craving for the drug has been reported in chronic users, as has the development of tolerance. Tolerance apparently develops quickly with frequent use.

Psilocybin is an ingredient of the *Psilocybe* mushroom indigenous to the United States and Mexico. Ingestion of these mushrooms produces an effect similar to that of

LSD but of a shorter duration. This hallucinogenic chemical can now be produced synthetically.

Mescaline is the only hallucinogenic compound used legally for religious purposes today by members of the Native American Church of the United States. It is the primary active ingredient of the peyote cactus. Neither physical nor psychological dependence occurs with the use of mescaline, although, as with other hallucinogens, tolerance can develop quickly with frequent use.

Among the very potent hallucinogens of the current drug culture are those that are categorized as derivatives of amphetamines. These include 2,5-dimethoxy-4-methylamphetamine (DOM, STP), MDMA, and MDA. At lower doses, these drugs produce the "high" associated with CNS stimulants. At higher doses, hallucinogenic effects occur. These drugs have existed for many years but were *rediscovered* only in the mid-1980s. Because of the rapid increase in recreational use, the Drug Enforcement Agency imposed an emergency classification of MDMA as a schedule I drug in 1985.

Effects on the Body

The effects produced by the various hallucinogenics are highly unpredictable. The variety of effects may be related to dosage, the mental state of the individual, and the environment in which the substance is used. Some common effects have been reported (APA, 2000; Julien, 2005; Sadock & Sadock, 2003):

PHYSIOLOGICAL EFFECTS

● Nausea and vomiting
● Chills
● Pupil dilation
● Increased pulse, blood pressure, and temperature
● Mild dizziness
● Trembling
● Loss of appetite
● Insomnia
● Sweating
● A slowing of respirations
● Elevation in blood sugar

PSYCHOLOGICAL EFFECTS

● Heightened response to color, texture, and sounds
● Heightened body awareness
● Distortion of vision
● Sense of slowing of time
● All feelings magnified: love, lust, hate, joy, anger, pain, terror, despair
● Fear of losing control
● Paranoia, panic
● Euphoria, bliss
● Projection of self into dreamlike images
● Serenity, peace

● Depersonalization
● Derealization
● Increased libido

The effects of hallucinogens are not always pleasurable for the user. Two types of toxic reactions are known to occur. The first is the *panic reaction*, or "bad trip." Symptoms include an intense level of anxiety, fear, and stimulation. The individual hallucinates and fears going insane. Paranoia and acute psychosis may be evident.

The second type of toxic reaction to hallucinogens is the *flashback*. This phenomenon refers to the transient, spontaneous repetition of a previous LSD-induced experience that occurs in the absence of the substance. Various studies have reported that a range from 15 to 80 percent of hallucinogen users report having experienced flashbacks (Sadock & Sadock, 2003).

Hallucinogen Intoxication

Symptoms of hallucinogen intoxication develop during, or shortly after (within minutes to a few hours) hallucinogen use (APA, 2000). Maladaptive behavioral or psychological changes include marked anxiety or depression, ideas of reference (a type of delusional thinking that all activity within one's environment is "referred to" [about] one's self), fear of losing one's mind, paranoid ideation, and impaired judgment. Perceptual changes occur in a state of full wakefulness and alertness and include intensification of perceptions, depersonalization, derealization, illusions, hallucinations, and synesthesias (APA, 2000). Physical symptoms include pupillary dilation, tachycardia, sweating, palpitations, blurring of vision, tremors, and incoordination (APA, 2000).

Symptoms of PCP intoxication develop within an hour of use (or less when it is smoked, snorted, or taken intravenously) (APA, 2000). Specific symptoms are dose related and include belligerence, assaultiveness, impulsiveness, unpredictability, psychomotor agitation, and impaired judgment. Physical symptoms include vertical or horizontal nystagmus, hypertension or tachycardia, numbness or diminished responsiveness to pain, ataxia, dysarthria, muscle rigidity, seizures or coma, and hyperacusis.

Cannabis Abuse and Dependence

A Profile of the Substance

Cannabis is second only to alcohol as the most widely abused drug in the United States. The major psychoactive ingredient of this class of substances is delta-9-tetrahydrocannabinol (THC). It occurs naturally in the plant *Cannabis sativa*, which grows readily in warm climates. Marijuana, the most prevalent type of cannabis preparation, is composed of the dried leaves, stems, and flowers of the plant. Hashish is a more potent concentrate of the resin derived from the flowering tops of the plant. Hash oil is a very concentrated form of THC made by boiling hashish in a solvent and filtering out the solid matter (*Street Drugs*, 2005). Cannabis products are usually smoked in the form of loosely rolled cigarettes. Cannabis can also be taken orally when it is prepared in food, but about two to three times the amount of cannabis must be ingested orally to equal the potency of that obtained by the inhalation of its smoke (Sadock & Sadock, 2003).

At moderate dosages, cannabis drugs produce effects resembling those of alcohol and other CNS depressants. By depressing higher brain centers, they release lower centers from inhibitory influences. There has been some controversy in the past over the classification of these substances. They are not narcotics, although they are legally classified as controlled substances. They are not hallucinogens, although in very high dosages they can induce hallucinations. They are not sedative-hypnotics, although they most closely resemble these substances. Like that of sedative-hypnotics, their action occurs in the ascending reticular activating system.

Psychological dependence has been shown to occur with cannabis and tolerance can occur. Controversy exists about whether physiological dependence occurs with cannabis. Sadock and Sadock (2003) state:

> Withdrawal symptoms in humans are limited to modest increases in irritability, restlessness, insomnia, and anorexia and mild nausea; all these symptoms appear only when a person abruptly stops taking high doses of cannabis. (p. 425)

Common cannabis preparations are presented in Table 27–6.

Historical Aspects

Products of *Cannabis sativa* have been used therapeutically for nearly 5000 years (Julien, 2005). Cannabis was first employed in China and India as an antiseptic and an analgesic. Its use later spread to the Middle East, Africa, and Eastern Europe.

In the United States, medical interest in the use of cannabis arose during the early part of the 19th century.

TABLE 27–6	Cannabinoids	
CATEGORY	COMMON PREPARATIONS	STREET NAMES
Cannabis	Marijuana	Joint, weed, pot, grass, Mary Jane, Texas tea, locoweed, MJ, hay, stick
	Hashish	Hash, bhang, ganja, charas

Many articles were published espousing its use for many and varied reasons. The drug was almost as commonly used for medicinal purposes as aspirin is today and could be purchased without a prescription in any drug store. It was purported to have antibacterial and anticonvulsant capabilities, decrease intraocular pressure, decrease pain, help in the treatment of asthma, increase appetite, and generally raise one's morale.

The drug went out of favor primarily because of the huge variation in potency within batches of medication caused by the variations in the THC content of different plants. Other medications were favored for their greater degree of solubility and faster onset of action than cannabis products. A federal law put an end to its legal use in 1937, after an association between marijuana and criminal activity became evident. In the 1960s, marijuana became the symbol of the "antiestablishment" generation, at which time it reached its peak as a drug of abuse.

Research continues in regard to the possible therapeutic uses of cannabis. It has been shown to be an effective agent for relieving the nausea and vomiting associated with cancer chemotherapy, when other antinausea medications fail. It has also been used in the treatment of chronic pain, glaucoma, multiple sclerosis, and acquired immune deficiency syndrome (Sadock & Sadock, 2003).

Advocates who praise the therapeutic usefulness and support the legalization of the cannabinoids persist within the United States today. Such groups as the Alliance for Cannabis Therapeutics (ACT) and the National Organization for the Reform of Marijuana Laws (NORML) have lobbied extensively to allow disease sufferers easier access to the drug. The medical use of marijuana has been legalized by a number of states. The U.S. Drug Enforcement Agency (DEA) (2003) states:

> Legalizing marijuana through the political process bypasses the safeguards established by the Food and Drug Administration to protect the public from dangerous or ineffective drugs. Every other prescribed drug must be tested according to scientifically rigorous protocols to ensure that it is safe and effective before it can be sold. The medical marijuana movement and its million-dollar media campaign have helped contribute to the changing attitude among our youth that marijuana use is harmless. Among marijuana's most harmful consequences is its role in leading to the use of other illegal drugs like heroin and cocaine. Long-term studies of students who use drugs show that very few young people use other illegal drugs without first trying marijuana. While not all people who use marijuana go on to use other drugs, using marijuana sometimes lowers inhibitions about drug use and exposes users to a culture that encourages use of other drugs.

A great deal more research is required to determine the long-term effects of the drug. Until results indicate otherwise, it is safe to assume that the harmful effects of the drug outweigh the benefits.

Patterns of Use/Abuse

In its 2003 National Survey on Drug Use and Health, SAMHSA (2005) reported that an estimated 19.5 million Americans aged 12 years or older were current illicit drug users, meaning they had used an illicit drug during the month before the survey interview. This estimate represents 8.2 percent of the population aged 12 years old or older. Marijuana is the most commonly used illicit drug. In 2003, it was used by 75 percent of current illicit drug users. This constitutes about 14.6 million users of marijuana in the United States in the year 2003.

Many people incorrectly regard cannabis as a substance of low abuse potential. This lack of knowledge has promoted use of the substance by some individuals who believe it is harmless. Tolerance, although it tends to decline rapidly, does occur with chronic use. As tolerance develops, physical dependence also occurs, resulting in a mild withdrawal syndrome (as previously described) upon cessation of drug use.

One controversy that exists regarding marijuana is whether its use leads to the use of other illicit drugs. Sadock and Sadock (2003) state:

> Marijuana is the most widely used illicit drug among high school students. It has been termed a "gateway drug," because the strongest predictor of future cocaine use is frequent marijuana use during adolescence. (p. 1286)

Effects on the Body

Following is a summary of some of the effects that have been attributed to marijuana in recent years. Undoubtedly, as research continues, evidence of additional physiological and psychological effects will be made available.

Cardiovascular Effects. Cannabis ingestion induces tachycardia and orthostatic hypotension (National Institutes of Health [NIH], 2003). With the decrease in blood pressure, myocardial oxygen supply is decreased. Tachycardia in turn increases oxygen demand.

Respiratory Effects. Marijuana produces a greater amount of "tar" than its equivalent weight in tobacco. Because of the method by which marijuana is smoked— that is, the smoke is held in the lungs for as long as possible to achieve the desired effect—larger amounts of tar are deposited in the lungs, promoting deleterious effects on the lungs.

Although the initial reaction to the marijuana is bronchodilatation, thereby facilitating respiratory function, chronic use results in obstructive airway disorders (NIH, 2003). Frequent marijuana users often have laryngitis, bronchitis, cough, and hoarseness. Cannabis smoke contains more carcinogens than tobacco smoke, so lung damage and cancer are real risks for heavy users (Goldstein, 2002).

Reproductive Effects. Some studies have shown a decrease in levels of serum testosterone and abnormalities in sperm count, motility, and structure correlated with heavy marijuana use (NIH, 2003). In women, heavy marijuana use has been correlated with failure to ovulate, difficulty with lactation, and an increased risk of spontaneous abortion.

CNS Effects. Acute CNS effects of marijuana are dose related. Many people report a feeling of being "high"— the equivalent of being "drunk" on alcohol. Symptoms include feelings of euphoria, relaxed inhibitions, disorientation, depersonalization, and relaxation. At higher doses, sensory alterations may occur, including impairment in judgment of time and distance, recent memory, and learning ability. Physiological symptoms may include tremors, muscle rigidity, and conjunctival redness. Toxic effects are generally characterized by panic reactions. Very heavy usage has been shown to precipitate an acute psychosis that is self limited and short lived once the drug is removed from the body (Julien, 2005).

Heavy long-term cannabis use is also associated with a syndrome called *amotivational syndrome*. When this syndrome occurs, the individual is preoccupied with using the substance. Symptoms include lethargy, apathy, social and personal deterioration, and lack of motivation. This syndrome appears to be more common in countries in which the most potent preparations are used and where the substance is more freely available than it is in the United States.

Sexual Functioning. Marijuana is reported to enhance the sexual experience in both men and women. The intensified sensory awareness and the subjective slowness of time perception are thought to increase sexual satisfaction. Marijuana also enhances the sexual functioning by releasing inhibitions for certain activities that would normally be restrained.

Cannabis Intoxication

Cannabis intoxication is evidenced by the presence of clinically significant maladaptive behavioral or psychological changes that develop during, or shortly after, cannabis use (APA, 2000). Symptoms include impaired motor coordination, euphoria, anxiety, a sensation of slowed time, and impaired judgment. Physical symptoms include conjunctival injection, increased appetite, dry mouth, and tachycardia. The impairment of motor skills lasts for 8 to 12 hours and interferes with the operation of motor vehicles. These effects are additive to those of alcohol, which is commonly used in combination with cannabis (Sadock & Sadock, 2003).

Tables 27–7 and 27–8 include summaries of the psychoactive substances, including symptoms of intoxication, withdrawal, use, overdose, possible therapeutic uses, and trade and common names by which they may be referred. The dynamics of substance use disorders using the Transactional Model of Stress/Adaptation are presented in Figure 27–2.

TABLE 27–7   Psychoactive Substances: A Profile Summary

CLASS OF DRUGS	SYMPTOMS OF USE	THERAPEUTIC USES	SYMPTOMS OF OVERDOSE	TRADE NAMES	COMMON NAMES
CNS Depressants					
Alcohol	Relaxation, loss of inhibitions, lack of concentration, drowsiness, slurred speech, sleep	Antidote for methanol consumption; ingredient in many pharmacological concentrates	Nausea, vomiting; shallow respirations; cold, clammy skin; weak, rapid pulse; coma; possible death	Ethyl alcohol, beer, gin, rum, vodka, bourbon, whiskey, liqueurs, wine, brandy, sherry, champagne	Booze, alcohol, liquor, drinks, cocktails, highballs, nightcaps, high-balls, nightcaps, moonshine, white lightening, firewater
Other (barbiturates and nonbarbiturates)	Same as alcohol	Relief from anxiety and insomnia; as anticonvulsants and anesthetics	Anxiety, fever, agitation, hallucinations, disorientation, tremors, delirium, convulsions, possible death	Seconal, Nembutal, Amytal Valium Librium Noctec Miltown	Red birds, yellow birds, blue birds Blues/yellows Green & whites Mickies Downers
CNS Stimulants					
Amphetamines and related drugs	Hyperactivity, agitation, euphoria, insomnia, loss of appetite	Management of narcolepsy, hyperkinesia, and weight control	Cardiac arrhythmias, headache, convulsions, hypertension, rapid heart rate, coma, possible death	Dexedrine, Didrex, Tenuate, Prelu-2, Ritalin, Focalin, Cylert, Meridia, Provigil	Uppers, pep pills, wakeups, bennies, eye-openers, speed, black beauties, sweet As
Cocaine	Euphoria, hyperactivity, restlessness, talkativeness, increased pulse, dilated pupils, rhinitis		Hallucinations, convulsions, pulmonary edema, respiratory failure, coma, cardiac arrest, possible death	Cocaine hydrochloride	Coke, flake, snow, dust, happy dust, gold dust, girl, cecil, C, toot, blow, crack
Opioids	Euphoria, lethargy, drowsiness, lack of motivation, constricted pupils	As analgesics; methadone in substitution therapy; heroin has no therapeutic use	Shallow breathing, slowed pulse, clammy skin, pulmonary edema, respiratory arrest, convulsions, coma, possible death	Heroin Morphine Codeine Dilaudid Demerol Dolophine Percodan Talwin Opium	Snow, stuff, H, harry, horse M, morph, Miss Emma Schoolboy Lords Doctors Dollies Perkies Ts Big O, black stuff
Hallucinogens	Visual hallucinations, disorientation, confusion, paranoid delusions, euphoria, anxiety, panic, increased pulse	LSD has been proposed in the treatment of chronic alcoholism, and in the reduction of intractable pain	Agitation, extreme hyperactivity, violence, hallucinations, psychosis, convulsions, possible death	LSD PCP Mescaline DMT STP	Acid, cube, big D Angel dust, hog, peace pill Mesc Businessman's trip Serenity and peace
Cannabinols	Relaxation, talkativeness, lowered inhibitions, euphoria, mood swings	Marijuana has been used for relief of nausea and vomiting associated with antineoplastic chemotherapy and to reduce eye pressure in glaucoma	Fatigue, paranoia, delusions, hallucinations, possible psychosis	Cannabis Hashish	Marijuana, pot, grass, joint, Mary Jane, MJ Hash, rope, Sweet Lucy

TABLE 27–8   **Summary of Symptoms Associated with the Syndromes of Intoxication and Withdrawal**

CLASS OF DRUGS	INTOXICATION	WITHDRAWAL	COMMENTS
Alcohol	Aggressiveness, impaired judgment, impaired attention, irritability, euphoria, depression, emotional lability, slurred speech, incoordination, unsteady gait, nystagmus, flushed face	Tremors, nausea/vomiting, malaise, weakness, tachycardia, sweating, elevated blood pressure, anxiety, depressed mood, irritability, hallucinations, headache, insomnia, seizures	Alcohol withdrawal begins within 4–6 hr after last drink. May progress to delirium tremens on 2nd or 3rd day. Use of Librium or Serax is common for substitution therapy.
Amphetamines and related substances	Fighting, grandiosity, hypervigilance, psychomotor agitation, impaired judgment, tachycardia, pupillary dilation, elevated blood pressure, perspiration or chills, nausea and vomiting.	Anxiety, depressed mood, irritability, craving for the substance, fatigue, insomnia or hypersomnia, psychomotor agitation, paranoid and suicidal ideation.	Withdrawal symptoms usually peak within 2–4 days, although depression and irritability may persist for months. Antidepressants may be used.
Caffeine	Restlessness, nervousness, excitement, insomnia, flushed face, diuresis, gastrointestinal complaints, muscle twitching, rambling flow of thought and speech, cardiac arrhythmia, periods of inexhaustibility, psychomotor agitation	Headache	Caffeine is contained in coffee, tea, colas, cocoa, chocolate, some over-the-counter analgesics, "cold" preparations, and stimulants.
Cannabis	Euphoria, anxiety, suspiciousness, sensation of slowed time, impaired judgment, social withdrawal, tachycardia, conjunctival redness, increased appetite, hallucinations	Restlessness, irritability, insomnia, loss of appetite	Intoxication occurs immediately and lasts about 3 hours. Oral ingestion is more slowly absorbed and has longer-lasting effects.
Cocaine	Euphoria, fighting, grandiosity, hypervigilance, psychomotor agitation, impaired judgment, tachycardia, elevated blood pressure, pupillary dilation, perspiration or chills, nausea/vomiting, hallucinations, delirium	Depression, anxiety, irritability, fatigue, insomnia or hypersomnia, psychomotor agitation, paranoid or suicidal ideation, apathy, social withdrawal	Large doses of the drug can result in convulsions or death from cardiac arrhythmias or respiratory paralysis.
Inhalants	Belligerence, assaultiveness, apathy, impaired judgment, dizziness, nystagmus, slurred speech, unsteady gait, lethargy, depressed reflexes, tremor, blurred vision, stupor or coma, euphoria, irritation around eyes, throat, and nose		Intoxication occurs within 5 minutes of inhalation. Symptoms last 60–90 min. Large doses can result in death from CNS depression or cardiac arrhythmia.
Nicotine		Craving for the drug, irritability, anger, frustration, anxiety, difficulty concentrating, restlessness, decreased heart rate, increased appetite, weight gain, tremor, headaches, insomnia	Symptoms of withdrawal begin within 24 hours of last drug use and decrease in intensity over days, weeks, or sometimes longer.
Opioids	Euphoria, lethargy, somnolence, apathy, dysphoria, impaired judgment, pupillary constriction, drowsiness, slurred speech, constipation, nausea, decreased respiratory rate and blood pressure	Craving for the drug, nausea/vomiting, muscle aches, lacrimation or rhinorrhea, pupillary dilation, piloerection or sweating, diarrhea, yawning, fever, insomnia	Withdrawal symptoms appear within 6–8 hours after last dose, reach a peak in the 2nd or 3rd day, and disappear in 7–10 days. Times are shorter with meperidine and longer with methadone.
Phencyclidine and related substances	Belligerence, assaultiveness, impulsiveness, psychomotor agitation, impaired judgment, nystagmus, increased heart rate and blood pressure, diminished pain response, ataxia, dysarthria, muscle rigidity, seizures, hyperacusis, delirium		Delirium can occur within 24 hours after use of phencyclidine, or may occur up to a week following recovery from an overdose of the drug.
Sedatives, hypnotics, and anxiolytics	Disinhibition of sexual or aggressive impulses, mood lability, impaired judgment, slurred speech, incoordination, unsteady gait, impairment in attention or memory disorientation, confusion	Nausea/vomiting, malaise, weakness, tachycardia, sweating, anxiety, irritability, orthostatic hypotension, tremor, insomnia, seizures	Withdrawal may progress to delirium, usually within 1 week of last use. Long-acting barbiturates or benzodiazepines may be used in withdrawal substitution therapy.

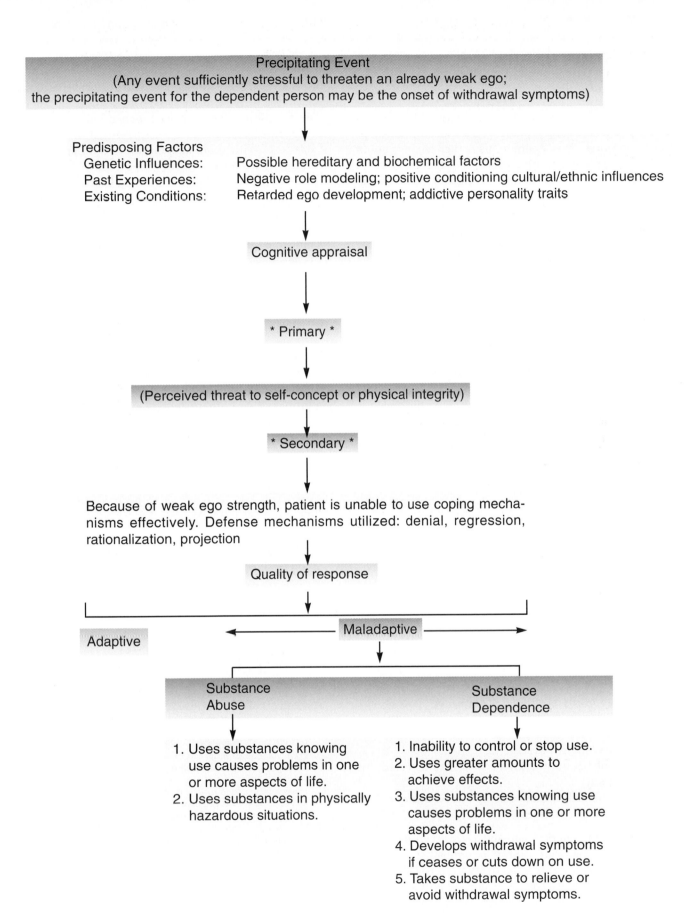

Precipitating Event
(Any event sufficiently stressful to threaten an already weak ego;
the precipitating event for the dependent person may be the onset of withdrawal symptoms)

Predisposing Factors
  Genetic Influences: Possible hereditary and biochemical factors
  Past Experiences: Negative role modeling; positive conditioning cultural/ethnic influences
  Existing Conditions: Retarded ego development; addictive personality traits

Cognitive appraisal

* Primary *

(Perceived threat to self-concept or physical integrity)

* Secondary *

Because of weak ego strength, patient is unable to use coping mechanisms effectively. Defense mechanisms utilized: denial, regression, rationalization, projection

Quality of response

Adaptive   Maladaptive

Substance   Substance
Abuse   Dependence

1. Uses substances knowing   1. Inability to control or stop use.
   use causes problems in one   2. Uses greater amounts to
   or more aspects of life.   achieve effects.
2. Uses substances in physically   3. Uses substances knowing use
   hazardous situations.   causes problems in one or more
                                        aspects of life.
                                     4. Develops withdrawal symptoms
                                        if ceases or cuts down on use.
                                     5. Takes substance to relieve or
                                        avoid withdrawal symptoms.

FIGURE 27–2   The dynamics of substance use disorders using the transactional model of stress/adaptation.

APPLICATION OF THE NURSING PROCESS

Assessment

In the pre-introductory phase of relationship development, the nurse must examine his or her feelings about working with a client who abuses substances. If these behaviors are viewed as morally wrong and the nurse has internalized these attitudes from very early in life, it may be very difficult to suppress judgmental feelings. The role that alcohol or other substances has played (or plays) in the life of the nurse will most certainly affect the way in which he or she approaches interaction with the substance-abusing client.

How are attitudes examined? Some individuals may have sufficient ability for introspection to be able to recognize on their own whether they have unresolved issues related to substance abuse. For others, it may be more helpful to discuss these issues in a group situation, where insight may be gained from feedback regarding the perceptions of others.

Whether alone or in a group, the nurse may gain a greater understanding about attitudes and feelings related to substance abuse by responding to the following types of questions. As written here, the questions are specific to alcohol, but they could be adapted for any substance.

What are my drinking patterns?
If I drink, why do I drink? When, where, and how much?
If I don't drink, why do I abstain?
Am I comfortable with my drinking patterns?
If I decided not to drink any more, would that be a problem for me?
What did I learn from my parents about drinking?
Have my attitudes changed as an adult?
What are my feelings about people who become intoxicated?
Does it seem more acceptable for some individuals than for others?
Do I ever use terms like "sot," "drunk," or "boozer," to describe some individuals who overindulge, yet overlook it in others?
Do I ever overindulge myself?
Has the use of alcohol (by myself or others) affected my life in any way?
Do I see alcohol/drug abuse as a sign of weakness? A moral problem? An illness?

Unless nurses fully understand and accept their own attitudes and feelings, they cannot be empathetic toward clients' problems. Clients in recovery need to know they are accepted for themselves, regardless of past behaviors. Nurses must be able to separate the client from the behavior and to accept that individual with unconditional positive regard.

Assessment Tools

Nurses are often the individuals who perform the admission interview. A variety of assessment tools are appropriate for use in chemical dependency units. A nursing history and assessment tool was presented in Chapter 9 of this text. With some adaptation, it is an appropriate instrument for creating a database on clients who abuse substances. Table 27–9 presents a drug history and assessment that could be used in conjunction with the general biopsychosocial assessment.

Other screening tools exist for determining whether an individual has a problem with substances. Two such tools developed by the American Psychiatric Association for the diagnosis of alcoholism include the Michigan Alcoholism Screening Test and the CAGE Questionnaire (Tables 27–10 and 27–11). Some psychiatric units administer these surveys to all clients who are admitted to help determine if there is a secondary alcoholism problem in addition to the psychiatric problem for which the client is being admitted (sometimes called **dual diagnosis**). It would be possible to adapt these tools to use in diagnosing problems with other drugs as well.

Dual Diagnosis

If it is determined that the client has a coexisting substance disorder and mental illness, he or she may be

---

TABLE 27–9	Drug History and Assessment*

1. When you were growing up, did anyone in your family drink alcohol or take other kinds of drugs?
2. If so, how did the substance use affect the family situation?
3. When did you have your first drink/drugs?
4. How long have you been drinking/taking drugs on a regular basis?
5. What is your pattern of substance use?
   a. When do you use substances?
   b. What do you use?
   c. How much do you use?
   d. Where are you and with whom when you use substances?
6. When did you have your last drink/drug? What was it and how much did you consume?
7. Does using the substance(s) cause problems for you? Describe. Include family, friends, job, school, other.
8. Have you ever experienced injury as a result of substance use?
9. Have you ever been arrested or incarcerated for drinking/using drugs?
10. Have you ever tried to stop drinking/using drugs? If so, what was the result? Did you experience any physical symptoms, such as tremors, headache, insomnia, sweating, or seizures?
11. Have you ever experienced loss of memory for times when you have been drinking/using drugs?
12. Describe a typical day in your life.
13. Are there any changes you would like to make in your life? If so, what?
14. What plans or ideas do you have for seeing that these changes occur?

*To be used in conjunction with general biopsychosocial nursing history and assessment tool (Chapter 9).

TABLE 27–10	Michigan Alcoholism Screening Test (MAST)		

Answer the following questions by placing an X under yes or no.*	Yes	No
1. Do you enjoy a drink now and then?	0	0
2. Do you feel you are a normal drinker? (By normal we mean you drink less than or as much as most people.)		2
3. Have you ever awakened the morning after some drinking the night before and found that you could not remember a part of the evening?	2	
4. Does your wife, husband, parent, or other near relative ever worry or complain about your drinking?	1	
5. Can you stop drinking without a struggle after one or two drinks?		2
6. Do you ever feel guilty about your drinking?	1	
7. Do friends or relatives think you are a normal drinker?		2
8. Are you able to stop drinking when you want to?		2
9. Have you ever attended a meeting of Alcoholics Anonymous (AA)?	5	
10. Have you gotten into physical fights when drinking?	1	
11. Has your drinking ever created problems between you and your wife, husband, a parent, or other relative?	2	
12. Has your wife, husband, or another family member ever gone to anyone for help about your drinking?	2	
13. Have you ever lost friends because of your drinking?	2	
14. Have you ever gotten into trouble at work or school because of drinking?	2	
15. Have you ever lost a job because of drinking?	2	
16. Have you ever neglected your obligations, your family, or your work for 2 or more days in a row because you were drinking?	2	
17. Do you drink before noon fairly often?	1	
18. Have you ever been told you have liver trouble? Cirrhosis?	2	
19. After heavy drinking have you ever had delirium tremens (DTs) or severe shaking or heard voices or seen things that really were not there?	5	
20. Have you ever gone to anyone for help about your drinking?	5	
21. Have you ever been in a hospital because of drinking?	5	
22. Have you ever been a patient in a psychiatric hospital or on a psychiatric ward of a general hospital where drinking was part of the problem that resulted in hospitalization?	2	
23. Have you ever been seen at a psychiatric or mental health clinic or gone to any doctor, social worker, or clergyman for help with any emotional problem, where drinking was part of the problem?	2	
24. Have you ever been arrested for drunk driving, driving while intoxicated, or driving under the influence of alcoholic beverages? (If yes, how many times?____)	2 ea	
25. Have you ever been arrested, or taken into custody, even for a few hours, because of other drunk behavior? (If yes, how many times?____)	2 ea	

*Items are scored under the response that would indicate a problem with alcohol.
Method of scoring: 0—3 points = no problem with alcohol
4 points = possible problem with alcohol
5 or more = indicates problem with alcohol

SOURCE: From Selzer, M.L.: The Michigan alcohol screening test: The quest for a new diagnostic instrument. *American Journal of Psychiatry* (1971), *127*, 1653–1658. With permission.

assigned to a special program that targets both problems. Counseling for the mentally ill person who abuses substances takes a different approach than that which is directed at individuals who abuse substances but are not mentally ill. In the latter, many counselors use direct confrontation of the substance use behaviors. This approach is thought to be detrimental to the treatment of a chronically mentally ill person (Mack, Franklin, & Frances, 2003). Most dual diagnosis programs take a more supportive and less confrontational approach.

Peer support groups are an important part of the treatment program. Group members offer encouragement and practical advice to each other. Psychodynamic therapy can be useful for some individuals with dual diagnosis by delving into the personal history of how psychiatric disorders and substance abuse have reinforced one another and how the cycle can be broken (Harvard Medical School, 2003). Cognitive and behavioral therapies are helpful in training clients to monitor moods and thought patterns that lead to substance abuse. With these therapies, clients also learn to avoid substance use and to cope with cravings and the temptation to relapse (Harvard Medical School, 2003).

Individuals with dual diagnoses should be encouraged to attend 12-step recovery programs (e.g., Alcoholics

TABLE 27–11	The CAGE Questionnaire

1. Have you ever felt you should *C*ut down on your drinking?
2. Have people *A*nnoyed you by criticizing your drinking?
3. Have you ever felt bad or *G*uilty about your drinking?
4. Have you ever had a drink first thing in the morning to steady your nerves or get rid of a hangover (*E*ye-opener)?

Scoring: 2 or 3 "yes" answers strongly suggest a problem with alcohol.

SOURCE: From Mayfield, D., McLeod, G., & Hall, P. (1974), with permission.

Anonymous or Narcotics Anonymous). Dual diagnosis clients are sometimes resistant to attending 12-step programs, and they often do better in groups specifically designed for people with psychiatric disorders.

Substance abuse groups are usually integrated into regular programming for the psychiatric client with a dual diagnosis. An individual in a psychiatric facility or day treatment program will attend a substance abuse group periodically in lieu of another scheduled activity therapy. Topics are directed toward areas that are unique to clients with a mental illness, such as mixing medications with other substances, as well as topics that are common to primary substances abusers. Individuals are encouraged to discuss their personal problems.

Mack, Franklin, and Frances (2003) state:

> The dual diagnosis patient often falls through the cracks of the treatment system. Severe psychiatric disorders often preclude full treatment in substance abuse clinics or self-help groups. The addition of other Axis I, II, and III disorders to a substance use disorder greatly complicates diagnosis and makes treatment more difficult. (p. 359)

Continued attendance at 12-step group meetings is encouraged on discharge from treatment. Family involvement is enlisted, and preventive strategies are outlined. Individual case management is common and success is often promoted by this close supervision.

Diagnosis/Outcome Identification

The next step in the nursing process is to identify appropriate nursing diagnoses by analyzing the data collected during the assessment phase. The individual who abuses or is dependent on substances undoubtedly has many unmet physical and emotional needs. Possible nursing diagnoses for clients with substance-related disorders include:

Ineffective denial related to weak, underdeveloped ego evidenced by "I don't have problem with (substance). I can quit any time I want to."

Ineffective coping related to inadequate coping skills and weak ego evidenced by use of substances as a coping mechanism.

Imbalanced nutrition: Less than body requirements/deficient fluid volume related to drinking or taking drugs instead of eating, evidenced by loss of weight, pale conjunctiva and mucous membranes, poor skin turgor, electrolyte imbalance, anemias, and other signs and symptoms of malnutrition/dehydration.

Risk for infection related to malnutrition and altered immune condition.

Low self-esteem related to weak ego, lack of positive feedback evidenced by criticism of self and others and use of substances as a coping mechanism (self-destructive behavior).

Deficient knowledge (effects of substance abuse on the body) related to denial of problems with substances evidenced by abuse of substances.

For the client in substance withdrawal, possible nursing diagnoses include:

Risk for injury related to CNS agitation (withdrawal from CNS depressants).

Risk for suicide related to depressed mood (withdrawal from CNS stimulants).

The following criteria may be used for measurement of outcomes in the care of the client with substance-related disorders.

The client:

1. Has not experienced physical injury.
2. Has not caused harm to self or others.
3. Accepts responsibility for own behavior.
4. Acknowledges association between personal problems and use of substance(s).
5. Demonstrates more adaptive coping mechanisms that can be used in stressful situations (instead of taking substances).
6. Shows no signs or symptoms of infection or malnutrition.
7. Exhibits evidence of increased self-worth by attempting new projects without fear of failure and by demonstrating less defensive behavior toward others.
8. Verbalizes importance of abstaining from use of substances in order to maintain optimal wellness.

Planning/Implementation

Table 27–12 provides a plan of care for the client with substance-related disorders. Selected nursing diagnoses are presented, along with outcome criteria, appropriate nursing interventions, and rationales for each.

Some institutions are using a case management model to coordinate care (see Chapter 9 for a more detailed explanation). In case management models, the plan of care may take the form of a critical pathway. Table 27–13 presents an example of a critical pathway of care for a client experiencing the alcohol withdrawal syndrome.

The concept map care plan is an innovative approach to planning and organizing nursing care (see Chapter 9). It is a diagrammatic teaching and learning strategy that allows visualization of interrelationships between medical diagnoses, nursing diagnoses, assessment data, and treatments. An example of a concept map care plan for a client with substance use disorder is presented in Figure 27–3.

Implementation with clients who abuse substances is a long-term process, often beginning with **detoxification** and progressing to total abstinence. The following common major treatment objectives have been identified for clients with substance-use disorders.

NURSING DIAGNOSIS: INEFFECTIVE DENIAL
RELATED TO: Weak, underdeveloped ego
EVIDENCED BY: Statements indicating no problem with substance use

OUTCOME CRITERIA	NURSING INTERVENTIONS	RATIONALE
Client will demonstrate acceptance of responsibility for own behavior and acknowledge association between substance use and personal problems.	1. Develop trust. Convey an attitude of acceptance. Ensure that client understands it is not the *person* but the *behavior* that is unacceptable. 2. Correct any misconceptions, such as, "I don't have a drinking problem. I can quit any time I want to." Do this in a matter-of-fact, nonjudgmental manner. 3. Identify recent maladaptive behaviors or situations that have occurred in the client's life, and discuss how use of substances may be a contributing factor. Say, "The lab report shows your blood alcohol level was 250 when you were involved in that automobile accident." 4. Do not allow client to rationalize or blame others for behaviors associated with substance use.	1. Unconditional acceptance promotes dignity and self-worth, qualities that this individual has been trying to achieve with substances. 2. These interventions help the client see the condition as an illness that requires help. 3. The first step in decreasing use of denial is for the client to see the relationship between substance use and personal problems. To confront issues with a caring attitude preserves self-esteem. 4. This only serves to prolong the denial.

NURSING DIAGNOSIS: INEFFECTIVE COPING
RELATED TO: Inadequate coping skills and weak ego
EVIDENCED BY: Use of substances as a coping mechanism

OUTCOME CRITERIA	NURSING INTERVENTIONS	RATIONALE
Client will be able to verbalize adaptive coping mechanisms to use, instead of substance abuse, in response to stress (and demonstrate, as applicable).	1. Set limits on manipulative behavior. Administer consequences when limits are violated. Obtain routine urine samples for laboratory analysis of substances. 2. Explore options available to assist with stress rather than resorting to substance use. Practice these techniques. 3. Give positive reinforcement for ability to delay gratification and respond to stress with adaptive coping strategies.	1. Because of weak ego and delayed development, client is unable to establish own limits or delay gratification. Client may obtain substances from various sources while in treatment. 2. Because gratification has been closely tied to oral needs, it is unlikely that client is aware of more adaptive coping strategies. 3. Because of weak ego, client needs lots of positive feedback to enhance self-esteem and promote ego development.

NURSING DIAGNOSIS: IMBALANCED NUTRITION: LESS THAN BODY REQUIREMENTS/DEFICIENT FLUID VOLUME
RELATED TO: Use of substances instead of eating
EVIDENCED BY: Loss of weight, pale conjunctiva and mucous membranes, poor skin turgor, electrolyte imbalance, anemias (and/or other signs and symptoms of malnutrition/dehydration)

OUTCOME CRITERIA	NURSING INTERVENTIONS	RATIONALE
Client will be free of signs/symptoms of malnutrition/dehydration.	1. Parenteral support may be required initially. 2. Encourage cessation of smoking.	1. To correct fluid and electrolyte imbalance, hypoglycemia, and some vitamin deficiencies. 2. To facilitate repair of damage to GI tract.

(Continued on following page)

OUTCOME CRITERIA	NURSING INTERVENTIONS	RATIONALE
	3. Consult dietitian. Determine the number of calories required based on body size and level of activity. Document intake and output and calorie count, and weigh client daily.	3. These interventions are necessary to maintain an ongoing nutritional assessment.
	4. Ensure that the amount of protein in the diet is correct for the individual client's condition. Protein intake should be adequate to maintain nitrogen equilibrium, but should be drastically decreased or eliminated if there is potential for hepatic coma.	4. Diseased liver may be incapable of properly metabolizing proteins, resulting in an accumulation of ammonia in the blood that circulates to the brain and can result in altered consciousness.
	5. Sodium may need to be restricted.	5. To minimize fluid retention (e.g., ascites and edema).
	6. Provide foods that are nonirritating to clients with esophageal varices.	6. To avoid irritation and bleeding of these swollen blood vessels.
	7. Provide small frequent feeding of client's favorite foods. Supplement nutritious meals with multiple vitamin and mineral tablet.	7. To encourage intake and facilitate client's achievement of adequate nutrition.

TABLE 27–13   Critical Pathway of Care for Client in Alcohol Withdrawal

Estimated Length of Stay: 7 Days—Variations from Designated Pathway Should Be Documented in Progress Notes

Nursing Diagnoses and Categories of Care	Time Dimension	Goals and/or Actions	Time Dimension	Goals and/or Actions	Time Dimension	Discharge Outcome
Risk for injury related to CNS agitation					Day 7	Client shows no evidence of injury obtained during ETOH withdrawal
Referrals	Day 1	Psychiatrist Assess need for: Neurologist Cardiologist Internist			Day 7	Discharge with follow-up appointments as required.
Diagnostic studies	Day 1	Blood alcohol level Drug screen (urine and blood) Chemistry profile Urinalaaysis Chest X–ray ECG	Day 4	Repeat of selected diagnostic studies as necessary.		
Additional assessments	Day 1 Days 1–5 Ongoing Ongoing	VS q4h I&O Restraints p.r.n. Assess withdrawal symptoms: tremors, nausea/vomiting, tachycardia, sweating, high blood pressure, seizures, insomnia, hallucinations	Days 2–3 Day 6 Day 4	VS q8h if stable DC I&O Marked decrease in objective withdrawal symptoms	Days 4–7 Day 7	VS bid; remain stable Discharge; absence of objective withdrawal symptoms
Medications	Day 1 Day 2 Days 1–6 Days 1–7	*Librium 200 mg in divided doses Librium 160 mg in divided doses Librium p.r.n. Maalox ac & hs *Note: Some physicians may elect to use Serax or Tegretol in the detoxification process	Day 3 Day 4	Librium 120 mg in divided doses Librium 80 mg in divided doses	Day 5 Day 6 Day 7	Librium 40 mg DC Librium Discharge; no withdrawal symptoms

(Continued on opposite page)

Estimated Length of Stay: 7 Days—Variations from Designated Pathway Should Be Documented in Progress Notes

Nursing Diagnoses and Categories of Care	Time Dimension	Goals and/or Actions	Time Dimension	Goals and/or Actions	Time Dimension	Discharge Outcome
Client education			Day 5	Discuss goals of AA and need for out-patient therapy	Day 7	Discharge with information regarding AA attendance or outpatient treatment
Imbalanced nutrition: Less than body requirements					Day 7	Nutritional condition has stabilized.
Referrals	Day 1	Consult dietitian	Days 1–7	Fulfill nutritional needs		
Diet	Day 1	Bland as tolerated; fluids as tolerated	Days 2–3	Frequent, small, meals; easily digested foods; advance as tolerated	Days 4–7	High–protein (unless contraindicated by diseased liver), high–carbohydrate diet
Additional assessments	Days 1–7	Weight I&O Skin turgor Color of mucous membranes				
Medications	Days 1–7	Thiamine 100 mg po (or injection, depending on condition of pt.) Multiple vitamin tablet Folate 1 mg po				
Client education			Day 4 Day 5	Principles of nutrition; foods for maintenance of wellness Reinforce teaching	Days 6–7	Client demonstrates ability to select appropriate foods for healthy diet

***NOTE:** With the advent of shorter hospital stays, adjustments may need to be made in the time dimensions. This CPC is intended to provide guidelines from which the student or practitioner can base client care.

Detoxification

1. Provide a safe and supportive environment for the detoxification process.
2. Administer **substitution therapy** as ordered.

Intermediate Care

1. Provide explanations of physical symptoms.
2. Promote understanding and identify the causes of substance dependency.
3. Provide education and assistance in course of treatment to client and family.

Rehabilitation

1. Encourage continued participation in long-term treatment.
2. Promote participation in outpatient support system (e.g., AA).

3. Assist client to identify alternative sources of satisfaction.
4. Provide support for health promotion and maintenance.

Client/Family Education

The role of client teacher is important in the psychiatric area, as it is in all areas of nursing. A list of topics for client/family education relevant to substance related disorders is presented in Table 27–14.

Evaluation

The final step of the nursing process involves reassessment to determine if the nursing interventions have been effective in achieving the intended goals of care. Evaluation of the client with a substance-related disorder may be accomplished by using information gathered from the following reassessment questions:

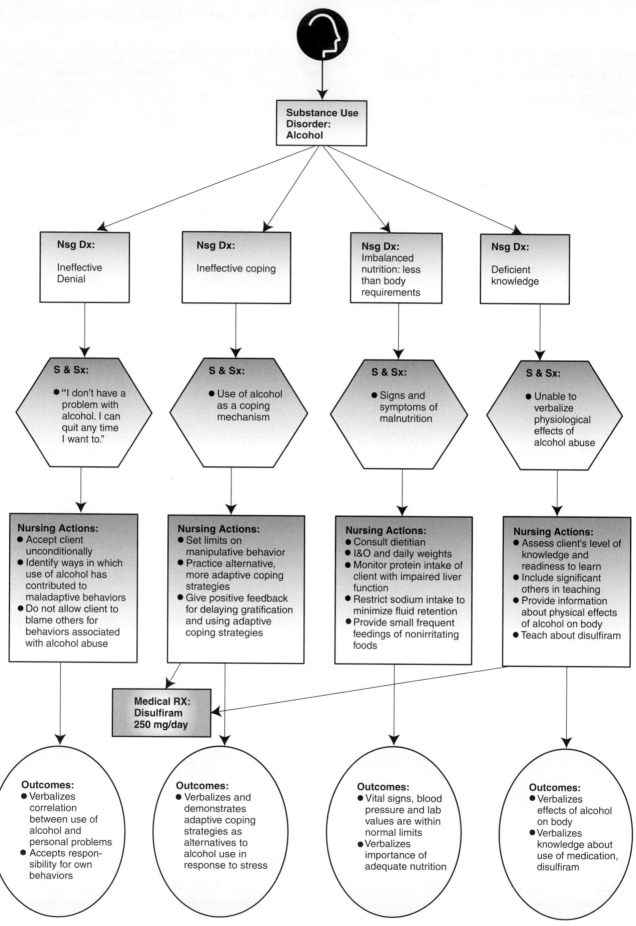

FIGURE 27–3 Concept map care plan for client with substance use disorder: alcohol.

TABLE 27–14 Topics for Client/Family Education Related to Substance Use Disorders

Nature of the Illness

1. Effects of (substance) on the body
   a. Alcohol
   b. Other CNS depressants
   c. CNS stimulants
   d. Hallucinogens
   e. Inhalants
   f. Opioids
   g. Cannabinols
2. Ways in which use of (substance) affects life.

Management of the Illness

1. Activities to substitute for (substance) in times of stress
2. Relaxation techniques
   a. Progressive relaxation
   b. Tense and relax
   c. Deep breathing
   d. Autogenics
3. Problem-solving skills
4. The essentials of good nutrition

Support Services

1. Financial assistance
2. Legal assistance
3. Alcoholics Anonymous (or other support group specific to another substance)
4. One-to-one support person

---

1. Has detoxification occurred without complications?
2. Is the client still in denial?
3. Does the client accept responsibility for his or her own behavior? Has he or she acknowledged a personal problem with substances?
4. Has a correlation been made between personal problems and the use of substances?
5. Does the client still make excuses or blame others for use of substances?
6. Has the client remained substance-free during hospitalization?
7. Does the client cooperate with treatment?
8. Does the client refrain from manipulative behavior and violation of limits?
9. Is the client able to verbalize alternative adaptive coping strategies to substitute for substance use? Has the use of these strategies been demonstrated? Does positive reinforcement encourage repetition of these adaptive behaviors?
10. Has nutritional status been restored? Does the client consume diet adequate for his or her size and level of activity? Is the client able to discuss the importance of adequate nutrition?
11. Has the client remained free of infection during hospitalization?
12. Is the client able to verbalize the effects of substance abuse on the body?
13. Does the client verbalize that he or she wants to recover and lead a life free of substances?

THE IMPAIRED NURSE

Substance abuse and dependency is a problem that has the potential for impairment in an individual's social, occupational, psychological, and physical functioning. This becomes an especially serious problem when the impaired person is responsible for the lives of others on a daily basis. Approximately 10 percent of the general population suffers from the disease of chemical dependency. It is estimated that 10 to 15 percent of nurses suffer from this disease (Raia, 2004a). Alcohol is the most widely abused drug, followed closely by narcotics. One study found a difference in the substances used based on specific nursing specialties (Trinkoff & Storr, 1998). Emergency and critical care nurses were more than three times as likely to use marijuana or cocaine as nurses in other specialties. Oncology and administration nurses were twice as likely to engage in binge drinking, while psychiatric nurses were most likely to smoke cigarettes.

In the past, the majority of disciplinary actions against nurses involved chemical dependency or substance abuse. In 2002, the number of practice-related issues surpassed those of drug- and alcohol-related issues, to make it second in number of grounds for complaints against nurses (National Council of State Boards of Nursing, 2002).

For years, the impaired nurse was protected, promoted, transferred, ignored, or fired. These types of responses promoted the growth of the problem. Programs are needed that involve early reporting and treatment of chemical dependency as a disease, with a focus on public safety and rehabilitation of the nurse.

How does one identify the impaired nurse? It is still easiest to overlook what *might* be a problem. Denial, on the part of the impaired nurse as well as nurse colleagues, is still the strongest defense for dealing with substance-abuse problems. Some states have mandatory reporting laws that require observers to report substance-abusing nurses to the state board of nursing. They are difficult laws to enforce, and hospitals are not always compliant with mandatory reporting. Some hospitals may choose not to report to the state board of nursing if the impaired nurse is actively seeking treatment and is not placing clients in danger.

A number of clues for recognizing substance impairment in nurses have been identified (Oklahoma Nurse Assistance Program, 2004; Raia, 2004b). They are not easy to detect and will vary according to the substance being used. There may be high absenteeism if the person's source is outside the work area, or the individual may rarely miss work if the substance source is at work. There may be an increase in "wasting" of drugs, higher incidences of incorrect narcotic counts, and a higher record of signing out drugs than for other nurses.

Poor concentration, difficulty in meeting deadlines, inappropriate responses, and poor memory or recall are usually late in the disease process. The person may also have problems with relationships. Some other possible signs are irritability, tendency to isolate, elaborate excuses for behavior, unkempt appearance, impaired motor coordination, slurred speech, flushed face, job shrinkage, and frequent use of the restroom. He or she may frequently medicate other nurses' patients, and there may be patient complaints of inadequate pain control. Discrepancies in documentation may occur.

If suspicious behavior occurs, it is important to keep careful, objective records. Confrontation with the impaired nurse will undoubtedly result in hostility and denial. Confrontation should occur in the presence of a supervisor or other nurse and should include the offer of assistance in seeking treatment. If a report is made to the state board of nursing, it should be a factual documentation of specific events and actions, not a diagnostic statement of impairment.

What will the state board do? Each case is generally decided on an individual basis. A state board may deny, suspend, or revoke a license based on a report of chemical abuse by a nurse. Several state boards of nursing have passed diversionary laws that allow impaired nurses to avoid disciplinary action by agreeing to seek treatment. Some of these state boards administer the treatment programs themselves, and others refer the nurse to community resources or state nurses' association assistance programs. This may require successful completion of inpatient, outpatient, group, or individual counseling treatment program(s); evidence of regular attendance at nurse support groups or 12-step program; random negative drug screens; and employment or volunteer activities during the suspension period. When a nurse is deemed safe to return to practice, he or she may be closely monitored for several years and required to undergo random drug screenings. The nurse also may be required to practice under specifically circumscribed conditions for a designated period of time.

In 1982, the ANA House of Delegates adopted a national resolution to provide assistance to impaired nurses. Since that time, the majority of state nurses' associations have developed (or are developing) programs for nurses who are impaired by substances or psychiatric illness. The individuals who administer these efforts are nurse members of the state associations, as well as nurses who are in recovery themselves. For this reason, they are called **peer assistance programs**.

The peer assistance programs strive to intervene early, to reduce hazards to clients, and increase prospects for the nurse's recovery. Most states provide either a hot-line number that the impaired nurse or intervening colleague may call or phone numbers of peer assistance committee members, which are made available for the same purpose. Typically, a contract is drawn up detailing the method of treatment, which may be obtained from various sources, such as employee assistance programs, Alcoholics Anonymous, Narcotics Anonymous, private counseling, or outpatient clinics. Guidelines for monitoring the course of treatment are established. Peer support is provided through regular contact with the impaired nurse, usually for a period of 2 years. Peer assistance programs serve to assist impaired nurses to recognize their impairment, to obtain necessary treatment, and to regain accountability within their profession.

CODEPENDENCY

Codependence is a term that has been given much attention in the last 20 years. The concept arose out of a need to define the dysfunctional behaviors that are evident among members of the family of a chemically dependent person. The term has been expanded to include all individuals from families that harbor secrets of physical or emotional abuse, other cruelties, or pathological conditions. Living under these conditions results in unmet needs for autonomy and self-esteem and a profound sense of powerlessness. The codependent person is able to achieve a sense of control only through fulfilling the needs of others.

A number of authors have proposed various definitions for codependence. Examples include the following:

An unhealthy dependence on another person leading to overinvolvement with the other and underinvolvement with the self. There is a loss of personal balance and power, confused identity, and blurred boundaries within relationships. This occurs and is nurtured in an atmosphere of denial and collusion. (Monahan, 2002)

An emotional, psychological, and behavioral condition that develops as a result of an individual's prolonged exposure to, and practice of, a set of oppressive rules – rules which prevent the open expression of feeling as well as direct discussion of personal and interpersonal problems. (Subby & Friel, 2002)

A popular term referring to all the effects that people who are dependent on alcohol or other substances have on those around them, including the attempts of those people to affect the dependent person. The term implies that codependence is a psychiatric disorder and hypothesizes that the family's actions tend to perpetuate (enable) the person's dependence. Empirical studies, however, support a stress and coping model for explanation of the family behavior. (Shahrokh & Hales, 2003)

The traits associated with a codependent personality are varied. The *DSM-IV-TR* (APA, 2000) states that personality traits become disorders only when they are "inflexible and maladaptive and cause significant functional impairment or subjective distress." To date, no diagnostic criteria exist for the diagnosis of codependent personality disorder.

A codependent individual is confused about his or her own identity. In a relationship, the codependent person derives self-worth from that of the partner, whose feelings and behaviors determine how the codependent should feel and behave. In order for the codependent to feel good, his or her partner must be happy and behave in appropriate ways. If the partner is not happy, the codependent feels responsible for *making* him or her happy. The codependent's home life is fraught with stress. Ego boundaries are weak and behaviors are often enmeshed with those of the pathological partner. Denial that problems exist is common. Feelings are kept in control, and anxiety may be released in the form of stress-related illnesses or compulsive behaviors such as eating, spending, working, or use of substances.

Wesson (2002) describes the following behaviors characteristic of codependency. She stated that codependents:

1. Have a long history of focusing thoughts and behavior on other people.
2. Are "people pleasers" and will do almost anything to get the approval of others.
3. Seem very competent on the outside but actually feel quite needy, helpless, or perhaps nothing at all.
4. Have experienced abuse or emotional neglect as a child.
5. Are outwardly focused toward others, and know very little about how to direct their own lives from their own sense of self.

The Codependent Nurse

Certain characteristics of codependence have been associated with the profession of nursing. A shortage of nurses combined with the increasing ranks of seriously ill clients may result in nurses providing care and fulfilling everyone's needs but their own. Many health care workers who are reared in homes with a chemically dependent person or otherwise dysfunctional family are at risk for having any unresolved codependent tendencies activated. Nurses who as children assumed the "fixer" role in their dysfunctional families of origin may attempt to resume that role in their caregiving professions. They are attracted to a profession in which they are needed, but they nurture feelings of resentment for receiving so little in return. Their emotional needs go unmet; however, they continue to deny that these needs exist. Instead, these unmet emotional needs may be manifested through use of compulsive behaviors, such as work or spending excessively, or addictions, such as to food or substances.

Codependent nurses have a need to be in control. They often strive for an unrealistic level of achievement. Their self-worth comes from the feeling of being needed by others and of maintaining control over their environment. They nurture the dependence of others and accept the responsibility for the happiness and contentment of others. They rarely express their true feelings, and do what is necessary to preserve harmony and maintain control. They are at high risk for physical and emotional burnout.

Treating Codependence

Cermak (1986) identified four stages in the recovery process for individuals with codependent personality.

Stage I: The Survival Stage. In this first stage, codependent persons must begin to let go of the denial that problems exist or that their personal capabilities are unlimited. This initiation of abstinence from blanket denial may be a very emotional and painful period.

Stage II: The Reidentification Stage. Reidentification occurs when the individuals are able to glimpse their true selves through a break in the denial system. They accept the label of codependent and take responsibility for their own dysfunctional behavior. Codependents tend to enter reidentification only after being convinced that it is more painful not to. They accept their limitations and are ready to face the issues of codependence.

Stage III: The Core Issues Stage. In this stage, the recovering codependent must face the fact that relationships cannot be managed by force of will. Each partner must be independent and autonomous. The goal of this stage is to detach from the struggles of life that exist because of prideful and willful efforts to control those things that are beyond the individual's power to control.

Stage IV: The Reintegration Stage. This is a stage of self-acceptance and willingness to change when codependents relinquish the power *over others* that was not rightfully theirs but reclaim the *personal* power that they do possess. Integrity is achieved out of awareness, honesty, and being in touch with one's spiritual consciousness. Control is achieved through self-discipline and self-confidence.

Self-help groups have been found to be helpful in the treatment of codependency. Groups developed for families of chemically dependent people, such as Al-Anon, may be of assistance. Groups specific to the problem of codependency also exist. Two of these groups include:

Co-Dependents Anonymous (CoDA)
P.O. Box 33577
Phoenix, AZ 85067-3577
602-277-7991

Co-Dependents Anonymous for Helping Professionals (CODAHP)
P.O. Box 42253
Mesa, AZ 85274-2253
602-644-8605

Both of these groups apply the Twelve Steps and Twelve Traditions developed by Alcoholics Anonymous to codependency (Tables 27–15 and 27–16).

Table 27–15 The Twelve Steps of Alcoholics Anonymous
1. We admitted we were powerless over alcohol—that our lives have become unmanageable.
2. Came to believe that a Power greater than ourselves could restore us to sanity.
3. Made a decision to turn our will and our lives over to the care of God as we understood Him.
4. Made a searching and fearless moral inventory of ourselves.
5. Admitted to God, to ourselves, and to another human being the exact nature of our wrongs.
6. Were entirely ready to have God remove all these defects of character.
7. Humbly asked Him to remove our shortcomings.
8. Made a list of all persons we had harmed and became willing to make amends to them all.
9. Made direct amends to such people wherever possible except when to do so would injure them or others.
10. Continued to take personal inventory and when we were wrong promptly admitted it.
11. Sought through prayer and meditation to improve our conscious contact with God as we understood Him, praying only for knowledge of His will for us and the power to carry that out.
12. Having had a spiritual awakening as the result of these steps, we tried to carry this message to alcoholics and to practice these principles in all our affairs.

The Twelve Steps and Twelve Traditions are reprinted with permission of Alcoholics Anonymous World Services, Inc. (AAWS). Permission to reprint the Twelve Steps and Twelve Traditions does not mean that AAWS has reviewed or approved the contents of this publication, or that AA necessarily agrees with the views expressed herein. AA is a program of recovery from alcoholism *only*. Use of the Twelve Steps and Twelve Traditions in connection with programs and activities which are patterned after AA, but which address other problems, or in any other non-AA context, does not imply otherwise.

Table 27–16 The Twelve Traditions of Alcoholics Anonymous
1. Our common welfare should come first; personal recovery depends upon AA unity.
2. For our group purpose there is but one ultimate authority—a loving God as He may express Himself in our group conscience. Our leaders are but trusted servants; they do not govern.
3. The one requirement for AA membership is a desire to stop drinking.
4. Each group should be autonomous except in matters affecting other groups or AA as a whole.
5. Each group has but one primary purpose—to carry its message to the alcoholic who still suffers.
6. An AA group ought never endorse, finance, or lend the AA name to any related facility or outside enterprise, lest problems of money, property, and prestige divert us from our primary purpose.
7. Every AA group ought to be fully self-supporting, declining outside contributions.
8. Alcoholics Anonymous should remain forever nonprofessional, but our service centers may employ special workers.
9. Alcoholics Anonymous, as such, ought never be organized; but we may create service boards of committees directly responsible to those they serve.
10. Alcoholics Anonymous has no opinion on outside issues; hence, the Alcoholics Anonymous name ought never be drawn into public controversy.
11. Our public relations policy is based on attraction rather than promotion; we need always maintain personal anonymity at the level of press, radio, and films.
12. Anonymity is the spiritual foundation of all our traditions, ever reminding us to place principles before personalities.

The Twelve Steps and Twelve Traditions are reprinted with permission of Alcoholics Anonymous World Services, Inc. (AAWS). Permission to reprint the Twelve Steps and Twelve Traditions does not mean that AAWS has reviewed or approved the contents of this publication, or that AA necessarily agrees with the views expressed herein. AA is a program of recovery from alcoholism *only*. Use of the Twelve Steps and Twelve Traditions in connection with programs and activities which are patterned after AA, but which address other problems, or in any other non-AA context, does not imply otherwise.

TREATMENT MODALITIES FOR SUBSTANCE-RELATED DISORDERS

Alcoholics Anonymous

Alcoholics Anonymous (AA) is a major self-help organization for the treatment of alcoholism. It was founded in 1935 by two alcoholics—a stockbroker, Bill Wilson, and a physician, Dr. Bob Smith—who discovered that they could remain sober through mutual support. This they accomplished not as professionals, but as peers who were able to share their common experiences. Soon they were working with other alcoholics, who in turn worked with others. The movement grew, and remarkably, individuals who had been treated unsuccessfully by professionals were able to maintain sobriety through helping one another.

Today AA chapters exist in virtually every community in the United States. The self-help groups are based on the concept of peer support—acceptance and understanding from others who have experienced the same problems in their lives. The only requirement for membership is a desire on the part of the alcoholic person to stop drinking. Each new member is assigned a support person from whom he or she may seek assistance when the temptation to drink occurs.

A survey by the General Service Office of Alcoholics Anonymous in 1998 (AA, 2002) revealed the following statistics: members ages 30 and younger comprised 11 percent of the membership; women comprised 34 percent; 88 percent were white; 5 percent were African American; 4 percent were Hispanic; 2 percent were Native American; and 1 percent were Asian American and other minorities. The highest percentage (13 percent) represented occupations in the professional and technical fields.

The sole purpose of AA is to help members stay sober. When sobriety has been achieved, they in turn are expected to help other alcoholic persons. The Twelve Steps that embody the philosophy of AA provide specific guidelines on how to attain and maintain sobriety (Table 27–15).

AA accepts alcoholism as an illness and promotes total abstinence as the only cure, emphasizing that the alco-

TABLE 27–17	Addiction Self-Help Groups
GROUP	**MEMBERSHIP**
Adult Children of Alcoholics (ACOA)	Adults who grew up with an alcoholic in the home
Al-Anon	Families of alcoholics
Alateen	Adolescent children of alcoholics
Children Are People	School-age children with an alcoholic family member
Cocaine Anonymous	Cocaine addicts
Families Anonymous	Parents of children who abuse substances
Fresh Start	Nicotine addicts
Narcotics Anonymous	Narcotics addicts
Nar-Anon	Families of narcotics addicts
Overeaters Anonymous	Food addicts
Pills Anonymous	Polysubstance addicts
Potsmokers Anonymous	Marijuana smokers
Smokers Anonymous	Nicotine addicts
Women for Sobriety	Female alcoholics

holic person can never safely return to social drinking. They encourage the members to seek sobriety, taking one day at a time. The Twelve Traditions are the statements of principles that govern the organization (Table 27–16).

AA has been the model for various other self-help groups associated with abuse or dependency problems. Some of these groups and the memberships for which they are organized are listed in Table 27–17. Nurses need to be fully and accurately informed about available self-help groups and their importance as a treatment resource on the health care continuum so that they can use them as a referral source for clients with substance-related disorders.

Pharmacotherapy

Disulfiram (Antabuse)

Disulfiram (**Antabuse**) is a drug that can be administered to individuals who abuse alcohol as a deterrent to drinking. Ingestion of alcohol while disulfiram is in the body results in a syndrome of symptoms that can produce a good deal of discomfort for the individual. It can even result in death if the blood alcohol level is high. The reaction varies according to the sensitivity of the individual and how much alcohol was ingested.

Disulfiram works by inhibiting the enzyme aldehyde dehydrogenase, thereby blocking the oxidation of alcohol at the stage when acetaldehyde is converted to acetate. This results in an accumulation of acetaldehyde in the blood, which is thought to produce the symptoms associated with the disulfiram–alcohol reaction. These symptoms persist as long as alcohol is being metabolized. The rate of alcohol elimination does not appear to be affected.

Symptoms of disulfiram–alcohol reaction can occur within 5 to 10 minutes of ingestion of alcohol. Mild reactions can occur at blood alcohol levels as low as 5 to 10 mg/dl. Symptoms are fully developed at approximately 50 mg/dl, and may include flushed skin, throbbing in the head and neck, respiratory difficulty, dizziness, nausea and vomiting, sweating, hyperventilation, tachycardia, hypotension, weakness, blurred vision, and confusion. With a blood alcohol level of approximately 125 to 150 mg/dl, severe reactions can occur, including respiratory depression, cardiovascular collapse, arrhythmias, myocardial infarction, acute congestive heart failure, unconsciousness, convulsions, and death.

Disulfiram should not be administered until it has been ascertained that the client has abstained from alcohol for at least 12 hours. If disulfiram is discontinued, it is important for the client to understand that the sensitivity to alcohol may last for as long as 2 weeks. Consuming alcohol or alcohol-containing substances during this 2-week period could result in the disulfiram–alcohol reaction.

The client receiving disulfiram therapy should be aware of the large number of alcohol-containing substances. These products, such as liquid cough and cold preparations, vanilla extract, aftershave lotions, colognes, mouthwash, nail polish removers, and isopropyl alcohol, if ingested or even rubbed on the skin, are capable of producing the symptoms described. The individual must read labels carefully and must inform any doctor, dentist, or other health care professional from whom assistance is sought that he or she is taking disulfiram. In addition, it is important that the client carry a card explaining participation in disulfiram therapy, possible consequences of the therapy, and symptoms that may indicate an emergency situation.

Obviously, the client must be assessed carefully before beginning disulfiram therapy. A thorough medical screening is performed before starting therapy, and written informed consent is usually required. The drug is contraindicated for clients who are at high risk for alcohol ingestion. It is also contraindicated for psychotic clients and clients with severe cardiac, renal, or hepatic disease.

Disulfiram therapy is not a cure for alcoholism. It provides a measure of control for the individual who desires to avoid impulse drinking. Clients receiving disulfiram therapy are encouraged to seek other assistance with their problem, such as AA or other support group, to aid in the recovery process.

Other Medications for Treatment of Alcoholism

The narcotic antagonist naltrexone (ReVia) was approved ● by the Food and Drug Administration (FDA) in 1994 for the treatment of alcohol dependence. Naltrexone, which was approved in 1984 for the treatment of heroin abuse, works on the same receptors in the brain that produce the feelings of pleasure when heroin or other opiates bind to them, but it does not produce the "narcotic high" and is not habit forming. Although alcohol does not bind to these same brain receptors, studies have shown that naltrexone works equally well against it (O'Malley et al., 1992; Volpicelli et al., 1992). In comparison to the placebo-treated clients, subjects on naltrexone therapy showed significantly lower overall relapse rates and fewer drinks per drinking day among those clients who did resume drinking. A study with an oral form of nalmefene (Revex) produced similar results (Mason et al., 1994).

The efficacy of selective serotonin reuptake inhibitors (SSRIs) in the decrease of alcohol craving among alcohol-dependent individuals has yielded mixed results (NIAAA, 2000). A greater degree of success was observed with moderate drinkers than with heavy drinkers.

In August 2004, the FDA approved acamprosate (Campral), which is indicated for the maintenance of abstinence from alcohol in patients with alcohol dependence who are abstinent at treatment initiation. The mechanism of action of acamprosate in maintenance of alcohol abstinence is not completely understood. It is hypothesized to restore the normal balance between neuronal excitation and inhibition by interacting with glutamate and gamma-aminobutyric acid (GABA) neurotransmitter systems. Acamprosate is ineffective in clients who have not undergone detoxification and not achieved alcohol abstinence prior to beginning treatment. It is recommended for concomitant use with psychosocial therapy.

Counseling

Counseling on a one-to-one basis is often used to help the client who abuses substances. The relationship is goal directed, and the length of the counseling may vary from weeks to years. The focus is on current reality, development of a working treatment relationship, and strengthening ego assets. The counselor must be warm, kind, and nonjudgmental, yet able to set limits firmly. Najavits and Weiss (1994) state, "The primary characteristic of counselors that influences treatment outcome appears to be interpersonal functioning, including therapists' empathy, genuineness, and respect for patients."

Counseling of the client who abuses substances passes through various phases, each of which is of indeterminate length. In the first phase, an assessment is conducted. Factual data are collected to determine whether the client does indeed have a problem with substances; that is, that substances are regularly impairing effective functioning in a significant life area.

Following the assessment, in the working phase of the relationship, the counselor assists the individual to work on acceptance of the fact that the use of substances causes problems in significant life areas and that he or she is not able to prevent it from occurring. The client states a desire to make changes. The strength of the denial system is determined by the duration and extent of substance-related adverse effects in the person's life. Thus, those individuals with rather minor substance-related problems of recent origin have less difficulty with this problem than those with long-term extensive impairment. The individual also works to gain self-control and abstain from substances.

Once the problem has been identified and sobriety is achieved, the client must have a concrete and workable plan for getting through the early weeks of abstinence. Anticipatory guidance through role-play helps the individual practice how he or she will respond when substances are readily obtainable and the impulse to partake is strong.

Counseling often includes the family or specific family members. In family counseling the therapist tries to help each member see how he or she has affected, and been affected by, the substance abuse behavior. Family strengths are mobilized, and family members are encouraged to move in a positive direction. Referrals are often made to self-help groups such as Al-Anon, Nar-Anon, Alateen, Families Anonymous, and Adult Children of Alcoholics.

Group Therapy

Group therapy with substance abusers has long been regarded as a powerful agent of change. In groups, individuals are able to share their experiences with others who are going through similar problems. They are able to "see themselves in others," and confront their defenses about giving up the substance. They may confront similar attitudes and defenses in others. Groups also give individuals the capacity for communicating needs and feelings directly.

Some groups may be task-oriented education groups in which the leader is charged with presenting material associated with substance abuse and its various effects on the person's life. Other educational groups that may be helpful with individuals who abuse substances include assertiveness techniques and relaxation training. Teaching groups differ from psychotherapy groups, whose focus is more on helping individuals understand and manage difficult feelings and situations, particularly as they relate to use of substances.

Therapy groups and self-help groups such as AA are complementary to each other. Whereas the self-help group focus is on achieving and maintaining sobriety, in the therapy group the individual may learn more adaptive ways of coping, how to deal with problems that may have arisen or were exacerbated by the former substance use, and ways to improve quality of life and to function more effectively without substances.

Psychopharmacology for Substance Intoxication and Substance Withdrawal

Various medications have been used to decrease the intensity of symptoms in an individual who is withdrawing from, or who is experiencing the effects of excessive use of, alcohol and other drugs. **Substitution therapy** may be required to reduce the life-threatening effects of intoxication or withdrawal from some substances. The severity of the withdrawal syndrome depends on the particular drug used, how long it has been used, the dose used, and the rate at which the drug is eliminated from the body.

Alcohol

Benzodiazepines are the most widely used group of drugs for substitution therapy in alcohol withdrawal. Chlordiazepoxide (Librium), oxazepam (Serax), and diazepam (Valium) are the most commonly used agents. Because of its ability to decrease the cardiovascular hyperactivity associated with alcohol withdrawal, the benzodiazepine alprazolam (Xanax) also is frequently being used (NIAAA, 2000). The approach to treatment with benzodiazepines for alcohol withdrawal is to start with relatively high doses and reduce the dosage by 20 to 25 percent each day until withdrawal is complete. In clients with liver disease, accumulation of the longer-acting agents (chlordiazepoxide and diazepam) may be problematic, and the use of the shorter-acting benzodiazepine, oxazepam, is more appropriate. Studies have also indicated that control of withdrawal symptoms with benzodiazepines on an "as needed" basis, rather than fixed schedule, resulted in the need for lower doses of the medication and less time in treatment (NIAAA, 2000).

Some physicians may order anticonvulsant medication (e.g., carbamazepine, valproic acid, or gabapentin) for management of withdrawal seizures. These drugs are particularly useful in individuals who undergo repeated episodes of alcohol withdrawal. Repeated episodes of withdrawal appear to "kindle" even more serious withdrawal episodes, including the production of withdrawal seizures that can result in brain damage (Julien, 2005). These anticonvulsants have been used successfully in both acute withdrawal and longer-term craving situations.

Multivitamin therapy, in combination with daily injections or oral administration of thiamine, is common protocol. Thiamine commonly is deficient in chronic alcoholics. Replacement therapy is required to prevent neuropathy, confusion, and encephalopathy.

Opioids

Examples of opioids are heroin, morphine, opium, meperidine, codeine, and methadone. Withdrawal symptoms generally begin within 8 to 12 hours after the last opioid dose and become most intense by 36 to 48 hours. The acute phase of withdrawal is over in approximately 10 days; however, symptoms of irritability and restlessness may persist for 2 to 3 months.

Opioid intoxication is treated with narcotic antagonists such as naloxone (Narcan), naltrexone (ReVia), or nalmefene (Revex). Withdrawal therapy includes rest, adequate nutritional support, and methadone substitution. Methadone is given on the first day in a dose sufficient to suppress withdrawal symptoms. The dose is then gradually tapered over a specified time. Federal regulations allow methadone detoxification in licensed facilities to last as long as 180 days (Mirin et al., 2002). As the dose of methadone diminishes, renewed abstinence symptoms may be ameliorated by the addition of clonidine.

In October 2002, the FDA approved two forms of the drug buprenorphine for treating opiate dependence. Buprenorphine is less powerful than methadone but is considered to be somewhat safer and causes fewer side effects, making it especially attractive for clients who are mildly or moderately addicted. Individuals will be able to access treatment with buprenorphine in office-based settings, providing a choice to methadone clinics. Physicians are deemed qualified to prescribe buprenorphine if they hold an addiction certification from the American Society of Addiction Medicine, the American Academy of Addiction Psychiatry, the American Psychiatric Association, or other associations deemed appropriate (Manisses Communications Group, 2002).

Clonidine (Catapres) also has been used to suppress opiate withdrawal symptoms. As monotherapy, it is not as effective as substitution with methadone, but it is nonaddicting and serves effectively as a bridge to enable the client to stay opiate-free long enough to facilitate termination of methadone maintenance.

Depressants

Substitution therapy for CNS depressant withdrawal (particularly barbiturates) is most commonly with the long-acting barbiturate phenobarbital (Luminal). The dosage required to suppress withdrawal symptoms is administered. When stabilization has been achieved, the dose is gradually decreased by 30 mg/day until withdrawal is complete. Long-acting benzodiazepines are commonly used for substitution therapy when the abused substance is a nonbarbiturate CNS depressant (Ashton, 2002).

Stimulants

Treatment of stimulant intoxication usually begins with minor tranquilizers such as chlordiazepoxide and progresses to major tranquilizers such as haloperidol (Haldol). Antipsychotics should be administered with caution because of their propensity to lower seizure threshold (Mack, Franklin, & Frances, 2003). Repeated seizures are treated with intravenous diazepam.

Withdrawal from CNS stimulants is not the medical emergency observed with CNS depressants. Treatment is usually aimed at reducing drug craving and managing severe depression. The client is placed in a quiet atmosphere and allowed to sleep and eat as much as is needed or desired. Suicide precautions may need to be instituted. Antidepressant therapy may be helpful in treating symptoms of depression. Desipramine has been especially successful with symptoms of cocaine withdrawal and abstinence (Mack, Franklin, & Frances, 2003).

Hallucinogens and Cannabinols

Substitution therapy is not required with these drugs. When adverse reactions, such as anxiety or panic, occur, benzodiazepines (e.g., diazepam or chlordiazepoxide) may be prescribed to prevent harm to the client or others. Psychotic reactions may be treated with antipsychotic medications.

SUMMARY

An individual is considered to be dependent on a substance when he or she is unable to control its use, even knowing that it interferes with normal functioning; when more and more of the substance is required to produce the desired effects; and when characteristic withdrawal symptoms develop upon cessation or drastic decrease in use of the substance. Abuse is considered when there is continued use of the substance despite having a persistent or recurrent problem that is caused or exacerbated by its use or when the substance is used in physically hazardous situations.

Substance intoxication is defined as the development of a reversible syndrome of maladaptive behavioral or psychological changes that are due to the direct physiological effects of a substance on the CNS and develop during or shortly after ingestion of (or exposure to) a substance. Substance withdrawal is the development of a substance-specific maladaptive behavioral change, with physiological and cognitive concomitants, that is due to the cessation of, or reduction in, heavy and prolonged substance use.

The etiology of substance-use disorders is unknown. Various contributing factors have been implicated, such as genetics, biochemical changes, developmental influences, personality factors, social learning, conditioning, and cultural and ethnic influences.

Seven classes of substances are presented in terms of a profile of the substance, historical aspects, patterns of use and abuse, and effects on the body. These six classes include alcohol, other CNS depressants, CNS stimulants, opioids, hallucinogens, inhalants, and cannabinols.

The nursing process is presented as the vehicle for delivery of care of the client with a substance-related disorder. The nurse must first examine his or her own feelings regarding personal substance use and the substance use by others. Only the nurse who can be accepting and nonjudgmental of substance-abuse behaviors will be effective in working with these clients. Care of clients with dual diagnoses of mental illness and substance use disorders was discussed.

Substance abuse by members of the nursing profession is discussed. Many state boards of nursing and state nurses' associations have established avenues for peer assistance to provide help to impaired members of the profession.

Individuals who are reared in families with chemically dependent persons learn patterns of dysfunctional behavior that carry over into adult life. These dysfunctional behavior patterns have been termed *codependence*. Codependent persons sacrifice their own needs for the fulfillment of others' in order to achieve a sense of control. Many nurses also have codependent traits.

Treatment modalities for substance-related disorders include self-help groups, deterrent therapy, individual counseling, and group therapy. Substitution pharmacotherapy is frequently implemented with clients experiencing substance intoxication or substance withdrawal. Treatment modalities are implemented on an inpatient basis or in outpatient settings, depending on the severity of the impairment.

REVIEW QUESTIONS

SELF-EXAMINATION/LEARNING EXERCISE

Select the answer that is most appropriate for each of the following questions:

Situation: Mr. White is admitted to the hospital after an extended period of binge alcohol drinking. His wife reports that he has been a heavy drinker for a number of years. Lab reports reveal he has a blood alcohol level of 250 mg/dl. He is placed on the chemical dependency unit for detoxification.

1. When would the first signs of alcohol withdrawal symptoms be expected to occur?
   a. Several hours after the last drink
   b. Two to 3 days after the last drink
   c. Four to 5 days after the last drink
   d. Six to 7 days after the last drink

2. Symptoms of alcohol withdrawal include:
   a. Euphoria, hyperactivity, and insomnia
   b. Depression, suicidal ideation, and hypersomnia
   c. Diaphoresis, nausea and vomiting, and tremors
   d. Unsteady gait, nystagmus, and profound disorientation

3. Which of the following medications is the physician most likely to order for Mr. White during his withdrawal syndrome?
   a. Haloperidol (Haldol)
   b. Chlordiazepoxide (Librium)
   c. Propoxyphene (Darvon)
   d. Phenytoin (Dilantin)

Situation: Dan, age 32, has been admitted for inpatient treatment of his alcoholism. He began drinking when he was 15 years old. Through the years, the amount of alcohol he consumes has increased. He and his wife report that for the last 5 years he has consumed at least a pint of bourbon a day. He also drinks beer and wine. He has been sneaking drinks at work, and his effectiveness has started to decline. His boss has told him he must seek treatment or he will be fired. This is his second week in treatment. The first week he experienced an uncomplicated detoxification.

4. Dan states, "I don't have a problem with alcohol. I can handle my booze better than anyone I know. My boss is a jerk! I haven't missed any more days than my coworkers." The nurse's best response is:
   a. "Maybe your boss is mistaken, Dan."
   b. "You are here because your drinking was interfering with your work, Dan."
   c. "Get real, Dan! You're a boozer and you know it!"
   d. "Why do you think your boss sent you here, Dan?"

5. The defense mechanism that Dan is using is:
   a. Denial
   b. Projection
   c. Displacement
   d. Rationalization

6. Dan's drinking buddies come for a visit, and when they leave, the nurse smells alcohol on Dan's breath. Which of the following would be the best intervention with Dan at this time?
   a. Search his room for evidence.
   b. Ask, "Have you been drinking alcohol, Dan?"
   c. Send a urine specimen from Dan to the lab for drug screening.
   d. Tell Dan, "These guys cannot come to the unit to visit you again."

7. Dan begins attendance at AA meetings. Which of the statements by Dan reflects the purpose of this organization?
   a. "They claim they will help me stay sober."
   b. "I'll dry out in AA, then I can have a social drink now and then."
   c. "AA is only for people who have reached the bottom."
   d. "If I lose my job, AA will help me find another."

The following general questions relate to substance abuse.

8. From which of the following symptoms might the nurse identify a chronic cocaine user?
   a. Clear, constricted pupils
   b. Red, irritated nostrils
   c. Muscle aches
   d. Conjunctival redness

9. An individual who is addicted to heroin is likely to experience which of the following symptoms of withdrawal?
   a. Increased heart rate and blood pressure
   b. Tremors, insomnia, and seizures
   c. Incoordination and unsteady gait
   d. Nausea and vomiting, diarrhea, and diaphoresis.

10. A polysubstance abuser makes the statement, "The green and whites do me good after speed." How might the nurse interpret the statement?
    a. The client abuses amphetamines and anxiolytics.
    b. The client abuses alcohol and cocaine.
    c. The client is psychotic.
    d. The client abuses narcotics and marijuana.

TEST YOUR CRITICAL THINKING SKILLS

Kelly, age 23, is a first-year law student. She is engaged to a surgical resident at the local university hospital. She has been struggling to do well in law school because she wants to make her parents, two prominent local attorneys, proud of her. She had never aspired to do anything but go into law, and that is also what her parents expected her to do.

Kelly's mid-term grades were not as high as she had hoped, so she increased the number of hours of study time, staying awake all night several nights a week to study. She started drinking large amounts of coffee to stay awake, but still found herself falling asleep as she tried to study at the library and in her apartment. As final exams approached, she began to panic that she would not be able to continue the pace of studying she felt she needed in order to make the grades she hoped for.

One of Kelly's classmates told her that she needed some "speed" to give her that extra energy to study. Her classmate said, "All the kids do it. Hardly anyone I know gets through law school without it." She gave Kelly the name of a source.

Kelly contacted the source, who supplied her with enough amphetamines to see her through final exams. Kelly was excited, because she had so much energy, did not require sleep, and was able to study the additional hours she thought she needed for the exams. However,

when the results were posted, Kelly had failed two courses and would have to repeat them in summer school if she was to continue with her class in the fall. She continued to replenish her supply of amphetamines from her "contact" until he told her he could not get her any more. She became frantic and stole a prescription blank from her fiancé and forged his name for more pills.

She started taking more and more of the medication in order to achieve the "high" she wanted to feel. Her behavior became erratic. Yesterday, her fiancé received a call from a pharmacy to clarify an order for amphetamines that Kelly had written. He insisted that she admit herself to the chemical dependency unit for detoxification.

On the unit, she appears tired, depressed, moves very slowly, and wants to sleep all the time. She keeps saying to the nurse, "I'm a real failure. I'll never be an attorney like my parents. I'm too dumb. I just wish I could die."

Answer the following questions related to Kelly:

1. What is the primary nursing diagnosis for Kelly?
2. Describe important nursing interventions to be implemented with Kelly.
3. In addition to physical safety, what would be the primary short-term goal the nurses would strive to achieve with Kelly?

IMPLICATIONS OF RESEARCH FOR EVIDENCE-BASED PRACTICE

Gaffney, K.F. (2001). Infant exposure to environmental tobacco smoke. *Journal of Nursing Scholarship*, *33*(4), 343–347.

Description of the Study: A review of 10 studies with a range of 100 to more than 1,000 participants was conducted. The studies took place in a variety of health care settings in the United States, Australia, and Europe. The studies measured infant exposure to environmental tobacco smoke (ETS). Parents of the infants completed the self-reports that inquired about number of people in the household who smoked and the proximity of the infant to the smoking. The studies focused on children in the first year of life.

Results of the Study: In one of the studies, questionnaire information was supported by hair analysis of the subjects. Median level of hair nicotine was more than 1.5 times higher among infants in homes reported by means of questionnaires to have smokers than among those in homes reported to have

no smokers. Eight of the 10 studies demonstrated increased risk for poor infant health outcomes associated with ETS exposure. Positive associations were found between infant ETS exposure and gastroesophageal reflux, colic, sudden infant death syndrome, lower respiratory tract infections, ear infections, and altered thyroid function.

Implications for Nursing Practice: The author suggests that nurses may use these results to document the need for identifying mothers who smoke as an important target group for clinical intervention. She states, "This review shows the importance of identifying and assisting mothers who smoke so that this critical proximity with their infants may provide optimal health promotion. Nurses who care for infants as part of the regular health maintenance visits conducted during the first year of life are particularly well-prepared and logically situated to advise and assist these mothers as they initiate the long-term process of smoking cessation."

REFERENCES

Alcoholics Anonymous [AA]. (2002). *Analysis of the 1998 survey of the membership of AA.* Retrieved on February 19, 2002 from the World Wide Web at http://www.aa.org/english/E FactFile/P-48_d1.html

American Insomnia Association. (2005). Medications: History. Retrieved March 14, 2005 from the World Wide Web at http://www.americaninsomniaassociation.org/medications.htm

American Psychiatric Association. (2000). *Diagnostic and statistical manual of mental disorders* (4th ed.) *Text revision.* Washington, DC: American Psychiatric Association.

Ashton, C.H. (2002). *Benzodiazepines: How they work and how to withdraw.* Newcastle upon Tyne, UK: University of Newcastle.

Barclay, L.L. (2005). *Alcohol-related neurologic disease.* Retrieved March 14, 2005 from the World Wide Web at http://www2.vhihealthe.com/article/gale/100085011

Behavioral Neuroscience Laboratory. (2002). *Tetrahydroisoquinolines and alcohol preference in rats.* Retrieved February 14, 2002 from the World Wide Web at http://www-org.usm.edu/~neurolab/research.htm

Bruckenthal, P. (2001). *Managing nonmalignant pain: Challenges for clinicians.* Paper presented April 19–22, 2001, at the 20th Annual Meeting of the American Pain Society.

Goldstein, A. (2002). *Addiction: From biology to drug policy* (2nd ed.). New York: Oxford University Press.

Greer, M. (2004, October). Statistics show mental health services still needed for native populations. *APA Online*, *35*(9). Retrieved March 13, 2005 from the World Wide Web at http://www.apa.org/monitor/oct04/services.html

Habal, R. (2004). Toxicity, barbiturate. Retrieved March 14, 2005 from the World Wide Web at http://www.emedicine.com/med/topic207.htm

Hanley, C.E. (2004). Navajos. In J.N. Giger and R.E. Davidhizar (Eds.). *Transcultural nursing* (4th ed.). St. Louis: C.V. Mosby.

Harvard Medical School. (2001). *Alcohol use and abuse.* Boston: Harvard Health Publications.

Harvard Medical School. (2003, September). Dual diagnosis: Part II. *Harvard Mental Health Letter, 20*(3), 1–5.

Jamal, M., Ameno, K., Kubota, T., Ameno, S., Zhang, X., Kumihashi, M., & Ijiri, I. (2003). In vivo formation of salsolinol induced by high acetaldehyde concentration in rat striatum employing microdialysis. *Alcohol and Alcoholism*, *38*(3), 197–201.

Julien, R.M. (2005). *A primer of drug action: A comprehensive guide to actions, uses and side effects of psychoactive drugs* (10th ed.). New York: Worth Publishers.

Knowles, J.A. (2003). Genetics. In R.E. Hales & S.C. Yudofsky (Eds.). *Textbook of Clinical Psychiatry* (4th ed.). Washington, DC: American Psychiatric Publishing.

Kuhn, M.A. (1998). Central nervous system stimulants. In M.A. Kuhn (Ed.). *Pharmacotherapeutics: A nursing process approach* (4th ed.). Philadelphia: F.A. Davis.

Mack, A.H., Franklin, J.E., & Frances, R.J. (2003). Substance Use Disorders. In R.E. Hales & S.C. Yudofsky (Eds.). *Textbook of clinical psychiatry* (4th ed.). Washington, DC: American Psychiatric Publishing.

Manisses Communications Group. (2002). Will buprenorphine usher in new era for opiate treatment? *Alcoholism and Drug Abuse Weekly*, *14*(48), 1, 6–7.

Mason, G.J., Ritvo, E.C., Morgan, R.O., Salvanto, F.R., Goldberg, G., Welch, B., & Mantero-Atienza, E. (1994). Double-blind, placebo-controlled pilot study to evaluate the efficacy and safety of oral nalmefene HCl for alcohol dependence. *Alcoholism, Clinical and Experimental Research*, *18*(5), 1162–1167.

Mayo Foundation for Medical Education and Research. (2005). Cirrhosis. Retrieved March 14, 2005 from the World Wide Web at http://www.ohiohealth.com/healthreference

Mirin, S.M., Batki, S.L., Buketein, O., Isbell, P.G., et al. (2002). Practice guidelines for the treatment of patients with substance use disorders: Alcohol, cocaine, opioids. In the *American Psychiatric Association Practice Guidelines for the Treatment of Psychiatric Disorders, Compendium 2002.* Washington, DC: American Psychiatric Association.

Monahan, M.J. (2002). *Definitions of codependence.* Adult Children Anonymous Online Meeting Manual. Retrieved on February 19, 2002 from the World Wide Web at http://www.intrepidsoftware.com/rec/defines.html

Najavits, L.M., & Weiss, R.D. (1994). Variations in therapist effectiveness in the treatment of patients with substance use disorders: An empirical review. *Addiction*, *89*(6), 679–688.

National Council on Alcoholism and Drug Dependence. (2005). *Alcohol and drug dependence are America's number one health problem.* Retrieved March 14, 2005 from the World Wide Web at http://www.ncadd.org/facts/numberoneprob.html

National Council of State Boards of Nursing (2002). *Commitment to public protection through excellence in nursing regulation.* Retrieved March 22, 2005 from the World Wide Web at http://www.ncsbn.org/pdfs/ResearchFinalAggregateReport/pdf

National Institute on Alcohol Abuse and Alcoholism (NIAAA).

(2000). *Tenth Special Report to the U.S. Congress on Alcohol and Health.* Bethesda, MD: The Institute.

National Institute on Alcohol Abuse and Alcoholism (NIAAA). (2005). Retrieved March 14, 2005 from the World Wide Web at http://www.niaaa.nih.gov/

National Institutes of Health (NIH) (2003). Workshop on the medical utility of marijuana. Retrieved March 21, 2005 from the World Wide Web at http://www.nih.gov/news/medmarijuana/Medical Marijuana.htm#CLINICAL

National Library of Medicine. (2002). *Hepatic encephalopathy.* Retrieved February 15, 2002 from the World Wide Web at http://www.nlm.nih.gov/medlineplus/ency/article/000302.htm

Newhouse, E. (1999, August 22). Bane of the Blackfeet. *Great Falls Tribune.* Retrieved February 14, 2002 from the World Wide Web at http://www.gannett.com/go/difference/greatfalls/pages/part8/blackfeet.html

Oklahoma Nurse Assistance Program (ONAP) (2004). *Substance abuse employment behaviors.* Oklahoma City, OK: Oklahoma Nurses Association.

O'Malley, S.S., Jaffe, A.J., Chang, G., Schottenfeld, R.S., Meyer, R.E., & Rounsaville, B. (1992). Naltrexone and coping skills therapy for alcohol dependence: A controlled study. *Archives of General Psychiatry, 49*(11), 881–887.

Raia, S. (2004a). The problem of impaired practice. *New Jersey Nurse, 34*(6), 8.

Raia, S. (2004b). Understanding chemical dependency. *New Jersey Nurse, 34*(7), 8.

Royal College of Physicians. (2000). *Nicotine addition in Britain.* London: Royal College of Physicians.

Sadock, B.J., & Sadock, V.A. (2003). *Synopsis of psychiatry: Behavioral sciences/ clinical psychiatry* (9th ed.). Philadelphia: Lippincott Williams & Wilkins.

Shahrokh, N.C., & Hales, R.E. (2003). *American psychiatric glossary* (8th ed.). Washington, DC: American Psychiatric Publishing.

Street Drugs. (2005). Plymouth, MN: The Publishers Group.

Subby, R., & Friel, J. (2002). *Definitions of codependency.* J.S. Allmond, Delaware Technical & Community College, Human Services Department. Retrieved February 19, 2002 from the World Wide Web at http://www.dtcc.edu/terry/hms/dept/codependency/sld001.htm

Substance Abuse and Mental Health Services Administration (SAMHSA). (2003). Office of Applied Studies. 2002 National Survey on Drug Use and Health. Washington, DC: U.S. Department of Health and Human Services.

Substance Abuse and Mental Health Services Administration (SAMHSA). (2005). *2003 National Survey on Drug Use & Health.* Retrieved March 14, 2005 from the World Wide Web at http://oas.samhsa.gov/NHSDA/2k3NSDUH/2k3results.htm

Tazbir, J., & Keresztes, P.A. (2005). Management of clients with functional cardiac disorders. In J.M. Black & J.H. Hawks (Eds.). *Medical-Surgical Nursing: Clinical management for positive outcomes* (7th ed.). St. Louis: W.B. Saunders.

Trinkoff, A.M., & Storr, C.L. (1998). Substance use among nurses: Differences between specialties. *American Journal of Public Health, 88*(4), 581–585.

United States Drug Enforcement Administration (USDEA). (2003). *Drug information: Cannabis.* Retrieved October 9, 2003 from the World Wide Web at http://www.dea.gov

Volpicelli, J.R., Alterman, A.I., Hayashida, M., & O'Brien, C.P. (1992). Naltrexone in the treatment of alcohol dependence. *Archives of General Psychiatry, 49*(11), 876–880.

Wesson, N. (2002). *Codependence: What is it? How do I know if I am codependent?* Retrieved February 19, 2002 from the World Wide Web at http://www.wespsych.com/codepend.html

C L A S S I C A L R E F E R E N C E S

Cermak, T.L. (1986). *Diagnosing and treating co-dependence.* Minneapolis: Johnson Institute Books.

Jellinek, E.M. (1952). Phases of alcohol addiction. *Quarterly Journal of Studies on Alcohol, 13,* 673–684.

Mayfield, D., McLeod, G., & Hall, P. (1974). The CAGE question-naire: Validation of a new alcoholism screening instrument. *American Journal of Psychiatry, 131,* 1121–1123.

Seltzer, M.L. (1971). The Michigan Alcoholism Screening Test: The quest for a new diagnostic instrument. *American Journal of Psychiatry, 127,* 1653–1658.

@ I N T E R N E T R E F E R E N C E S

Additional information on addictions may be located at the following Web sites:

- http://www.recovery-works.com/
- http://www.samhsa.gov/index.aspx
- http://www.ccsa.ca/index.asp
- http://www.well.com/user/woa/

Additional information on self-help organizations may be located at the following Web sites:

- http://www.ca.org (Cocaine Anonymous)
- http://www.aa.org (Alcoholics Anonymous)
- http://www.na.org (Narcotics Anonymous)
- http://www.al-anon.org

Additional information about medications for treatment of alcohol and drug dependence may be located at the following Web sites:

- http://www.fadavis.com/Townsend
- http://www.nlm.nih.gov/medlineplus/
- http://www.nimh.nih.gov/publicat/medicate.cfm

SCHIZOPHRENIA AND OTHER PSYCHOTIC DISORDERS

CHAPTER OUTLINE

OBJECTIVES

NATURE OF THE DISORDER

PREDISPOSING FACTORS

TYPES OF SCHIZOPHRENIA AND OTHER PSYCHOTIC DISORDERS

APPLICATION OF THE NURSING PROCESS

TREATMENT MODALITIES FOR SCHIZOPHRENIA AND OTHER PSYCHOTIC DISORDERS

SUMMARY

REVIEW QUESTIONS

KEY TERMS

anhedonia
associative looseness
autism
catatonic
circumstantiality
clang association
delusions
echolalia
echopraxia
hallucinations
illusion

magical thinking
neologism
neuroleptics
paranoia
perseveration
religiosity
social skills training
tangentiality
waxy flexibility
word salad

CORE CONCEPT

psychosis

OBJECTIVES

After reading this chapter, the student will be able to:

1. Discuss the concepts of schizophrenia and related psychotic disorders.
2. Identify predisposing factors in the development of these disorders.
3. Describe various types of schizophrenia and related psychotic disorders.
4. Identify symptomatology associated with these disorders and use this information in client assessment.
5. Formulate nursing diagnoses and outcomes of care for clients with schizophrenia and other psychotic disorders.
6. Identify topics for client and family teaching relevant to schizophrenia and other psychotic disorders.
7. Describe appropriate nursing interventions for behaviors associated with these disorders.
8. Describe relevant criteria for evaluating nursing care of clients with schizophrenia and related psychotic disorders.
9. Discuss various modalities relevant to treatment of schizophrenia and related psychotic disorders.

he term *schizophrenia* was coined in 1908 by the Swiss psychiatrist Eugen Bleuler. The word was derived from the Greek *skhizo* (split) and *phren* (mind).

Over the years, much debate has surrounded the concept of schizophrenia. Various definitions of the disorder have evolved, and numerous treatment strategies have been proposed, but none has proven to be uniformly effective or sufficient.

Although the controversy lingers, two general factors appear to be gaining acceptance among clinicians. The first is that schizophrenia is probably not a homogeneous disease entity with a single cause but results from a variable combination of genetic predisposition, biochemical dysfunction, physiological factors, and psychosocial stress. The second factor is that there is not now and probably never will be a single treatment that cures the disorder. Instead, effective treatment requires a comprehensive, multidisciplinary effort, including pharmacotherapy and various forms of psychosocial care, such as living skills and **social skills training**, rehabilitation, and family therapy.

Of all the mental illnesses responsible for suffering in society, schizophrenia probably causes more lengthy hospitalizations, more chaos in family life, more exorbitant costs to individuals and governments, and more fears than any other. Because it is such an enormous threat to life and happiness and because its causes are an unsolved puzzle, it has probably been studied more than any other mental disorder.

Ho, Black, and Andreasen (2003) have stated:

> Schizophrenia is perhaps the most enigmatic and tragic disease that psychiatrists treat, and perhaps also the most devastating. It is one of the leading causes of disability among young adults. Schizophrenia strikes at a young age so that, unlike patients with cancer or heart disease, patients with schizophrenia usually live many years after onset of the disease and continue to suffer its effects, which prevent them from leading fully normal lives—attending school, working, having a close network of friends, marrying, or having children. Apart from its effect on individuals and families, schizophrenia creates a huge economic burden for society. A study at the National Institute of Mental Health calculated the total cost of schizophrenia in 1991 at $65 billion. Despite its emotional and economic costs, schizophrenia has yet to receive sufficient recognition as a major health concern or the necessary research support to investigate its causes, treatments, and prevention. (p. 379)

This chapter explores various theories of predisposing factors that have been implicated in the development of schizophrenia. Symptomatology associated with different diagnostic categories of the disorder is discussed. Nursing care is presented in the context of the six steps of the nursing process. Various dimensions of medical treatment are explored.

NATURE OF THE DISORDER

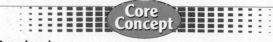

Psychosis

A severe mental condition in which there is disorganization of the personality, deterioration in social functioning, and loss of contact with, or distortion of, reality. There may be evidence of hallucinations and delusional thinking. Psychosis can occur with or without the presence of organic impairment.

Perhaps no psychological disorder is more crippling than schizophrenia. Characteristically, disturbances in thought processes, perception, and affect invariably result in a severe deterioration of social and occupational functioning.

In the United States, the lifetime prevalence of schizophrenia is about 1 percent (Sadock & Sadock, 2003). Symptoms generally appear in late adolescence or early adulthood, although they may occur in middle or late adult life (American Psychiatric Association [APA], 2000). Some studies have indicated that symptoms occur earlier in men than in women. The premorbid personality often indicates social maladjustment or schizoid or other personality disturbances (Ho, Black, & Andreasen, 2003). This premorbid behavior is often a predictor in the pattern of development of schizophrenia, which can be viewed in four phases.

Phase I: The Schizoid Personality

The *DSM-IV-TR* (APA, 2000) describes these individuals as indifferent to social relationships and having a very limited range of emotional experience and expression. They do not enjoy close relationships and prefer to be "loners." They appear cold and aloof. Not all individuals who demonstrate the characteristics of schizoid personality will progress to schizophrenia. However, most individuals with schizophrenia show evidence of having had these characteristics in the premorbid condition.

Phase II: The Prodromal Phase

Characteristics of this phase include social withdrawal; impairment in role functioning; behavior that is peculiar or eccentric; neglect of personal hygiene and grooming; blunted or inappropriate affect; disturbances in communication; bizarre ideas; unusual perceptual experiences; and lack of initiative, interests, or energy. The length of this phase is highly variable, and may last for many years before deteriorating to the schizophrenic state.

Phase III: Schizophrenia

In the active phase of the disorder, psychotic symptoms are prominent. Following are the *DSM-IV-TR* (APA, 2000) diagnostic criteria for schizophrenia:

1. **Characteristic Symptoms:** Two (or more) of the following, each present for a significant portion of time during a 1-month period (or less if successfully treated):
   a. **Delusions**
   b. **Hallucinations**
   c. Disorganized speech (e.g., frequent derailment or incoherence)
   d. Grossly disorganized or **catatonic behavior**
   e. Negative symptoms (i.e., affective flattening, alogia, or avolition)
2. **Social/Occupational Dysfunction:** For a significant portion of the time since the onset of the disturbance, one or more major areas of functioning such as work, interpersonal relations, or self-care are markedly below the level achieved before the onset (or when the onset is in childhood or adolescence, failure to achieve expected level of interpersonal, academic, or occupational achievement).
3. **Duration:** Continuous signs of the disturbance persist for at least 6 months. This 6-month period must include at least 1 month of symptoms (or less if successfully treated) that meet criterion 1 (i.e., active-phase symptoms) and may include periods of prodromal or residual symptoms. During these prodromal or residual periods, the signs of the disturbance may be manifested by only negative symptoms or two or more symptoms listed in criterion1 present in an attenuated form (e.g., odd beliefs, unusual perceptual experiences).
4. **Schizoaffective and Mood Disorder Exclusion:** Schizoaffective disorder and mood disorder with psychotic features have been ruled out because (1) no major depressive, manic, or mixed episodes have occurred concurrently with the active-phase symptoms; or (2) if mood episodes have occurred during active-phase symptoms, their total duration has been brief relative to the duration of the active and residual periods.
5. **Substance/General Medical Condition Exclusion:** The disturbance is not due to the direct physiological effects of a substance (e.g., a drug of abuse, a medication) or a general medical condition.
6. **Relationship to a Pervasive Developmental Disorder:** If there is a history of autistic disorder or another pervasive developmental disorder, the additional diagnosis of schizophrenia is made only if prominent delusions or hallucinations are also present for at least 1 month (or less if successfully treated).

Phase IV: Residual Phase

Schizophrenia is characterized by periods of remission and exacerbation. A residual phase usually follows an active phase of the illness. Symptoms during the residual phase are similar to those of the prodromal phase, with flat affect and impairment in role functioning being prominent. Residual impairment often increases between episodes of active psychosis.

Prognosis

A return to full premorbid functioning is not common (APA, 2000). However, several factors have been associated with a more positive prognosis. These include good premorbid adjustment, later age at onset, female gender, abrupt onset of symptoms precipitated by a stressful event (as opposed to gradual insidious onset of symptoms), associated mood disturbance, brief duration of active-phase symptoms, good interepisode functioning, minimal residual symptoms, absence of structural brain abnormalities, normal neurological functioning, a family history of mood disorder, and no family history of schizophrenia (APA, 2000).

PREDISPOSING FACTORS

The cause of schizophrenia is still uncertain. Most likely no single factor can be implicated in the etiology; rather, the disease probably results from a combination of influences including biological, psychological, and environmental factors.

Biological Influences

Refer to Chapter 4 for a more thorough review of the biological implications of psychiatric illness.

Genetics

The body of evidence for genetic vulnerability to schizophrenia is growing. Studies show that relatives of individuals with schizophrenia have a much higher probability of developing the disease than does the general population. Whereas the lifetime risk for developing schizophrenia is about 1 percent in most population studies, the siblings or offspring of an identified client have a 5 to 10 percent risk of developing schizophrenia (Ho, Black, & Andreasen, 2003).

How schizophrenia is inherited is uncertain. No reliable biological marker has as yet been found. It is unknown which genes are important in the vulnerability to schizophrenia, or whether one or many genes are implicated. Some individuals have a strong genetic link to the illness, whereas others may have only a weak genetic basis. This theory gives further credence to the notion of multiple causations.

Twin Studies. The rate of schizophrenia among monozygotic (identical) twins is four times that of dizygotic (fraternal) twins and approximately 50 times that of the general population (Sadock & Sadock, 2003). Identical twins reared apart have the same rate of development of the illness as do those reared together. Because in about half of the cases only one of a pair of monozygotic twins develops schizophrenia, some investigators believe environmental factors interact with genetic ones.

Adoption Studies. In studies conducted by both American and Danish investigators, adopted children born of schizophrenic mothers were compared with adopted children whose mothers had no psychiatric disorder. It was found that the children who were born of schizophrenic mothers were more likely to develop the illness than the comparison control groups (Ho, Black, & Andreasen, 2003). Studies also indicate that children born of nonschizophrenic parents, but reared by schizophrenic parents, do not seem to suffer more often from schizophrenia than general controls. These findings provide additional evidence for the genetic basis of schizophrenia.

Biochemical Influences

The oldest and most thoroughly explored biological theory in the explanation of schizophrenia attributes a pathogenic role to abnormal brain biochemistry. Notions of a "chemical disturbance" as an explanation for insanity were suggested by some theorists as early as the mid-19th century.

The Dopamine Hypothesis. This theory suggests that schizophrenia (or schizophrenia-like symptoms) may be caused by an excess of dopamine-dependent neuronal activity in the brain. (See Figure 28–1.) This excess activity may be related to increased production or release of the substance at nerve terminals, increased receptor sensitivity, too many dopamine receptors, or a combination of these mechanisms (Sadock & Sadock, 2003).

Pharmacological support for this hypothesis exists. Amphetamines, which increase levels of dopamine, induce psychotomimetic symptoms. The **neuroleptics** (e.g., chlorpromazine or haloperidol) lower brain levels of dopamine by blocking dopamine receptors, thus reducing the schizophrenic symptoms, including those induced by amphetamines.

Postmortem studies of schizophrenic brains have reported a significant increase in the average number of dopamine receptors in approximately two thirds of the brains studied. This suggests that an increased dopamine response may not be important in *all* schizophrenic clients. Clients with acute manifestations (e.g., delusions and hallucinations) respond with greater efficacy to neuroleptic drugs than do clients with chronic manifestations (e.g., apathy, poverty of ideas, and loss of drive). The current position, in terms of the dopamine hypothesis, is that manifestations of acute schizophrenia may be related to increased numbers of dopamine receptors in the brain and respond to neuroleptic drugs that block these receptors. Manifestations of chronic schizophrenia are probably unrelated to numbers of dopamine receptors, and neuroleptic drugs are unlikely to be as effective in treating these chronic symptoms.

Other Biochemical Hypotheses. Various other biochemicals have been implicated in the predisposition to schizophrenia. Abnormalities in the neurotransmitters norepinephrine, serotonin, acetylcholine, and gamma-aminobutyric acid and in the neuroregulators, such as prostaglandins and endorphins, have been suggested.

Physiological Influences

A number of physical factors of possible etiological significance have been identified in the medical literature. Their specific mechanisms in the implication of schizophrenia are, however, unclear.

Viral Infection. Sadock and Sadock (2003) report that epidemiological data indicate a high incidence of schizophrenia after prenatal exposure to influenza. They state:

> Other data supporting a viral hypothesis are an increased number of physical anomalies at birth, an increased rate of pregnancy and birth complications, seasonality of birth consistent with viral infection, geographical clusters of adult cases, and seasonality of hospitalizations. (p. 482)

Another study found an association between viral infections of the central nervous system during childhood and adult-onset schizophrenia (Rantakallio et al., 1997).

Anatomical Abnormalities. With the use of neuroimaging technologies, structural brain abnormalities have been observed in individuals with schizophrenia. Ventricular enlargement is the most consistent finding; however, sulci enlargement and cerebellar atrophy are also reported. Ho, Black, and Andreasen (2003) state:

> There is substantial evidence to suggest that ventricular enlargement is associated with poor premorbid functioning, negative symptoms, poor response to treatment, and cognitive impairment. CT scan abnormalities may have some clinical significance, but they are not diagnostically specific; similar abnormalities are seen in other disorders such as Alzheimer's disease or alcoholism. (p. 405)

Magnetic resonance imaging (MRI) provides a greater ability to image in multiple planes. Studies with MRI have revealed a possible decrease in cerebral and intracranial size in clients with schizophrenia. Studies have also revealed a decrease in frontal lobe size, but this has been less consistently replicated. MRI has been used

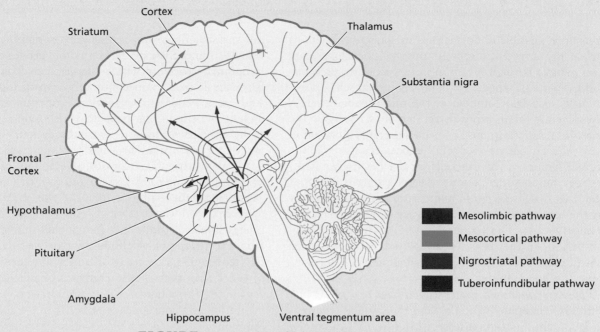

FIGURE 28–1 Neurobiology of schizophrenia.

Neurotransmitters
A number of neurotransmitters have been implicated in the etiology of schizophrenia. These include dopamine, norepinephrine, serotonin, glutamate, and GABA. The dopaminergic system has been most widely studied and closely linked to the symptoms associated with the disease.

Areas of the Brain Affected
- Four major dopaminergic pathways have been identified:
  - *Mesolimbic pathway*: Originates in the ventral tegmentum area and projects to areas of the limbic system, including the nucleus accumbens, amygdala, and hippocampus. The mesolimbic pathway is associated with functions of memory, emotion, arousal, and pleasure. Excess activity in the mesolimbic tract has been implicated in the positive symptoms of schizophrenia (e.g., hallucinations, delusions).
  - *Mesocortical pathway*: originates in the ventral tegmentum area and has projections into the cortex. The mesocortical pathway is concerned with cognition, social behavior, planning, problem solving, motivation, and reinforcement in learning. Negative symptoms of schizophrenia (e.g., flat affect, apathy, lack of motivation, and anhedonia) have been associated with diminished activity in the mesocortical tract.
  - *Nigrostriatal pathway*: originates in the substantia nigra and terminates in the striatum of the basal ganglia. This pathway is associated with the function of motor control. Degeneration in this pathway is associated with Parkinson's disease and involuntary psychomotor symptoms of schizophrenia.
  - *Tuberoinfundibular pathway*: originates in the hypothalamus and projects to the pituitary gland. It is associated with endocrine function, digestion, metabolism, hunger, thirst, temperature control, and sexual arousal. Implicated in certain endocrine abnormalities associated with schizophrenia.
- Two major groups of dopamine receptors and their highest tissue locations include:
  - The D_1 Family:
        D_1 receptors: basal ganglia, nucleus accumbens, and cerebral cortex
        D_5 receptors: hippocampus and hypothalamus, with lower concentrations in the cerebral cortex and basal ganglia
  - The D_2 Family:
        D_2 receptors: basal ganglia, anterior pituitary, cerebral cortex, limbic structures
        D_3 receptors: limbic regions, with lower concentrations in basal ganglia
        D_4 receptors: frontal cortex, hippocampus, amygdala

Antipsychotic Medications

Type	Receptor Affinity	Associated Side Effects
Conventional (typical) antipsychotics: Phenothiazines Haloperidol Provide relief of psychosis, improvement in positive symptoms, worsening of negative symptoms.	Strong D_2 (dopamine) Varying degrees of affinity for: (cholinergic) Ach α_1 (norepinephrine) H_1 (histamine) Weak 5-HT (serotonin)	EPS, hyperprolactinemia, Neuroleptic Malignant Syndrome Anticholinergic effects Tachycardia, tremors, insomnia, postural hypotension Weight gain, sedation Low potential for ejaculatory difficulty
Novel (atypical) antipsychotics: Clozapine, Olanzapine, Quetiapine, Aripiprazole, Risperidone, Ziprasidone Provide relief of psychosis, improvement in positive symptoms, improvement in negative symptoms.	Strong 5-HT Low to Moderate D_2 Varying degrees of affinity for: Ach α adrenergic H_1	Sexual dysfunction, GI disturbance, headache Low potential for EPS Anticholinergic effects Tachycardia, tremors, insomnia, postural hypotension Weight gain, sedation

457

to explore possible abnormalities in specific subregions such as the amygdala, hippocampus, temporal lobes, and basal ganglia in the brains of people with schizophrenia.

Histological Changes. Cerebral changes in schizophrenia have also been studied at the microscopic level. A "disordering" or disarray of the pyramidal cells in the area of the hippocampus has been suggested (Jonsson et al., 1997). This disarray of cells has been compared to the normal alignment of the cells in the brains of clients without the disorder. Some researchers have hypothesized that this alteration in hippocampal cells occurs during the second trimester of pregnancy and may be related to an influenza virus encountered by the mother during this period. Further research is required to determine the possible link between this birth defect and the development of schizophrenia.

Physical Conditions. Some studies have reported a link between schizophrenia and epilepsy (particularly temporal lobe), Huntington's disease, birth trauma, head injury in adulthood, alcohol abuse, cerebral tumor (particularly in the limbic system), cerebrovascular accidents, systemic lupus erythematosus, myxedema, Parkinsonism, and Wilson's disease.

Psychological Influences

Early conceptualizations of schizophrenia focused on family relationship factors as major influences in the development of the illness. This probably occurred in light of the conspicuous absence of information related to a biological connection. These early theories related to poor parent–child relationships and dysfunctional family systems as the cause of schizophrenia.

Can family interaction patterns cause schizophrenia? The answer is most probably not. Researchers are now focusing their studies more in terms of schizophrenia as a brain disorder. Nevertheless, Sadock and Sadock (2003) state:

> Clinicians should consider the psychosocial factors affecting schizophrenia. Although, historically, theorists have attributed the development of schizophrenia to psychosocial factors, contemporary clinicians can benefit from using the relevant theories and guidelines of these past observations and hypotheses. Although many psychodynamic theories about the pathogenesis of schizophrenia seem out of date, perceptive clinical observations can help contemporary clinicians understand how the disease may affect a patient's psyche. (p. 483)

Environmental Influences
Sociocultural Factors

Many studies have been conducted that have attempted to link schizophrenia to social class. Indeed epidemiolog-

ical statistics have shown that greater numbers of individuals from the lower socioeconomic classes experience symptoms associated with schizophrenia than do those from the higher socioeconomic groups (Ho, Black, & Andreasen, 2003). Explanations for this occurrence include the conditions associated with living in poverty, such as congested housing accommodations, inadequate nutrition, absence of prenatal care, few resources for dealing with stressful situations, and feelings of hopelessness for changing one's lifestyle of poverty.

An alternative view is that of the *downward drift hypothesis* (Sadock & Sadock, 2003). This hypothesis relates the schizophrenic individual's move into, or failure to move out of, the low socioeconomic group to the tendency for social isolation and the segregation of self from others—characteristics of the disease process itself. Proponents of this notion view poor social conditions as a consequence rather than a cause of schizophrenia.

Stressful Life Events

Studies have been conducted in an effort to determine whether psychotic episodes may be precipitated by stressful life events. There is no scientific evidence to indicate that stress causes schizophrenia. It is very probable, however, that stress may contribute to the severity and course of the illness. It is known that extreme stress can precipitate psychotic episodes (Goff, 2002). Stress may indeed precipitate symptoms in an individual who possesses a genetic vulnerability to schizophrenia. Sadock and Sadock (2003) state:

> The stress can be biological, environmental, or both. The environmental component can be either biological (e.g., an infection) or psychological (e.g., a stressful family situation). (p. 477)

Stressful life events may be associated with exacerbation of schizophrenic symptoms and increased rates of relapse.

The Transactional Model

The etiology of schizophrenia remains unclear. No single theory or hypothesis has been postulated that substantiates a clear-cut explanation for the disease. Indeed, it seems the more research that is conducted, the more evidence is compiled to support the concept of multiple causation in the development of schizophrenia. The most current theory seems to be that schizophrenia is a biologically based disease, the onset of which is influenced by factors within the environment (either internal or external). The dynamics of schizophrenia using the Transactional Model of Stress/Adaptation are presented in Figure 28–2.

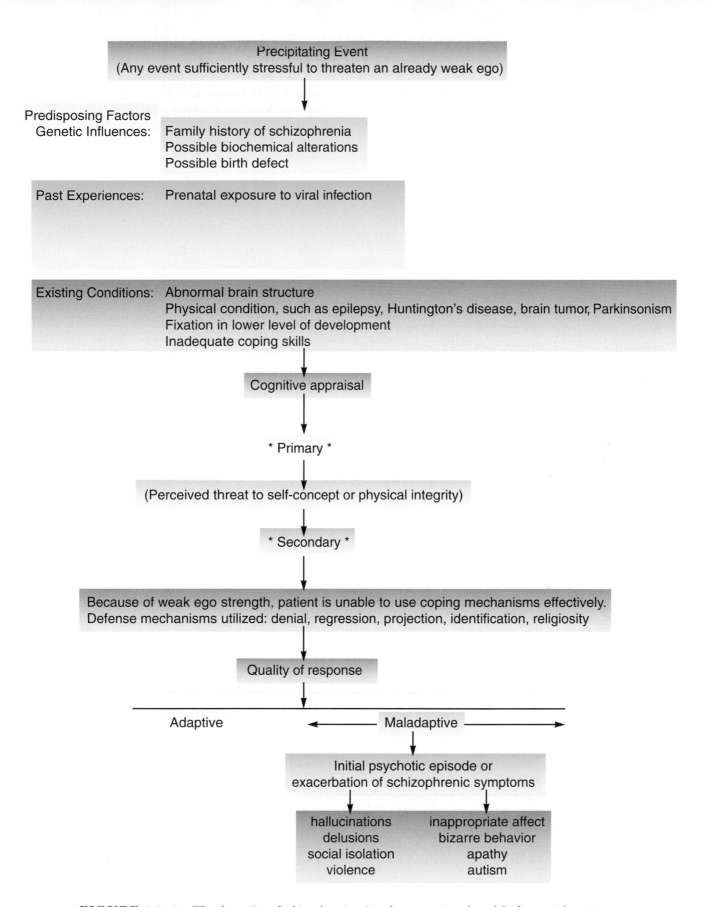

FIGURE 28–2 The dynamics of schizophrenia using the transactional model of stress/adaptation.

TYPES OF SCHIZOPHRENIA AND OTHER PSYCHOTIC DISORDERS

The *DSM-IV*-TR (APA, 2000) identifies various types of schizophrenia and other psychotic disorders. Differential diagnosis is made according to the total symptomatic clinical picture presented.

Disorganized Schizophrenia

This type previously was called *hebephrenic schizophrenia*. Onset of symptoms is usually before age 25, and the course is commonly chronic. Behavior is markedly regressive and primitive. Contact with reality is extremely poor. Affect is flat or grossly inappropriate, often with periods of silliness and incongruous giggling. Facial grimaces and bizarre mannerisms are common, and communication is consistently incoherent. Personal appearance is generally neglected, and social impairment is extreme.

Catatonic Schizophrenia

Catatonic schizophrenia is characterized by marked abnormalities in motor behavior and may be manifested in the form of *stupor* or *excitement* (Sadock & Sadock, 2003).

Catatonic stupor is characterized by extreme psychomotor retardation. The individual exhibits a pronounced decrease in spontaneous movements and activity. Mutism (i.e., absence of speech) is common, and negativism (i.e., an apparently motiveless resistance to all instructions or attempts to be moved) may be evident. **Waxy flexibility** may be exhibited. This term describes a type of "posturing," or voluntary assumption of bizarre positions, in which the individual may remain for long periods. Efforts to move the individual may be met with rigid bodily resistance.

Catatonic excitement is manifested by a state of extreme psychomotor agitation. The movements are frenzied and purposeless, and are usually accompanied by continuous incoherent verbalizations and shouting. Clients in catatonic excitement urgently require physical and medical control because they are often destructive and violent to others, and their excitement may cause them to injure themselves or to collapse from complete exhaustion.

Catatonic schizophrenia was quite common before the advent of antipsychotic medications for use in psychiatry. The illness is now rare in Europe and North America (Sadock & Sadock, 2003).

Paranoid Schizophrenia

Paranoid schizophrenia is characterized mainly by the presence of delusions of persecution or grandeur and auditory hallucinations related to a single theme. The individual is often tense, suspicious, and guarded, and may be argumentative, hostile, and aggressive. Onset of symptoms is usually later (perhaps in the late 20s or 30s), and less regression of mental faculties, emotional response, and behavior is seen than in the other subtypes of schizophrenia. Social impairment may be minimal, and there is some evidence that prognosis, particularly with regard to occupational functioning and capacity for independent living, is promising (APA, 2000).

Undifferentiated Schizophrenia

Sometimes clients with schizophrenic symptoms do not meet the criteria for any of the subtypes, or they may meet the criteria for more than one subtype. These individuals may be given the diagnosis of undifferentiated schizophrenia. The behavior is clearly psychotic; that is, there is evidence of delusions, hallucinations, incoherence, and bizarre behavior. However, the symptoms cannot be easily classified into any of the previously listed diagnostic categories.

Residual Schizophrenia

This diagnostic category is used when the individual has a history of at least one previous episode of schizophrenia with prominent psychotic symptoms. Residual schizophrenia occurs in an individual who has a chronic form of the disease and is the stage that follows an acute episode (prominent delusions, hallucinations, incoherence, bizarre behavior, and violence). In the residual stage, there is continuing evidence of the illness, although there are no prominent psychotic symptoms. Residual symptoms may include social isolation, eccentric behavior, impairment in personal hygiene and grooming, blunted or inappropriate affect, poverty of or overly elaborate speech, illogical thinking, or apathy.

Schizoaffective Disorder

This disorder is manifested by schizophrenic behaviors, with a strong element of symptomatology associated with the mood disorders (depression or mania). The client may appear depressed, with psychomotor retardation and suicidal ideation, or symptoms may include euphoria, grandiosity, and hyperactivity. However, the decisive factor in the diagnosis of schizoaffective disorder is the presence of characteristic schizophrenic symptoms. For example, in addition to the dysfunctional mood, the individual exhibits bizarre delusions, prominent hallucinations, incoherent speech, catatonic behavior, or blunted or inappropriate affect. The prognosis for schizoaffective disorder is generally better than that for other schizophrenic disorders but worse than that for mood disorders alone (Sadock & Sadock, 2003).

Brief Psychotic Disorder

The essential feature of this disorder is the sudden onset of psychotic symptoms that may or may not be preceded by a severe psychosocial stressor. These symptoms last at least 1 day but less than 1 month, and there is an eventual full return to the premorbid level of functioning (APA, 2000). The individual experiences emotional turmoil or overwhelming perplexity or confusion. Evidence of impaired reality testing may include incoherent speech, delusions, hallucinations, bizarre behavior, and disorientation. Individuals with preexisting personality disorders (most commonly, histrionic, narcissistic, paranoid, schizotypal, and borderline personality disorders) appear to be susceptible to this disorder (Sadock & Sadock, 2003).

Schizophreniform Disorder

The essential features of this disorder are identical to those of schizophrenia, with the exception that the duration, including prodromal, active, and residual phases, is at least 1 month but less than 6 months (APA, 2000). If the diagnosis is made while the individual is still symptomatic but has been so for less than 6 months, it is qualified as "provisional." The diagnosis is changed to schizophrenia if the clinical picture persists beyond 6 months.

Schizophreniform disorder is thought to have a good prognosis if at least two of the following features are present:

1. Onset of prominent psychotic symptoms within 4 weeks of first noticeable change in usual behavior or functioning
2. Confusion or perplexity at the height of the psychotic episode
3. Good premorbid social and occupational functioning
4. Absence of blunted or flat affect (APA, 2000)

Delusional Disorder

The essential feature of this disorder is the presence of one or more nonbizarre delusions that persist for at least 1 month (APA, 2000). If present at all, hallucinations are not prominent, and apart from the delusions, behavior is not bizarre. The subtype of delusional disorder is based on the predominant delusional theme.

Erotomanic Type

With this type of delusion, the individual believes that someone, usually of a higher status, is in love with him or her. Famous persons are often the subjects of erotomanic delusions. Sometimes the delusion is kept secret, but some individuals may follow, contact, or otherwise try to pursue the object of their delusion.

Grandiose Type

Individuals with grandiose delusions have irrational ideas regarding their own worth, talent, knowledge, or power. They may believe that they have a special relationship with a famous person, or even assume the identity of a famous person (believing that the actual person is an imposter). Grandiose delusions of a religious nature may lead to assumption of the identity of a deity or religious leader.

Jealous Type

The content of jealous delusions centers on the idea that the person's sexual partner is unfaithful. The idea is irrational and without cause, but the deluded individual searches for evidence to justify the belief. The sexual partner is confronted (and sometimes physically attacked) regarding the imagined infidelity. The imagined "lover" of the sexual partner may also be the object of the attack. Attempts to restrict the autonomy of the sexual partner in an effort to stop the imagined infidelity are common.

Persecutory Type

In persecutory delusions, which are the most common type, individuals believe they are being malevolently treated in some way. Frequent themes include being conspired against, cheated, spied on, followed, poisoned or drugged, maliciously maligned, harassed, or obstructed in the pursuit of long-term goals (APA, 2000). The individual may obsess about and exaggerate a slight rebuff (either real or imagined) until it becomes the focus of a delusional system. Repeated complaints may be directed at legal authorities, lack of satisfaction from which may result in violence toward the object of the delusion.

Somatic Type

Individuals with somatic delusions believe they have some physical defect, disorder, or disease. The *DSM-IV-TR* (APA, 2000) identifies the most common types of somatic delusions as those in which the individual believes that he or she:

1. Emits a foul odor from the skin, mouth, rectum, or vagina.
2. Has an infestation of insects in or on the skin.
3. Has an internal parasite.
4. Has misshapen and ugly body parts.
5. Has dysfunctional body parts.

Shared Psychotic Disorder

The essential feature of this disorder, also called *folie à deux*, is a delusional system that develops in a second person as a result of a close relationship with another person who already has a psychotic disorder with prominent delusions (APA, 2000). The person with the primary delusional disorder is usually the dominant person in the relationship, and the delusional thinking is gradually imposed on the more passive partner. This occurs within the context of a long-term close relationship, particularly when the couple has been socially isolated from other people. The course is usually chronic, and is more common in women than in men.

Psychotic Disorder Due to a General Medical Condition

The essential features of this disorder are prominent hallucinations and delusions that can be directly attributed to a general medical condition (APA, 2000). The diagnosis is not made if the symptoms occur during the course of a delirium or chronic, progressing dementia. A number of medical conditions can cause psychotic symptoms. Common ones identified by the *DSM-IV-TR* (APA, 2000) are presented in Table 28–1.

Substance-Induced Psychotic Disorder

The essential features of this disorder are the presence of prominent hallucinations and delusions that are judged to be directly attributable to the physiological effects of a substance (i.e., a drug of abuse, a medication, or toxin exposure) (APA, 2000). The diagnosis is made in the absence of reality testing and when history, physical examination, or laboratory findings indicate use of substances. When reality testing has been retained in the presence of substance-induced psychotic symptoms, the diagnosis would be substance-related disorder (Sadock & Sadock, 2003). Substances identified by the *DSM-IV-TR*

TABLE 28–1	General Medical Conditions that May Cause Psychotic Symptoms
Neurological conditions	Neoplasms
	Cerebrovascular disease
	Huntington's disease
	Epilepsy
	Auditory nerve injury
	Deafness
	Migraine headache
	CNS infections
Endocrine conditions	Hyperthyroidism
	Hypothyroidism
	Hyperparathyroidism
	Hypoparathyroidism
	Hypoadrenocorticism
Metabolic conditions	Hypoxia
	Hypercarbia
	Hypoglycemia
Autoimmune disorders	Systemic lupus erythematosus
Others	Fluid or electrolyte imbalances
	Hepatic or renal diseases

TABLE 28–2	Substances that May Cause Psychotic Disorders
Drugs of abuse	Alcohol
	Amphetamines and related substances
	Cannabis
	Cocaine
	Hallucinogens
	Inhalants
	Opioids
	Phencyclidine and related substances
	Sedatives, hypnotics, and anxiolytics
Medications	Anesthetics and analgesics
	Anticholinergic agents
	Anticonvulsants
	Antidepressant medication
	Antihistamines
	Antihypertensive agents
	Cardiovascular medications
	Antimicrobial medications
	Antiparkinsonian agents
	Chemotherapeutic agents
	Corticosteroids
	Disulfiram
	Gastrointestinal medications
	Muscle relaxants
	Nonsteroidal anti-inflammatory agents
Toxins	Anticholinesterase
	Organophosphate insecticides
	Nerve gases
	Carbon monoxide
	Carbon dioxide
	Volatile substances (e.g., fuel or paint)

(APA, 2000) that are believed to induce psychotic disorders are presented in Table 28–2.

APPLICATION OF THE NURSING PROCESS

Background Assessment Data

In the first step of the nursing process, the nurse gathers a database from which nursing diagnoses are derived and a plan of care is formulated. This first step of the nursing process is extremely important because without an accurate assessment, problem identification, objectives of care, and outcome criteria cannot be accurately determined.

Assessment of the client with schizophrenia may be a complex process, based on information gathered from a number of sources. Clients in an acute episode of their illness are seldom able to make a significant contribution to their history. Data may be obtained from family members, if possible; from old records, if available; or from other individuals who have been in a position to report on the progression of the client's behavior.

The nurse must be familiar with behaviors common to the disorder to be able to obtain an adequate assessment of the client with schizophrenia. Previous editions of the *Diagnostic and Statistical Manual of Mental Disorders* presented behavioral disturbances in eight areas of functioning: content of thought, form of thought, perception, affect, sense of self, volition, impaired interpersonal functioning and relationship to the external world, and psychomotor behavior. These areas of functioning are employed to facilitate the presentation of background information on which to base the initial assessment of the client with schizophrenia. Additional impairments outside the limits of these eight areas are also presented.

Content of Thought

Delusions. Delusions are false personal beliefs that are inconsistent with the person's intelligence or cultural background. The individual continues to have the belief in spite of obvious proof that it is false or irrational. Delusions are subdivided according to their content. Some of the more common ones are listed here.

Delusion of Persecution. The individual feels threatened and believes that others intend harm or persecution toward him or her in some way (e.g., "The FBI has 'bugged' my room and intends to kill me." "I can't take a shower in this bathroom; the nurses have put a camera in there so that they can watch everything I do").

Delusion of Grandeur. The individual has an exaggerated feeling of importance, power, knowledge, or identity (e.g., "I am Jesus Christ").

Delusion of Reference. All events within the environment are referred by the psychotic person to himself or herself (e.g., "Someone is trying to get a message to me through the articles in this magazine [or newspaper or TV program]; I must break the code so that I can receive the message"). *Ideas* of reference are less rigid than delusions of reference. An example of an idea of reference is irrationally thinking that one is being talked about or laughed at by other people.

Delusion of Control or Influence. The individual believes certain objects or persons have control over his or her behavior (e.g., "The dentist put a filling in my tooth; I now receive transmissions through the filling that control what I think and do").

Somatic Delusion. The individual has a false idea about the functioning of his or her body (e.g., "I'm 70 years old and I will be the oldest person ever to give birth. The doctor says I'm not pregnant, but I know I am").

Nihilistic Delusion. The individual has a false idea that the self, a part of the self, others, or the world is nonexistent (e.g., "The world no longer exists." "I have no heart.").

Religiosity. Religiosity is an excessive demonstration of or obsession with religious ideas and behavior. Because individuals vary greatly in their religious beliefs and level of spiritual commitment, religiosity is often difficult to assess. The individual with schizophrenia may use religious ideas in an attempt to provide rational meaning and structure to his or her behavior. Religious preoccupation in this vein may therefore be considered a manifestation of the illness. However, clients who derive comfort from their religious beliefs should not be discouraged from employing this means of support. An example of religiosity is the individual who believes the voice he or she hears is God and incessantly searches the Bible for interpretation.

Paranoia. Individuals with **paranoia** have extreme suspiciousness of others and of their actions or perceived intentions (e.g., "I won't eat this food. I know it has been poisoned.").

Magical Thinking. With **magical thinking**, the person believes that his or her thoughts or behaviors have control over specific situations or people (e.g., the mother who believed if she scolded her son in any way he would be taken away from her). Magical thinking is common in children. (For example, "Step on a crack and you break your mother's back." "An apple a day keeps the doctor away.")

Form of Thought

Associative Looseness. Thinking is characterized by speech in which ideas shift from one unrelated subject to another. With **associative looseness**, the individual is unaware that the topics are unconnected. When the condition is severe, speech may be incoherent. (For example, "We wanted to take the bus, but the airport took all the traffic. Driving is the ticket when you want to get somewhere. No one needs a ticket to heaven. We have it all in our pockets.")

Neologisms. The psychotic person invents new words, or **neologisms,** that are meaningless to others but have symbolic meaning to the psychotic person (e.g., "She wanted to give me a ride in her new *uniphorum*").

Concrete Thinking. Concreteness, or literal interpretations of the environment, represents a regression to an earlier level of cognitive development. Abstract thinking is very difficult. For example, the client with schizophrenia would have great difficulty describing the abstract meaning of sayings such as "I'm climbing the walls," or "It's raining cats and dogs."

Clang Associations. Choice of words is governed by sounds. **Clang associations** often take the form of rhyming. For instance, "It is very cold. I am cold and bold. The gold has been sold."

Word Salad. A word salad is a group of words that are put together randomly, without any logical connection (e.g., "Most forward action grows life double plays circle uniform").

Circumstantiality. With **circumstantiality**, the individual is delayed in reaching the point of a communication because of unnecessary and tedious details. The point or goal is usually met but only with numerous interruptions by the interviewer to keep the person on track of the topic being discussed.

Tangentiality. Tangentiality differs from circumstantiality in that the person never really gets to the point of the communication. Unrelated topics are introduced, and the original discussion is lost.

Mutism. This is an individual's inability or refusal to speak.

Perseveration. The individual who exhibits **perseveration** persistently repeats the same word or idea in response to different questions.

Perception

Hallucinations. Hallucinations, or false sensory perceptions not associated with real external stimuli, may involve any of the five senses. Types of hallucinations include the following:

Auditory. Auditory hallucinations are false perceptions of sound. Most commonly they are of voices, but the individual may report clicks, rushing noises, music, and other noises. Command hallucinations may place the individual or others in a potentially dangerous situation. "Voices" that issue commands for violence to self or others may or may not be heeded by the psychotic person. Auditory hallucinations are the most common type in psychiatric disorders.

Visual. These are false visual perceptions. They may consist of formed images, such as of people, or of unformed images, such as flashes of light.

Tactile. Tactile hallucinations are false perceptions of the sense of touch, often of something on or under the skin. One specific tactile hallucination is formication, the sensation that something is crawling on or under the skin.

Gustatory. This type is a false perception of taste. Most commonly, gustatory hallucinations are described as unpleasant tastes.

Olfactory. Olfactory hallucinations are false perceptions of the sense of smell.

Illusions. Illusions are misperceptions or misinterpretations of real external stimuli.

Affect

Affect describes the behavior associated with an individual's feeling state or emotional tone.

Inappropriate Affect. Affect is inappropriate when the individual's emotional tone is incongruent with the circumstances (e.g., a young woman who laughs when told of the death of her mother).

Bland or Flat Affect. Affect is described as bland when the emotional tone is very weak. The individual with flat affect appears to be void of emotional tone (or overt expression of feelings).

Apathy. The client with schizophrenia often demonstrates an indifference to or disinterest in the environment. The bland or flat affect is a manifestation of the emotional apathy.

Sense of Self

Sense of self describes the uniqueness and individuality a person feels. Because of extremely weak ego boundaries, the individual with schizophrenia lacks this feeling of uniqueness and experiences a great deal of confusion regarding his or her identity.

Echolalia. The client with schizophrenia may repeat words that he or she hears, which is called **echolalia**. This is an attempt to identify with the person speaking. (For instance, the nurse says, "John, it's time for lunch." The client may respond, "It's time for lunch, it's time for lunch" or sometimes, "Lunch, lunch, lunch, lunch").

Echopraxia. The client who exhibits **echopraxia** may purposelessly imitate movements made by others.

Identification (on an Unconscious Level) and Imitation (on a Conscious Level). These ego defense mechanisms are used by individuals with schizophrenia and reflect their confusion regarding self-identity. Because they have difficulty knowing where their ego boundaries end and another person's begins, their behavior often takes on the form of that which they see in the other person.

Depersonalization. The unstable self-identity of an individual with schizophrenia may lead to feelings of unreality (e.g., feeling that one's extremities have changed in size; or a sense of seeing oneself from a distance).

Volition

Volition has to do with impairment in the ability to initiate goal-directed activity. In the individual with schizophrenia, this may take the form of inadequate interest, motivation, or ability to choose a logical course of action in a given situation.

Emotional Ambivalence. Ambivalence in the client with schizophrenia refers to the coexistence of opposite emotions toward the same object, person, or situation. These opposing emotions may interfere with the person's ability to make even a very simple decision (e.g., whether to have coffee or tea with lunch). Underlying the ambivalence in the schizophrenic client is the difficulty he or she has in fulfilling a satisfying human relationship. This difficulty is based on the *need–fear dilemma*—the simultaneous need for and fear of intimacy.

Impaired Interpersonal Functioning and Relationship to the External World

Some clients with acute schizophrenia cling to others and intrude on the personal space of others, exhibiting behaviors that are not socially and culturally acceptable. Impairment in social functioning may also be reflected in social isolation, emotional detachment, and lack of regard for social convention.

Autism. Autism describes the condition created by the person with schizophrenia who focuses inward on a fantasy world, while distorting or excluding the external environment.

Deteriorated Appearance. Personal grooming and self-care activities may become minimal. The client with schizophrenia may appear disheveled and untidy and may need to be reminded of the need for personal hygiene.

Psychomotor Behavior

Anergia. Anergia is a deficiency of energy. The individual with schizophrenia may lack sufficient energy to carry out activities of daily living or to interact with others.

Waxy Flexibility. Waxy flexibility describes a condition in which the client with schizophrenia allows body parts to be placed in bizarre or uncomfortable positions. Once placed in position, the arm, leg, or head remains in that position for long periods, regardless of how uncomfortable it is for the client. For example, the nurse may position the client's arm in an outward position to take a blood pressure measurement. When the cuff is removed, the client may maintain the arm in the position in which it was placed to take the reading.

Posturing. This symptom is manifested by the voluntary assumption of inappropriate or bizarre postures.

Pacing and Rocking. Pacing back and forth and body rocking (a slow, rhythmic, backward-and-forward swaying of the trunk from the hips, usually while sitting) are common psychomotor behaviors of the client with schizophrenia.

Associated Features

Anhedonia. **Anhedonia** is the inability to experience pleasure. This is a particularly distressing symptom that compels some clients to attempt suicide.

Regression. Regression is the retreat to an earlier level of development. Regression, a primary defense mechanism of schizophrenia, is a dysfunctional attempt to reduce anxiety. It provides the basis for many of the behaviors associated with schizophrenia.

Positive and Negative Symptoms

Some clinicians find it useful to describe symptoms of schizophrenia as positive or negative. Positive symptoms tend to reflect an excess or distortion of normal functions, whereas negative symptoms reflect a diminution or loss of normal functions (APA, 2000). Most clients exhibit a mixture of both types of symptoms.

Positive symptoms are associated with normal brain structures on CT scan and relatively good responses to treatment. Individuals who exhibit mostly negative symptoms often show structural brain abnormalities on CT scans and respond poorly to treatment (Sadock & Sadock, 2003). Examples of positive and negative symptoms are presented in Table 28–3.

Diagnosis/Outcome Identification

From analysis of the assessment data, appropriate nursing diagnoses are formulated for the psychotic client and

TABLE 28–3	Positive and Negative Symptoms of Schizophrenia
POSITIVE SYMPTOMS	**NEGATIVE SYMPTOMS**
Hallucinations Auditory Visual Olfactory Gustatory Tactile	**Affective Flattening** Unchanging facial expression Poor eye contact Reduced body language Inappropriate affect Diminished emotional expression
Delusions Persecution Grandeur Reference Control or influence Somatic	**Alogia (Poverty of Speech)** Brief, empty responses Decreased fluency of speech Decreased content of speech
Disorganized Thinking/Speech Loose associations Incoherence Clang associations Word salad Neologisms Concrete thinking Echolalia Tangentiality Circumstantiality	**Avolition/Apathy** Inability to initiate goal-directed activity Little or no interest in work or social activities Impaired grooming/hygiene **Anhedonia** Absence of pleasure in social activities Diminished intimacy/sexual interest
Disorganized Behavior Disheveled appearance Inappropriate sexual behavior Restless, agitated behavior Waxy flexibility	**Social Isolation**

SOURCES: Adapted from *DSM-IV-TR* (APA, 2000) and Sadock & Sadock, 2003.

his or her family. From these identified problems, accurate planning of nursing care is executed. Possible nursing diagnoses for clients with psychotic disorders include:

Disturbed thought processes related to inability to trust, panic anxiety, possible hereditary or biochemical factors, evidenced by delusional thinking; inability to concentrate; impaired volition; inability to problem solve, abstract, or conceptualize; extreme suspiciousness of others.

Disturbed sensory perception: auditory/visual related to panic anxiety, extreme loneliness and withdrawal into the self, evidenced by inappropriate responses, disordered thought sequencing, rapid mood swings, poor concentration, disorientation.

Social isolation related to inability to trust, panic anxiety, weak ego development, delusional thinking, regression evidenced by withdrawal, sad dull affect, need–fear dilemma, preoccupation with own thoughts, expression of feelings of rejection or of aloneness imposed by others.

Risk for violence: Self-directed or other-directed related to extreme suspiciousness, panic anxiety, catatonic excitement, rage reactions, command hallucinations evidenced by overt and aggressive acts, goal-directed destruction of objects in the environment, self-destructive behavior, or active aggressive suicidal acts.

Impaired verbal communication related to panic anxiety, regression, withdrawal, and disordered, unrealistic thinking evidenced by loose association of ideas, neologisms, word salad, clang associations, echolalia, verbalizations that reflect concrete thinking, and poor eye contact.

Self-care deficit related to withdrawal, regression, panic anxiety, perceptual or cognitive impairment, inability to trust evidenced by difficulty carrying out tasks associated with hygiene, dressing, grooming, eating, and toileting.

Disabled family coping: related to difficulty coping with client's illness evidenced by neglectful care of the client in regard to basic human needs or illness treatment, extreme denial or prolonged over concern regarding client's illness.

Ineffective health maintenance related to disordered thinking or delusions evidenced by reported or observed inability to take responsibility for meeting basic health practices in any or all functional pattern areas.

Impaired home-maintenance management related to regression, withdrawal, lack of knowledge or resources, or impaired physical or cognitive functioning evidenced by unsafe, unclean, disorderly home environment.

The following criteria may be used for measurement of outcomes in the care of the client with schizophrenia.

The client:

1. Demonstrates an ability to relate satisfactorily with others.
2. Recognizes distortions of reality.
3. Has not harmed self or others.
4. Perceives self realistically.
5. Demonstrates the ability to perceive the environment correctly.
6. Maintains anxiety at a manageable level.
7. Relinquishes the need for delusions and hallucinations.
8. Demonstrates the ability to trust others.
9. Uses appropriate verbal communication in interactions with others.
10. Performs self-care activities independently.

Planning/Implementation

Table 28–4 provides a plan of care for the client with schizophrenia. Selected nursing diagnoses are presented,

TABLE 28–4	Care Plan for the Client with Schizophrenia

NURSING DIAGNOSIS: DISTURBED THOUGHT PROCESSES
RELATED TO: Inability to trust, panic anxiety, possible hereditary or biochemical factors
EVIDENCED BY: Delusional thinking; inability to concentrate; impaired volition; inability to problem solve, abstract, or conceptualize; extreme suspiciousness of others

OUTCOME CRITERIA	NURSING INTERVENTIONS	RATIONALE
Client will eliminate pattern of delusional thinking. Client will demonstrate trust in others.	1. Convey acceptance of client's need for the false belief, but indicate that you do not share the belief.	1. Client must understand that you do not view the idea as real.
	2. Do not argue or deny the belief. Use 'reasonable doubt' as a therapeutic technique: "I find that hard to believe."	2. Arguing or denying the belief serves no useful purpose, as delusional ideas are not eliminated by this approach, and the development of a trusting relationship may be impeded.
	3. Reinforce and focus on reality. Discourage long ruminations about the irrational thinking. Talk about real events and real people.	3. Discussions that focus on the false ideas are purposeless and useless, and may even aggravate the psychosis.
	4. If client is highly suspicious, the following interventions may help:	4. To decrease client's suspiciousness:
	a. Use same staff as much as possible; be honest and keep all promises.	a. Promotes trust.
	b. Avoid physical contact; avoid laughing, whispering, or talking quietly where client can see but cannot hear what is being said; provide canned food with can opener or serve food family style; avoid competitive activities; use assertive, matter-of-fact, yet friendly approach.	b. Prevents the client from feeling threatened.

(Continued on opposite page)

NURSING DIAGNOSIS: DISTURBED SENSORY PERCEPTION: AUDITORY/VISUAL

RELATED TO: Panic anxiety, extreme loneliness and withdrawal into the self

EVIDENCED BY: Inappropriate responses, disordered thought sequencing, rapid mood swings, poor concentration, disorientation

OUTCOME CRITERIA	NURSING INTERVENTIONS	RATIONALE
Client will be able to define and test reality, eliminating the occurrence of hallucinations.	1. Observe client for signs of hallucinations (listening pose, laughing or talking to self, stopping in midsentence).	1. Early intervention may prevent aggressive response to command hallucinations.
	2. Avoid touching the client without warning.	2. Client may perceive touch as threatening and may respond in an aggressive manner.
	3. An attitude of acceptance will encourage the client to share the content of the hallucination with you.	3. This is important to prevent possible injury to the client or others from command hallucinations.
	4. Do not reinforce the hallucination. Use "the voices" instead of words like "they" that imply validation. Let client know that you do not share the perception. Say, "Even though I realize the voices are real to you, I do not hear any voices."	4. Client must accept the perception as unreal before hallucinations can be eliminated.
	5. Help the client understand the connection between anxiety and hallucinations.	5. If client can learn to interrupt escalating anxiety, hallucinations may be prevented.
	6. Try to distract the client from the hallucination.	6. Involvement in interpersonal activities and explanation of the actual situation will help bring the client back to reality.

NURSING DIAGNOSIS: SOCIAL ISOLATION

RELATED TO: Inability to trust, panic anxiety, weak ego development, delusional thinking, regression

EVIDENCED BY: Withdrawal, sad, dull affect, need-fear dilemma, preoccupation with own thoughts, expression of feelings of rejection or of aloneness imposed by others

OUTCOME CRITERIA	NURSING INTERVENTIONS	RATIONALE
Client will voluntarily spend time with other clients and staff members in group therapeutic activities.	1. Convey an accepting attitude by making brief, frequent contacts. Show unconditional positive regard.	1. An accepting attitude increases feelings of self-worth and facilitates trust.
	2. Offer to be with client during group activities that he or she finds frightening or difficult.	2. The presence of a trusted individual provides emotional security for the client.
	3. Give recognition and positive reinforcement for client voluntary interactions with others.	3. Positive reinforcement enhances self-esteem and encourages repetition of acceptable behaviors.

NURSING DIAGNOSIS: RISK FOR VIOLENCE: SELF-DIRECTED OR OTHER-DIRECTED

RELATED TO: Extreme suspiciousness, panic anxiety, catatonic excitement, rage reactions, command hallucinations

EVIDENCED BY: Overt and aggressive acts, goal-directed destruction of objects in the environment, self-destructive behavior or active aggressive suicidal acts

OUTCOME CRITERIA	NURSING INTERVENTIONS	RATIONALE
Client will not harm self or others.	1. Maintain low level of stimuli in client's environment (low lighting, few people, simple decor, low noise level).	1. Anxiety level rises in stimulating environment. Individuals may be perceived as threatening by a suspicious, agitated client.

(Continued on following page)

TABLE 28–4   **Care Plan for the Client with Schizophrenia** *(Continued)*

OUTCOME CRITERIA	NURSING INTERVENTIONS	RATIONALE
	2. Observe client behavior frequently. Do this while carrying out routine activities.	2. Observation during routine activities avoids creating suspiciousness on the part of the client. Close observation is necessary so that intervention can occur if required to ensure client (and others') safety.
	3. Remove all dangerous objects from client's environment.	3. Removal of dangerous objects prevents client, in an agitated, confused state, from harming self or others.
	4. Redirect violent behavior with physical outlets for the anxiety.	4. Physical exercise is a safe and effective way of relieving pent-up tension.
	5. Staff should maintain a calm attitude toward client.	5. Anxiety is contagious and can be transmitted from staff to client.
	6. Have sufficient staff available to indicate a show of strength to client if it becomes necessary.	6. This shows the client evidence of control over the situation and provides some physical security for staff.
	7. Administer tranquilizing medications as ordered by physician. If client is not calmed by "talking down" or by medication, use of mechanical restraints may be necessary.	7. The avenue of the "least restrictive alternative" must be selected when planning interventions for a violent client.

NURSING DIAGNOSIS: IMPAIRED VERBAL COMMUNICATION

RELATED TO: Panic anxiety, regression, withdrawal, disordered, unrealistic thinking

EVIDENCED BY: Loose association of ideas, neologisms, word salad, clang association, echolalia, verbalizations that reflect concrete thinking, poor eye contact

OUTCOME CRITERIA	NURSING INTERVENTIONS	RATIONALE
Client will be able to communicate appropriately and comprehensibly with others.	1. Attempt to decode incomprehensible communication patterns. Seek validation and clarification by stating, "Is it that you mean…?" or "I don't understand what you mean by that. Would you please clarify it for me?"	1. These techniques reveal how the client is being perceived by others, while the responsibility for not understanding is accepted by the nurse.
	2. Facilitate trust and understanding by maintaining staff assignments as consistently as possible. The technique of *verbalizing the implied* is used with the client who is mute (unable or unwilling to speak). Example: "That must have been a very difficult time for you when your mother left. You must have felt very alone."	2. This approach conveys empathy and may encourage the client to disclose painful issues.
	3. Anticipate and fulfill client's needs until functional communication pattern returns.	3. Client safety and comfort are nursing priorities.
	4. Orient client to reality as required. Call the client by name. Validate those aspects of communication that help differentiate between what is real and not real.	4. These techniques may facilitate restoration of functional communication patterns in the client.

(Continued on opposite page)

NURSING DIAGNOSIS: SELF-CARE DEFICIT
RELATED TO: Withdrawal, regression, panic anxiety, perceptual or cognitive impairment, inability to trust
EVIDENCED BY: Difficulty carrying out tasks associated with hygiene, dressing, grooming, eating, toileting

OUTCOME CRITERIA	NURSING INTERVENTIONS	RATIONALE
Client will demonstrate ability to meet self-care needs independently.	1. Provide assistance with self-care needs as required. Some clients who are severely withdrawn may require total care. 2. Encourage client to perform independently as many activities as possible. Provide positive reinforcement for independent accomplishments. 3. Use concrete communication to show client what is expected. Example: "Pick up the spoon, scoop some mashed potatoes into it, and put it in your mouth." 4. Creative approaches may need to be taken with the client who is not eating, such as allowing client to open own canned or packaged foods; family-style serving may also be an option. 5. If toileting needs are not being met, establish a structured schedule for the client.	1. Client safety and comfort are nursing priorities. 2. Independent accomplishment and positive reinforcement enhance self-esteem and promote repetition of desirable behaviors. 3. Because concrete thinking prevails, explanations must be provided at the client's concrete level of comprehension. 4. This technique may be helpful with the client who is paranoid and may be suspicious that he or she is being poisoned with food or medication. 5. A structured schedule will help the client establish a pattern so that he or she can develop an independent habit of toileting independently.

NURSING DIAGNOSIS: DISABLED FAMILY COPING
RELATED TO: Difficulty coping with client's illness
EVIDENCED BY: Neglectful care of the client in regard to basic human needs or illness treatment, extreme denial or prolonged overconcern regarding client's illness

OUTCOME CRITERIA	NURSING INTERVENTIONS	RATIONALE
Family will identify more adaptive coping strategies for dealing with client's illness and treatment regimen.	1. Identify level of family functioning. Assess communication patterns, interpersonal relationships between members, role expectations, problem-solving skills, and availability of outside support systems. 2. Provide information for the family about the client's illness, what will be required in the treatment regimen, and long-term prognosis. 3. With family members, practice how to respond to bizarre behavior and communication patterns and in the event that the client becomes violent.	1. These factors will help to identify how successful the family is in dealing with stressful situations, and areas where assistance is required. 2. Knowledge and understanding about what to expect may facilitate the family's ability to successfully integrate the client into the system. 3. A plan of action will assist the family to respond adaptively in the face of what they may consider to be a crisis situation.

along with outcome criteria; appropriate nursing interventions, and rationales for each.

Some institutions are using a case management model to coordinate care (see Chapter 9 for more detailed explanation). In case management models, the plan of care may take the form of a critical pathway. Table 28–5 depicts an example of a critical pathway of care for a client experiencing an exacerbation of schizophrenic psychosis.

The concept map care plan is an innovative approach to planning and organizing nursing care (see Chapter 9).

Estimated Length of Stay: 7 Days—Variations from Designated Pathway Should Be Documented in Progress Notes

Nursing Diagnoses and Categories of Care	Time Dimension	Goals and/or Actions	Time Dimension	Goals and/or Actions	Time Dimension	Discharge Outcome
Disturbed thought processes/Disturbed sensory perception			Day 5	Client is able to differentiate between what is real and what is not real	Day 7	Client experiences no delusional thinking or hallucinations
Referrals	Day 1	Psychiatrist Psychologist Social worker Clinical nurse specialist Music therapist Occupational therapist Recreational therapist			Day 7	Discharge with follow-up appointments as required.
Diagnostic studies	Day 1 Days 3–5	Drug screen Chemistry profile CT scan, MRI, PET, EEG. (These may be ordered to examine structure and function of the brain.)				
Additional assessments	Day 1 Day 1	VS every shift. Assess for: delusions, hallucinations, loose associations, inappropriate affect, excitement/stupor, panic anxiety, suspiciousness.	Days 2–7 Days 2–5	Ongoing assessments Establish trust with at least one person.	Days 2–7 Day 7	VS daily if stable. No evidence of delusions, hallucinations, loose associations, inappropriate affect, excitement/stupor, panic anxiety, suspiciousness.
Medications	Day 1	Antipsychotic medication (scheduled and p.r.n.). May need order for concentrate and injectable form. Antiparkinsonian medication (p.r.n.)	Days 1–7	Assess for effectiveness and side effects of medications.	Day 7	Client is discharged with medications.
Client education			Day 5 Day 6	Discuss correlation between increased anxiety and psychotic symptoms. Discuss ways to de-escalate anxiety. Discuss importance of taking medications regularly, even when feeling well. Discuss possible side effects of medications and when to see the doctor.	Day 7 Day 7	Reinforce teaching. Client verbalizes understanding of information presented prior to discharge.
Risk for violence: Self-directed or other-directed	Day 1	Environment is made safe for client and others.	Ongoing	Client does not harm self or others.	Day 7	Client is discharged without harm to self or others.
Referrals	Day 1	Alert hostility management team of the admission of a potentially violent client. For relaxation therapy: Music therapist Clinical nurse specialist Stress management specialist			Day 7	Discharge with follow-up appointments as required.

(Continued on opposite page)

Nursing Diagnoses and Categories of Care	Time Dimension	Goals and/or Actions	Time Dimension	Goals and/or Actions	Time Dimension	Discharge Outcome
		Psychiatrist: May give order for mechanical restraints to be used if needed.				
Additional assessments	Day 1	Assess for signs of impending violent behavior: increase in psychomotor activity; angry affect; verbalized persecutory delusions or frightening hallucinations.	Days 2–7	Ongoing assessments.		
Medications	Day 1	Antipsychotic medications (p.r.n.) when signs of agitation begin.	Days 1–7	Use of medications, isolation/seclusion, or mechanical restraints. If client refuses medications, administer following application of restraints.	Day 7	Client is discharged with medications.
Client education			Days 3–6	Teach relaxation techniques; discuss activities in which client could participate to relieve pent-up tension; discuss signs and symptoms of escalating anxiety.	Day 7 Day 7	Reinforce teaching. Client verbalizes understanding of information presented prior to discharge.

CT = computed tomography; EEG = electroencephalogram; MRI = magnetic resonance imaging; PET = positron emission tomography.

It is a diagrammatic teaching and learning strategy that allows visualization of interrelationships between medical diagnoses, nursing diagnoses, assessment data, and treatments. An example of a concept map care plan for a client with schizophrenia is presented in Figure 28–3.

Client/Family Education

The role of client teacher is important in the psychiatric area, as it is in all areas of nursing. A list of topics for client/family education relevant to schizophrenia is presented in Table 28–6.

Evaluation

In the final step of the nursing process, a reassessment is conducted in order to determine if the nursing actions have been successful in achieving the objectives of care. Evaluation of the nursing actions for the client with exacerbation of schizophrenic psychosis may be facilitated by gathering information utilizing the following types of questions:

1. Has the client established trust with at least one staff member?
2. Is the anxiety level maintained at a manageable level?
3. Is delusional thinking still prevalent?
4. Is hallucinogenic activity evident? Does the client share content of hallucinations, particularly if commands are heard?
5. Is the client able to interrupt escalating anxiety with adaptive coping mechanisms?
6. Is the client easily agitated?
7. Is the client able to interact with others appropriately?
8. Does the client voluntarily attend therapy activities?
9. Is verbal communication comprehensible?
10. Is the client compliant with medication? Does the client verbalize the importance of taking medication regularly and on a long-term basis? Does he or she verbalize understanding of possible side effects, and when to seek assistance from the physician?
11. Does the client spend time with others rather than isolating self?
12. Is the client able to carry out all activities of daily living independently?
13. Is the client able to verbalize resources from which he or she may seek assistance outside the hospital?
14. Does the family have information regarding support groups in which they may participate, and from which they may seek assistance in dealing with their family member who is ill?

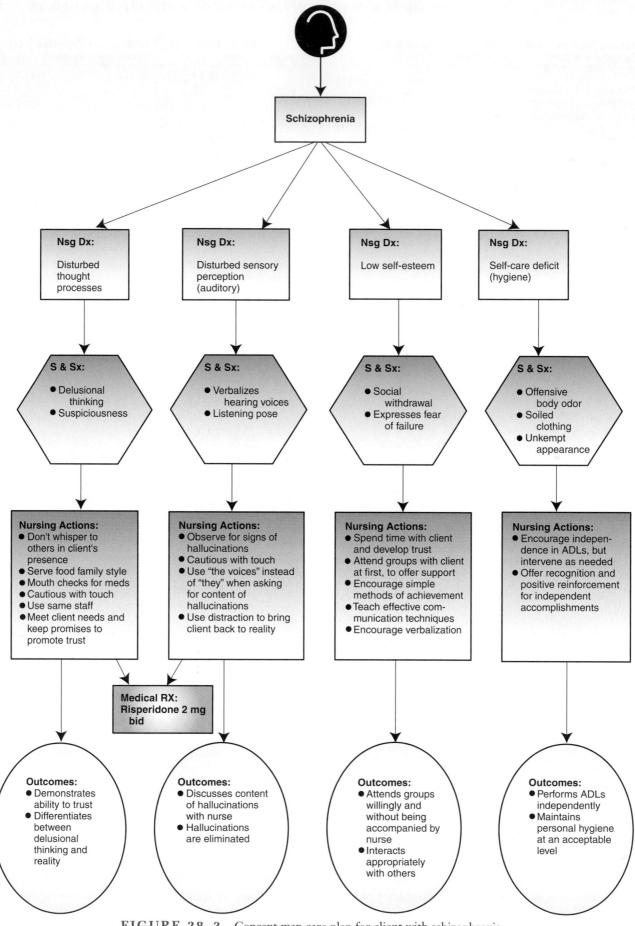

FIGURE 28–3 Concept map care plan for client with schizophrenia.

TABLE 28–6   Topics for Client/Family Education Related to Schizophrenia

Nature of the Illness
1. What to expect as the illness progresses
2. Symptoms associated with the illness
3. Ways for family to respond to behaviors associated with the illness

Management of the Illness
1. Connection of exacerbation of symptoms to times of stress
2. Appropriate medication management
3. Side effects of medications
4. Importance of not stopping medications
5. When to contact health-care provider
6. Relaxation techniques
7. Social skills training
8. Daily living skills training

Support Services
1. Financial assistance
2. Legal assistance
3. Caregiver support groups
4. Respite care
5. Home health care

15. If the client lives alone, does he or she have a source for assistance with home maintenance and health management?

TREATMENT MODALITIES FOR SCHIZOPHRENIA AND OTHER PSYCHOTIC DISORDERS

Psychological Treatments

Individual Psychotherapy

Ho, Black, and Andreasen (2003) state:

> Although intensive psychodynamic- and insight-oriented psychotherapy is generally not recommended, the form of individual psychotherapy that psychiatrists employ when providing pharmacological treatment typically involves a synthesis of various psychotherapeutic strategies and interventions. These include problem solving, reality testing, psychoeducation, and supportive and cognitive-behavioral techniques anchored on an empathetic therapeutic alliance with the patient. The goals of such individual psychotherapy are to improve medication compliance, enhance social and occupational functioning, and prevent relapse. (p. 419)

Reality-oriented individual therapy is the most suitable approach to individual psychotherapy for schizophrenia. The primary focus in all cases must reflect efforts to decrease anxiety and increase trust.

Establishing a relationship is often particularly difficult because the individual with schizophrenia is desperately lonely yet defends against closeness and trust. He or she is likely to respond to attempts at closeness with suspiciousness, anxiety, aggression, or regression. Successful intervention may be achieved with honesty, simple directness, and a manner that respects the client's privacy and human dignity. Exaggerated warmth and professions of friendship are likely to be met with confusion and suspicion.

Once a therapeutic interpersonal relationship has been established, reality orientation is maintained through exploration of the client's behavior within relationships. Education is provided to help the client identify sources of real or perceived danger and ways of reacting appropriately. Methods for improving interpersonal communication, emotional expression, and frustration tolerance are attempted.

Individual psychotherapy for clients with schizophrenia is seen as a long-term endeavor that requires patience on the part of the therapist, as well as the ability to accept that a great deal of change may not occur. Some cases report treatment durations of many years before clients regain some degree of independent functioning.

Group Therapy

Group therapy with individuals with schizophrenia has been shown to be effective, particularly with outpatients and when combined with drug treatment. Sadock and Sadock (2003) state:

> Group therapy for people with schizophrenia generally focuses on real-life plans, problems, and relationships. Some investigators doubt that dynamic interpretation and insight therapy are valuable for typical patients with schizophrenia. But group therapy is effective in reducing social isolation, increasing the sense of cohesiveness, and improving reality testing for patients with schizophrenia. (p. 501)

Group therapy in inpatient settings is less productive. Inpatient treatment usually occurs when symptomatology and social disorganization are at their most intense. At this time, the least amount of stimuli possible is most beneficial for the client. Because group therapy can be an intensive and highly stimulating environment, it may be counterproductive early in treatment.

Group therapy for schizophrenia has been most useful over the long-term course of the illness. The social interaction, sense of cohesiveness, identification, and reality testing achieved within the group setting have proven to be highly therapeutic processes for these clients. Groups led in a supportive manner, rather than in an interpretative way, appear to be most helpful for schizophrenic patients (Sadock & Sadock, 2003).

Behavior Therapy

Behavior modification has a history of qualified success in reducing the frequency of bizarre, disturbing, and deviant behaviors and increasing appropriate behaviors. Features that have led to the most positive results include:

1. Clearly defining goals and how they will be measured.
2. Attaching positive, negative, and aversive reinforcements to adaptive and maladaptive behavior.
3. Using simple, concrete instructions and prompts to elicit the desired behavior.

Behavior therapy can be a powerful treatment tool for helping clients change undesirable behaviors. In the treatment setting, the therapist can use praise and other positive reinforcements to help the schizophrenic person reduce the frequency of maladaptive or deviant behaviors. A limitation of this type of treatment is the inability of some individuals with schizophrenia to generalize what they have learned to the community setting following discharge from therapy.

Social Skills Training

Social skills training has become one of the most widely used psychosocial interventions in the treatment of schizophrenia. Mueser, Bond, and Drake (2001) state:

> The basic premise of social skills training is that complex interpersonal skills involve the smooth integration of a combination of simpler behaviors, including *nonverbal behaviors* (e.g., facial expression, eye contact); *paralinguistic features* (e.g., voice loudness and affect); *verbal content* (i.e., the appropriateness of what is said); and *interactive balance* (e.g., response latency, amount of time talking). These specific skills can be systematically taught, and, through the process of *shaping* (i.e., rewarding successive approximations toward the target behavior), complex behavioral repertoires can be acquired.

Social dysfunction is a hallmark of schizophrenia. Indeed, impairment in social functioning is included as one of the defining diagnostic criteria for schizophrenia in the *DSM-IV-TR* (APA, 2000). Considerable attention is now being given to enhancement of social skills in these clients.

The educational procedure in social skills training focuses on role-play. A series of brief scenarios are selected. These should be typical of situations clients experience in their daily lives and be graduated in terms of level of difficulty. The therapist may serve as a role model for some behaviors. For example, "See how I sort of nod my head up and down and look at your face while you talk." The therapist's demonstration is followed by the client's role-playing. Immediate feedback is provided regarding the client's presentation. Only by countless repetitions does the response gradually become smooth and effortless.

Progress is geared toward the client's needs and limitations. The focus is on small units of behavior, and the training proceeds very gradually. Highly threatening issues are avoided, and emphasis is placed on functional skills that are relevant to activities of daily living.

Social Treatment

Milieu Therapy

Some clinicians believe that milieu therapy can be an appropriate treatment for the client with schizophrenia. Research suggests that psychotropic medication is more effective at all levels of care when used along with milieu therapy and that milieu therapy is more successful if used in conjunction with these medications.

Sadock and Sadock (2003) state:

> Most milieu therapy programs emphasize group and social interaction; rules and expectations are mediated by peer pressure for normalization of adaptation. When patients are viewed as responsible human beings, the patient role becomes blurred. Milieu therapy stresses a patient's rights to goals and to have freedom of movement and informal relationship with staff; it also emphasizes interdisciplinary participation and goal-oriented, clear communication. (p. 966)

Individuals with schizophrenia who are treated with milieu therapy alone require longer hospital stays than do those treated with drugs and psychosocial therapy. Other economic considerations, such as the need for a high staff-to-client ratio, in addition to the longer admission, limit the use of milieu therapy in the treatment of schizophrenia.

Family Therapy

Some therapists treat schizophrenia as an illness not of the client alone, but of the entire family. Even when families appear to cope well, there is a notable impact on the mental health status of relatives when a family member has the illness. Safier (1997) states:

> When a family member has a serious mental illness, the family must deal with a major upheaval in their lives, a terrible event that causes great pain and grief for the loss of a once-promising child or relationship. (p. 5)

The importance of the expanded role of family in the aftercare of relatives with schizophrenia has been recognized, thereby stimulating interest in family intervention programs designed to support the family system, prevent or delay relapse, and help to maintain the client in the community. These psychoeducational programs treat the family as a resource rather than a stressor, with the focus on concrete problem solving and specific helping behaviors for coping with stress. Many of these programs recognize a biological basis for the illness and the impact that stress has on the client's ability to function. By providing the family with information about the illness and suggestions for effective coping, psychoeducational programs reduce the likelihood of the client's relapse and the possible emergence of mental illness in previously nonaffected relatives.

Dixon and Lehman (1995) state that although studies of family interventions with schizophrenia differ in their characteristics and methods, they tend to share a common set of assumptions:

1. Schizophrenia is regarded as an illness.
2. The family environment is not implicated in the etiology of the illness.
3. Support is provided and families are enlisted as therapeutic agents.
4. The interventions are part of a treatment package used in conjunction with routine drug treatment and outpatient clinical management.

Asen (2002) suggests the following interventions with families of individuals with schizophrenia:

1. Forming a close alliance with the caregivers
2. Lowering the emotional intrafamily climate by reducing stress and burden on relatives
3. Increasing the capacity of relatives to anticipate and solve problems
4. Reducing the expressions of anger and guilt by family members
5. Maintaining reasonable expectations for how the ill family member should perform
6. Encouraging relatives to set appropriate limits while maintaining some degree of separateness
7. Promoting desirable changes in the relatives' behaviors and belief systems

Family therapy typically consists of a brief program of family education about schizophrenia, and a more extended program of family contact designed to reduce overt manifestations of conflict and to alter patterns of family communication and problem solving. The response to this type of therapy has been very dramatic. Ho, Black, and Andreasen (2003) report on several studies, clearly revealing that a more positive outcome in the treatment of the client with schizophrenia can be achieved by including the family system in the program of care.

Assertive Community Treatment (ACT)

Assertive Community Treatment (ACT) is a program of case management that takes a team approach in providing comprehensive, community-based psychiatric treatment, rehabilitation, and support to persons with serious and persistent mental illness such as schizophrenia. Aggressive programs of treatment are individually tailored for each client and include the teaching of basic living skills, helping clients work with community agencies, and assisting clients in developing a social support network (Ho, Black, & Andreasen, 2003). There is emphasis on vocational expectations, and supported work settings (i.e., sheltered workshops) are an important part of the treatment program. Other services include substance abuse treatment, psychoeducational programs, family support and education, mobile crisis intervention, and attention to health care needs.

Responsibilities are shared by multiple team members, including psychiatrists, nurses, social workers, vocational rehabilitation therapists, and substance abuse counselors. Services are provided in the person's home, within the neighborhood, in local restaurants, parks, stores, or wherever assistance by the client is required. These services are available to the client 24 hours a day, 365 days a year. The National Alliance for the Mentally Ill (NAMI) (2003) lists the primary goals of ACT as follows:

1. To meet basic needs and enhance quality of life
2. To improve functioning in adult social and employment roles
3. To enhance an individual's ability to live independently in his or her own community
4. To lessen the family's burden of providing care
5. To lessen or eliminate the debilitating symptoms of mental illness
6. To minimize or prevent recurrent acute episodes of the illness

Individuals best served by ACT are identified by the Assertive Community Treatment Association (ACTA) (2005) as follows:

> Clients served by ACT are individuals with serious and persistent mental illness or personality disorders, with severe functional impairments, who have avoided or not responded well to traditional outpatient mental health care and psychiatric rehabilitation services. Persons served by ACT often have co-existing problems such as homelessness, substance abuse problems, or involvement with the judicial system.

ACT has been shown to reduce the number of hospitalizations and decrease costs of care for these clients. Although it has been called "paternalistic" and "coercive" by its critics, ACT has provided a much-needed service and increased quality of life to many clients who are unable to manage in a less-structured environment.

Organic Treatment

Psychopharmacology

Chlorpromazine (Thorazine) was first introduced in the United States in 1952. At that time, it was used in conjunction with barbiturates in surgical anesthesia. With increased use, the drug's psychic properties were recognized, and by 1954 it was marketed as an antipsychotic medication in the United States. The manufacture and sale of other antipsychotic drugs followed in rapid succession. (See Chapter 21 for a detailed discussion of antipsychotic medications.)

Antipsychotic medications are very effective in treating the symptoms of schizophrenia. Unfortunately, substantiated evidence of long-term recovery with antipsychotic medications is notably lacking. *The Merck Manual of Diagnosis and Therapy (MMDT)* (2002) reports:

> Over a short period (1 year), the prognosis of schizophrenia is closely related to how well a person follows a drug treatment plan. Without drug treatment, 70 to 80 percent of the people who have experienced a schizophrenic episode will relapse over the next 12 months and experience a subsequent episode. Drugs taken continuously can reduce the relapse rate to about 30 percent.

The prognosis of schizophrenia is often reported in the paradigm of thirds. One third of the people achieve significant and lasting improvement. They may never experience another episode of psychosis following the initial occurrence. One third may achieve some improvement with intermittent relapses and residual disability. Their occupational level may have decreased because of their illness, or they may be socially isolated. Finally, one third experiences severe and permanent incapacity. They often do not respond to medication and remain chronically ill for much of their lives. Men have poorer outcomes than women do; women respond better to treatment with antipsychotic medications (*MMDT*, 2002).

As mentioned earlier, the efficacy of antipsychotic medications is enhanced by adjunct psychosocial therapy. Because the psychotic manifestations of the illness subside with use of the drugs, clients are generally more cooperative with the psychosocial therapies.

Antipsychotic drugs, also called neuroleptics or major tranquilizers, are effective in the treatment of acute and chronic manifestations of schizophrenia and in maintenance therapy to prevent exacerbation of schizophrenic symptoms. However, because of a number of unpleasant and even dangerous side effects, the advisability of long-term use may be questionable. Common side effects include anticholinergic manifestations (dry mouth, blurred vision, constipation, urinary retention), nausea, gastrointestinal upset, skin rash, sedation, orthostatic hypotension, photosensitivity, decreased libido, retrograde ejaculation, gynecomastia, amenorrhea, weight gain, reduction in seizure threshold, agranulocytosis, extrapyramidal symptoms (pseudoparkinsonism, akinesia, akathisia, dystonia, oculogyric crisis), tardive dyskinesia, and neuroleptic malignant syndrome.

Antiparkinsonian agents may be prescribed to counteract the extrapyramidal symptoms associated with antipsychotic medications. These drugs are cholinergic blockers, producing the same anticholinergic side effects as the antipsychotic medications. Some physicians routinely prescribe the antiparkinsonian drug to be given on a scheduled basis with the antipsychotic medication. Others prefer to order the drug on an as-needed basis, to be administered only if the neurological symptoms appear, thus reducing the compounded anticholinergic effects of the two drugs together. When the drug is given as needed, it is extremely important for the nurse to be able to recognize the symptoms associated with extrapyramidal side effects so that he or she can administer the antiparkinsonian drug without delay (see Chapter 21). Many physicians are choosing to prescribe the newer atypical antipsychotics (e.g., clozapine, risperidone, olanzapine, quetiapine, ziprasidone, aripiprazole) that cause few, if any, extrapyramidal symptoms.

For those clients with schizophrenia who do not respond to antipsychotic medications, a number of other pharmacological options have been tried, with various degrees of success. Use of the following medication alternatives have been reported (Ho, Black, & Andreasen, 2003; Sadock & Sadock, 2003):

1. Reserpine, a dopamine receptor antagonist, has been used as an antihypertensive agent and as an antipsychotic. It has produced severe depression in humans and for this reason is now rarely used for either purpose.
2. Lithium carbonate can ameliorate schizophrenic symptoms or suppress episodic violence in clients with schizophrenia but is seldom an adequate drug therapy alone.
3. Carbamazepine ameliorates symptoms in some treatment-resistant psychotic clients, but it alone is not an adequate therapy for schizophrenia.
4. Valium, in high dosages, was shown to control psychotic symptoms of schizophrenia, such as agitation, thought disorder, delusions, and hallucinations. It has also been used to relieve akathisia associated with some antipsychotic medication. The best use of benzodiazepines appears to be as adjunct therapy with antipsychotic medication in the management of psychotic agitation (Ho, Black, & Andreasen, 2003).
5. Propranolol may be useful in controlling temper outbursts in aggressive or violent psychotic clients.

The advent of antipsychotic medications in the 1950s was hailed as a medical breakthrough for psychiatry. At last the physician could do something substantive for the client with schizophrenia. No one knows exactly how the antipsychotic effect is achieved or why it takes several weeks for these effects to be observed. Scientists cannot yet explain why clients do not become tolerant to antipsychotics, or why discontinuing the drug does not make the disease worse than it was before treatment. By studying the action of antipsychotic drugs, however, progress has been made toward understanding what is wrong with the schizophrenic brain. Continual refinement of the research methods and investigation of other transmitter systems may reveal more precisely how the schizophrenic brain differs from the healthy one. A summary of medications used in the treatment of schizophrenia is presented in Table 28–7.

TABLE 28–7	**Medications Used in the Treatment of Schizophrenia**		
CLASSIFICATION	**GENERIC (TRADE) NAME**	**DAILY DOSAGE RANGE (MG)**	**SIDE EFFECTS**
Phenothiazines	Chlorpromazine (Thorazine)	75–400	For all phenothiazines: Anticholinergic side effects, nausea, skin rash, sedation, orthostatic hypotension, tachycardia, photosensitivity, decreased libido, amenorrhea, retrograde ejaculation, gynecomastia, weight gain, reduction of seizure threshold, agranulocytosis, EPS, tardive dyskinesia, NMS
	Fluphenazine (Prolixin)	2.5–10	
	Perphenazine (Trilafon)	12–64	
	Prochlorperazine (Compazine)	15–150	
	Thioridazine (Mellaril)	150–800	
	Trifluoperazine (Stelazine)	4–40	
Thioxanthenes	Thiothixene (Navane)	6–30	Refer to side effects of phenothiazines
Benzisoxazole	Risperidone (Risperdal)	1–6	Anxiety, agitation, insomnia, sedation, EPS, dizziness, headache, constipation, nausea, rhinitis, rash, tachycardia, hyperglycemia
Butyrophenone	Haloperidol (Haldol)	1–100	Refer to side effects of phenothiazines
Dibenzoxazepine	Loxapine (Loxitane)	20–250	Refer to side effects of phenothiazines
Dihydroindolone	Molindone (Moban)	15–225	Refer to side effects of phenothiazines
Dibenzodiazepine	Clozapine (Clozaril)	300–900	Drowsiness, dizziness, agranulocytosis, seizures, sedation, hypersalivation, tachycardia, constipation, fever, weight gain, orthostatic hypotension, NMS, hyperglycemia
Thienobenzodiazepine	Olanzapine (Zyprexa)	5–20	Asthenia, somnolence, headache, fever, dizziness, dry mouth, constipation, weight gain, orthostatic hypotension, tachycardia, EPS (high-dose dependent), hyperglycemia
Dibenzothiazepine	Quetiapine (Seroquel)	150–750	Somnolence, dizziness, headache, constipation, dry mouth, dyspepsia, weight gain, orthostatic hypotension, NMS, EPS, tardive dyskinesia, cataracts, lowered seizure threshold, hyperglycemia
Benzothiazolylpiperazine	Ziprasidone (Geodon)	40–160	Somnolence, headache, nausea, dyspepsia, constipation, dizziness, diarrhea, restlessness, EPS, prolonged QT interval, orthostatic hypotension, rash, hyperglycemia
Dihydrocarbostyril	Aripiprazole (Abilify)	10–30	Headache, nausea and vomiting, constipation, anxiety, restlessness, insomnia, lightheadedness, somnolence, weight gain, blurred vision, increased salivation, EPS, hyperglycemia

EPS = extrapyramidal symptoms; NMS = neuroleptic malignant syndrome.

SUMMARY

Of all mental illness, schizophrenia undoubtedly results in the greatest amount of personal, emotional, and social costs. It presents an enormous threat to life and happiness, yet it remains a puzzle to the medical community. In fact, for many years there was little agreement as to a definition of the concept of schizophrenia. The *DSM-IV-TR* (APA, 2000) identifies specific criteria for diagnosis of the disorder, which were presented in this chapter.

The initial symptoms of schizophrenia most often occur in early adulthood. Development of the disorder can be viewed in four phases: (1) the schizoid personality, (2) the prodromal phase, (3) the active phase of schizophrenia, and (4) the residual phase.

The cause of schizophrenia remains unclear. Research continues, and most contemporary psychiatrists are giving more credence to the biological theories and placing little emphasis on psychosocial influences. The transactional view, however, supports the idea that no single factor can be implicated in the etiology, but that the disease most likely results from a combination of influences including genetics, biochemical dysfunction, and physiological and environmental factors.

Various types of schizophrenic and related psychotic disorders have been identified. They are differentiated by their total picture of clinical symptomatology. They include disorganized schizophrenia, catatonic schizophrenia, paranoid schizophrenia, undifferentiated schizophrenia, residual schizophrenia, schizoaffective disorder, brief psychotic disorder, schizophreniform disorder, delusional disorder, shared psychotic disorder, psychotic disorder caused by a general medical condition, and substance-induced psychotic disorder.

Care of the client with schizophrenia was presented in the context of the six steps of the nursing process. Nursing assessment is based on knowledge of symptomatology related to thought content and form, perception, affect, sense of self, volition, impaired interpersonal functioning and relationship to the external world, and psychomotor behavior. Nursing diagnoses were formulated from the assessment data, and a plan of care was developed. A critical pathway of care for

the client with schizophrenia was included as a guideline for nurses who follow a program of case management. A concept map care plan, an additional model for organizing nursing care, was also included. Guide lines for evaluation of client outcomes were presented.

Various treatment modalities for schizophrenia were discussed, including individual psychotherapy, group therapy, behavior therapy, social skills training, milieu therapy, family therapy, assertive community treatment, and psychopharmacology. For the majority of clients, the most effective treatment appears to be a combination of psychotropic medication and psychosocial therapy.

REVIEW QUESTIONS

SELF-EXAMINATION/LEARNING EXERCISE

Situation: Tony, age 20 years, quit college 2 months ago and returned to live at his parents' home. He has become increasingly withdrawn, suspicious, and isolated since his return, and his parents have taken him to the emergency department. His parents report that he has been looking at them strangely as if he did not know them, refusing to talk to anyone, spending a lot of time in his room alone, refusing all help. The father brought the client to the hospital against his will following a verbal argument during the course of which the client attempted to stab the father with a kitchen knife. The father had successfully subdued him and removed the weapon. On arrival at the emergency department, the client was agitated and exhibiting acutely psychotic symptoms. He reports that "they" told him to kill his father before his father kills him. Verbalizations are often incoherent. Affect is flat, and he continuously scans the environment. He is admitted to the psychiatric unit with a diagnosis of schizophreniform disorder, provisional.

Based on the above situation, select the answer that is most appropriate for each of the following questions:

1. The *initial* nursing intervention for Tony is to:
   a. Give him an injection of Thorazine.
   b. Ensure a safe environment for him and others.
   c. Place him in restraints.
   d. Order him a nutritious diet.

2. The primary goal in working with Tony would be to:
   a. Promote interaction with others.
   b. Decrease his anxiety and increase trust.
   c. Improve his relationship with his parents.
   d. Encourage participation in therapy activities.

3. Orders from the physician include 100 mg chlorpromazine (Thorazine) STAT and then 50 mg b.i.d.; 2 mg benztropine (Cogentin) b.i.d. p.r.n. Why is chlorpromazine ordered?
   a. To reduce extrapyramidal symptoms
   b. To prevent neuroleptic malignant syndrome
   c. To decrease psychotic symptoms
   d. To induce sleep

4. Benztropine was ordered on a p.r.n. basis. Which of the following assessments by the nurse would convey a need for this medication?
   a. The client's level of agitation increases.
   b. The client complains of a sore throat.
   c. The client's skin has a yellowish cast.
   d. The client develops tremors and a shuffling gait.

5. Tony begins to tell the nurse about how the CIA is looking for him and will kill him if they find him. The most appropriate response by the nurse is:
   a. "That's ridiculous, Tony. No one is going to hurt you."
   b. "The CIA isn't interested in people like you, Tony."
   c. "Why do you think the CIA wants to kill you?"
   d. "I find that very hard to believe, Tony."

6. Tony's belief about the CIA is an example of a:
   a. Delusion of persecution
   b. Delusion of reference
   c. Delusion of control or influence
   d. Delusion of grandeur

7. Tony tilts his head to the side, stops talking in midsentence, and listens intently. The nurse recognizes from these signs that Tony is likely experiencing:
   a. Somatic delusions
   b. Catatonic stupor
   c. Auditory hallucinations
   d. Pseudoparkinsonism

8. The most appropriate nursing intervention for the symptom just described is to:
   a. Ask the client to describe his physical symptoms.
   b. Ask the client to describe what he is hearing.
   c. Administer a dose of benztropine.
   d. Call the physician for additional orders.

9. Should Tony suddenly become aggressive and violent on the unit, which of the following approaches would be best for the nurse to use first?
   a. Provide large motor activities to relieve Tony's pent-up tension.
   b. Administer a large dose of sedative to keep Tony calm.
   c. Call for sufficient help to control the situation safely.
   d. Convey to Tony that his behavior is unacceptable and will not be permitted.

10. Tony and his parents attend a weekly family therapy group. The primary focus of this type of group is:
    a. To discuss concrete problem solving and adaptive behaviors for coping with stress
    b. To introduce the family to others with the same problem
    c. To keep the client and family in touch with the health care system
    d. To promote family interaction and increase understanding of the illness

---

TEST YOUR CRITICAL THINKING SKILLS

Sara, a 23-year-old single woman, has just been admitted to the psychiatric unit by her parents. They explain that over the past few months she has become more and more withdrawn. She stays in her room alone, but lately has been heard talking and laughing to herself.

Sara left home for the first time at age 18 to attend college. She performed well during her first semester, but when she returned after Christmas, she began to accuse her roommate of stealing her possessions. She started writing to her parents that her roommate wanted to kill her and that her roommate was turning everyone against her. She said she feared for her life. She started missing classes and stayed in her bed most of the time. Sometimes she locked herself in her closet. Her parents took her home, and she was hospitalized and diagnosed with paranoid schizophrenia. She has since been maintained on antipsychotic medication while taking a few classes at the local community college.

Sara tells the admitting nurse that she quit taking her medication 4 weeks ago because the pharmacist who fills the prescriptions is plotting to have her killed. She believes he is trying to poison her. She says she got this information from a television message. As Sara speaks, the nurse notices that she sometimes stops in midsentence and listens; sometimes she cocks her head to the side and moves her lips as though she is talking.

Answer the following questions related to Sara:

1. From the assessment data, what would be the most immediate nursing concern in working with Sara?
2. What is the nursing diagnosis related to this concern?
3. What interventions must be accomplished before the nurse can be successful in working with Sara?

IMPLICATIONS OF RESEARCH FOR EVIDENCE-BASED PRACTICE

Trygstad, L., Buccheri, R., Dowling, G., Zin, R., White, K., Griffin, J.J., Henderson, S., Suciu, L., Hippe, S., Kaas, M.J., Covert, C., & Hebert, P. (2002). Behavioral management of persistent auditory hallucinations in schizophrenia: Outcomes from a 10–week course. *Journal of the American Psychiatric Nurses Association, 8*(3), 84–91.

Description of the Study: The purpose of this study was to examine the effects of a 10-week course in which behavior management strategies were taught to participants with schizophrenia who experienced persistent auditory hallucinations. The primary aim was to examine the effects of the intervention on seven specific characteristics of auditory hallucinations: frequency, loudness, self-control, clarity, tone, distractibility, and distress. The secondary aim was to examine level of anxiety and depression. The sample consisted of 62 subjects who had been diagnosed with schizophrenia by a board-certified psychiatrist using *DSM-IV* diagnostic criteria. They all reported having persistent auditory hallucinations for at least 10 minutes a day for the past 3 months; reported a desire to learn new strategies to manage their auditory hallucinations; were taking stable doses of antipsychotic medication for at least 4 weeks before entry into the study; were able to read and write in English; and did not have a severe cognitive deficit. The 10-week course was taught in nine different outpatient settings by nurses who had experience caring for patients with schizophrenia and were knowledgeable in group facilitation skills. In each class, participants were taught and practiced one behavior strategy. The following strategies were taught in the course: self-monitoring, talking with someone, listening to music with or without earphones, watching television, saying "stop"/ignoring what the voices say to do, using ear plugs, learning relaxation techniques, keeping busy with an enjoyable activity and/or helping others, and practicing communication related to taking medication and not using drugs and alcohol. Measurement of the outcomes were based on subjects' scores on the Characteristics of Auditory Hallucinations Questionnaire (CAHQ), the Profile of Mood States (POMS) scale, and the Beck Depression Inventory, second edition (BDI-II).

Results of the Study: The outcome of this study strongly supported the expectation that subjects who attended the behavior-management strategy classes for auditory hallucinations would experience improvement in the characteristics of their auditory hallucinations and have less anxiety and depression. Post-intervention scores on the POMS and BDI-II were significantly lower than pre-intervention scores, indicating an overall decrease in anxiety and depression. Post-intervention mean scores on the CAHQ were significantly lower than pre-intervention on all hallucination characteristics, with the exception of loudness, which did not change significantly. In a 5-point self-report rating helpfulness of the course, 25% of the participants reported that the course was *extremely helpful*, 42% reported that it was *helpful*, 23% *moderately helpful*, 8% *minimally helpful*, and 2% *not helpful*.

Implications for Nursing Practice: This study shows that individuals can manage their auditory hallucinations by learning and using specific behavioral strategies. The group setting also proved to be beneficial, as clients were able to have their own experiences validated, to see that others had similar experiences, and to learn how others managed them. They gained encouragement and hope from learning that certain strategies were effective for others in the group. The authors state, "This low cost, low-tech intervention could be incorporated into the practice of psychiatric nurses or other mental health professionals who have group training and experience facilitating groups with people who have schizophrenia. Teaching behavior management of persistent auditory hallucinations to clients who wish to learn has minimal risks and could be easily incorporated into existing outpatient programs."

REFERENCES

American Psychiatric Association. (2000). *Diagnostic and statistical manual of mental disorders* (4th ed.) *Text revision.* Washington, DC: American Psychiatric Association.

Asen, E. (2002). Outcome research in family therapy: Family intervention for psychosis. *Advances in Psychiatric Treatment, 8,* 230–238.

Assertive Community Treatment Association (ACTA). (2005). *ACT Model.* Retrieved March 28, 2005 from the World Wide Web at http://www.actassociation.org/actModel

Dixon, L.B., & Lehman, A.F. (1995). Family interventions for schizophrenia. National Institute of Mental Health. *Schizophrenia Bulletin, 21*(4), 631–643.

Goff, D. (2002). *Psychosis.* MerckMedicus. Retrieved March 27, 2005 from the World Wide Web at http://merck.micromedex.com/

Ho, B.C., Black, D.W., & Andreasen, N.C. (2003). Schizophrenia and other psychotic disorders. In R.E. Hales & S.C. Yudofsky (Eds.). *Textbook of clinical psychiatry* (4th ed.). Washington, DC: American Psychiatric Publishing.

Jonsson, S.A., Luts, A., Guldberg-Kjaer, N., & Brun, A. (1997). Hippocampal pyramidal cell disarray correlates negatively to cell number: Implications for the pathogenesis of schizophrenia. *European Archives of Psychiatry and Clinical Neuroscience, 247*(3), 120–127.

The Merck Manual of Diagnosis and Therapy (MMDT)(2002). Schizophrenia. Retrieved from the World Wide Web on February 25, 2002 at http://www.merck.com/pubs/mmanual/section15/chapter193/193b.htm

Mueser, K.T., Bond, G.R., & Drake, R.E. (2001). Community based treatment of schizophrenia and other severe mental disorders: Treatment outcomes. *Medscape Psychiatry & Mental Health eJournal 6*(1). Retrieved March 28, 2005 from the World Wide Web at http://www.medscape.com/viewarticle/430529

National Alliance for the Mentally Ill (NAMI). (2003). *Assertive Community Treatment (ACT).* Retrieved March 28, 2005 from the World Wide Web at http://www.nami.org/

Rantakallio, P., Jones, P., Moring, J., & VonWendt, L. (1997). Association between central nervous system infections during childhood and adult onset schizophrenia and other psychoses: A 28–year follow-up. *International Journal of Epidemiology, 26,* 837–843.

Sadock, B.J., & Sadock, V.A. (2003). *Synopsis of psychiatry: Behavioral sciences/clinical psychiatry* (9th ed.). Philadelphia: Lippincott Williams & Wilkins.

Safier, E. (1997). Our families, the context of our lives. *Menninger Perspective, 28(1),* 4–9.

INTERNET REFERENCES

Additional information about Schizophrenia may be located at the following Web sites:

- http://www.schizophrenia.com
- http://www.nimh.nih.gov
- http://schizophrenia.nami.org
- http://mentalhealth.com
- http://www.narsad.org/

Additional information about medications to treat Schizophrenia may be located at the following Web sites:

- http://www.medicinenet.com/medications/article.htm
- http://www.fadavis.com/townsend
- http://www.nlm.nih.gov/medlineplus

MOOD DISORDERS

CHAPTER OUTLINE

OBJECTIVES

HISTORICAL PERSPECTIVE

EPIDEMIOLOGY

TYPES OF MOOD DISORDERS

DEPRESSIVE DISORDERS

APPLICATION OF THE NURSING PROCESS
TO DEPRESSIVE DISORDERS

BIPOLAR DISORDER (MANIA)

APPLICATION OF THE NURSING PROCESS
TO BIPOLAR DISORDER (MANIA)

TREATMENT MODALITIES FOR MOOD
DISORDERS

SUMMARY

REVIEW QUESTIONS

KEY TERMS

bipolar disorder
cognitive therapy
cyclothymic disorder
delirious mania
dysthymic disorder
hypomania
melancholia

postpartum depression
premenstrual
    dysphoric disorder
psychomotor
    retardation
tyramine

CORE CONCEPTS

depression
mania
mood

OBJECTIVES

After reading this chapter, the student will be able to:

1. Recount historical perspectives of mood disorders.
2. Discuss epidemiological statistics related to mood disorders.
3. Describe various types of mood disorders.
4. Identify predisposing factors in the development of mood disorders.
5. Discuss implications of mood disorders related to developmental stage.
6. Identify symptomatology associated with mood disorders and use this information in client assessment.
7. Formulate nursing diagnoses and goals of care for clients with mood disorders.
8. Identify topics for client and family teaching relevant to mood disorders.
9. Describe appropriate nursing interventions for behaviors associated with mood disorders.
10. Describe relevant criteria for evaluating nursing care of clients with mood disorders.
11. Discuss various modalities relevant to treatment of mood disorders.

epression is likely the oldest and still one of the most frequently diagnosed psychiatric illnesses. Symptoms of depression have been described almost as far back as there is evidence of written documentation.

An occasional bout with the "blues," a feeling of sad-ness or downheartedness, is common among healthy people and considered to be a normal response to everyday disappointments in life. These episodes are short-lived as the individual adapts to the loss, change, or failure (real or perceived) that has been experienced. Pathological depression occurs when adaptation is ineffective.

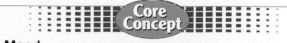

Mood
Also called *affect*. Mood is a pervasive and sustained emotion that may have a major influence on a person's perception of the world. Examples of mood include depression, joy, elation, anger, and anxiety. *Affect* is described as the emotional reaction associated with an experience (Taber's, 2005).

This chapter focuses on the consequences of dysfunctional grieving, as it is manifested by mood disorders. Mood disorders are classified as depressive or bipolar.

A historical perspective and epidemiological statistics related to mood disorders are presented here. Predisposing factors that have been implicated in the etiology of mood disorders provide a framework for studying the dynamics of depression and **bipolar disorder**.

The implications of mood disorders relevant to individuals of various developmental stages are discussed. An explanation of the symptomatology is presented as background knowledge for assessing the client with a mood disorder. Nursing care is described in the context of the six steps of the nursing process, and critical pathways of care are included as guidelines for use in a case management approach. Various medical treatment modalities are explored.

Depression
An alteration in mood that is expressed by feelings of sadness, despair, and pessimism. There is a loss of interest in usual activities, and somatic symptoms may be evident. Changes in appetite and sleep patterns are common.

Mania
An alteration in mood that is expressed by feelings of elation, inflated self-esteem, grandiosity, hyperactivity, agitation, and accelerated thinking and speaking. Mania can occur as a biological (organic) or psychological disorder, or as a response to substance use or a general medical condition.

HISTORICAL PERSPECTIVE

Many ancient cultures (e.g., Babylonian, Egyptian, Hebrew) believed in the supernatural or divine origin of depression and mania. The Old Testament states in the Book of Samuel that King Saul's depression was inflicted by an "evil spirit" sent from God to "torment" him.

A clearly nondivine point of view regarding depressive and manic states was held by the Greek medical community from the 5th century B.C. through the 3rd century A.D. This represented the thinking of Hippocrates, Celsus, and Galen, among others. They strongly rejected the idea of divine origin and considered the brain as the seat of all emotional states. Hippocrates believed that **melancholia** was caused by an excess of black bile, a heavily toxic substance produced in the spleen or intestine, which affected the brain.

During the Renaissance, several new theories evolved. Depression was viewed by some as being the result of obstruction of vital air circulation, excessive brooding, or helpless situations beyond the individual's control. These strong emotions of depression and mania were reflected in major literary works of the time, including Shakespeare's *King Lear*, *Macbeth*, and *Hamlet*.

In the 19th century, the definition of mania was narrowed down from the concept of total madness to that of a disorder of affect and action. The old notion of melancholia was refurnished with meaning, and emphasis was placed on the primary affective nature of the disorder. Finally, an introduction was made to the possibility of an alternating pattern of affective symptomatology associated with the disorders.

Contemporary thinking has been shaped a great deal by the works of Sigmund Freud, Emil Kraepelin, and Adolf Meyer. Having evolved from these early 20th-century models, current thinking about mood disorders generally encompasses the intrapsychic, behavioral, and biological perspectives. These various perspectives support the notion of multiple causation in the development of mood disorders.

EPIDEMIOLOGY

Major depression is one of the leading causes of disability in the United States. It affects almost 10 percent of the population, or 19 million Americans, in a given year (International Society for Mental Health Online, 2004). During their lifetimes, 10 to 25 percent of women and 5 to 12 percent of men will become clinically depressed.

This preponderance has led to the consideration of depression by some researchers as "the common cold of psychiatric disorders" and this generation as an "age of melancholia."

Bipolar disorder affects approximately 2.3 million American adults, or about 1.2 percent of the U.S. population age 18 and older in a given year (National Institute of Mental Health [NIMH], 2001).

Gender

Studies indicate that the incidence of depressive disorder is higher in women than it is in men by about 2 to 1. The

TABLE 29–2   Diagnostic Criteria for Dysthymic Disorder

A. Depressed mood for most of the day, more days than not, as indicated either by subjective account or observation by others, for at least 2 years
   NOTE: In children and adolescents, mood can be irritable and duration must be at least 1 year.
B. Presence, while depressed, of two (or more) of the following:
   1. Poor appetite or overeating
   2. Insomnia or hypersomnia
   3. Low energy or fatigue
   4. Low self-esteem
   5. Poor concentration or difficulty making decisions
   6. Feelings of hopelessness
C. During the 2-year period (1 year for children or adolescents) of the disturbance, the person has never been without the symptoms in A or B for more than 2 months at a time.
D. No major depressive disorder has been present during the first 2 years of the disturbance (1 year for children and adolescents)
E. There has never been a manic, mixed, or hypomanic episode, and criteria have never been met for cyclothymic disorder.
F. The disturbance does not occur exclusively during the course of a chronic psychotic disorder, such as schizophrenia or delusional disorder.
G. The symptoms are not due to the direct physiological effects of a substance (e.g., a drug of abuse, a medication) or a general medical condition (e.g., hypothyroidism).
H. The symptoms cause clinically significant distress or impairment in social, occupational, or other important areas of functioning.
   Specify if:
   Early onset: Before age 21 years
   Late onset: Age 21 years or older

SOURCE: American Psychiatric Association (2000), with permission.

TABLE 29–3   Research Criteria for Premenstrual Dysphoric Disorder

A. In most menstrual cycles during the past year, five (or more) of the following symptoms were present for most of the time during the last week of the luteal phase, began to remit within a few days after the onset of the follicular phase, and were absent in the week postmenses, with at least one of the symptoms being 1, 2, 3, or 4:
   1. Markedly depressed mood, feelings of hopelessness, or self-deprecating thoughts
   2. Marked anxiety, tension, feelings of being "keyed up," or "on edge"
   3. Marked affective lability (e.g., feeling suddenly sad or tearful or increased sensitivity to rejection)
   4. Persistent and marked anger or irritability or increased interpersonal conflicts
   5. Decreased interest in usual activities (e.g., work, school, friends, hobbies)
   6. Subjective sense of difficulty in concentrating
   7. Lethargy, easy fatigability, or marked lack of energy
   8. Marked change in appetite, overeating, or specific food cravings
   9. Hypersomnia or insomnia
   10. A subjective sense of being overwhelmed or out of control
   11. Other physical symptoms, such as breast tenderness or swelling, headaches, joint or muscle pain, a sensation of "bloating," weight gain
B. The disturbance markedly interferes with work or school or with usual social activities and relationships with others (e.g., avoidance of social activities, decreased productivity and efficiency at work or school).
C. The disturbance is not merely an exacerbation of the symptoms of another disorder, such as major depressive disorder, panic disorder, dysthymic disorder, or a personality disorder (although it may be superimposed on any of these disorders).
D. Criteria A, B, and C must be confirmed by prospective daily ratings during at least two consecutive symptomatic cycles.

SOURCE: American Psychiatric Association (2000), with permission.

require hospitalization to prevent harm to self or others. Motor activity is excessive and frenzied. Psychotic features may be present.

A somewhat milder degree of this clinical symptom picture is called **hypomania**. Hypomania is not severe enough to cause marked impairment in social or occupational functioning or to require hospitalization, and it does not include psychotic features. The *DSM-IV-TR* diagnostic criteria for mania are presented in Table 29–4.

The diagnostic picture for depression associated with bipolar disorder is identical to that described for major depressive disorder, with one addition: the client must have a history of one or more manic episodes.

When the symptom presentation includes rapidly alternating moods (sadness, irritability, euphoria) accompanied by symptoms associated with both depression and mania, the individual is given a diagnosis of *bipolar disorder, mixed*. This disturbance is severe enough to cause marked impairment in social or occupational functioning or to require hospitalization. Psychotic features may be evident.

Bipolar I Disorder

Bipolar I disorder is the diagnosis given to an individual who is experiencing, or has experienced, a full syndrome of manic or mixed symptoms. The client may also have experienced episodes of depression. This diagnosis is further specified by the current or most recent behavioral episode experienced. For example, the specifier might be single manic episode (to describe individuals having a first episode of mania) or current (or most recent) episode manic, hypomanic, mixed, or depressed (to describe individuals who have had recurrent mood episodes).

Bipolar II Disorder

This diagnostic category is characterized by recurrent bouts of major depression with episodic occurrence of hypomania. The individual who is assigned this diagnosis may present with symptoms (or history) of depression or hypomania. The client has never experienced an episode that meets the full criteria for mania or mixed symptomatology.

Cyclothymic Disorder

The essential feature of **cyclothymic disorder** is a chronic mood disturbance of at least 2-year duration,

TABLE 29–4   Diagnostic Criteria for Manic Episode

A. A distinct period of abnormally and persistently elevated, expansive, or irritable mood, lasting 1 week (or any duration if hospitalization is necessary).

B. During the period of mood disturbance, three (or more) of the following symptoms have persisted (four if the mood is only irritable) and have been present to a significant degree:
1. Inflated self-esteem or grandiosity
2. Decreased need for sleep (e.g., feels rested after only 3 hours of sleep)
3. More talkative than usual or pressure to keep talking
4. Flight of ideas or subjective experience that thoughts are racing
5. Distractibility (i.e., attention too easily drawn to unimportant or irrelevant external stimuli)
6. Increase in goal-directed activity (either socially, at work or school, or sexually) or psychomotor agitation
7. Excessive involvement in pleasurable activities that have a high potential for painful consequences (e.g., engaging in unrestrained buying sprees, sexual indiscretions, or foolish business investments)

C. The mood disturbance is sufficiently severe to cause marked impairment in occupational functioning or in usual social activities or relationships with others, or to necessitate hospitalization to prevent harm to self or others, or there are psychotic features.

D. The symptoms are not due to the direct physiological effects of a substance (e.g., a drug of abuse, a medication, or other treatment) or a general medical condition (e.g., hyperthyroidism).

SOURCE: American Psychiatric Association (2000), with permission.

involving numerous episodes of hypomania and depressed mood of insufficient severity or duration to meet the criteria for either bipolar I or II disorder. The individual is never without hypomanic or depressive symptoms for more than 2 months. The *DSM-IV-TR* criteria for cyclothymic disorder are presented in Table 29–5.

Other Mood Disorders

Mood Disorder Due to a General Medical Condition

This disorder is characterized by a prominent and persistent disturbance in mood that is judged to be the result of direct physiological effects of a general medical condition (APA, 2000). The mood disturbance may involve depression or elevated, expansive, or irritable mood, and causes clinically significant distress or impairment in social, occupational, or other important areas of functioning. Types of physiological influences are included in the discussion of predisposing factors to mood disorders.

Substance-Induced Mood Disorder

The disturbance of mood associated with this disorder is considered to be the direct result of physiological effects

TABLE 29–5   Diagnostic Criteria for Cyclothymic Disorder

A. For at least 2 years, the presence of numerous periods with hypomanic symptoms and numerous periods with depressive symptoms that do not meet the criteria for major depressive disorder.
   NOTE: In children and adolescents, the duration must be at least 1 year.

B. During the 2-year period (1 year in children and adolescents), the person has not been without the symptoms in criterion A for more than 2 months at a time.

C. No major depressive episode, manic episode, or mixed episode has been present during the first 2 years of the disturbance.

D. The symptoms in criterion A are not better accounted for by schizoaffective disorder and are not superimposed on schizophrenia, schizophreniform disorder, delusional disorder, or psychotic disorder not otherwise specified.

E. The symptoms are not due to the direct physiological effects of a substance (e.g., a drug of abuse, a medication) or a general medical condition (e.g., hyperthyroidism).

F. The symptoms cause clinically significant distress or impairment in social, occupational, or other important areas of functioning.

SOURCE: American Psychiatric Association (2000), with permission.

of a substance (e.g., a drug of abuse, a medication, or toxin exposure). The mood disturbance may involve depression or elevated, expansive, or irritable mood, and causes clinically significant distress or impairment in social, occupational, or other important areas of functioning.

Mood disturbances are associated with *intoxication* from substances such as alcohol, amphetamines, cocaine, hallucinogens, inhalants, opioids, phencyclidine, sedatives, hypnotics, and anxiolytics. Symptoms can occur with *withdrawal* from substances such as alcohol, amphetamines, cocaine, sedatives, hypnotics, and anxiolytics. Heavy metals and toxins, such as gasoline, paint, organophosphate insecticides, nerve gases, carbon monoxide, and carbon dioxide, may also cause mood symptoms (APA, 2000).

A number of medications have been known to evoke mood symptoms. Classifications include anesthetics, analgesics, anticholinergics, anticonvulsants, antihypertensives, antiparkinsonian agents, antiulcer agents, cardiac medications, oral contraceptives, psychotropic medications, muscle relaxants, steroids, and sulfonamides. Some specific examples are included in the discussion of predisposing factors to mood disorders.

DEPRESSIVE DISORDERS

Predisposing Factors

Biological Theories

Genetics

Affective illness has been the subject of considerable research on the relevance of hereditary factors. A genetic link has been suggested in numerous studies; however, no definitive mode of genetic transmission has yet to be demonstrated.

Twin Studies. Twin studies suggest a genetic factor in the illness because about 50 percent of monozygotic twins are concordant for the illness (concordant refers to twins who are both affected with the illness). Similar results were revealed in studies of monozygotic twins raised apart. The concordance rate in dizygotic twins is 10 to 25 percent (Sadock & Sadock, 2003).

Family Studies. Most family studies have shown that major depression is 1.5 to 3 times more common among first-degree biological relatives of people with the disorder than among the general population (APA, 2000). Indeed, the evidence to support an increased risk of depressive disorder in individuals with positive family history is quite compelling. It is unlikely that random environmental factors could cause the concentration of illness that is seen within families.

Adoption Studies. Further support for heritability as an etiological influence in depression comes from studies of the adopted offspring of affectively ill biological parents. Sadock and Sadock (2003) state:

> Adoption studies have shown that the biological children of affected parents remain at increased risk of a mood disorder, even if they are reared in nonaffected, adoptive families. (p. 540)

Biochemical Influences

Biogenic Amines. It has been hypothesized that depressive illness may be related to a deficiency of the neurotransmitters norepinephrine, serotonin, and dopamine, at functionally important receptor sites in the brain. Historically, the biogenic amine hypothesis of mood disorders grew out of the observation that reserpine, which depletes the brain of amines, was associated with the development of a depressive syndrome (Slattery, Hudson, & Nutt, 2004). The catecholamine norepinephrine has been identified as a key component in the mobilization of the body to deal with stressful situations. Neurons that contain serotonin are critically involved in the regulation of many psychobiological functions, such as mood, anxiety, arousal, vigilance, irritability, thinking, cognition, appetite, aggression, and circadian rhythm (Dubovsky, Davies, & Dubovsky, 2003). Tryptophan, the amino acid precursor of serotonin, has been shown to enhance the efficacy of antidepressant medications and, on occasion, to be effective as an antidepressant itself. The level of dopamine in the mesolimbic system of the brain is thought to exert a strong influence over human mood and behavior. A diminished supply of these biogenic amines inhibits the transmission of impulses from one neuronal fiber to another, causing a failure of the cells to fire or become charged (see Figure 29–1).

More recently, the biogenic amine hypothesis has been expanded to include another neurotransmitter, acetylcholine. Because cholinergic agents do have profound effects on mood, electroencephalogram, sleep, and neuroendocrine function, it has been suggested that the problem in depression and mania may be an imbalance between the biogenic amines and acetylcholine. Cholinergic transmission is thought to be excessive in depression and inadequate in mania (Dubovsky, Davies, & Dubovsky, 2003).

The precise role that any of the neurotransmitters plays in the etiology of depression is unknown. As the body of research grows, there is no doubt that increased knowledge regarding the biogenic amines will contribute to a greater capacity for understanding and treating affective illness.

Neuroendocrine Disturbances

Neuroendocrine disturbances may play a role in the pathogenesis or persistence of depressive illness. This notion has arisen in view of the marked disturbances in mood observed with the administration of certain hormones or in the incidence of endocrine disease.

Hypothalamic–Pituitary–Adrenocortical Axis. In clients who are depressed, the normal system of hormonal inhibition fails, resulting in a hypersecretion of cortisol. This elevated serum cortisol is the basis for the dexamethasone suppression test that is sometimes used to determine if an individual has somatically treatable depression.

Hypothalamic–Pituitary–Thyroid Axis. Thyrotropin-releasing factor (TRF) from the hypothalamus stimulates the release of thyroid-stimulating hormone (TSH) from the anterior pituitary gland. In turn, TSH stimulates the thyroid gland. Diminished TSH response to administered TRF is observed in approximately 25 percent of depressed persons. This laboratory test has future potential for identifying clients at high risk for affective illness.

Physiological Influences

Depressive symptoms that occur as a consequence of a non-mood disorder or as an adverse effect of certain medications are called *secondary* depression. Secondary depression may be related to medication side effects, neurological disorders, electrolyte or hormonal disturbances, nutritional deficiencies, and other physiological or psychological conditions.

Medication Side Effects. A number of drugs, either alone or in combination with other medications, can produce a depressive syndrome. Most common among these drugs are those that have a direct effect on the central nervous system. Examples of these include the anxiolytics, antipsychotics, and sedative-hypnotics. Certain antihypertensive medications, such as propranolol and reserpine, have been known to produce depressive symptoms. Depressed mood may also occur with any of the

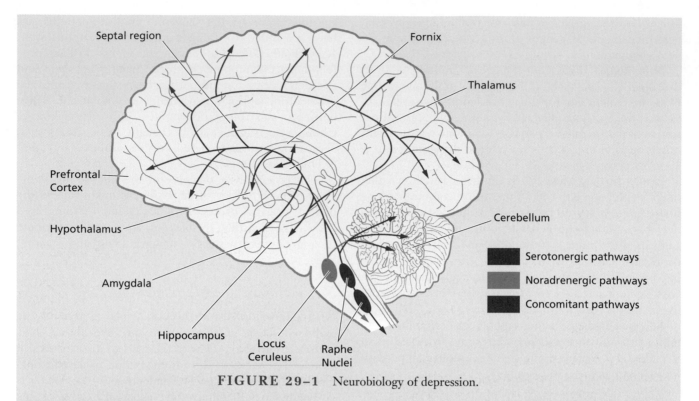

FIGURE 29–1   Neurobiology of depression.

Neurotransmitters

Although other neurotransmitters have also been implicated in the pathophysiology of depression, disturbances in serotonin and norepinephrine have been the most extensively scrutinized.

Cell bodies of origin for the serotonin pathways lie within the raphe nuclei located in the brain stem. Those for norepinephrine originate in the locus ceruleus. Projections for both neurotransmitters extend throughout the forebrain, prefrontal cortex, cerebellum, and limbic system.

Areas of the Brain Affected

Areas of the brain affected by depression and the symptoms that they mediate include the following:

- Hippocampus: Memory impairments, feelings of worthlessness, hopelessness, and guilt
- Amygdala: Anhedonia, anxiety, reduced motivation
- Hypothalamus: Increased or decreased sleep and appetite; decreased energy and libido
- Other limbic structures: Emotional alterations
- Frontal cortex: Depressed mood; problems concentrating
- Cerebellum: Psychomotor retardation/agitation

Medications and Their Effects on the Brain

All medications that increase serotonin, norepinephrine, or both can improve the emotional and vegetative symptoms of depression. Medications that produce these effects include those that block the presynaptic reuptake of the neurotransmitters or block receptors at nerve endings (tricyclics; SSRIs) and those that inhibit monoamine oxidase, an enzyme that is involved in the metabolism of the monoamines serotonin, norepinephrine, and dopamine (MAOIs).

Side effects of these medications relate to their specific neurotransmitter receptor-blocking action. Tricyclic and tetracyclic drugs (e.g., imipramine, amitriptyline, mirtazapine) block reuptake and/or receptors for serotonergic, noradrenergic, anticholinergic, and histamine. SSRIs are selective serotonergic reuptake inhibitors. Others, such as bupropion, venlafaxine, and duloxetine block serotonin and norepinephrine reuptake, and also are weak inhibitors of dopamine.

Blockade of norepinephrine reuptake results in side effects of tremors, cardiac arrhythmias, sexual dysfunction, and hypertension. Blockade of serotonin reuptake results in side effects of GI disturbances, increased agitation, and sexual dysfunction. Blockade of dopamine reuptake results in side effects of psychomotor activation. Blockade of acetylcholine reuptake results in dry mouth, blurred vision, constipation, and urinary retention. Blockade of histamine reuptake results in sedation and hypotension.

following medications, although the list is by no means all-inclusive (Sadock & Sadock, 2003):

Steroids: prednisone and cortisone
Hormones: estrogen and progesterone
Sedatives: barbiturates and benzodiazepines

Antibacterial and antifungal drugs: ampicillin, cycloserine, tetracycline, and sulfonamides
Antineoplastics: vincristine and zidovudine
Analgesics and anti-inflammatory drugs: opiates, ibuprofen, and phenylbutazone
Antiulcer: cimetidine

Neurological Disorders. An individual who has suffered a cardiovascular accident (CVA) may experience a despondency unrelated to the severity of the CVA. These are true mood disorders, and antidepressant drug therapy may be indicated. Brain tumors, particularly in the area of the temporal lobe, often cause symptoms of depression. Agitated depression may be part of the clinical picture associated with Alzheimer's disease, Parkinson's disease, and Huntington's disease. Agitation and restlessness may also represent an underlying depression in the individual with multiple sclerosis.

Electrolyte Disturbances. Excessive levels of sodium bicarbonate or calcium can produce symptoms of depression, as can deficits in magnesium and sodium. Potassium is also implicated in the syndrome of depression. Symptoms have been observed with excesses of potassium in the body, as well as in instances of potassium depletion.

Hormonal Disturbances. Depression is associated with dysfunction of the adrenal cortex and is commonly observed in both Addison's disease and Cushing's syndrome. Other endocrine conditions that may result in symptoms of depression include hypoparathyroidism, hyperparathyroidism, hypothyroidism, and hyperthyroidism.

An imbalance of the hormones estrogen and progesterone has been implicated in the predisposition to premenstrual dysphoric disorder. It is postulated that excess estrogen or a high estrogen-to-progesterone ratio during the luteal phase of the menstrual cycle is responsible for the symptoms associated with premenstrual syndrome (Sadock & Sadock, 2003).

Nutritional Deficiencies. Deficiencies in vitamin B_1 (thiamine), vitamin B_6 (pyridoxine), vitamin B_{12}, niacin, vitamin C, iron, folic acid, zinc, calcium, and potassium may produce symptoms of depression (Schimelpfening, 2002). A number of nutritional alterations have also been indicated in the etiology of premenstrual dysphoric disorder. They include deficiencies in the B vitamins, calcium, magnesium, manganese, vitamin E, and linolenic acid (Frackiewicz & Shiovitz, 2001). Glucose tolerance fluctuations, abnormal fatty acid metabolism, and sensitivity to caffeine and alcohol may also play a role in bringing about the symptoms associated with this disorder. No definitive evidence exists to support any specific nutritional alteration in the etiology of these symptoms.

Other Physiological Conditions. Other conditions that have been associated with secondary depression include collagen disorders, such as systemic lupus erythematosus (SLE) and polyarteritis nodosa; cardiovascular disease, such as cardiomyopathy, congestive heart failure, myocardial infarction, and cerebrovascular accident (stroke); infections, such as encephalitis, hepatitis, mononucleosis, pneumonia, and syphilis; and metabolic disorders, such as diabetes mellitus and porphyria.

Psychosocial Theories

Psychoanalytical Theory

Freud (1957) presented his classic paper "Mourning and Melancholia" in 1917. He defined the distinguishing features of melancholia as:

> …a profoundly painful dejection, cessation of interest in the outside world, loss of the capacity to love, inhibition of all activity, and a lowering of the self-regarding feelings to a degree that finds utterances in self-reproaches and self-revilings, and culminates in a delusional expectation of punishment.

He observed that melancholia occurs after the loss of a loved object, either actually by death or emotionally by rejection, or the loss of some other abstraction of value to the individual. Freud indicated that in melancholic clients, the depressed patient's rage is internally directed because of identification with the lost object (Sadock & Sadock, 2003).

Freud believed that the individual predisposed to melancholia experienced ambivalence in love relationships. He postulated, therefore, that once the loss had been incorporated into the self (ego), the hostile part of the ambivalence that had been felt for the lost object is then turned inward against the ego.

Learning Theory

The model of "learned helplessness" arises out of Seligman's (1973) experiments with dogs. The animals were exposed to electrical stimulation from which they could not escape. Later, when they were given the opportunity to avoid the traumatic experience, they reacted with helplessness and made no attempt to escape. A similar state of helplessness exists in humans who have experienced numerous failures (either real or perceived). The individual abandons any further attempt to succeed. Seligman theorized that learned helplessness predisposes individuals to depression by imposing a feeling of lack of control over their life situation. They become depressed because they feel helpless; they have learned that whatever they do is futile. This can be especially damaging very early in life, because the sense of mastery over one's environment is an important foundation for future emotional development.

Object Loss Theory

The theory of object loss suggests that depressive illness occurs as a result of having been abandoned by or otherwise separated from a significant other during the first six months of life. Because during this period the mother represents the child's main source of security, she is the "object." The response occurs not only with a physical loss. This absence of attachment, which may be either

Psalm 12:6 The words of the Lord are pure words: as silver in a furnace of earth [absolutely trustworthy] purified seven times — (fullest sense of the limit)

492   UNIT IV ● NURSING CARE OF CLIENTS WITH ALTERATIONS IN PSYCHOSOCIAL ADAPTATION

physical or emotional, leads to feelings of helplessness and despair that contribute to lifelong patterns of depression in response to loss.

The concept of "anaclitic depression" was introduced in 1946 by psychiatrist René Spitz to refer to children who became depressed after being separated from their mothers for and extended period of time during the first year of life (Cartwright, 2004). The condition included behaviors such as excessive crying, anorexia, withdrawal, psychomotor retardation, stupor, and a generalized impairment in the normal process of growth and development. Some researchers suggest that loss in adult life afflicts people much more severely in the form of depression if the subjects have suffered early childhood loss.

Cognitive Theory

Beck and colleagues (1979) proposed a theory suggesting that the primary disturbance in depression is cognitive rather than affective. The underlying cause of the depressive affect is seen as cognitive distortions that result in negative, defeated attitudes. Beck identifies three cognitive distortions that he believes serve as the basis for depression:

1. Negative expectations of the environment
2. Negative expectations of the self
3. Negative expectations of the future

These cognitive distortions arise out of a defect in cognitive development, and the individual feels inadequate, worthless, and rejected by others. The outlook for the future is one of pessimism and hopelessness.

Cognitive theorists believe that depression is the product of negative thinking. This is in contrast to the other theorists, who suggest that negative thinking occurs when an individual is depressed. **Cognitive therapy** focuses on helping the individual to alter mood by changing the way he or she thinks. The individual is taught to control negative thought distortions that lead to pessimism, lethargy, procrastination, and low self-esteem (see Chapter 20).

The Transactional Model

The etiology of depression remains unclear. No single theory or hypothesis has been postulated that substantiates a clear-cut explanation for the disorder. Evidence continues to mount in support of multiple causation. The transactional model recognizes the combined effects of genetic, biochemical, and psychosocial influences on an individual's susceptibility to depression. The dynamics of depression using the transactional model of stress/adaptation are presented in Figure 29–2.

Developmental Implications

Childhood

Only in recent years has a consensus developed among investigators identifying major depressive disorder as an entity in children and adolescents that can be identified using criteria similar to those used for adults (APA, 2000; Dubovsky, Davies, & Dubovsky, 2003). It is not uncommon, however, for the symptoms of depression to be manifested differently in childhood, and the picture changes with age (Harvard Medical School, 2002):

1. Up to age 3: Signs may include feeding problems, tantrums, and lack of playfulness and emotional expressiveness.
2. From ages 3 to 5: Common symptoms may include accident proneness, phobias, and excessive self-reproach for minor infractions.
3. From ages 6 to 8: There may be vague physical complaints and aggressive behavior. Children may cling to parents and avoid new people and challenges.
4. At ages 9 to 12: Common symptoms include morbid thoughts and excessive worrying. Children may reason that they are depressed because they have disappointed their parents in some way.

Other symptoms of childhood depression may include hyperactivity, delinquency, school problems, psychosomatic complaints, sleeping and eating disturbances, social isolation, and suicidal thoughts or actions.

Children may become depressed for various reasons. In many depressed children, there is a genetic predisposition toward the condition, which is then precipitated by a stressful situation. Common precipitating factors include physical or emotional detachment by the primary caregiver, parental separation or divorce, death of a loved one (person or pet), a move, academic failure, or physical illness. In any event, the common denominator is loss.

The focus of therapy with depressed children is to alleviate the child's symptoms and strengthen the child's coping and adaptive skills, with the hope of possibly preventing future psychological problems. Some studies have shown that untreated childhood depression may lead to subsequent problems in adolescence and adult life. Most children are treated on an outpatient basis. Hospitalization of the depressed child usually occurs only if he or she is actively suicidal, when the home environment precludes adherence to a treatment regimen, or if the child needs to be separated from the home for psychosocial deprivation.

Parental and family therapy are commonly used to help the younger depressed child. Recovery is facilitated by emotional support and guidance to family members.

Psalm 42:11 Why art thou cast down, O my soul? and why art thou disquieted within me? hope thou in God; for I shall yet praise him, who is the health of my countenance, and my God.

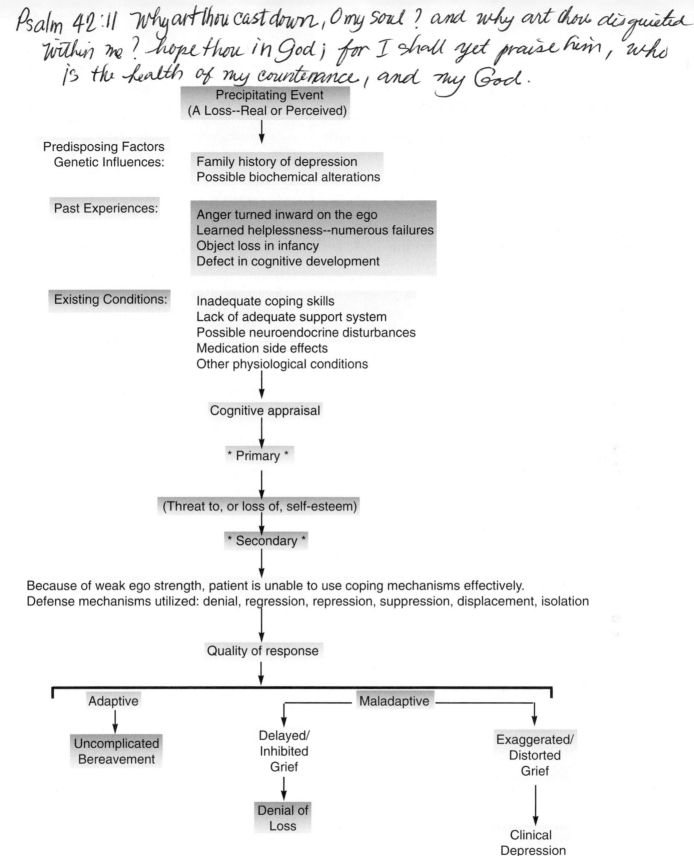

FIGURE 29–2   The dynamics of depression using the transactional model of stress/adaptation.

Children older than age 8 years usually participate in family therapy. In some situations, individual treatment may be appropriate for older children. Medications, such as antidepressants or lithium, can be important in the treatment of children, especially for the more serious and recurrent forms of depression.

Adolescence

Depression may be even harder to recognize in an adolescent than in a younger child. Feelings of sadness, loneliness, anxiety, and hopelessness associated with depression may be perceived as the normal emotional stresses of growing up. Therefore, many young people whose symptoms are attributed to the "normal adjustments" of adolescence do not get the help they need. Depression is a major cause of suicide among teens. During the past three decades, the rate of suicide for persons ages 15 to 24 has tripled, and it is the third leading cause of death in this age group (National Center for Health Statistics, 2004).

Common symptoms of depression in the adolescent are inappropriately expressed anger, aggressiveness, running away, delinquency, social withdrawal, sexual acting out, substance abuse, restlessness, and apathy. Loss of self-esteem, sleeping and eating disturbances, and psychosomatic complaints are also common.

Bipolar disorder, which often emerges during adolescence, is manifested by episodes of impulsivity, irritability, and loss of control, sometimes alternating with periods of withdrawal. These behaviors are often confused with the emotional cycles of adolescence, delaying necessary treatment.

What, then, is the indicator that differentiates mood disorder from the typical stormy behavior of adolescence? A visible manifestation of *behavioral change that lasts for several weeks* is the best clue for a mood disorder. Examples include the normally outgoing and extroverted adolescent who has become withdrawn and antisocial; the good student who previously received consistently high marks but is now failing and skipping classes; the usually self-confident teenager who is now inappropriately irritable and defensive with others.

Adolescents become depressed for all the same reasons that were considered in the discussion of childhood depression. In adolescence, however, depression is a common manifestation of the stress and independence conflicts associated with the normal maturation process. Depression may also be the response to death of a parent, other relative, or friend, or to a breakup with a boyfriend or girlfriend. This perception of abandonment by parents or closest peer relationship is thought to be the most frequent immediate precipitant to adolescent suicide.

Treatment of the depressed adolescent is often conducted on an outpatient basis. Hospitalization may be required in cases of severe depression or threat of imminent suicide, when a family situation is such that treatment cannot be carried out in the home, when the physical condition precludes self-care of biological needs, or when the adolescent has indicated possible harm to self or others in the family.

In addition to supportive psychosocial intervention, antidepressant therapy is part of the treatment of adolescent mood disorders. However, in October 2004, the U.S. Food and Drug Administration (FDA) issued a public health advisory warning the public about the increased risk of suicidal thoughts and behavior in children and adolescents being treated with antidepressant medications. The agency directed drug manufacturers to add a "black box" warning to the labeling of all antidepressant medications describing this risk and emphasizing the need for close monitoring of clients started on these medications. The new warning language does not prohibit the use of antidepressants in children and adolescents. Rather, it warns of the risk of suicidality and encourages prescribers to balance this risk with clinical need.

Fluoxetine (Prozac) is currently the only medication approved to treat depression in children and adolescents. The other selective serotonin reuptake inhibitor (SSRI) medications, such as sertraline, citalopram, and paroxetine, and the SSRI-related antidepressant venlafaxine, have not been approved for treatment of depression in children or adolescents, although they have been prescribed to children by physicians in "off-label use"—a use other than the FDA-approved use. In June 2003, the FDA recommended that paroxetine not be used in children and adolescents for the treatment of major depressive disorder.

Senescence

Depression is the most common psychiatric disorder of the elderly, who make up 12.3 percent of the general population of the United States (Administration on Aging, 2003). This is not surprising considering the disproportionate value our society places on youth, vigor, and uninterrupted productivity. These societal attitudes continually nurture the feelings of low self-esteem, helplessness, and hopelessness that become more pervasive and intensive with advanced age. Further, the aging individual's adaptive coping strategies may be seriously challenged by major stressors, such as financial problems, physical illness, changes in bodily functioning, and an increasing awareness of approaching death. The problem is often intensified by the numerous losses individuals experience during this period in life, such as spouse, friends, children, home, and independence. A phenomenon called *bereavement overload* occurs when individuals experience so many losses in their lives that they are not able to resolve one grief response before another one begins. Bereavement overload predisposes elderly individuals to depressive illness.

Although they make up less than 13 percent of the population, the elderly account for about 18 percent of the suicides in the United States (National Institute of Mental Health, 2004). The highest number of suicides are among white men 85 years of age and older, at more than 5 times the national rate.

Symptoms of depression in the elderly are not very different from those in younger adults. Depressive syndromes are often confused by other illnesses associated with the aging process, however. Symptoms of depression are often misdiagnosed as senile dementia, when in fact the memory loss, confused thinking, or apathy symptomatic of senility actually may be the result of depression. The early awakening and reduced appetite typical of depression are common among many older people who are not depressed. Compounding this situation is the fact that many medical conditions, such as endocrinological, neurological, nutritional, and metabolic disorders, often present with classic symptoms of depression. Many medications commonly used by the elderly, such as antihypertensives, corticosteroids, and analgesics, can also produce a depressant effect.

Depression does accompanies many of the illnesses that afflict older people, such as Parkinson's disease, cancer, arthritis, and the early stages of Alzheimer's disease. Treating depression in these situations can reduce unnecessary suffering and help afflicted individuals cope with their medical problems.

The most effective treatment of depression in the elderly individual is thought to be a combination of psychosocial and biological approaches. Antidepressant medications are administered with consideration for age-related physiological changes in absorption, distribution, elimination, and brain receptor sensitivity. Because of these changes, plasma concentrations of these medications can reach very high levels despite moderate oral doses.

Electroconvulsive therapy (ECT) remains one of the safest and most effective treatments for major depression in the elderly. The response to ECT appears to be slower with advancing age, and the therapeutic effects are of limited duration. However, it may be considered the treatment of choice for the elderly individual who is an acute suicidal risk or is unable to tolerate antidepressant medications.

Other therapeutic approaches include interpersonal, behavioral, cognitive, group, and family psychotherapies. Appropriate treatment of the depressed elderly individual can bring relief from suffering and offer a new lease on life with a feeling of renewed productivity.

Postpartum Depression

The severity of depression in the postpartum period varies from a feeling of the "blues," to moderate depression, to psychotic depression or melancholia. Of women who give birth, approximately 50 to 80 percent experience the "blues" following delivery (Kennedy & Suttenfield, 2002). The incidence of moderate depression is 10 to 16 percent. Severe, or psychotic, depression occurs rarely, in about 1 or 2 out of 1000 postpartum women.

Symptoms of the "maternity blues" include tearfulness, despondency, anxiety, and subjectively impaired concentration appearing in the early puerperium. The symptoms usually begin 3 to 4 days after delivery, worsen by days 5 to 7, and tend to resolve by day 12 (Kennedy & Suttenfield, 2002).

Symptoms of moderate **postpartum depression** have been described as depressed mood varying from day to day, with more bad days than good, tending to be worse toward evening and associated with fatigue, irritability, loss of appetite, sleep disturbances, and loss of libido. In addition, the new mother expresses a great deal of concern about her inability to care for her baby. These symptoms begin somewhat later than those described for "maternity blues," and take from a few weeks to several months to abate.

Postpartum melancholia, or depressive psychosis, is characterized by depressed mood, agitation, indecision, lack of concentration, guilt, and an abnormal attitude toward bodily functions. There may be lack of interest in, or rejection of, the baby, or a morbid fear that the baby may be harmed. Risks of suicide and infanticide should not be overlooked. These symptoms usually develop within 2 to 3 weeks following delivery, but sometimes they occur as early as 48 to 72 hours postpartum (Kennedy & Suttenfield, 2002).

The etiology of postpartum depression remains unclear. "Maternity blues" may be associated with hormonal changes, tryptophan metabolism, or alterations in membrane transport during the early postpartum period. Besides being exposed to these same somatic changes, the woman who experiences moderate to severe symptoms probably possesses a vulnerability to depression related to heredity, upbringing, early life experiences, personality, or social circumstances. Some women with this disorder complain of lack of support from their husbands and dissatisfaction with their marriage. The etiology of postpartum depression may very likely be a combination of hormonal, metabolic, and psychosocial influences.

Treatment of postpartum depression varies with the severity of the illness. Psychotic depression may be treated with antidepressant medication, along with supportive psychotherapy, group therapy, and possibly family therapy. Moderate depression may be relieved with supportive psychotherapy and continuing assistance with home management until the symptoms subside. "Maternity blues" usually need no treatment beyond a word of reassurance from the physician or nurse that these feelings are common and will soon pass. Extra support and comfort from significant others also is important.

APPLICATION OF THE NURSING PROCESS TO DEPRESSIVE DISORDERS

Background Assessment Data

Symptomatology of depression can be viewed on a continuum according to severity of the illness. All individuals become depressed from time to time. These are the transient symptoms that accompany the everyday disappointments of life. Examples of the disappointments include failing an examination or breaking up with a boyfriend or girlfriend. Transient symptoms of depression subside relatively quickly as the individual advances toward other goals and achievements.

Mild depressive episodes occur when the grief process is triggered in response to the loss of a valued object. This can occur with the loss of a loved one, pet, friend, home, or significant other. As one is able to work through the stages of grief, the loss is accepted, symptoms subside, and activities of daily living are resumed within a few weeks. If this does not occur, grief is prolonged or exaggerated, and symptoms intensify.

Moderate depression occurs when grief is prolonged or exaggerated. The individual becomes fixed in the anger stage of the grief response, and the anger is turned inward on the self. All of the feelings associated with normal grieving are exaggerated out of proportion, and the individual is unable to function without assistance. Dysthymic disorder is an example of moderate depression.

Severe depression is an intensification of the symptoms associated with the moderate level. The individual who is severely depressed may also demonstrate a loss of contact with reality. This level is associated with a complete lack of pleasure in all activities, and ruminations about suicide are common. Major depressive disorder is an example of severe depression. A continuum of depression is presented in Figure 29–3.

Symptoms of depression can be described as alterations in four spheres of human functioning: (1) affective,

(2) behavioral, (3) cognitive, and (4) physiological. Alterations within these spheres differ according to degree of severity of symptomatology.

Transient Depression

Symptoms at this level of the continuum are not necessarily dysfunctional. Alterations include:

1. **Affective**: sadness, dejection, feeling downhearted, having the "blues"
2. **Behavioral**: some crying possible
3. **Cognitive**: some difficulty getting mind off of one's disappointment
4. **Physiological**: feeling tired and listless

Mild Depression

Symptoms at the mild level of depression are identified by those associated with normal grieving. Alterations at the mild level include:

1. **Affective**: denial of feelings, anger, anxiety, guilt, helplessness, hopelessness, sadness, despondency
2. **Behavioral**: tearfulness, regression, restlessness, agitation, withdrawal
3. **Cognitive**: preoccupation with the loss, self-blame, ambivalence, blaming others
4. **Physiological**: anorexia or overeating, insomnia or hypersomnia, headache, backache, chest pain, or other symptoms associated with the loss of a significant other

Moderate Depression

This level of depression represents a more problematic disturbance. Symptoms associated with dysthymic disorder include:

1. **Affective**: feelings of sadness, dejection, helplessness, powerlessness, hopelessness; gloomy and pessimistic outlook; low self-esteem; difficulty experiencing pleasure in activities
2. **Behavioral**: slowed physical movements (i.e., psychomotor retardation); slumped posture; slowed speech; limited verbalizations, possibly consisting of ruminations about life's failures or regrets; social iso-

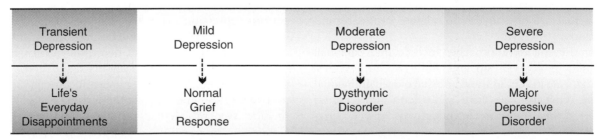

Transient Depression	Mild Depression	Moderate Depression	Severe Depression
↓	↓	↓	↓
Life's Everyday Disappointments	Normal Grief Response	Dysthymic Disorder	Major Depressive Disorder

FIGURE 29–3   A continuum of depression.

lation with a focus on the self; increased use of substances possible; self-destructive behavior possible; decreased interest in personal hygiene and grooming.
3. **Cognitive**: retarded thinking processes; difficulty concentrating and directing attention; obsessive and repetitive thoughts, generally portraying pessimism and negativism; verbalizations and behavior reflecting suicidal ideation
4. **Physiological**: anorexia or overeating; insomnia or hypersomnia; sleep disturbances; amenorrhea; decreased libido; headaches; backaches; chest pain; abdominal pain; low energy level; fatigue and listlessness; feeling best early in the morning and continually worse as the day progresses. This may be related to the diurnal variation in the level of neurotransmitters that affect mood and level of activity.

Severe Depression

Severe depression is characterized by an intensification of the symptoms described for moderate depression. Examples of severe depression include major depressive disorder and bipolar depression. Symptoms at the severe level of depression include:

1. **Affective**: feelings of total despair, hopelessness, and worthlessness; flat (unchanging) affect, appearing devoid of emotional tone; prevalent feelings of nothingness and emptiness; apathy; loneliness; sadness; inability to feel pleasure
2. **Behavioral**: psychomotor retardation so severe that physical movement may literally come to a standstill, or psychomotor behavior manifested by rapid, agitated, purposeless movements; slumped posture; sitting in a curled-up position; walking slowly and rigidly; virtually nonexistent communication (when verbalizations do occur, they may reflect delusional thinking); no personal hygiene and grooming; social isolation is common, with virtually no inclination toward interaction with others
3. **Cognitive**: prevalent delusional thinking, with delusions of persecution and somatic delusions being most common; confusion, indecisiveness, and an inability to concentrate; hallucinations reflecting misinterpretations of the environment; excessive self-deprecation, self-blame, and thoughts of suicide
   NOTE: Because of the low energy level and retarded thought processes, the individual may be unable to follow through on suicidal ideas. However, the desire is strong at this level.
4. **Physiological**: a general slowdown of the entire body, reflected in sluggish digestion, constipation, and urinary retention; amenorrhea; impotence; diminished libido; anorexia; weight loss; difficulty falling asleep and awakening very early in the morning; feeling worse early in the morning and somewhat better as the day progresses. As with moderate depression, this

may reflect the diurnal variation in the level of neurotransmitters that affect mood and activity.

Diagnosis/Outcome Identification

From the assessment data, the nurse formulates the appropriate nursing diagnoses for the depressed client. From these identified problems, care planning is executed, nursing actions are implemented, and relevant criteria for evaluation are established. Possible nursing diagnoses for depressed clients include:

Risk for suicide related to depressed mood, feelings of worthlessness, anger turned inward on the self, misinterpretations of reality.

Dysfunctional grieving related to real or perceived loss, bereavement overload, evidenced by denial of loss, inappropriate expression of anger, idealization of or obsession with the lost object, inability to carry out activities of daily living.

Low self-esteem related to learned helplessness, feelings of abandonment by significant other, or impaired cognition fostering negative view of self, evidenced by expressions of worthlessness, hypersensitivity to a slight or criticism, and a negative, pessimistic outlook.

Powerlessness related to dysfunctional grieving process or lifestyle of helplessness, evidenced by feelings of lack of control over life situation, overdependence on others to fulfill needs.

Spiritual distress related to dysfunctional grieving over loss of valued object evidenced by anger toward God, questioning meaning of own existence, inability to participate in usual religious practices.

Social isolation/impaired social interaction related to developmental regression, egocentric behaviors, fear of rejection or failure of the interaction, evidenced by being uncommunicative and withdrawn, seeking to be alone, and dysfunctional interaction with peers, family, or others.

Disturbed thought processes related to withdrawal into the self, underdeveloped ego, punitive superego, impaired cognition fostering negative perception of self or environment, evidenced by delusional thinking, confusion, difficulty concentrating, and impaired problem-solving ability.

Imbalanced nutrition, less than body requirements related to depressed mood, loss of appetite, or lack of interest in food, evidenced by weight loss, poor muscle tone, pale conjunctiva and mucous membranes, poor skin turgor, and weakness.

Disturbed sleep pattern related to depressed mood, anxiety, and fears, evidenced by difficulty falling asleep, awakening earlier or later than desired, verbal complaints of not feeling well rested.

Self-care deficit (hygiene, grooming) related to depressed mood, feelings of worthlessness, evidenced by uncombed hair, disheveled clothing, offensive body odor.

The following criteria may be used for measurement of outcomes in the care of the depressed client.

The client:

1. Has experienced no physical harm to self.
2. Discusses the loss with staff and family members.
3. No longer idealizes or obsesses about the lost object.
4. Sets realistic goals for self.
5. Is no longer afraid to attempt new activities.
6. Is able to identify aspects of self-control over life situation.
7. Expresses personal satisfaction and support from spiritual practices.
8. Interacts willingly and appropriately with others.
9. Is able to maintain reality orientation.
10. Is able to concentrate, reason, and solve problems.
11. Eats a well-balanced diet with snacks, to prevent weight loss and maintain nutritional status.
12. Sleeps 6 to 8 hours per night and reports feeling well rested.
13. Bathes, washes and combs hair, and dresses in clean clothing without assistance.

Planning/Implementation

Table 29–6 provides a plan of care for the depressed client. Selected nursing diagnoses are presented, along with outcome criteria, appropriate nursing interventions, and rationales for each.

TABLE 29–6   Care Plan for the Depressed Client

NURSING DIAGNOSIS: RISK FOR SUICIDE
RELATED TO: Depressed mood, feelings of worthlessness, anger turned inward on the self, misinterpretations of reality

OUTCOME CRITERIA	NURSING INTERVENTIONS	RATIONALE
Client will not harm self.	1. Ask client directly: "Have you thought about harming yourself in any way? If so, what do you plan to do? Do you have the means to carry out this plan?"	1. The risk of suicide is greatly increased if the client has developed a plan and particularly if means exist for the client to execute the plan.
	2. Create a safe environment for the client. Remove all potentially harmful objects from client's access (sharp objects, straps, belts, ties, glass items, alcohol). Supervise closely during meals and medication administration. Perform room searches as deemed necessary.	2. Client safety is a nursing priority.
	3. Formulate a short-term verbal or written contract that the client will not harm self. When time is up, make another, and so forth. Secure a promise that the client will seek out staff when feeling suicidal.	3. A degree of the responsibility for his or her safety is given to the client. Increased feelings of self-worth may be experienced when client feels accepted unconditionally regardless of thoughts or behavior.
	4. Maintain close observation of client. Depending on level of suicide precaution, provide one-to-one contact, constant visual observation, or every-15-minute checks. Place in room close to nurse's station; do not assign to private room. Accompany to off-ward activities if attendance is indicated. May need to accompany to bathroom.	4. Close observation is necessary to ensure that client does not harm self in any way. Being alert for suicidal and escape attempts facilitates being able to prevent or interrupt harmful behavior.
	5. Maintain special care in administration of medications.	5. Prevents saving up to overdose or discarding and not taking.
	6. Make rounds at frequent, *irregular* intervals (especially at night, toward early morning, at change of shift, or other predictably busy times for staff).	6. Prevents staff surveillance from becoming predictable. To be aware of client's location is important, especially when staff is busy, unavailable, or less observable
	7. Encourage client to express honest feelings, including anger. Provide hostility release if needed.	7. Depression and suicidal behaviors may be viewed as anger turned inward on the self. If this anger can be verbalized in a nonthreatening environment, the client may be able to eventually resolve these feelings.

(Continued on opposite page)

NURSING DIAGNOSIS: DYSFUNCTIONAL GRIEVING
RELATED TO: Real or perceived loss, bereavement overload
EVIDENCED BY: Denial of loss, inappropriate expression of anger, idealization of or obsession with lost object, inability to carry out activities of daily living

OUTCOME CRITERIA	NURSING INTERVENTIONS	RATIONALE
Client will be able to verbalize normal behaviors associated with grieving and begin progression toward resolution.	1. Assess stage of fixation in grief process. 2. Develop trust. Show empathy, concern, and unconditional positive regard. 3. Explore feelings of anger and help client direct them toward the intended object or person. Promote the use of large motor activities for relieving pent-up tension. 4. Teach normal behaviors associated with grieving. 5. Help client with honest review of relationship with lost object.	1. Accurate baseline data is required in order to plan accurate care. 2. Developing trust provides the basis for a therapeutic relationship. 3. Until client can recognize and accept personal feelings regarding the loss, grief work cannot progress. Physical exercise is a safe and effective way of relieving internalized anger. 4. Understanding of the grief process will help prevent feelings of guilt generated by these responses. 5. Only when the client is able to see both positive and negative aspects related to the lost object will the grieving process be complete.

NURSING DIAGNOSIS: LOW SELF-ESTEEM
RELATED TO: Learned helplessness, feelings of abandonment by significant other, impaired cognition fostering negative view of self
EVIDENCED BY: Expressions of worthlessness, hypersensitivity to slights or criticism, negative and pessimistic outlook

OUTCOME CRITERIA	NURSING INTERVENTIONS	RATIONALE
Client will be able to attempt new activities without fear of failure. Client will be able to verbalize positive aspects about self.	1. Be accepting of client and spend time with him or her even though pessimism and negativism may seem objectionable. Focus on strengths and accomplishments and minimize failures. 2. Promote attendance in therapy groups that offer client simple methods of accomplishment. Encourage client to be as independent as possible. 3. Encourage client to recognize areas of change and provide assistance toward this effort. 4. Teach assertiveness and communication techniques.	1. Interventions that focus on the positive contribute toward feelings of self-worth. 2. Success and independence promote feelings of self-worth. 3. Client will need assistance with problem solving. 4. Effective communication and assertiveness techniques enhance self-esteem.

NURSING DIAGNOSIS: POWERLESSNESS
RELATED TO: Dysfunctional grieving process, lifestyle of helplessness
EVIDENCED BY: Feelings of lack of control over life situation, overdependence on others to fulfill needs

OUTCOME CRITERIA	NURSING INTERVENTIONS	RATIONALE
Client will be able to solve problems to take control of life situation.	1. Allow client to participate in goal setting and decision-making regarding own care. 2. Ensure that goals are realistic and that client is able to identify areas of life situation that are realistically under his or her control. 3. Encourage client to verbalize feelings about areas that are not within his or her ability to control.	1. Providing client with choices will increase his or her feelings of control. 2. Realistic goals will avoid setting client up for further failures. 3. Verbalization of unresolved issues may help client accept what cannot be changed.

(Continued on following page)

TABLE 29–6	Care Plan for the Depressed Client *(Continued)*

NURSING DIAGNOSIS: SPIRITUAL DISTRESS
RELATED TO: Dysfunctional grieving over loss of valued object
EVIDENCED BY: Anger toward God, questioning meaning of own existence, inability to participate in usual religious practices

OUTCOME CRITERIA	NURSING INTERVENTIONS	RATIONALE
Client will express achievement of support and personal satisfaction from spiritual practices.	1. Be accepting and nonjudgmental when client expresses anger and bitterness toward God. Stay with client.	1. The nurse's presence and nonjudgmental attitude increase the client's feelings of self-worth and promote trust in the relationship.
	2. Encourage client to ventilate feelings related to meaning of own existence in the face of current loss.	2. Client may believe he or she cannot go on living without lost object. Catharsis can provide relief and put life back into realistic perspective.
	3. Encourage client as part of grief work to reach out to previous religious practices for support. Encourage client to discuss these practices and how they provided support in the past.	3. Client may find comfort in religious rituals with which he or she is familiar.
	4. Ensure client that he or she is not alone when feeling inadequate in the search for life's answers.	4. Validation of client's feelings and the assurance that others share them offers reassurance and an affirmation of acceptability.
	5. Contact spiritual leader of client's choice, if he or she requests.	5. These individuals serve to provide relief from spiritual distress and often can do so when other support persons cannot.

Some institutions are using a case management model to coordinate care (see Chapter 9 for more detailed explanation). In case management models, the plan of care may take the form of a critical pathway. Table 29–7 depicts an example of a critical pathway of care for a depressed client.

The concept map care plan is an innovative approach to planning and organizing nursing care (see Chapter 9). It is a diagrammatic teaching and learning strategy that allows visualization of interrelationships between medical diagnoses, nursing diagnoses, assessment data, and treatments. An example of a concept map care plan for a client with depression is presented in Figure 29–4.

Client/Family Education

The role of client teacher is important in the psychiatric area, as it is in all areas of nursing. A list of topics for client/family education relevant to depression is presented in Table 29–8.

Evaluation of Care for the Depressed Client

In the final step of the nursing process, a reassessment is conducted to determine if the nursing actions have been successful in achieving the objectives of care. Evaluation of the nursing actions for the depressed client may be facilitated by gathering information using the following types of questions:

1. Has self-harm to the individual been avoided?
2. Have suicidal ideations subsided?
3. Does the individual know where to seek assistance outside the hospital when suicidal thoughts occur?
4. Has the client discussed the recent loss with staff and family members?
5. Is he or she able to verbalize feelings and behaviors associated with each stage of the grieving process and recognize own position in the process?
6. Have obsession with and idealization of the lost object subsided?
7. Is anger toward the lost object expressed appropriately?
8. Does the client set realistic goals for him- or herself?
9. Is he or she able to verbalize positive aspects about self, past accomplishments, and future prospects?
10. Can the client identify areas of life situation over which he or she has control?
11. Is the client able to participate in usual religious practices and feel satisfaction and support from them?
12. Is the client seeking out interaction with others in an appropriate manner?

TABLE 29–7   **Critical Pathway of Care for the Depressed Client**

Estimated Length of Stay: 7 Days—Variations from Designated Pathway Should Be Documented in Progress Notes

Nursing Diagnoses and Categories of Care	Time Dimension	Goals and/or Actions	Time Dimension	Goals and/or Actions	Time Dimension	Discharge Outcome
Risk for suicide	Day 1	Environment is made safe for client.	Ongoing	Client does not harm self.	Day 7	Client is discharged without harm to self.
Referrals	Day 1	Psychiatrist: May give order to isolate if risk is great or may do ECT For relaxation therapy: Music therapist Clinical nurse specialist Stress management specialist			Day 7	Discharge with follow-up appointments as required.
Additional assessments	Day 1 Day 1	Suicidal assessment: • ideation • gestures • threats • plan • means • anxiety level • thought disorder Secure no-suicide contract.	Days 2–7	Ongoing assessments.	Day 7	Client discharged. Denies suicidal ideations.
Medications	Day 1	Antidepressant medication, as ordered. Antianxiety agents p.r.n.	Days 1–7	Assess for effectiveness and side effects of medications. Be alert for sudden lifts in mood.	Day 7	Discharged with antidepressant medications.
Client education	Days 3–6	Teach relaxation techniques. Discuss resources outside the hospital from whom client may seek assistance when feeling suicidal.	Days 6–7	Reinforce teaching.	Day 7	Discharge with understanding of instruction given.
Dysfunctional grieving	Day 1	Assess stage of fixation in grief process.			Day 7	Discharge with evidence of progression toward resolution of grief.
Referrals	Day 1	Psychiatrist Psychologist Social worker Clinical nurse specialist Music therapist Occupational therapist Recreational therapist Chaplain			Day 7	Discharge with follow-up appointments as required.
Diagnostic studies	Day 1 Days 2–3	Any of the following tests *may* be ordered: Drug screen Chemistry profile Urine test for norepinephrine and serotonin Dexamethasone-suppression test A measure of TSH response to administered TRH Serum and urine studies for nutritional deficiencies.				
Medications	Day 1	Antidepressant medication, as ordered. Antianxiety agent p.r.n.	Days 1–7	Assess for effectiveness and side effects of medications.	Day 7	Client is discharged with medications.

(Continued on following page)

TABLE 29–7	Critical Pathway of Care for the Depressed Client *(Continued)*					

Estimated Length of Stay: 7 Days—Variations from Designated Pathway Should Be Documented in Progress Notes

Nursing Diagnoses and Categories of Care	Time Dimension	Goals and/or Actions	Time Dimension	Goals and/or Actions	Time Dimension	Discharge Outcome
Diet	Day 1	If antidepressant medication is MAO inhibitor: low tyramine			Day 7	Client has experienced no symptoms of hypertensive crisis.
Additional assessments	Day 1	VS every shift Assess: • mental status • mood, affect • thought disorder • communication patterns • level of interest in environment • participation in activities • weight	Days 2–7 Days 2–7	VS daily if stable. Ongoing assessments.	Day 7	Mood and affect appropriate. No evidence of thought disorder. Participates willingly and appropriately in activities.
Client education	Day 1	Orient to unit	Day 4 Days 5–6	Discuss importance of taking medications regularly, even when feeling well or if feeling medication is not helping. Discuss possible side effects of medication and when to see the physician. Teach which foods to eliminate from diet if taking MAO inhibitor. Reinforce teaching.	Day 7	Client is discharged. Verbalizes understanding of information presented prior to discharge.

TABLE 29–8	Topics for Client/Family Education Related to Depression

Nature of the Illness

1. Stages of grief and symptoms associated with each stage.
2. What is depression?
3. Why do people get depressed?
4. What are the symptoms of depression?

Management of the Illness

1. Medication management
   a. Nuisance side effects
   b. Side effects to report to physician
   c. Importance of taking regularly
   d. Length of time to take effect
   e. Diet (related to MAO inhibitors)
2. Assertiveness techniques
3. Stress-management techniques
4. Ways to increase self-esteem
5. Electroconvulsive therapy

Support Services

1. Suicide hotline
2. Support groups
3. Legal/financial assistance

13. Does the client maintain reality orientation with no evidence of delusional thinking?
14. Is he or she able to concentrate and make decisions concerning own self-care?
15. Is the client selecting and consuming foods sufficiently high in nutrients and calories to maintain weight and nutritional status?
16. Does the client sleep without difficulty and wake feeling rested?
17. Does the client show pride in appearance by attending to personal hygiene and grooming?
18. Have somatic complaints subsided?

BIPOLAR DISORDER (MANIA)

Predisposing Factors

Biological Theories

Genetics

Twin Studies. Twin studies have indicated a concordance rate for bipolar disorder among monozygotic twins at 60

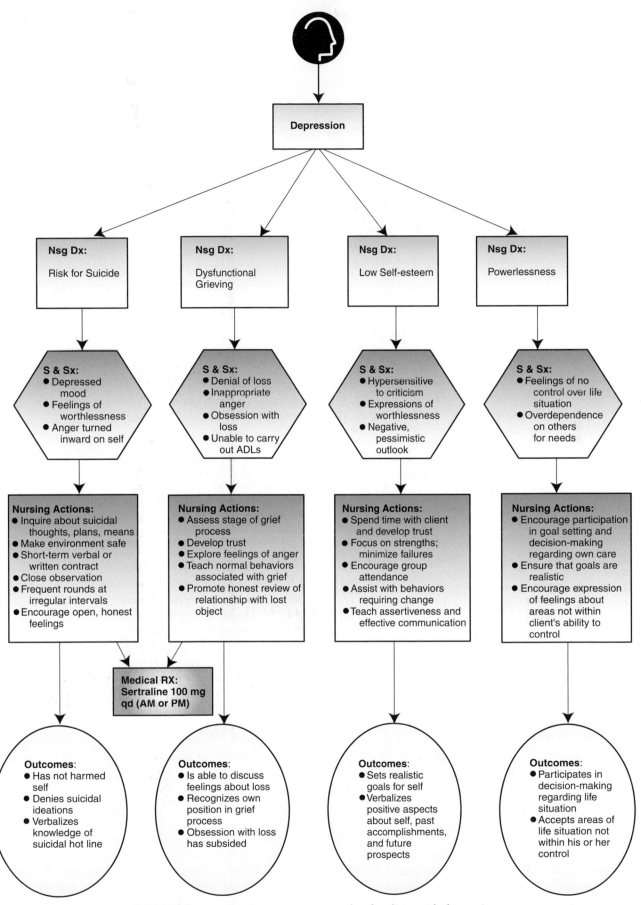

FIGURE 29–4 Concept map care plan for client with depression.

503

to 80 percent compared to 20 percent in dizygotic twins (Harvard Medical School, 2001). Because monozygotic twins have identical genes and dizygotic twins share only approximately half their genes, this is strong evidence that genes play a major role in the etiology.

Family Studies. Family studies have shown that if one parent has bipolar disorder, the risk that a child will have the disorder is around 28 percent (Dubovsky, Davies, & Dubovsky, 2003). If both parents have the disorder, the risk is two to three times as great. This has also been shown to be the case in studies of children born to parents with bipolar disorder who were adopted at birth and reared by adoptive parents without evidence of the disorder. These results strongly indicate that genes play a role separate from that of the environment.

Biochemical Influences

Biogenic Amines. Early studies have associated symptoms of depression with a functional deficiency of norepinephrine and dopamine and mania with a functional excess of these amines. The neurotransmitter serotonin appears to remain low in both states. A recent study at the University of Michigan using a presynaptic marker and positron emission tomography (PET) revealed an increased density in the amine-releasing cells in the brains of people with bipolar disorder compared to control subjects (Zubieta et al., 2000). It was hypothesized that these excess cells result in the altered brain chemistry that is associated with the symptoms of bipolar disorder. Some support of this neurotransmitter hypothesis has been demonstrated by the effects of neuroleptic drugs that influence the levels of these biogenic amines to produce the desired effect.

Electrolytes. Some studies have suggested possible alterations in normal electrolyte transfer across cell membranes in bipolar disorder resulting in elevated levels of intracellular sodium and calcium (Bohrer, 2001). The link between increased intracellular calcium and symptoms of bipolar disorder may be substantiated by the effectiveness of calcium channel blockers (e.g., verapamil; amlodipine) in some cases of refractory bipolar illness.

Physiological Influences

Neuroanatomical Factors. Right-sided lesions in the limbic system, temporobasal areas, basal ganglia, and thalamus have been shown to induce secondary mania. Magnetic resonance imaging (MRI) studies have revealed enlarged third ventricles and subcortical white matter and periventricular hyperintensities in clients with bipolar disorder (Dubovsky, Davies, & Dubovsky, 2003).

Medication Side Effects. Certain medications used to treat somatic illnesses have been known to trigger a manic response. The most common of these are the steroids frequently used to treat chronic illnesses such as multiple sclerosis and systemic lupus erythematosus

(SLE). Some clients whose first episode of mania occurred during steroid therapy have reported spontaneous recurrence of manic symptoms years later. Amphetamines, antidepressants, and high doses of anticonvulsants and narcotics also have the potential for initiating a manic episode (Dubovsky, Davies, & Dobovsky, 2003).

Psychosocial Theories

The credibility of psychosocial theories has declined in recent years. Conditions such as schizophrenia and bipolar disorder are being viewed by many as diseases of the brain with biological etiologies. The etiology of these illnesses remains unclear, however, and it is possible that both biological and psychosocial factors (such as environmental stressors) are influential (NIMH, 2000).

The Transactional Model

Bipolar disorder most likely results from an interaction between genetic, biological, and psychosocial determinants. Kaplan and Sadock (1998) state:

> The causative factors (of mood disorders) can be artificially divided into biological, genetic, and psychosocial, but this division is artificial because the three realms likely interact among themselves. Psychosocial and genetic factors can affect biological factors, such as concentrations of a certain neurotransmitter. Biological and psychosocial factors can also affect gene expression, and biological and genetic factors can affect a person's response to psychosocial factors. (p. 524)

The transactional model takes into consideration these various etiological influences, as well as those associated with past experiences, existing conditions, and the individual's perception of the event. Figure 29–5 depicts the dynamics of bipolar disorder, mania, using the transactional model of stress/adaptation.

Developmental Implications
Childhood and Adolescence

The lifetime prevalence of pediatric and adolescent bipolar disorders is estimated to be about 1 percent, but children and adolescents are often difficult to diagnose (Allen, 2003). The developmental courses and symptom profiles of psychiatric disorders in children are unique from those of adults; therefore, approaches to diagnosis and treatment cannot merely rely on strategies examined and implemented in a typical adult population.

A working group sponsored by the Child and Adolescent Bipolar Foundation (CABF) has developed consensus guidelines for the diagnosis and treatment of children with bipolar disorder. These guidelines were

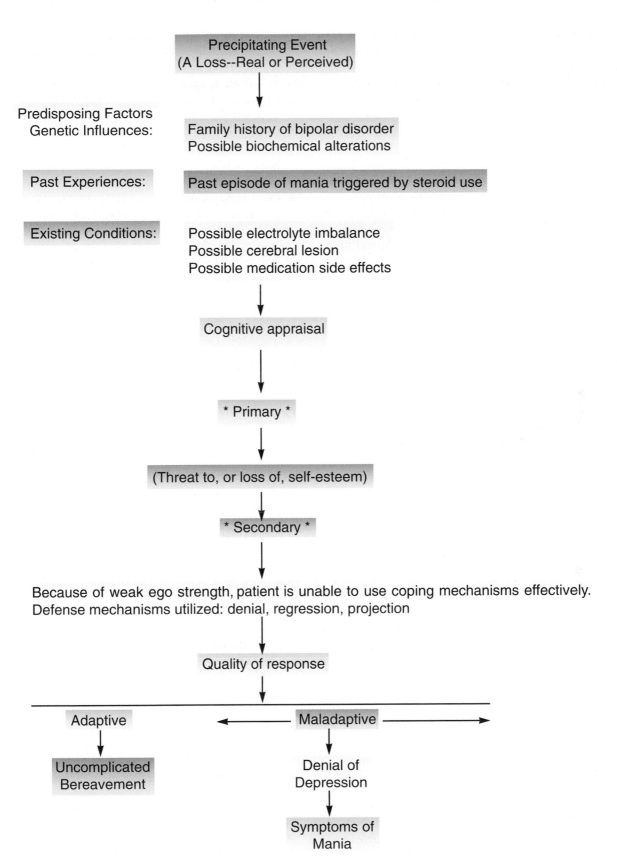

FIGURE 29–5 The dynamics of bipolar disorder, mania, using the transactional model of stress/adaptation.

presented in the March 2005 issue of the *Journal of the American Academy of Child and Adolescent Psychiatry* and address diagnosis, comorbidity, acute treatment, and maintenance treatment (Kowatch et al., 2005).

Symptoms of bipolar disorder are often difficult to assess in children, and they may also present with comorbid conduct disorders or attention-deficit hyperactivity disorder (ADHD). Because there is a genetic component and children of bipolar adults are at higher risk, family history may be particularly important (Allen, 2003). To differentiate between occasional spontaneous behaviors of childhood and behaviors associated with bipolar disorder, the Consensus Group recommends that clinicians use the FIND (frequency, intensity, number, and duration) strategy (Kowatch et al., 2005):

● Frequency: Symptoms occur most days in a week.
● Intensity: Symptoms are severe enough to cause extreme disturbance in one domain or moderate disturbance in two or more domains.
● Number: Symptoms occur three or four times a day.
● Duration: Symptoms occur 4 or more hours a day.

The symptoms associated with mania in children and adolescents are as follows. Regarding these symptoms, Kowatch and associates (2005) state:

For any of these symptoms to be counted as a manic symptom, they must exceed the FIND threshold. Additionally, they must occur in concert with other manic symptoms because no one symptom is diagnostic of mania. (p. 215)

● **Euphoric/Expansive Mood.** Extremely happy, silly, or giddy
● **Irritable Mood.** Hostility and rage, often over trivial matters. The irritability may be accompanied by aggressive and/or self-injurious behavior.
● **Grandiosity.** Believing that his or her abilities are better than everyone else's.
● **Decreased Need for Sleep.** May sleep only 4 or 5 hours per night and wake up fresh and full of energy the next day. Or he or she may get up in the middle of the night and wander around the house looking for things to do.
● **Pressured Speech.** Rapid speech that is loud, intrusive, and difficult to interrupt.
● **Racing Thoughts.** Topics of conversation change rapidly, in a manner confusing to anyone listening.
● **Distractibility.** To consider distractibility a manic symptom, it needs to reflect a change from baseline functioning, needs to occur in conjunction with a "manic" mood shift, and cannot be accounted for exclusively by another disorder, particularly ADHD (Kowatch et al., 2005). Distractibility during a manic episode may be reflected in a child who is normally a B or C student but is unable to focus on any school lessons.
● **Increase in Goal-Directed Activity/Psychomotor Agitation.** A child who is not usually highly produc-

tive becomes very project oriented during a manic episode, increasing goal-directed activity to an obsessive level. Psychomotor agitation represents a distinct change from baseline behavior.
● **Excessive Involvement in Pleasurable or Risky Activities.** Children with bipolar disorder are often hypersexual, exhibiting behavior that has an erotic, pleasure-seeking quality about it (Kowatch et al., 2005). Adolescents may seek out sexual activity multiple times in a day.
● **Psychosis.** In addition to core symptoms of mania, psychotic symptoms, including hallucinations and delusions, are frequently present in children with bipolar disorder (Geller et al., 2002; Kafantaris et al., 2001).
● **Suicidality.** Although not a core symptom of mania, children with bipolar disorder are at risk of suicidal ideation, intent, plans, and attempts during a depressed or mixed episode or when psychotic (Geller et al., 2002).

Treatment Strategies

Psychopharmacology

Lithium is currently the only medication approved by the FDA for children and adolescents with bipolar disorder (Allen, 2003). Monotherapy with the traditional mood stabilizers (e.g., lithium, divalproex, carbamazepine) or atypical antipsychotics (e.g., olanzapine, quetiapine, risperidone) was determined to be the first-line treatment (Kowatch et al., 2005). In the event of inadequate response to initial monotherapy, an alternate monotherapeutic agent is suggested. Augmentation with a second medication is indicated when monotherapy fails.

ADHD has been identified as the most common comorbid condition in children and adolescents with bipolar disorder. Because stimulants can exacerbate mania (Allen, 2003), it is suggested that medication for ADHD be initiated only after bipolar symptoms have been controlled with a mood stabilizer (Kowatch et al., 2005). Nonstimulant medications indicated for ADHD (e.g., atomoxetine, bupropion, the tricyclic antidepressants) may also induce switches to mania or hypomania.

Bipolar disorder in children and adolescents appears to be a chronic condition with a high risk of relapse (Kowatch et al., 2005). Maintenance therapy is with the same medications used to treat acute symptoms, although few research studies exist that deal with long-term maintenance of bipolar disorder in children. The Consensus Group recommends that medication tapering or discontinuation be considered after remission has been achieved for a minimum of 12 to 24 consecutive months. It was acknowledged, however, that some clients may require long-term or even lifelong pharmacotherapy (Kowatch et al., 2005).

Family Interventions

Although pharmacologic treatment is acknowledged as the primary method of stabilizing an acutely ill bipolar client, adjunctive psychotherapy has been recognized as playing an important role in preventing relapses and improving adjustment. Allen (2003) suggests that involving the family in postepisode stabilization of bipolar disorder is important and helps family members:

● Integrate their experience of the mood disorder.
● Know the symptoms of bipolar disorder and what precipitates episodes.
● Understand the client's vulnerability to future episodes.

Family support is also important in helping the client accept the necessity of ongoing medication administration. Family dynamics and attitudes can play a crucial role in the outcome of a client's recovery. Interventions with family members must include education that promotes understanding that at least part of the client's negative behaviors are attributable to an illness that must be managed, as opposed to being willful and deliberate.

Studies show that family-focused psychoeducational treatment (FFT) is an effective method of reducing relapses and increasing medication adherence in bipolar clients (Miklowitz, 2003). FFT includes sessions that deal with psychoeducation about bipolar disorder (i.e., symptoms, early recognition, etiology, treatment, self-management), communication training, and problem-solving skills training. Allen (2003) states:

> There are several important goals of FFT, which include: improving communication within the family, teaching the family to recognize the early warning signs of a relapse, teaching the family how to respond to these warning signs, and educating them regarding the necessary treatments. This education helps families gain some control over the conflict that occurs in the postepisode phases.

There is evidence to suggest that the addition of psychosocial therapy enhances the effectiveness of psychopharmacological therapy in the maintenance of bipolar disorder in children and adolescents.

APPLICATION OF THE NURSING PROCESS TO BIPOLAR DISORDER (MANIA)

Background Assessment Data

Symptoms of manic states can be described according to three stages: hypomania, acute mania, and **delirious mania**. Symptoms of mood, cognition and perception, and activity and behavior are presented for each stage.

Stage I: Hypomania

At this stage the disturbance is not sufficiently severe to cause marked impairment in social or occupational functioning or to require hospitalization (APA, 2000).

Mood. The mood of a hypomanic person is cheerful and expansive. There is an underlying irritability that surfaces rapidly when the person's wishes and desires go unfulfilled, however. The nature of the hypomanic person is very volatile and fluctuating.

Cognition and Perception. Perceptions of the self are exalted—ideas of great worth and ability. Thinking is flighty, with a rapid flow of ideas. Perception of the environment is heightened, but the individual is so easily distracted by irrelevant stimuli that goal-directed activities are difficult.

Activity and Behavior. Hypomanic individuals exhibit increased motor activity. They are perceived as being very extroverted and sociable, and because of this they attract numerous acquaintances. They lack the depth of personality and warmth to formulate close friendships, however. They talk and laugh a great deal, usually very loudly and often inappropriately. Increased libido is common. Some individuals experience anorexia and weight loss. The exalted self-perception leads some hypomanic individuals to engage in inappropriate behaviors, such as phoning the President of the United States, or buying huge amounts on a credit card without having the resources to pay.

Stage II: Acute Mania

Symptoms of acute mania may be a progression in intensification of those experienced in hypomania, or they may be manifested directly. Most individuals experience marked impairment in functioning and require hospitalization.

Mood. Acute mania is characterized by euphoria and elation. The person appears to be on a continuous "high." The mood is always subject to frequent variation, however, easily changing to irritability and anger or even to sadness and crying.

Cognition and Perception. Cognition and perception become fragmented and often psychotic in acute mania. Rapid thinking proceeds to racing and disjointed thinking (flight of ideas) and may be manifested by a continuous flow of accelerated, pressured speech (loquaciousness), with abrupt changes from topic to topic. When flight of ideas is severe, speech may be disorganized and incoherent. Distractibility becomes all-pervasive. Attention can be diverted by even the smallest of stimuli. Hallucinations and delusions (usually paranoid and grandiose) are common.

Activity and Behavior. Psychomotor activity is excessive. Sexual interest is increased. There is poor impulse control, and the individual who is normally discreet may become socially and sexually uninhibited. Excessive spending is common. Individuals with acute mania have the ability to manipulate others to carry out their wishes, and if things go wrong, they can skillfully project responsibility for the failure onto others. Energy seems inexhaustible, and the need for sleep is diminished. They may go for many days without sleep and still not feel tired. Hygiene and grooming may be neglected. Dress may be disorganized, flamboyant, or bizarre, and the use of excessive make-up or jewelry is common.

Stage III: Delirious Mania

Delirious mania is a grave form of the disorder characterized by severe clouding of consciousness and an intensification of the symptoms associated with acute mania. This condition has become relatively rare since the availability of antipsychotic medication.

Mood. The mood of the delirious person is very labile. He or she may exhibit feelings of despair, quickly converting to unrestrained merriment and ecstasy or becoming irritable or totally indifferent to the environment. Panic anxiety may be evident.

Cognition and Perception. Cognition and perception are characterized by a clouding of consciousness, with accompanying confusion, disorientation, and sometimes stupor. Other common manifestations include religiosity, delusions of grandeur or persecution, and auditory or visual hallucinations. The individual is extremely distractible and incoherent.

Activity and Behavior. Psychomotor activity is frenzied and characterized by agitated, purposeless movements. The safety of these individuals is at stake unless this activity is curtailed. Exhaustion, injury to self or others, and eventually death could occur without intervention.

Diagnosis/Outcome Identification

Nursing diagnoses are formulated from the assessment data, and the plan of care is devised. Possible nursing diagnoses for the client with bipolar disorder (mania) include:

Risk for injury related to extreme hyperactivity evidenced by increased agitation and lack of control over purposeless and potentially injurious movements.

Risk for violence: self-directed or other-directed related to manic excitement, delusional thinking, hallucinations.

Imbalanced nutrition: less than body requirements related to refusal or inability to sit still long enough to eat evidenced by loss of weight, amenorrhea.

Disturbed thought processes related to biochemical alterations in the brain evidenced by delusions of grandeur and persecution.

Disturbed sensory perception related to biochemical

alterations in the brain, possible sleep deprivation, evidenced by auditory and visual hallucinations.

Impaired social interaction related to egocentric and narcissistic behavior evidenced by inability to develop satisfying relationships and manipulation of others for own desires.

Disturbed sleep pattern related to excessive hyperactivity and agitation evidenced by difficulty falling asleep and sleeping only short periods.

The following criteria may be used for measuring outcomes in the care of the manic client.

The client:

1. Exhibits no evidence of physical injury.
2. Has not harmed self or others.
3. Is no longer exhibiting signs of physical agitation.
4. Eats a well-balanced diet with snacks to prevent weight loss and maintain nutritional status.
5. Verbalizes an accurate interpretation of the environment.
6. Verbalizes that hallucinatory activity has ceased and demonstrates no outward behavior indicating hallucinations.
7. Accepts responsibility for own behaviors.
8. Does not manipulate others for gratification of own needs.
9. Interacts appropriately with others.
10. Is able to fall asleep within 30 minutes of retiring.
11. Is able to sleep 6 to 8 hours per night without medication.

Planning/Implementation

Table 29–9 provides a plan of care for the manic client. Selected nursing diagnoses are presented, along with outcome criteria, appropriate nursing interventions, and rationales for each.

Some institutions are using a case management model to coordinate care (see Chapter 9 for a more detailed explanation). In case management models, the plan of care may take the form of a critical pathway. Table 29–10 depicts an example of a critical pathway of care for a manic client.

The concept map care plan is an innovative approach to planning and organizing nursing care (see Chapter 9). It is a diagrammatic teaching and learning strategy that allows visualization of interrelationships between medical diagnoses, nursing diagnoses, assessment data, and treatments. An example of a concept map care plan for a client with bipolar disorder, mania, is presented in Figure 29–6.

Client/Family Education

The role of client teacher is important in the psychiatric area, as it is in all areas of nursing. A list of topics for

TABLE 29–9   Care Plan for the Client Experiencing a Manic Episode

NURSING DIAGNOSIS: RISK FOR INJURY
RELATED TO: Extreme hyperactivity
EVIDENCED BY: Increased agitation and lack of control over purposeless and potentially injurious movements

OUTCOME CRITERIA	NURSING INTERVENTIONS	RATIONALE
Client will not experience injury.	1. Reduce environmental stimuli. Assign private room with simple decor, on quiet unit if possible. Keep lighting and noise level low. 2. Remove hazardous objects and substances (including smoking materials). 3. Stay with the client who is hyperactive and agitated. 4. Provide physical activities. 5. Administer tranquilizing medication as ordered by physician.	1. Client is extremely distractible and responses to even the slightest stimuli are exaggerated. A milieu unit may be too stimulating. 2. Rationality is impaired, and client may harm self inadvertently. 3. Nurse's presence may offer support and provide feeling of security for the client. 4. Physical activities help relieve pent-up tension. 5. Antipsychotics are common, and are very effective for providing rapid relief from symptoms of hyperactivity.

NURSING DIAGNOSIS: RISK FOR VIOLENCE: SELF-DIRECTED OR OTHER-DIRECTED
RELATED TO: Manic excitement, delusional thinking, hallucinations

OUTCOME CRITERIA	NURSING INTERVENTIONS	RATIONALE
Client will not harm self or others.	1. Maintain low level of stimuli in client's environment 2. Observe client's behavior at least every 15 minutes. 3. Ensure that all sharp objects, glass or mirrored items, belts, ties, smoking materials have been removed from client's environment. 4. Redirect violent behavior with physical outlets. 5. Maintain and convey a calm attitude to client. Respond matter-of-factly to verbal hostility. 6. Have sufficient staff to indicate a show of strength to client if necessary. 7. Offer tranquilizing medication. If client refuses, use of mechanical restraints may be necessary. 8. Medication may then be administered following application of mechanical restraints. Observe client every 15 minutes. 9. Remove restraints gradually, one at a time.	1. To minimize anxiety, agitation, and suspiciousness. 2. This is important so that intervention can occur if required to ensure client's (and others') safety. 3. These objects must be removed so that client cannot use them to harm self or others. 4. Physical activity is good for relieving pent-up tension and hostility. 5. Anxiety is contagious and can be transmitted from staff to client. 6. This conveys evidence of control over the situation and provides some physical security for staff. 7. Client should be offered an avenue of the "least restrictive alternative." 8. This ensures that needs for circulation, nutrition, hydration, and elimination are met. Client safety is a nursing priority. 9. Gradual removal of restraints minimizes potential for injury to client and staff.

NURSING DIAGNOSIS: IMBALANCED NUTRITION: LESS THAN BODY REQUIREMENTS
RELATED TO: Refusal or inability to sit still long enough to eat
EVIDENCED BY: Weight loss, amenorrhea

OUTCOME CRITERIA	NURSING INTERVENTIONS	RATIONALE
Client will exhibit no signs or symptoms of malnutrition.	1. Provide high-protein, high-calorie, nutritious finger foods and drinks that can be consumed "on the run."	1. Client has difficulty sitting still long enough to eat a meal.

(Continued on following page)

TABLE 29–9   **Care Plan for the Client Experiencing a Manic Episode** *(Continued)*

OUTCOME CRITERIA	NURSING INTERVENTIONS	RATIONALE
	2. Have juice and snacks on the unit at all times.	2. Nutritious intake is required on a regular basis to compensate for increased caloric requirement as a result of hyperactivity.
	3. Maintain accurate record of intake, output, calorie count, and weight. Monitor daily laboratory values.	3. These are important nutritional assessment data.
	4. Provide favorite foods.	4. This encourages eating.
	5. Supplement diet with vitamins and minerals.	5. To improve nutritional status.
	6. Walk or sit with client while he or she eats.	6. The nurse's presence offers support and encouragement to client to eat food that will maintain physical wellness.

NURSING DIAGNOSIS: IMPAIRED SOCIAL INTERACTION
RELATED TO: Egocentric and narcissistic behavior
EVIDENCED BY: Inability to develop satisfying relationships and manipulation of others for own desires

OUTCOME CRITERIA	NURSING INTERVENTIONS	RATIONALE
Client will interact appropriately with others.	1. Recognize that manipulative behaviors help to reduce feelings of insecurity by increasing feelings of power and control.	1. Understanding the motivation behind the behavior may facilitate greater acceptance of the individual.
	2. Set limits on manipulative behaviors. Explain what is expected and the consequences if limits are violated. Terms of the limitations must be agreed on by all staff who will be working with the client.	2. Consequences for violation of limits must be consistently administered, or behavior will not be eliminated.
	3. Ignore attempts by client to argue, bargain, or charm his or her way out of the limit setting.	3. Lack of feedback may decrease these behaviors.
	4. Give positive reinforcement for non-manipulative behaviors.	4. Positive reinforcement enhances self-esteem and promotes repetition of desirable behaviors.
	5. Discuss consequences of client's behavior and how attempts are made to attribute them to others.	5. Client must accept responsibility for own behavior before adaptive change can occur.
	6. Help client identify positive aspects about self, recognize accomplishments, and feel good about them.	6. As self-esteem is increased, client will feel less need to manipulate others for own gratification.

client/family education relevant to bipolar disorder is presented in Table 29–11.

Evaluation of Care for the Manic Client

In the final step of the nursing process, a reassessment is conducted to determine if the nursing actions have been successful in achieving the objectives of care. Evaluation of the nursing actions for the manic client may be facilitated by gathering information using the following types of questions.

1. Has the individual avoided personal injury?
2. Has violence to client or others been prevented?
3. Has agitation subsided?
4. Have nutritional status and weight been stabilized? Is the client able to select foods to maintain adequate nutrition?
5. Have delusions and hallucinations ceased? Is the client able to interpret the environment correctly?
6. Is the client able to make decisions about own self-care? Has hygiene and grooming improved?
7. Is behavior socially acceptable? Is the client able to interact with others in a satisfactory manner? Has the client stopped manipulating others to fulfill own desires?
8. Is the client able to sleep 6 to 8 hours per night and awaken feeling rested?
9. Does the client understand the importance of maintenance medication therapy? Does he or she under-

Estimated Length of Stay: 7 Days—Variations from Designated Pathway Should Be Documented in Progress Notes

Nursing Diagnoses and Categories of Care	Time Dimension	Goals and/or Actions	Time Dimension	Goals and/or Actions	Time Dimension	Discharge Outcome
Risk for injury/ violence	Day 1	Environment is made safe for client and others.	Ongoing	Client does not harm self or others.	Day 7	Client has not harmed self or others.
Referrals	Day 1	Psychiatrist Clinical nurse specialist Internist (may need to determine if symptoms are caused by other illness or medication side effects) Neurologist (may want to check for brain lesion) Alert hostility management team			Day 7	Discharge with follow-up appointments as required.
Diagnostic studies	Day 1	Drug screen Electrolytes Lithium level Chemistry profile	Day 5	Lithium level	Day 7	Lithium level and discharge with instructions to return monthly to have level drawn
Additional assessments	Day 1 Ongoing Ongoing	VS q4h Restraints p.r.n. Assess for signs of impending violent behavior: increase in psychomotor activity, angry affect, verbalized persecutory delusions or frightening hallucinations.	Days 2–7	Ongoing assessments		
Medications	Day 1	Antipsychotic medications, scheduled and p.r.n. *Lithium carbonate 600 mg t.i.d. or q.i.d. *Note: Physician may elect to use an anticonvulsant (e.g., valproic acid; carbamazepine)	Days 2–7	Administer medications as ordered and observe for effectiveness and side effects.	Day 7	Client is discharged on maintenance dose lithium carbonate (or other mood stabilizing agent).
Client education			Day 4	Teach about lithium: Continue to take medication even when feeling okay. Teach symptoms of toxicity. Emphasize importance of monthly blood levels. Teach about other medications client may be taking.	Day 7	Client is discharged with written instructions and verbalizes understanding of material presented.
			Day 6	Reinforce teaching		

(Continued on following page)

TABLE 29–10   **Critical Pathway of Care for the Client Experiencing a Manic Episode** *(Continued)*

Estimated Length of Stay: 7 Days—Variations from Designated Pathway Should Be Documented in Progress Notes

Nursing Diagnoses and Categories of Care	Time Dimension	Goals and/or Actions	Time Dimension	Goals and/or Actions	Time Dimension	Discharge Outcome
Imbalanced nutrition: Less than body requirements					Day 7	Nutritional condition and weight have stabilized.
Referrals	Day 1	Consult dietitian	Days 1–7	Fulfill nutritional needs.		
Diet	Day 1	High-protein, high-calorie nutritious finger foods. Juice and snacks as tolerated.	As mania subsides	Regular diet with foods of client's choice.		
Diagnostic studies	Day 1	Chemistry profile Urinalysis	Days 2–7	Repeat of selected diagnostic studies as required.		
Additional assessments	Days 1–7	Weight I&O Skin turgor Color of mucous membranes				
Medications	Days 1–7	Multiple vitamin/ mineral tab				
Client education			Day 4	Principles of nutrition; foods for maintenance of wellness; adequate sodium; 6–8 glasses of water/day. Contact dietitian if weight gain becomes a problem.	Days 5–7	Client demonstrates ability to select appropriate foods for healthy diet and verbalizes understanding of material presented.
			Day 6	Reinforce teaching		

stand that symptoms may return if medication is discontinued?

10. Can the client taking lithium verbalize early signs of lithium toxicity? Does he or she understand the necessity for monthly blood level checks?

TREATMENT MODALITIES FOR MOOD DISORDERS

Psychological Treatments

Individual Psychotherapy

For Depression

Research has documented both the importance of close and satisfactory attachments in the prevention of depression and the role of disrupted attachments in the development of depression. With this concept in mind, interpersonal psychotherapy focuses on the client's current interpersonal relationships. Interpersonal psychotherapy with the depressed person proceeds through the following phases and interventions:

Phase I. During the first phase, the client is assessed to determine the extent of the illness. Complete information is then given to the individual regarding the nature of depression, symptom pattern, frequency, clinical course, and alternative treatments. If the level of depression is severe, interpersonal psychotherapy has been shown to be more effective if conducted in combination with antidepressant medication. The client is encouraged to continue working and participating in regular activities during therapy. A mutually agreeable therapeutic contract is negotiated.

Phase II. Treatment at this phase focuses on helping the client resolve dysfunctional grief reactions. This may include resolving the ambivalence with a lost relationship, serving as a temporary substitute for the lost relationship, and assistance with establishing new relationships. Other areas of treatment focus may include interpersonal disputes between the client and a signifi-

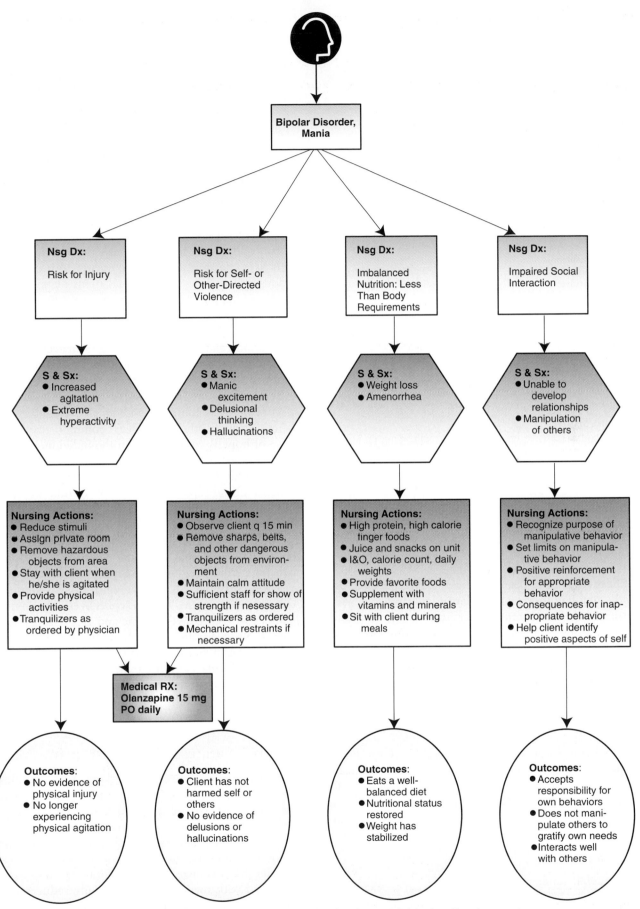

FIGURE 29–6   Concept map care plan for client with bipolar disorder, mania.

TABLE 29–11 Topics for Client/Family Education Related to Bipolar Disorder

Nature of the Illness
1. Causes of bipolar disorder
2. Cyclic nature of the illness
3. Symptoms of depression
4. Symptoms of mania

Management of the Illness
1. Medication management
   a. Lithium
   b. Others
      (1) Carbamazepine
      (2) Valproic acid
      (3) Clonazepam
      (4) Verapamil
      (5) Lamotrigine
      (6) Gabapentin
      (7) Topiramate
      (8) Olanzapine
      (9) Risperidone
   c. Side effects
   d. Symptoms of lithium toxicity
   e. Importance of regular blood tests
   f. Adverse effects
   g. Importance of not stopping medication, even when feeling well
2. Assertive techniques
3. Anger management

Support Services
1. Crisis hotline
2. Support groups
3. Individual psychotherapy
4. Legal and/or financial assistance

cant other, difficult role transitions at various developmental life cycles, and correction of interpersonal deficits that may interfere with the client's ability to initiate or sustain interpersonal relationships.

Phase III. During the final phase of interpersonal psychotherapy, the therapeutic alliance is terminated. With emphasis on reassurance, clarification of emotional states, improvement of interpersonal communication, testing of perceptions, and performance in interpersonal settings, interpersonal psychotherapy has been successful in helping depressed persons recover enhanced social functioning.

For Mania

Manic clients traditionally have been difficult candidates for psychotherapy. They form a therapeutic relationship easily because they are eager to please and grateful for the therapist's interest. The relationship often tends to remain shallow and rigid, however. Some reports have indicated that psychotherapy (in conjunction with medication maintenance treatment) and counseling may indeed be useful with these individuals. Goldberg and Hoop (2004) state:

> Interpersonal and social rhythm therapy is a form of interpersonal therapy tailored to bipolar patients. In addition to

focusing on grief, role conflicts, role transitions, and interpersonal deficiencies, it includes psychoeducation about bipolar disorder and encourages treatment adherence. Studies have suggested that bipolar patients receiving the treatment were more often euthymic [stable mood] than patients receiving only clinical management.

Group Therapy for Depression and Mania

Group therapy forms an important dimension of multimodal treatment of the manic or depressed client. Once an acute phase of the illness is passed, groups can provide an atmosphere in which individuals may discuss issues in their lives that cause, maintain, or arise out of having a serious affective disorder. The element of peer support provides a feeling of security, as troublesome or embarrassing issues are discussed and resolved. Some groups have other specific purposes, such as helping to monitor medication-related issues or serving as an avenue for promoting education related to the affective disorder and its treatment.

Support groups help members gain a sense of perspective on their condition and tangibly encourage them to link up with others who have common problems. A sense of hope is conveyed when the individual is able to see that he or she is not alone or unique in experiencing affective illness.

Self-help groups offer another avenue of support for the depressed or manic client. These groups are usually peer led and are not meant to substitute for, or compete with, professional therapy. They offer supplementary support that frequently enhances compliance with the medical regimen. Examples of self-help groups are the National Depressive and Manic–Depressive Association (NDMDA), Depressives Anonymous, Families of Depressives, Manic and Depressive Support Group, Recovery Inc., and New Images for Widows. Although self-help groups are not psychotherapy groups, they do provide important adjunctive support experiences, which often have therapeutic benefit for participants.

Family Therapy for Depression and Mania

The ultimate objectives in working with families of clients with mood disorders are to resolve the symptoms and initiate or restore adaptive family functioning. As with group therapy, the most effective approach appears to be with a combination of psychotherapeutic and pharmacotherapeutic treatments. Some studies with bipolar disorder have shown that behavioral family treatment combined with medication substantially reduces relapse rate compared with medication therapy alone.

Sadock and Sadock, (2003) state:

Family therapy is indicated if the disorder jeopardizes the patient's marriage or family functioning or if the mood disorder is promoted or maintained by the family situation. Family therapy examines the role of the mood-disordered member in the overall psychological well-being of the whole family; it also examines the role of the entire family in the maintenance of the patient's symptoms. (p. 565)

Cognitive Therapy for Depression and Mania

In cognitive therapy, the individual is taught to control thought distortions that are considered to be a factor in the development and maintenance of mood disorders. In the cognitive model, depression is characterized by a triad of negative distortions related to expectations of the environment, self, and future. The environment and activities within it are viewed as unsatisfying, the self is unrealistically devalued, and the future is perceived as hopeless. In the same model, mania is characterized by exaggeratedly positive cognitions and perceptions. The individual perceives the self as highly valued and powerful. Life is experienced with overstated self-assurance, and the future is viewed with unrealistic optimism.

The general goals in cognitive therapy are to obtain symptom relief as quickly as possible, to assist the client in identifying dysfunctional patterns of thinking and behaving, and to guide the client to evidence and logic that effectively tests the validity of the dysfunctional thinking. Therapy focuses on changing "automatic thoughts" that occur spontaneously and contribute to the distorted affect. Examples of automatic thoughts in depression include:

1. **Personalizing**: "I'm the only one who failed."
2. **All or nothing**: "I'm a complete failure."
3. **Mind reading**: "He thinks I'm foolish."
4. **Discounting positives**: "The other questions were so easy. Any dummy could have gotten them right."

Examples of automatic thoughts in mania include:

1. **Personalizing**: "She's this happy only when she's with me."
2. **All or nothing**: "Everything I do is great."
3. **Mind reading**: "She thinks I'm wonderful."
4. **Discounting negatives**: "None of those mistakes are really important."

The client is asked to describe evidence that both supports and disputes the automatic thought. The logic underlying the inferences is then reviewed with the client. Another technique involves evaluating what would most likely happen if the client's automatic thoughts were true. Implications of the consequences are then discussed.

Clients should not become discouraged if one technique seems not to be working. No single technique works with all clients. He or she should be reassured that any of a number of techniques may be used, and both therapist and client may explore these possibilities.

Finally, the use of cognitive therapy does not preclude the value of administering medication. Particularly in the treatment of mania, cognitive therapy should be considered a secondary treatment to pharmacological treatment. Cognitive therapy alone has offered encouraging results in the treatment of depression. In fact, the results of several studies with depressed clients show that in some cases cognitive therapy may be equally or even more effective than antidepressant medication (Hollon, DeRubeis, & Evans, 1992; Wright & Thase, 1992). Cognitive therapy is discussed at length in Chapter 20.

Organic Treatments

Psychopharmacology

For Depression

For more than 40 years, the tricyclic antidepressants (TCAs) have been widely used to treat depression. Since the initial discovery of their antidepressant properties, the tricyclic drugs have been subjected to hundreds of controlled trials, and their efficacy in treating depressive illness is now firmly established (see Chapter 21 for a detailed discussion of antidepressant medications).

A subsiding of symptoms may not occur for up to 4 weeks after beginning therapy with antidepressant medications. It is important, therefore, for clients to understand that although it may seem the medication is not producing the desired effects, he or she must continue taking it for at least a month to determine efficacy. The greater effectiveness of one medication over another with any given client is not yet fully understood. Choice of drug may be based on symptoms. For example, anxious clients may be started on TCAs with the most sedative properties and clients with psychomotor retardation may be prescribed those antidepressants with the least sedative properties. When possible, selection of the appropriate drug is based on a history of previous responses to antidepressant therapy.

Common side effects of the TCAs include sedation, tachycardia, dry mouth, constipation, urinary retention, blurred vision, orthostatic hypotension, lowering of the seizure threshold, weight gain, and changes in sexual functioning. Elderly individuals may be particularly sensitive to these medications, and adjustments in dosage must be considered. TCAs are absolutely contraindicated in cases of severe heart disease and untreated narrow-angle glaucoma.

Monoamine oxidase inhibitors (MAOIs) have a unique place in the history of antidepressant medications. They were originally used in the treatment of tuberculosis. Evidence that individuals who were treated with the medication experienced a sense of well-being, without bacteriological improvement, led to the discovery of their enzyme inhibition properties and the subsequent hypothesis that monoamines have a function in regulating mood.

Following the initial enthusiasm about MAOIs, they fell into relative disuse for nearly two decades because of a perceived poor risk-to-benefit ratio. They have now regained widespread acceptance as a viable alternative to TCAs because it has been shown that some individuals respond more beneficially to MAOIs than to any other antidepressant medication.

The greatest concern with using MAOIs is the potential for hypertensive crisis, which is considered a medical emergency. Hypertensive crisis occurs in clients receiving MAOI therapy who consume foods or drugs high in **tyramine** content (see Table 21–5). Typically, symptoms develop within 2 hours after ingestion of a food or drug high in tyramine, and include severe occipital and/or temporal pounding headaches with occasional photophobia. Sensations of choking, palpitations, and a feeling of "dread" are common. Marked systolic and diastolic hypertension occurs, sometimes with neck stiffness. In addition to hypertensive crisis, side effects are similar to those associated with the TCAs.

A second generation of antidepressants has been marketed in the United States during the last two decades. These include maprotiline (Ludiomil), amoxapine (Asendin), trazodone (Desyrel), bupropion (Wellbutrin), and mirtazapine (Remeron). Although most of these newer antidepressants were initially touted as being better than drugs used in the past, accumulated evidence and experience have dampened some of this initial enthusiasm.

The most recent classification of antidepressants on the market includes the selective serotonin reuptake inhibitors (SSRIs) and the nonselective reuptake inhibitors. The SSRIs include fluoxetine (Prozac), paroxetine (Paxil), sertraline (Zoloft), fluvoxamine (Luvox), citalopram (Celexa), and escitalopram (Lexapro). The nonselective reuptake inhibitors include venlafaxine (Effexor), nefazodone (Serzone), and duloxetine (Cymbalta). These drugs have fewer anticholinergic and cardiovascular side effects than the TCAs and often work faster. Although long-term studies are not yet available, these agents appear to be just as effective in alleviating symptoms of depression as the older antidepressants.

A summary of medications used in the treatment of depression is presented in Table 29–12.

TABLE 29–12 Medications Used in the Treatment of Depression

CHEMICAL CLASS	GENERIC (TRADE) NAME	DAILY ADULT DOSAGE RANGE (MG)ᴬ	SIDE EFFECTS
Tricyclics	Amitriptyline (Elavil; Endep)	50–300	With all TCAs: Dry mouth, drowsiness, blurred vision, urinary retention, constipation, arrhythmias, tachycardia, changes in AV conduction, lowered seizure threshold, nausea and vomiting, photosensitivity, blood dyscrasias, exacerbation of mania, orthostatic hypotension.
	Amoxapine (Asendin)	50–600	
	Clomipramine (Anafranil)	25–250	
	Desipramine (Norpramin)	25–300	
	Doxepin (Sinequan)	25–300	
	Imipramine (Tofranil)	30–300	
	Nortriptyline (Aventyl; Pamelor)	30–100	
	Protriptyline (Vivactil)	15–60	
	Trimipramine (Surmontil)	50–300	
Selective serotonin reuptake inhibitors (SSRIs)	Citalopram (Celexa)	20–60	With all SSRIs: Headache, insomnia, nausea, diarrhea, constipation, sexual dysfunction, somnolence, agitation, dry mouth, asthenia, serotonin syndrome (if taken concurrently with other medications that increase levels of serotonin).
	Fluoxetine (Prozac; Serafem)	20–80	
	Fluvoxamine (Luvox)	50–300	
	Escitalopram (Lexapro)	10–20	
	Paroxetine (Paxil)	10–50	
	Sertraline (Zoloft)	50–200	
Monoamine oxidase inhibitors (MAOIs)	Isocarboxazid (Marplan)	20–60	With all MAOIs: Dizziness, headache, orthostatic hypotension, constipation, nausea, dry mouth, tachycardia, palpitations, hypomania
	Phenelzine (Nardil)	45–90	
	Tranylcypromine (Parnate)	30–60	
Heterocyclics	Bupropion (Zyban; Wellbutrin)	200–450	With heterocyclics: Dry mouth, sedation, dizziness, tachycardia, headache, nausea/vomiting, constipation, priapism (trazodone), seizures (maprotiline; bupropion)
	Maprotiline (Ludiomil)	50–225	
	Mirtazapine (Remeron)	15–45	
	Trazodone (Desyrel)	150–600	
Nonselective reuptake inhibitors (NRIs)	Nefazodone (Serzone)	200–600	With NRIs: Nausea, dry mouth, constipation, dizziness, somnolence, insomnia, headache, sexual dysfunction, hepatic failure (warning with nafazodone)
	Venlafaxine (Effexor)	75–375	
	Duloxetine (Cymbalta)	40–60	

*Dosage requires slow titration; onset of therapeutic response may be 1 to 4 weeks.

For Mania

Lithium carbonate was the first drug approved by the U.S. Food and Drug Administration (FDA) for acute manic episodes and for maintenance therapy to prevent or diminish the intensity of subsequent manic episodes. Its mode of action in the control of manic symptoms is unclear. It has also been indicated for treatment of bipolar depression (see Chapter 21 for a detailed discussion of lithium carbonate).

Common side effects of lithium therapy include drowsiness, dizziness, headache, dry mouth, thirst, gastrointestinal upset, fine hand tremors, pulse irregularities, polyuria, and weight gain. In initiating lithium therapy with an acutely manic individual, physicians commonly order an antipsychotic as well. Because normalization of symptoms with lithium may not be achieved for 1 to 3 weeks, the antipsychotic medication is used to calm the excessive hyperactivity of the manic client until the lithium reaches a therapeutic level.

The therapeutic level of lithium carbonate is 1.0 to 1.5 mEq/L for acute mania and 0.6 to 1.2 mEq/L for maintenance therapy. There is a narrow margin between the therapeutic and toxic levels. Lithium levels should be drawn weekly until the therapeutic level is reached, and then monthly during maintenance therapy. Because lithium toxicity is a life-threatening condition, monitoring of lithium levels is critical. The initial signs of lithium toxicity include ataxia, blurred vision, severe diarrhea, persistent nausea and vomiting, and tinnitus. Symptoms intensify as toxicity increases and include excessive output of dilute urine, psychomotor retardation, mental confusion, tremors and muscular irritability, seizures, impaired consciousness, oliguria or anuria, arrhythmias, coma, and eventually death.

Pretreatment assessments should include adequacy of renal functioning because 95 percent of ingested lithium is eliminated via the kidneys. Use of lithium during pregnancy is not recommended. Results of studies have indicated a greater number of cardiac anomalies in babies born to mothers who consumed lithium, particularly in the first trimester.

A number of other medications are used for the treatment of mania, with varying degrees of success. Examples include anticonvulsants (e.g., carbamazepine, clonazepam, valproic acid, lamotrigine, gabapentin, oxcarbazepine, and topiramate) and calcium channel blockers (verapamil). These drugs have been used as alternate or adjunctive approaches to management of clients with bipolar illness refractory to lithium. Several antipsychotic medications have been approved by the FDA for the treatment of bipolar mania. These include chlorpromazine and the newer atypical antipsychotics olanzapine, risperidone, aripiprazole, ziprasidone, and quetiapine. Chlorpromazine is gradually becoming obsolete in the treatment of bipolar mania because of the more favorable side effect profile of the atypical antipsychotics. Depending on the severity of the symptoms, these medications may be used alone or in combination with lithium. Another atypical antipsychotic, clozapine, has also been used in the treatment of acute mania; however, its usefulness is limited by the potential for seizures and agranulocytosis (Goldberg & Hoop, 2004).

A summary of medications used in the treatment of bipolar mania is presented in Table 29–13.

TABLE 29–13	**Medications Used in the Treatment of Bipolar Mania**	
CLASSIFICATION: GENERIC (TRADE) NAME	**DAILY ADULT DOSAGE RANGE (MG)**	**SIDE EFFECTS**
Antimanic		
Lithium carbonate (Eskalith, Lithane; Lithobid)	Acute mania: 1800–2400 Maintenance: 900–1200	Drowsiness, dizziness, headache, dry mouth, thirst, GI upset, nausea and vomiting, fine hand tremors, hypotension, arrhythmias, polyuria, weight gain.
Anticonvulsants		
Clonazepam (Klonopin)	0.75–16	Nausea and vomiting, somnolence, dizziness, blood dyscrasias, diplopia, headache, prolonged bleeding time (with valproic acid), risk of severe rash (with lamotrigine), decreased efficacy with oral contraceptives (with topiramate).
Carbamazepine (Tegretol)	200–1200	
Valproic acid (Depakene; Depakote)	500–1500	
Gabapentin (Neurontin)	900–1800	
Lamotrigine (Lamictal)	100–200	
Topiramate (Topamax)	50–400	
Oxcarbazepine (Trileptal)	600–1200	
Calcium Channel Blocker		
Verapamil (Calan; Isoptin)	80–320	Drowsiness, dizziness, hypotension, bradycardia, nausea, constipation
Antipsychotics		
Chlorpromazine (Thorazine)	75–400	Drowsiness, dizziness, dry mouth, constipation, increased appetite, weight gain, ECG changes, hyperglycemia, headache (aripiprazole, risperidone, quetiapine), extrapyramidal symptoms (chlorpromazine, risperidone)
Olanzapine (Zyprexa)	5–20	
Aripiprazole (Abilify)	10–30	
Quetiapine (Seroquel)	400–800	
Risperidone (Risperdal)	1–6	
Ziprasidone (Geodon)	40–160	

Electroconvulsive Therapy for Depression and Mania

Electroconvulsive therapy (ECT) is the induction of a grand mal (generalized) seizure through the application of electrical current to the brain. ECT is effective with clients who are acutely suicidal and in the treatment of severe depression, particularly in those clients who are also experiencing psychotic symptoms and those with psychomotor retardation and neurovegetative changes, such as disturbances in sleep, appetite, and energy. It is often considered for treatment only after a trial of therapy with antidepressant medication has proved ineffective.

Episodes of acute mania are occasionally treated with ECT, particularly when the client does not tolerate or fails to respond to lithium or other drug treatment, or when life is threatened by dangerous behavior or exhaustion (see Chapter 22 for a detailed discussion of ECT).

SUMMARY

Depression is one of the oldest recognized psychiatric illnesses that is still prevalent today. It is so common, in fact that it has been referred to as the "common cold of psychiatric disorders."

The cause of depressive disorders is not entirely known. A number of factors, including genetics, bio-chemical influences, and psychosocial experiences likely enter into the development of the disorder. Secondary depression occurs in response to other physiological disorders. Symptoms occur along a continuum according to the degree of severity from transient to severe. The disorder occurs in all developmental levels, including childhood, adolescence, senescence, and during the puerperium.

Bipolar disorder, mania, is a maladaptive response to loss and has been referred to as the "mirror image of depression." Genetic influences have been strongly implicated in the development of the disorder. Various other physiological factors, such as biochemical and electrolyte alterations, as well as cerebral structural changes, have been implicated. Side effects of certain medications may also induce symptoms of mania. No single theory can explain the etiology of bipolar disorder, and it is likely that the illness is caused by a combination of factors. Symptoms of mania may be observed on a continuum of three phases, each identified by the degree of severity: phase I, hypomania; phase II, acute mania; and phase III, delirious mania. A review of bipolar disorder in children and adolescents was also presented.

Treatment of mood disorders includes individual, group, family, and cognitive therapies. Somatic therapies include psychopharmacology and ECT. Nursing care is accomplished using the six steps of the nursing process.

REVIEW QUESTIONS

SELF-EXAMINATION/LEARNING EXERCISE

Situation: Margaret, age 68, was brought to the emergency department of a large regional medical center by her sister-in-law who stated, "She does nothing but sit and stare into space. I can't get her to eat or anything!" Upon assessment, it was found that 6 months ago Margaret's husband of 45 years had died of a massive myocardial infarction. They had no children and had been inseparable. Since her husband's death, Margaret has visited the cemetery every day, changing the flowers often on his grave. She has not removed any of his clothes from the closet or chest of drawers. His shaving materials still occupy the same space in the bathroom. Over the months, Margaret has become more and more socially isolated. She refuses invitations from friends, preferring instead to make her daily trips to the cemetery. She has lost 15 pounds and her sister-in-law reports that there is very little food in the house. Today she said to her sister-in-law, "I don't really want to live anymore. My life is nothing without Frank." Her sister-in-law became frightened and, with forceful persuasion, was able to convince Margaret she needed to see a doctor. Margaret is admitted to the psychiatric unit.

Based on the above situation, select the answer that is most appropriate for each of the following questions:

1. The *priority* nursing diagnosis for Margaret would be:
   a. Imbalanced nutrition: less than body requirements
   b. Dysfunctional grieving
   c. Risk for suicide
   d. Social isolation

2. The physician orders sertraline (Zoloft) 50 mg b.i.d. for Margaret. After 3 days of taking the medication, Margaret says to the nurse, "I don't think this medicine is doing any good. I don't feel a bit better." What is the most appropriate response by the nurse?
   a. "Cheer up, Margaret. You have so much to be happy about."
   b. "Sometimes it takes a few weeks for the medicine to bring about an improvement in symptoms."
   c. "I'll report that to the physician, Margaret. Maybe he will order something different."
   d. "Try not to dwell on your symptoms, Margaret. Why don't you join the others down in the dayroom?"

After being stabilized on her medication, Margaret was released from the hospital with directions to continue taking the sertraline as ordered. A week later her sister-in-law found Margaret in bed and was unable to awaken her. An empty prescription bottle was by her side. She was revived in the emergency department and transferred to the psychiatric unit in a state of severe depression. The physician determines that ECT may help Margaret. Consent is obtained.

3. About 30 minutes prior to the first treatment the nurse administers atropine sulfate 0.4 mg IM. The rationale for this order is:
   a. To decrease secretions and increase heart rate
   b. To relax muscles
   c. To produce a calming effect
   d. To induce anesthesia

4. When Margaret is in the treatment room, the anesthesiologist administers thiopental sodium (Pentothal) followed by IV succinylcholine (Anectine). The purposes of these medications are to:
   a. Decrease secretions and increase heart rate
   b. Prevent nausea and induce a calming effect
   c. Minimize memory loss and stabilize mood
   d. Induce anesthesia and relax muscles

5. After three ECTs, Margaret's mood begins to lift and she tells the nurse, "I feel so much better, but I'm having trouble remembering some things that happened this last week." The nurse's best response would be:
   a. "Don't worry about that. Nothing important happened."
   b. "Memory loss is just something you have to put up with in order to feel better."
   c. "Memory loss is a side effect of ECT, but it is only temporary. Your memory should return within a few weeks."
   d. "Forget about last week, Margaret. You need to look forward from here."

A year later, Margaret presents in the emergency department, once again accompanied by her sister-in-law. This time Margaret is agitated, pacing, demanding, and speaking very loudly. "I didn't want to come here! My sister-in-law is just jealous, and she's trying to make it look like I'm insane!" On assessment, the sister-in-law reports that Margaret has become engaged to a 25-year-old construction worker to whom she has willed her sizable inheritance and her home. Margaret loudly praises her fiancé's physique and sexual abilities. She has been spending large sums of money on herself and giving her fiancé $500 a week. The sister-in-law tells the physician, "I know it is Margaret's business what she does with her life, but I'm really worried about her. She is losing weight again. She eats very little and almost never sleeps. I'm afraid she's going to just collapse!" Margaret is once again admitted to the psychiatric unit.

6. The *priority* nursing diagnosis for Margaret is:
   a. Imbalanced nutrition: less than body requirements related to not eating
   b. Risk for injury related to hyperactivity
   c. Disturbed sleep pattern related to agitation
   d. Ineffective coping related to denial of depression

7. One way to promote adequate nutritional intake for Margaret is to:
   a. Sit with her during meals to ensure that she eats everything on her tray.
   b. Have her sister-in-law bring all her food from home because she knows Margaret's likes and dislikes.
   c. Provide high-calorie, nutritious finger foods and snacks that Margaret can eat "on the run."
   d. Tell Margaret that she will be on room restriction until she starts gaining weight.

8. The physician orders lithium carbonate 600 mg t.i.d. for Margaret. There is a narrow margin between the therapeutic and toxic levels of lithium. The therapeutic range for acute mania is:
   a. 1.0 to 1.5 mEq/L
   b. 10 to 15 mEq/L
   c. 0.5 to 1.0 mEq/L
   d. 5 to 10 mEq/L

9. After an appropriate length of time, the physician determines that Margaret does not respond satisfactorily to lithium therapy. He changes her medication to another drug that has been found to be effective in the treatment of bipolar mania. This drug is:
   a. Molindone (Moban)
   b. Paroxetine (Paxil)
   c. Carbamazepine (Tegretol)
   d. Tranylcypromine (Parnate)

10. Margaret's statement, "My sister-in-law is just jealous, and she's trying to make it look like I'm insane!" is an example of:
    a. A delusion of grandeur
    b. A delusion of persecution
    c. A delusion of reference
    d. A delusion of control or influence

TEST YOUR CRITICAL THINKING SKILLS

Alice, age 29, had been working in the typing pool of a large corporation for 6 years. Her immediate supervisor recently retired and Alice was promoted to supervisor, in charge of 20 people in the department. Alice was flattered by the promotion but anxious about the additional responsibility of the position. Shortly after the promotion, she overheard two of her former coworkers saying, "Why in the world did they choose her? She's not the best one for the job. I know *I* certainly won't be able to respect her as a boss!" Hearing these comments added to Alice's anxiety and self-doubt.

Shortly after Alice began her new duties, her friends and coworkers noticed a change. She had a great deal of energy and worked long hours on her job. She began to speak very loudly and rapidly. Her roommate noticed that Alice slept very little, yet seldom appeared tired. Every night she would go out to bars and dances. Sometimes she brought men she had just met home to the apartment, something she had never done before. She bought lots of clothes and make-up and had her hair restyled in a more youthful look. She failed to pay her share of the rent and bills but came home with a brand new convertible. She lost her temper and screamed at her roommate to "Mind your own business!" when asked to pay her share.

She became irritable at work, and several of her subordinates reported her behavior to the corporate manager. When the manager confronted Alice about her behavior, she lost control, shouting, cursing, and striking out at anyone and anything that happened to be within her reach. The security officers restrained her and took her to the emergency department of the hospital, where she was admitted to the psychiatric unit. She had no previous history of psychiatric illness.

The psychiatrist assigned a diagnosis of Bipolar I disorder and wrote orders for olanzapine (Zyprexa) 15 mg PO STAT, olanzapine 15 mg PO qd, and lithium carbonate 600 mg q.i.d.

Answer the following questions related to Alice:

1. What are the most important considerations with which the nurse who is taking care of Alice should be concerned?
2. Why was Alice given the diagnosis of Bipolar I disorder?
3. The doctor should order a lithium level drawn after 4 to 6 days. For what symptoms should the nurse be on the alert?
4. Why did the physician order olanzapine in addition to the lithium carbonate?

REFERENCES

Administration on Aging. (2003). A profile of older Americans: 2003. Washington, DC: U.S. Department of Health and Human Services.

Allen, M.H. (2003). Approaches to the treatment of mania. *Medscape Psychiatry.* Retrieved September 23, 2003 from the World Wide Web at http://www.medscape.com/viewprogram/2639_pnt

American Psychiatric Association. (2000). *Diagnostic and statistical manual of mental disorders* (4th ed.) *Text Revision.* Washington, DC: American Psychiatric Association.

Bohrer, G.J. (2001). *Going to extremes: The difficulties of living with bipolar illness.* Retrieved October 24, 2003 from the World Wide Web at http://www.nurseweek.com/ce/ce1230a.html

Cartwright, L. (2004). Emergencies of survival: Moral spectatorship and the new vision of the child in postwar child psychoanalysis. *Journal of Visual Culture, 3*(1), 35–49.

Davidson, L. (2005). *Suicide and season.* New York: American Foundation for Suicide Prevention.

Dubovsky, S.L., Davies, R., & Dubovsky, A.M. (2003). Mood disorders. In R.E. Hales & S.C. Yudofsky (Eds.). *Textbook of clinical psychiatry* (4th ed.). Washington, DC: American Psychiatric Publishing.

Frackiewicz, E.J., & Shiovitz, T.M. (2001). Evaluation and management of premenstrual syndrome. *Journal of the American Pharmaceutical Association, 41*(3), 437–447.

Geller, B., Zimerman, B., Williams, M., Delbello, M.P., Frazier, J., & Beringer, L. (2002). Phenomenology of prepubertal and early adolescent bipolar disorder: Examples of elated mood, grandiose behaviors, decreased need for sleep, racing thoughts, and hypersexuality. *Journal of Child and Adolescent Psychopharmacology, 12,* 3–9.

Goldberg, J.F., & Hoop, J. (2004). Bipolar depression: Long-term challenges for the clinician. *Medscape Psychiatry.* Retrieved August 25, 2004 from the World Wide Web at http://www.medscape.com/viewprogram/3350

Harvard Medical School. (2001, April). Bipolar disorder—Part I. *The Harvard Mental Health Letter.* Boston, MA: Harvard Medical School Publications Group.

Harvard Medical School. (2002, February). Depression in Children—Part I. *The Harvard Mental Health Letter.* Boston, MA: Harvard Medical School Publications Group.

Hollon, S.D., DeRubeis, R.J., & Evans, M.D. (1992). Cognitive therapy and pharmacotherapy for depression: singly and in combination. *Archives of General Psychiatry, 49,* 774–781.

International Society for Mental Health Online [ISMHO]. (2004). *All about depression.* Retrieved on March 31, 2005 from the WorldWide Web at http://www.allaboutdepression.com/gen_01.html#3

Kafantaris, V., Dicker, R., Coletti, D.J., & Kane, J.M. (2001). Adjunctive antipsychotic treatment is necessary for adolescents with psychotic mania. *Journal of Child and Adolescent Psychopharmacology, 11,* 409–413.

Kaplan, H.I., & Sadock, B.J. (1998). *Synopsis of psychiatry: Behavioral sciences/clinical psychiatry* (8th ed.). Baltimore: Williams & Wilkins.

Kennedy, R., & Suttenfield, K. (2002). *Postpartum depression.* Retrieved on March 1, 2002 from the World Wide Web at http://www.medscape.com/viewarticle/408688

Kowatch, R.A., Fristad, M., Birmaher, B., Wagner, K.D., Findling, R.L., & Hellander, M. (2005). Treatment guidelines for children and adolescents with bipolar disorder. *Journal of the American Academy of Child and Adolescent Psychiatry, 44*(3), 213–235.

Merck Manual of Diagnosis and Therapy. (2005). Mood Disorders. Retrieved March 31, 2005 from the World Wide Web at http://www.merck.com/

Miklowitz, D.J., George, E.L., Richards, J.A., Simoneau, T.L., & Suddath, R.L. (2003). A randomized study of family-focused psychoeducation and pharmacotherapy in the outpatient management of bipolar disorder. *Archives of General Psychiatry, 60*(9), 904–912.

National Center for Health Statistics. (2004). *Health, United States, 2004.* Library of Congress Catalog Number 76–641496. Washington, DC: U.S. Government Printing Office.

National Institute of Mental Health (NIMH). (2000). Bipolar disorder research fact sheet. NIH Publication No. 00–4502. Washington, DC: Department of Health and Human Services.

National Institute of Mental Health (NIMH). (2001). *Mental disorders in America: The numbers count.* Bethesda, MD: National Institutes of Health.

National Institute of Mental Health (NIMH). (2004). *"Care managers" help depressed elderly reduce suicidal thoughts.* Retrieved April 4, 2005 from the World Wide Web at http://www.nimh.nih.gov/

Sadock, B.J., & Sadock, V.A. (2003). *Synopsis of psychiatry: Behavioral sciences/clinical psychiatry* (9th ed.). Philadelphia: Lippincott Williams & Wilkins.

Schimelpfening, N. (2002). *A vitamin a day keeps depression away.* Retrieved on February 28, 2002 from the World Wide Web at http://depression.about.com/library/weekly/aa051799.htm

Slattery, D.A., Hudson, A.L., & Nutt, D.J. (2004). Invited review: The evolution of antidepressant mechanisms. *Fundamental & Clinical Pharmacology, 18*(1), 1–21.

Taber's Cyclopedic Medical Dictionary (20th ed.). (2005). Philadelphia: F.A. Davis.

Wright, J.H., & Thase, M.E. (1992). Cognitive and biological therapies: A synthesis. *Psychiatric Annals, 22,* 451–458.

Zubieta, J.K., Huguelet, P., Koeppe, R.A., Kilbourn, M.R., Carr, J.M., Giordani, B.J., & Frey, K.A. (2000). High vesicular monoamine transporter binding in asymptomatic bipolar I disorder: Sex differences and cognitive correlates. *American Journal of Psychiatry, 157,* 1619–1628.

CLASSICAL REFERENCES

Beck, A.T., Rush, A.J., Shaw, B.F., & Emery, G. (1979). *Cognitive theory of depression.* New York: Guilford Press.

Freud, S. (1957). *Mourning and melancholia,* vol. 14 (standard ed.). London: Hogarth Press. (Original work published 1917.)

Seligman, M.E.P. (1973). Fall into helplessness. *Psychology Today, 7,* 43–48.

 ## INTERNET REFERENCES

Additional information about mood disorders, including psychosocial and pharmacological treatment of these disorders, may be located at the following Web sites:

- http://www.pslgroup.com/depression.htm
- http://depression.miningco.com/
- http://www.ndmda.org
- http://www.fadavis.com/townsend
- http://www.laurus.com
- www.mentalhealth.com/p.html
- www.mhsource.com/bipolar
- www.mhsource.com/depression
- www.mental-health-matters.com/mood.html
- www.mentalhelp.net
- http://www.nlm.nih.gov/medlineplus

IMPLICATIONS OF RESEARCH FOR EVIDENCE-BASED PRACTICE

Dimeo, F., Bauer, M., Varahram, I., Proest, G., & Halter, U. (2001). Benefits from Aerobic Exercise in Patients with Major Depression: A Pilot Study. *British Journal of Sports Medicine, 35*(2), 114–117.

Description of the Study: The literature search for this study revealed that physical activity can reduce the severity of symptoms in depressed patients. Some data suggested that even a single exercise bout could result in substantial mood improvement. This study was conducted to evaluate the short-term effects of a training program on patients with moderate to severe major depression. The study participants included 5 men and 7 women with a mean age of 49 years. They each had been diagnosed with major depressive episode according to the *DSM-IV* criteria. The mean duration of the depressive episode was 35 weeks (range 12–96 weeks). Training consisted of walking on a treadmill following an interval-training pattern and was carried out for 30 minutes a day for 10 days. Objective depression scores were measured using the Hamilton Rating Scale for

Depression. Subjective self-assessment reports were also considered.

Results of the Study: At the end of the training program, there was a clinically relevant and statistically significant reduction in mean depression scores, as follows:

Hamilton Rating Scores:	Before: 19.5	After: 13
Self-assessment Scores:	Before: 23.2	After: 17.7

Subjective and objective changes in depression scores correlated strongly.

Implications for Nursing Practice: This study concludes that aerobic exercise can produce substantial improvement in mood in patients with major depressive disorders in a short time. Psychiatric nurses can be instrumental in educating depressed clients to these benefits and encourage participation in aerobic exercise programs. They can also be influential in supporting strategy to establish aerobic exercise guidelines and equipment into psychiatric treatment programs.

30

ANXIETY DISORDERS

CHAPTER OUTLINE

OBJECTIVES
HISTORICAL ASPECTS
EPIDEMIOLOGICAL STATISTICS
HOW MUCH IS TOO MUCH?

APPLICATION OF THE NURSING PROCESS
POSTTRAUMATIC STRESS DISORDER
TREATMENT MODALITIES
SUMMARY
REVIEW QUESTIONS

KEY TERMS

agoraphobia
flooding
generalized anxiety
   disorder
implosion therapy
obsessive–compulsive
   disorder
panic disorder

posttraumatic stress
   disorder
ritualistic behavior
social phobia
specific phobia
systematic
   desensitization

CORE CONCEPTS

anxiety
compulsions
obsessions
panic
phobia

OBJECTIVES

After reading this chapter, the student will be able to:

1. Differentiate among the terms *stress*, *anxiety*, and *fear*.
2. Discuss historical aspects and epidemiological statistics related to anxiety disorders.
3. Differentiate between normal anxiety and psychoneurotic anxiety.
4. Describe various types of anxiety disorders and identify symptomatology associated with each. Use this information in client assessment.
5. Identify predisposing factors in the development of anxiety disorders.

6. Formulate nursing diagnoses and outcome criteria for clients with anxiety disorders.
7. Describe appropriate nursing interventions for behaviors associated with anxiety disorders.
8. Identify topics for client and family teaching relevant to anxiety disorders.
9. Evaluate nursing care of clients with anxiety disorders.
10. Discuss various modalities relevant to treatment of anxiety disorders.

*T*he following is an account by singer-songwriter Michael Johnson (1994) relating his experience with performance anxiety:

You've got your Jolly Roger clothes on, you've got the microphone, the lights are on you, the owner has just told the crowd to shut up, and you are getting that kind of "show and tell" sickness that you used to get at grade school

pageants or college recitals. Suddenly your mouth is so dry that your lips are sticking to your teeth and you find yourself gesturing oddly with your shoulder and wondering if they think that maybe something unfortunate happened to you. And they're trying to cope with the whole thing. It is now, of course, it hits you that you started with the second verse, you're doing a live rewrite, and you have no idea how this song is going to end. Your vocal range has shrunk and

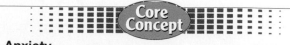

Anxiety

An emotional response (e.g., apprehension, tension, uneasiness) to anticipation of danger, the source of which is largely unknown or unrecognized. Anxiety may be regarded as pathologic when it interferes with effectiveness in living, achievement of desired goals or satisfaction, or reasonable emotional comfort (Shahrokh & Hales, 2003).

your heartbeat is interfering with your vibrato. Your palms are wet and your mouth is dry—a great combination!

Individuals face anxiety on a daily basis. Anxiety, which provides the motivation for achievement, is a necessary force for survival. The term *anxiety* is often used interchangeably with the word *stress*; however, they are not the same. Stress, or more properly, a *stressor*, is an external pressure that is brought to bear on the individual. Anxiety is the subjective emotional response to that stressor. (See Chapter 2 for an overview of anxiety as a psychological response to stress.)

Anxiety may be distinguished from *fear* in that the former is an emotional process, whereas fear is a cognitive one. Fear involves the intellectual appraisal of a threatening stimulus; anxiety involves the emotional response to that appraisal.

This chapter focuses on disorders that are characterized by exaggerated and often disabling anxiety reactions. Historical aspects and epidemiological statistics are presented. Predisposing factors that have been implicated in the etiology of anxiety disorders provide a framework for studying the dynamics of phobias, **obsessive–compulsive disorder (OCD), generalized anxiety disorder, panic disorder, posttraumatic stress disorder (PTSD)**, and other anxiety disorders. Various theories of causation are presented, although it is most likely that a combination of factors contribute to the etiology of anxiety disorders. The neurobiology of anxiety disorders is presented in Figure 30-1.

An explanation of the symptomatology is presented as background knowledge for assessing the client with an anxiety disorder. Nursing care is described in the context of the nursing process, and a critical pathway of care is included as a guideline for use in a case management approach. Various medical treatment modalities are explored.

HISTORICAL ASPECTS

Individuals have experienced anxiety throughout the ages. Yet anxiety, like fear, was not clearly defined or isolated as a separate entity by psychiatrists or psychologists until the 19th and 20th centuries. In fact, what we now

know as anxiety was once solely identified by its physiological symptoms, focusing largely on the cardiovascular system. A myriad of diagnostic terms were used in attempts to identify these symptoms. For example, cardiac neurosis, DaCosta's syndrome, irritable heart, nervous tachycardia, neurocirculatory asthenia, soldier's heart, vasomotor neurosis, and vasoregulatory asthenia are just a few of the names under which anxiety has been concealed over the years (Sadock & Sadock, 2003).

Freud first introduced the term *anxiety neurosis* in 1895. Freud wrote, "I call this syndrome 'anxiety neurosis' because all its components can be grouped round the chief symptom of anxiety" (Freud, 1959). This notion attempted to negate the previous concept of the problem as strictly physical, although it was some time before physicians of internal medicine were ready to accept the psychological implications for the symptoms. In fact, it was not until the years during World War II that the psychological dimensions of these various functional heart conditions were recognized.

For many years, anxiety disorders were viewed as purely psychological or purely biological in nature. Researchers have begun to focus on the interrelatedness of mind and body, and anxiety disorders provide an excellent example of this complex relationship. It is likely that various factors, including genetic, developmental, environmental, and psychological, play a role in the etiology of anxiety disorders.

EPIDEMIOLOGICAL STATISTICS

Anxiety disorders are the most common of all psychiatric illnesses and result in considerable functional impairment and distress (Hollander & Simeon, 2003). Statistics vary widely, but most agree that anxiety disorders are more common in women than in men by at least 2 to 1. Prevalence rates have been given at 1.5 to 5 percent for panic disorder; 2 to 3 percent for OCD; 8 percent for PTSD, and 0.6 to 6 percent for **agoraphobia** (Sadock & Sadock, 2003). A review of the literature revealed a wide range of reports regarding the prevalence of anxiety disorders in children (2 percent to 43 percent). Epidemiological studies suggest that the symptoms are more prevalent among girls than boys (American Psychiatric Association [APA], 2000) and that minority children and children from low socioeconomic environments may be at greater risk for all emotional illness (National Mental Health Association [NMHA], 2005). Studies of familial patterns suggest that a familial predisposition to anxiety disorders probably exists.

HOW MUCH IS TOO MUCH?

Anxiety is usually considered a normal reaction to a realistic danger or threat to biological integrity or self-

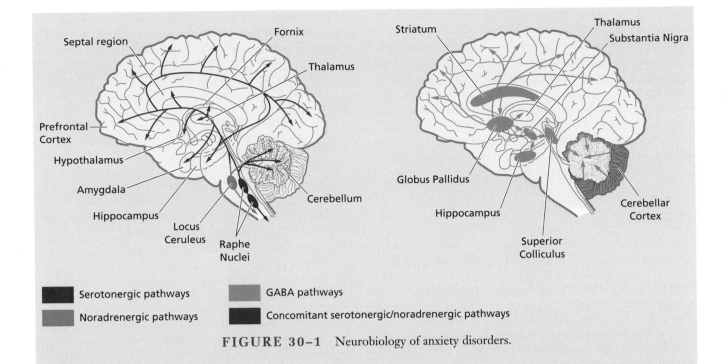

FIGURE 30–1 Neurobiology of anxiety disorders.

Neurotransmitters

Although other neurotransmitters have also been implicated in the pathophysiology of anxiety disorders, disturbances in serotonin, norepinephrine, and gamma-aminobutyric acid (GABA) appear to be most significant.

Cell bodies of origin for the serotonin pathways lie within the raphe nuclei located in the brain stem. Serotonin is thought to be decreased in anxiety disorders. Cell bodies for norepinephrine originate in the locus ceruleus. Norepinephrine is thought to be increased in anxiety disorders. GABA is the major inhibitory neurotransmitter in the brain. It is involved in the reduction and slowing of cellular activity. It is synthesized from glutamic acid, with vitamin B_6 as a cofactor. It is found in almost every region of the brain. GABA is thought to be decreased in anxiety disorders (allowing for increased cellular excitability).

Areas of the Brain Affected

Areas of the brain affected by anxiety disorders and the symptoms that they mediate include the following:
- Amygdala: Fear. Particularly important in panic and phobic disorders.
- Hippocampus: Associated with memory related to fear responses.
- Locus ceruleus: Arousal
- Brain stem: Respiratory activation; heart rate
- Hypothalamus: Activation of stress response
- Frontal cortex: Cognitive interpretations
- Thalamus: Integration of sensory stimuli
- Basal ganglia: Tremor

Anxiolytic Agents	Action	Side Effects
Benzodiazepines	Increases the affinity of the $GABA_A$ receptor for GABA	Sedation, dizziness, weakness, ataxia, decreased motor performance, dependence, withdrawal
SSRIs	Blocks reuptake of serotonin into the presynaptic nerve terminal, increasing synaptic concentration of serotonin	Nausea, diarrhea, headache, insomnia, somnolence, sexual dysfunction
Noradrenergic agents (e.g., propranolol, clonidine)	Propranolol: blocks beta adrenergic receptor activity Clonidine: stimulates alpha-adrenergic receptors	Propranolol: bradycardia, hypotension, weakness, fatigue, impotence, GI upset, bronchospasm Clonidine: dry mouth, sedation, fatigue, hypotension
Barbiturates	CNS depression. Also produces effects in the hepatic and cardiovascular systems	Somnolence, agitation, confusion, ataxia, dizziness, bradycardia, hypotension, constipation
Buspirone	Partial agonist of $5-HT_{1A}$ receptor	Dizziness, drowsiness, dry mouth, headache, nervousness, nausea, insomnia

concept. Normal anxiety dissipates when the danger or threat is no longer present.

It is difficult to draw a precise line between normal and abnormal anxiety. Normality is determined by societal standards; what is considered normal in Chicago, Illinois may not be considered so in Cairo, Egypt. There may even be regional differences within a country or cultural differences within a region. So what criteria can be used to determine if an individual's anxious response is normal? Anxiety can be considered abnormal or pathological if:

1. It is out of proportion to the situation that is creating it.

EXAMPLE:

Mrs. K. witnessed a serious automobile accident 4 weeks ago when she was out driving in her car, and since that time refuses to drive even to the grocery store a few miles from her house. When he is available, her husband must take her wherever she needs to go.

2. The anxiety interferes with social, occupational, or other important areas of functioning.

EXAMPLE:

Because of the anxiety associated with driving her car, Mrs. K. has been forced to quit her job in a downtown bank for lack of transportation.

APPLICATION OF THE NURSING PROCESS

Panic Disorder

Background Assessment Data

This disorder is characterized by recurrent panic attacks, the onsets of which are unpredictable, and manifested by intense apprehension, fear, or terror, often associated with feelings of impending doom and accompanied by intense physical discomfort. The symptoms come on unexpectedly; that is, they do not occur immediately before or on exposure to a situation that usually causes anxiety (as in specific phobia). They are not triggered by situations in which the person is the focus of others' attention (as in social phobia). Organic factors in the role of etiology have been ruled out.

At least four of the following symptoms must be pres-

Core Concept

Panic
A sudden overwhelming feeling of terror or impending doom. This most severe form of emotional anxiety is usually accompanied by behavioral, cognitive, and physiological signs and symptoms considered to be outside the expected range of normalcy.

---

ent to identify the presence of a panic attack. When fewer than four symptoms are present, the individual is diagnosed as having a limited-symptom attack.

1. Palpitations, pounding heart, or accelerated heart rate
2. Sweating
3. Trembling or shaking
4. Sensations of shortness of breath or smothering
5. Feeling of choking
6. Chest pain or discomfort
7. Nausea or abdominal distress
8. Feeling dizzy, unsteady, lightheaded, or faint
9. Derealization (feelings of unreality) or depersonalization (being detached from oneself)
10. Fear of losing control or going crazy
11. Fear of dying
12. Paresthesias (numbness or tingling sensations)
13. Chills or hot flashes

The attacks usually last minutes, or more rarely, hours. The individual often experiences varying degrees of nervousness and apprehension between attacks. Symptoms of depression are common.

The average age of onset of panic disorder is the late 20s. Frequency and severity of the panic attacks vary widely (APA, 2000). Some individuals may have attacks of moderate severity weekly; others may have less severe or limited-symptom attacks several times a week. Still others may experience panic attacks that are separated by weeks or months. The disorder may last for a few weeks or months or for a number of years. Sometimes the individual experiences periods of remission and exacerbation. In times of remission, the person may have recurrent limited-symptom attacks. Panic disorder may or may not be accompanied by agoraphobia.

Panic Disorder with Agoraphobia. Panic disorder with agoraphobia is characterized by the symptoms described for panic disorder. In addition, the individual experiences a fear of being in places or situations from which escape might be difficult (or embarrassing) or in which help might not be available in the event that a panic attack should occur (APA, 2000). This fear severely restricts travel and the individual may become nearly or completely housebound or unable to leave the house unaccompanied. Common agoraphobic situations include being outside the home alone; being in a crowd or standing in a line; being on a bridge; and traveling in a bus, train, or car.

Generalized Anxiety Disorder

Background Assessment Data

Generalized anxiety disorder is characterized by chronic, unrealistic, and excessive anxiety and worry. The symptoms have existed for 6 months or longer and cannot be attributed to specific organic factors, such as caffeine intoxication or hyperthyroidism.

The *DSM-IV-TR* identifies the following symptoms associated with generalized anxiety disorder. The symptoms must have occurred more days than not for at least 6 months and must cause clinically significant distress or impairment in social, occupational, or other important areas of functioning.

1. Excessive anxiety and worry about a number of events that the individual finds difficult to control
2. Restlessness or feeling keyed up or on edge
3. Being easily fatigued
4. Difficulty concentrating or mind "going blank"
5. Irritability
6. Muscle tension
7. Sleep disturbance (difficulty falling or staying asleep, or restless unsatisfying sleep)

The disorder may begin in childhood or adolescence, but onset is not uncommon after age 20. Depressive symptoms are common, and numerous somatic complaints may also be a part of the clinical picture. Generalized anxiety disorder tends to be chronic, with frequent stress-related exacerbations and fluctuations in the course of the illness.

Predisposing Factors for Panic and Generalized Anxiety Disorders

Psychodynamic Theory

The psychodynamic view focuses on the inability of the ego to intervene when conflict occurs between the id and the superego, producing anxiety. For various reasons (unsatisfactory parent–child relationship; conditional love or provisional gratification), ego development is delayed. When developmental defects in ego functions compromise the capacity to modulate anxiety, the individual resorts to unconscious mechanisms to resolve the conflict. Overuse or ineffective use of ego defense mechanisms results in maladaptive responses to anxiety.

Cognitive Theory

The main thesis of the cognitive view is that faulty, distorted, or counterproductive thinking patterns accompany or precede maladaptive behaviors and emotional disorders (Sadock & Sadock, 2003). When there is a disturbance in this central mechanism of cognition, there is a consequent disturbance in feeling and behavior. Because of distorted thinking, anxiety is maintained by erroneous or dysfunctional appraisal of a situation. There is a loss of ability to reason regarding the problem, whether it is physical or interpersonal. The individual feels vulnerable in a given situation, and the distorted thinking results in an irrational appraisal, fostering a negative outcome.

Biological Aspects

Research investigations into the psychobiological correlation of panic and generalized anxiety disorders have implicated a number of possibilities.

Genetics. Panic disorder has a strong genetic element (Harvard Medical School, 2001). The concordance rate for identical twins is 30 percent, and the risk for the disorder in a close relative is 10 to 20 percent. The Harvard Medical School (2001) reports:

> A possible hereditary basis is suggested by some new research on a protein called cholecystokinin, which can induce panic attacks when it is injected. In a recent study, investigators found an association between panic disorder and a variant of the gene that controls the manufacture of this protein. (p. 2)

Neuroanatomical. Modern theory on the physiology of emotional states places the key in the lower brain centers, including the limbic system, the diencephalon (thalamus and hypothalamus), and the reticular formation. Structural brain imaging studies in patients with panic disorder have implicated pathological involvement in the temporal lobes, particularly the hippocampus (Sadock & Sadock, 2003).

Biochemical. Abnormal elevations of blood lactate have been noted in clients with panic disorder. Likewise, infusion of sodium lactate into clients with anxiety neuroses produced symptoms of panic disorder. Although several laboratories have replicated these findings of increased lactate sensitivity in panic-prone individuals, no specific mechanism that triggers the panic symptoms can be explained (Hollander & Simeon, 2003).

Neurochemical. Stronger evidence exists for the involvement of the neurotransmitter norepinephrine in the etiology of panic disorder (Daniels & Yerkes, 2004). Norepinephrine is known to mediate arousal, and it causes hyperarousal and anxiety. This fact has been demonstrated by a notable increase in anxiety following the administration of drugs that increase the synaptic availability of norepinephrine, such as yohimbine.

Medical Conditions. The following medical conditions have been associated to a greater degree with individuals who suffer panic and generalized anxiety disorders than in the general population:

1. Abnormalities in the hypothalamic–pituitary–adrenal and hypothalamic–pituitary–thyroid axes
2. Acute myocardial infarction
3. Pheochromocytomas
4. Substance intoxication and withdrawal (cocaine, alcohol, marijuana, opioids)
5. Hypoglycemia
6. Caffeine intoxication
7. Mitral valve prolapse
8. Complex partial seizures

Transactional Model of Stress/Adaptation. Panic and generalized anxiety disorders are most likely caused by multiple factors. In Figure 30–2, a graphic depiction of this theory of multiple causation is presented in the transactional model of stress/adaptation.

Diagnosis/Outcome Identification

Nursing diagnoses are formulated from the data gathered during the assessment phase and with background knowledge regarding predisposing factors to the disorder. Some common nursing diagnoses for clients with panic disorder and generalized anxiety disorder include:

Panic anxiety related to real or perceived threat to biological integrity or self-concept evidenced by any or all of the physical symptoms identified by the *DSM-IV-TR* as being descriptive of panic or generalized anxiety disorder.

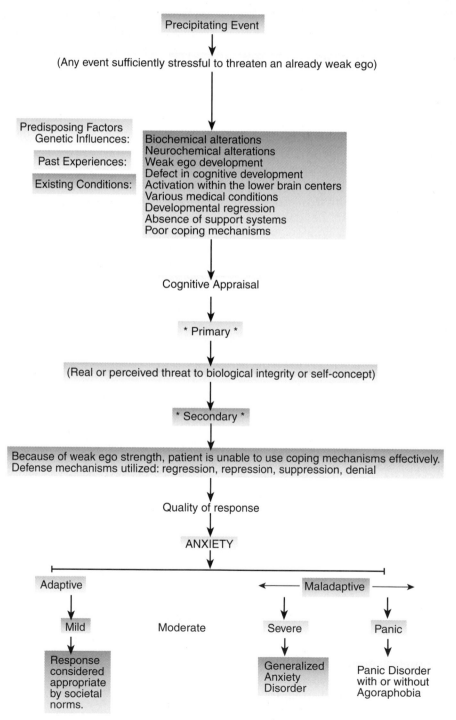

FIGURE 30–2 The dynamics of panic and generalized anxiety disorders using the transactional model of stress/adaptation.

Powerlessness related to impaired cognition evidenced by verbal expressions of no control over life situation and nonparticipation in decision making related to own care or life situation.

The following criteria may be used for measurement of outcomes in the care of the client with panic disorder or generalized anxiety disorder.

The client:

1. Is able to recognize signs of escalating anxiety.
2. Is able to intervene so that anxiety does not reach the panic level.
3. Is able to discuss long-term plan to prevent panic anxiety when stressful situation occurs.
4. Practices techniques of relaxation daily.
5. Engages in physical exercise three times a week.
6. Performs activities of daily living independently.
7. Expresses satisfaction with independent functioning.
8. Is able to maintain anxiety at manageable level without use of medication.
9. Is able to participate in decision making, thereby maintaining control over life situation.
10. Verbalizes acceptance of life situations over which he or she has no control.

Planning/Implementation

Table 30–1 provides a plan of care for the client with panic disorder or generalized anxiety disorder. Nursing diagnoses are presented, along with outcome criteria, appropriate nursing interventions, and rationales for each.

The concept map care plan is an innovative approach to planning and organizing nursing care (see Chapter 9). It is a diagrammatic teaching and learning strategy that allows visualization of interrelationships between medical diagnoses, nursing diagnoses, assessment data, and treatments. An example of a concept map care plan for a client with panic or generalized anxiety disorder is presented in Figure 30–3.

Evaluation

Reassessment determines if the nursing actions have been successful in achieving the objectives of care. Evaluation of the nursing actions for the client with panic disorder or generalized anxiety disorder may be facilitated by gathering information using the following types of questions:

TABLE 30–1	Care Plan for the Client with Panic Disorder or Generalized Anxiety Disorder

NURSING DIAGNOSIS: PANIC ANXIETY
RELATED TO: Real or perceived threat to biological integrity or self-concept
EVIDENCED BY: Any or all of the physical symptoms identified by the *DSM-IV-TR*

OUTCOME CRITERIA	NURSING INTERVENTIONS	RATIONALE
Client will be able to recognize symptoms of onset of anxiety and to intervene before reaching panic level.	1. Stay with the client and offer reassurance of safety and security.	1. The client may fear for his or her life. Presence of a trusted individual provides a feeling of security and assurance of personal safety.
	2. Maintain a calm, nonthreatening, matter-of-fact approach.	2. Anxiety is contagious and may be transferred from staff to client or vice versa. Client develops a feeling of security in the presence of a calm staff person.
	3. Use simple words and brief messages, spoken calmly and clearly, to explain hospital experiences.	3. In an intensely anxious situation, the client is unable to comprehend anything but the most elemental communication.
	4. Keep immediate surroundings low in stimuli (dim lighting, few people, simple decor).	4. A stimulating environment may increase level of anxiety.
	5. Administer tranquilizing medication, as ordered by physician. Assess for effectiveness and for side effects.	5. Antianxiety medication provides relief from the immobilizing effects of anxiety.
	6. When level of anxiety has been reduced, explore possible reasons for occurrence.	6. Recognition of precipitating factor(s) is the first step in teaching client to interrupt escalation of anxiety.
	7. Teach signs and symptoms of escalating anxiety, and ways to interrupt its progression (relaxation techniques, deep-breathing exercises, and meditation, or physical exercise, brisk walks, and jogging).	7. Relaxation techniques result in a physiological response opposite that of the anxiety response. Physical activities discharge excess energy in a healthful manner.

(Continued on following page)

| TABLE 30–1 | Care Plan for the Client with Panic Disorder or Generalized Anxiety Disorder (Continued) | |

NURSING DIAGNOSIS: POWERLESSNESS
RELATED TO: Impaired cognition
EVIDENCED BY: Verbal expressions of no control over life situation and nonparticipation in decision making related to own care or life situation

OUTCOME CRITERIA	NURSING INTERVENTIONS	RATIONALE
Client will be able to effectively problem solve ways to take control of life situation, thereby decreasing feelings of powerlessness and anxiety.	1. Allow client to take as much responsibility as possible for self-care practices. Examples include: a. Allow client to establish own schedule for self-care activities. b. Include client in setting goals of care. c. Provide client with privacy as need is determined. d. Provide positive feedback for decisions made. Respect client's right to make those decisions independently, and refrain from attempting to influence him or her toward those that may seem more logical.	1. Providing choices will increase client's feelings of control.
	2. Assist client to set realistic goals.	2. Unrealistic goals set the client up for failure and reinforce feelings of powerlessness.
	3. Help identify areas of life situation that client can control.	3. Client's emotional condition interferes with the ability to solve problems. Assistance is required to perceive the benefits and consequences of available alternatives accurately.
	4. Help client identify areas of life situation that are not within his or her ability to control. Encourage verbalization of feelings related to this inability.	4. This will assist the client to deal with unresolved issues and learn to accept what cannot be changed.

1. Can the client recognize signs and symptoms of escalating anxiety?
2. Can the client use skills learned to interrupt the escalating anxiety before it reaches the panic level?
3. Can the client demonstrate the activities most appropriate for him or her that can be used to maintain anxiety at a manageable level (e.g., relaxation techniques; physical exercise)?
4. Can the client maintain anxiety at a manageable level without medication?
5. Can the client verbalize a long-term plan for preventing panic anxiety in the face of a stressful situation?
6. Does the client perform activities of daily living independently?
7. Does the client exercise control over life situation by participating in the decision-making process?
8. Can the client verbalize resources outside the hospital from which he or she can seek assistance during times of extreme stress?

Phobias

Background Assessment Data

Agoraphobia Without History of Panic Disorder

Agoraphobia without accompanying panic disorder is less common than the type that precipitates panic attacks. In this disorder, there is a fear of being in places or situa-

---

Core Concept

Phobia

Fear cued by the presence or anticipation of a specific object or situation, exposure to which almost invariably provokes an immediate *anxiety* response or *panic attack* even though the subject recognizes that the fear is excessive or unreasonable. The phobic stimulus is avoided or endured with marked distress (Shahrokh & Hales, 2003).

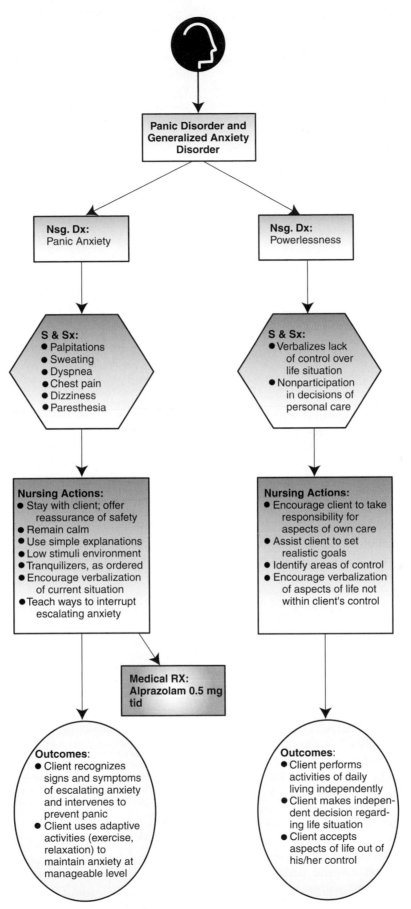

FIGURE 30–3 Concept map care plan for panic disorder and generalized anxiety disorder.

TABLE 30–2 Diagnostic Criteria for Agoraphobia Without History of Panic Disorder

A. The presence of agoraphobia related to fear of developing panic-like symptoms. Agoraphobia is the fear of being in places or situations from which escape might be difficult (or embarrassing) or in which help might not be available in the event of suddenly developing a symptom(s) that could be incapacitating or extremely embarrassing. Examples include: dizziness or falling, depersonalization or derealization, loss of bladder or bowel control, vomiting, or cardiac distress. As a result of this fear, the person either restricts travel or needs a companion when away from home, or else endures agoraphobic situations despite intense anxiety. Common agoraphobic situations include being outside the home alone, being in a crowd or standing in a line, being on a bridge, and traveling in a bus, train, or car.
B. Criteria for panic disorder have never been met.
C. The disturbance is not due to the direct physiological effects of a substance (e.g., a drug of abuse, a medication) or a general medical condition.
D. If an associated general medical condition is present, the fear is clearly in excess of that usually associated with the condition.

SOURCE: From the American Psychiatric Association (2000), with permission.

tions from which escape might be difficult, or in which help might not be available if a limited-symptom attack or panic-like symptoms (rather than full panic attacks) should occur (APA, 2000). It is possible that the individual may have experienced the symptom(s) in the past and is preoccupied with fears of their recurrence. The *DSM-IV-TR* diagnostic criteria for agoraphobia without history of panic disorder is presented in Table 30–2.

Onset of symptoms most commonly occurs in the 20s and 30s and persists for many years. It is diagnosed more commonly in women than in men. Impairment can be very severe. In extreme cases the individual is unable to leave his or her home without being accompanied by a friend or relative. If this is not possible the person may become totally confined to his or her home.

Social Phobia

Social phobia is an excessive fear of situations in which a person might do something embarrassing or be evaluated negatively by others. The individual has extreme concerns about being exposed to possible scrutiny by others and fears social or performance situations in which embarrassment may occur (APA, 2000). In some instances, the fear may be very defined, such as the fear of speaking or eating in a public place, fear of using a public restroom, or fear of writing in the presence of others. In other cases, the social phobia may involve general social situations, such as saying things or answering questions in a manner that would provoke laughter on the part of others. Exposure to the phobic situation usually results in feelings of panic anxiety, with sweating, tachycardia, and dyspnea.

Onset of symptoms of this disorder often begins in late childhood or early adolescence and runs a chronic,

sometimes lifelong, course. It appears to be equally common among men and women (APA, 2000). Impairment interferes with social or occupational functioning, or causes marked distress. The *DSM-IV-TR* diagnostic criteria for social phobia are presented in Table 30–3.

Specific Phobia

Specific phobia was formerly called simple phobia. The essential feature of this disorder is a marked, persistent, and excessive or unreasonable fear when in the presence of, or when anticipating an encounter with, a specific object or situation (APA, 2000).

Specific phobias frequently occur concurrently with other anxiety disorders, but are rarely the focus of clinical attention in these situations (APA, 2000). Treatment is generally aimed at the primary diagnosis because it usually produces the greatest distress and interferes with functioning more so than does a specific phobia.

TABLE 30–3 Diagnostic Criteria for Social Phobia

A. A marked and persistent fear of one or more social or performance situations in which the person is exposed to unfamiliar people or to possible scrutiny by others. The individual fears that he or she will act in a way (or show anxiety symptoms) that will be humiliating or embarrassing.
NOTE: In children, there must be evidence of the capacity for age-appropriate social relationships with familiar people and the anxiety must occur in peer settings, not just in interactions with adults.
B. Exposure to the feared social situation almost invariably provokes anxiety, which may take the form of a situationally bound or situationally predisposed panic attack.
NOTE: In children, the anxiety may be expressed by crying, tantrums, freezing, or shrinking from social situations with unfamiliar people.
C. The person recognizes that the fear is excessive or unreasonable.
NOTE: In children, this feature may be absent.
D. The feared social or performance situations are avoided or else are endured with intense anxiety or distress.
E. The avoidance, anxious anticipation, or distress in the feared social or performance situation(s) interferes significantly with the person's normal routine, occupational (academic) functioning, or social activities or relationships, or there is marked distress about having the phobia.
F. In individuals under age 18 years, the duration is at least 6 months.
G. The fear or avoidance is not due to the direct physiological effects of a substance (e.g., a drug of abuse, a medication) or a general medical condition and is not better accounted for by another mental disorder (e.g., panic disorder with or without agoraphobia, separation anxiety disorder, body dysmorphic disorder, a pervasive developmental disorder, or schizoid personality disorder).
H. If a general medical condition or another mental disorder is present, the fear in criterion A is unrelated to it (e.g., the fear is not of stuttering, trembling in Parkinson's disease, or exhibiting abnormal eating behavior in anorexia nervosa or bulimia nervosa).

The diagnosis is further specified as *generalized* if the fears include most social situations.

SOURCE: From the APA (2000), with permission.

The phobic person may be no more (or less) anxious than anyone else until exposed to the phobic object or situation. Exposure to the phobic stimulus produces overwhelming symptoms of panic, including palpitations, sweating, dizziness, and difficulty breathing. In fact, these symptoms may occur in response to the individual's merely *thinking* about the phobic stimulus. Invariably the person recognizes that his or her fear is excessive or unreasonable, but is powerless to change, even though the individual may occasionally endure the phobic stimulus when experiencing intense anxiety.

Phobias may begin at almost any age. Those that begin in childhood often disappear without treatment, but those that begin or persist into adulthood usually require assistance with therapy. The disorder is diagnosed more often in women than in men.

Even though the disorder is common among the general population, people seldom seek treatment unless the phobia interferes with ability to function. Obviously the individual who has a fear of snakes, but who lives on the 23rd floor of an urban, high-rise apartment building, is not likely to be bothered by the phobia unless he or she decides to move to an area where snakes are prevalent. On the other hand, a fear of elevators may very well interfere with this individual's daily functioning.

Specific phobias have been classified according to the phobic stimulus. A list of some of the more common ones appears in Table 30–4. This list is by no means all-inclusive. People can become phobic about almost any object or situation, and anyone with a little knowledge of Greek or Latin can produce a phobia classification, thereby making possibilities for the list almost infinite.

The *DSM-IV-TR* identifies subtypes of the most common specific phobias. They include the following:

1. **Animal type.** This subtype would be identified as part of the diagnosis if the fear is of animals or insects.
2. **Natural environment type.** Examples of this subtype include objects or situations that occur within the natural environment, such as heights, storms, or water.
3. **Blood-injection-injury type.** This diagnosis should be specified if the individual has a fear of seeing blood or an injury or of receiving an injection or other invasive medical or dental procedure.
4. **Situational type.** This subtype is designated if the fear involves a specific situation, such as public transportation, tunnels, bridges, elevators, flying, driving, or enclosed places.
5. **Other type.** This category covers all other excessive or irrational fears. It may include fear of contracting a serious illness, fear of situations that might lead to vomiting or choking, fear of loud noises, or fear of driving.

The *DSM-IV-TR* diagnostic criteria for specific phobia are presented in Table 30–5.

TABLE 30–4	**Classifications of Specific Phobias**
CLASSIFICATION	**FEAR**
Acrophobia	Height
Ailurophobia	Cats
Algophobia	Pain
Anthophobia	Flowers
Anthropophobia	People
Aquaphobia	Water
Arachnophobia	Spiders
Astraphobia	Lightning
Belonephobia	Needles
Brontophobia	Thunder
Claustrophobia	Closed spaces
Cynophobia	Dogs
Dementophobia	Insanity
Equinophobia	Horses
Gamophobia	Marriage
Herpetophobia	Lizards, reptiles
Homophobia	Homosexuality
Murophobia	Mice
Mysophobia	Dirt, germs, contamination
Numerophobia	Numbers
Nyctophobia	Darkness
Ochophobia	Riding in a car
Ophidiophobia	Snakes
Pyrophobia	Fire
Scoleciphobia	Worms
Siderodromophobia	Railroads or train travel
Taphophobia	Being buried alive
Thanatophobia	Death
Trichophobia	Hair
Triskaidekaphobia	The number 13
Xenophobia	Strangers
Zoophobia	Animals

TABLE 30–5   Diagnostic Criteria for Specific Phobia

A. Marked and persistent fear that is excessive or unreasonable, cued by the presence or anticipation of a specific object or situation (e.g., flying, heights, animals, receiving an injection, seeing blood).
B. Exposure to the phobic stimulus almost invariably provokes an immediate anxiety response, which may take the form of a situationally bound or situationally predisposed panic attack. **NOTE:** In children, the anxiety may be expressed by crying, tantrums, freezing, or clinging.
C. The person recognizes that the fear is excessive or unreasonable. **NOTE:** In children, this feature may be absent.
D. The phobic situation(s) is avoided or else is endured with intense anxiety or distress.
E. The avoidance, anxious anticipation, or distress in the feared situation(s) interferes significantly with the person's normal routine, occupational (academic) functioning, or social activities or relationships, or there is marked distress about having the phobia.
F. In individuals under 18 years, the duration is at least 6 months.
G. The anxiety, panic attacks, or phobic avoidance associated with the specific object or situation are not better accounted for by another mental disorder.

The diagnosis may be further specified as:
Animal type
Natural environment type (e.g., heights, storms, water)
Blood-injection-injury type
Situational type (e.g., airplanes, elevators, enclosed places)
Other type

SOURCE: From the APA (2000), with permission.

Predisposing Factors to Phobias

The cause of phobias is unknown. However, various theories exist that may offer insight into the etiology.

Psychoanalytical Theory

Freud believed that phobias developed when a child experiences normal incestual feelings toward the opposite-sex parent (Oedipal/Electra complex) and fears aggression from the same-sex parent (castration anxiety). To protect themselves, these children *repress* this fear of hostility from the same-sex parent, and *displace* it onto something safer and more neutral, which becomes the phobic stimulus. The phobic stimulus becomes the symbol for the parent, but the child does not realize this.

Modern-day psychoanalysts believe in the same concept of phobic development, but believe that castration anxiety is not the sole source of phobias. They believe that other unconscious fears may also be expressed in a symbolic manner as phobias. For example, a female child who was sexually abused by an adult male family friend when he was taking her for a ride in his boat grew up with an intense, irrational fear of all water vessels. Psychoanalytical theory postulates that fear of the man was repressed and displaced onto boats. Boats became an unconscious symbol for the feared person, but one that the young girl viewed as safer since her fear of boats prevented her from having to confront the real fear.

Learning Theory

Classic conditioning in the case of phobias may be explained as follows: a stressful stimulus produces an "unconditioned" response of fear. When the stressful stimulus is repeatedly paired with a harmless object, eventually the harmless object alone produces a "conditioned" response: fear. This becomes a phobia when the individual consciously avoids the harmless object to escape fear.

Some learning theorists hold that fears are conditioned responses and, thus, they are learned by imposing rewards for appropriate behaviors. In the instance of phobias, when the individual avoids the phobic object, he or she escapes fear, which is indeed a powerful reward.

Phobias also may be acquired by direct learning or imitation (modeling) (e.g., a mother who exhibits fear toward an object will provide a model for the child, who may also develop a phobia toward the same object).

Cognitive Theory

Cognitive theorists espouse that anxiety is the product of faulty cognitions or anxiety-inducing self-instructions. Two types of faulty thinking have been investigated: negative self-statements and irrational beliefs. Cognitive theorists believe that some individuals engage in negative and irrational thinking that produces anxiety reactions.

The individual begins to seek out avoidance behaviors to prevent the anxiety reactions, and phobias result.

Somewhat related to the cognitive theory is the involvement of locus of control. Johnson and Sarason (1978) suggested that individuals with internal locus of control and those with external locus of control might respond differently to life change. These researchers proposed that locus of control orientation may be an important variable in the development of phobias. Individuals with an external control orientation experiencing anxiety attacks in a stressful period are likely to mislabel the anxiety and attribute it to external sources (e.g., crowded areas) or to a disease (e.g., heart attack). They may perceive the experienced anxiety as being outside of their control. Figure 30–4 depicts a graphic model of the relationship between locus of control and the development of phobias.

Biological Aspects

Temperament. Children experience fears as a part of normal development. Most infants are afraid of loud noises. Common fears of toddlers and preschoolers include strangers, animals, darkness, and fears of being separated from parents or attachment figures. During the school-age years, there is fear of death and anxiety about school achievement. Fears of social rejection and sexual anxieties are common among adolescents.

Innate fears represent a part of the overall characteristics or tendencies with which one is born that influence how he or she responds throughout life to specific situations. Innate fears usually do not reach phobic intensity but may have the capacity for such development if reinforced by events in later life. For example, a 4-year-old girl is afraid of dogs. By age 5, however, she has overcome her fear and plays with her own dog and the neighbors' dogs without fear. Then, when she is 19, she is bitten by a stray dog and develops a dog phobia.

Life Experiences

Certain early experiences may set the stage for phobic reactions later in life. Some researchers believe that phobias, particularly specific phobias, are symbolic of original anxiety-producing objects or situations that have been repressed. Examples include:

1. A child who is punished by being locked in a closet develops a phobia for elevators or other closed places.
2. A child who falls down a flight of stairs develops a phobia for high places.
3. A young woman who, as a child, survived a plane crash in which both her parents were killed has a phobia of airplanes.

Transactional Model of Stress/Adaptation. The etiology of phobic disorders is most likely influenced by multiple factors. In Figure 30–5, a graphic depiction of this theory

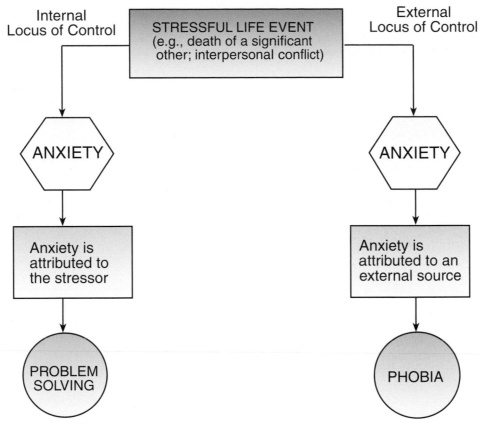

FIGURE 30–4 Locus of control as a variable in the etiology of phobias.

of multiple causation is presented in the transactional model of stress/adaptation.

Diagnosis/Outcome Identification

Nursing diagnoses are formulated from the data gathered during the assessment phase and with background knowledge regarding predisposing factors to the disorder. Some common nursing diagnoses for clients with phobias include:

Fear related to causing embarrassment to self in front of others; to being in a place from which one is unable to escape; or to a specific stimulus, evidenced by behavior directed toward avoidance of the feared object or situation.

Social isolation related to fears of being in a place from which one is unable to escape, evidenced by staying alone, refusing to leave room or home.

The following criteria may be used for measurement of outcomes in the care of the client with phobic disorders.

The client:

1. Functions adaptively in the presence of the phobic object or situation without experiencing panic anxiety.
2. Demonstrates techniques that can be used to maintain anxiety at a manageable level.
3. Voluntarily attends group activities and interacts with peers.
4. Discusses feelings that may have contributed to irrational fears.
5. Verbalizes a future plan of action for responding in the presence of the phobic object or situation without developing panic anxiety.

Planning/Implementation

Table 30–6 provides a plan of care for the client with phobic disorder. Nursing diagnoses are presented, along with outcome criteria, appropriate nursing interventions, and rationales for each.

The concept map care plan is an innovative approach to planning and organizing nursing care (see Chapter 9). It is a diagrammatic teaching and learning strategy that allows visualization of interrelationships between medical diagnoses, nursing diagnoses, assessment data, and treatments. An example of a concept map care plan for a client with phobic disorder is presented in Figure 30–6.

Evaluation

Reassessment is conducted to determine if the nursing actions have been successful in achieving the objectives of

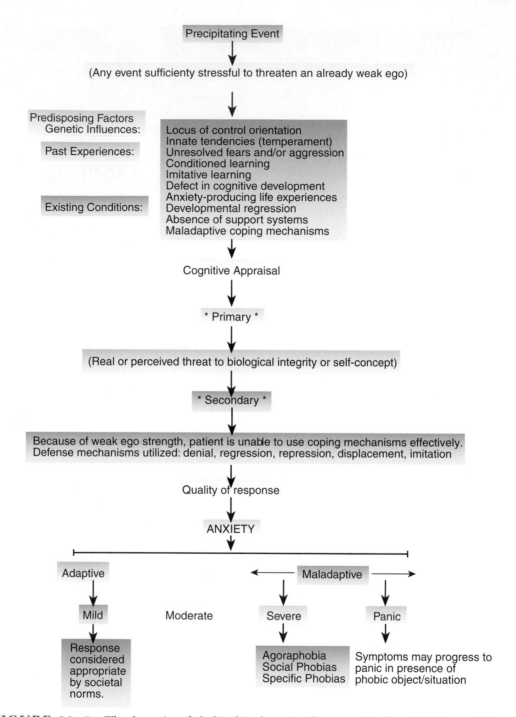

FIGURE 30–5   The dynamics of phobic disorder using the transactional model of stress/adaptation.

care. Evaluation of the nursing actions for the client with a phobic disorder may be facilitated by gathering information using the following types of questions:

1. Can the client discuss the phobic object or situation without becoming anxious?
2. Can the client function in the presence of the phobic object or situation without experiencing panic anxiety?

3. Does the client voluntarily leave the room or home to attend group activities?
4. Is the client able to verbalize the signs and symptoms of escalating anxiety?
5. Is the client able to demonstrate techniques that he or she may use to prevent the anxiety from escalating to the panic level?
6. Can the client verbalize the thinking process that promoted the irrational fears?

TABLE 30–6 Care Plan for Clients with Phobic Disorders

NURSING DIAGNOSIS: FEAR

RELATED TO: Causing embarrassment to self in front of others, being in a place from which one is unable to escape, or a specific stimulus

EVIDENCED BY: Behavior directed toward avoidance of the feared object or situation

OUTCOME CRITERIA	NURSING INTERVENTIONS	RATIONALE
Client will be able to function in presence of phobic object or situation without experiencing panic anxiety.	1. Reassure client that he or she is safe.	1. At the panic level of anxiety, client may fear for his or her own life.
	2. Explore client's perception of the threat to physical integrity or threat to self-concept.	2. It is important to understand client's perception of the phobic object or situation to assist with the desensitization process.
	3. Discuss reality of the situation with client to recognize aspects that can be changed and those that cannot.	3. Client must accept the reality of the situation (aspects that cannot change) before the work of reducing the fear can progress.
	4. Include client in making decisions related to selection of alternative coping strategies (e.g., client may choose either to avoid the phobic stimulus or to attempt to eliminate the fear associated with it).	4. Allowing the client choices provides a measure of control and serves to increase feelings of self-worth.
	5. If client elects to work on elimination of the fear, techniques of desensitization or implosion therapy may be employed. (See explanation of these techniques under "Treatment Modalities" at the end of this chapter.)	5. Fear is decreased as the physical and psychological sensations diminish in response to repeated exposure to the phobic stimulus under nonthreatening conditions.
	6. Encourage client to explore underlying feelings that may be contributing to irrational fears, and to face them rather than suppress them.	6. Exploring underlying feelings may help the client to confront unresolved conflicts and develop more adaptive coping abilities.

NURSING DIAGNOSIS: SOCIAL ISOLATION

RELATED TO: Fears of being in a place from which one is unable to escape

EVIDENCED BY: Staying alone; refusing to leave room or home

OUTCOME CRITERIA	NURSING INTERVENTIONS	RATIONALE
Client will voluntarily participate in group activities with peers.	1. Convey an accepting attitude and unconditional positive regard. Make brief, frequent contacts. Be honest and keep all promises.	1. These interventions increase feelings of self-worth and facilitate a trusting relationship.
	2. Attend group activities with client if it may be frightening for him or her.	2. The presence of a trusted individual provides emotional security.
	3. Be cautious with touch. Allow client extra space and an avenue for exit if anxiety becomes overwhelming.	3. A person in panic anxiety may perceive touch as threatening.
	4. Administer tranquilizing medications as ordered by physician. Monitor for effectiveness and adverse side effects.	4. Antianxiety medications, such as diazepam, chlordiazepoxide, or alprazolam, help to reduce level of anxiety in most individuals, thereby facilitating interactions with others.
	5. Discuss with client signs and symptoms of increasing anxiety and techniques to interrupt the response (e.g., relaxation exercises, "thought stopping").	5. Maladaptive behaviors, such as withdrawal and suspiciousness, are manifested during times of increased anxiety.
	6. Give recognition and positive reinforcement for voluntary interactions with others.	6. This enhances self-esteem and encourages repetition of acceptable behaviors.

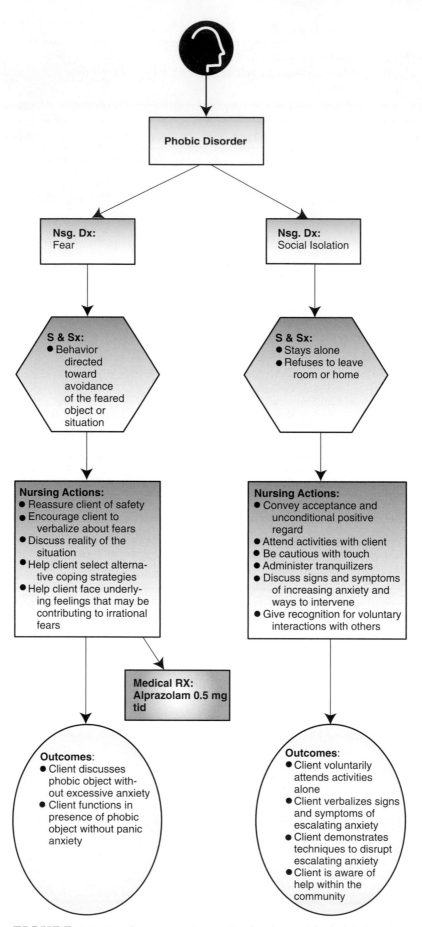

FIGURE 30-6 Concept map care plan for client with phobic disorder.

7. Is the client capable of creating change in his or her life to confront (or eliminate or avoid) the phobic situation?

8. Is the client able to verbalize resources within the community from which he or she can seek assistance during times of extreme stress?

Obsessive–Compulsive Disorder

Background Assessment Data

The *DSM-IV-TR* describes obsessive-compulsive disorder (OCD) as recurrent obsessions or compulsions that are severe enough to be time consuming or to cause marked distress or significant impairment (APA, 2000). The individual recognizes that the behavior is excessive or unreasonable but, because of the feeling of relief from discomfort that it promotes, is compelled to continue the act. The most common compulsions involve washing and cleaning, counting, checking, requesting or demanding assurances, repeating actions, and ordering (APA, 2000). The *DSM-IV-TR* diagnostic criteria for OCD are presented in Table 30–7.

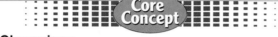

Obsessions
Unwanted, intrusive, persistent ideas, thoughts, impulses, or images that cause marked anxiety or distress. The most common ones include repeated thoughts about contamination, repeated doubts, a need to have things in a particular order, aggressive or horrific impulses, and sexual imagery (APA, 2000).

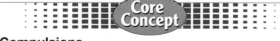

Compulsions
Unwanted repetitive behavior patterns or mental acts (e.g., praying, counting, repeating words silently) that are intended to reduce anxiety, not to provide pleasure or gratification (APA, 2000). They may be performed in response to an obsession or in a stereotyped fashion.

The disorder is equally common among men and women. It may begin in childhood, but more often begins in adolescence or early adulthood. The course is usually chronic, and may be complicated by depression or substance abuse. Single people are affected by OCD more often than are married people (Sadock & Sadock, 2003).

Predisposing Factors to Obsessive–Compulsive Disorder

Psychoanalytical Theory

Psychoanalytical theorists propose that individuals with OCD have weak, underdeveloped egos (for any of a vari-

TABLE 30–7 Diagnostic Criteria for Obsessive–Compulsive Disorder

A. Either obsessions or compulsions:

Obsessions as defined by 1, 2, 3, and 4:
1. Recurrent and persistent thoughts, impulses, or images that are experienced at some time during the disturbance as intrusive and inappropriate and that cause marked anxiety or distress.
2. The thoughts, impulses, or images are not simply excessive worries about real-life problems.
3. The person attempts to ignore or suppress such thoughts, impulses, or images, or to neutralize them with some other thought or action.
4. The person recognizes that the obsessional thoughts, impulses, or images are a product of his or her own mind (not imposed from without as in thought insertion).

Compulsions as defined by 1 and 2:
1. Repetitive behaviors (e.g., hand washing, ordering, checking) or mental acts (e.g., praying, counting, repeating words silently) that the person feels driven to perform in response to an obsession, or according to rules that must be applied rigidly.
2. The behaviors or mental acts are aimed at preventing or reducing distress or preventing some dreaded event or situation; however, these behaviors or mental acts either are not connected in a realistic way with what they are designed to neutralize or prevent or are clearly excessive.

B. At some point during the course of the disorder, the person has recognized that the obsessions or compulsions are excessive or unreasonable. **NOTE:** This does not apply to children.

C. The obsessions or compulsions cause marked distress, are time consuming (take more than 1 hr a day), or significantly interfere with the person's normal routine, occupational (or academic) functioning, or usual social activities or relationships.

D. If another axis I disorder is present, the content of the obsessions or compulsions is not restricted to it (e.g., preoccupation with food in the presence of an eating disorder; hair pulling in the presence of trichotillomania; concern with appearance in the presence of body dysmorphic disorder; preoccupation with having a serious illness in the presence of hypochondriasis; preoccupation with sexual urges or fantasies in the presence of a paraphilia; or guilty ruminations in the presence of major depressive disorder).

E. This disturbance is not due to the direct physiological effects of a substance (e.g., drug of abuse, a medication) or a general medical condition.

SOURCE: From the APA (2000), with permission.

ety of reasons: unsatisfactory parent–child relationship, conditional love, or provisional gratification). The psychoanalytical concept views clients with OCD as having regressed to earlier developmental stages of the infantile superego—the harsh, exacting, punitive characteristics that now reappear as part of the psychopathology. Regression to the pre-oedipal anal–sadistic phase, combined with use of specific ego defense mechanisms (isolation, undoing, displacement, reaction formation), produces the clinical symptoms of obsessions and compulsions (Sadock & Sadock, 2003). Aggressive impulses (common during the anal–sadistic developmental phase) are channeled into thoughts and behaviors that prevent the feelings of aggression from surfacing and producing intense anxiety fraught with guilt (generated by the punitive superego).

Learning Theory

Learning theorists explain obsessive–compulsive behavior as a conditioned response to a traumatic event. The traumatic event produces anxiety and discomfort, and the individual learns to prevent the anxiety and discomfort by avoiding the situation with which they are associated. This type of learning is called *passive avoidance* (staying away from the source). When passive avoidance is not possible, the individual learns to engage in behaviors that provide relief from the anxiety and discomfort associated with the traumatic situation. This type of learning is called *active avoidance* and describes the behavior pattern of the individual with OCD (Sadock & Sadock, 2003).

According to this classic conditioning interpretation, a traumatic event should mark the beginning of the obsessive–compulsive behaviors. In a significant number of cases, however, the onset of the behavior is gradual and the clients relate the onset of their problems to life stress in general rather than to one or more traumatic events.

Biological Aspects

Recent findings suggest that neurobiological disturbances may play a role in the pathogenesis and maintenance of OCD.

Neuroanatomy. Abnormalities in various regions of the brain have been implicated in the neurobiology of OCD. Functional neuroimaging techniques have shown abnormal metabolic rates in the basal ganglia and orbital–frontal cortex of individuals with the disorder (Hollander & Simeon, 2003).

Physiology. Electrophysiological, sleep electroencephalogram, and neuroendocrine studies have suggested that there are commonalities between depressive disorders and OCD (Sadock & Sadock, 2003). Neuroendocrine commonalities were suggested in studies in which about one third of OCD clients show nonsuppression on the dexamethasone suppression test and decreased growth hormone secretion with clonidine infusions.

Biochemical. A number of studies have implicated the neurotransmitter serotonin as influential in the etiology of obsessive–compulsive behaviors. Drugs that have been used successfully in alleviating the symptoms of OCD are clomipramine and the selective serotonin reuptake inhibitors (SSRIs), all of which are believed to block the neuronal reuptake of serotonin, thereby potentiating serotoninergic activity in the central nervous system.

Transactional Model of Stress Adaptation

The etiology of obsessive–compulsive disorder is most likely influenced by multiple factors. In Figure 30–7 a graphic depiction of this theory of multiple causation is presented in the transactional model of stress/adaptation.

Diagnosis/Outcome Identification

Nursing diagnoses are formulated from the data gathered during the assessment phase and with background knowledge regarding predisposing factors to the disorder. Some common nursing diagnoses for clients with OCD include:

Ineffective coping related to underdeveloped ego, punitive superego; avoidance learning; possible biochemical changes evidenced by **ritualistic behavior** and/or obsessive thoughts.

Ineffective role performance related to need to perform rituals evidenced by inability to fulfill usual patterns of responsibility.

The following criteria may be used to measure outcomes in the care of the client with OCD.

The client:

1. Is able to maintain anxiety at a manageable level without resorting to the use of ritualistic behavior.
2. Is able to perform activities of daily living independently.
3. Verbalizes understanding of relationship between anxiety and ritualistic behavior.
4. Verbalizes specific situations that in the past have provoked anxiety and resulted in seeking relief through rituals.
5. Demonstrates more adaptive coping strategies to deal with stress, such as thought stopping, relaxation techniques, and physical exercise.
6. Is able to resume role-related responsibilities because of decreased need for ritualistic behaviors.

Planning/Implementation

Table 30–8 provides a plan of care for the client with OCD. Nursing diagnoses are presented, along with outcome criteria, appropriate nursing interventions, and rationales for each.

The concept map care plan is an innovative approach to planning and organizing nursing care (see Chapter 9). It is a diagrammatic teaching and learning strategy that allows visualization of interrelationships between medical diagnoses, nursing diagnoses, assessment data, and treatments. An example of a concept map care plan for a client with OCD is presented in Figure 30–8.

Evaluation

Reassessment is conducted in order to determine if the nursing actions have been successful in achieving the objectives of care. Evaluation of the nursing actions for the client with OCD may be facilitated by gathering information using the following types of questions:

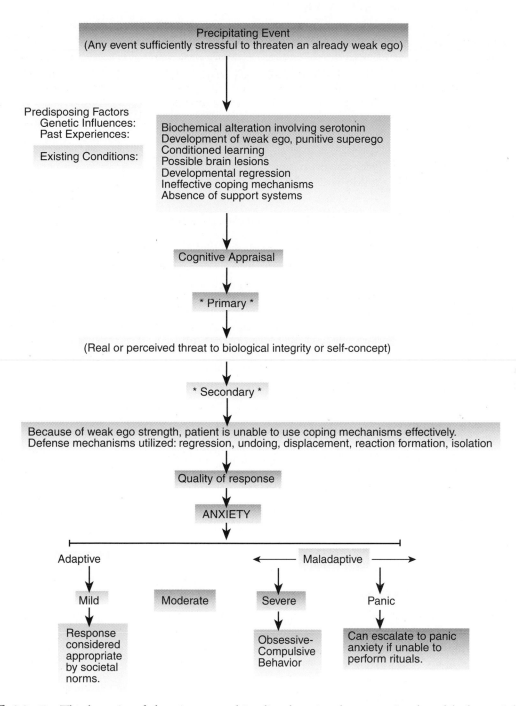

FIGURE 30–7   The dynamics of obsessive–compulsive disorder using the transactional model of stress/adaptation.

1. Can the client refrain from performing rituals when anxiety level rises?
2. Can the client demonstrate substitute behaviors to maintain anxiety at a manageable level?
3. Does the client recognize the relationship between escalating anxiety and the dependence on ritualistic behaviors for relief?
4. Can the client verbalize situations that occurred in the past during which this strategy was used?
5. Can the client verbalize a plan of action for dealing with these stressful situations in the future?
6. Can client perform self-care activities independently?
7. Can the client demonstrate an ability to fulfill role-related responsibilities?

TABLE 30–8 Care Plan for the Client with Obsessive–Compulsive Disorder

NURSING DIAGNOSIS: INEFFECTIVE COPING
RELATED TO: Underdeveloped ego, punitive superego; avoidance learning; possible biochemical changes
EVIDENCED BY: Ritualistic behavior or obsessive thoughts

OUTCOME CRITERIA	NURSING INTERVENTIONS	RATIONALE
Client will demonstrate ability to cope effectively without resorting to obsessive-compulsive behaviors or increased dependency.	1. Work with client to determine types of situations that increase anxiety and result in ritualistic behaviors. 2. Initially meet the client's dependency needs as required. Encourage independence and give positive reinforcement for independent behaviors. 3. In the beginning of treatment, allow plenty of time for rituals. Do not be judgmental or verbalize disapproval of the behavior. 4. Support client's efforts to explore the meaning and purpose of the behavior. 5. Provide structured schedule of activities for client, including adequate time for completion of rituals. 6. Gradually begin to limit amount of time allotted for ritualistic behavior as client becomes more involved in other activities. 7. Give positive reinforcement for nonritualistic behaviors. 8. Help client learn ways of interrupting obsessive thoughts and ritualistic behavior with techniques such as thought stopping, relaxation, and physical exercise.	1. Recognition of precipitating factors is the first step in teaching the client to interrupt the escalating anxiety. 2. Sudden and complete elimination of all avenues for dependency would create intense anxiety on the part of the client. Positive reinforcement enhances self-esteem and encourages repetition of desired behaviors. 3. To deny client this activity may precipitate panic anxiety. 4. Client may be unaware of the relationship between emotional problems and compulsive behaviors. Recognition is important before change can occur. 5. Structure provides a feeling of security for the anxious client. 6. Anxiety is minimized when client is able to replace ritualistic behaviors with more adaptive ones. 7. Positive reinforcement enhances self-esteem and encourages repetition of desired behaviors. 8. Knowledge and practice of coping techniques that are more adaptive will help client change and let go of maladaptive responses to anxiety.

NURSING DIAGNOSIS: INEFFECTIVE ROLE PERFORMANCE
RELATED TO: Need to perform rituals
EVIDENCED BY: Inability to fulfill usual patterns of responsibility

OUTCOME CRITERIA	NURSING INTERVENTIONS	RATIONALE
Client will be able to resume role-related responsibilities.	1. Determine client's previous role within the family and extent to which this role is altered by the illness. Identify roles of other family members. 2. Discuss client's perception of role expectations. 3. Encourage client to discuss conflicts evident within the family system. Identify how client and other family members have responded to this conflict. 4. Explore available options for changes or adjustments in role. Practice through role-play. 5. Encourage family participation in the development of plans to effect positive change, and work to resolve the cause of the anxiety from which the client seeks relief through use of ritualistic behaviors. 6. Give client lots of positive reinforcement for ability to resume role responsibilities by decreasing need for ritualistic behaviors.	1. This is important assessment data for formulating an appropriate plan of care. 2. Determine if client's perception of his or her role expectations are realistic. 3. Identifying specific stressors, as well as adaptive and maladaptive responses within the system, is necessary before assistance can be provided in an effort to create change. 4. Planning and rehearsal of potential role transitions can reduce anxiety. 5. Input from the individuals who will be directly involved in the change will increase the likelihood of a positive outcome. 6. Positive reinforcement enhances self-esteem and promotes repetition of desired behaviors.

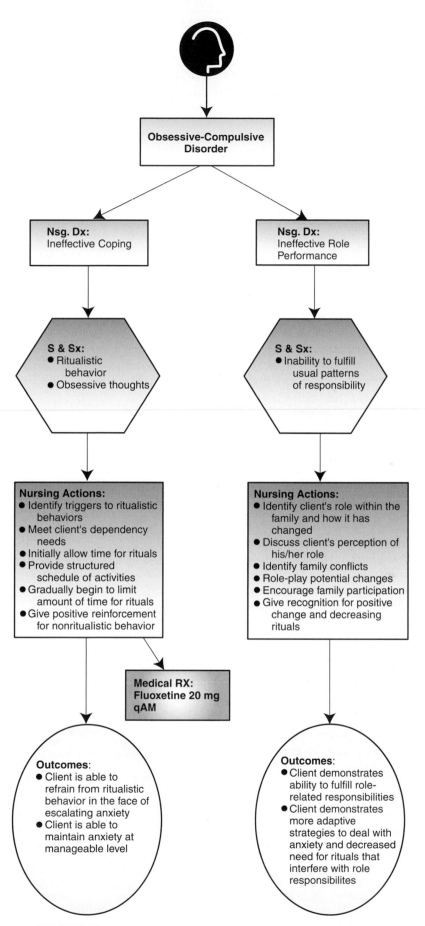

FIGURE 30–8 Concept map care plan for client with OCD.

8. Can the client verbalize resources from which he or she can seek assistance during times of extreme stress?

POSTTRAUMATIC STRESS DISORDER

Background Assessment Data

Posttraumatic stress disorder (PTSD) is described by the *DSM-IV-TR* as the development of characteristic symptoms following exposure to an extreme traumatic stressor involving a personal threat to physical integrity or to the physical integrity of others. The symptoms may occur after learning about unexpected or violent death, serious harm, or threat of death or injury of a family member or other close associate (APA, 2000). These symptoms are not related to common experiences such as uncomplicated bereavement, marital conflict, or chronic illness, but are associated with events that would be markedly distressing to almost anyone. The individual may experience the trauma alone or in the presence of others. Examples of some experiences that may produce this type of response include participation in military combat, experiencing violent personal assault, being kidnapped or taken hostage, being tortured, being incarcerated as a prisoner of war, experiencing natural or manmade disasters, surviving severe automobile accidents, or being diagnosed with a life-threatening illness (APA, 2000).

Characteristic symptoms include re-experiencing the traumatic event, a sustained high level of anxiety or arousal, or a general numbing of responsiveness. Intrusive recollections or nightmares of the event are common. Some individuals may be unable to remember certain aspects of the trauma.

Symptoms of depression are common with this disorder and may be severe enough to warrant a diagnosis of a depressive disorder. In the case of a life-threatening trauma shared with others, survivors often describe painful guilt feelings about surviving when others did not or about the things they had to do to survive (APA, 2000). Substance abuse is common.

The full symptom picture must be present for more than 1 month and cause significant interference with social, occupational, and other areas of functioning. If the symptoms have not been present for more than 1 month, the diagnosis assigned is acute stress disorder (APA, 2000).

The disorder can occur at any age. Symptoms may begin within the first 3 months after the trauma, or there may be a delay of several months or even years. The *DSM-IV-TR* diagnostic criteria for PTSD are presented in Table 30–9.

Studies reveal a lifetime prevalence for PTSD of approximately 8 percent of the adult population in the United States (APA, 2000). About 30 percent of Vietnam veterans have experienced PTSD, and an additional 25 percent encountered subclinical forms of the disorder (Sadock & Sadock, 2003).

TABLE 30–9 Diagnostic Criteria for Posttraumatic Stress Disorder

A. The person has been exposed to a traumatic event in which both of the following were present:
  1. The person experienced, witnessed, or was confronted with an event or events that involved actual or threatened death or serious injury, or a threat to the physical integrity of self or others.
  2. The person's response involved intense fear, helplessness, or horror.
    NOTE: In children, this may be expressed instead by disorganized or agitated behavior.
B. The traumatic event is persistently re-experienced in one (or more) of the following ways:
  1. Recurrent and intrusive distressing recollections of the event, including images, thoughts, or perceptions.
    NOTE: In young children, repetitive play may occur in which themes or aspects of the trauma are expressed.
  2. Recurrent distressing dreams of the event.
    NOTE: In children, there may be frightening dreams without recognizable content.
  3. Acting or feeling as if the traumatic event were recurring (includes a sense of reliving the experience, illusions, hallucinations, and dissociative flashback episodes, including those that occur on awakening or when intoxicated).
    NOTE: In young children, trauma-specific reenactment may occur.
  4. Intense psychological distress at exposure to internal or external cues that symbolize or resemble an aspect of the traumatic event.
  5. Physiological reactivity on exposure to internal or external cues that symbolize or resemble an aspect of the traumatic event.
C. Persistent avoidance of stimuli associated with the trauma and numbing of general responsiveness (not present before the trauma), as indicated by three (or more) of the following:
  1. Efforts to avoid thoughts or feelings associated with the trauma
  2. Efforts to avoid activities, places, or people that arouse recollections of the trauma
  3. Inability to recall an important aspect of the trauma
  4. Markedly diminished interest or participation in significant activities
  5. Feeling of detachment or estrangement from others
  6. Restricted range of affect (e.g., unable to have loving feelings)
  7. Sense of a foreshortened future (e.g., does not expect to have a career, marriage, children, or a normal life span)
D. Persistent symptoms of increased arousal (not present before the trauma), as indicated by two (or more) of the following:
  1. Difficulty falling or staying asleep
  2. Irritability or outbursts of anger
  3. Difficulty concentrating
  4. Hypervigilance
  5. Exaggerated startle response
E. Duration of the disturbance more than 1 month
F. Disturbance that causes clinically significant distress or impairment in social, occupational, or other important areas of functioning
    Specify if acute (symptoms less than 3 months), chronic (symptoms 3 months or more), or delayed onset (onset of symptoms at least 6 months after the stressor).

SOURCE: From APA (2000), with permission.

Predisposing Factors to Posttraumatic Stress Disorder

Reports of symptoms and syndromes with PTSD-like features have existed in writing throughout the centuries. In the early part of the 20th century, traumatic neurosis was viewed as the ego's inability to master the degree of disorganization brought about by a traumatic experience. Very little was written about posttraumatic neurosis during the years between 1950 and 1970. This absence was followed in the 1970s and 1980s with an explosion in the amount of research and writing on the subject. Many of the papers written during this time were about Vietnam veterans. Clearly, the renewed interest in PTSD was linked to the psychological casualties of the Vietnam War.

The diagnostic category of PTSD did not appear until the third edition of the *Diagnostic and Statistical Manual of Mental Disorders* (*DSM-III*) in 1980, after a need was indicated by increasing numbers of problems with Vietnam veterans and victims of multiple disasters.

Psychosocial Theory

One psychosocial model that has become widely accepted seeks to explain why certain persons exposed to massive trauma develop PTSD and others do not. Variables include characteristics that relate to (1) the traumatic experience, (2) the individual, and (3) the recovery environment.

The Traumatic Experience. Specific characteristics relating to the trauma have been identified as crucial elements in the determination of an individual's long-term response to stress. They include:

1. Severity and duration of the stressor
2. Degree of anticipatory preparation for the event
3. Exposure to death
4. Numbers affected by life threat
5. Amount of control over recurrence
6. Location where the trauma was experienced (e.g., familiar surroundings, at home, in a foreign country)

The Individual. Variables that are considered important in determining an individual's response to trauma include:

1. Degree of ego-strength
2. Effectiveness of coping resources
3. Presence of preexisting psychopathology
4. Outcomes of previous experiences with stress/trauma
5. Behavioral tendencies (temperament)
6. Current psychosocial developmental stage
7. Demographic factors (e.g., age, socioeconomic status, education)

The Recovery Environment. It has been suggested that the quality of the environment in which the individual attempts to work through the traumatic experience is correlated with the outcome. Environmental variables include:

1. Availability of social supports
2. The cohesiveness and protectiveness of family and friends
3. The attitudes of society regarding the experience
4. Cultural and subcultural influences

In research with Vietnam veterans, it was shown that the best predictors of PTSD were the severity of the stressor and the degree of psychosocial isolation in the recovery environment.

Learning Theory

Learning theorists view negative reinforcement as behavior that leads to a reduction in an aversive experience, thereby reinforcing and resulting in repetition of the behavior. The avoidance behaviors and psychic numbing in response to a trauma are mediated by negative reinforcement (behaviors that decrease the emotional pain of the trauma). Behavioral disturbances, such as anger and aggression and drug and alcohol abuse, are the behavioral patterns that are reinforced by their capacity to reduce objectionable feelings.

Cognitive Theory

These models take into consideration the cognitive appraisal of an event and focus on assumptions that an individual makes about the world. Epstein (1991) outlines three fundamental beliefs that most people construct within a personal theory of reality. They include:

1. The world is benevolent and a source of joy.
2. The world is meaningful and controllable.
3. The self is worthy (e.g., lovable, good, and competent).

As life situations occur, some disequilibrium is expected to occur until accommodation for the change has been made and it has become assimilated into one's personal theory of reality. An individual is vulnerable to PTSD when the fundamental beliefs are invalidated by a trauma that cannot be comprehended and a sense of helplessness and hopelessness prevail. One's appraisal of the environment can be drastically altered.

Biological Aspects

It has been suggested that an individual who has experienced previous trauma is more likely to develop symptoms after a stressful life event (Hollander & Simeon, 2003). These individuals with previous traumatic experiences may be more likely to become exposed to future traumas, as they can be inclined to reactivate the behaviors associated with the original trauma.

Hollander and Simeon (2003) also report on studies that suggest an endogenous opioid peptide response may assist in the maintenance of chronic PTSD. The hypothesis supports a type of "addiction to the trauma," which is explained in the following manner.

Opioids, including endogenous opioid peptides, have the following psychoactive properties:

1. Tranquilizing action
2. Reduction of rage/aggression
3. Reduction of paranoia

4. Reduction of feelings of inadequacy
5. Antidepressant action

These studies suggest that physiological arousal initiated by reexposure to trauma-like situations enhances production of endogenous opioid peptides and results in increased feelings of comfort and control. When the stressor terminates, the individual may experience opioid withdrawal, the symptoms of which bear strong resemblance to those of PTSD.

Other biological systems have also been implicated in the symptomatology of PTSD. Hageman and associates (2001) state:

It is reasonable to suggest that any disorder such as PTSD that can persist for decades (e.g., Holocaust survivors and Vietnam veterans) is associated with measurable biological features. Evidence suggests that biological dysregulation of the opioid, glutamatergic, noradrenergic, serotonergic, and neuroendocrine pathways are involved in the pathophysiology of PTSD. (p. 412)

Transactional Model of Stress/Adaptation

The etiology of PTSD is most likely influenced by multiple factors. In Figure 30–9, a graphic depiction of this theory of multiple causation is presented in the transactional model of stress/adaptation.

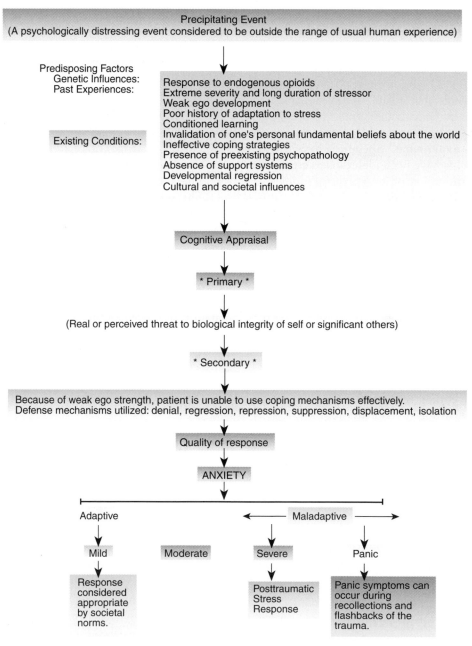

FIGURE 30–9   The dynamics of posttraumatic stress disorder using the transactional model of stress/adaptation.

Diagnosis/Outcome Identification

Nursing diagnoses are formulated from the data gathered during the assessment phase and with background knowledge regarding predisposing factors to the disorder. Some common nursing diagnoses for clients with PTSD include:

Posttrauma syndrome related to distressing event considered to be outside the range of usual human experience evidenced by flashbacks, intrusive recollections, nightmares, psychological numbness related to the event, dissociation, or amnesia.

Dysfunctional grieving related to loss of self as perceived before the trauma or other actual or perceived losses incurred during or after the event evidenced by irritability and explosiveness, self-destructiveness, substance abuse, verbalization of survival guilt, or guilt about behavior required for survival.

The following criteria may be used for measurement of outcomes in the care of the client with PTSD.

The client:

1. Can acknowledge the traumatic event and the impact it has had on his or her life.
2. Is experiencing fewer flashbacks, intrusive recollections, and nightmares than he or she was on admission (or at the beginning of therapy).
3. Can demonstrate adaptive coping strategies (e.g., relaxation techniques, mental imagery, music, art).
4. Can concentrate and has made realistic goals for the future.
5. Includes significant others in the recovery process and willingly accepts their support.
6. Verbalizes no ideas or intent of self-harm.
7. Has worked through feelings of survivor's guilt.
8. Gets enough sleep to avoid risk of injury.
9. Verbalizes community resources from whom he or she may seek assistance in times of stress.
10. Attends support group of individuals who have recovered or are recovering from similar traumatic experiences.
11. Verbalizes desire to put the trauma in the past and progress with his or her life.

Planning/Implementation

Table 30–10 provides a plan of care for the client with PTSD. Nursing diagnoses are presented, along with outcome criteria, appropriate nursing interventions, and rationales for each.

TABLE 30–10   Care Plan for the Client with Posttraumatic Stress Disorder

NURSING DIAGNOSIS: POSTTRAUMA SYNDROME
RELATED TO: Distressing event considered to be outside the range of usual human experience
EVIDENCED BY: Flashbacks, intrusive recollections, nightmares, psychological numbness related to the event, dissociation, or amnesia

OUTCOME CRITERIA	NURSING INTERVENTIONS	RATIONALE
The client will integrate the traumatic experience into his or her persona, renew significant relationships, and establish meaningful goals for the future.	1. a. Assign the same staff as often as possible. b. Use a nonthreatening, matter-of-fact, but friendly approach. c. Respect client's wishes regarding interaction with individuals of opposite sex at this time (especially important if the trauma was rape). d. Be consistent; keep all promises; convey acceptance; spend time with client. 2. Stay with client during periods of flashbacks and nightmares. Offer reassurance of safety and security and that these symptoms are not uncommon following a trauma of the magnitude he or she has experienced. 3. Obtain accurate history from significant others about the trauma and the client's specific response.	1. All of these interventions serve to facilitate a trusting relationship. 2. Presence of a trusted individual may calm fears for personal safety and reassure client that he or she is not "going crazy." 3. Various types of traumas elicit different responses in clients (e.g., human-engendered traumas often generate a greater degree of humiliation and guilt in victims than trauma associated with natural disasters).

(Continued on following page)

OUTCOME CRITERIA	NURSING INTERVENTIONS	RATIONALE
	4. Encourage the client to talk about the trauma at his or her own pace. Provide a nonthreatening, private environment, and include a significant other if the client wishes. Acknowledge and validate client's feelings as they are expressed.	4. This debriefing process is the first step in the progression toward resolution.
	5. Discuss coping strategies used in response to the trauma, as well as those used during stressful situations in the past. Determine those that have been most helpful, and discuss alternative strategies for the future. Include available support systems, including religious and cultural influences. Identify maladaptive coping strategies (e.g., substance use, psychosomatic responses) and practice more adaptive coping strategies for possible future post-trauma responses.	5. Resolution of the post-trauma response is largely dependent on the effectiveness of the coping strategies employed.
	6. Assist the individual to try to comprehend the trauma if possible. Discuss feelings of vulnerability and the individual's "place" in the world following the trauma.	6. Post-trauma response is largely a function of the shattering of basic beliefs the victim holds about self and world. Assimilation of the event into one's persona requires that some degree of meaning associated with the event be incorporated into the basic beliefs, which will affect how the individual eventually comes to reappraise self and world (Epstein, 1991).

NURSING DIAGNOSIS: DYSFUNCTIONAL GRIEVING

RELATED TO: Loss of self as perceived prior to the trauma or other actual/perceived losses incurred during/following the event

EVIDENCED BY: Irritability and explosiveness, self-destructiveness, substance abuse, verbalization of survival guilt or guilt about behavior required for survival

OUTCOME CRITERIA	NURSING INTERVENTIONS	RATIONALE
Client will demonstrate progress in dealing with stages of grief and will verbalize a sense of optimism and hope for the future.	1. Acknowledge feelings of guilt or self-blame that client may express.	1. Guilt at having survived a trauma in which others died is common. The client needs to discuss these feelings and recognize that he or she is not responsible for what happened but must take responsibility for own recovery.
	2. Assess stage of grief in which the client is fixed. Discuss normalcy of feelings and behaviors related to stages of grief.	2. Knowledge of grief stage is necessary for accurate intervention. Guilt may be generated if client believes it is unacceptable to have these feelings. Knowing they are normal can provide a sense of relief.
	3. Assess impact of the trauma on client's ability to resume regular activities of daily living. Consider employment, marital relationship, and sleep patterns.	3. Following a trauma, individuals are at high risk for physical injury because of disruption in ability to concentrate and problem solve and because of lack of sufficient sleep. Isolation and avoidance behaviors may interfere with interpersonal relatedness.
	4. Assess for self-destructive ideas and behavior.	4. The trauma may result in feelings of hopelessness and worthlessness, leading to high risk for suicide.
	5. Assess for maladaptive coping strategies, such as substance abuse.	5. These behaviors interfere with and delay the recovery process.
	6. Identify available community resources from which the individual may seek assistance if problems with dysfunctional grieving persist.	6. Support groups for victims of various types of traumas exist within most communities. The presence of support systems in the recovery environment has been identified as a major predictor in the successful recovery from trauma.

Some institutions are using a case management model to coordinate care (see Chapter 9 for a more detailed explanation). In case management models, the plan of care may take the form of a critical pathway. Table 30–11 depicts an example of a critical pathway of care for a client with PSTD.

The concept map care plan is an innovative approach to planning and organizing nursing care (see Chapter 9). It is a diagrammatic teaching and learning strategy that allows visualization of interrelationships between medical diagnoses, nursing diagnoses, assessment data, and treatments. An example of a concept map care plan for a client with PTSD is presented in Figure 30–10.

Evaluation

Reassessment is conducted to determine if the nursing actions have been successful in achieving the objectives of care. Evaluation of the nursing actions for the client with

---

TABLE 30–11	Critical Pathway of Care for the Posttrauma Client

Estimated Length of Stay: 7 Days—Variations from Designated Pathway Should Be Documented in Progress Notes

Nursing Diagnoses and Categories of Care	Time Dimension	Goals and/or Actions	Time Dimension	Goals and/or Actions	Time Dimension	Discharge Outcome
Posttrauma syndrome	Day 1	Reassurance of client safety.	Ongoing	Environment is made safe for client.	Day 7	Client is able to carry out activities of daily living. Fewer flashbacks, nightmares.
Referrals	Day 1	Psychiatrist Psychologist Social worker Clinical nurse specialist Music therapist Occupational therapist Recreational therapist Chaplain			Day 7	Discharged with follow-up appointments as required.
Diagnostic studies	Day 1 Days 2–5	Drug screen; EKG; EEG; Chemistry profile MMPI Impact of event scale (IES)				
Medications	Day 1	Antidepressant medication, as ordered (SSRIs, tricyclics or MAO inhibitors). Antianxiety medication, as ordered (benzodiazepines); may be given p.r.n. because of addictive quality. Clonidine or propranolol (for intrusive thoughts and hyperarousal). Sedative/hypnotics for sleep disturbances, may be given p.r.n.	Days 1–7	Assess for effectiveness and side effects of medications. Administer addictive medications judiciously and taper dosage.	Day 7	Discharged with scripts as ordered by physician (e.g., antidepressants; clonidine; propranolol).
Additional assessments	Day 1	VS every shift Assess: • Mental status • Mood swings • Anxiety level • Social interaction • Ability to carry out activities of daily living • Suicide ideation • Sleep disturbances • "Flashbacks" • Presence of guilt feelings	Days 2–7	VS daily if stable Ongoing assessments	Day 7	Anxiety is maintained at manageable level. Mood is appropriate. Interacts with others. Carries out activities of daily living independently. Denies suicide ideation. Sleeps without medication. Is able to interrupt flashbacks with adaptive, coping strategies. Has worked through feelings of guilt.

(Continued on following page)

TABLE 30-11   Critical Pathway of Care for the Posttrauma Client *(Continued)*

Estimated Length of Stay: 7 Days—Variations from Designated Pathway Should Be Documented in Progress Notes

Nursing Diagnoses and Categories of Care	Time Dimension	Goals and/or Actions	Time Dimension	Goals and/or Actions	Time Dimension	Discharge Outcome
Diet	Day 1	Client's choice or low-tyramine if taking MAO inhibitor (MAOI)	Days 2–7	Same	Day 7	Client eats well-balanced diet.
Client education	Day 1	Orient to unit	Days 3–4	Stages of grief Side effects of medications Coping strategies Low-tyramine diet Community resources Support group Importance of not mixing drugs and alcohol.	Day 7	Client is discharged. Verbalizes understanding of information presented before discharge.
			Day 6	Reinforce teaching.		

PTSD may be facilitated by gathering information using the following types of questions:

1. Can the client discuss the traumatic event without experiencing panic anxiety?
2. Does the client voluntarily discuss the traumatic event?
3. Can the client discuss changes that have occurred in his or her life because of the traumatic event?
4. Does the client have "flashbacks?"
5. Can the client sleep without medication?
6. Does the client have nightmares?
7. Has the client learned new, adaptive coping strategies for assistance with recovery?
8. Can the client demonstrate successful use of these new coping strategies in times of stress?
9. Can the client verbalize stages of grief and the normal behaviors associated with each?
10. Can the client recognize his or her own position in the grieving process?
11. Is guilt being alleviated?
12. Has the client maintained or regained satisfactory relationships with significant others?
13. Can the client look to the future with optimism?
14. Does the client attend a regular support group for victims of similar traumatic experiences?
15. Does the client have a plan of action for dealing with symptoms, if they return?

Anxiety Disorder Due to a General Medical Condition

Background Assessment Data

The symptoms of this disorder are judged to be the direct physiological consequence of a general medical condition. Symptoms may include prominent generalized anxiety

symptoms, panic attacks, or obsessions or compulsions (APA, 2000). History, physical examination, or laboratory findings must be evident to substantiate the diagnosis.

The *DSM-IV-TR* (APA, 2000) lists the following types and examples of medical conditions that may cause anxiety symptoms:

Endocrine conditions:	Hyperthyroidism and hypothyroidism, pheochromocytoma, hypoglycemia, hyperadrenocorticism
Cardiovascular conditions:	Congestive heart failure, pulmonary embolism, arrhythmia
Respiratory conditions:	Chronic obstructive pulmonary disease, pneumonia, hyperventilation
Metabolic conditions:	Vitamin B_{12} deficiency, porphyria
Neurological conditions:	Neoplasms, vestibular dysfunction, encephalitis

Care of clients with this disorder must take into consideration the underlying cause of the anxiety. Holistic nursing care is essential to ensure that the client's physiological and psychosocial needs are met. Nursing actions appropriate for the specific medical condition must be considered. Actions for dealing with the symptoms of anxiety were discussed previously.

Substance-Induced Anxiety Disorder

Background Assessment Data

The *DSM-IV-TR* (APA, 2000) describes the essential features of this disorder as prominent anxiety symptoms that are judged to be due to the direct physiological effects of

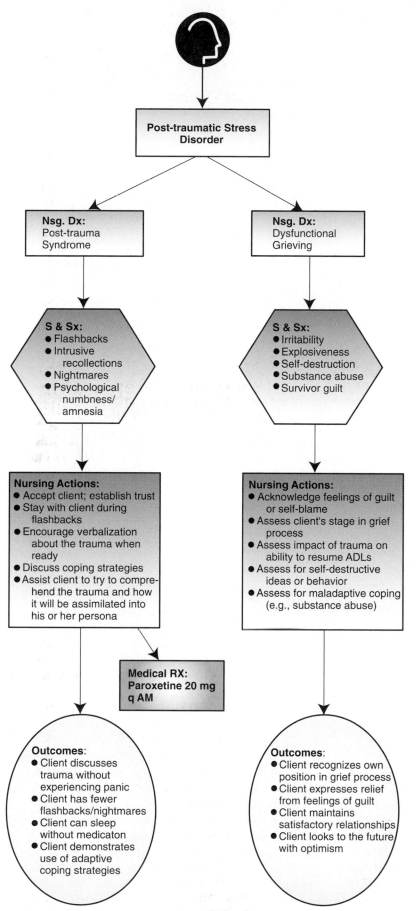

FIGURE 30–10 Concept map care plan for client with PTSD.

a substance (i.e., a drug of abuse, a medication, or toxin exposure). The symptoms may occur during substance intoxication or withdrawal, and may involve prominent anxiety, panic attacks, phobias, or obsessions or compulsions. Diagnosis of this disorder is made only if the anxiety symptoms are in excess of those usually associated with the intoxication or withdrawal syndrome and warrant independent clinical attention. Evidence of intoxication or withdrawal must be available from history, physical examination, or laboratory findings to substantiate the diagnosis. See Chapter 27 for a discussion of the types of substances that may produce these symptoms.

Nursing care of the client with substance-induced anxiety disorder must take into consideration the nature of the substance and the context in which the symptoms occur; that is, intoxication or withdrawal (see Chapter 27). Nursing actions for dealing with anxiety symptoms were discussed previously.

TREATMENT MODALITIES

Individual Psychotherapy

Most clients experience a marked lessening of anxiety when given the opportunity to discuss their difficulties with a concerned and sympathetic therapist. Sadock and Sadock (2003) state:

[Insight-oriented psychotherapy] focuses on helping patients understand the hypothesized unconscious meaning of the anxiety, the symbolism of the avoided situation, the need to repress impulses, and the secondary gains of the symptoms. (p. 608)

With continuous and regular contact with an interested, sympathetic, and encouraging professional person, patients may be able to function by virtue of this help, without which their symptoms would incapacitate them. (p. 623)

The psychotherapist also can use logical and rational explanations to increase the client's understanding about various situations that create anxiety in his or her life. Educational topics for client and family are presented in Table 30–12.

Cognitive Therapy

The cognitive model relates how individuals respond in stressful situations to their subjective cognitive appraisal of the event. Anxiety is experienced when the cognitive appraisal is one of danger with which the individual perceives that he or she is unable to cope. Impaired cognition can contribute to anxiety disorders when the individual's appraisals are chronically negative. Automatic negative appraisals provoke self-doubts, negative evalua-

TABLE 30–12 Topics for Client/Family Education Related to Anxiety Disorders

Nature of the Illness
1. What is anxiety?
2. To what might it be related?
3. What is OCD?
4. What is PTSD?
5. Symptoms of anxiety disorders

Management of the Illness
1. Medication management:
   - Possible adverse effects
   - Length of time to take effect
   - What to expect from the medication
   a. For panic disorder and generalized anxiety disorder
      (1) Benzodiazepines
      (2) Buspirone (Buspar)
      (3) Tricyclics
      (4) SSRIs
      (5) Propranolol
      (6) Clonidine
   b. For phobic disorders
      (1) Benzodiazepines
      (2) Tricyclics
      (3) Propranolol
      (4) SSRIs
   c. For OCD
      (1) SSRIs
      (2) Clomipramine
   d. For PTSD
      (1) Tricyclics
      (2) SSRIs
      (3) MAOIs
      (4) Trazodone
      (5) Propranolol
      (6) Carbamazepine
      (7) Valproic acid
      (8) Lithium carbonate
2. Stress management
   a. Teach ways to interrupt escalating anxiety
      (1) Relaxation techniques (see Chapter 14)
         (a) Progressive muscle relaxation
         (b) Imagery
         (c) Music
         (d) Meditation
         (e) Yoga
         (f) Physical exercise

Support Services
1. Crisis hotline
2. Support groups
3. Individual psychotherapy

tions, and negative predictions. Anxiety is maintained by this dysfunctional appraisal of a situation.

Cognitive therapy strives to assist the individual to reduce anxiety responses by altering cognitive distortions. Anxiety is described as being the result of exaggerated, *automatic* thinking.

Cognitive therapy for anxiety is brief and time limited, usually lasting from 5 to 20 sessions. Brief therapy discourages the client's dependency on the therapist, which is prevalent in anxiety disorders, and encourages the client's self-sufficiency.

A sound therapeutic relationship is a necessary condition for effective cognitive therapy. The client must be able to talk openly about fears and feelings for the therapeutic process to occur. A major part of treatment consists of encouraging the client to face frightening situations to be able to view them realistically, and talking about them is one way of achieving this. Treatment is a collaborative effort between client and therapist.

Rather than offering suggestions and explanations, the therapist uses questions to encourage the client to correct his or her anxiety-producing thoughts. The client is encouraged to become aware of the thoughts, examine them for cognitive distortions, substitute more balanced thoughts, and eventually develop new patterns of thinking.

Cognitive therapy is very structured and orderly, which is important for the anxious client who is often confused and lacks self-assurance. The focus is on solving current problems. Together, the client and therapist work to identify and correct maladaptive thoughts and behaviors that maintain a problem and block its solution.

Cognitive therapy is based on education. The premise is that one develops anxiety because he or she has learned inappropriate ways of handling life experiences. The belief is that with practice individuals can learn more effective ways of responding to these experiences. Homework assignments, a central feature of cognitive therapy, provide an experimental, problem-solving approach to overcoming long-held anxieties. Through fulfillment of these personal "experiments," the effectiveness of specific strategies and techniques is determined.

Behavior Therapy

Two common forms of behavior therapy include **systematic desensitization** and **implosion therapy (flooding)**. They are commonly used to treat clients with phobic disorders and to modify stereotyped behavior of clients with PTSD. They have also been shown to be effective in a variety of other anxiety-producing situations.

Systematic Desensitization

In systematic desensitization, the client is gradually exposed to the phobic stimulus, either in a real or imagined situation. The concept was introduced by Joseph Wolpe in 1958, and is based on behavioral conditioning principles. Emphasis is placed on reciprocal inhibition or counterconditioning.

Reciprocal inhibition is described as the restriction of anxiety prior to the effort of reducing avoidance behavior. The rationale behind this concept is that because relaxation is antagonistic to anxiety, individuals cannot be anxious and relaxed at the same time.

Systematic desensitization with reciprocal inhibition involves two main elements:

1. Training in relaxation techniques
2. Progressive exposure to a hierarchy of fear stimuli while in the relaxed state

The individual is instructed in the art of relaxation using techniques most effective for him or her (e.g., progressive relaxation, mental imagery, tense and relax, meditation). When the individual has mastered the relaxation technique, exposure to the phobic stimulus is initiated. He or she is asked to present a hierarchal arrangement of situations pertaining to the phobic stimulus in order from most disturbing to least disturbing. While in a state of maximum relaxation, the client may be asked to imagine the phobic stimulus. Initial exposure is focused on a concept of the phobic stimulus that produces the least amount of fear or anxiety. In subsequent sessions, the individual is gradually exposed to stimuli that are more fearful. Sessions may be executed in fantasy, in real-life (*in vivo*) situations, or sometimes in a combination of both.

CASE STUDY

John was afraid to ride on elevators. He had been known to climb 24 flights of stairs in an office building to avoid riding the elevator. John's own insurance office had plans for moving the company to a high-rise building soon, with offices on the 32nd floor. John sought assistance from a therapist for help to treat this fear. He was taught to achieve a sense of calmness and well-being by using a combination of mental imagery and progressive relaxation techniques. In the relaxed state, John was initially instructed to imagine the entry level of his office building, with a clear image of the bank of elevators. In subsequent sessions, and always in the relaxed state, John progressed to images of walking onto an elevator, having the elevator door close after he had entered, riding the elevator to the 32nd floor, and emerging from the elevator once the doors were opened. The progression included being accompanied in the activities by the therapist and eventually accomplishing them alone.

Therapy for John also included *in vivo* sessions in which he was exposed to the phobic stimulus in real-life situations (always after achieving a state of relaxation). This technique, combining imagined and *in vivo* procedures, proved successful for John, and his employment in the high-rise complex was no longer in jeopardy because of claustrophobia.

Implosion Therapy (Flooding)

Implosion therapy, or *flooding*, is a therapeutic process in which the client must imagine situations or participate in real-life situations that he or she finds extremely frightening, for a prolonged period of time. Relaxation training is not a part of this technique. Plenty of time must be allowed for these sessions because brief periods may be ineffective or even harmful. A session is terminated when the client responds with considerably less anxiety than at the beginning of the session.

In flooding, the therapist "floods" the client with information concerning situations that trigger anxiety in him or her. The therapist describes anxiety-provoking situations in vivid detail and is guided by the client's response; the more anxiety provoked, the more expedient is the therapeutic endeavor. The same theme is continued as long as it arouses anxiety. The therapy is continued until a topic no longer elicits inappropriate anxiety on the part of the client. Sadock and Sadock (2003) state:

> Many patients refuse flooding because of the psychological discomfort involved. It is also contraindicated in patients for whom intense anxiety would be hazardous (e.g., patients with heart disease or fragile psychological adaptation). The technique works best with specific phobias. (p. 952)

Group/Family Therapy

Group therapy has been strongly advocated for clients with PTSD. It has proved especially effective with Vietnam veterans (Sadock & Sadock, 2003). The importance of being able to share their experiences with empathetic fellow veterans, to talk about problems in social adaptation, and to discuss options for managing their aggression toward others has been emphasized. Some groups are informal and leaderless, such as veterans' "rap" groups, and some are led by experienced group therapists who may have had some first-hand experience with the trauma. Some groups involve family members, thereby recognizing that the symptoms of PTSD may also severely affect them. Hollander and Simeon (2003) state:

> Because of past experiences, [clients with PTSD] are often mistrustful and reluctant to depend on authority figures, whereas the identification, support, and hopefulness of peer settings can facilitate therapeutic change. (p. 606)

Psychopharmacology

For Panic and Generalized Anxiety Disorders

Anxiolytics

The benzodiazepines have been used with success in the treatment of generalized anxiety disorder. They can be prescribed on an as-needed basis when the client is feeling particularly anxious. Alprazolam, lorazepam, and clonazepam have been particularly effective in the treatment of panic disorder. The major risks with benzodiazepine therapy are physical dependence and tolerance, which may encourage abuse. Because withdrawal symptoms can be life threatening, clients must be warned against abrupt discontinuation of the drug and should be tapered off the medication at the end of therapy.

The antianxiety agent buspirone (Buspar) is effective in about 60 to 80 percent of clients with generalized anxiety disorder (Sadock & Sadock, 2003). One disadvantage of buspirone is its 10- to 14-day delay in alleviating symptoms. However, the benefit of lack of physical dependence and tolerance with buspirone may make it the drug of choice in the treatment of generalized anxiety disorder.

Antidepressants

Several antidepressants are effective as major antianxiety agents. The tricyclics clomipramine and imipramine have been used with success in clients experiencing panic disorder. However, since the advent of SSRIs, the tricyclics are less widely used because of their tendency to produce severe side effects at the high doses required to relieve symptoms of panic disorder (Sadock & Sadock, 2003).

The SSRIs have been effective in the treatment of panic disorder. Paroxetine, fluoxetine, and sertraline have been approved by the Food and Drug Administration (FDA) for this purpose. The dosage of these drugs must be titrated slowly because clients with panic disorder appear to be sensitive to the overstimulation caused by SSRIs.

The use of antidepressants in the treatment of generalized anxiety disorder is still being investigated. Some success has been reported with the tricyclic imipramine and with the SSRIs. The FDA has approved paroxetine and venlafaxine extended-release in the treatment of generalized anxiety disorder.

Antihypertensive Agents

Several studies have called attention to the effectiveness of beta blockers (e.g., propranolol) and alpha$_2$-receptor agonists (e.g., clonidine) in the amelioration of anxiety symptoms (Hollander & Simeon, 2003). Propranolol has potent effects on the somatic manifestations of anxiety (e.g., palpitations, tremors), with less dramatic effects on the psychic component of anxiety. It appears to be most effective in the treatment of acute situational anxiety (e.g., performance anxiety; test anxiety), but it is not the first-line drug of choice in the treatment of panic disorder and generalized anxiety disorder.

Clonidine is effective in blocking the acute anxiety effects in conditions such as opioid and nicotine withdrawal. However, it has had limited usefulness in the long-term treatment of panic and generalized anxiety disorders, particularly because of the development of tolerance to its antianxiety effects.

For Phobic Disorders

Anxiolytics

The benzodiazepines have been successful in the treatment of social phobia (Hollander & Simeon, 2003). Controlled studies have shown the efficacy of alprazolam and clonazepam in reducing symptoms of social anxiety. They both are well tolerated and have a rapid onset of action. However, because of their potential for abuse and dependence, they are not considered first-line choice of treatment for social phobia.

Antidepressants

The tricyclic imipramine and the monoamine oxidase (MAO) inhibitor phenelzine have been effective in diminishing symptoms of agoraphobia and social phobia. In recent years, the SSRIs have become the first-line treatment of choice for social phobia. The SSRIs paroxetine and sertraline have been approved by the FDA for the treatment of social anxiety disorder. Additional clinical trials have also indicated efficacy with other antidepressants, including nefazodone, venlafaxine, and bupropion. Specific phobias are generally not treated with medication unless panic attacks accompany the phobia.

Antihypertensive Agents

The beta-blockers propranolol and atenolol have been tried with success in clients experiencing anticipatory performance anxiety or "stage fright" (Hollander & Simeon, 2003). This type of phobic response produces symptoms such as sweaty palms, racing pulse, trembling hands, dry mouth, labored breathing, nausea, and memory loss. The beta-blockers appear to be quite effective in reducing these symptoms in some individuals.

For Obsessive–Compulsive Disorder

Antidepressants

The SSRIs fluoxetine, paroxetine, sertraline, and fluvoxamine have been approved by the FDA for the treatment of OCD. Doses in excess of what is effective for treating depression may be required for OCD. Common side effects include sleep disturbances, headache, and restlessness. These effects are often transient, and are less troublesome than those of the tricyclics.

The tricyclic antidepressant clomipramine was the first drug approved by the FDA in the treatment of OCD. Clomipramine is more selective for serotonin reuptake than any of the other tricyclics. Its efficacy in the treatment of OCD is well established, although the adverse effects, such as those associated with all the tricyclics, may make it less desirable than the SSRIs.

For Posttraumatic Stress Disorder

Antidepressants

The SSRIs are now considered first-line treatment of choice for PTSD because of their efficacy, tolerability, and safety ratings (Sadock & Sadock, 2003). Paroxetine and sertraline have been approved by the FDA for this purpose. The tricyclic antidepressants (e.g., amitriptyline and imipramine), the MAO inhibitors (e.g., phenelzine), and trazodone have also been effective in the treatment of PTSD.

Anxiolytics

Alprazolam has been prescribed for PTSD clients for its antidepressant and antipanic effects. Other benzodiazepines have also been used, despite the absence of controlled studies demonstrating their efficacy in PTSD. Kaplan and Sadock (1998) state:

> Although some anecdotal reports point to the effectiveness of alprazolam in posttraumatic stress disorder, the use of that drug is complicated by the high association of substance-related disorders in patients with the disorder and by the emergence of withdrawal symptoms on discontinuation of the drug. (p. 622)

One study with buspirone showed significant reduction in PTSD symptoms (Sadock & Sadock, 2003). Further controlled trials with this drug are needed to validate its efficacy in treating PTSD.

Antihypertensives

The beta-blocker propranolol and alpha$_2$-receptor agonist clonidine have been successful in alleviating some of the symptoms associated with PTSD. In clinical trials, marked reductions in nightmares, intrusive recollections, hypervigilance, insomnia, startle responses, and angry outbursts were reported with the use of these drugs (Hollander & Simeon, 2003).

Other Drugs

Carbamazepine, valproic acid, and lithium carbonate have been reported to alleviate symptoms of intrusive recollections, flashbacks, nightmares, impulsivity, irritability, and violent behavior in PTSD clients. Sadock and Sadock (2003) report that little positive evidence exists concerning the use of antipsychotics in PTSD. They suggest that these drugs "should be reserved for the short-term control of severe aggression and agitation."

SUMMARY

Anxiety is a necessary force for survival and has been experienced by humanity throughout the ages. It was first described as a physiological disorder and identified by its physical symptoms, particularly the cardiac symptoms. The psychological implications for the symptoms were not recognized until the early 1900s.

Anxiety is considered a normal reaction to a realistic danger or threat to biological integrity or self-concept. Normality of the anxiety experienced in response to a stressor is defined by societal and cultural standards.

Anxiety disorders are more common in women than in men by at least two to one. Studies of familial patterns suggest that a familial predisposition to anxiety disorders probably exists.

The *DSM-IV-TR* identifies several broad categories of anxiety disorders. They include panic and generalized anxiety disorders, phobic disorders, OCD, PTSD, anxiety disorder due to a general medical condition, and substance-induced anxiety disorder. A number of ele-

ments, including psychosocial factors, biological influences, and learning experiences most likely contribute to the development of these disorders.

Treatment of anxiety disorders include individual psychotherapy, cognitive therapy, behavior therapy, group and family therapy, and psychopharmacology. Common behavior therapies include systematic desensitization and implosion therapy (flooding). Nursing care is accomplished using the six steps of the nursing process.

Nurses encounter clients experiencing anxiety in virtually all types of health care settings. Nurses should be able to recognize the symptoms of anxiety and help clients understand that these symptoms are normal and acceptable.

Clients with anxiety disorders are usually seen in emergency departments or psychiatric facilities. There, nurses help clients to gain insight and increase self-awareness in relation to their illness. Intervention focuses on assisting clients to learn techniques with which they may interrupt the escalation of anxiety before it reaches unmanageable proportions. Maladaptive behavior patterns are replaced by new, more adaptive, coping skills.

REVIEW QUESTIONS

SELF-EXAMINATION/LEARNING EXERCISE

Select the answer that is *most* appropriate for each of the following questions.

Situation: Ms. T. has been diagnosed with agoraphobia.

1. Which behavior would be most characteristic of this disorder?
   a. Ms. T. experiences panic anxiety when she encounters snakes.
   b. Ms. T. refuses to fly in an airplane.
   c. Ms. T. will not eat in a public place.
   d. Ms. T. stays in her home for fear of being in a place from which she cannot escape.

2. The therapist who works with Ms. T. would likely choose which of the following therapies for her?
   a. 10 mg Valium q.i.d
   b. Group therapy with other agoraphobic individuals
   c. Facing her fear in gradual step progression
   d. Hypnosis

3. Should the therapist choose to use implosion therapy, Ms. T. would be:
   a. Taught relaxation exercises
   b. Subjected to graded intensities of the fear
   c. Instructed to stop the therapeutic session as soon as anxiety is experienced
   d. Presented with massive exposure to a variety of stimuli associated with the phobic object/situation

Situation: Sandy is a 29-year-old woman who has been admitted to the psychiatric unit with a diagnosis of obsessive–compulsive disorder. She spends many hours during the day and night washing her hands.

4. The most likely reason Sandy washes her hands so much is that it:
   a. Relieves her anxiety.
   b. Reduces the probability of infection.
   c. Gives her a feeling of control over her life.
   d. Increases her self-concept.

5. The *initial* care plan for Sandy would include which of the following nursing interventions?
   a. Keep Sandy's bathroom locked so she cannot wash her hands all the time.
   b. Structure Sandy's schedule so that she has plenty of time for washing her hands.
   c. Put Sandy in isolation until she promises to stop washing her hands so much.
   d. Explain Sandy's behavior to her, since she is probably unaware that it is maladaptive.

6. On Sandy's fourth hospital day, she says to the nurse, "I'm feeling better now. I feel comfortable on this unit, and I'm not ill at ease with the staff or other patients anymore." In light of this change, which nursing intervention is most appropriate?
   a. Give attention to the ritualistic behaviors each time they occur and point out their inappropriateness.
   b. Ignore the ritualistic behaviors, and they will be eliminated for lack of reinforcement.
   c. Set limits on the amount of time Sandy may engage in the ritualistic behavior.
   d. Continue to allow Sandy all the time she wants to carry out the ritualistic behavior.

Situation: John is a 28-year-old high-school science teacher whose Army Reserve unit was called to fight in Operation Desert Storm. John did not want to fight. He admits that he joined the reserves to help pay off his college loans. In Saudi Arabia, he participated in combat and witnessed the wounding of several from his unit, as well as the death of his best friend. He has been experiencing flashbacks, intrusive recollections, and nightmares. His wife reports he is afraid to go to sleep, and his work is suffering. Sometimes he just sits as though he is in a trance. John is diagnosed with PTSD.

7. John says to the nurse, "I can't figure out why God took my buddy instead of me." From this statement, the nurse assesses which of the following in John?
   a. Repressed anger
   b. Survivor's guilt
   c. Intrusive thoughts
   d. Spiritual distress

8. John experiences a nightmare during his first night in the hospital. He explains to the nurse that he was dreaming about gunfire all around and people being killed. The nurse's most appropriate *initial* intervention is:
   a. Administer alprazolam as ordered p.r.n. for anxiety.
   b. Call the physician and report the incident.
   c. Stay with John and reassure him of his safety.
   d. Have John listen to a tape of relaxation exercises.

9. Which of the following therapy regimens would most appropriately be ordered for John?
   a. Paroxetine and group therapy
   b. Diazepam and implosion therapy
   c. Alprazolam and behavior therapy
   d. Carbamazepine and cognitive therapy

10. Which of the following may be influential in the predisposition to PTSD?
   a. Unsatisfactory parent–child relationship
   b. Excess of the neurotransmitter serotonin
   c. Distorted, negative cognitions
   d. Severity of the stressor and availability of support systems

---

TEST *YOUR* CRITICAL THINKING SKILLS

Sarah, age 25, was taken to the emergency room by her friends. They were at a dinner party when Sally suddenly clasped her chest and started having difficulty breathing. She complained of nausea and was perspiring profusely. She had calmed down some by the time they reached the hospital. She denied any pain, and electrocardiogram and laboratory results were unremarkable.

Sarah told the admitting nurse that she had a history of these "attacks." She began having them in her sophomore year of college. She knew her parents had expectations that she should follow in their footsteps and become an attorney. They also expected her to earn grades that would promote acceptance by a top Ivy League university. Sarah experienced her first attack when she made a "B" in English during her third semester of college. Since that time, she has experienced these symptoms sporadically, often in conjunction with her perception of the need to excel. She graduated with top honors from Harvard.

Last week Sarah was promoted within her law firm. She was assigned her first solo case of representing a couple whose baby had died at birth and who were suing the physician for malpractice. She has experienced these panic symptoms daily for the past week, stating, "I feel like I'm going crazy!"

Sarah is transferred to the psychiatric unit. The psychiatrist diagnoses panic disorder without agoraphobia.
Answer the following questions related to Sarah:

1. What would be the priority nursing diagnosis for Sarah?
2. What is the priority nursing intervention with Sarah?
3. What medical treatment might you expect the physician to prescribe?

REFERENCES

American Psychiatric Association. (2000). *Diagnostic and statistical manual of mental disorders* (4th ed.) *Text revision*. Washington, DC: American Psychiatric Association.

Daniels, C.Y., & Yerkes, S. (2004). Panic disorder. Retrieved April 11, 2005 from the World Wide Web at http://www.emedicine.com/med/topic1725.htm

Epstein, S. (1991). Beliefs and symptoms in maladaptive resolutions of the traumatic neurosis. In D. Ozer, J.M. Healy, Jr., & A.J. Stewart (Eds.). *Perspectives on personality* (Vol. 3). London: Jessica Kingsley.

Hageman, I., Anderson, H.S., & Jergensen, M.B. (2001). Post-traumatic stress disorder: A review of psychobiology and pharmacotherapy. *ACTA Psychiatrica Scandinavica, 104*, 411–422.

Harvard Medical School. (2001, March). Panic disorder. *The Harvard Mental Health Letter*. Boston, MA: Harvard Medical School Publications Group.

Hollander, E., & Simeon, D. (2003). Anxiety Disorders. In R.E. Hales & S.C. Yudofsky (Eds.). *Textbook of clinical psychiatry* (4th ed.). Washington, DC: American Psychiatric Publishing.

Johnson, M. (1994, May/June). Stage fright. From *Performing Songwriter 1*(6). Retrieved March 2, 2002 from the World Wide Web at http://www.mjblue.com/pfright.html

Kaplan, H.I., & Sadock (1998). *Synopsis of psychiatry: Behavioral sciences/clinical psychiatry* (8th ed.). Baltimore: Williams & Wilkins.

National Mental Health Association (NMHA). (2005). *Children with emotional disorders in the juvenile justice system*. Alexandria, VA: NMHA.

Sadock, B.J., & Sadock, V.A. (2003). *Synopsis of psychiatry: Behavioral sciences/clinical psychiatry* (9th ed.). Philadelphia: Lippincott Williams & Wilkins.

Shahrokh, N.C., & Hales, R.E. (2003). *American psychiatric glossary*. Washington, DC: American Psychiatric Publishing.

CLASSICAL REFERENCES

Freud, S. (1959). On the grounds for detaching a particular syndrome from neurasthenia under the description 'anxiety neurosis.' In *The standard edition of the complete psychological works of Sigmund Freud* (Vol. 3). London: Hogarth Press.

Johnson, J.H., & Sarason, I.B. (1978). Life stress, depression and anxiety: Internal-external control as moderator variable. *Journal of Psychosomatic Research, 22*, 205–208.

IMPLICATIONS OF RESEARCH FOR EVIDENCE-BASED PRACTICE

Johnson, J.G., Cohen, P., Pine, D.S., Klein, D.F., Kasen, S., & Brook, J.S. (2000). Association between cigarette smoking and anxiety disorders during adolescence and early adulthood. *Journal of the American Medical Association, 284*(18), 2348–2351.

Description of the Study: The main objective of this study was to investigate the longitudinal association between cigarette smoking and anxiety disorders among adolescents and young adults. The study sample included 688 teenagers (51 percent female and 49 percent male) from upstate New York. The youths were interviewed at a mean age of 16 years, during the years 1985 to 1986, and again at a mean age of 22 years, during the years 1991 to 1993. At age 16, 6 percent of the participants smoked 20 or more cigarettes a day. The number increased to 15 percent by age 22.

Results of the Study: Of the participants who smoked 20 cigarettes or more a day during adolescence, a significant number developed an anxiety disorder during young adulthood: 20.5 percent developed generalized anxiety disorder, 10.3 percent developed agoraphobia, and 7.7 percent developed panic disorder. According to the researchers, cigarette smoking does not appear to increase the risk of developing OCD or social anxiety disorder.

Implications for Nursing Practice: The results of this study present just one more reason why adolescents should be encouraged not to smoke or not to begin smoking. The implications for nursing practice are serious. Nurses can initiate and become involved in educational programs to discourage cigarette smoking. Many negative health concerns are related to smoking, and this study provides additional information to include in educational programs designed specifically for adolescents.

 INTERNET REFERENCES

Additional information about anxiety disorders and medications to treat these disorders may be located at the following Web sites:

- http://www.adaa.org
- http://www.mentalhealth.com
- http://www.psychweb.com/disorders/index.htm

- http://www.nimh.nih.gov/
- http://www.anxietynetwork.com/pdhome.html
- http://www.psychiatrymatters.md/index.asp?sec=sres&criteria=anxiolytics
- http://www.fadavis.com/townsend

31
CHAPTER

SOMATOFORM AND SLEEP DISORDERS

CHAPTER OUTLINE

OBJECTIVES

SOMATOFORM DISORDERS

APPLICATION OF THE NURSING PROCESS TO SOMATOFORM DISORDERS

SLEEP DISORDERS

APPLICATION OF THE NURSING PROCESS TO SLEEP DISORDERS

TREATMENT MODALITIES

SUMMARY

REVIEW QUESTIONS

KEY TERMS

anosmia
aphonia
hypersomnia
hypochondriasis
insomnia
la belle indifference

narcolepsy
parasomnias
primary gain
pseudocyesis
secondary gains
tertiary gain

CORE CONCEPTS

hysteria
somatization

OBJECTIVES

After reading this chapter, the student will be able to:

1. Define the term *hysteria*.
2. Discuss historical aspects and epidemiological statistics related to somatoform and sleep disorders.
3. Describe various types of somatoform and sleep disorders and identify symptomatology associated with each; use this information in client assessment.
4. Identify predisposing factors in the development of somatoform and sleep disorders.
5. Formulate nursing diagnoses and goals of care for clients with somatoform and sleep disorders.
6. Describe appropriate nursing interventions for behaviors associated with somatoform and sleep disorders.
7. Identify topics for client and family teaching relevant to somatoform and sleep disorders.
8. Evaluate the nursing care of clients with somatoform and sleep disorders.
9. Discuss various modalities relevant to treatment of somatoform and sleep disorders.

 omatoform disorders are characterized by physical symptoms suggesting medical disease, but without demonstrable organic pathology or known pathophysiological mechanism to account for them. They are classified as mental disorders because pathophysiological processes are not demonstrable or understandable by existing laboratory procedures, and there is either evidence or strong presumption that psychological factors are the major cause of the symptoms. Somatization refers to all those mechanisms by which anxiety is translated into physical illness or bodily complaints.

It is now well documented that a large proportion of clients in general medical outpatient clinics and private medical offices do not have organic disease requiring medical treatment. It is likely that many of these clients have somatoform disorders, but they do not perceive themselves as having a psychiatric problem and thus do not seek treatment from psychiatrists.

Disordered sleep is a problem for a great many individuals. For some, the problem may be a temporary one related to stress or anxiety; for others, the cause could be physiological. The study of sleep physiology in psychiatric disorders remains a powerful tool in the research of brain function (Neylan, Reynolds, & Kupfer, 2003).

This chapter focuses on the process of nursing clients exhibiting symptoms of disordered sleep and those who are characterized by repressed anxiety that is being expressed in the form of physiological symptoms. Historical and epidemiological statistics are presented. Predisposing factors that have been implicated in the etiology of somatoform and sleep disorders provide a framework for studying the dynamics of somatization disorder, pain disorder, hypochondriasis, conversion disorder, body dysmorphic disorder, and sleep disorders.

An explanation of the symptomatology is presented as background knowledge for assessing clients with these disorders. Nursing care is described in the context of the nursing process. Various medical treatment modalities are explored.

SOMATOFORM DISORDERS

Historical Aspects

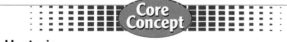

Hysteria

A polysymptomatic disorder that usually begins in adolescence (rarely after the 20s), chiefly affects women, and is characterized by recurrent multiple somatic complaints that are unexplained by organic pathology. It is thought to be associated with repressed anxiety.

The concept of hysteria is at least 4000 years old and probably originated in Egypt. The name has been in use since the time of Hippocrates. In the Middle Ages, hysteria was associated with witchcraft, demonology, and sorcery. Mysterious symptoms and unusual behavior were frequently considered manifestations of supernatural, evil influences, with the client being considered as either the evil spirit itself or the victim of the evil force.

In the 19th century, the French physician Paul Briquet defined a disorder that has come to be known as somatization disorder. He described the disorder as "multiple dramatic and excessive medical complaints in the absence of demonstrable organic pathology" (Yutzy, 2003). Another French physician, Jean Martin Charcot, proposed an essentially physical theory for the disorder,

attributing the symptoms to a hereditary degenerative process of the nervous system. Despite his feelings about a physical basis for hysteria, he became famous for his use of hypnosis in the treatment of the disorder (Goodwin & Guze, 1997).

Freud, whose interest in hysterical disorders had developed while he was working in Paris with Charcot, observed that under hypnosis, clients could recall past memories and emotional experiences that would relieve their symptoms. This led to his proposal that unexpressed emotion can be "converted" into physical symptoms.

In the 1960s a series of studies originated with a subgroup of hysteria clients who presented with multiple somatic symptoms, a chronic course, and excessive amounts of medical and surgical care. The disorder that delineated this homogeneous group came to be known as Briquet's syndrome, and was referred to by this name until the *DSM-III* was introduced in 1980. Somatization disorder, as it is described in the *DSM-IV-TR*, is a simplified version of Briquet's syndrome.

Epidemiological Statistics

The lifetime prevalence rate for somatization disorder in the general population is estimated at 0.2 to 2 percent in women and 0.2 percent in men (Sadock & Sadock, 2003). Tendencies toward somatization are apparently more common in those who are poorly educated and from the lower socioeconomic classes.

Lifetime prevalence rates of conversion disorder vary widely. Statistics within the general population have ranged from 5 to 30 percent. The disorder occurs more frequently in women than in men and more frequently in adolescents and young adults than in other age groups. A higher prevalence exists in lower socioeconomic groups, rural populations, and among those with less education (Sadock & Sadock, 2003).

Hypochondriasis affects 1 to 5 percent of the general population (APA, 2000). The disorder is equally common among men and women, and the most common age at onset is in early adulthood (Sadock & Sadock, 2003).

Pain is likely the most frequent presenting complaint in medical practice today. Pain disorder (previously called *somatoform pain disorder*) is diagnosed more frequently in women than in men by about 2 to 1. Its onset can occur at any age, with the peak ages of onset in the 40s and 50s. It is more common among people in so-called blue-collar occupations, perhaps because of increased likelihood of job-related injuries (Sadock & Sadock, 2003).

Body dysmorphic disorder is rare, although it may be more common than once believed. In the practices of plastic surgery and dermatology, reported rates of body dysmorphic disorder range from 6 to 15 percent (APA, 2000). Psychiatrists see only a small fraction of the cases. A profile of these clients reveals that they are usually in the late teens or 20s and unmarried. Co-morbidity with another psychiatric disorder, such as major depression, anxiety disorder, or even a psychotic disorder, is not uncommon with body dysmorphic disorder (Sadock & Sadock, 2003).

APPLICATION OF THE NURSING PROCESS TO SOMATOFORM DISORDERS

Core Concept

Somatization
The process by which psychological needs are expressed in the form of physical symptoms. Somatization is thought to be associated with repressed anxiety.

Somatization Disorder

Background Assessment Data

Somatization disorder is a syndrome of multiple somatic symptoms that cannot be explained medically and are associated with psychosocial distress and long-term seeking of assistance from health care professionals. Symptoms may be vague, dramatized, or exaggerated in their presentation. The disorder is chronic, with symptoms beginning before age 30. The symptoms are identified as pain (in at least four different sites), gastrointestinal symptoms (e.g., nausea, vomiting, diarrhea), sexual symptoms (e.g., irregular menses, erectile or ejaculatory dysfunction), and symptoms suggestive of a neurological condition (e.g., paralysis, blindness, deafness) (APA, 2000). Anxiety and depression are frequently manifested, and suicidal threats and attempts are not uncommon.

The disorder usually runs a fluctuating course, with periods of remission and exacerbation. Clients often receive medical care from several physicians, sometimes concurrently, leading to the possibility of dangerous combinations of treatments (APA, 2000). They have a tendency to seek relief through overmedicating with prescribed analgesics or antianxiety agents. Drug abuse and dependence are common complications of somatization disorder. When suicide results, it is usually in association with substance abuse (Sadock & Sadock, 2003).

It has been suggested that in somatization disorder there may be some overlapping of personality characteristics and features associated with histrionic personality disorder. This would include heightened emotionality, impressionistic thought and speech, seductiveness, strong dependency needs, and a preoccupation with symptoms and oneself.

The *DSM-IV-TR* diagnostic criteria for somatization disorder is presented in Table 31–1.

TABLE 31–1	Diagnostic Criteria for Somatization Disorder

A. A history of many physical complaints beginning before age 30 years that occur over a period of several years and result in treatment being sought or significant impairment in social, occupational, or other important areas of functioning.
B. Each of the following criteria must have been met, with individual symptoms occurring at any time during the course of the disturbance:
　1. *Four Pain Symptoms*: A history of pain related to at least four different sites or functions (e.g., head, abdomen, back, joints, extremities, chest, rectum, during menstruation, during sexual intercourse, or during urination).
　2. *Two Gastrointestinal Symptoms*: A history of at least two gastrointestinal symptoms other than pain (e.g., nausea, bloating, vomiting other than during pregnancy, diarrhea, or intolerance of several different foods).
　3. *One Sexual Symptom*: A history of at least one sexual or reproductive symptom other than pain (e.g., sexual indifference, erectile or ejaculatory dysfunction, irregular menses, excessive menstrual bleeding, vomiting throughout pregnancy).
　4. *One Pseudoneurological Symptom*: A history of at least one symptom of deficit suggesting a neurological condition not limited to pain (e.g., conversion symptoms such as impaired coordination or balance, paralysis or localized weakness, difficulty swallowing or lump in throat, aphonia, urinary retention, hallucinations, loss of touch or pain sensation, double vision, blindness, deafness, seizures; dissociative symptoms such as amnesia; or loss of consciousness other than fainting).
C. Either 1 or 2:
　1. After appropriate investigation, each of the symptoms in criterion B cannot be fully explained by a known general medical condition or the direct effects of a substance (e.g., a drug of abuse or a medication).
　2. When there is a related general medical condition, the physical complaints or resulting social or occupational impairment are in excess of what would be expected from the history, physical examination, or laboratory findings.
D. The symptoms are not intentionally produced or feigned (as in factitious disorder or malingering).

SOURCE: American Psychiatric Association (2000), with permission.

Predisposing Factors to Somatization Disorder

Theory of Family Dynamics

In some families, the family members are unable to express emotions openly and resolve conflicts verbally. They tend to deny psychological problems in general. In these "psychosomatic families," when the child becomes ill, the focus shifts from the open conflict to the child's illness, leaving unresolved the underlying issues that the family cannot confront openly. Thus, somatization by the child brings some stability to the family, as harmony replaces discord and the child's welfare becomes the common concern. The child in turn receives positive reinforcement for the illness.

Somatization may also have its roots in the family system because of parental teaching and parental example. The effectiveness of learning through role modeling has been well established and may be instrumental in teaching children to respond to anxious situations with somatization.

An additional theory related to family dynamics suggests that in families in which nurturing is provided on a conditional basis, the child fails to develop feelings of self-security. These children defend themselves against this insecurity by learning to gain affection and care through illness.

Cultural and Environmental Factors

Some cultures and religions carry implicit sanctions against verbalizing or directly expressing emotional states, thereby indirectly encouraging "more acceptable" somatic behaviors. Cross-cultural studies have shown that the somatization symptoms associated with depression are relatively similar, but the "cognitive" or emotional symptoms such as guilt are seen predominantly in Western societies. In Middle Eastern and Asian cultures, depression is almost exclusively manifested by somatic or vegetative symptoms.

Environmental influences may be significant in the predisposition to somatization disorder. Some studies have suggested that a tendency toward somatization appears to be more common in individuals who have low socioeconomic, occupational, and educational status.

Genetic Factors

Studies have shown a 10- to 20-fold increased incidence in female first-degree relatives of persons with the disorder (Sadock & Sadock, 2003). These statistics may imply a possible inheritable predisposition. Studies with monozygotic and dizygotic twins have also provided information that suggests a possible genetic influence.

Transactional Model of Stress/Adaptation

The etiology of somatization disorder is most likely influenced by multiple factors. In Figure 31–1 a graphic depiction of this theory of multiple causation is presented in the transactional model of stress/adaptation.

Diagnosis/Outcome Identification

Nursing diagnoses are formulated from the data gathered during the assessment phase and with background knowledge regarding predisposing factors to the disorder. Some common nursing diagnoses for clients with somatization disorder include:

Ineffective coping related to repressed anxiety and unmet dependency needs, evidenced by verbalization of numerous physical complaints in the absence of any pathophysiological evidence; focus on the self and physical symptoms.
Deficient knowledge (psychological causes for physical symptoms) related to strong denial defense system evi-

denced by history of "doctor shopping" for evidence of organic pathology to substantiate physical symptoms and by statements such as, "I don't know why the doctor put me on the psychiatric unit. I have a physical problem."

The following criteria may be used for measurement of outcomes in the care of the client with somatization disorder.

The client:

1. Demonstrates adaptive coping strategies.
2. Effectively uses adaptive coping strategies during stressful situations without resorting to physical symptoms.
3. Identifies stressors that cause anxiety level to rise.
4. Verbalizes understanding of correlation between times of increased anxiety and onset of physical symptoms.
5. Demonstrates control over life situation by meeting needs in an assertive manner.

Planning/Implementation

In Table 31–2, these nursing diagnoses are presented in a plan of care for the client with somatization disorder. Nursing diagnoses are included, along with outcome criteria, appropriate nursing interventions, and rationales for each.

The concept map care plan is an innovative approach to planning and organizing nursing care (see Chapter 9). It is a diagrammatic teaching and learning strategy that allows visualization of interrelationships between medical diagnoses, nursing diagnoses, assessment data, and treatments. An example of a concept map care plan for a client with somatization disorder is presented in Figure 31–2.

Evaluation

Reassessment is conducted to determine if the nursing actions have been successful in achieving the objectives of care. Evaluation of the nursing actions for the client with somatization disorder may be facilitated by gathering information using the following types of questions:

1. Can the client recognize signs and symptoms of escalating anxiety?
2. Can the client intervene with adaptive coping strategies to interrupt the escalating anxiety before physical symptoms are exacerbated?
3. Can the client verbalize an understanding of the correlation between physical symptoms and times of escalating anxiety?
4. Does the client have a plan for dealing with increased stress to prevent exacerbation of physical symptoms?
5. Can the client demonstrate assertiveness skills?
6. Does the client exercise control over life situation by participating in the decision-making process?

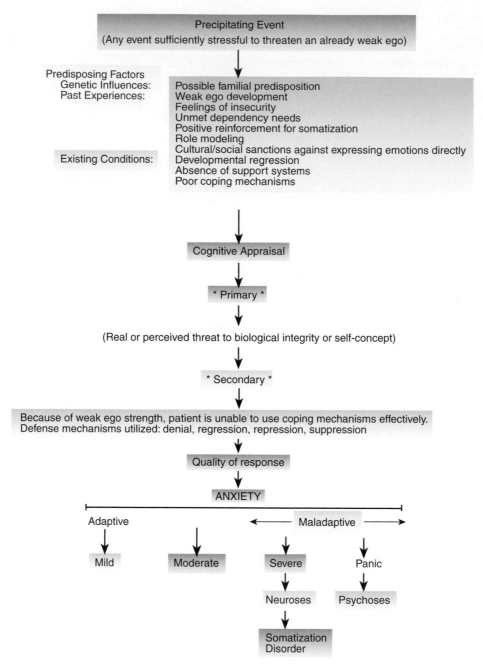

FIGURE 31–1 The dynamics of somatization disorder using the transactional model of stress/adaptation.

7. Can the client verbalize resources outside the hospital from whom he or she may seek assistance during times of extreme stress?

Pain Disorder

Background Assessment Data

The essential feature of pain disorder is severe and prolonged pain that causes clinically significant distress or impairment in social, occupational, or other important areas of functioning (APA, 2000). This diagnosis is made when psychological factors have been judged to have a major role in the onset, severity, exacerbation, or maintenance of the pain, even when the physical examination reveals pathology that is associated with the pain. Psychological implications in the etiology of the pain complaint may be evidenced by the correlation of a stressful situation with the onset of the symptom. Additional psychological implications may be supported by the facts that (1) appearance of the pain enables the client to avoid some unpleasant activity [**primary gain**], and (2) the pain promotes emotional support or attention that the client might not otherwise receive [**secondary gain**].

TABLE 31-2 Care Plan for the Client with Somatization Disorder

NURSING DIAGNOSIS: INEFFECTIVE COPING

RELATED TO: Repressed anxiety and unmet dependency needs

EVIDENCED BY: Verbalization of numerous physical complaints in the absence of any pathophysiological evidence; total focus on the self and physical symptoms

OUTCOME CRITERIA	NURSING INTERVENTIONS	RATIONALE
Client will demonstrate ability to cope with stress by means other than preoccupation with physical symptoms.	1. Monitor physician's ongoing assessments, laboratory reports, and other data to maintain assurance that possibility of organic pathology is clearly ruled out. Review findings with client. 2. Recognize and accept that the physical complaint is real to the client, even though no organic etiology can be identified. 3. Identify gains that the physical symptoms are providing for the client: increased dependency, attention, distraction from other problems. 4. Initially, fulfill the client's most urgent dependency needs, but gradually withdraw attention to physical symptoms. Minimize time given in response to physical complaints. 5. Explain to client that any new physical complaints will be referred to the physician and give no further attention to them. Ensure physician's assessment of the complaint. 6. Encourage client to verbalize fears and anxieties. Explain that attention will be withdrawn if rumination about physical complaints begins. Follow through. 7. Discuss possible alternative coping strategies client may use in response to stress (e.g., relaxation exercises; physical activities; assertiveness skills). Give positive reinforcement for use of these alternatives. 8. Help client identify ways to achieve recognition from others without resorting to physical complaints.	1. Accurate medical assessment is vital for the provision of adequate and appropriate care. Honest explanation may help client understand psychological implications. 2. Denial of the client's feelings is nontherapeutic and interferes with establishment of a trusting relationship. 3. Identification of underlying motivation is important in assisting the client with problem resolution. 4. Anxiety and maladaptive behaviors will increase if dependency needs are ignored initially. Gradual withdrawal of positive reinforcement will discourage repetition of maladaptive behaviors. 5. The possibility of organic pathology must always be considered. Failure to do so could jeopardize client safety. 6. Without consistency of limit setting, change will not occur. 7. Client may need help with problem solving. Positive reinforcement encourages repetition. 8. Positive recognition from others enhances self-esteem and minimizes the need for attention through maladaptive behaviors.

NURSING DIAGNOSIS: DEFICIENT KNOWLEDGE (PSYCHOLOGICAL CAUSES FOR PHYSICAL SYMPTOMS)

RELATED TO: Strong denial defense system

EVIDENCED BY: History of doctor shopping for evidence of organic pathology to substantiate physical symptoms and statements such as, "I don't know why the doctor put me on the psychiatric unit. I have a physical problem."

OUTCOME CRITERIA	NURSING INTERVENTIONS	RATIONALE
Client will verbalize psychological implications for physical symptoms.	1. Assess client's level of knowledge regarding effects of psychological problems on the body. Assess level of anxiety and readiness to learn. 2. Discuss results of laboratory tests and physical examinations with client.	1. An adequate database is necessary for the development of an effective teaching plan. Learning does not occur beyond the moderate level of anxiety. 2. Objective information about physical condition may help to break through the strong denial defense.

(Continued on following page)

TABLE 31–2	Care Plan for the Client with Somatization Disorder *(Continued)*	
OUTCOME CRITERIA	NURSING INTERVENTIONS	RATIONALE
	3. Have client keep a diary of appearance, duration, and intensity of physical symptoms. A separate record of situations that the client finds especially stressful should also be kept.	3. Comparison of these records may provide objective data from which to observe the relationship between physical symptoms and stress.
	4. Help client identify needs that are being met through the sick role. Formulate a more adaptive means for fulfilling these needs. Practice by role-playing.	4. Change cannot occur until the client realizes that physical symptoms are used to fulfill unmet needs. Anxiety is relieved by role-playing, because the client is then able to anticipate responses to stressful situations.
	5. Have client demonstrate adaptive methods of stress management, such as relaxation exercises, meditation, deep-breathing exercises, autogenics, mental imagery, and assertiveness techniques.	5. Demonstration by the client provides a measurable means of evaluating the effectiveness of what has been taught.

Characteristic behaviors include frequent visits to physicians in an effort to obtain relief, excessive use of analgesics, and requests for surgery (Sadock & Sadock, 2003). Symptoms of depression are common and often severe enough to warrant a diagnosis of major depression. Dependence on addictive substances is not an uncommon complication of pain disorder. *DSM-IV-TR* diagnostic criteria for this disorder are presented in Table 31–3.

Predisposing Factors to Pain Disorder

Psychodynamic Theory

Sadock and Sadock (2003) state, "Patients who experience bodily aches and pains without identifiable and adequate physical causes may be symbolically expressing an intrapsychic conflict through the body." Individuals who have difficulty expressing emotions verbally are expressing feelings and emotions with bodily sensations. Some individuals may feel that emotional pain is not as authentic as physical pain and therefore not worthy of the kind of attention that will be rendered to the individual with physical pain.

Sadock and Sadock (2003) explain the psychoanalytical view in the following manner:

The symbolic meaning of body disturbances may also relate to atonement for perceived sin, to expiation of guilt, or to suppressed aggression. Many patients have intractable and unresponsive pain because they are convinced that they deserve to suffer. Pain can function as a method of obtaining love, a punishment for wrongdoing, and a way of expiating guilt and of atoning for an innate sense of badness. (p. 655)

Behavioral Theory

In behavioral terminology, psychogenic pain is explained as a response that is learned through operant and classi-

cal conditioning. In classical conditioning, a previously neutral stimulus may become a trigger for pain-related behaviors when it becomes associated in the mind of the individual with a painful stimulus. For example, the room where a painful event occurred may itself alone evoke pain-related behaviors because it has become associated with the painful event.

In operant conditioning, learning occurs when pain behaviors are positively or negatively reinforced. When pain behavior elicits attention, sympathy, and nurturing, this positive reinforcement increases the probability of

TABLE 31–3	Diagnostic Criteria for Pain Disorder

A. Pain in one or more anatomical sites is the predominant focus of the clinical presentation and is of sufficient severity to warrant clinical attention.
B. The pain causes clinically significant distress or impairment in social, occupational, or other important areas of functioning.
C. Psychological factors are judged to have an important role in the onset, severity, exacerbation, or maintenance of the pain.
D. The symptom or deficit is not intentionally produced or feigned (as in factitious disorder or malingering).
E. The pain is not better accounted for by a mood, anxiety, or psychotic disorder and does not meet criteria for dyspareunia.
May be coded as:
Pain Disorder Associated with Psychological Factors: Psychological factors are judged to have the major role in the onset, severity, exacerbation, or maintenance of the pain.
  Acute: Duration of less than 6 months
  Chronic: Duration of 6 months or longer
Pain Disorder Associated with Both Psychological Factors and a General Medical Condition: Both psychological factors and a general medical condition are judged to have important roles in the onset, severity, exacerbation, or maintenance of the pain.
  Acute: Duration of less than 6 months
  Chronic: Duration of 6 months or longer
Pain Disorder Associated with a General Medical Condition: A general medical condition has a major role in the onset, severity, exacerbation, or maintenance of the pain.

SOURCE: American Psychiatric Association (2000), with permission.

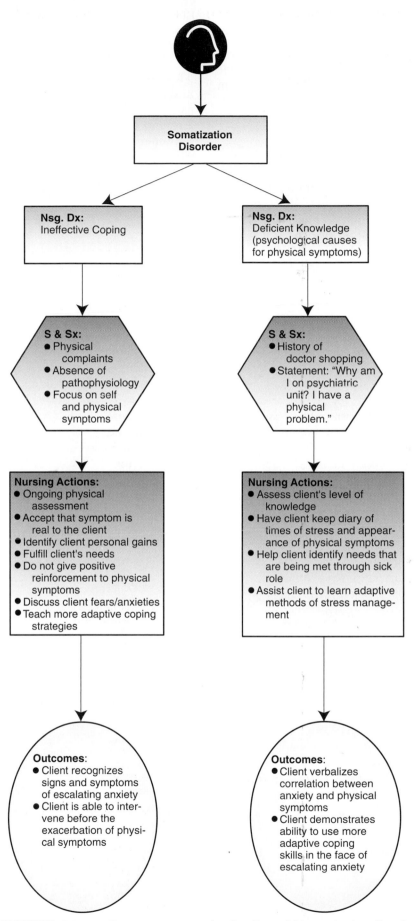

FIGURE 31–2 Concept map care plan for client with somatization disorder.

the pain behavior continuing. Negative reinforcement results when the pain behavior prevents an undesirable response from occurring (e.g., provides relief from responsibilities for the client).

Theory of Family Dynamics

"Pain games" may be played in families burdened by conflict. Pain may be used by a family member to control and coerce others and to manipulate and gain the advantage in interpersonal relationships. Pain may also serve as a **tertiary gain** for a family in conflict, which maintains the identified client in such a position that the real issue is disregarded and remains unresolved, even though some of the conflict is relieved.

Neurophysiological Theory

This theory postulates that the cerebral cortex and medulla are involved in inhibiting the firing of afferent pain fibers. Serotonin and the endorphins probably play a role in the central modulation of pain. The levels of serotonin and endorphins are believed to be decreased in clients with chronic, intractable pain. This deficiency seems to correlate with the augmentation of incoming sensory (pain) stimuli (Sadock & Sadock, 2003).

Transactional Model of Stress/Adaptation

The etiology of pain disorder is most likely influenced by multiple factors. Figure 31–3 presents a graphic depic-

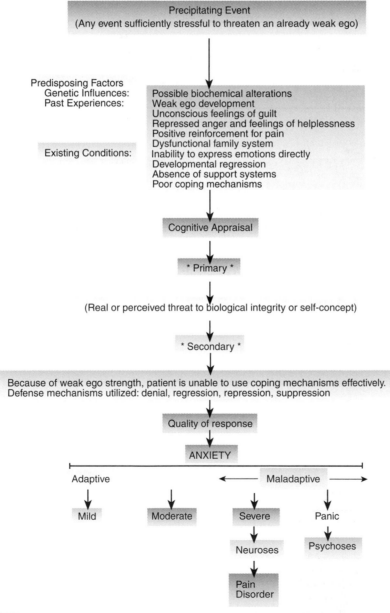

FIGURE 31–3 The dynamics of pain disorder using the transactional model of stress/adaptation.

tion of this theory of multiple causation in the transactional model of stress/adaptation.

Diagnosis/Outcome Identification

Nursing diagnoses are formulated from the data gathered during the assessment phase and with background knowledge regarding predisposing factors to the disorder. Some common nursing diagnoses for clients with pain disorder include:

Chronic pain related to repressed anxiety and learned maladaptive coping skills, evidenced by verbal complaints of pain, with evidence of psychological contributing factors, and excessive use of analgesics.
Social isolation related to preoccupation with self and pain, evidenced by seeking to be alone; refusal to participate in therapeutic activities.

The following criteria may be used for measurement of outcomes in the care of the client with pain disorder.

The client:

1. Demonstrates adaptive coping strategies.
2. Verbalizes relief from pain.
3. Effectively uses adaptive coping strategies during stressful situations to prevent the onset of pain.
4. Has identified stressors that raise the anxiety level.
5. Verbalizes understanding of correlation between times of increased anxiety and onset of pain.
6. Demonstrates control over life situation by meeting needs assertively.
7. Interacts with others appropriately.
8. Demonstrates the ability to focus on the needs of others rather than focusing on the self and pain.

Planning/Implementation

Table 31–4 provides a plan of care for the client with pain disorder. Nursing diagnoses are included, along with outcome criteria, appropriate nursing interventions, and rationales for each.

TABLE 31–4   **Care Plan for the Client with Pain Disorder**

NURSING DIAGNOSIS: CHRONIC PAIN
RELATED TO: Repressed anxiety and learned maladaptive coping skills
EVIDENCED BY: Verbal complaints of pain, with evidence of psychological contributing factors, and excessive use of analgesics

OUTCOME CRITERIA	NURSING INTERVENTIONS	RATIONALE
Client will verbalize relief from pain while demonstrating more adaptive coping strategies for dealing with life situation.	1. Monitor physician's ongoing assessments and laboratory reports. 2. Recognize and accept that the pain is indeed real to the client even though no organic etiology can be identified. 3. Observe and record the duration and intensity of the pain. Note factors that precipitate the onset of pain. 4. Provide pain medication as prescribed by physician. 5. Provide nursing comfort measures (e.g., backrub, warm bath, heating pad) with a matter-of-fact approach that does not reinforce the pain behavior. 6. Offer attention at times when client is not focusing on pain. 7. Identify activities that serve to distract client from focus on self and pain. 8. Encourage verbalization of feelings. Explore meaning that pain holds for client. Help client connect symptoms of pain to times of increased anxiety and to identify specific situations that cause anxiety to rise. 9. Encourage client to identify alternative methods of coping with stress.	1. Organic pathology must be clearly ruled out. 2. Denying the client's feelings is nontherapeutic and hinders the development of a trusting relationship 3. Identification of the precipitating stressor is important for assessment and care planning. 4. Client comfort and safety are nursing priorities. 5. Comfort measures may provide some relief from pain. Secondary gains from physical symptoms may prolong maladaptive behaviors. 6. Positive reinforcement encourages repetition of adaptive behaviors. 7. These distracters serve in a therapeutic manner as a transition from focus on self and pain to focus on unresolved psychological issues. 8. Verbalization of feelings in a nonthreatening environment facilitates expression and resolution of disturbing emotional issues. 9. Alternative stress management techniques may avert the use of pain as a maladaptive response to stress.

(Continued on following page)

TABLE 31–4	Care Plan for the Client with Pain Disorder *(Continued)*	
OUTCOME CRITERIA	**NURSING INTERVENTIONS**	**RATIONALE**
	10. Explore ways to intervene as symptoms begin to intensify (e.g., visual or auditory distractions, mental imagery, deep-breathing exercises, application of hot or cold compresses, relaxation exercises).	10. These techniques are adaptive ways of preventing the pain from becoming disabling.
	11. Provide positive reinforcement for times when client is not focusing on pain.	11. Positive reinforcement, in the form of the nurse's presence and attention, may encourage a continuation of these more adaptive behaviors.

NURSING DIAGNOSIS: SOCIAL ISOLATION
RELATED TO: Preoccupation with self and pain
EVIDENCED BY: Seeking to be alone; refusal to participate in therapeutic activities

OUTCOME CRITERIA	**NURSING INTERVENTIONS**	**RATIONALE**
Client will voluntarily spend time with other clients and staff members in group activities.	1. Spend more time with the client after setting limits on attention-seeking behaviors. Withdraw presence if ruminations about pain begin.	1. The nurse's presence conveys a sense of worthiness to the client. Lack of reinforcement of maladaptive behaviors may help to decrease their repetition.
	2. Increase amount of attention given during times when client is not focusing on pain.	2. This separates the person from the behavior. The client experiences unconditional acceptance without a need for the pain behavior.
	3. Describe to the client how the focus on pain and self discourages others from wanting to spend time with him or her.	3. Client may not realize how own behavior is perceived and may result in alienation from others.
	4. Teach client to recognize the differences among passive, assertive, and aggressive behaviors and the importance of respecting the human rights of others while protecting one's own basic human rights.	4. These assertive techniques enhance self-esteem and facilitate communication and mutual acceptance in interpersonal relationships.
	5. Provide positive feedback for any attempts at social interaction in which the client's focus is on others rather than on self or pain.	5. Positive feedback enhances self-esteem and encourages repetition of desirable behaviors.

The concept map care plan is an innovative approach to planning and organizing nursing care (see Chapter 9). It is a diagrammatic teaching and learning strategy that allows visualization of interrelationships between medical diagnoses, nursing diagnoses, assessment data, and treatments. An example of a concept map care plan for a client with pain disorder is presented in Figure 31–4.

Evaluation

Reassessment is conducted to determine if the nursing actions have been successful in achieving the objectives of care. Evaluation of the nursing actions for the client with pain disorder may be facilitated by gathering information using the following types of questions:

1. Can the client recognize signs and symptoms of escalating anxiety?

2. Can the client intervene with adaptive coping strategies to interrupt the escalating anxiety before pain becomes unmanageable?

3. Can the client verbalize an understanding of the correlation between onset of pain and times of escalating anxiety?

4. Does the client have a plan for dealing with increased stress so that the pain response can be diminished?

5. Can the client demonstrate assertiveness skills?

6. Does the client exercise control over life situations by participating in the decision-making process?

7. Is the client willingly and voluntarily interacting with others in an appropriate manner?

8. Does the client verbalize understanding of how pain behaviors interfere with the development of satisfactory interpersonal relationships?

9. Does the client show concern for the needs of others and focus less on self and pain?

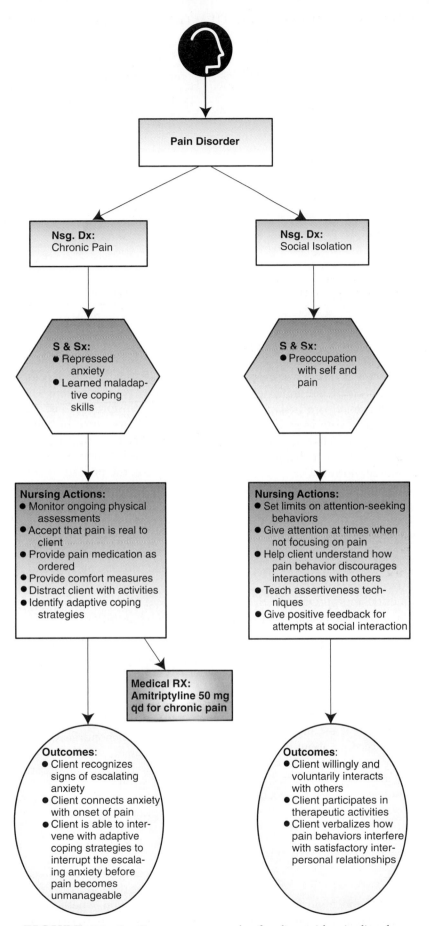

FIGURE 31–4 Concept map care plan for client with pain disorder.

10. Can the client verbalize resources outside the hospital from whom he or she may seek assistance during times of extreme stress?

Hypochondriasis

Background Assessment Data

Hypochondriasis may be defined as an unrealistic or inaccurate interpretation of physical symptoms or sensations, leading to preoccupation and fear of having a serious disease. The fear becomes disabling and persists despite appropriate reassurance that no organic pathology can be detected. Occasionally medical disease may be present, but in the individual with hypochondriasis, the symptoms are excessive in relation to the degree of pathology.

The preoccupation may be with a specific organ or disease (e.g., cardiac disease), with bodily functions, such as peristalsis or heartbeat, or even with minor physical alterations, such as a small sore or an occasional cough (APA, 2000). Individuals with hypochondriasis may become convinced that a rapid heart rate indicates they have heart disease or that the small sore is skin cancer. They are profoundly preoccupied with their bodies and are totally aware of even the slightest change in feeling or sensation. Their response to these small changes is usually unrealistic and exaggerated, however.

Individuals with hypochondriasis often have a long history of "doctor shopping" and are convinced that they are not receiving the proper care. Anxiety and depression are common, and obsessive–compulsive traits frequently accompany the disorder.

Preoccupation with the fear of serious disease may interfere with social or occupational functioning. Some individuals are able to function appropriately on the job, however, while limiting their physical complaints to non-work time.

Individuals with hypochondriasis are so totally convinced that their symptoms are related to organic pathology that they adamantly reject, and are often irritated by, any implication that stress or psychosocial factors play any role in their condition. They are so apprehensive and fearful that they become alarmed at the slightest intimation of serious illness. Even reading about a disease or hearing that someone they know has been diagnosed with an illness precipitates alarm on their part.

The *DSM-IV-TR* diagnostic criteria for hypochondriasis is presented in Table 31–5.

Predisposing Factors to Hypochondriasis

Psychodynamic Theory

Some psychodynamicists view hypochondriasis as an ego defense mechanism. Physical complaints are the expression of low self-esteem and feelings of worthlessness,

TABLE 31–5 Diagnostic Criteria for Hypochondriasis
A. Preoccupation with fears of having, or the idea that one has, a serious disease, based on the person's misinterpretation of bodily symptoms.
B. The preoccupation persists despite appropriate medical evaluation and reassurance.
C. The belief in criterion A is not of delusional intensity (as in delusional disorder, somatic type) and is not restricted to a circumscribed concern about appearance (as in body dysmorphic disorder).
D. The preoccupation causes clinically significant distress or impairment in social, occupational, or other important areas of functioning.
E. The duration of the disturbance is at least 6 months.
F. The preoccupation is not better accounted for by generalized anxiety disorder, obsessive–compulsive disorder, panic disorder, a major depressive episode, separation anxiety, or another somatoform disorder.

SOURCE: American Psychiatric Association (2000), with permission.

because it is easier to feel something is wrong with the body than to feel something is wrong with the self.

Another psychodynamic view explains hypochondriasis as the transformation of aggressive and hostile wishes toward others into physical complaints to others. Repressed anger, originating from past disappointments and unfulfilled needs for nurturing and caring, is expressed in the present by soliciting other people's help and concern and then thwarting and rejecting them as ineffective.

Still other psychodynamicists have viewed hypochondriasis as a defense against guilt (Sadock & Sadock, 2003). The individual views the self as "bad," based on real or imagined past misconduct, and views physical suffering as the deserved punishment required for atonement.

Cognitive Theory

Studies show that noxious sensory input undergoes a cognitive screening process involving assessment and clarification, which may amplify or reduce the sensations. Cognitive theorists view hypochondriasis as arising out of perceptual and cognitive abnormalities. This theory suggests that bodily sensations are intensified in individuals with hypochondriasis. When emotional arousal precipitates somatic symptoms, they are incorrectly assessed and misinterpreted, and negative cognitive meanings are attached to them. All future somatic perceptions are interpreted to fit this cognitive schema that the individual has established.

Social Learning Theory

Somatic complaints are often reinforced when the sick role relieves the individual from the need to deal with a stressful situation, whether it be within society or within the family. When the sick person is allowed to avoid stressful obligations and postpone unwelcome challenges, is excused from troublesome duties, or becomes the prominent focus of attention because of the illness, positive reinforcement virtually guarantees repetition of the response.

Past Experiences with Physical Illness

Personal experience, particularly in childhood, or the experience of close family members, with serious or life-threatening illness can predispose an individual to hypochondriasis. Once an individual has experienced a threat to biological integrity, he or she may develop a fear of recurrence. Increased bodily sensitivity develops, and the individual becomes strongly in tune to changes that may occur. The fear of recurring illness generates an exaggerated response leading to hypochondriacal behaviors.

Genetic Influences

Although little is known about the inheritance of hypochondriasis, some evidence indicates an increased prevalence of hypochondriasis among identical twins and other first-degree relatives (Noyes, Holt, & Happel, 1997).

Transactional Model of Stress/Adaptation

The etiology of hypochondriasis is most likely influenced by multiple factors. In Figure 31–5, a graphic depiction of this theory of multiple causation is presented in the transactional model of stress/adaptation.

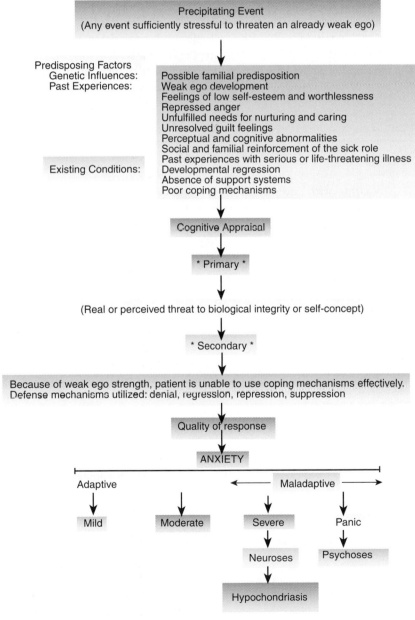

FIGURE 31–5   The dynamics of hypochondriasis using the transactional model of stress/adaptation.

Diagnosis/Outcome Identification

Nursing diagnoses are formulated from the data gathered during the assessment phase and with background knowledge regarding predisposing factors to the disorder. Common nursing diagnoses for clients with hypochondriasis include:

Fear (of having serious disease) related to past experience with life-threatening illness (of self or significant others) evidenced by preoccupation with and unrealistic interpretation of bodily signs and sensations.

Chronic low self-esteem related to unfulfilled childhood needs for nurturing and caring evidenced by transformation of internalized anger into physical complaints and hostility toward others.

The following criteria may be used to measure outcomes in the care of the client with hypochondriasis.

The client:

1. Interprets bodily sensations rationally.
2. Verbalizes significance the irrational fear held for him or her.

3. Has decreased the number and frequency of physical complaints.
4. Has identified the correlation between increased anxiety and the exacerbation of physical symptoms.
5. Has identified life situations that precipitate anxiety.
6. Demonstrates more adaptive ways of coping with stress than with physical symptoms.
7. Demonstrates acceptance of self as a worthwhile person.
8. Expresses self-confidence in dealing with stressful life situations.
9. Makes life changes for improvement and accepts situations that cannot be changed.
10. Sets realistic goals for the future.

Planning/Implementation

Table 31–6 provides a plan of care for the client with hypochondriasis. Nursing diagnoses are included, along with outcome criteria, appropriate nursing interventions, and rationales for each.

TABLE 31–6	Care Plan for the Client with Hypochondriasis

NURSING DIAGNOSIS: FEAR (OF HAVING A SERIOUS DISEASE)
RELATED TO: Past experience with life-threatening illness of self or significant others
EVIDENCED BY: Preoccupation with and unrealistic interpretation of bodily signs and sensations

OUTCOME CRITERIA	NURSING INTERVENTIONS	RATIONALE
Client will verbalize irrationality of fear and interpret bodily sensations correctly.	1. Monitor physician's ongoing assessments and laboratory reports. 2. Refer all new physical complaints to physician. 3. Assess function client's illness is fulfilling for him or her (e.g., unfulfilled needs for dependency, nurturing, caring, attention, or control). 4. Identify times during which preoccupation with physical symptoms is worse. Determine extent of correlation of physical complaints with times of increased anxiety. 5. Convey empathy. Let client know that you understand how a specific symptom may conjure up fears of previous life-threatening illness. 6. Initially allow client a limited amount of time (e.g., 10 minutes each hour) to discuss physical symptoms. 7. Help client determine what techniques may be most useful for him or her to implement when fear and anxiety are exacerbated (e.g., relaxation techniques; mental imagery; thought-stopping techniques; physical exercise).	1. Organic pathology must be clearly ruled out. 2. To assume that all physical complaints are hypochondriacal would place client's safety in jeopardy. 3. This information may provide insight into reasons for maladaptive behavior and provide direction for planning client care. 4. Client is unaware of the psychosocial implications of the physical complaints. Knowledge of the relationship is the first step in the process for creating change. 5. Unconditional acceptance and empathy promote a therapeutic nurse/client relationship. 6. Because this has been his or her primary method of coping for so long, complete prohibition of this activity would likely raise client's anxiety level significantly, further exacerbating the hypochondriacal behavior. 7. All of these techniques are effective in reducing anxiety and may assist client in the transition from focusing on fear of physical illness to the discussion of honest feelings.

(Continued on opposite page)

OUTCOME CRITERIA	NURSING INTERVENTIONS	RATIONALE
	8. Gradually increase the limit on amount of time spent each hour in discussing physical symptoms. If client violates the limits, withdraw attention.	8. Lack of positive reinforcement may help to extinguish maladaptive behavior.
	9. Encourage client to discuss feelings associated with fear of serious illness.	9. Verbalization of feelings in a nonthreatening environment facilitates expression and resolution of disturbing emotional issues. When the client can express feelings directly, there is less need to express them through physical symptoms.
	10. Role-play the client's plan for dealing with the fear the next time it assumes control and before it becomes disabling through the exacerbation of physical symptoms.	10. Anxiety and fears are minimized when client has achieved a degree of comfort through practicing a plan for dealing with stressful situations in the future.

NURSING DIAGNOSIS: CHRONIC LOW SELF-ESTEEM
RELATED TO: Unfulfilled childhood needs for nurturing and caring
EVIDENCED BY: Transformation of internalized anger into physical complaints and hostility toward others

OUTCOME CRITERIA	NURSING INTERVENTIONS	RATIONALE
Client will demonstrate acceptance of self as a person of worth, as evidenced by setting realistic goals, limiting physical complaints and hostility toward others, and verbalizing positive prospects for the future.	1. Convey acceptance, unconditional positive regard, and remain nonjudgmental at all times.	1. Offering the client respect and dignity adds to feelings of self-worth.
	2. Encourage client to participate in decision making regarding care as well as life situations.	2. Feelings of personal control decreases feelings of powerlessness.
	3. Help client to recognize and focus on strengths and accomplishments. Minimize attention given to past (real or perceived) failures.	3. Lack of attention may help to eliminate negative ruminations.
	4. Encourage participation in group activities.	4. Through participation in these activities, client may receive positive feedback and support from peers.
	5. Ensure that client is not becoming increasingly dependent. Withdraw attention at times when client is focusing on physical symptoms.	5. Independent functioning increases feelings of self-worth. Lack of reinforcement may help to extinguish maladaptive behaviors.
	6. Ensure that therapy groups offer client simple methods of achievement. Offer recognition and positive feedback for actual accomplishments.	6. Successes and recognition increase self-esteem.
	7. Teach assertiveness techniques and effective communication techniques.	7. Self-esteem is enhanced by the ability to interact with others in an effective manner.
	8. Offer positive feedback when client responds to stressful situation with coping strategies other then physical complaints.	8. Positive feedback enhances self-esteem and encourages repetition of desirable behaviors.

The concept map care plan is an innovative approach to planning and organizing nursing care (see Chapter 9). It is a diagrammatic teaching and learning strategy that allows visualization of interrelationships between medical diagnoses, nursing diagnoses, assessment data, and treatments. An example of a concept map care plan for a client with hypochondriasis is presented in Figure 31–6.

Evaluation

Reassessment is conducted to determine if the nursing actions have been successful in achieving the objectives of care. Evaluation of the nursing actions for the client with hypochondriasis may be facilitated by gathering information using the following types of questions:

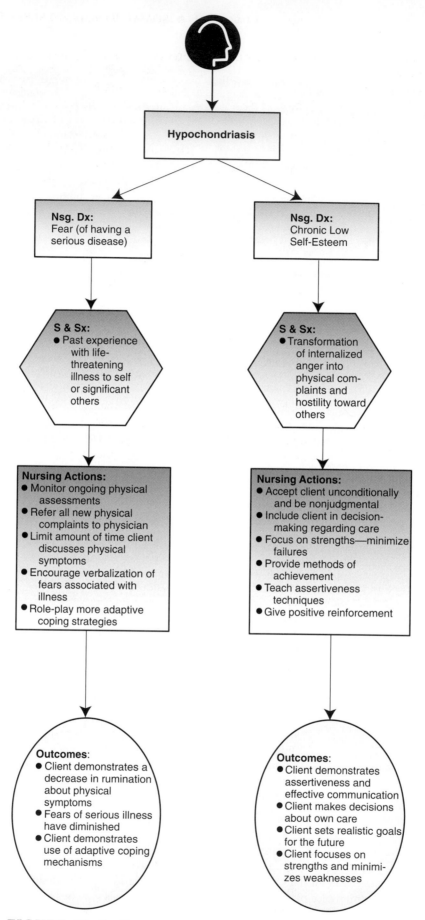

FIGURE 31–6 Concept map care plan for a client with hypochondriasis.

1. Does the client demonstrate a decrease in ruminations about physical symptoms?
2. Have fears of serious illness diminished?
3. Can the client correlate the exacerbation of physical symptoms to times of escalating anxiety?
4. Can the client use more adaptive coping mechanisms to interrupt the anxiety response?
5. Can the client demonstrate assertiveness and effective communication skills?
6. Does the client exercise control over life situation by participating in the decision-making process?
7. Does the client set realistic goals for the future?
8. Can the client maximize his or her potential by making the most of personal strengths?
9. Can the client verbalize resources outside the hospital from whom he or she may seek assistance during times of extreme stress?

Conversion Disorder

Background Assessment Data

Conversion disorder is a loss of or change in body function resulting from a psychological conflict, the physical symptoms of which cannot be explained by any known medical disorder or pathophysiological condition. Clients are unaware of the psychological basis and therefore are unable to control their symptoms.

Conversion symptoms affect voluntary motor or sensory functioning suggestive of neurological disease and therefore are sometimes called "pseudoneurological" (APA, 2000). Examples include paralysis, **aphonia**, seizures, coordination disturbance, difficulty swallowing, urinary retention, akinesia, blindness, deafness, double vision, **anosmia**, loss of pain sensation, and hallucinations. **Pseudocyesis** (false pregnancy) is a conversion symptom and may represent a strong desire to be pregnant.

Precipitation of conversion symptoms must be explained by psychological factors, and this may be evidenced by the presence of primary or secondary gain. When an individual achieves primary gain, the conversion symptoms serve to prevent internal conflicts or painful issues or events from attaining awareness. Conversion symptoms promote secondary gain for the individual by enabling him or her to avoid difficult situations or to obtain support that might not otherwise be forthcoming.

The symptom usually occurs after a situation that produces extreme psychological stress for the individual. The symptom appears suddenly, and often the person expresses a relative lack of concern that is out of keeping with the severity of the impairment (APA, 2000). This lack of concern is identified as **la belle indifference** and is often a clue to the physician that the problem may be psychological rather than physical. Other individuals, however, may present symptoms in a dramatic or histrionic fashion (APA, 2000).

Most symptoms of conversion disorder resolve within a few weeks. About 75 percent of people who experience conversion symptoms will never experience another episode (Sadock & Sadock, 2003). The other 25 percent have additional episodes during periods of extreme stress. Symptoms of blindness, aphonia, and paralysis are associated with good prognosis, whereas seizures and tremor are associated with poorer prognosis (APA, 2000). The *DSM-IV-TR* diagnostic criteria for conversion disorder are presented in Table 31–7.

Predisposing Factors to Conversion Disorder

Psychoanalytical Theory

This theory proposes that emotions associated with a traumatic event that the individual cannot express because of moral or ethical unacceptability are "converted" into physical symptoms. The unacceptable emotions are repressed and converted to a somatic hysterical symptom that is symbolic in some way of the original emotional trauma. An example might be the young soldier who, knowing that at daybreak he will be sent to the front lines to participate in battle, develops a paralysis of his arms and is unable to pick up his rifle.

Familial Factors

Some data have suggested that conversion disorder occurs more often in relatives of individuals with the disorder. Studies show an increased risk in monozygotic twins, but not in dizygotic twins (Soares & Grossman,

---

TABLE 31–7 Diagnostic Criteria for Conversion Disorder

A. One or more symptoms or deficits affecting voluntary motor or sensory function that suggest a neurological or other general medical condition.
B. Psychological factors are judged to be associated with the symptom or deficit because the initiation or exacerbation of the symptom or deficit is preceded by conflicts or other stressors.
C. The symptom or deficit is not intentionally produced or feigned (as in factitious disorder or malingering).
D. The symptom or deficit cannot, after appropriate investigation, be fully explained by a general medical condition, by the direct effects of a substance, or as a culturally sanctioned behavior or experience.
E. The symptom or deficit causes clinically significant distress or impairment in social, occupational, or other important areas of functioning or warrants medical evaluation.
F. The symptom or deficit is not limited to pain or sexual dysfunction, does not occur exclusively during the course of somatization disorder, and is not better accounted for by another mental disorder.
    Specify type of symptom or deficit:
       With motor symptom or deficit
       With sensory symptom or deficit
       With seizures or convulsions
       With mixed presentation

SOURCE: American Psychiatric Association (2000), with permission.

2003). Nongenetic familial factors, such as incestuous sexual abuse in childhood, also may be associated with an increased risk for conversion disorder.

Neurophysiological Theory

This theory suggests that some clients with conversion disorder have a disturbance in central nervous system (CNS) arousal. Symptoms are thought to be derived from an excessive cortical arousal creating a negative feedback loop between the cerebral cortex and the brainstem reticular formation (Sadock & Sadock, 2003). This activity diminishes the awareness of bodily sensation and would explain the observed sensory deficits in some conversion disorder clients and their apparently low levels of anxiety and relative indifference to their impairment.

Behavioral Theory

Behavioral theorists believe that conversion symptoms are learned through positive reinforcement from cultural, social, and interpersonal influences. The individual uses physical symptoms to communicate helplessness and, in return, gains attention and support from the environment. These secondary gains reinforce the perpetuation of symptoms during times of stress or conflict.

Transactional Model of Stress/Adaptation

The etiology of conversion disorder is most likely influenced by multiple factors. In Figure 31–7, a graphic depiction of this theory of multiple causation is presented in the transactional model of stress/adaptation.

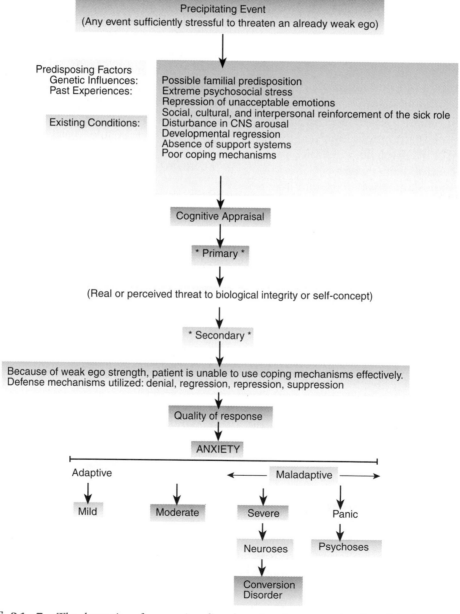

FIGURE 31–7 The dynamics of conversion disorder using the transactional model of stress/adaptation.

Diagnosis/Outcome Identification

Nursing diagnoses are formulated from the data gathered during the assessment phase and with background knowledge regarding predisposing factors to the disorder. Common nursing diagnoses for clients with conversion disorder include:

Disturbed sensory perception related to repressed severe anxiety evidenced by loss or alteration in physical functioning without evidence of organic pathology, and "la belle indifference."

Self-care deficit related to loss or alteration in physical functioning evidenced by the need for assistance to carry out self-care activities such as eating, dressing, maintaining hygiene, and toileting.

The following criteria may be used for measurement of outcomes in the care of the client with conversion disorder.

The client:

1. Is free of physical disability.
2. Verbalizes the correlation between the loss of or alteration in function and extreme emotional stress.
3. Is able to identify the stressful situation that precipitated the physical disability.
4. Verbalizes the purpose the disability serves for him or her.
5. Demonstrates more adaptive coping strategies for dealing with stress in the future.
6. Performs all self-care activities without assistance.

Planning/Implementation

Table 31–8 provides a plan of care for the client with conversion disorder. Nursing diagnoses are presented, along with outcome criteria, appropriate nursing interventions, and rationales.

TABLE 31–8   Care Plan for the Client with Conversion Disorder

NURSING DIAGNOSIS: DISTURBED SENSORY PERCEPTION
RELATED TO: Repressed severe anxiety
EVIDENCED BY: Loss or alteration in physical functioning, without evidence of organic pathology; "la belle indifference"

OUTCOME CRITERIA	NURSING INTERVENTIONS	RATIONALE
Client will demonstrate recovery of lost or altered function.	1. Monitor physician's ongoing assessments, laboratory reports, and other data to ensure that possibility of organic pathology is clearly ruled out.	1. Failure to do so may jeopardize client safety.
	2. Identify primary or secondary gains that the physical symptom is providing for the client (e.g., increased dependency, attention, protection from experiencing a stressful event).	2. These are considered to be etiological factors and will be used to assist in problem resolution.
	3. Do not focus on the disability, and encourage client to be as independent as possible. Intervene only when client requires assistance.	3. Positive reinforcement would encourage continual use of the maladaptive response for secondary gains, such as dependency.
	4. Do not allow the client to use the disability as a manipulative tool to avoid participation in therapeutic activities. Withdraw attention if client continues to focus on physical limitation.	4. Lack of reinforcement may help to extinguish the maladaptive response.
	5. Encourage client to verbalize fears and anxieties. Help identify physical symptoms as a coping mechanism that is used in times of extreme stress.	5. Clients with conversion disorder are usually unaware of the psychological implications of their illness.
	6. Help client identify coping mechanisms that he or she could use when faced with stressful situations, rather than retreating from reality with a physical disability.	6. Client needs assistance with problem solving at this severe level of anxiety.
	7. Give positive reinforcement for identification or demonstration of alternative, more adaptive coping strategies.	7. Positive reinforcement enhances self-esteem and encourages repetition of desirable behaviors.

(Continued on following page)

TABLE 31–8	Care Plan for the Client with Conversion Disorder *(Continued)*

NURSING DIAGNOSIS: SELF-CARE DEFICIT
RELATED TO: Loss or alteration in physical functioning
EVIDENCED BY: Need for assistance to carry out self-care activities, such as eating, dressing, hygiene, and toileting

OUTCOME CRITERIA	NURSING INTERVENTIONS	RATIONALE

Client will be able to perform self-care activities independently.	1. Assess client's level of disability. Note areas of strength and impairment.
	2. Encourage client to perform self-care to his or her level of ability. Intervene when client is unable to perform.
	3. Maintain nonjudgmental attitude when providing assistance to the client. The physical symptom is not within the client's conscious control and is very real to him or her.
	4. Assist as required with self-care deficits:
	  a. Feed client, if necessary, or provide assistance with containers, positioning, and so forth.
	  b. Bathe client, or assist with bath, as required.
	  c. Assist with dressing, oral hygiene, combing hair, applying make-up.
	  d. Provide bedpan, commode, or assistance to bathroom, as required.
	5. Avoid fostering dependency by intervening when client is capable of performing independently. Allow ample time to complete these activities to the best of client's ability without assistance. Provide positive reinforcement for independent accomplishments.
	6. Help client understand the purpose this disability is serving for him or her. Discuss honest feelings.
		1. This information will be used to plan care for the client.
		2. Successful performance of independent activities enhances self-esteem.
		3. A judgmental attitude interferes with the nurse's ability to provide therapeutic care for the client.
		
		4. Client comfort and safety are nursing priorities.
		
		5. Success and positive reinforcement enhance self-esteem and encourage repetition of desirable behaviors.
		
		6. Self-disclosure and exploration of feelings with a trusted individual may help client fulfill unmet needs and confront unresolved issues.

The concept map care plan is an innovative approach to planning and organizing nursing care (see Chapter 9). It is a diagrammatic teaching and learning strategy that allows visualization of interrelationships between medical diagnoses, nursing diagnoses, assessment data, and treatments. An example of a concept map care plan for a client with conversion disorder is presented in Figure 31–8.

Evaluation

Reassessment is conducted to determine if the nursing actions have been successful in achieving the objectives of care. Evaluation of the nursing actions for the client with conversion disorder may be facilitated by gathering information using the following types of questions:

1. Does the client demonstrate full recovery from previous physical disability?
2. Can the client perform all self-care activities independently?
3. Can the client verbalize why the disability occurred?
4. Can the client verbalize the relationship between loss of function and the stressful event?
5. Does the client recognize what unfulfilled need the loss of function was serving?
6. Can the client openly discuss feelings associated with the stressful event?
7. Can the client directly confront the conflict that was previously repressed and somaticized?
8. Can the client demonstrate more adaptive coping skills for dealing with stress or conflict?
9. Does he or she have a plan for coping with future stressful situations?
10. Can the client verbalize resources outside the hospital to whom he or she may turn when feeling the need for assistance?

Body Dysmorphic Disorder

Background Assessment Data

This disorder, formerly called dysmorphophobia, is characterized by the exaggerated belief that the body is deformed or defective in some specific way. The most common complaints involve imagined or slight flaws of the face or head, such as thinning hair, acne, wrinkles,

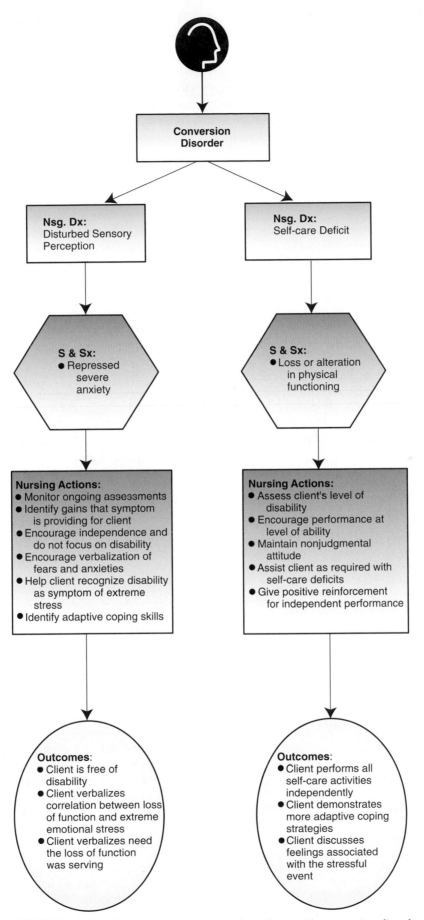

FIGURE 31–8 Concept map care plan for a client with conversion disorder.

scars, vascular markings, facial swelling or asymmetry, or excessive facial hair (APA, 2000). Other complaints may have to do with some aspect of the nose, ears, eyes, mouth, lips, or teeth. Some clients may present with complaints involving other parts of the body, and in some instances a true defect is present. The significance of the defect is unrealistically exaggerated, however, and the person's concern is grossly excessive.

Symptoms of depression and characteristics associated with obsessive–compulsive personality are common in individuals with body dysmorphic disorder. Social and occupational impairment may occur because of the excessive anxiety experienced by the individual in relation to the imagined defect. The person's medical history may reflect numerous visits to plastic surgeons and dermatologists in an unrelenting drive to correct the imagined defect. He or she may undergo unnecessary surgical procedures toward this effort.

This disorder has been closely associated with delusional thinking, and the *DSM-IV-TR* suggests that if the perceived body defect is in fact of delusional intensity, the appropriate diagnosis would be delusional disorder, somatic type (APA, 2000). Traits associated with schizoid, obsessive–compulsive, and narcissistic personality disorders are not uncommon (Sadock & Sadock, 2003).

The *DSM-IV-TR* diagnostic criteria for body dysmorphic disorder are presented in Table 31–9.

Predisposing Factors to Body Dysmorphic Disorder

The etiology of body dysmorphic disorder is unknown. In some clients the belief is due to another more pervasive psychiatric disorder, such as schizophrenia. A high incidence of comorbidity with major mood disorder and anxiety disorder and the responsiveness of the condition to the serotonin-specific drugs may indicate some involvement of the serotonergic system.

Body dysmorphic disorder has been classified as one of several *monosymptomatic hypochondriacal syndromes*. Each of these syndromes is characterized by a single hypo-

---

TABLE 31–9   Diagnostic Criteria for Body Dysmorphic Disorder

A. Preoccupation with an imagined defect in appearance. If a slight physical anomaly is present, the person's concern is markedly excessive.

B. The preoccupation causes clinically significant distress or impairment in social, occupational, or other important areas of functioning.

C. The preoccupation is not better accounted for by another mental disorder (e.g., dissatisfaction with body shape and size in anorexia nervosa).

SOURCE: American Psychiatric Association (2000), with permission

---

chondriacal belief about one's body. Body dysmorphic disorder is one of the most common such syndromes. Others include delusions of parasitosis (i.e., false belief that one is infested with some parasite or vermin) and of bromosis (i.e., false belief that one is emitting an offensive body odor).

Body dysmorphic disorder has also been defined as the fear of some physical defect thought to be noticeable to others although the client appears normal. These interpretations suggest that the disorder may be related to predisposing factors similar to those associated with hypochondriasis or phobias. The psychodynamic view suggests that unresolved emotional conflict is displaced onto a body part through symbolization and projection (Sadock & Sadock, 2003). Repression of morbid anxiety is undoubtedly an underlying factor, and it is very likely that multiple factors are involved in the predisposition to body dysmorphic disorder.

Diagnosis/Outcome Identification

Nursing diagnoses are formulated from the data gathered during the assessment phase and with background knowledge regarding predisposing factors to the disorder. Nursing diagnoses for clients with body dysmorphic disorder may include:

Disturbed body image related to repressed severe anxiety, evidenced by preoccupation with imagined defect; verbalizations that are out of proportion to any actual physical abnormality that may exist; and numerous visits to plastic surgeons or dermatologists seeking relief.

The following criteria may be used for measurement of outcomes in the care of the client with body dysmorphic disorder.

The client:

1. Verbalizes a realistic perception of his or her appearance.
2. Expresses feelings of self-worth that reflect a positive body image and acceptance of personal appearance.
3. Verbalizes fears and anxieties that may contribute to altered body image.
4. Verbalizes adaptive strategies for dealing with fears and anxieties more effectively.
5. Expresses satisfaction with accomplishments unrelated to physical appearance.
6. Verbalizes intent to participate in a support group.

Planning/Implementation

Table 31–10 provides a plan of care for the client with body dysmorphic disorder. The nursing diagnosis is presented, along with outcome criterion, appropriate nursing interventions and rationales.

TABLE 31-10	Care Plan for the Client with Body Dysmorphic Disorder

NURSING DIAGNOSIS: DISTURBED BODY IMAGE

RELATED TO: Repressed severe anxiety

EVIDENCED BY: Preoccupation with imagined defect; verbalizations that are out of proportion to any actual physical abnormality that may exist; and numerous visits to plastic surgeons or dermatologists seeking relief

OUTCOME CRITERIA	NURSING INTERVENTIONS	RATIONALE
Client will verbalize realistic perception of body appearance.	1. Assess client's perception of his or her body image. Keep in mind that this image is real to the client.	1. Assessment information is necessary in developing an accurate plan of care. Denial of the client's feelings impedes the development of a trusting, therapeutic relationship.
	2. Help client to see that his or her body image is distorted or that it is out of proportion in relation to the significance of an actual physical anomaly.	2. Recognition that a misperception exists is necessary before the client can accept reality and reduce the significance of the imagined defect.
	3. Encourage verbalization of fears and anxieties associated with identified stressful life situations. Discuss alternative adaptive coping strategies.	3. Verbalization of feelings with a trusted individual may help the client come to terms with unresolved issues. Knowledge of alternative coping strategies may help the client respond to stress more adaptively in the future.
	4. Involve client in activities that reinforce a positive sense of self not based on appearance.	4. When the client is able to develop self-satisfaction based on accomplishments and unconditional acceptance, significance of the imagined defect or minor physical anomaly will diminish.
	5. Make referrals to support groups of individuals with similar histories (e.g., Adult Children of Alcoholics [ACOA], Victims of Incest, Survivors of Suicide [SOS], Adults Abused as Children).	5. Having a support group of understanding, empathic peers can help the client accept the reality of the situation, correct distorted perceptions, and make adaptive life changes.

Evaluation

Reassessment is conducted in order to determine if the nursing actions have been successful in achieving the objectives of care. Evaluation of the nursing actions for the client with body dysmorphic disorder may be facilitated by gathering information using the following types of questions:

1. Does the client demonstrate a decrease in ruminations about the imagined defect?
2. Can the client maximize his or her potential by making the most of personal strengths?
3. Has the client verbalized a realistic perception of personal appearance?
4. Does he or she demonstrate satisfactory acceptance of personal appearance?
5. Does the client interact with others comfortably?
6. Does the client focus attention on activities or personal accomplishments rather than on personal appearance?
7. Does the client demonstrate a positive self-worth not based on appearance?
8. Has he or she expressed fears and anxieties that may have provided the foundation for preoccupation with the imagined defect?
9. Can the client demonstrate strategies for coping more adaptively with stress in the future?
10. Can the client verbalize resources from whom he or she may seek assistance during times of extreme stress (including regular attendance in a support group)?

SLEEP DISORDERS

The main purposes of sleep are to restore homeostatic function, maintain normal thermoregulation, and conserve energy (Sadock & Sadock, 2003). Some individuals require fewer than 6 hours, whereas others need more than 9 hours of sleep per night to function adequately. Individuals who require less sleep are generally efficient, ambitious, socially adept, and content. The longer sleepers tend to be mildly depressed, anxious, and socially withdrawn (Sadock & Sadock, 2003). The need for sleep increases with physical activity, illness, pregnancy, emotional stress, and increased mental activity.

According to a survey by the National Sleep Foundation (2005):

● Approximately 75 percent of adult Americans report experiencing a sleep problem a few nights a week or more during the last year.
● More than two thirds of all children (69%) experience one or more sleep problems at least a few nights a week.
● The prevalence of sleep disorders appears to increase with advancing age to age 64, and then decreases with advancing age
● Indirect costs of insomnia to the national health care bill are estimated to be $28 billion annually.

Common types of sleep disorders include **insomnia**, **hypersomnia**, **parasomnias**, and circadian rhythm sleep disorders.

APPLICATION OF THE NURSING PROCESS TO SLEEP DISORDERS

Background Assessment Data

Insomnia

Insomnia is defined as difficulty with initiating or maintaining sleep (Sadock & Sadock, 2003). The *DSM-IV-TR* identifies this disorder as primary insomnia, to differentiate it from insomnia that is secondary to another sleep disorder. The *DSM-IV-TR* specifies that the symptom must be of at least 1 month's duration; must cause significant impairment in social, occupational, or other important areas of functioning; and must not be due to the direct effects of a substance, a general medical condition, or a mental disorder (APA, 2000).

Primary insomnia may be manifested by a combination of difficulty falling asleep and intermittent wakefulness during sleep. The disorder often becomes a vicious cycle when the individual becomes more and more distressed by the inability to achieve sleep, and the additional stress in turn contributes to the insomnia.

Individuals with this disorder often have an anxious overconcern with their general health. Depression and anxiety are not uncommon. Lack of sleep results in daytime irritability and problems with attention and concentration. Inappropriate use of substances, both hypnotics for sleep and stimulants to counteract fatigue, often occurs.

Primary insomnia typically begins in early to middle adulthood and increases with age. It is more common in women than in men.

Hypersomnia

Hypersomnia, or *somnolence*, can be defined as excessive sleepiness or seeking excessive amounts of sleep. Primary hypersomnia refers to the condition when no other cause for the symptom can be found. The term should be used for individuals who have difficulty staying awake during what should be considered the waking hours of the sleep–wake cycle; it should not be used for those who are simply physically tired or weary (Sadock & Sadock, 2003). The *DSM-IV-TR* specifies that the symptom must be for at least 1 month's duration; must be severe enough to interfere with social, occupational, or other important areas of functioning; and must not be due to the direct physiological effects of a substance or a general medical condition (APA, 2000).

Excessive sleepiness interferes with attention, concentration, memory, and productivity. It can also lead to disruption in social and family relationships. Depression is a common side effect of hypersomnia, as are substance-related disorders, particularly those related to self-medication with stimulants (APA, 2000).

Approximately 5 to 10 percent of individuals who present to sleep disorders clinics with complaints of daytime sleepiness are diagnosed as having primary hypersomnia (APA, 2000). The disorder usually begins in late adolescence or early adulthood and is more common in men than in women.

Narcolepsy is a disorder similar to hypersomnia. Both produce excessive sleepiness, have similar age at onset, and run the same stable course over time. The characteristic manifestation of narcolepsy is sleep attacks. The individual cannot prevent falling asleep. He or she may be in the middle of a task or even in the middle of a sentence when the attack occurs. Associated with the attack in 50 to 70 percent of the cases is cataplexy, a sudden loss of muscle tone, such as jaw drop, head drop, weakness of the knees, or paralysis of all skeletal muscles with collapse (Sadock & Sadock, 2003). The episode is followed by full return of muscle strength. Individuals with narcolepsy are at risk for injury to self or others if they participate in dangerous activities, such as driving an automobile or operating dangerous machinery.

The onset of narcolepsy occurs most frequently in late adolescence or early adulthood. Clinical history may reveal, however, that excessive sleepiness may have been present in childhood. The disorder is equally common in men and women.

Parasomnias

Parasomnias are unusual to undesirable behaviors that occur during sleep. Examples of parasomnias include nightmares, sleep terrors, and sleepwalking.

Nightmare Disorder. Nightmares are frightening dreams that lead to awakenings from sleep (APA, 2000). Nightmare disorder is diagnosed when there is a repeated occurrence of the frightening dreams, which interferes with social or occupational functioning.

Content of the nightmares usually relates to imminent physical danger to the individual, personal failure or embarrassment, or the replication of a traumatic experience. They occur during rapid eye movement (REM) sleep and can occur at any time during that sleep episode. The individual is usually fully alert upon awakening from the nightmare and, because of lingering fear or anxiety, may have difficulty returning to sleep.

Nightmares are not uncommon between the ages of 3 and 6 years, and most children outgrow the phenomenon. Many adults report an occasional nightmare, but the incidence of nightmare disorder is not known.

Sleep Terror Disorder. The manifestations of sleep terrors include abrupt arousal from sleep with a piercing scream or cry. The individual is difficult to awaken or comfort, and if wakefulness does occur, the individual is usually disoriented and expresses a sense of intense fear but cannot recall the dream episode. On awakening in the morning, the individual has amnesia for the whole experience.

Sleep terrors are closely associated with sleepwalking, and often a night terror episode progresses into a sleepwalking episode (Sadock & Sadock, 2003). Approximately 1 to 6 percent of children experience sleep terrors, and the incidence appears to be more common in boys than in girls. Resolution usually occurs spontaneously during adolescence (APA, 2000). If the disorder begins in adulthood, it usually runs a chronic course.

Sleepwalking. The disorder of sleepwalking is characterized by the performance of motor activity initiated during sleep in which the individual may leave the bed and walk about, dress, go to the bathroom, talk, scream, or even drive (Sadock & Sadock, 2003). Episodes may last from a few minutes to a half hour. Most often the person returns to bed and has no memory of the event upon awakening. Occasionally, the individual may awaken during the episode, experiencing several minutes of confusion and disorientation. Individuals with sleepwalking disorder are at risk of injuring themselves or others.

The incidence of sleepwalking disorder among children ranges from 1 to 5 percent. Onset most commonly occurs between ages 4 and 8 years and usually subsides spontaneously during adolescence. The disorder is equally common in boys and girls. Sleepwalking episodes can occur as isolated behaviors at any age.

Circadian Rhythm Sleep Disorders

Circadian rhythm sleep disorders can be described as a misalignment between sleep and waking behaviors. The normal sleep–wake schedule is disrupted from its usual circadian rhythm. The individual is unable to sleep (or be awake) when he or she wants to sleep (or be awake), but can do so at other times. Sleep–wake schedule disturbances are common among shift workers and airplane travelers.

Shift Work Type. The disorder is common in shift workers who experience rapid and repeated changes in their work schedules. Many rotating-shift workers sleep fewer hours and have more disturbances in their sleep patterns than those shift workers who maintain a night or evening routine. Social and family demands, as well as environmental disturbances (e.g., telephone, traffic noise), during intended sleep times also interfere with these individuals' ability to achieve adequate sleep (APA, 2000).

Jet Lag Type. Airplane travel contributes to sleep–wake schedule disturbances when individuals travel through a number of time zones in a short period of time. This phenomenon is commonly called *jet lag*, which arises from conflict between the pattern of sleep and wakefulness generated by the circadian system and the pattern of sleep and wakefulness required by a new time zone (APA, 2000). Advancing the sleep–wake cycle (travel from west to east) appears to be more difficult for most people than delaying the sleep–wake cycle (travel from east to west).

Delayed Sleep Phase Type. In this type of circadian rhythm disorder, the individual's sleep and wake times are later than usual or than desired. He or she is unable to fall asleep at what would be considered the conventional time. Symptoms may mimic sleep onset insomnia. The individual has no difficulty maintaining sleep once it has begun. However, even with multiple alarm clocks, he or she has a great deal of difficulty awakening at a conventional time or at a time required to meet social or occupational obligations (APA, 2000).

Predisposing Factors to Sleep Disorders

Various factors have been shown to predispose individuals to sleep disorders. Genetic or familial patterns are thought to play a contributing role in primary insomnia, primary hypersomnia, narcolepsy, sleep terror disorder, and sleepwalking.

A number of medical conditions, as well as aging, have been implicated in the etiology of insomnia. They include pain; sleep apnea syndrome; restless leg syndrome; the use of, or withdrawal from, substances (including alcohol); endocrine or metabolic disorders; infectious, neoplastic, or other diseases; and CNS lesions (Sadock & Sadock, 2003).

Medical conditions associated with hypersomnia include metabolic and encephalitic conditions, the use of alcohol or other CNS depressants, withdrawal from stimulants, sleep apneas, and hypoventilation syndromes (Sadock & Sadock, 2003).

Psychiatric or environmental conditions that can contribute to insomnia or hypersomnia include anxiety, depression, environmental changes, circadian rhythm sleep disturbances, posttraumatic stress disorder, and schizophrenia (Sadock & Sadock, 2003).

Night terrors may be related to minor neurological abnormalities, particularly in the temporal lobe. Onset of sleep terror episodes in adolescence or early adulthood often prove to be the initial symptoms of temporal lobe epilepsy (Sadock & Sadock, 2003). The use of alcohol or other CNS depressants, sleep deprivation, sleep–wake disruptions, fatigue, and physical or emotional stress increase the incidence of episodes of night terrors (APA, 2000). Episodes of sleepwalking are exacerbated by extreme fatigue and sleep deprivation.

Activities that interfere with the 24-hour circadian rhythm of hormonal and neurotransmitter functioning within the body predispose individuals to sleep–wake schedule disturbances. See Chapter 4 for a more detailed explanation of the relationship between circadian rhythm and sleep.

Diagnosis/Outcome Identification

Nursing diagnoses are formulated from the data gathered during the assessment phase and with background knowledge regarding predisposing factors to the disorder. Common nursing diagnoses for clients with sleep disorders include:

Disturbed sleep pattern related to (specific medical condition); use of, or withdrawal from, substances; anxiety or depression; circadian rhythm disruption; familial patterns; evidenced by insomnia, hypersomnia, nightmares, sleep terrors, or sleepwalking.

Risk for injury related to excessive sleepiness, sleep terrors, or sleepwalking.

The following criteria may be used to measure outcomes in the care of the client with sleep disorders.

The client:

1. Has not experienced injury.
2. Verbalizes understanding of the sleep disorder.
3. Demonstrates individually appropriate interventions that promote sleep.
4. Adjusts lifestyle to accommodate alteration in biological rhythms.
5. Demonstrates improvement in sleep patterns.
6. Reports increased sense of well-being and feeling rested.

Planning/Implementation

Table 31–11 provides a plan of care for the client with a sleep disorder. Nursing diagnoses are presented, along with outcome criteria, appropriate nursing interventions, and rationales.

The concept map care plan is an innovative approach to planning and organizing nursing care (see Chapter 9). It is a diagrammatic teaching and learning strategy that allows visualization of interrelationships between medical diagnoses, nursing diagnoses, assessment data, and treatments. An example of a concept map care plan for a client with a sleep disorder is presented in Figure 31–9.

TABLE 31–11	Care Plan for the Client with a Sleep Disorder

NURSING DIAGNOSIS: DISTURBED SLEEP PATTERN
RELATED TO: Use of, or withdrawal from, substances; anxiety or depression; circadian rhythm disruption; familial patterns; or specific medical condition
EVIDENCED BY: Insomnia, hypersomnia, nightmares, sleep terrors, or sleepwalking

OUTCOME CRITERIA	NURSING INTERVENTIONS	RATIONALE
Client will be able to achieve adequate, uninterrupted sleep. Client will report feeling rested and demonstrate a sensation of well-being.	1. To promote sleep: a. Encourage activities that prepare one for sleep: soft music, relaxation exercises, warm bath. b. Discourage strenuous exercise within 1 hr of bedtime. c. Control intake of caffeine-containing substances within 4 hr of bedtime (e.g., coffee, tea, colas, chocolate, and certain analgesic medications). d. Provide a high-carbohydrate snack before bedtime.	a. These activities promote relaxation. b. Strenuous exercise can be stimulating and keep one awake. c. Caffeine is a CNS stimulant and can interfere with the promotion of sleep. d. Carbohydrates increase the levels of the amino acid tryptophan, a precursor to the neurotransmitter serotonin. Serotonin is thought to play a role in the promotion of sleep.

(Continued on opposite page)

	e. Keep the temperature of the room between 68° and 72° F.	e. This range provides the temperature most conducive to sleep.
	f. Instruct the client not to use alcoholic beverages to relax.	f. Although alcohol may initially induce drowsiness and promote falling asleep, a rebound stimulation occurs in the CNS within several hours after drinking alcohol. The individual may fall asleep, only to be wide awake a few hours later.
	g. Discourage smoking and use of other tobacco products near sleep time.	g. Tobacco products produce a stimulant effect on the CNS.
	h. Discourage daytime napping. Increase program of activities to keep the person busy.	h. Sleeping during the day can interfere with the ability to achieve sleep at night.
	i. Individuals with chronic insomnia should use sleeping medications judiciously.	i. Sedatives and hypnotics have serious side effects and are highly addicting. Life-threatening symptoms can occur with abrupt withdrawal and discontinuation should be tapered under a physician's supervision. Long-term use can result in rebound insomnia.
	2. To prevent "jet lag" circadian rhythm disruption:	
	a. If time permits, use a preventive strategy of altering mealtimes and sleep times in the appropriate direction.	a. This strategy will prepare the body for the oncoming change.
	b. If preventive measures are impossible, increase the amount of sleep upon arrival.	b. This may help to reduce fatigue and restore the rested feeling.
	c. Provide short-term use of sleep medication by physician's order.	c. May provide restful sleep when other measures are unsuccessful.

NURSING DIAGNOSIS: RISK FOR INJURY
RELATED TO: Excessive sleepiness, sleep terrors, or sleepwalking

OUTCOME CRITERIA	NURSING INTERVENTIONS	RATIONALE
Client will not experience injury.	1. Ensure that siderails are up on the bed.	1. An individual who experiences serious nightmares or night terrors can fall from the bed during an episode.
	2. Keep the bed in a low position.	2. To diminish the risk of injury by the person who gets out of bed during a sleepwalking episode.
	3. Equip the bed with a bell (or other audible device) that is activated when the bed is exited.	3. This may alert the caretaker so that supervision to prevent accidental injury can be instituted.
	4. Keep a night light on and arrange the furniture in the bedroom in a manner that promotes safety.	4. To provide a safe environment for the individual who awakens (fully or partially) during the night.
	5. Administer drug therapy as ordered (see "Treatment Modalities"). For the child who experiences nightmares, encourage him or her to talk about the dream. Tell the child that all people have dreams. Validate his or her feeling of fearfulness while ensuring safety. Keep a light on in the room or give the child a flashlight.	5. Talking about the dream helps to promote the unreality of the dream and to differentiate between what is real and what is not real. Light gives the child a feeling of control over the darkness within the room.

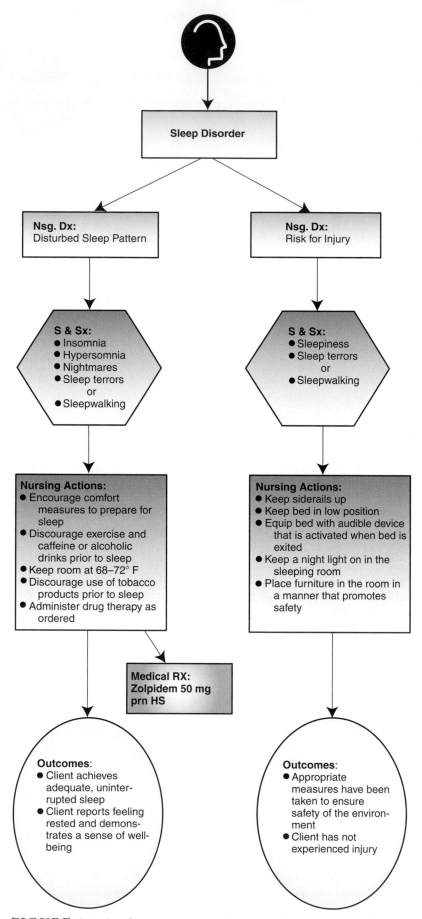

FIGURE 31–9 Concept map care plan for a client with a sleep disorder.

Evaluation

Reassessment is conducted in order to determine if the nursing actions have been successful in achieving the objectives of care. Evaluation of the nursing actions for the client with a sleep disorder may be facilitated by gathering information using the following types of questions.

1. Is the client free from injury?
2. Have appropriate measures been taken to ensure that the environment has been made as risk-free from injury as possible?
3. Can the client verbalize knowledge about his or her sleep disorder and understand possible causes?
4. Does the client demonstrate appropriate interventions that promote sleep? Can he or she verbalize activities and behaviors that may interfere with the promotion of sleep?
5. Does the pattern of sleep indicate improvement since the beginning of treatment?
6. Does the client report feeling rested and demonstrate a noticeable sense of well- being?

Table 31–12 presents topics for client/family education related to somatoform and sleep disorders.

TREATMENT MODALITIES

Somatoform Disorders

Clients with somatoform disorders are difficult to treat. The typical clinical picture of recurrent, multiple, vague symptoms combined with "doctor-shopping" and frequent requests for time and attention may generate frustration and anger in the physician. Many clients with these disorders ignore referrals to psychiatrists, and those who do follow through rarely persist with the treatment. Thus, the majority of care for these clients continues to rest with other physicians, even though psychiatric consultation has been shown to reduce both extent and cost of medical care.

Individual Psychotherapy

The goal of psychotherapy is to help clients develop healthy and adaptive behaviors, encourage them to move beyond their somatization, and manage their lives more effectively. The focus is on personal and social difficulties that the client is experiencing in daily life as well as the achievement of practical solutions for these difficulties.

Treatment is initiated with a complete physical examination to rule out organic pathology. Once this has been ensured, the physician turns his or her attention to the client's social and personal problems and away from the somatic complaints.

In the case of conversion disorder, the therapist will attempt to identify precipitating stressors and conflicts.

TABLE 31–12   Topics for Client/Family Education Related to Somatoform and Sleep Disorders

Nature of the Illness
1. Define and describe symptoms of:
   a. Somatization disorder
   b. Pain disorder
   c. Hypochondriasis
   d. Conversion disorder
   e. Body dysmorphic disorder
   f. Primary insomnia or hypersomnia
   g. Parasomnias
   h. Circadian rhythm sleep disorders
2. Discuss etiologies of above disorders

Management of the Illness
1. Ways to identify onset of escalating anxiety
2. Ways to intervene to prevent exacerbation of physical symptom
3. Assertiveness techniques
4. Relaxation techniques
5. Physical activities
6. Ways to increase feelings of control and decrease feelings of powerlessness
7. Pain management
8. Family: How to prevent reinforcing the illness
9. Ways to minimize sleep–wake circadian rhythm cycle
10. Activities to promote sleep
    a. Soft music
    b. Relaxation exercises
    c. Warm bath
    d. Control caffeine intake
    e. Pre-bedtime high carbohydrate snack
    f. Control temperature of bedroom.
    g. Discourage use of alcohol and tobacco.
    h. Discourage daytime napping.
    i. Encourage regular daytime exercise.
11. Family with member who sleepwalks: Ways to prevent injury.
12. Pharmacology:
    a. For pain:
       (1) Aspirin
       (2) Nonsteroidal anti-inflammatory agents (NSAIDs)
       (3) Some antidepressants
    b. For insomnia:
       (1) Benzodiazepines
       (2) Zaleplon
       (3) Zolpidem
       (4) Eszopiclone
    c. For hypersomnia/narcolepsy:
       (1) CNS stimulants
       (2) Selective serotonin reuptake inhibitors (SSRIs)

Support Services
1. Support groups
2. Individual psychotherapy
3. Biofeedback

He or she may be assisted in this effort by the use of hypnosis and narcoanalysis (Amytal interview). These techniques consist of placing the client in a relaxed state and, through questioning and suggestion, allowing him or her to re-experience the precipitating stress and fully reliving the repressed emotions, thereby freeing the client of the psychological need for the symptom.

Psychotherapy appears to be useful with very few hypochondriacal clients. Treatment consists of a complete medical examination by the primary physician to rule out organic pathology. Because most people with hypochondriasis are opposed to psychiatric treatment, the best approach seems to be a supportive and accepting relationship with a general medical practitioner who tolerates the client's behavior without judgment and who is available during periods of distress and increased symptoms. This type of support can help to minimize incapacitating anxiety, "doctor-shopping," and further regression.

Group Psychotherapy

Group therapy may be helpful for somatoform disorders because it provides a setting where clients can share their experiences of illness, can learn to verbalize thoughts and feelings, and can be confronted by group members and leaders when they reject responsibility for maladaptive behaviors. It has been reported to be the treatment of choice for both somatization disorder and hypochondriasis, in part because it provides the social support and social interaction that these clients need.

Behavior Therapy

Behavior therapy is more likely to be successful in instances when secondary gain is prominent. This may involve working with the client's family or other significant others who may be perpetuating the physical symptoms by rewarding passivity and dependency and by being overly solicitous and helpful. Behavioral therapy focuses on teaching these individuals to reward the client's autonomy, self-sufficiency, and independence. This process becomes more difficult when the client is very regressed and the sick role well established.

Psychopharmacology

Tricyclic antidepressants (TCAs) are often used with somatoform pain disorder. All of the TCAs appear to be equally analgesic; however, amitriptyline, with its strong sedative effect, may be of benefit for clients with chronic pain whose sleep is significantly impaired by the pain (King, 2003). They often provide pain relief at a dosage below that used to treat depression. The selective serotonin reuptake inhibitors (SSRIs) paroxetine (Paxil), fluoxetine (Prozac), sertraline (Zoloft), and fluvoxamine (Luvox) have been studied for their analgesic effects, but have been found to be somewhat less efficacious than the tricyclics with which they were compared (King, 2003). Extended-release venlafaxine (Effexor XR) has been efficacious as an analgesic, and King (2003) states:

> Extended-release venlafaxine (Effexor XR) [may be considered] the second-line antidepressant for analgesia for patients who are unable to tolerate TCAs or for whom these medications are contraindicated because of the presence of other medical conditions, such as cardiac disease. (p. 1038)

Anticonvulsants such as phenytoin (Dilantin), carbamazepine (Tegretol), and clonazepam (Klonopin) have been reported to be effective in treating neuropathic and neuralgic pain, at least for short periods. Their efficacy in other somatoform pain disorders is less clear.

Sleep Disorders

Primary Insomnia

Relaxation Therapy

Relaxation therapies can be helpful in the treatment of chronic insomnia. Self-hypnosis, meditation, deep breathing, and progressive muscle relaxation are effective (Karren et al., 2002). Success with these interventions requires a great deal of practice and motivation on the part of the client.

Biofeedback

Biofeedback has been used with success in some clients (Neylan, Reynolds, & Kupfer, 2003). The use of a biological variable, such as electromyography or electroencephalography, helps these clients increase sensitivity to their internal state of arousal.

Pharmacotherapy

The efficacy of medications in the treatment of insomnia cannot be disputed. When used judiciously, sedatives and hypnotics produce the calming effect needed for many individuals to achieve much needed sleep. These medications are CNS depressants that, with long-term use, have the capacity for psychological and physiological dependence. The most commonly used group is the benzodiazepines. Some of those most frequently used include flurazepam (Dalmane), temazepam (Restoril), and triazolam (Halcion). Nonbenzodiazepines frequently used include zolpidem (Ambien), zaleplon (Sonata), and eszopiclone (Lunesta). Common side effects of these medications include headache, dizziness, confusion, impairment of cognitive and psychomotor skills, and nausea. Caution is required in using these drugs with elderly clients, since they have reduced clearance of hypnotics and hence experience more sedation and cognitive side effects than younger clients (Sadock & Sadock, 2003). Gradual discontinuation and tapering of the dosage is required with all long-term users to diminish the risk of withdrawal symptoms and rebound insomnia.

Primary Hypersomnia/Narcolepsy

Pharmacotherapy

The usual treatment for hypersomnolence is with CNS stimulants such as amphetamines (Sadock & Sadock,

2003). In some instances, the nonsedating SSRIs may be helpful with this problem.

Narcolepsy is also treated with CNS stimulants, such as amphetamine or methylphenidate. Tricyclic antidepressants have been effective in the treatment of symptoms of cataplexy.

Parasomnias

Treatment of parasomnias usually centers around measures to relieve obvious stress within the family. Individual or family therapy is sometimes useful. Interventions to prevent injury are required. In severe cases, pharmacological intervention may be instituted with tricyclic antidepressants or low-dose benzodiazepines.

Sleep–Wake Schedule Disturbances

Disturbances of the sleep–wake cycle are usually treated with behavior modification; that is, the individual trains himself or herself to adapt to the change in schedule. Phototherapy (also called "bright light" therapy) has been shown to be effective in treating delayed sleep phase disorder and jet lag (Sadock & Sadock, 2003). Typically, individuals require 30 minutes to 2 hours of daily exposure to bright light to achieve a therapeutic response.

SUMMARY

Somatoform disorders, known historically as hysteria, affect about 1 or 2 percent of the female population. There is a higher prevalence rate among the lower socioeconomic groups and the less educated. Somatoform disorders include somatization disorder, pain disorder, hypochondriasis, conversion disorder, and body dysmorphic disorder.

The person with somatization disorder has physical symptoms that may be vague, dramatized, or exaggerated in their presentation. No evidence of organic pathology can be identified. In pain disorder, the predominant symptom is pain, for which there is either no medical explanation or for which the symptom is exaggerated out of proportion to what would be the expected reaction.

Psychological factors can be identified as contributing to the symptom. Individuals with these disorders commonly have long histories of "doctor shopping" in search of validation of their symptoms.

Hypochondriasis is an unrealistic preoccupation with fear of having a serious illness. This disorder may follow a personal experience, or the experience of a close family member, with serious or life-threatening illness.

The individual with conversion disorder experiences a loss of or alteration in bodily functioning, unsubstantiated by medical or pathophysiological explanation. Psychological factors are evident by the primary or secondary gains the individual achieves from experiencing the physiological manifestation. A relative lack of concern regarding the symptom is identified as "la belle indifference."

Body dysmorphic disorder, formerly called dysmorphophobia, is the exaggerated belief that the body is deformed or defective in some way. It may be related to more serious psychiatric illness.

Sleep disorders include primary insomnia, primary hypersomnia, parasomnias, and sleep–wake schedule disturbances. Clients with primary insomnia have difficulty initiating or maintaining sleep. Primary hypersomnia manifests as excessive amounts of sleep and excessive daytime sleepiness.

Parasomnias include nightmare disorder, sleep terror disorder, and sleepwalking. These disorders primarily begin in childhood but can also affect adults.

Circadian rhythm sleep disorders occur when there is a disruption in an individual's regular pattern of fluctuation in physiology that is linked to the 24-hour light–dark cycle. This commonly occurs in individuals whose jobs require rotating shifts and in those who frequently travel long distances over a short period of time (commonly called "jet lag").

Various modalities have been implemented in the treatment of somatoform and sleep disorders, including individual psychotherapy, group psychotherapy, behavior therapy, and psychopharmacology. Nursing care is accomplished using the steps of the nursing process. Nurses can assist clients with these disorders by helping them to understand their problems and identify and establish new, more adaptive behavior patterns.

INTERNET REFERENCES

Additional information about sleep disorders may be located at the following Web sites:

- http://www.sleepnet.com/disorder.htm
- http://sleepdisorders.about.com/
- http://www.nhlbi.nih.gov/about/ncsdr/

Information about medications for sleep disorders may be located at the following Web sites:

- http://www.laurus.com/library/healthguide/en-us/drug-guide/default.htm

- http://www.nlm.nih.gov/medlineplus
- http://www.fadavis.com/townsend

Additional information about somatoform disorders may be located at the following Web sites:

- http://www.psyweb.com/Mdisord/somatd.html
- http://www.uib.no/med/avd/med_a/gastro/wilhelms/hypochon.html
- http://www.emedicine.com/EMERG/topic112.Htm
- http://www.findarticles.com/cf_dls/g2601/0012/2601001276/p1/article.jhtml

---

IMPLICATIONS OF RESEARCH FOR EVIDENCE-BASED PRACTICE

Tworoger, S.S., Yasui, Y., Vitiello, M.V., Schwartz, R.S., Ulrich, C.M., Aiello, E.J., Irwin, M.L., Bowen, D., Potter, J.D., & McTierman, A. (2003). Effects of a year-long moderate-intensity exercise and a stretching intervention on sleep quality in postmenopausal women. *Sleep 26(7), 830–836.*

Description of the Study: The objective of this study was to examine the effects of a moderate-intensity exercise or stretching intervention and changes in fitness, body mass index, or time spent outdoors, on self-reported sleep quality and to examine the relationship between the amount and timing of exercise and sleep quality. The study took place in a cancer research center in Seattle, Washington. The participants included 173 postmenopausal, overweight or obese, sedentary women not taking hormone replacement therapy recruited from the Seattle metropolitan area. Ages ranged from 50 to 75 years. Eighty-seven participated in the exercise program (usually a 30-minute brisk walk) and 86 participated in the stretching intervention.

Results of the Study: Among the participants who exercised during the morning hours, those who exercised at least 225 minutes per week had less trouble falling asleep compared

with those who exercised less than 180 minutes per week. Conversely, among participants who exercised during the evening hours, those who exercised at least 225 minutes per week had more trouble falling asleep compared with those who exercised less than 180 minutes per week. Individuals who participated in the stretching intervention were less likely to use sleep medication or have trouble falling asleep during the intervention compared with baseline. Reductions in body mass index and increases in time spent outdoors had inconsistent effects on sleep quality.

Implications for Nursing Practice: The authors suggest that both stretching and moderate exercise may improve sleep quality in sedentary, overweight, postmenopausal women. In this study, increased fitness was associated with improvements in sleep. However, the effect of moderate-intensity exercise appears to depend on the amount of exercise and time of day it is performed. This study has nursing implications for educating individuals about the importance of a regular exercise program, not only on fitness but also on quality of sleep. It is important that clients understand that exercise is more beneficial to sleep if undertaken earlier in the day rather than in the evening hours.

IMPLICATIONS OF RESEARCH FOR EVIDENCE-BASED PRACTICE

Visser, S., & Bouman, T.K. (2001). The treatment of hypochondriasis: Exposure plus response prevention vs cognitive therapy. *Behavior Research and Therapy 39,* 423–442.

Description of the Study: This study was conducted to determine whether short-term cognitive-behavioral therapy can help clients with hypochondriasis. Two treatments were employed: (1) exposure plus response prevention (exposure to hypochondriacal fears; prevention of reassurance seeking, checking, and avoidance), and (2) cognitive therapy (systematic monitoring, evaluation, and testing of hypochondriacal beliefs and interpretations of bodily sensations). Seventy-eight outpatients with primary diagnoses of hypochondriasis were randomized into three groups: a control group or one of the two treatment groups. Medications were discontinued or held at constant dosages during the study.

Results of the Study: No changes in outcome scores were observed in the control group. Compared with controls, active-treatment clients achieved significant reductions in hypochondriacal concerns and behaviors, depression, and overall mood disruption. No significant differences were found between the two treatment groups.

Implications for Nursing Practice: Some nurses, particularly Advanced Practice Nurses, practice cognitive-behavioral therapy (CBT). These nurses should understand the importance of this type of therapy with clients who have hypochondriasis. It is also important for generalist nurses to understand the concepts of CBT, so that they may use these concepts in their therapeutic interactions with clients with hypochondriasis. This study has important implications for nursing practice.

TEST YOUR CRITICAL THINKING SKILLS

Ricky, age 11, was recently hospitalized on the psychiatric unit for evaluation. His parents stated to the nurse, "We are beside ourselves about what to do with him." They explained that Ricky has been sleepwalking almost nightly for the last 2 months. Before that, he had experienced an occasional episode (perhaps three per year at the most) beginning at about age 7. During sleepwalking, Ricky seldom awakens, and when he does, he appears confused and just returns to bed and sleep. In the morning he has no memory of the episode. Several times his parents have found him wandering around the front yard. They called the physician today after finding him riding his bicycle down the middle of the street in the middle of the night last night. Ricky says he cannot remember the incident. His parents are afraid for Ricky's safety.

Answer the following questions related to Ricky:

1. What is the *priority* nursing consideration when caring for Ricky?
2. Describe some nursing interventions that may be implemented for the consideration in Question 1.
3. What treatment might you expect the physician to prescribe for Ricky?

REVIEW QUESTIONS

SELF-EXAMINATION/LEARNING EXERCISE

For each situation select the answer that is most appropriate for the questions that follow.

Situation: Amy, age 24, was selected to represent the local children's home in the upcoming 26-mile marathon. If she wins, the children's home gets the new playground equipment they want so badly. If she loses, they will have to wait until another financial source can be located. Amy wants desperately to win for them. The morning of the race, she falls when she tries to get out of bed. She discovers her right leg is paralyzed.

1. Amy's mother takes her to the emergency department. Her physician is notified. It is likely that his initial intervention will be to:
   a. Prescribe an antianxiety medication.
   b. Rule out organic pathology.
   c. Refer her to the rehabilitation clinic.
   d. Refer her to a psychiatrist.

2. Amy shows a relative lack of concern for her sudden paralysis, even though her athletic abilities have always been a source of pride to her. This manifestation is known as:
   a. Tardive dyskinesia.
   b. Secondary gain.
   c. Malingering.
   d. "La belle indifference."

3. Amy is admitted to the psychiatric unit with a diagnosis of conversion disorder. The primary nursing diagnosis for Amy would be:
   a. Self-care deficit related to inability to walk without assistance.
   b. Severe anxiety related to fear of losing the race.
   c. Ineffective coping related to severe anxiety.
   d. Fear related to lack of confidence in her athletic ability.

4. Which of the following nursing interventions would be most appropriate for Amy?
   a. Promote Amy's dependence, so that unfulfilled dependency needs can be met.
   b. Encourage her to discuss her feelings about the paralysis.
   c. Explain to her that the paralysis is not "real."
   d. Promote independence and withdraw attention when she continues to focus on the paralysis.

5. Conversion symptoms provide primary and secondary gains for the individuals experiencing them. Which of the following is an example of a primary gain for Amy?
   a. Allows her to receive additional personal attention.
   b. Allows her to be totally dependent on others.
   c. Allows her an acceptable excuse for not running in the race.
   d. Allows her to feel more accepted and cared for by others.

Situation: Lorraine is a frequent visitor to the outpatient clinic. She has been diagnosed with somatization disorder.

6. Which of the following symptom profiles would you expect when assessing Lorraine?
   a. Multiple somatic symptoms in several body systems
   b. Fear of having a serious disease
   c. Loss or alteration in sensorimotor functioning
   d. Belief that the body is deformed or defective in some way

7. Which of the following ego defense mechanisms describes the underlying dynamics of somatization disorder?
   a. Denial of depression
   b. Repression of anxiety
   c. Suppression of grief
   d. Displacement of anger

8. Nursing care for Lorraine would focus on helping her to:
   a. Eliminate the stress in her life.
   b. Discontinue her numerous physical complaints.
   c. Take her medication only as prescribed.
   d. Learn more adaptive coping strategies.

9. Lorraine states, "My doctor thinks I should see a psychiatrist. I can't imagine why he would make such a suggestion?" What is the basis for Lorraine's statement?
   a. She thinks her doctor wants to get rid of her as a client.
   b. She does not understand the correlation of symptoms and stress.
   c. She thinks psychiatrists are only for "crazy" people.
   d. She thinks her doctor has made an error in diagnosis.

10. Lorraine tells the nurse about a pain in her side. She says she has not experienced it before. Which is the most appropriate response by the nurse?
   a. "I don't want to hear about another physical complaint. You know they are all in your head. It's time for group therapy now."
   b. "Let's sit down here together and you can tell me about this new pain you are experiencing. You'll just have to miss group therapy today."
   c. "I will report this pain to your physician. In the meantime, group therapy starts in 5 minutes. You must leave now to be on time."
   d. "I will call your physician and see if he will order a new pain medication for your side. The one you have now doesn't seem to provide relief. Why don't you get some rest for now?"

REFERENCES

American Psychiatric Association. (2000). *Diagnostic and statistical manual of mental disorders.* (4th ed.) *Text revision.* Washington, DC: American Psychiatric Association.

Goodwin, D.W., & Guze, S.B. (1997). *Psychiatric diagnosis* (5th ed.). New York: Oxford University Press.

Karren, K.J., Hafen, B.Q., Smith, N.L., & Frandsen, K.J. (2002). *Mind/body health: The effects of attitudes, emotions, and relationships.* San Francisco: Benjamin Cummings.

King, S.A. (2003). Pain disorders. In R.E. Hales and S.C. Yudofsky (Eds.). *Textbook of clinical psychiatry.* Washington, DC: American Psychiatric Publishing.

National Sleep Foundation (NSF). (2005). 2002–2005 Sleep in America Polls. Washington, DC: NSF.

Neylan, T.C., Reynolds, C.F., & Kupfer, D.J. (2003). Sleep disorders. In R.E. Hales and S.C. Yudofsky (Eds.). *Textbook of clinical psychiatry* (4th ed.). Washington, DC: American Psychiatric Publishing.

Noyes, R., Holt, C.S., & Happel, R.L. (1997). A family study of hypochondriasis. *Journal of Nervous and Mental Disease, 185*(4), 223–232.

Sadock, B.J., & Sadock, V.A. (2003). *Synopsis of psychiatry: Behavioral sciences/clinical psychiatry* (9th ed.). Philadelphia: Lippincott Williams & Wilkins.

Soares, N., & Grossman, L. (2003, February 7). Somatoform disorder: Conversion. *Emedicine Journal, 2*(9). Retrieved April 17, 2005 from the World Wide Web at http://www.emedicine.com/PED/topic2780.htm

Yutzy, S.H. (2003). Somatoform disorders. In R.E. Hales & S.C. Yudofsky (Eds.). *Textbook of clinical psychiatry* (4th ed.). Washington, DC: American Psychiatric Publishing.

32
CHAPTER

DISSOCIATIVE DISORDERS

CHAPTER OUTLINE

KEY TERMS

abreaction
depersonalization
derealization
directed association

free association
fugue
hypnosis
integration

CORE CONCEPTS

amnesia
dissociation

OBJECTIVES

After reading this chapter, the student will be able to:

1. Discuss historical aspects and epidemiological statistics related to dissociative disorders.
2. Describe various types of dissociative disorders and identify symptomatology associated with each; use this information in client assessment.
3. Identify predisposing factors in the development of dissociative disorders.
4. Formulate nursing diagnoses and goals of care for clients with dissociative disorders.

5. Describe appropriate nursing interventions for clients with dissociative disorders.
6. Identify topics for client and family teaching relevant to dissociative disorders.
7. Evaluate nursing care of clients with dissociative disorders.
8. Discuss various modalities relevant to treatment of dissociative disorders.

he *DSM-IV-TR* describes the essential feature of dissociative disorders as a disruption in the usually integrated functions of consciousness, memory, identity, or perception (American Psychiatric Association [APA], 2000). Dissociative responses occur when anxiety becomes overwhelming and the personality becomes disorganized. Defense mechanisms that normally govern consciousness, identity, and memory break down, and behavior occurs with little or no participation on the part of the conscious personality. Four types of dissociative disorders are described by the *DSM-IV-TR*: dissociative amnesia, dissociative fugue, dissociative identity disorder, and depersonalization disorder.

This chapter focuses on disorders characterized by severe anxiety that has been repressed and is being expressed in the form of dissociative behavior. In these clients, certain mental contents are removed from consciousness to protect the ego from experiencing the painful anxiety. Historical and epidemiological statistics are presented. Predisposing factors that have been implicated in the etiology of dissociative disorders provide a framework for studying the dynamics of dissociative amnesia, dissociative fugue, dissociative identity disorder, and depersonalization disorder.

An explanation of the symptomatology is presented as background knowledge for assessing the client with a dissociative disorder. Nursing care is described in the con-

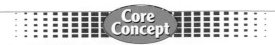

Dissociation
The splitting off of clusters of mental contents from conscious awareness, a mechanism central to hysterical conversion and dissociative disorder (Shahrokh & Hales, 2003).

text of the nursing process. Various medical treatment modalities are explored.

HISTORICAL ASPECTS

There was a great deal of interest in the phenomena of dissociative processes during the 19th century when the concept of dissociation was first formulated by the French physician and psychologist Pierre Janet. He used it to explain the myriad bizarre symptoms of hysteria, which he characterized as "a form of mental disintegration characterized by a tendency toward the permanent and complete undoubling of consciousness" (Janet, 1907).

Freud (1962) viewed dissociation as a type of repression, an active defense mechanism used to remove threatening or unacceptable mental contents from conscious awareness. He also described the defense of splitting of the ego in the management of incompatible mental contents.

Professional interest in the dissociative disorders waned after the turn of the century but has recently been revived, with the study of dissociative identity disorder in particular achieving a level surpassing all previous periods. Despite the fact that Janet pioneered the study of dissociative processes in the 1890s, scientists still know remarkably little about the phenomena. Are dissociative disorders psychopathological processes or ego-protective devices? Are dissociative processes under voluntary control, or are they a totally unconscious effort? The wide scope of current studies concerning the dissociative syndromes promises to lead to a more accurate picture of their scope, etiology, and underlying mechanisms.

EPIDEMIOLOGICAL STATISTICS

Dissociative syndromes are statistically quite rare, but when they do occur they may present very dramatic clinical pictures of severe disturbances in normal personality functioning. Dissociative amnesia is relatively rare, occurring most frequently under conditions of war or during natural disasters. However, in recent years, there has been an increase in the number of reported cases, possibly attributed to increased awareness of the phenomenon, and identification of cases that were previously

undiagnosed (APA, 2000). It appears to be more common in women than in men and in young than in older adults (Sadock & Sadock, 2003). Dissociative amnesia can occur at any age but is difficult to diagnose in children because it is easily confused with inattention or oppositional behavior.

Dissociative fugue is also rare and occurs most often under conditions of war, natural disasters, or intense psychosocial stress. Information regarding gender distribution and familial patterns of occurrence is not available.

Estimates of the prevalence of dissociative identity disorder (DID) vary widely. Sadock and Sadock (2003) report that perhaps as many as 5 percent of all patients with psychiatric disorders meet the criteria for DID. The disorder occurs from three to nine times more frequently in women than in men, and onset likely occurs in childhood, although manifestations of the disorder may not be recognized until much later (APA, 2000). Clinical symptoms usually are not recognized until late adolescence or early adulthood, although they have probably existed for a number of years prior to diagnosis (Sadock & Sadock, 2003). There appears to be some evidence that the disorder is more common in first-degree biological relatives of people with the disorder than in the general population.

The prevalence of severe episodes of depersonalization disorder is unknown, although single brief episodes of depersonalization may occur at some time in as many as half of all adults, particularly in the event of severe psychosocial stress (APA, 2000). Symptoms usually begin in adolescence or early adulthood. The disorder is chronic, with periods of remission and exacerbation. The incidence of depersonalization disorder is high under conditions of sustained traumatization, such as in military combat or prisoner-of-war camps. It has also been reported in many individuals who endure near-death experiences.

APPLICATION OF THE NURSING PROCESS

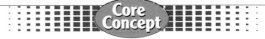

Amnesia
Pathologic loss of memory; a phenomenon in which an area of experience becomes inaccessible to conscious recall. The loss in memory may be organic, emotional, dissociative, or of mixed origin, and may be permanent or limited to a sharply circumscribed period of time (Shahrokh & Hales, 2003).

Dissociative Amnesia

Background Assessment Data

Dissociative amnesia is an inability to recall important personal information, usually of a traumatic or stressful nature, that is too extensive to be explained by ordinary forgetfulness and is not due to the direct effects of substance use or a neurological or other general medical condition (APA, 2000). Five types of disturbance in recall have been described. In the following examples, the individual is involved in a traumatic automobile accident in which a loved one is killed.

1. **Localized Amnesia.** The inability to recall all incidents associated with the traumatic event for a specific time period following the event (usually a few hours to a few days).

EXAMPLE:

The individual cannot recall events of the automobile accident and events occurring during a period after the accident (a few hours to a few days).

2. **Selective Amnesia.** The inability to recall only certain incidents associated with a traumatic event for a specific period after the event.

EXAMPLE:

The individual may not remember events leading to the impact of the accident but may remember being taken away in the ambulance.

3. **Continuous Amnesia.** The inability to recall events occurring after a specific time up to and including the present.

EXAMPLE:

The individual cannot remember events associated with the automobile accident and anything that has occurred since. That is, the individual cannot form new memories, even though apparently alert and aware.

4. **Generalized Amnesia.** The rare phenomenon of not being able to recall anything that has happened during the individual's entire lifetime, including his or her personal identity.

5. **Systematized Amnesia.** With this type of amnesia, the individual cannot remember events that relate to a specific category of information (e.g., one's family) or to one particular person or event.

The individual with amnesia usually appears alert and may give no indication to observers that anything is wrong, although at the onset of the episode there may be a brief period of disorganization or clouding of consciousness (Sadock & Sadock, 2003). Clients suffering from amnesia are often brought to general hospital emergency departments by police who have found them wandering confusedly around the streets.

Onset of an amnestic episode usually follows severe psychosocial stress. Termination is typically abrupt and followed by complete recovery. Recurrences are unusual. *DSM-IV-TR* diagnostic criteria for dissociative amnesia are presented in Table 32–1.

TABLE 32–1   Diagnostic Criteria for Dissociative Amnesia

A. The predominant disturbance is one or more episodes of inability to recall important personal information, usually of a traumatic or stressful nature, that is too extensive to be explained by ordinary forgetfulness.
B. The disturbance does not occur exclusively during the course of dissociative identity disorder, dissociative fugue, posttraumatic stress disorder, acute stress disorder, or somatization disorder and is not due to the direct physiological effect of a substance (e.g., a drug of abuse, a medication) or a neurological or other general medical condition (e.g., amnestic disorder due to head trauma).
C. The symptoms cause clinically significant distress or impairment in social, occupational, or other important areas of functioning.

SOURCE: American Psychiatric Association (2000), with permission.

Predisposing Factors to Dissociative Amnesia

Psychodynamic Theory

Freud (1962) described amnesia as the result of repression of distressing mental contents from conscious awareness. He believed the unconscious was a dynamic entity in which repressed mental contents were stored and unavailable to conscious recall. Current psychodynamic explanations of dissociation are based on Freud's concepts. The repression of mental contents is perceived as a coping mechanism for protecting the client from emotional pain that has arisen from either disturbing external circumstances or anxiety-provoking internal urges and feelings (Maldonado & Spiegel, 2003).

Behavioral Theory

Dissociative amnesia may also be explained by potential gains derived from the response. Reinforcement, in the form of primary and secondary gains for the individual, may contribute to the maladaptive functioning associated with this disorder. Primary gain from the amnesia would be protection from a painful emotional experience. Secondary gains may be derived from the gratifying responses of others that fulfill certain psychological needs and thus serve to maintain the amnesia after it is established.

Biological Theory

Some efforts have been made to explain dissociative amnesia on the basis of neurophysiological dysfunction. Areas of the brain that have been associated with memory include the hippocampus, amygdala, fornix, mammillary bodies, thalamus, and frontal cortex. Brunet, Holowka, and Laurence (2001) state:

Given the intimate relationship between dissociation, memory, and trauma, researchers have begun to investigate the brain structures and neurochemical systems that mediate functions. Several substances such as sodium-lactate, yohimbine, and metachlorophenylpiperazine have been shown to elicit dissociative symptoms in patients with PTSD or panic disorder, but not in normal controls. Such findings suggest a role for the locus coeruleus/noradrenergic system, which is implicated in fear and arousal regulation and influence a number of cortical structures such as the prefrontal, sensory and parietal cortex, the hippocampus, the hypothalamus, the amygdala, and the spinal cord. Still the relationship between trauma exposure, cortisol, hippocampus damage, memory, and dissociation is tentative at best, and remains to be thoroughly investigated. (p. 26)

Transactional Model of Stress/Adaptation

The etiology of dissociative amnesia is most likely influenced by multiple factors. In Figure 32–1 a graphic depiction of this theory of multiple causation is presented in the transactional model of stress/adaptation.

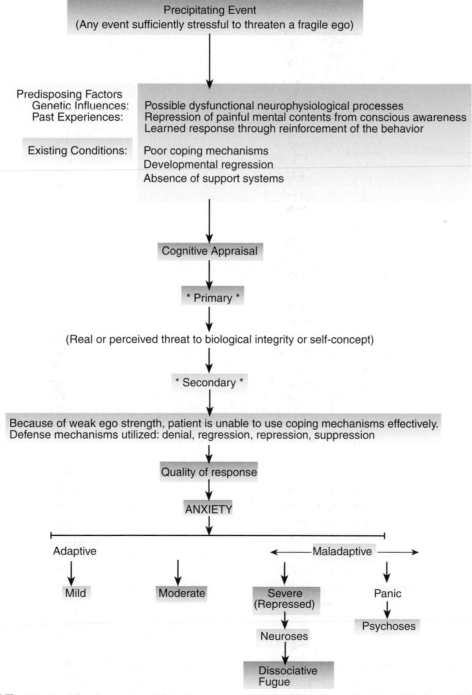

FIGURE 32-1   The dynamics of dissociative amnesia using the transactional model of stress/adaptation.

Diagnosis/Outcome Identification

Nursing diagnoses are formulated from the data gathered during the assessment phase and with background knowledge regarding predisposing factors to the disorder. The following nursing diagnoses may be used for the client with dissociative amnesia:

Disturbed thought processes related to severe psychological stress and repression of anxiety evidenced by loss of memory.

Powerlessness related to inability to cope effectively with severe anxiety evidenced by verbalizations of frustration over lack of control and dependence on others.

The following criteria may be used for measurement of outcomes in the care of the client with dissociative amnesia.

The client:

1. Can recall events associated with a traumatic or stressful situation.
2. Can recall all events of past life.
3. Can demonstrate more adaptive coping strategies to avert amnestic behaviors in the face of severe anxiety.
4. Verbalizes control over certain life situations.

5. Verbalizes acceptance of certain life situations over which he or she has no control.
6. Sets realistic goals and expresses a sense of control over outcomes for the future.

Planning/Implementation

Table 32–2 provides a plan of care for the client with dissociative amnesia. Nursing diagnoses are included, along with outcome criteria, appropriate nursing interventions, and rationales.

The concept map care plan is an innovative approach to planning and organizing nursing care (see Chapter 9). It is a diagrammatic teaching and learning strategy that allows visualization of interrelationships between medical diagnoses, nursing diagnoses, assessment data, and treatments. An example of a concept map care plan for a client with dissociative amnesia is presented in Figure 32–2.

Evaluation

Reassessment is conducted to determine if the nursing actions have been successful in achieving the objectives of care. Evaluation of the nursing actions for the client with

TABLE 32–2	Care Plan for the Client with Dissociative Amnesia

NURSING DIAGNOSIS: DISTURBED THOUGHT PROCESSES
RELATED TO: Severe psychological stress and repression of anxiety
EVIDENCED BY: Loss of memory

OUTCOME CRITERIA	NURSING INTERVENTIONS	RATIONALE
Client will recover deficits in memory and develop more adaptive coping mechanisms to deal with stress.	1. Obtain as much information as possible about the client from family and significant others if possible. Consider likes, dislikes, important people, activities, music, pets. 2. Do not flood client with data regarding his or her past life. 3. Instead, expose client to stimuli that represent pleasant experiences from the past such as smells associated with enjoyable activities, beloved pets, and music known to have been pleasurable to the client. As memory begins to return, engage client in activities that may provide additional stimulation. 4. Encourage client to discuss situations that have been especially stressful and to explore the feelings associated with those times. 5. Identify specific conflicts that remain unresolved, and assist client to identify possible solutions. Provide instruction regarding more adaptive ways to respond to anxiety.	1. A comprehensive baseline assessment is important for the development of an effective plan of care. 2. Individuals who are exposed to painful information from which the amnesia is providing protection may decompensate even further into a psychotic state. 3. Recall may occur during activities that simulate life experiences. 4. Verbalization of feelings in a non-threatening environment may help client come to terms with unresolved issues that may be contributing to the dissociative process. 5. Unless these underlying conflicts are resolved, any improvement in coping behaviors must be viewed as only temporary.

(Continued on opposite page)

NURSING DIAGNOSIS: POWERLESSNESS
RELATED TO: Inability to cope effectively with severe anxiety
EVIDENCED BY: Verbalizations of frustration over lack of control and dependence on others

OUTCOME CRITERIA	NURSING INTERVENTIONS	RATIONALE
Client will be able to effectively problem solve ways to take control of life situation.	1. Allow client to take as much responsibility as possible for own self-care practices. 2. Provide positive feedback for decisions made. Respect client's right to make those decisions independently, and refrain from attempting to influence him or her toward those that may seem more logical. 3. Assist client to set realistic goals for the future. 4. Help client identify areas of life situation that he or she can control. 5. Help client identify areas of life situation that are not within his or her ability to control. Encourage verbalization of feelings related to this inability. 6. Identify ways in which client can achieve. Encourage participation in these activities, and provide positive reinforcement for participation, as well as for achievement. 7. Encourage client's participation in supportive self-help groups.	1. Providing client with choices will increase feelings of control. 2. Positive feedback encourages repetition of desirable behaviors. 3. Unrealistic goals set client up for failure and reinforce feelings of powerlessness. 4. Client's memory deficits may interfere with his or her ability to solve problems. Assistance is required to perceive the benefits and consequences of available alternatives accurately. 5. This intervention helps client learn to deal with unresolved issues and accept what cannot be changed. 6. Positive reinforcement enhances self-esteem and encourages repetition of desirable behaviors. 7. In support groups, client can learn ways to achieve greater control over life situation through direct feedback and by hearing about the experiences of others.

dissociative amnesia may be facilitated by gathering information using the following types of questions:

1. Has the client's memory been restored?
2. Can the client connect occurrence of psychological stress to loss of memory?
3. Can the client verbalize more adaptive methods of coping with stress?
4. Can the client demonstrate use of these more adaptive coping strategies?
5. Can the client carry out activities of daily living independently?
6. Can the client identify aspects of life situation over which control can be achieved?
7. Does he or she verbalize acceptance of aspects of life situation over which control is not possible?
8. Does the client set realistic goals for the future?
9. Does he or she express positive outcomes for the future?
10. Can the client verbalize the names of support groups of which he or she may become a member in an effort to deal successfully with stressful life situations?
11. Does he or she express an intention to become affiliated with one of these self-help groups?

Dissociative Fugue

Background Assessment Data

The characteristic feature of dissociative **fugue** is a sudden, unexpected travel away from home or customary place of daily activities, with inability to recall some or all of one's past (APA, 2000). An individual in a fugue state cannot recall personal identity and often assumes a new identity. Sadock and Sadock (2003) state:

> During [the fugue] they have complete amnesia for their past lives and associations, but, unlike patients with dissociative amnesia, they are generally unaware that they have forgotten anything. Only when they suddenly return to their former selves do they recall the time antedating the onset of fugue, but then they remain amnesic for the period of the fugue itself. (p. 680)

Individuals in a fugue state do not appear to be behaving in any way out of the ordinary. Contacts with other people are minimal. The assumed identity may be simple and incomplete or complex and elaborate. If a complex identity is established, the individual may engage in intricate interpersonal and occupational activities. A divergent perception regarding the assumption of a new identity in

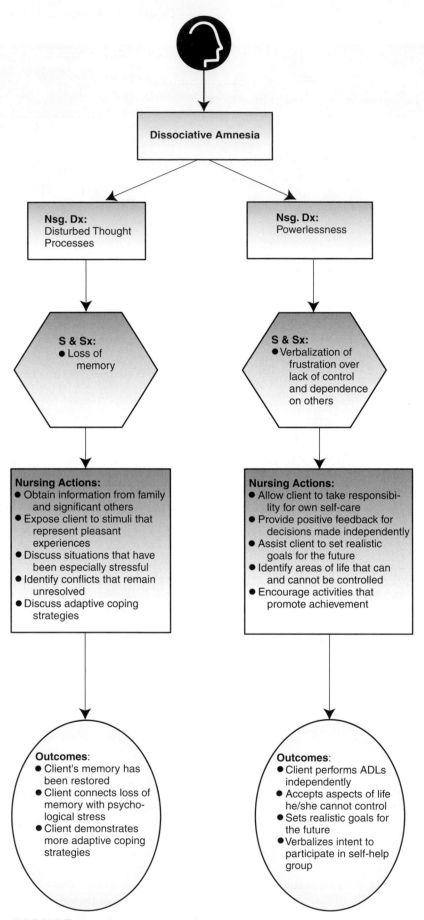

FIGURE 32–2 Concept care map for a client with dissociative amnesia.

dissociative fugue is reported by Maldonado and Spiegel (2003):

> It was thought that the assumption of a new identity was typical of dissociative fugue. However, [studies have] documented that in most cases, there is a loss of personal identity but no clear assumption of a new identity. (p. 718)

Clients with dissociative fugue often are picked up by the police when they are found wandering in a somewhat confused and frightened condition after emerging from the fugue in unfamiliar surroundings. They are usually presented to emergency departments of general hospitals. On assessment, they are able to provide details of their earlier life situation but have no recall from the beginning of the fugue state. Information from other sources usually reveals that the occurrence of severe psychological stress or excessive alcohol use precipitated the fugue behavior.

Duration is usually brief—that is, hours to days or more rarely, months—and recovery is rapid and complete. Recurrences are not common. *DSM-IV-TR* diagnostic criteria for dissociative fugue are presented in Table 32–3.

Predisposing Factors to Dissociative Fugue

The theoretical models described as predisposing factors to dissociative amnesia also have relevance for dissociative fugue. Psychodynamic features, behavioral aspects, and possible biological factors have etiological implications for both disorders. Sadock and Sadock (2003) identify some additional factors that may play a role in the predisposition to dissociative fugue. They include:

1. A history of substance abuse
2. Marital, financial, or occupational stressors
3. War-related stressors
4. Depression and suicidal ideation
5. Certain personality disorders (e.g., borderline, histrionic, and schizoid)
6. Organic disorders (especially epilepsy)

TABLE 32–3 Diagnostic Criteria for Dissociative Fugue

A. The predominant disturbance is sudden, unexpected travel away from home or one's customary place of work, with inability to recall one's past.
B. Confusion about personal identity or assumption of a new identity (partial or complete).
C. The disturbance does not occur exclusively during the course of dissociative identity disorder and is not due to the direct physiological effects of a substance (e.g., a drug of abuse, a medication) or a general medical condition (e.g., temporal lobe epilepsy).
D. The symptoms cause clinically significant distress or impairment in social, occupational, or other important areas of functioning.

SOURCE: American Psychiatric Association (2000), with permission.

Transactional Model of Stress/Adaptation

The etiology of dissociative fugue is most likely influenced by multiple factors. In Figure 32–3, a graphic depiction of this theory of multiple causation is presented in the transactional model of stress/adaptation.

Diagnosis/Outcome Identification

Nursing diagnoses are formulated from the data gathered during the assessment phase and with background knowledge regarding predisposing factors to the disorder. Some common nursing diagnoses for clients with dissociative fugue include:

Risk for other-directed violence related to fear of unknown circumstances surrounding emergence from the fugue state.
Ineffective coping related to severe psychosocial stressor or substance abuse and repressed severe anxiety evidenced by sudden travel away from home with inability to recall previous identity.

The following criteria may be used for measurement of outcomes in the care of the client with dissociative fugue.

The client:

1. Has not harmed self or others.
2. Can maintain anxiety at a level at which he or she feels no need for aggression.
3. Can discuss fears and anxieties with staff.
4. Can verbalize the extreme anxiety that precipitated the fugue state.
5. Can demonstrate more adaptive coping strategies in the face of extreme anxiety.
6. Can verbalize resources from whom he or she may seek assistance in times of extreme anxiety.

Planning/Implementation

Table 32–4 provides a plan of care for the client with dissociative fugue. Nursing diagnoses are included, along with outcome criteria, appropriate nursing interventions, and rationales.

The concept map care plan is an innovative approach to planning and organizing nursing care (see Chapter 9). It is a diagrammatic teaching and learning strategy that allows visualization of interrelationships between medical diagnoses, nursing diagnoses, assessment data, and treatments. An example of a concept map care plan for a client with dissociative fugue is presented in Figure 32–4.

Evaluation

Reassessment is conducted in order to determine if the nursing actions have been successful in achieving the objectives of care. Evaluation of the nursing actions

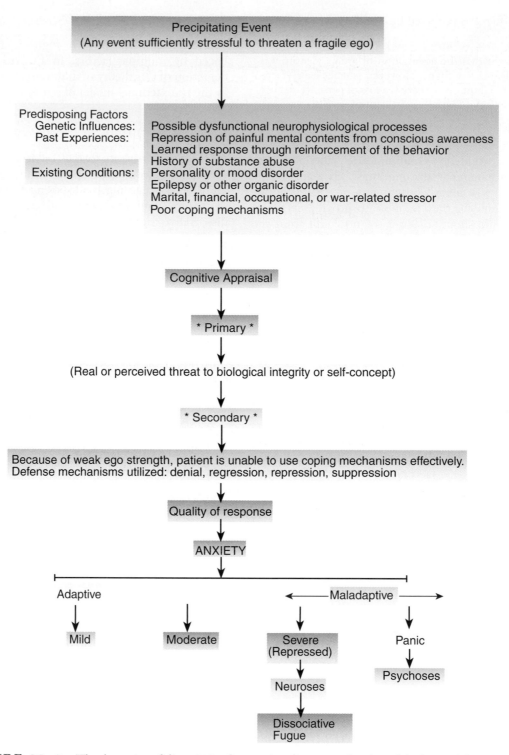

FIGURE 32–3   The dynamics of dissociative fugue using the transactional model of stress/adaptation.

for the client with dissociative fugue may be facilitated by gathering information using the following types of questions:

1. Can the client control anxiety without using violence?
2. Can he or she demonstrate strategies for relieving anxiety without resorting to aggression?

3. Does the client discuss fears and anxieties with members of the staff?
4. Has he or she confronted these fears and anxieties and dealt with them in an effort toward resolution?
5. Can the client verbalize and demonstrate adaptive coping strategies for dealing with extreme stress without resorting to dissociation?

TABLE 32–4 Care Plan for the Client with Dissociative Fugue

NURSING DIAGNOSIS: RISK FOR OTHER-DIRECTED VIOLENCE

RELATED TO: Fear of unknown circumstances surrounding emergence from fugue state

OUTCOME CRITERIA	NURSING INTERVENTIONS	RATIONALE
Client will not harm self or others.	1. Maintain low level of stimuli in client's environment (low lighting, few people, simple decor, low noise level).	1. Anxiety level rises in stimulating environment. Individuals may be perceived as threatening by a fearful and agitated client.
	2. Observe client's behavior frequently.	2. Close observation is necessary so that intervention can occur if required to ensure client's (and others') safety.
	3. Remove all dangerous objects from client's environment.	3. This will prevent the confused and agitated client from using them to harm self or others.
	4. Try to redirect violent behavior with physical outlets for the client's anxiety (e.g., punching bag).	4. Physical exercise is a safe and effective way of relieving pent-up tension.
	5. Staff should maintain and convey a calm attitude to client.	5. Anxiety is contagious and can be transmitted from staff to client.
	6. Have sufficient staff available to indicate a show of strength to client if it becomes necessary.	6. This shows the client evidence of control over the situation and provides some physical security for staff.
	7. Administer tranquilizing medications as ordered by physician. Monitor medication for its effectiveness and for any adverse side effects.	7. The avenue of the "least restrictive alternative" (see Chapter 5) must be selected when planning intervention for a psychiatric client.
	8. If the client is not calmed by "talking down" or by medication, use of mechanical restraints may be necessary. Be sure to have sufficient staff available to assist. Follow protocol established by the institution in executing this intervention. The Joint Commission on Accreditation of Healthcare Organizations (JCAHO) requires that the physician re-evaluate and issue a new order for restraints every 4 hr for adults age 18 and older. If the client has previously refused medication, administer it after restraints have been applied. Most states consider this intervention appropriate in emergency situations or in the event that a client is likely to harm self or others. Never use restraints as a punitive measure; they should be used as a protective measure for a client who is out of control. Observe the client in restraints every 15 minutes (or according to institutional policy). Ensure that circulation to extremities is not compromised (check temperature, color, pulse). Assist client with needs related to nutrition, hydration, and elimination. Position client so that comfort is facilitated and aspiration can be prevented.	8. Client safety is a nursing priority.
	9. As agitation decreases, assess client's readiness for restraint removal or reduction. Remove one restraint at a time, while assessing client's response.	9. This minimizes risk of injury to client and staff.

(Continued on following page)

TABLE 32–4	Care Plan for the Client with Dissociative Fugue *(Continued)*	

NURSING DIAGNOSIS: INEFFECTIVE COPING
RELATED TO: Severe psychosocial stressor or substance abuse and repressed severe anxiety
EVIDENCED BY: Sudden travel away from home with inability to recall previous identity

OUTCOME CRITERIA	NURSING INTERVENTIONS	RATIONALE
Client will demonstrate more adaptive ways of coping in stressful situations than resorting to dissociation.	1. Reassure client of safety and security through your presence. Dissociative behaviors may be frightening to the client.	1. Presence of a trusted individual provides feeling of security and assurance of freedom from harm.
	2. Identify stressor that precipitated severe anxiety.	2. This information is necessary for the development of an effective plan of client care and problem resolution.
	3. Explore feelings that client experienced in response to the stressor. Help client understand that the disequilibrium felt is acceptable in times of severe stress.	3. Client's self-esteem is preserved by the knowledge that others may experience these behaviors under similar circumstances.
	4. As anxiety level decreases and memory returns, use exploration and an accepting, nonthreatening environment to encourage client to identify repressed traumatic experiences that contribute to chronic anxiety.	4. Client must confront and deal with painful issues to achieve resolution.
	5. Have client identify methods of coping with stress in the past and determine whether the response was adaptive or maladaptive.	5. In times of extreme anxiety, client is unable to evaluate appropriateness of response. This information is necessary for client to develop a plan of action for the future.
	6. Help client define more adaptive coping strategies. Make suggestions of alternatives that might be tried. Examine benefits and consequences of each alternative. Assist client in the selection of those that are most appropriate for him or her.	6. Depending on current level of anxiety, client may require assistance with problem solving and decision making.
	7. Provide positive reinforcement for client's attempts to change.	7. Positive reinforcement enhances self-esteem and encourages repetition of desired behaviors.
	8. Identify community resources to which the individual may go for support if past maladaptive coping patterns return.	8. Knowledge alone that this type of support exists may provide the client with a feeling of security. Use of the resources may help to keep the client from decompensating.

6. Does the client recall the extreme stressor that precipitated the fugue state?
7. Does he or she have a plan for dealing with the stressor should it recur in the future?
8. Can he or she verbalize resources for seeking assistance in the face of extreme stress?

Dissociative Identity Disorder

Background Assessment Data

Dissociative identity disorder (DID) was formerly called multiple personality disorder. This disorder is characterized by the existence of two or more personalities in a single individual. Only one of the personalities is evident at any given moment, and one of them is dominant most of the time over the course of the disorder. Each personality is unique and composed of a complex set of memories, behavior patterns, and social relationships that surface during the dominant interval. The transition from one personality to another is usually sudden, often dramatic, and usually precipitated by stress. The *DSM-IV-TR* (APA, 2000) states:

> The time required to switch from one identity to another is usually a matter of seconds but, less frequently, may be gradual. Behavior that may be frequently associated with identity switches include rapid blinking, facial changes, changes in voice or demeanor, or disruption in the individual's train of thought. (p. 527)

Before therapy, the original personality usually has no knowledge of the other personalities, but when there are two or more subpersonalities, they are usually aware of

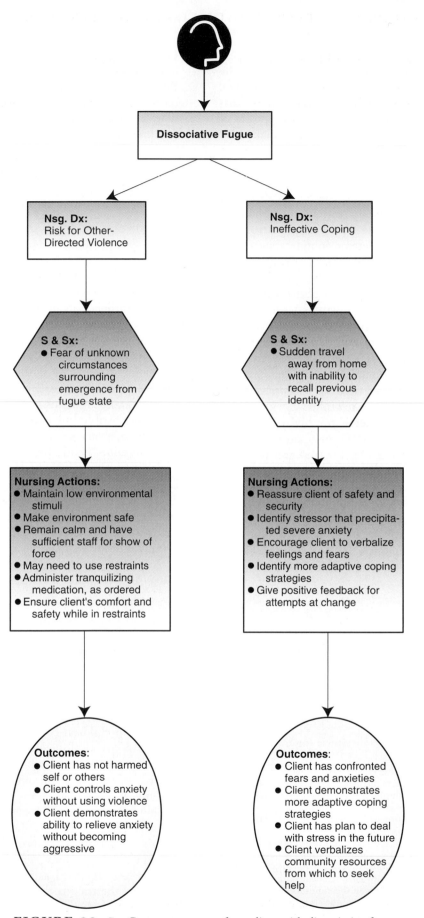

FIGURE 32–4 Concept care map for a client with dissociative fugue.

each other's existence. Most often, the various subpersonalities have different names, but they may be unnamed and may be of a different sex, race, and age. The various personalities are almost always quite disparate and may even appear to be the exact opposite of the original personality. For example, a normally shy, socially withdrawn, faithful husband may become a gregarious womanizer and heavy drinker with the emergence of another personality.

Generally, there is amnesia for the events that took place when another personality was in the dominant position. Often, however, one personality state is not bound by such amnesia and retains complete awareness of the existence, qualities, and activities of the other personalities (Sadock & Sadock, 2003). Subpersonalities that are amnestic for the other subpersonalities experience the periods when others are dominant as "lost time" or blackouts. They may "wake up" in unfamiliar situations with no idea where they are, how they got there, or who the people around them are. They may frequently be accused of lying when they deny remembering or being responsible for events or actions that occurred while another personality controlled the body.

Dissociative identity disorder is not always incapacitating. Some individuals with DID maintain responsible positions, complete graduate degrees, and are successful spouses and parents before diagnosis and while in treatment. Before they are diagnosed with DID, many individuals are misdiagnosed with depression, borderline and antisocial personality disorders, schizophrenia, epilepsy, or bipolar disorder.

The *DSM-IV-TR* diagnostic criteria for dissociative identity disorder are presented in Table 32–5.

Predisposing Factors to Dissociative Identity Disorder

Sadock and Sadock (2003) describe four types of causative factors associated with a predisposition to DID. These include:

TABLE 32–5   **Diagnostic Criteria for Dissociative Identity Disorder**

A. The presence of two or more distinct personality states (each with its own relatively enduring pattern of perceiving, relating to, and thinking about the environment and self).
B. At least two of these identities or personality states recurrently take control of the person's behavior.
C. Inability to recall important personal information that is too extensive to be explained by ordinary forgetfulness.
D. The disturbance is not due to the direct physiological effects of a substance (e.g., blackouts or chaotic behavior during alcohol intoxication) or a general medical condition (e.g., complex partial seizures). **NOTE:** In children, the symptoms are not attributable to imaginary playmates or other fantasy play.

SOURCE: American Psychiatric Association (2000), with permission.

---

1. Having experienced a traumatic life event, most often in childhood
2. Possessing a vulnerability for the disorder to develop (either biological or psychological)
3. The existence of formulative environmental factors (e.g., negative role models or the absence of adaptive coping ability)
4. The absence of external support from significant other(s)

These four factors may be explained by the following theories.

Biological Theories

Genetics. Several studies have indicated that DID is more common in first-degree biological relatives of people with the disorder than in the general population (APA, 2000). The disorder is often seen in more than one generation of a family. Some clinicians believe this may reflect a genetic component of DID, perhaps linked to a psychobiological capacity for dissociation.

Organic. The role of organic influences in the development of DID remains unclear. Some studies have suggested a possible link between DID and certain neurological conditions, such as temporal lobe epilepsy and severe migraine headaches. Electroencephalographic abnormalities have been observed in some clients with DID (Sadock & Sadock, 2003).

The majority of individuals with these organic alterations show no signs of DID. Based on the body of present knowledge, the hypothesis of organic dysfunction as a determinant of DID should be approached with caution.

Psychological Influences

History of Traumatic Experience. A growing body of evidence points to the etiology of DID as a set of traumatic experiences that overwhelms the individual's capacity to cope by any means other than dissociation. These experiences usually take the form of severe physical, sexual, or psychological abuse by a parent or significant other in the child's life. The most widely accepted etiological explanation for DID is that it begins as a survival strategy that serves to help children cope with the horrifying sexual, physical, or psychological abuse. In this traumatic environment, the child uses dissociation to become a passive victim of the cruel and unwanted experience. He or she creates a new being who is able to endure the overwhelming pain of the cruel reality, while the primary self can then escape awareness of the pain. Each new personality has as its nucleus a means of responding without anxiety and distress to various painful or dangerous stimuli.

Studies have revealed a great diversity in the nature and scope of the trauma that individuals with DID have suffered. *Sexual* abuse has included rape, incest, and sodomy. Some individuals report being forced to witness the physical or sexual abuse of other children. Individuals with the disorder have given such examples of *psychological* abuse as being compelled to participate in murders, including cult activities involving ritual murders. *Physical* abuse has included being buried, tortured, beaten, given excessive enemas and massive doses of cathartics, as well as enduring total neglect. It has been suggested that the number of an individual's alternate personalities may be related to the number of different types of abuse he or she suffered as a child. Individuals with many personalities have usually been severely abused well into adolescence.

Theory of Family Dynamics. Sadock and Sadock (2003) have indicated that individuals with DID do not find the necessary healing support in their environment. A profile of the family of origin of the individual with DID reveals the following characteristics:

1. Upholding rigid religious or mystical beliefs
2. Presenting a united front to the community, while internally riddled with conflict
3. Isolation from the community and lack of cooperation regarding intervention or assistance
4. At least one caretaker who exhibits severe psychopathology
5. Subjecting the child to contradictory communications
6. Polarization by one overadequate parent (the abuser) and one underadequate parent (the enabler)

The individual who is not given the opportunity to heal following abuse and dissociation adopts this defense as a routine strategy for dealing with life problems.

Transactional Model of Stress/Adaptation

The etiology of DID is most likely influenced by multiple factors. In Figure 32–5, a graphic depiction of this theory of multiple causation is presented in the transactional model of stress/adaptation.

Diagnosis/Outcome Identification

Nursing diagnoses are formulated from the data gathered during the assessment phase and with background knowledge regarding predisposing factors to the disorder. Some common nursing diagnoses for clients with dissociative identity disorder include:

Risk for suicide related to unresolved grief and self-blame associated with childhood abuse.

Disturbed personal identity related to childhood trauma/abuse evidenced by the presence of more than one personality within the individual.

The following criteria may be used for measurement of outcomes in the care of the client with dissociative identity disorder.

The client:

1. Has not harmed self or others.
2. Seeks out staff when aggressive feelings emerge.

3. Verbalizes understanding of the existence of multiple personalities.
4. Verbalizes understanding of the purpose the various personalities serve.
5. Verbalizes understanding that transition from one personality to another occurs in times of stress.
6. Verbalizes knowledge of various situations that precipitate stress.
7. Verbalizes understanding of and willingness to participate in integration therapy.

Planning/Implementation

Table 32–6 provides a plan of care for the client with DID. Nursing diagnoses are included, along with outcome criteria, appropriate nursing interventions, and rationales.

The concept map care plan is an innovative approach to planning and organizing nursing care (see Chapter 9). It is a diagrammatic teaching and learning strategy that allows visualization of interrelationships between medical diagnoses, nursing diagnoses, assessment data, and treatments. An example of a concept map care plan for a client with panic or generalized anxiety disorder is presented in Figure 32–6.

Evaluation

Hospitalization of the client with DID usually occurs only in an acute situation (e.g., an attempted suicide, or an attempt to integrate a personality that the therapist is anticipating may precipitate violence and requires a more structured setting). In these cases, the nursing interventions would be directed toward the most critical issues.

Reassessment is ongoing, to determine if the nursing actions have been successful in achieving the stated objectives of care. Evaluation of the nursing actions for the client with DID may be facilitated by gathering information using the following types of questions:

1. Can the client maintain control over hostile impulses?
2. Has injury to client and others been avoided?
3. Does the client seek support from staff when aggressive feelings emerge?
4. Can the client discuss the presence of various personalities within the self?
5. Can he or she verbalize why these personalities exist?
6. Can the client verbalize situations that precipitate transition from one personality to another?
7. Can the client demonstrate alternative, more adaptive coping strategies?
8. Does the client verbalize understanding of the process of **integration**?
9. Is he or she willing to undergo the lengthy therapy required for integration?
10. Do the alternate personalities resist integration?

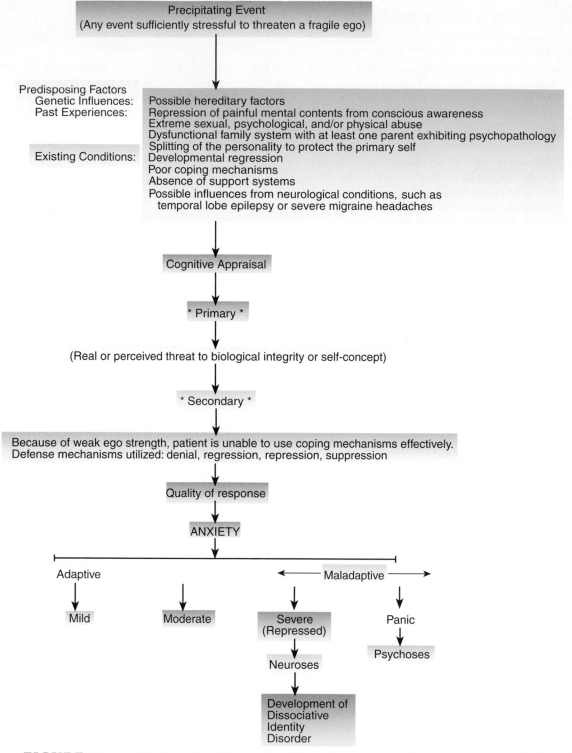

FIGURE 32–5   The dynamics of dissociative identity disorder using the transactional model of stress/adaptation.

11. Do the alternate personalities understand that integration means not extinction, but rather instead a "coming together" of all the personalities into one identity?

12. Does the client have a plan for dealing with stress outside the therapy setting, particularly those situations that provoke feelings of violence to self or others? If so, has the plan been demonstrated (e.g., through role-play)?

13. Can the client verbalize resources outside the hospital from whom he or she may seek assistance during times of extreme stress?

NURSING DIAGNOSIS: RISK FOR SUICIDE
RELATED TO: Unresolved grief and self-blame associated with childhood abuse

OUTCOME CRITERIA	NURSING INTERVENTIONS	RATIONALE
Client will not harm self.	1. Assess suicidal or harmful intent. Discuss consideration of a plan and availability of means. Assess sudden changes in behavior.	1. Impulse control may be impaired. Sudden changes may signal a switch to the "suicidal" personality.
	2. Help client identify stressful precipitating factors that initiate emergence of the "suicidal" personality.	2. Early detection allows time to manipulate the environment to reduce the possibility of injury.
	3. Establish trust and secure a promise that client seek out support when self-destructive impulses are present.	3. This allows the client to assume some of the responsibility for his or her behavior, while still offering assistance if self-control is lacking.
	4. Seek assistance from another, strong-willed personality.	4. A strong-willed personality may help to control the behavior of the "suicidal" personality.
	5. Assist the client in identifying alternative behaviors to self-destructive behaviors (e.g., verbal or written expression; physical activity).	5. These activities may provide a nondestructive alternative in the face of overwhelming aggressive impulses.
	6. If necessary, place in isolation or provide physical restraint in a non-punitive manner.	6. External controls will ensure client safety when internal controls fail.
	7. Assess physical and emotional status every 15 minutes while in restraints.	7. Client safety and security are nursing priorities.
	8. Administer antidepressant and antianxiety medications as ordered by physician.	8. Depression is common and the client may become frustrated with the long-term treatment (sometimes in excess of 10 years). Anxiolytics may be required to reduce anxiety until internal controls are achieved.

NURSING DIAGNOSIS: DISTURBED PERSONAL IDENTITY
RELATED TO: Childhood trauma/abuse
EVIDENCED BY: The presence of more than one personality within the individual

OUTCOME CRITERIA	NURSING INTERVENTIONS	RATIONALE
Client will verbalize understanding about the existence of multiple personalities, the reason for their existence, and the importance of eventual integration of the personalities into one.	1. The nurse must develop a trusting relationship with the original personality and with each of the subpersonalities.	1. Trust is the basis of a therapeutic relationship. Each of the personalities views itself as a separate entity and must initially be treated as such.
	2. Help client understand the existence of the subpersonalities and the need each serves in the personal identity of the individual.	2. Client may initially be unaware of the dissociative response. Knowledge of the needs each personality fulfills is the first step in the integration process.
	3. Help client identify stressful situations that precipitate transition from one personality to another. Carefully observe and record these transitions.	3. Identification of stressors is required to assist client in responding more adaptively and to eliminate the need for transition to another personality.
	4. Use nursing interventions necessary to deal with maladaptive behaviors associated with individual subpersonalities. For example, if one personality is suicidal, precautions must be taken to guard against client's self-harm. If another personality has a tendency toward physical hostility, precautions must be taken to protect others.	4. The safety of client and others is a nursing priority.
	5. Help subpersonalities to understand that their "being" will not be destroyed but rather integrated into a unified identity within the individual.	5. Because subpersonalities function as separate entities, the idea of total elimination generates fear and defensiveness.
	6. Provide support during disclosure of painful experiences and reassurance when client becomes discouraged with lengthy treatment.	6. Positive reinforcement may encourage repetition of desirable behaviors.

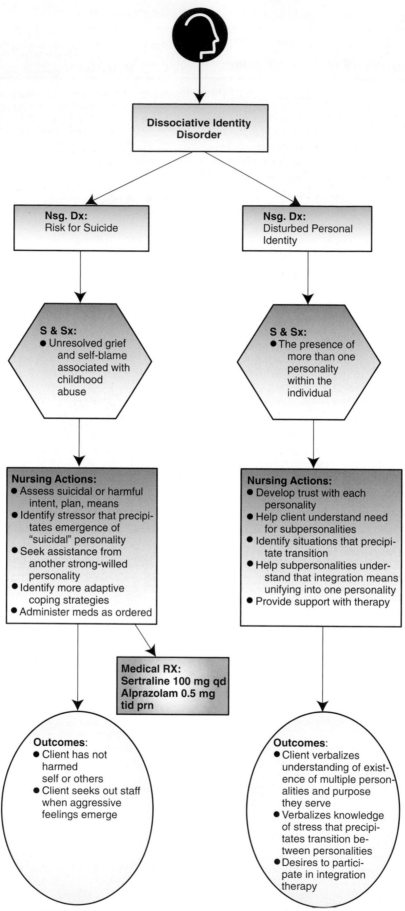

FIGURE 32–6 Concept care map for a client with DID.

Depersonalization Disorder

Background Assessment Data

Depersonalization disorder is characterized by a temporary change in the quality of self-awareness, which often takes the form of feelings of unreality, changes in body image, feelings of detachment from the environment, or a sense of observing oneself from outside the body. Depersonalization (a disturbance in the perception of oneself) is differentiated from **derealization**, which describes an alteration in the perception of the external environment. Both of these phenomena also occur in a variety of psychiatric illnesses such as schizophrenia, depression, anxiety states, and organic mental disorders. As previously stated, the symptom of depersonalization is very common. It is estimated that approximately half of all adults experience transient episodes of depersonalization (APA, 2000). The diagnosis of depersonalization disorder is made only if the symptom causes significant distress or impairment in functioning.

The *DSM-IV-TR* describes this disorder as the persistence or recurrence of episodes of depersonalization characterized by a feeling of detachment or estrangement from one's self (APA, 2000). There may be a mechanical or dreamlike feeling, or belief that the body's physical characteristics have changed. If derealization is present, objects in the environment are perceived as altered in size or shape. Other people in the environment may seem automated or mechanical.

These altered perceptions are experienced as disturbing, and are often accompanied by anxiety, depression, fear of going insane, obsessive thoughts, somatic complaints, and a disturbance in the subjective sense of time (APA, 2000). The disorder has been found to occur at least twice as often in women as in men, and is a disorder of younger people, rarely occurring in individuals older than 40 years of age (Sadock & Sadock, 2003). The diagnostic criteria for depersonalization disorder are presented in Table 32–7.

Predisposing Factors to Depersonalization Disorder

Physiological Theories

A variety of empirical observations have led some investigators to suggest that the phenomenon of depersonalization has a neurophysiological basis. Clients with diseases of the central nervous system, such as brain tumors and epilepsy, and individuals subjected to severe sensory deprivation, have reported episodes of depersonalization (Sadock & Sadock, 2003). Electrical stimulation of the cortex of the temporal lobes has produced the same effect. Some psychotomimetic drugs, such as lysergic acid diethylamide (LSD) and mescaline, create distortions of perception and alterations in the sense of reality.

TABLE 32–7 Diagnostic Criteria for Depersonalization Disorder
A. Persistent or recurrent experiences of feeling detached from, and as if one is an outside observer of, one's mental processes or body (e.g., feeling like one is in a dream).
B. During the depersonalization experience, reality testing remains intact.
C. The depersonalization causes clinically significant distress or impairment in social, occupational, or other important areas of functioning.
D. The depersonalization experience does not occur exclusively during the course of another mental disorder, such as schizophrenia, panic disorder, acute stress disorder, or another dissociative disorder, and is not due to the direct physiological effects of a substance (e.g., a drug of abuse, a medication) or a general medical condition (e.g., temporal lobe epilepsy).

SOURCE: American Psychiatric Association (2000), with permission.

Psychodynamic Theories

Psychodynamic explanations emphasize psychological conflict and disturbances of ego structure in the predisposition to depersonalization disorder.

Perceiving the self as "not real" serves as a defense mechanism and offers protection or escape from anxiety or some other unpleasant emotion resulting from internal psychological conflict. For example, an individual who experiences extreme anxiety after a severe automobile accident perceives himself or herself (or the situation) as "not real" and therefore escapes the emotional pain associated with the incident.

Theories related to disturbances in ego structure focus on problems with personal identity and ego boundaries. Depersonalization occurs in response to psychological conflicts in the ego itself. Psychodynamic theory suggests that the conflict results in a split in the ego between an observing self and an acting self or a split between conflicting identifications. Proponents of this theory believe that explanation of depersonalization lay primarily in understanding the pathology of the structure and function of the ego.

Transactional Model of Stress/Adaptation

The etiology of depersonalization disorder is most likely influenced by multiple factors. In Figure 32–7, a graphic depiction of this theory of multiple causation is presented in the transactional model of stress/adaptation.

Diagnosis/Outcome Identification

Nursing diagnoses are formulated from the data gathered during the assessment phase and with background knowledge regarding predisposing factors to the disorder. Some common nursing diagnoses for clients with depersonalization disorder include:

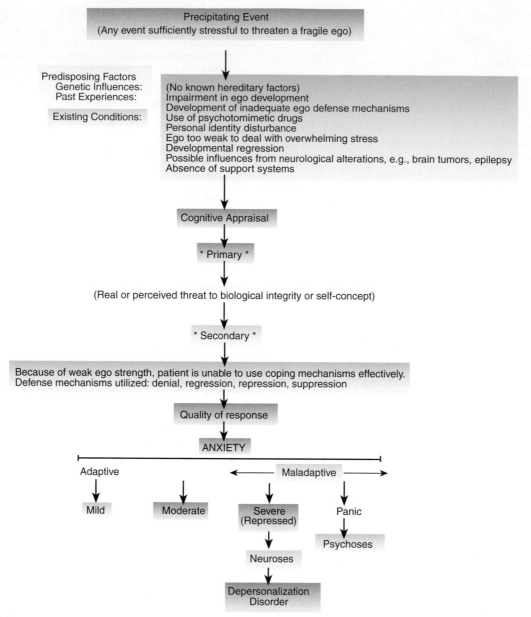

FIGURE 32–7 The dynamics of depersonalization disorder using the transactional model of stress/adaptation.

Disturbed sensory perception (visual and kinesthetic) related to repressed severe anxiety and underdeveloped ego evidenced by alteration in the perception or experience of the self or the environment.

Anxiety (severe to panic) related to fears of losing control or going insane evidenced by somatic complaints, obsessive thoughts, and disturbances in the sense of time.

The following criteria may be used for measurement of outcomes in the care of the client with depersonalization disorder.

The client:

1. Maintains a sense of reality during stressful situations.
2. Perceives self and environment accurately.

3. Verbalizes correlation between severe anxiety and symptoms of depersonalization.
4. Can maintain anxiety at a manageable level.
5. Verbalizes an understanding of the role depersonalization behaviors play in the management of anxiety.
6. Can verbalize more adaptive strategies for coping with stress.

Planning/Implementation

Table 32–8 provides a plan of care for the client with depersonalization disorder. Nursing diagnoses are included, along with outcome criteria, appropriate nursing interventions, and rationales.

NURSING DIAGNOSIS: DISTURBED SENSORY PERCEPTION (VISUAL/KINESTHETIC)
RELATED TO: Repressed severe anxiety and underdeveloped ego
EVIDENCED BY: Alteration in the perception or experience of the self or the environment

OUTCOME CRITERIA	NURSING INTERVENTIONS	RATIONALE
Client will demonstrate the ability to perceive stimuli correctly and maintain a sense of reality during stressful situations.	1. Provide support and encouragement during times of depersonalization. Clients manifesting these symptoms may express fear and anxiety at experiencing such behaviors. They do not understand the response and may express a fear of going insane. 2. Explain the depersonalization behaviors and the purpose they usually serve for the client. 3. Explain the relationship between severe anxiety and depersonalization behaviors. Help relate these behaviors to times of severe psychological stress that client has experienced. 4. Explore past experiences and possibly repressed painful situations, such as trauma or abuse. 5. Discuss these painful experiences with client, and encourage him or her to deal with the feelings associated with these situations. Work to resolve the conflicts these repressed feelings have nurtured. 6. Discuss ways the client may more adaptively respond to stress, and use role-play to practice using these new methods.	1. Support and encouragement from a trusted individual provide a feeling of security when fears and anxieties are manifested. 2. This knowledge may help to minimize fears and anxieties associated with their occurrence. 3. The client may be unaware that the occurrence of depersonalization behaviors is related to severe anxiety. Knowledge of this relationship is the first step in the process of behavioral change. 4. Traumatic experiences may predispose individuals to dissociative disorders. 5. Conflict resolution will serve to decrease the need for the dissociative response to anxiety. 6. Having practiced through role-play helps to prepare client to face stressful situations by using these new behaviors when they occur in real life.

NURSING DIAGNOSIS: ANXIETY (SEVERE TO PANIC)
RELATED TO: Fears of losing control or going insane
EVIDENCED BY: Somatic complaints, obsessive thoughts, and disturbances in the sense of time

OUTCOME CRITERIA	NURSING INTERVENTIONS	RATIONALE
Client will verbalize understanding of purpose depersonalization behaviors fulfill, thereby decreasing fears and anxieties associated with experiencing them.	1. Maintain a calm, nonthreatening manner while working with the client. 2. Reassure client of his or her safety and security. This can be conveyed by the physical presence of the nurse. Do not leave the client alone at this time. 3. Use simple words and brief messages, spoken calmly and clearly. 4. Explain to client what is happening. Assure the client that the experiencing of depersonalization behaviors does not mean that he or she is going crazy. 5. When depersonalization behaviors have diminished and anxiety has been reduced, explore with the client the stressful situation that may have precipitated the response.	1. Anxiety is contagious and may be transferred from staff to a client or vice versa. Client develops feeling of security in presence of calm staff person. 2. The client may fear for his or her life. The presence of a trusted individual provides client with a feeling of security and assurance of personal safety. 3. In an intensely anxious situation, the client is unable to comprehend anything but the most elemental communication. 4. The feeling of a lack of control over behavior he or she does not understand will contribute to anxiety. Explanations should offer some relief. 5. The client may be unaware that the occurrence of depersonalization behaviors is related to severe anxiety.

(Continued on following page)

TABLE 32–8	Care Plan for the Client with Depersonalization Disorder *(Continued)*	
OUTCOME CRITERIA	NURSING INTERVENTIONS	RATIONALE
	6. Discuss with the client ways in which he or she might respond to stressful situations that would be less likely to result in depersonalization behaviors. 7. Use role-play to practice new, more adaptive coping strategies.	6. This may have been the client's way of dealing with stress for a long time. He or she may need help to identify alternative coping strategies. 7. Role-play allows the client to practice and be better prepared to deal with the stressful situation should it recur. Being prepared provides a feeling of security and offers a sense of control to the client.

The concept map care plan is an innovative approach to planning and organizing nursing care (see Chapter 9). It is a diagrammatic teaching and learning strategy that allows visualization of interrelationships between medical diagnoses, nursing diagnoses, assessment data, and treatments. An example of a concept map care plan for a client with depersonalization disorder is presented in Figure 32–8.

Evaluation

Reassessment is conducted in order to determine if the nursing actions have been successful in achieving the objectives of care. Evaluation of the nursing actions for the client with depersonalization disorder may be facilitated by gathering information using the following types of questions:

1. Does the client demonstrate the ability to perceive stimuli correctly?
2. Does he or she maintain a sense of reality during stressful situations?
3. Can the client verbalize the purpose depersonalization behaviors serve?
4. Can the client verbalize a correlation between stressful situations and the onset of depersonalization behaviors?
5. Can the client demonstrate more adaptive coping strategies for dealing with stress without resorting to dissociation?
6. Has the client role-played these strategies in preparation for use in real-life situations?
7. Can the client verbalize types of situations that precipitate extreme stress?
8. Can the client discuss more adaptive ways that he or she plans to deal with these times of extreme stress in the future?
9. Can the client verbalize resources outside the hospital to whom he or she may turn when feeling the need for assistance?

Table 32–9 presents topics for client/family education related to dissociative disorders.

TABLE 32–9	Topics for Client/Family Education Related to Dissociative Disorders

Nature of the Illness

1. Define and describe symptoms of:
   a. Dissociative amnesia
   b. Dissociative fugue
   c. Dissociative identity disorder
   d. Depersonalization disorder
2. Discuss etiologies of the above disorders.
3. Discuss possibility of long-term course, particularly in the case of DID.

Management of the Illness

1. Discuss ways to identify onset of escalating anxiety.
2. Discuss ways to intervene to prevent exacerbation of symptoms.
3. Teach relaxation techniques.
4. Teach assertiveness techniques.
5. Discuss pharmacology:
   a. Teach about any medications that may be used to treat symptoms associated with dissociative disorders or disorders of comorbidity. For example:
      (1) Anxiolytics
      (2) Antipsychotics
      (3) Antidepressants

Support Services

1. Support groups
2. Individual psychotherapy

TREATMENT MODALITIES

Dissociative Amnesia

Many cases of dissociative amnesia resolve spontaneously when the individual is removed from the stressful situation. For other, more refractory conditions, intravenous administration of amobarbital is useful in the retrieval of lost memories. Most clinicians recommend supportive psychotherapy also to reinforce adjustment to the psychological impact of the retrieved memories and the emotions associated with them.

In some instances, psychotherapy is used as the primary treatment. Techniques of persuasion and **free** or **directed association** are used to help the client remember. In other cases, **hypnosis** may be required to mobilize the memories. Once the memories are obtained

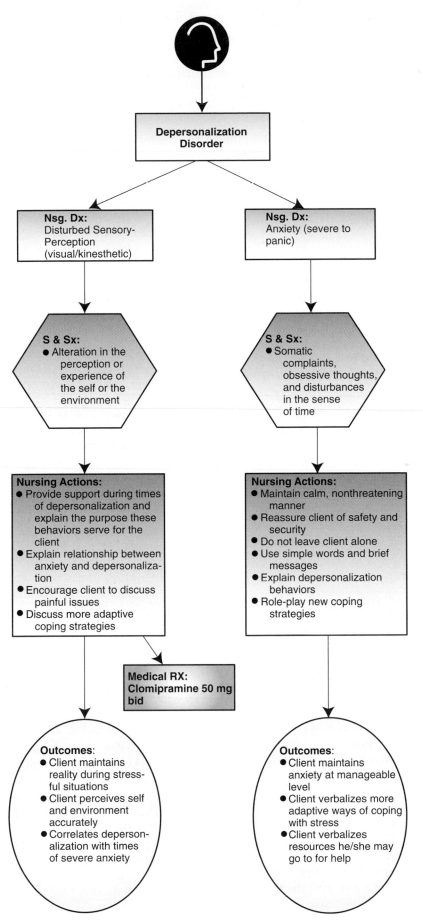

FIGURE 32–8 Client care map for a client with depersonalization disorder.

through hypnosis, psychotherapy may be employed to help the client integrate the memories into his or her conscious state (Sadock & Sadock, 2003).

Dissociative Fugue

Recovery from dissociative fugue is usually rapid, spontaneous, and complete. In some instances, manipulation of the environment or psychotherapeutic support may help to diminish stress or help the client adapt to stress in the future. When the fugue is prolonged, techniques of gentle encouragement, persuasion, or directed association may be helpful, either alone or in combination with hypnosis or amobarbital interviews. Ford-Martin (2001) states:

> Treatment for dissociative fugue should focus on helping the patient come to terms with the traumatic event or stressor that caused the disorder. This can be accomplished through various kinds of interactive therapies that explore the trauma and work on building the patient's coping mechanisms to prevent further recurrence.

Cognitive therapy may be useful in helping the client attempt a change in inappropriate or irrational thinking patterns. Creative therapies (e.g., art therapy, music therapy) are also constructive in allowing clients to express and explore thoughts and emotions in "safe" ways (Ford-Martin, 2001). Group therapy can be helpful in providing the client with ongoing support from supportive peers. Family therapy sessions may be used to explore the trauma that precipitated the fugue episode and to educate family members about the dissociative disorder.

Dissociative Identity Disorder

The goal of therapy for the client with DID is to optimize the client's function and potential. The achievement of integration (a blending of all the personalities into one) is usually considered desirable, but some clients choose not to pursue this lengthy therapeutic regimen. In these cases resolution, or a smooth collaboration among the subpersonalities, may be all that is realistic.

Intensive, long-term psychotherapy with the DID client is directed toward uncovering the underlying psychological conflicts, helping him or her gain insight into these conflicts, and striving to synthesize the various identities into one integrated personality. Clients are assisted to recall past traumas in detail. They must mentally re-experience the abuse that caused their illness. This process, called **abreaction**, or "remembering with feeling," is so painful that clients may actually cry, scream, and feel the pain that they felt at the time of the abuse. Some individuals even experience sights, sounds, and smells that were associated with the original traumatic situation. Hypnosis is commonly used to identify

previously unrecognized personalities and for fostering abreaction (Sadock & Sadock, 2003).

The individual with DID may exhibit considerable resistance to the process of integration. Most clients view the dissociation as their only means of protection. Maldonado and Spiegel (2003) state:

> [The client] may experience efforts of integration as an attempt on the part of the therapist to "kill" personalities. These fears must be worked through and the patient shown how to control the degree of integration, giving the patient a sense of gradually being able to control his or her dissociative processes in the service of working through traumatic memories. (p. 727)

During therapy, each personality must be actively explored and encouraged to become aware of the others across previously amnestic barriers. Traumatic memories associated with the different personality manifestations, especially those related to childhood abuse, are examined. The course of treatment is often difficult and anxiety-provoking to client and therapist alike, especially when aggressive or suicidal personalities are in the dominant role. In these instances, brief periods of hospitalization may be necessary as an interim supportive measure.

When integration is achieved, the individual becomes a total of all the feelings, experiences, memories, skills, and talents that were previously in the command of the various personalities. He or she learns how to function effectively without the necessity for creating new personalities to cope with life. This is possible only after years of intense psychotherapy, and even then, recovery is often incomplete.

Depersonalization Disorder

Information about the treatment of depersonalization disorder is sparse and inconclusive. Various regimens have been tried, although none has proven widely successful. Anxiolytics provide symptomatic relief if anxiety is an important element of the clinical condition (Sadock & Sadock, 2003). If other psychiatric disorders, such as schizophrenia, are evident, they too may be treated pharmacologically. A study by Simeon, Stein, and Hollander (1998) found the antidepressant clomipramine (Anafranil) to be a promising pharmacological treatment for primary depersonalization disorder. For clients with evident intrapsychic conflict, analytically oriented insight psychotherapy may be useful. Specific recommendations for the management of depersonalization disorder need to await more extensive clinical investigation.

SUMMARY

A dissociative response has been described as a defense mechanism to protect the ego in the face of overwhelming anxiety. Dissociative responses result in an alteration in the normally integrative functions of identity, memory, or consciousness. Classification of dissociative disorders includes dissociative amnesia, dissociative fugue, dissociative identity disorder, and depersonalization disorder.

In comparison to other primary psychiatric disorders, dissociative disorders are relatively rare. Dissociative behaviors are commonly observed in clients with other disorders, however.

The individual with dissociative amnesia is unable to recall important personal information that is too extensive to be explained by ordinary forgetfulness. The memory deficit may be described as *localized*, *selective*, *generalized*, *continuous*, or *systematized*. Dissociative fugue is characterized by a sudden, unexpected travel away from home with an inability to recall the past, including personal identity. Duration of the fugue is usually brief, and once it is over the individual recovers memory of the past life but is amnestic for the time period covered by the fugue. The prominent feature of DID is the existence of two or more personalities within a single individual. An individual may have many personalities, each of which serves a purpose for that individual of enduring painful stimuli that the original personality is too weak to face. Depersonalization disorder is characterized by an alteration in the perception of oneself (sometimes described as a feeling of having separated from the body and watching the activities of the self from a distance).

Nursing care of individuals with dissociative disorders is accomplished using the steps of the nursing process. Background assessment data and nursing diagnoses common to each disorder were presented. Interventions appropriate to each nursing diagnosis and relevant outcome criteria for each were included. An overview of current medical treatment modalities was discussed.

Nurses in all areas of clinical practice should be aware of client potential for dissociative responses and be able to recognize these behaviors should they occur. Clients exhibiting dissociative behaviors often receive health care initially in areas other than psychiatry.

REVIEW QUESTIONS

SELF-EXAMINATION/LEARNING EXERCISE

Select the answer that is *most* appropriate for the questions that follow the situation.

Situation: Ellen, age 32, was diagnosed as having DID at age 28. Since that time she has been in therapy with a psychiatrist, who has detected the presence of 12 personalities and identified a history of childhood abuse. Yesterday, Beth, the personality with suicidal ideations, swallowed a bottle of 20 alprazolam (Xanax). Ellen's roommate found her when she returned from work and called the emergency medical service. She was stabilized in the emergency department and 48 hours later transferred to the psychiatric unit.

1. The primary nursing diagnosis for Ellen would be:
   a. Disturbed personal identity related to childhood abuse.
   b. Disturbed sensory perception related to repressed anxiety.
   c. Disturbed thought processes related to memory deficit.
   d. Risk for suicide related to unresolved grief.

2. In establishing trust with Ellen, the nurse must:
   a. Try to relate to Ellen as though she did not have multiple personalities.
   b. Establish a relationship with each of the personalities separately.
   c. Ignore behaviors that Ellen attributes to Beth.
   d. Explain to Ellen that he or she will work with her only if she maintains the status of the primary personality.

3. The ultimate goal of therapy for Ellen is:
   a. Integration of the personalities into one.
   b. Being able to switch from one personality to another voluntarily.
   c. To select which personality she wants to be her dominant self.
   d. To recognize that the various personalities exist.

4. The ultimate goal of therapy will most likely be achieved through:
   a. Crisis intervention and directed association.
   b. Psychotherapy and hypnosis.
   c. Psychoanalysis and free association.
   d. Insight psychotherapy and dextroamphetamines.

5. Which of the following is an appropriate nursing intervention for controlling the behavior of the "suicidal personality," Beth?
   a. When Beth emerges, put the client in restraints.
   b. Keep Ellen in isolation during her hospitalization.
   c. Make a verbal contract with Ellen that Beth will do no harm.
   d. Elicit the help of another, strong-willed personality to help control Beth's behavior.

The following are general questions related to dissociative disorders:

6. Which of the following nursing interventions is most appropriate for the nurse working with the client experiencing dissociative amnesia?
   a. Use the technique of implosion therapy (flooding) to help the client remember.
   b. Use hypnosis to help the client remember.
   c. Expose the client to stimuli that represent pleasant memories from the past.
   d. Expose the client to stimuli that represent the painful stimuli for which the amnesia is providing the protection.

7. It is important for the nurse to understand that, when an individual awakens from a fugue state, he or she:
   a. Will have no memory for what occurred during the fugue.
   b. Will remember everything that occurred during the fugue.
   c. Will have no memory for life before the fugue occurred.
   d. Will have total recall of the time before and during the fugue.

8. Bob was driving his automobile when it was involved in an accident in which his wife and child were killed. Unable to carry on with his life, he has sought emotional help. He says to the nurse, "I don't know how I managed to make all the funeral arrangements. At times it seemed as though I was an outside observer of everything that was happening." What is this phenomenon called?
   a. Derealization
   b. Abreaction
   c. Depersonalization
   d. Psychosis

9. Bob continues, "At other times, when I was with a group of people, it would appear as though everyone was moving in slow motion." What is this phenomenon called?
   a. Derealization
   b. Abreaction
   c. Depersonalization
   d. Psychosis

10. Which of the following examples of Bob's situation describes selective amnesia?
    a. Bob was unable to remember anything having to do with the accident until 3 days following the accident.
    b. Bob could not remember the accident, but remembered hearing the ambulance siren and being admitted to the emergency room.
    c. Bob is unable to remember anything that has happened during his entire lifetime.
    d. Bob can remember nothing since the time of the accident.

TEST YOUR CRITICAL THINKING SKILLS

Sam was admitted to the psychiatric unit from the emergency department of a general hospital in the Midwest. The owner of a local bar called the police when Sam suddenly seemed to "lose control. He just went ballistic." The police reported that Sam did not know where he was or how he got there. He kept saying, "My name is John Brown, and I live in Philadelphia." When the police ran an identity check on Sam, they found that he was indeed John Brown from Philadelphia and his wife had reported him missing a month ago. Mrs. Brown explained that about 12 months before his disappearance, her husband, who was a shop foreman at a large manufacturing plant, had been having considerable difficulty at work. He had been passed over for a promotion, and his supervisor had been very critical of his work. Several of his staff had left the company for other jobs, and without enough help,

Sam had been unable to meet shop deadlines. Work stress made him very difficult to live with at home. Previously an easygoing, extroverted individual, he became withdrawn and extremely critical of his wife and children. Immediately preceding his disappearance, he had had a violent argument with his 18-year-old son, who called Sam a "loser" and stormed out of the house to stay with some friends. It was the day after this argument that Sam disappeared. The psychiatrist assigns a diagnosis of dissociative fugue.

Answer the following questions related to Sam:

1. Describe the priority nursing intervention with Sam as he is admitted to the psychiatric unit.
2. What approach should be taken to help Sam with his problem?
3. What is the long-term goal of therapy for Sam?

@ **INTERNET REFERENCES**

Additional information about dissociative disorders may be located at the following Web sites:

- http://www.human-nature.com/odmh/dissociative.html
- http://www.nami.org/helpline/dissoc.htm
- http://www.mental-health-matters.com/disorders/
- http://www.issd.org/
- http://www.findarticles.com/cf_dls/g2601/0004/ 2601000438/p1/article.jhtml
- http://www.sidran.org/didbr.html
- http://www.merck.com/mrkshared/mmanual section15/chapter188/188a.jsp

IMPLICATIONS OF RESEARCH FOR EVIDENCE-BASED PRACTICE

Brunner, R., Parzer, P., Schuld, V., & Resch, F. (2000). Dissociative symptomatology and traumatogenic factors in adolescent psychiatric patients. *The Journal of Nervous and Mental Disease, 188*(2), 71–77.

Description of the Study: This study describes the relationship between different types of childhood trauma to the degree of dissociative experiences. Subjects were 198 consecutively admitted adolescent psychiatric patients, 11 to 19 years old (89 inpatients and 109 outpatients). All patients completed the Adolescent Dissociative Experiences Scale (ADES), a self-administered questionnaire with 30 items that quantifies the frequency of dissociative experiences on an 11-point scale ranging from 0 (never) to 10 (always). The instrument has been shown to discriminate patients with dissociative disorders from patients in several other diagnostic categories, as well as from adolescents in the general population. Subjects' therapists were asked to complete the Checklist of Traumatic Childhood Events, based on assessments, client self-reports, and reports by caregivers and custodial and social services. The checklist covered four main areas of traumatic experiences: sexual abuse, physical abuse, neglect, and stressful life events. Each area was further categorized by experiences considered from minor to severe. Examples of these abuse extremes included:

- Sexual: From sexualized communication to fondling to masturbation to penetration
- Physical: From being hit with a hand to punching, kicking, lacerations, burns, fractures

- Neglect: From physical and educational neglect to social/ environmental neglect to emotional and psychological involvement (rejection; hostility)
- Stressful life events: From loss related to family members to physical/mental illness of family members to "others" (e.g., personal physical illness, witnessing an accident or violence, institutional placement)

Results of the Study: All mean scores by traumatized adolescents were elevated in comparison to those of the control (nontraumatized) group. Increased dissociative symptomatology was unrelated to the degree of severity of sexual abuse experiences. Interestingly, the study found an increased amount of dissociative symptomatology associated with minor forms of physical abuse, as compared to the severe forms. Only severe forms of stressful life events contributed significantly to a higher degree of dissociative experiences. The study revealed that emotional neglect appears to be the best predictor of dissociative symptoms.

Implications for Nursing Practice: The authors state: "In contrast to the current psychopathogenic model of dissociation which maintains that particularly severe traumatic events lead to dissociative symptomatology, moderate but chronic emotional stress may be equal or even more important in the development of dissociation." This is important information for the nursing database. Nurses should be aware that even less severe forms of abuse and neglect may have a significant impact on the development of dissociative psychopathology in adolescents.

REFERENCES

American Psychiatric Association. (2000). *Diagnostic and statistical manual of mental disorders* (4th ed.) *Text revision*. Washington, DC: American Psychiatric Association.

Brunet, A., Holowka, D.W., & Laurence, J.R. (2003). Dissociation. In M.J. Aminoff & R.B. Daroff (Eds.). *Encyclopedia of the neurological sciences* (vol. 2). New York: Elsevier.

Ford-Martin, P. (2001). Fugue. *Gale Encyclopedia of Psychology*. Retrieved April 23, 2005 from the World Wide Web at http://www. findarticles.com/p/articles/mi_g2699/is_0004/ai_2699000474/print

Maldonado J.R., & Spiegel, D. (2003). Dissociative disorders. In R.E.

Hales & S.C. Yudofsky (Eds.). *Textbook of clinical psychiatry* (4th ed.). Washington, DC: American Psychiatric Publishing.

Sadock, B.J., & Sadock, V.A. (2003). *Synopsis of psychiatry: Behavioral sciences/clinical psychiatry* (9th ed.). Philadelphia: Lippincott Williams & Wilkins.

Shahrokh, N.C., & Hales, R.E. (2003). *American psychiatric glossary* (8th ed.). Washington, DC: American Psychiatric Publishing.

Simeon, D., Stein, D.J., & Hollander, E. (1998). Treatment of deper-sonalization disorder with clomipramine. *Biological Psychiatry, 44*(4), 302–303.

CLASSICAL REFERENCES

Freud, S. (1962). The neuro-psychoses of defense (1894). In J. Strachey (Ed.). *Standard edition of the complete psychological works of*

Sigmund Freud (vol. 3). London: Hogarth Press. (Original work published 1894).

Janet, P. (1907). *The major symptoms of hysteria*. New York: Macmillan.

SEXUAL AND GENDER IDENTITY DISORDERS

CHAPTER OUTLINE

OBJECTIVES

DEVELOPMENT OF HUMAN SEXUALITY

SEXUAL DISORDERS

GENDER IDENTITY DISORDER

VARIATIONS IN SEXUAL ORIENTATION

SEXUALLY TRANSMITTED DISEASES

SUMMARY

REVIEW QUESTIONS

KEY TERMS

anorgasmia
dyspareunia
exhibitionism
fetishism
frotteurism
homosexuality
lesbianism
masochism
orgasm
paraphilia

pedophilia
premature ejaculation
retarded ejaculation
sadism
sensate focus
transsexualism
transvestic fetishism
vaginismus
voyeurism

CORE CONCEPTS

gender
sexuality

OBJECTIVES

After reading this chapter, the student will be able to:

1. Describe developmental processes associated with human sexuality.
2. Discuss historical and epidemiological aspects of paraphilias and sexual dysfunction disorders.
3. Identify various types of paraphilias, sexual dysfunction disorders, and gender identity disorders.
4. Discuss predisposing factors associated with the etiology of paraphilias, sexual dysfunction disorders, and gender identity disorders.
5. Describe the physiology of the human sexual response.
6. Conduct a sexual history.
7. Formulate nursing diagnoses and goals of

care for clients with sexual and gender identity disorders.
8. Identify appropriate nursing interventions for clients with sexual disorders and gender identity disorders.
9. Identify topics for client/family education relevant to sexual disorders.
10. Evaluate care of clients with sexual and gender identity disorders.
11. Describe various medical treatment modalities for clients with sexual and gender identity disorders.
12. Discuss variations in sexual orientation.
13. Identify various types of sexually transmitted diseases and discuss the consequences of each.

uman beings are sexual beings. Sexuality is a basic human need and an innate part of the total personality. It influences our thoughts, actions, and interactions, and is involved in aspects of physical and mental health.

Society's attitude toward sexuality is changing. Clients are more open to seeking assistance in matters that pertain to sexuality. Although not all nurses need to be educated as sex therapists, they can readily integrate information on sexuality into the care they give by focusing on preventive, therapeutic, and educational interventions to assist individuals to attain, regain, or maintain sexual wellness.

This chapter focuses on disorders associated with sexual functioning and gender identity. Primary consideration is given to the categories of **paraphilias**, sexual dysfunction, and gender identity disorders as classified in the *DSM-IV-TR* (American Psychiatric Association [APA], 2000). An overview of human sexual development throughout the life span is presented. Historical and epidemiological information associated with sexual disorders is included. Predisposing factors that have been implicated in the etiology of sexual and gender identity disorders provide a framework for studying the dynamics of these disorders. Various medical treatment modalities are explored. A discussion of variations in sexual orientation is included. Various types of sexually transmitted diseases (STDs) are described, and an explanation of the consequences of each is presented.

Symptomatology of each disorder is presented as background knowledge for assessing clients with sexual and gender identity disorders. A tool for acquiring a sexual history is included. Nursing care is described in the context of the nursing process.

Core Concept

Sexuality

Sexuality is the constitution and life of an individual relative to characteristics regarding intimacy. It reflects the totality of the person and does not relate exclusively to the sex organs or sexual behavior.

DEVELOPMENT OF HUMAN SEXUALITY

Birth Through Age 12

Although the sexual identity of an infant is determined before birth by chromosomal factors and physical appearance of the genitals, postnatal factors can greatly influence the way developing children perceive themselves sexually. Masculinity and femininity, as well as gender roles, are for the most part culturally defined. For example, differentiation of roles may be initiated at birth by painting a child's room pink or blue and by clothing the child in frilly, delicate dresses or tough, sturdy rompers.

It is not uncommon for infants to touch and explore their genitals. In fact, research on infantile sexuality indicates that both male and female infants are capable of sexual arousal and **orgasm** (Berman & Berman, 2001).

By age 2 or 2½, children know what gender they are. They know that they are like the parent of the same gender and different from the parent of the opposite gender and from other children of the opposite gender. They become acutely aware of anatomical sex differences during this time period (Masters, Johnson, & Kolodny, 1995).

By age 4 or 5, children engage in heterosexual play. "Playing doctor" can be a popular game at this age. In this way, children form a concept of marriage to a member of the opposite gender.

Children increasingly gain experience with masturbation during childhood, although certainly not all children masturbate during this period. Most children begin self-exploration and genital self-stimulation at about 15 to 19 months of age (Sadock & Sadock, 2003).

Late childhood and preadolescence may be characterized by heterosexual or homosexual play. Generally the activity involves no more than touching the other's genitals, but may include a wide range of sexual behaviors (Masters, Johnson, & Kolodny, 1995). Girls at this age become interested in menstruation, and members of both sexes are interested in learning about fertility, pregnancy, and birth. Interest in the opposite sex increases. Children of this age become self-conscious about their bodies and are concerned with physical attractiveness.

Children ages 10 to 12 are preoccupied with pubertal changes and the beginnings of romantic interest in the opposite gender. Prepubescent boys may engage in group sexual activities such as genital exhibition or group masturbation. Homosexual sex play is not uncommon. Prepubescent girls may engage in some genital exhibition but are usually not as preoccupied with the genitalia as are boys of this age.

Adolescence

Adolescence represents an acceleration in terms of biological changes and psychosocial and sexual development. This time of turmoil is nurtured by awakening endocrine forces and a new set of psychosocial tasks to undertake (Bell, 1998). Included in these tasks are issues relating to sexuality, such as how to deal with new or more powerful sexual feelings, whether to participate in various types of sexual behavior, how to recognize love, how to prevent unwanted pregnancy, and how to define age-appropriate sex roles.

Biologically, puberty begins for the female adolescent with breast enlargement, widening of the hips, and growth of pubic and ancillary hair. The onset of menstruation usually occurs between the ages of 11 and 13 years. In the male adolescent, growth of pubic hair and enlargement of the testicles begin at 12 to 16 years of age. Penile growth and the ability to ejaculate usually occur from the ages of 13 to 17. There is a marked growth of the body between ages 11 and 17, accompanied by the growth of body and facial hair, increased muscle mass, and a deeper voice.

Sexuality is slower to develop in the female than in the male adolescent. Women show steady increases in sexual responsiveness that peak in their middle 20s or early 30s. Sexual maturity for men is usually reached in the late teens, but their sexual drive remains high through young adulthood (Murray & Zentner, 2001). Masturbation is a common sexual activity among male and female adolescents.

Many individuals have their first experience with sexual intercourse during the adolescent years. Although studies indicate a variety of statistics related to incidence of adolescent coitus, three notable trends have become evident during the past two decades. According to Sadock and Sadock (2003), the trends are:

1. More adolescents are engaging in premarital intercourse.
2. The incidence of premarital intercourse for girls has increased.
3. The average age at first intercourse is decreasing.

The American culture has ambivalent feelings toward adolescent sexuality. Psychosexual development is desired, but most parents want to avoid anything that may encourage teenage sex. The rise in number of cases of STDs, some of which are life threatening, also contributes to fears associated with unprotected sexual activity in all age groups.

Adulthood

This period of the life cycle begins at approximately 20 years of age and continues to age 65. Sexuality associated with ages 65 and older is discussed in Chapter 38.

Marital Sex

Choosing a marital partner or developing a sexual relationship with another individual is one of the major tasks in the early years of this life-cycle stage. Current cultural perspective reflects that the institution of marriage has survived. About 80 percent to 90 percent of all people in the United States marry, and of those who divorce, a high percentage remarries. Intimacy in marriage is one of the most common forms of sexual expressions for adults. The average American couple has coitus about two or three times per week when they are in their 20s, with the frequency gradually declining to about once weekly for those aged 45 and over (Sinclair Intimacy Institute, 2002). Many adults continue to masturbate even though they are married and have ready access to heterosexual sex. This behavior is perfectly normal, although it often evokes feelings of guilt and may be kept secret.

Extramarital Sex

About half of married men and women have engaged in extramarital sex at some time during their marriages (Atwood & Schwartz, 2002). Although the incidence of extramarital sex for men seems to be holding constant, some evidence exists to suggest that the incidence for women may be increasing.

Although attitudes toward premarital sex have changed substantially during the last several decades, attitudes toward extramarital sex have remained relatively stable. Most women and men say they believe sexual exclusivity should be a goal in marriage, although they were less certain about what would happen if their partner did not live up to that ideal. Some studies place the incidence of divorce caused by infidelity or adultery at around 20 percent of all divorce cases.

Sex and the Single Person

Attitudes about sexual intimacy among singles—never married, divorced, or widowed—vary from individual to individual. Some single people will settle for any kind of relationship, casual or committed, that they believe will enrich their lives. Others deny any desire for marriage or sexual intimacy, cherishing instead the independence they retain by being "unattached." Still others may desperately search for a spouse, with the desperation increasing as the years wear on.

Most divorced men and women return to having an active sex life following separation from their spouse. More widowed men than widowed women return to an active sex life after the loss of their partner. This may have in part to do with the fact that men choose women partners younger than themselves, and because widows outnumber widowers by more than 4 to 1 (Administration on Aging, 2003).

The "Middle" Years—40 to 65

With the advent of the middle years, a decrease in hormonal production initiates a number of changes in the sex organs, as well as the rest of the body. The average age of onset of menopause for the woman is around 50, although changes can be noted from about 40 to 60 years of age. Approximately 1 percent of women experience symptoms as early as age 35 (Murray & Zentner, 2001). The decrease in the amount of estrogen can result in loss of vaginal lubrication, making intercourse painful. Other symptoms may include insomnia, "hot flashes," headaches, heart palpitations, and depression. Hormonal supplements may alleviate some of these symptoms, although controversy currently exists within the medical community regarding the safety of hormone replacement therapy.

With the decrease of androgen production during these years, men also experience sexual changes. The amount of ejaculate may decrease, and ejaculation may be less forceful. The testes decrease in size, and erections may be less frequent and less rigid. By age 50, the refractory period increases, and men may require 8 to 24 hours after orgasm before another erection can be achieved.

Biological drives decrease, and interest in sexual activity may decrease during these "middle" years. Although men need longer stimulation to reach orgasm and intensity of pleasure may decrease, women stabilize at the same level of sexual activity as at the previous stage in the life cycle and often have a greater capacity for orgasm in middle adulthood than in young adulthood (Sadock & Sadock, 2003). Murray and Zentner (2001) state:

> The enjoyment of sexual relations in younger years, rather than the frequency, is a key factor for maintenance of desire and activity in women, whereas frequency of relations and enjoyment are important factors for men. (p. 690)

SEXUAL DISORDERS

Paraphilias

The term **paraphilia** is used to identify repetitive or preferred sexual fantasies or behaviors that involve any of the following:

1. The preference for use of a nonhuman object
2. Repetitive sexual activity with humans that involves real or simulated suffering or humiliation
3. Repetitive sexual activity with nonconsenting partners

The *DSM-IV-TR* specifies that these sexual fantasies or behaviors are recurrent over a period of at least 6 months and cause the individual clinically significant distress or impairment in social, occupational, or other important areas of functioning (APA, 2000).

Historical Aspects

Historically, it seems, some restrictions on human sexual expression have always existed. Under the code of Orthodox Judaism, masturbation was punishable by death. In ancient Catholicism it was considered a carnal sin. In the late 19th century this activity was viewed as a major cause of insanity.

The sexual exploitation of children was condemned in ancient cultures, as it continues to be today. Incest remains the one taboo that crosses cultural barriers. It was punishable by death in Babylonia, Judea, and ancient China, and offenders were given the death penalty as late as 1650 in England.

Oral–genital, anal, homosexual, and animal sexual contacts were viewed by the early Christian church as unnatural and, in fact, were considered greater transgressions than extramarital sexual activity because they did not lead to biological reproduction. Today, of these church-condemned behaviors, only sex with animals (zoophilia) retains its classification as a paraphilia in the *DSM-IV-TR*.

Epidemiological Statistics

Relatively limited data exist on the prevalence or course of the paraphilias. Most information that is available has been obtained from studies of incarcerated sex offenders. Another source of information has been from outpatient psychiatric services for paraphiliacs outside the criminal justice system.

Because few paraphiliacs experience personal distress from their behavior, most individuals come for treatment because of pressure from their partners or the authorities (Becker & Johnson, 2003). Data suggest that the most people with paraphilias who seek outpatient treatment do so for **pedophilia** (45 percent), **exhibitionism** (25 percent), or **voyeurism** (12 percent).

Most individuals with paraphilias are men, and more than 50 percent of these individuals develop the onset of their paraphilic arousal before age 18 (Sadock & Sadock, 2003). The behavior peaks between ages 15 and 25 and gradually declines so that, by age 50, the occurrence of paraphilic acts is very low, except for those paraphilic behaviors that occur in isolation or with a cooperative partner. Some individuals with these disorders experience multiple paraphilias.

Types of Paraphilias

The following types of paraphilias are identified by the *DSM-IV-TR*:

Exhibitionism

Exhibitionism is characterized by recurrent, intense, sexual urges, behaviors, or sexually arousing fantasies, of at least 6 months' duration, involving the exposure of one's genitals to an unsuspecting stranger (APA, 2000). Masturbation may occur during the exhibitionism. In almost 100 percent of cases of exhibitionism, the perpetrators are men and the victims are women (Sadock & Sadock, 2003).

The urges for genital exposure intensify when the exhibitionist has excessive free time or is under significant stress. Most people who engage in exhibitionism have rewarding sexual relationships with adult partners but concomitantly expose themselves to others.

Fetishism

Fetishism involves recurrent, intense, sexual urges or behaviors, or sexually arousing fantasies, of at least 6 months' duration, involving the use of nonliving objects (APA, 2000). The sexual focus is commonly on objects intimately associated with the human body (e.g., shoes, gloves, stockings) (Sadock & Sadock, 2003). The fetish object is usually used during masturbation or incorporated into sexual activity with another person in order to produce sexual excitation.

When the fetish involves cross-dressing, the disorder is called **transvestic fetishism**. The individual is a heterosexual man who keeps a collection of women's clothing that he intermittently uses to dress in when alone. The sexual arousal may be produced by an accompanying fantasy of the individual as a woman with female genitalia, or merely by the view of himself fully clothed as a woman without attention to the genitalia (APA, 2000).

Requirement of the fetish object for sexual arousal may become so intense in some individuals that to be without it may result in impotence. Onset of the disorder usually occurs during adolescence.

The disorder is chronic, and the complication arises when the individual becomes progressively more intensely aroused by sexual behaviors that exclude a sexual partner. The person with the fetish and his partner may become so distant that the partner eventually terminates the relationship.

Frotteurism

Frotteurism is the recurrent preoccupation with intense sexual urges, behaviors, or fantasies of at least 6 months' duration involving touching and rubbing against a nonconsenting person (APA, 2000). Sexual excitement is derived from the actual touching or rubbing, not from the coercive nature of the act. Almost without exception, the gender of the frotteur is male.

The individual usually chooses to commit the act in crowded places, such as on buses or subways during rush hour. In this way, he can provide rationalization for his behavior should someone complain, and more easily escape arrest. The frotteur waits in a crowd until he identifies a victim, then he follows her and allows the rush of the crowd to push him against her. He fantasizes a relationship with his victim while rubbing his genitals against her thighs and buttocks or touching her genitalia or breasts with his hands. He often escapes detection owing

to the victim's initial shock and denial that such an act has been committed in this public place.

Pedophilia

The *DSM-IV-TR* describes the essential feature of pedophilia as recurrent sexual urges, behaviors, or sexually arousing fantasies, of at least 6 months' duration, involving sexual activity with a prepubescent child. The age of the molester is at least 16 and at least 5 years older than the child. This category of paraphilia is the most common of sexual assaults.

Most child molestations involve genital fondling or oral sex. Vaginal or anal penetration of the child is most common in cases of incest. Others may limit their activity to undressing the child and looking, exposing themselves, masturbating in the presence of the child, or gently touching and fondling the child (APA, 2000). Onset usually occurs during adolescence, and the disorder often runs a chronic course, particularly with male pedophiles who demonstrate a preference for young boys.

Sexual Masochism

The identifying feature of sexual **masochism** is recurrent, intense, sexual urges, behaviors, or sexually arousing fantasies, of at least 6 months' duration, involving the act (real, not simulated) of being humiliated, beaten, bound, or otherwise made to suffer (APA, 2000). These masochistic activities may be fantasized (e.g., being raped) and may be performed alone (e.g., self-inflicted pain) or with a partner (e.g., being restrained, spanked, or beaten by the partner). Some masochistic activities have resulted in death, in particular those that involve sexual arousal by oxygen deprivation. The disorder is usually chronic and can progress to the point at which the individual cannot achieve sexual satisfaction without masochistic fantasies or activities.

Sexual Sadism

The *DSM-IV-TR* identifies the essential feature of sexual sadism as recurrent, intense, sexual urges, behaviors, or sexually arousing fantasies, of at least 6 months' duration, involving acts (real, not simulated) in which the psychological or physical suffering (including humiliation) of the victim is sexually exciting to the person (APA, 2000). The sadistic activities may be fantasized or acted on with a consenting or nonconsenting partner. In all instances, sexual excitation occurs in response to the suffering of the victim. Examples of sadistic acts include restraint, beating, burning, rape, cutting, torture, and even killing.

The course of the disorder is usually chronic, with the severity of the sadistic acts often increasing over time. Activities with nonconsenting partners are usually terminated by legal apprehension.

Voyeurism

This disorder is identified by recurrent, intense, sexual urges, behaviors, or sexually arousing fantasies, of at least 6 months' duration, involving the act of observing an unsuspecting person who is naked, in the process of disrobing, or engaging in sexual activity (APA, 2000). Sexual excitement is achieved through the act of looking, and no contact with the person is attempted. Masturbation usually accompanies the "window peeping" but may occur later as the individual fantasizes about the voyeuristic act.

Onset of voyeuristic behavior is usually before age 15, and the disorder is often chronic. Most voyeurs enjoy satisfying sexual relationships with an adult partner. Few apprehensions occur because most targets of voyeurism are unaware that they are being observed.

Predisposing Factors to Paraphilias

Biological Factors

Various studies have implicated several organic factors in the etiology of paraphilias. Destruction of parts of the limbic system in animals has been shown to cause hypersexual behavior (Becker & Johnson, 2003). Temporal lobe diseases, such as psychomotor seizures or temporal lobe tumors, have been implicated in some individuals with paraphilias. Abnormal levels of androgens also may contribute to inappropriate sexual arousal. The majority of studies have involved violent sex offenders, and the results cannot accurately be generalized.

Psychoanalytical Theory

The psychoanalytical approach defines a paraphiliac as one who has failed the normal developmental process toward heterosexual adjustment (Sadock & Sadock, 2003). This occurs when the individual fails to resolve the Oedipal crisis and either identifies with the parent of the opposite gender or selects an inappropriate object for libido cathexis. Becker and Johnson (2003) offer the following explanation:

> Severe castration anxiety during the Oedipal phase of development leads to the substitution of a symbolic object (inanimate or an anatomic part) for the mother, as in fetishism and transvestitism. Similarly, anxiety over arousal to the mother can lead to the choice of "safe," inappropriate sexual partners, as in pedophilia and zoophilia, or safe sexual behaviors in which there is no sexual contact, as in exhibitionism and voyeurism. (p. 758)

Behavioral Theory

The behavioral model hypothesizes that whether or not an individual engages in paraphiliac behavior depends on the type of reinforcement he or she receives following the behavior. The initial act may be committed for vari-

ous reasons. Some examples include recalling memories of experiences from an individual's early life (especially the first shared sexual experience), modeling behavior of others who have carried out paraphilic acts, mimicking sexual behavior depicted in the media, and recalling past trauma such as one's own molestation (Sadock & Sadock, 2003).

Once the initial act has been committed, the paraphiliac consciously evaluates the behavior and decides whether to repeat it. A fear of punishment or perceived harm or injury to the victim, or a lack of pleasure derived from the experience, may extinguish the behavior. When negative consequences do not occur, however, when the act itself is highly pleasurable, or when the person with the paraphilia immediately escapes and thereby avoids seeing any negative consequences experienced by the victim, the activity is more likely to be repeated.

Transactional Model of Stress/Adaptation

One model alone is probably not sufficient to explain the etiology of paraphilias. It is most likely that the integration of learning experiences, sociocultural factors, and biologic processes must occur to account for these deviant sexual behaviors. A combination of biological inheritance, hormonal variations, poor parenting, sociocultural attitudes, and aspects of the learning paradigm previously described probably provides the most comprehensive etiological explanation for paraphilias to date (Abel, Rouleau, & Osborn, 1994). In Figure 33–1, a graphic depiction of the theory of multiple causation is presented in the transactional model of stress/adaptation.

Treatment Modalities

Biological Treatment

Biological treatment of individuals with paraphilias has focused on blocking or decreasing the level of circulating androgens. The most extensively used of the antiandrogenic medications are the progestin derivatives that block testosterone synthesis or block androgen receptors (Becker & Johnson, 2003). They do not influence the direction of sexual drive toward appropriate adult partners. Instead they act to decrease libido and thus break the individual's pattern of compulsive deviant sexual behavior (Becker & Johnson, 2003). They are not meant to be the sole source of treatment and work best when given in conjunction with participation in individual or group psychotherapy.

Psychoanalytical Therapy

Psychoanalytical approaches have been tried in the treatment of paraphilias. In this type of therapy, the therapist helps the client to identify unresolved conflicts and traumas from early childhood. The therapy focuses on help-

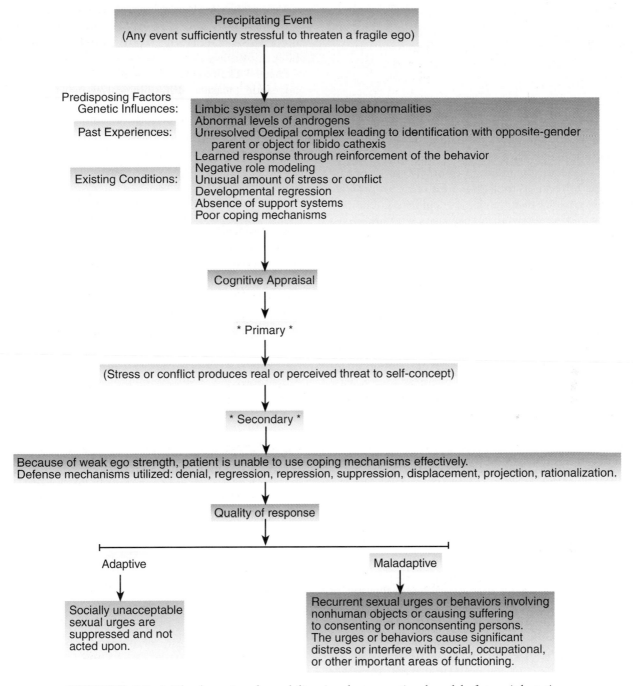

FIGURE 33–1 The dynamics of paraphilia using the transactional model of stress/adaptation.

ing the individual resolve these early conflicts, thus relieving the anxiety that prevents him or her from forming appropriate sexual relationships. In turn the individual has no further need for paraphilic fantasies.

Behavioral Therapy

Aversion techniques have been used to modify undesirable behavior. Aversion therapy methods in the treatment of paraphilias involve paring noxious stimuli, such as electric shocks and bad odors, with the impulse, which

then diminishes. Behavioral therapy also includes skills training and cognitive restructuring in an effort to change the individual's maladaptive beliefs (Becker & Johnson, 2003).

Other behavioral approaches to decreasing inappropriate sexual arousal have included covert sensitization and satiation. With covert sensitization, the individual combines inappropriate sexual fantasies with aversive, anxiety-provoking scenes under the guidance of the therapist (Becker & Johnson, 2003). Satiation is a technique in which the postorgasmic individual repeatedly fantasizes deviant behaviors to the point of saturation with the deviant stimuli, consequently making the fantasies and behavior unexciting.

Role of the Nurse

Treatment of the person with a paraphilia is often very frustrating for both the client and the therapist. Most individuals with paraphilias deny that they have a problem and seek psychiatric care only after their inappropriate behavior comes to the attention of others. In secondary prevention, the focus is to diagnose and treat the problem as early as possible to minimize difficulties. These individuals should be referred to specialists who are accustomed to working with this very special population.

Nursing may best become involved in the primary prevention process. The focus of primary prevention in sexual disorders is to intervene in home life or other facets of childhood in an effort to prevent problems from developing. An additional concern of primary prevention is to assist in the development of adaptive coping strategies to deal with stressful life situations.

Three major components of sexual development have been identified: (1) gender identity (one's sense of maleness or femaleness), (2) sexual responsiveness (arousal to appropriate stimuli), and (3) the ability to establish relationships with others. A disturbance in one or more of these components may lead to a variety of sexual deviations.

Different developmental components seem to be disturbed in the various sexual deviations. For example, gender identity may be disturbed in transvestitism or **transsexualism**. The second component, sexual responsiveness to appropriate stimuli, is disturbed in the case of the fetishist. In the case of the exhibitionist or the frotteur, the ability to form relationships may be disturbed.

Nurses can participate in the regular evaluation of these developmental components to ensure that as children mature, their development in each of these three components is healthy, thereby preventing deviant sexual behaviors. Nurses who work in pediatrics, psychiatry, public health, ambulatory clinics, schools, and any other facility requiring contact with children must be knowledgeable about human sexual development. Accurate assessment and early intervention by these nurses can contribute a great deal toward primary prevention of sexual disorders.

Sexual Dysfunctions

The Sexual Response Cycle

Because sexual dysfunctions occur as disturbances in any of the phases of the sexual response cycle, an understanding of anatomy and physiology is a prerequisite to considerations of pathology and treatment.

Phase I. Desire. During this phase, the desire to have sexual activity occurs in response to verbal, physical, and/or visual stimulation. Sexual fantasies can also bring about this desire.

Phase II. Excitement. This is the phase of sexual arousal and erotic pleasure. Physiological changes occur. The male responds with penile tumescence and erection. Female changes include vasocongestion in the pelvis, vaginal lubrication and expansion, and swelling of the external genitalia (APA, 2000).

Phase III. Orgasm. Orgasm is identified as a peaking of sexual pleasure, with release of sexual tension and rhythmic contraction of the perineal muscles and reproductive organs (APA, 2000). Orgasm in women is marked by simultaneous rhythmic contractions of the uterus, the lower third of the vagina, and the anal sphincter. In men, a forceful emission of semen occurs in response to rhythmic spasms of the prostate, seminal vesicles, vas, and urethra (APA, 2000; Sadock & Sadock, 2003).

Phase IV: Resolution. If orgasm has occurred, this phase is characterized by disgorgement of blood from the genitalia (detumescence), creating a sense of general relaxation, well-being, and muscular relaxation. If orgasm does not occur, resolution may take 2 to 6 hours and be associated with irritability and discomfort (Sadock & Sadock, 2003).

After orgasm, men experience a refractory period that may last from several minutes to many hours, during which time they cannot be stimulated to further orgasm. Commonly, the length of the refractory period increases with age. Women experience no refractory period and may be able to respond to additional stimulation almost immediately (APA, 2000).

Historical and Epidemiological Aspects Related to Sexual Dysfunction

Concurrent with the cultural changes occurring during the sexual revolution of the 1960s and 1970s came an increase in scientific research into sexual physiology and sexual dysfunctions. Masters and Johnson (1966, 1970) pioneered this work with their studies on human sexual response and the treatment of sexual dysfunctions. Spear (2001) reports:

> Sex therapy, the treatment of sexual disorders, has evolved from early studies on sexual behavior made over 50 years ago. During these 50 years, the approach to sex therapy has changed immensely. When William Masters and Virginia Johnson published *Human Sexual Inadequacy* in 1970, the sexual revolution, born in the 1960s, was not yet in full force. Due in part to the development of the oral contraceptive known as 'the pill' and the rise in the politics of feminism, society began to take a different, more open view of sexuality. The rise in sex therapy addressed [sexual] issues as they had never been addressed before, in the privacy of a doctor's office.

Sexual dysfunction consists of an impairment or disturbance in any of the phases of the sexual response cycle. No one knows exactly how many people experience sexual dysfunctions. Knowledge exists only about those who seek some kind of treatment for the problem, and they may be few in number compared with those who have a dysfunction but suffer quietly and never seek therapy.

In 1970, Masters and Johnson reported that 50 percent of all American couples suffered from some type of sexual dysfunction. In 1984, Robins and coworkers estimated that 24 percent of the U.S. population will experience a sexual dysfunction at some time in their lives. The *DSM-IV-TR* reports on the most comprehensive survey to date, conducted on a representative sample of the U.S. population of individuals between ages 18 and 59, regarding the prevalence of the various sexual dysfunctions. These data are presented in Table 33–1.

Types of Sexual Dysfunction

Sexual Desire Disorders

Hypoactive Sexual Desire Disorder. This disorder is defined by the *DSM-IV-TR* (APA, 2000) as a persistent or recurrent deficiency or absence of sexual fantasies and desire for sexual activity. The judgment of deficiency or absence is made by the clinician, taking into account factors that affect sexual functioning, such as age and the context of the person's life.

An individual's absolute level of sexual desire may not be the problem; rather, the problem may be a discrepancy between the partners' levels. The conflict may occur if one partner wants to have sexual relations more often than the other. Care must be taken not to label one partner as pathological when the problem actually lies in the discrepancy of sexual desire between the partners.

An estimated 20 percent of the total population has hypoactive sexual desire disorder (Sadock & Sadock, 2003). The complaint is more common in women than in men.

Sexual Aversion Disorder. This disorder is characterized by a persistent or recurrent extreme aversion to, and

avoidance of, all (or almost all) genital sexual contact with a sexual partner (APA, 2000). Whereas individuals displaying hypoactive desire are often neutral or indifferent toward sexual interaction, sexual aversion implies anxiety, fear, or disgust in sexual situations.

Sexual Arousal Disorders

Female Sexual Arousal Disorder. Female sexual arousal disorder is identified in the *DSM-IV-TR* as a persistent or recurrent inability to attain, or to maintain until completion of the sexual activity, an adequate lubrication/swelling response of sexual excitement.

Male Erectile Disorder. Male erectile disorder is characterized by persistent or recurrent inability to attain, or to maintain until completion of the sexual activity, an adequate erection (APA, 2000). *Primary erectile dysfunction* refers to cases in which the man has never been able to have intercourse; *secondary erectile dysfunction* refers to cases in which the man has difficulty getting or maintaining an erection but has been able to have vaginal or anal intercourse at least once.

Orgasmic Disorders

Female Orgasmic Disorder. Female orgasmic disorder is defined by the *DSM-IV-TR* as persistent or recurrent delay in, or absence of, orgasm following a normal sexual excitement phase. This condition is sometimes referred to as **anorgasmia**. Women who can achieve orgasm through noncoital clitoral stimulation but are not able to experience it during coitus in the absence of manual clitoral stimulation are not necessarily categorized as anorgasmic (Sadock & Sadock, 2003).

A woman is considered to have *primary orgasmic dysfunction* when she has never experienced orgasm by any kind of stimulation. *Secondary orgasmic dysfunction* exists if the woman has experienced at least one orgasm, regardless of the means of stimulation, but no longer does so.

Male Orgasmic Disorder. Male orgasmic disorder, sometimes referred to as **retarded ejaculation**, is characterized by persistent or recurrent delay in, or absence of, orgasm following a normal sexual excitement phase during sexual activity that the clinician, taking into account the person's age, judges to be adequate in focus, intensity, and duration (APA, 2000). With this disorder, the man is unable to ejaculate, even though he has a firm erection and has had more than adequate stimulation. The severity of the problem may range from only occasional problems ejaculating (*secondary disorder*) to a history of never having experienced an orgasm (*primary disorder*). In the most common version, the man cannot ejaculate during coitus but may be able to ejaculate as a result of other types of stimulation.

Premature Ejaculation. The *DSM-IV-TR* describes **premature ejaculation** as persistent or recurrent ejacu-

TABLE 33–1	Estimates of Prevalence Rates* for Sexual Dysfunctions	
DISORDER	**MEN (%)**	**WOMEN (%)**
Dyspareunia	3	15
Orgasm problems	10	25
Hypoactive sexual desire	—	33
Premature ejaculation	27	—
Arousal problems	—	20
Erectile difficulties	10	—

*Prevalence rate refers to an estimate of the number of people who have a disorder at any given time.
SOURCE: Adapted from the *DSM-IV-TR* (APA, 2000).

lation with minimal sexual stimulation before, on, or shortly after penetration and before the person wishes it. Diagnosis should take into account factors that affect duration of the excitement phase, such as age, novelty of the sexual partner or situation, and recent frequency of sexual activity (APA, 2000).

An estimated 27 percent of the male population has this dysfunction, and 35 to 40 percent of men treated for sexual disorders have premature ejaculation as the chief complaint (Becker & Johnson, 2003; Sadock & Sadock, 2003). It is particularly common among young men who have a very high sex drive and have not yet learned to control ejaculation.

Sexual Pain Disorders

Dyspareunia. **Dyspareunia** is recurrent or persistent genital pain associated with sexual intercourse in either a man or a woman (APA, 2000). It is not caused by **vaginismus**, lack of lubrication, other general medical conditions, or physiological effects of substance use. In women, the pain may be felt in the vagina, around the vaginal entrance and clitoris, or deep in the pelvis. In men, the pain is felt in the penis. Dyspareunia makes intercourse very unpleasant and may even lead to abstention from sexual activity.

Prevalence studies of dyspareunia have provided estimates of 15 percent in women and 3 percent in men (APA, 2000). Dyspareunia in men is often associated with urinary tract infection, with pain being experienced during urination as well as during ejaculation.

Vaginismus. Vaginismus is an involuntary constriction of the outer one third of the vagina that prevents penile insertion and intercourse (APA, 2000). Vaginismus is less prevalent than female orgasmic disorder, and the disorder most often afflicts highly educated women and those in the high socioeconomic groups (Sadock & Sadock, 2003). It is estimated that 12 to 17 percent of women presenting to sexual therapy clinics do so with the complaint of vaginismus (Leiblum, 1999).

Sexual Dysfunction Due to a General Medical Condition and Substance-Induced Sexual Dysfunction

With these disorders, the sexual dysfunction is judged to be caused by the direct physiological effects of a general medical condition or use of a substance. The dysfunction may involve pain, impaired desire, impaired arousal, or impaired orgasm. Types of medical conditions that are associated with sexual dysfunction include neurological (e.g., multiple sclerosis, neuropathy), endocrine (e.g., diabetes mellitus, thyroid dysfunctions), vascular (e.g., atherosclerosis), and genitourinary (e.g., testicular disease, urethral or vaginal infections). Some substances that can interfere with sexual functioning include alcohol,

amphetamines, cocaine, opioids, sedatives, hypnotics, anxiolytics, antidepressants, antipsychotics, and antihypertensives.

Predisposing Factors to Sexual Dysfunctions

Biological Factors

Sexual Desire Disorders. Studies have correlated decreased levels of serum testosterone with hypoactive sexual desire disorder in men. Evidence also exists that suggests a relationship between serum testosterone and increased female libido (Leiblum, 1999). Diminished libido has been observed in men with elevated levels of serum prolactin (Shenenberger & Knee, 2004). Various medications have also been implicated in the etiology of hypoactive sexual desire disorder. Some examples include antihypertensives, antipsychotics, antidepressants, anxiolytics, and anticonvulsants. Alcohol and cocaine have also been associated with impaired desire, especially after chronic use.

Sexual Arousal Disorders. Postmenopausal women require a longer period of stimulation for lubrication to occur, and there is generally less vaginal transudate after menopause (Altman & Hanfling, 2003). Various medications, particularly those with antihistaminic and anticholinergic properties, may also contribute to decreased ability for arousal in women. Arteriosclerosis is a common cause of male erectile disorder as a result of arterial insufficiency (Brosman & Leslie, 2004). Various neurological disorders can contribute to erectile dysfunctions as well. The most common neurologically based cause may be diabetes, which places men at high risk for neuropathy (Brosman & Leslie, 2004). Others include temporal lobe epilepsy and multiple sclerosis. Trauma (e.g., spinal cord injury, pelvic cancer surgery) can also result in erectile dysfunction. Several medications have been implicated in the etiology of this disorder, including antihypertensives, antipsychotics, antidepressants, and anxiolytics. Chronic use of alcohol has also been shown to be a contributing factor.

Orgasmic Disorders. Some women report decreased ability to achieve orgasm following hysterectomy. Conversely, some report increased sexual activity and decreased sexual dysfunction following hysterectomy (Rhodes et al., 1999). Studies of the use of transdermal testosterone for sexual dysfunction in women after hysterectomy have revealed mixed results (Nappi et al., 2005). Some medications (e.g., selective serotonin reuptake inhibitors) may inhibit orgasm. Medical conditions, such as depression, hypothyroidism, and diabetes mellitus, may cause decreased sexual arousal and orgasm.

Biological factors associated with inhibited male orgasm include surgery of the genitourinary tract (e.g., prostatectomy), various neurological disorders (e.g., Parkinson's disease), and other diseases (e.g., diabetes mellitus). Medications that have been implicated include opioids, antihypertensives, antidepressants, and antipsychotics (Altman & Hanfling, 2003). Transient cases of the disorder may occur with excessive alcohol intake.

Although premature ejaculation is commonly caused by psychological factors, general medical conditions or substance use may also be contributing influences. Particularly in cases of secondary dysfunction, in which a man at one time had ejaculatory control but later lost it, physical factors may be involved. Examples include a local infection such as prostatitis or a degenerative neural disorder such as multiple sclerosis.

Sexual Pain Disorders. A number of organic factors can contribute to painful intercourse in women, including intact hymen, episiotomy scar, vaginal or urinary tract infection, ligament injuries, endometriosis, or ovarian cysts or tumors. Painful intercourse in men may also be caused by various organic factors. For example, infection caused by poor hygiene under the foreskin of an uncircumsized man can cause pain. Phimosis, a condition in which the foreskin cannot be pulled back, can also cause painful intercourse. An allergic reaction to various vaginal spermicides or irritation caused by vaginal infections may be a contributing factor. Finally, various prostate problems may cause pain on ejaculation.

Psychosocial Factors

Sexual Desire Disorders. Phillips (2000) has identified a number of individual and relationship factors that may contribute to hypoactive sexual desire disorder. Individual causes include religious orthodoxy; sexual identity conflicts; past sexual abuse; financial, family, or job problems; depression; and aging-related concerns (e.g., changes in physical appearance). Among the relationship causes are interpersonal conflicts; current physical, verbal, or sexual abuse; extramarital affairs; and desire or practices that differ from those of the partner.

Regarding sexual aversion disorder, Leiblum (1999) states:

> Many clinicians believe that this disorder might best be viewed as a phobia and removed from the sexual desire category. In general, sexual aversion is associated with a past history of sexual or gynecologic trauma.

Sexual Arousal Disorders. A number of psychological factors have been cited as possible impediments to female arousal. They include doubt, guilt, fear, anxiety, shame, conflict, embarrassment, tension, disgust, irritation, resentment, grief, hostility toward partner, and a puritanical or moralistic upbringing. It is well documented that sexual abuse is a significant risk factor

for desire and arousal disorders in women (Lieblum, 1999).

The etiology of male erectile disorder may be related to chronic stress, anxiety, or depression (Sadock & Sadock, 2003). Developmental factors that hinder the ability to be intimate, that lead to a feeling of inadequacy or distrust, or that develop a sense of being unloving or unlovable may also result in impotence. Relationship factors that may affect erectile functioning include lack of attraction to one's partner, anger toward one's partner, or being in a relationship that is not characterized by trust (Altman & Hanfling, 2003). Unfortunately, regardless of the etiology of the impotence, once it occurs, the man may become increasingly anxious about his next sexual encounter. This anticipatory anxiety about achieving and maintaining an erection may then perpetuate the problem.

Orgasmic Disorders. Numerous psychological factors are associated with inhibited female orgasm. They include fears of becoming pregnant, rejection by the sexual partner, damage to the vagina, hostility toward men, and feelings of guilt regarding sexual impulses (Sadock & Sadock, 2003). Negative cultural conditioning ("nice girls don't enjoy sex") may also influence the adult female's sexual response. Various developmental factors also have relevance to orgasmic dysfunction. Examples include childhood exposure to rigid religious orthodoxy, negative family attitudes toward nudity and sex, and traumatic sexual experiences during childhood or adolescence, such as incest or rape (Clayton, 2002; Phillips, 2000).

Psychological factors are also associated with inhibited male orgasm. In the primary disorder (never experienced prior orgasm), the man often comes from a rigid, puritanical background. He perceives sex as sinful and the genitals as dirty, and he may have conscious or unconscious incest wishes and guilt (Sadock & Sadock, 2003). In the case of secondary disorder (previously experienced orgasms that have now stopped), interpersonal difficulties are usually implicated. There may be some ambivalence about commitment, fear of pregnancy, or unexpressed hostility.

Premature ejaculation may be related to a lack of physical awareness on the part of a sexually inexperienced man. The ability to control ejaculation occurs as a gradual maturing process with a sexual partner in which foreplay becomes more give-and-take "pleasuring," rather than strictly goal oriented. The man becomes aware of the sensations and learns to delay the point of ejaculatory inevitability. Relationship problems such as a stressful marriage, negative cultural conditioning, anxiety over intimacy, and lack of comfort in the sexual relationship may also contribute to this disorder (Sadock & Sadock, 2003).

Sexual Pain Disorders. Vaginismus may occur in response to having experienced dyspareunia (painful intercourse) for various organic reasons stated in the "biological factors" section. Involuntary constriction within the vagina occurs in response to anticipatory pain, making intercourse impossible. The diagnosis does not apply if the cause of the vaginismus is determined to be organic. A variety of psychosocial factors have been implicated, including negative childhood conditioning of sex as dirty, sinful, and shameful. Early traumatic sexual experiences (e.g., rape or incest) may also cause vaginismus. Other factors that may be important in the etiology of vaginismus include homosexual orientation, traumatic experience with an early pelvic examination, pregnancy phobia, STD phobia, or cancer phobia (Dreyfus, 1998; Leiblum, 1999; Phillips, 2000; Sadock & Sadock, 2003).

Transactional Model of Stress/Adaptation

The etiology of sexual dysfunction is most likely influenced by multiple factors. In Figure 33–2, a graphic depiction of the theory of multiple causation is presented in the transactional model of stress/adaptation.

Application of the Nursing Process to Sexual Disorders

Assessment

Most assessment tools for taking a general nursing history contain some questions devoted to sexuality. Although many nurses feel uncomfortable obtaining information about the subject, accurate data must be collected if problems are to be identified and resolutions attempted. Sexual health is an integral part of physical and emotional well-being. The nursing history is incomplete if items directed toward sexuality are not included.

Indeed, most nurses are not required to obtain a sexual history as in-depth as the one presented in this chapter. However, certain clients require a more extensive sexual history than that which is included in the general nursing history. These include clients who have medical or surgical conditions that may affect their sexuality; clients with infertility problems, STDs, or complaints of sexual inadequacy; clients who are pregnant, or have gynecological problems; those seeking information on abortion or family planning; and individuals in premarital, marital, and psychiatric counseling.

The best approach for taking a sexual history is a nondirective one; that is, it is best to use the sexual history outline as a guideline but allow the interview to progress in a less restrictive manner than the outline permits (with one question immediately following the other). The order of the questions should be adjusted according to the client's needs as they are identified dur-

ing the interview. A nondirective approach allows time for the client to interject information related to feelings or concerns about his or her sexuality.

The language used should be understandable to the client. If he or she uses terminology that is unfamiliar, ask for clarification. Take level of education and cultural influences into consideration.

The nurse's attitude must convey warmth, openness, honesty, and objectivity. Personal feelings, attitudes, and values should be clarified and should not interfere with acceptance of the client. The nurse must remain nonjudgmental. This is conveyed by listening in an interested matter-of-fact manner without overreacting to any information the client may present.

The content outline for a sexual history presented in Table 33–2 is not intended to be used as a rigid questionnaire but as guidelines from which the nurse may select appropriate topics for gathering information about the client's sexuality. The outline should be individualized according to client needs.

Diagnosis/Outcome Identification

Nursing diagnoses are formulated from the data gathered during the assessment phase and with background knowledge regarding predisposing factors to the disorder. The following nursing diagnoses may be used for the client with sexual disorders:

Sexual dysfunction related to depression and conflict in relationship or certain biological or psychological contributing factors to the disorder evidenced by loss of sexual desire or function.
Ineffective sexuality patterns related to conflicts with sexual orientation or variant preferences, evidenced by expressed dissatisfaction with sexual behaviors (e.g., voyeurism, transvestitism).

The following criteria may be used for measurement of outcomes in the care of the client with sexual disorders.

The client:

1. Can correlate stressful situations that decrease sexual desire.
2. Can communicate with partner about sexual situation without discomfort.
3. Can verbalize ways to enhance sexual desire.
4. Verbalizes resumption of sexual activity at level satisfactory to self and partner.
5. Can correlate variant behaviors with times of stress.
6. Can verbalize fears about abnormality and inappropriateness of sexual behaviors.
7. Expresses desire to change variant sexual behavior.
8. Participates and cooperates with extended plan of behavior modification.
9. Expresses satisfaction with own sexuality pattern.

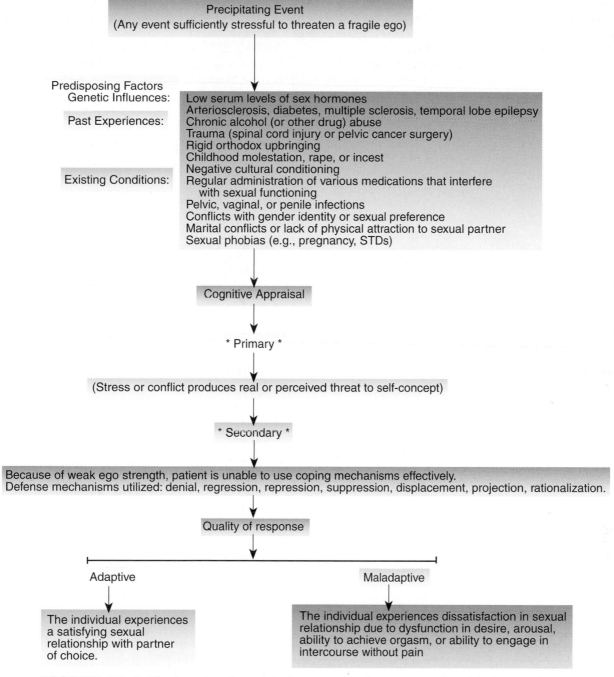

Precipitating Event
(Any event sufficiently stressful to threaten a fragile ego)

Predisposing Factors
Genetic Influences:

Past Experiences:

Existing Conditions:

Low serum levels of sex hormones
Arteriosclerosis, diabetes, multiple sclerosis, temporal lobe epilepsy
Chronic alcohol (or other drug) abuse
Trauma (spinal cord injury or pelvic cancer surgery)
Rigid orthodox upbringing
Childhood molestation, rape, or incest
Negative cultural conditioning
Regular administration of various medications that interfere
    with sexual functioning
Pelvic, vaginal, or penile infections
Conflicts with gender identity or sexual preference
Marital conflicts or lack of physical attraction to sexual partner
Sexual phobias (e.g., pregnancy, STDs)

Cognitive Appraisal

* Primary *

(Stress or conflict produces real or perceived threat to self-concept)

* Secondary *

Because of weak ego strength, patient is unable to use coping mechanisms effectively.
Defense mechanisms utilized: denial, regression, repression, suppression, displacement, projection, rationalization.

Quality of response

Adaptive

The individual experiences
a satisfying sexual
relationship with partner
of choice.

Maladaptive

The individual experiences dissatisfaction in sexual
relationship due to dysfunction in desire, arousal,
ability to achieve orgasm, or ability to engage in
intercourse without pain

FIGURE 33–2 The dynamics of sexual dysfunction using the transactional model of stress/adaptation.

Planning/Implementation

Table 33–3 provides a plan of care for the client with sexual disorders. Nursing diagnoses are presented, along with outcome criteria, appropriate nursing interventions, and rationales.

The concept map care plan is an innovative approach to planning and organizing nursing care (see Chapter 9). It is a diagrammatic teaching and learning strategy that allows visualization of interrelationships between medical diagnoses, nursing diagnoses, assessment data, and treatments. An example of a concept map care plan for a client with a sexual disorder is presented in Figure 33–3.

Client/Family Education

The role of client teacher is important in the psychiatric area, as it is in all areas of nursing. A list of topics for

TABLE 33–2 **Sexual History: Content Outline**

I. Identify data
  A. Client
    1. Age
    2. Gender
    3. Marital status
  B. Parents
    1. Ages
    2. Dates of death and ages at death
    3. Birthplace
    4. Marital status
    5. Religion
    6. Education
    7. Occupation
    8. Congeniality
    9. Demonstration of affection
    10. Feelings toward parents
  C. Siblings (same information as above)
  D. Marital partner (same information as above)
  E. Children
    1. Ages
    2. Gender
    3. Strengths
    4. Identified problems
II. Childhood sexuality
  A. Family attitudes about sex
    1. Parents' openness about sex
    2. Parents' attitudes about nudity
  B. Learning about sex
    1. Asking parents about sex
    2. Information volunteered by parents
    3. At what age and how did client learn about:
      pregnancy, birth, intercourse, masturbation,
      nocturnal emissions, menstruation, homosexuality, STDs
  C. Childhood sex activity
    1. First sight of nude body:
      a. Same gender
      b. Opposite gender
    2. First genital self-stimulation
      a. Age
      b. Feelings
      c. Consequences
    3. First sexual exploration at play with another child
      a. Age (of self and other child)
      b. Gender of other child
      c. Nature of the activity
      d. Feelings and consequences
    4. Sexual activity with older persons
      a. Age (of self and other person)
      b. Gender of other person
      c. Nature of the activity
      d. Client willingness to participate
      e. Feelings and consequences
  D. Did you ever see your parents (or others) having intercourse?
     Describe your feelings.
  E. Childhood sexual theories or myths:
    1. Thoughts about conception and birth.
    2. Roles of male/female genitals and other body parts in sexuality.
III. Onset of adolescence
  A. In girls:
    1. Information about menstruation:
      a. How received: from whom
      b. Age received
      c. Feelings
    2. Age:
      a. Of first period
      b. When breasts began to develop
      c. At appearance of ancillary and pubic hair
    3. Menstruation
      a. Regularity; discomfort; duration
      b. Feelings about first period

  B. In boys:
    1. Information about puberty:
      a. How received; from whom
      b. Age received
      c. Feelings
    2. Age
      a. Of appearance of ancillary and pubic hair
      b. Change of voice
      c. First orgasm (with or without ejaculation); emotional
         reaction
IV. Orgastic experiences
  A. Nocturnal emissions (male) or orgasms (female) during
     sleep.
    1. Frequency
  B. Masturbation
    1. Age begun; ever punished?
    2. Frequency; methods used.
    3. Marital partner's knowledge
    4. Practiced with others? Spouse?
    5. Emotional reactions.
    6. Accompanying fantasies.
  C. Necking and petting ("making out")
    1. Age when begun.
    2. Frequency.
    3. Number of partners.
    4. Types of activity.
  D. Premarital intercourse.
    1. Frequency.
    2. Relationship with and number of partners.
    3. Contraceptives used.
    4. Feelings
  E. Orgasmic frequency
    1. Past
    2. Present.
V. Feelings about self as masculine/feminine
  A. The male client:
    1. Does he feel masculine?
    2. Accepted by peers?
    3. Sexually adequate?
    4. Feelings/concerns about body:
      a. Size
      b. Appearance
      c. Function
  B. The female client:
    1. Does she feel feminine?
    2. Accepted by peers?
    3. Sexually adequate?
    4. Feelings/concerns about body:
      a. Size
      b. Appearance
      c. Function
VI. Sexual fantasies and dreams
  A. Nature of sex dreams
  B. Nature of fantasies
    1. During masturbation
    2. During intercourse.
VII. Dating
  A. Age and feelings about:
    1. First date
    2. First kissing
    3. First petting or "making out"
    4. First going steady
VIII. Engagement
  A. Age
  B. Sex activity during engagement period:
    1. With fiancee
    2. With others
IX. Marriage
  A. Date of marriage
  B. Age at marriage: Spouse:

(Continued on opposite page)

C. Spouse's occupation
D. Previous marriages: Spouse:
E. Reason for termination of previous marriages:
    Client: Spouse:
F. Children from previous marriages:
    Client: Spouse:
G. Wedding trip (honeymoon):
    1. Where? How long?
    2. Pleasant or unpleasant?
    3. Sexual considerations?
H. Sex in marriage:
    1. General satisfaction/dissatisfaction.
    2. Thoughts about spouse's general satisfaction/dissatisfaction
I. Pregnancies
    1. Number: Ages of couple:
    2. Results (normal birth; cesarean delivery; miscarriage; abortion).
    3. Planned or unplanned.
    4. Effects on sexual adjustment.
    5. Sex of child wanted or unwanted.
X. Extramarital sex
A. Emotional attachments
    1. Number; frequency; feelings
B. Sexual intercourse
    1. Number; frequency; feelings
C. Postmarital masturbation
    1. Frequency; feelings
D. Postmarital homosexuality
    1. Frequency; feelings
E. Multiple sex ("swinging")
    1. Frequency; feelings
XI. Sex after widowhood, separation, or divorce:
A. Outlet
    1. Orgasms in sleep
    2. Masturbation
    3. Petting
    4. Intercourse
    5. Homosexuality
    6. Other
B. Frequency; feelings
XII. Variation in sexual orientation:
A. Homosexuality
    1. First experience; describe circumstances.
    2. Frequency since adolescence
XIII. Paraphilias
A. Sexual contact with animals
    1. First experience; describe nature of contact
    2. Frequency and recent contact.
    3. Feelings
B. Voyeurism
    1. Describe types of observation experienced
    2. Feelings

C. Exhibitionism
    1. To whom? When?
    2. Feelings
D. Fetishes; transvestitism
    1. Nature of fetish
    2. Nature of transvestite activity
    3. Feelings
E. Sadomasochism
    1. Nature of activity
    2. Sexual response
    3. Frequency; recency
    4. Consequences
F. Seduction and rape
    1. Has client seduced/raped another?
    2. Has client ever been seduced/raped?
G. Incest
    1. Nature of the sexual activity
    2. With whom?
    3. When occurred? Frequency; recency.
    4. Consequences
XIV. Prostitution
A. Has client ever accepted/paid
    money for sex?
B. Type of sexual activity engaged in.
C. Feelings about prostitution.
XV. Certain effects of sex activities
A. STDs
    1. Age at learning about STDs
    2. Type of STD contracted
    3. Age and treatment received.
B. Illegitimate pregnancy
    1. At what age(s)
    2. Outcome of the pregnancy(ies)
    3. Feelings
C. Abortion
    1. Why performed?
    2. At what age(s)?
    3. How often?
    4. Before or after marriage?
    5. Circumstance: who, where, how?
    6. Feelings about abortion: at the time; in retrospect; anniversary reaction.
XVI. Use of erotic material
A. Personal response to erotic material
    1. Sexual pleasure—arousal
    2. Mild pleasure
    3. Disinterest; disgust
B. Use in connection with sexual activity
    1. Type and frequency of use
    2. To accompany what type of sexual activity

SOURCE: Adapted from an outline prepared by the Group for Advancement of Psychiatry, based on the Sexual Performance Evaluation Questionnaire of the Marriage Council of Philadelphia. Used with permission.

client/family education relevant to sexual disorders is presented in Table 33–4.

Evaluation

Reassessment is necessary to determine if selected interventions have been successful in helping the client overcome problems with sexual functioning. Evaluation may be facilitated by gathering information using the following types of questions.

For the client with sexual dysfunction:

1. Has the client identified life situations that promote feelings of depression and decreased sexual desire?
2. Can he or she verbalize ways to deal with this stress?
3. Can the client satisfactorily communicate with sexual partner about the problem?
4. Have the client and sexual partner identified ways to enhance sexual desire and the achievement of sexual satisfaction for both?
5. Are client and partner seeking assistance with relationship conflict?
6. Do both partners agree on what the major problem is? Do they have the motivation to attempt change?

TABLE 33-3 Care Plan for the Client with a Sexual Disorder

NURSING DIAGNOSIS: SEXUAL DYSFUNCTION

RELATED TO: Depression and conflict in relationship; biological or psychological contributing factors to the disorder

EVIDENCED BY: Loss of sexual desire or function

OUTCOME CRITERIA	NURSING INTERVENTIONS	RATIONALE
Client identifies stressors that contribute to loss of sexual desire or function. Client resumes sexual activity at level satisfactory to self and partner.	1. Assess client's sexual history and previous level of satisfaction in sexual relationship. 2. Assess client's perception of the problem. 3. Help client determine time dimension associated with the onset of the problem and discuss what was happening in life situation at that time. 4. Assess client's level of energy. 5. Review medication regimen; observe for side effects. 6. Provide information regarding sexuality and sexual functioning. 7. Refer for additional counseling or sex therapy if required.	1. Client history establishes a database from which to work and provides a foundation for goal setting. 2. Client's idea of what constitutes a problem may differ from that of the nurse. It is the client's perception on which the goals of care must be established. 3. Stress in all areas of life will affect sexual functioning. Client may be unaware of correlation between stress and sexual dysfunction. 4. Fatigue decreases client's desire and enthusiasm for participation in sexual activity. 5. Many medications can affect libido. Evaluation of drug and individual response is important to ascertain whether drug is responsible for the problem. 6. Increasing knowledge and correcting misconceptions can decrease feelings of powerlessness and anxiety and facilitate problem resolution. 7. Client and partner may need additional or more in-depth assistance if problems in sexual relationship are severe or remain unresolved.

NURSING DIAGNOSIS: INEFFECTIVE SEXUALITY PATTERNS

RELATED TO: Conflicts with sexual orientation or variant preferences

EVIDENCED BY: Expressed dissatisfaction with sexual behaviors (e.g., voyeurism; transvestism)

OUTCOME CRITERIA	NURSING INTERVENTIONS	RATIONALE
Client will express satisfaction with own sexuality pattern.	1. Take sexual history, noting client's expression of areas of dissatisfaction with sexual pattern. 2. Assess areas of stress in client's life and examine relationship with sexual partner. 3. Note cultural, social, ethnic, racial, and religious factors that may contribute to conflicts regarding variant sexual practices. 4. Be accepting and nonjudgmental. 5. Assist therapist in plan of behavior modification to help client decrease variant behaviors. 6. Teach client that sexuality is a normal human response and is not synonymous with any one sexual act; that it reflects the totality of the person and does not relate exclusively to the sex organs or sexual behavior. Client must understand that *sexual* feelings are *human* feelings.	1. Knowledge of what client perceives as the problem is essential for providing the type of assistance he or she may need. 2. Sexual variant behaviors are often associated with added stress in the client's life. 3. Client may be unaware of the influence these factors exert in creating feelings of shame and guilt. 4. Sexuality is a very personal and sensitive subject. The client is more likely to share this information if he or she does not fear being judged by the nurse. 5. Individuals with paraphilias are treated by specialists who have experience in modifying variant sexual behaviors. Nurses can intervene by providing assistance with implementation of the plan for behavior modification. 6. If client feels abnormal or very unlike everyone else, the self-concept is likely to be very low—even worthless. Helping him or her to see that even though the behavior is variant, feelings and motivations are common may help to increase feelings of self-worth and desire to change behavior.

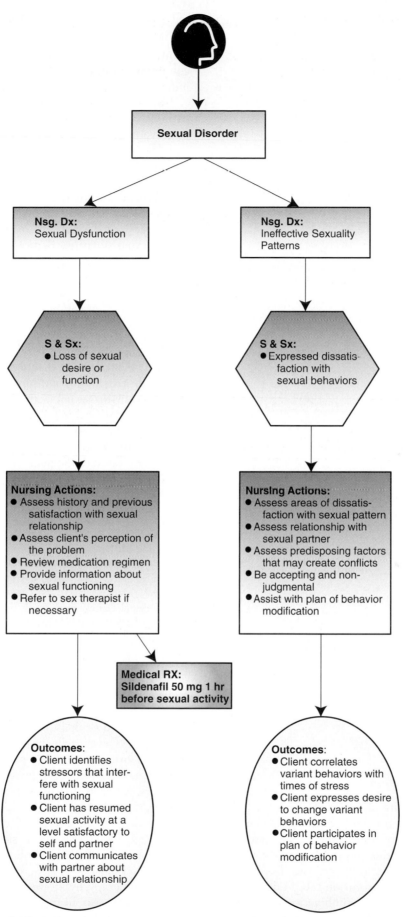

FIGURE 33–3 Concept map care plan for client with a sexual disorder.

TABLE 33–4 Topics for Client/Family Education Related to Sexual Disorders

Nature of the Illness

1. The human sexual response cycle
2. What is "normal" and "abnormal?"
3. Types of sexual dysfunctions
4. Causes of sexual dysfunctions
5. Types of paraphilias
6. Causes of paraphilias
7. Symptoms associated with sexual dysfunctions and paraphilias

Management of the Disorder

1. Teach practices and ways of sexual expression.
2. Teach relaxation techniques.
3. Teach side effects of medications that may be contributing to sexual dysfunction.
4. Teach effects of alcohol consumption on sexual functioning.
5. Teach about STDs (see Table 33–6).

Support Services

1. Provide appropriate referral for assistance from sex therapist.
2. One national association to which many qualified sex therapists belong is:
   American Association of Sex Educators, Counselors and Therapists
   435 N. Michigan Avenue, Suite 1717
   Chicago, IL 60611–4067
   (312) 644–0828

7. Do client and partner verbalize an increase in sexual satisfaction?

For the client with variant sexual behaviors:

1. Can the client correlate an increase in variant sexual behavior to times of severe stress?
2. Has the client been able to identify those stressful situations and verbalize alternative ways to deal with them?
3. Does the client express a desire to change variant sexual behavior and a willingness to cooperate with extended therapy to do so?
4. Does the client express an understanding about the normalcy of sexual feelings, aside from the inappropriateness of his or her behavior?
5. Are expressions of increased self-worth evident?

Treatment Modalities for Sexual Dysfunctions

Sexual Desire Disorders

Hypoactive Sexual Desire Disorder. Hypoactive sexual desire disorder has been treated in both men and women with the administration of testosterone. The masculinizing side effects makes this approach unacceptable to women, and the evidence that it increases libido in men is inconclusive. Becker and Johnson (2003) describe the most effective treatment as a combination of cognitive therapy to deal with maladaptive beliefs; behavioral treat-

ment, such as exercises to enhance sexual pleasuring and communication; and relationship therapy to deal with the individual's use of sex as a method of control.

Low sexual desire is often the result of partner incompatibility. If this is the case, the therapist may choose to shift from the sexual issue to helping a couple identify and deal with their incompatibility.

Sexual Aversion Disorder. Systematic desensitization (see Chapter 30) is often the treatment of choice for sexual aversion disorder, to reduce the client's fear and avoidance of sex (Becker & Johnson 2003). Gradual exposure, under relaxed conditions, to imagined and actual sexual situations decreases the amount of anxiety generated by these experiences. Successful treatment of sexual phobias has also been reported using tricyclic medications and psychosexual therapy aimed at developing insight into unconscious conflicts.

Sexual Arousal Disorders

Female Sexual Arousal Disorder. The goal of treatment for female sexual arousal disorder is to reduce the anxiety associated with sexual activity. Masters and Johnson (1970) reported successful results using their behaviorally oriented **sensate focus** exercises to treat this disorder. The objective is to reduce the goal-oriented demands of intercourse on both the man and the woman, thus reducing performance pressures and anxiety associated with possible failure. Altman and Hanfling (2003) state:

> The cornerstone of sex therapy is a series of behavioral exercises called sensate focus exercises. These highly structured touching activities are designed to help overcome performance anxiety and increase comfort with physical intimacy. Initially, the couple agrees to refrain from intercourse or genital stimulation until the later stages of treatment. This helps dispel anxiety that's built up around sexual performance and allows establishment of new patterns of relating. (pp. 38–39)

The couple is instructed to take turns caressing each other's bodies. Initially, they are to avoid touching breasts and genitals, and to focus on the sensations of being touched. The caressing progresses to include touching of the breasts and genitals, to touching each other simultaneously, and eventually to include intercourse. These non–goal-oriented exercises promote the sensual side of sexual interaction in a nonpressured, nonevaluative way (Masters, Johnson, & Kolodny, 1995).

Male Erectile Disorder. Sensate focus has been used effectively for male erectile disorder as well. Clinicians widely agree that even when significant organic factors have been identified, psychological factors may also be present and must be considered in treatment.

Group therapy, hypnotherapy, and systematic desensitization have also been used successfully in reducing the anxiety that may contribute to erectile difficulties.

Psychodynamic interventions may help alleviate intrapsychic conflicts contributing to performance anxiety (Becker & Johnson, 2003).

Various medications, including testosterone and yohimbine have been used to treat male erectile dysfunction. Penile injections of papaverine or prostaglandin have been used to produce an erection lasting from 1 to 4 hours. However, this treatment is unacceptable to many men because of pain of the injection and side effects, such as priapism and fibrotic nodules in the penis (Becker & Johnson, 2003).

Several new medications have recently been approved by the U.S. Food and Drug Administration for the treatment of erectile dysfunction. They include sildenafil (Viagra), tadalafil (Cialis), and vardenafil (Levitra). These new impotence agents block the action of phosphodiesterase (PDE5), an enzyme that breaks down cyclic guanosine monophosphate (cGMP), a compound that is required to produce an erection. This action, however, occurs only in the presence of nitric oxide (NO), which is released during sexual arousal. PDE5 inhibitors do not result in sexual arousal. They work to achieve penile erection in the presence of sexual arousal. Adverse effects include headache, facial flushing, indigestion, nasal congestion, dizziness, and visual changes (mild color tinges and blurred vision) (Noviasky, Masood, & Lo, 2004).

Two other oral medications for erectile dysfunction, apomorphine and phentolamine, are being investigated at this time. Phentolamine has been used in combination with papaverine in an injectable form. Both of these medications increase blood flow to the penis, resulting in an erection.

For erectile dysfunction refractory to other treatment methods, penile prostheses may be implanted. Two basic types are currently available: a bendable silicone implant and an inflatable device. The bendable variety requires a relatively simple surgical technique for insertion of silicone rods into the erectile areas of the penis. This results in a perpetual state of semierection for the client. The inflatable penile prosthesis produces an erection only when it is desired, and the appearance of the penis in both the flaccid and erect states is completely normal. Potential candidates for penile implantation should undergo careful psychological and physical screening. Although penile implants do not enable the client to recover the ability to ejaculate or to have an orgasm, men with prosthetic devices have generally reported satisfaction with their subsequent sexual functioning (Becker & Johnson, 2003).

Female Orgasmic Disorder. Because anxiety may contribute to the lack of orgasmic ability in women, sensate focus is often advised to reduce anxiety, increase awareness of physical sensations, and transfer communication skills from the verbal to the nonverbal domain. Phillips (2000) provides the following description of therapy for the anorgasmic woman:

Treatment relies on maximizing stimulation and minimizing inhibition. Stimulation may include masturbation with prolonged stimulation (initially up to one hour) and/or the use of a vibrator as needed, and muscular control of sexual tension (alternating contraction and relaxation of the pelvic muscles during high sexual arousal). The latter is similar to Kegal exercises. Methods to minimize inhibition include distraction by "spectatoring" (observing oneself from a third-party perspective), fantasizing, or listening to music.

Treatment for secondary anorgasmia (in which the client has had orgasms in the past, but is now unable to achieve them) focuses on the couple and their relationship. Therapy with both partners is essential to the success of this disorder.

Male Orgasmic Disorder. Treatment for male orgasmic disorder is very similar to that described for the anorgasmic woman. A combination of sensate focus and masturbatory training has been used with a high degree of success in the Masters and Johnson clinic. Treatment for male orgasmic disorder almost always includes the sexual partner.

Premature Ejaculation. Masters, Johnson, and Kolodny (1995) advocate what they suggest is a highly successful technique for the treatment of premature ejaculation. Sensate focus is used, with progression to genital stimulation. When the man reaches the point of imminent ejaculation, the woman is instructed to apply the "squeeze" technique: applying pressure at the base of the glans penis with her thumb and first two fingers. Pressure is held for about 4 seconds and then released. This technique is continued until the man is no longer on the verge of ejaculating. This technique is practiced during subsequent periods of sexual stimulation.

Sexual Pain Disorders

Dyspareunia. Treatment for the pain of intercourse begins with a thorough physical and gynecological examination. When organic pathology has been eliminated, the client's fears and anxieties underlying sexual functioning are investigated (Becker & Johnson, 2003). Systematic desensitization has been used successfully to decrease fears and anxieties associated with painful intercourse.

Vaginismus. Treatment of this disorder begins with education of the woman and her sexual partner regarding the anatomy and physiology of the disorder (i.e., what exactly is occurring during the vaginismus reflex and possible etiologies). The involuntary nature of the disorder is stressed in an effort to alleviate the perception on the part of the sexual partner that this occurrence is an act of willful withholding by the woman.

The second phase of treatment involves systematic desensitization. The client is taught a series of tensing and relaxing exercises aimed at relaxation of the pelvic musculature. Relaxation of the pelvic muscles is followed by a procedure involving the systematic insertion of dilators of graduated sizes until the woman is able to accept the penis into the vagina without discomfort. This physical therapy, combined with treatment of any identified relationship problems, has been used by the Masters and Johnson clinic with a high degree of success (Masters, Johnson, & Kolodny, 1995).

GENDER IDENTITY DISORDER

Gender identity is the sense of knowing to which sex one belongs—that is, the awareness of one's masculinity or femininity. Gender identity disorders occur when there is incongruence between anatomical sex and gender identity. The *DSM-IV-TR* categorizes diagnosis of the disorder according to the client's current age: gender identity disorder in children and gender identity disorder in adolescents or adults. Although most cases of the disorder begin in childhood, persons who present clinically with gender identity problems may be of any age. It is for this reason that they are categorized together.

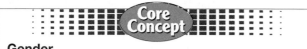

Gender
The condition of being either male or female.

For purposes of this text, differentiation between the age groups will be discussed, but the major focus will be on the disorder as it emerges in childhood. Nurses who work in areas of primary prevention with children can have the greatest effect in terms of treating this disorder. Treatment aimed at reversal in behavior is considered cautiously optimistic if initiated in childhood. After establishment of a core gender identity, it is difficult later in life to instill attributes of an opposite identity.

Predisposing Factors

Biological Influences

Abel, Rouleau, and Osborn (1994) report the results of a study with girls and women diagnosed with congenital adrenal hyperplasia (CAH). The data are interesting but inconclusive. They state:

> In this condition, the adrenal gland does not produce normal amounts of corticosteroids, which causes an increase in testosterone production and the subsequent masculinization of the external genitalia. Although the girls with CAH are more masculine in gender role behavior, the evidence of frank identity disorder is not clear. (p. 260)

Because the incidence of gender identity disorder is relatively low, genetic studies have been difficult to conduct. Meston and Frohlich (2002) report on a case of

18-year-old monozygotic female twins requesting gender reassignment surgery, which they suggest may indicate a possible genetic component for gender identity disorder.

An additional study reports on possible effects of testosterone on brain differentiation (Zhou et al., 1995). The researchers found that the red nucleus of the stria terminalis (a region of the hypothalamus) in male-to-female transsexuals corresponded to that of typical females, rather than of typical males. This was the case whether the individual was heterosexual or homosexual, and was not accounted for by hormone therapy.

Family Dynamics

It appears that family dynamics plays the most influential role in the etiology of gender disorders. Sadock and Sadock (2003) state, "Children develop a gender identity consonant with their sex of rearing (also known as assigned sex)." Gender roles are culturally determined, and parents encourage masculine or feminine behaviors in their children. Although "temperament" may play a role with certain behavioral characteristics being present at birth, mothers usually foster a child's pride in their gender. Sadock and Sadock (2003) state:

> The father's role is also important in the early years, and his presence normally helps the separation-individuation process. Without a father, mother and child may remain overly close. For a girl, the father is normally the prototype of future love objects; for a boy, the father is a model for male identification. (p. 731)

Psychoanalytical Theory

The psychoanalytical theory suggests that gender identity problems begin during the struggle of the Oedipal conflict. Problems may reflect both real family events and those created in the child's imagination. These conflicts, whether real or imagined, interfere with the child's loving of the opposite-gender parent and identifying with the same-gender parent, and ultimately with normal gender identity.

Application of the Nursing Process to Gender Identity Disorders

Background Assessment Data (Symptomatology)

Gender Identity Disorder in Children

The *DSM-IV-TR* describes the manifestations of this disorder as the presence of four (or more) of the following:

1. Repeatedly stated desire to be, or insistence that he or she is, the opposite gender
2. In boys, preference for cross-dressing or simulating

female attire; in girls, insistence on wearing only stereotypical masculine clothing

3. Strong and persistent preferences for cross-gender roles in make-believe play or persistent fantasies of being the opposite gender
4. Intense desire to participate in the stereotypical games and pastimes of the opposite gender
5. Strong preference for playmates of the opposite gender

They may be subjected to teasing and rejection by their peers and disapproval from family members. This occurs early in childhood for boys, but often does not occur before adolescence in girls. Because of this rejection, interpersonal relationships are hampered. The disorder is not common but occurs more frequently in boys than in girls.

Gender Identity Disorder in Adolescents and Adults

The *DSM-IV-TR* describes this disorder as one in which there is a strong and persistent cross-gender identification (not merely a desire for any perceived cultural advantages of being the opposite gender) (APA, 2000). Symptomatic manifestations include a stated desire to be of the opposite gender, frequently passing as the opposite gender, a desire to live or be treated as the opposite gender, or the conviction that he or she has the typical feelings and reactions of the opposite gender (APA, 2000). These symptoms are accompanied by a persistent discomfort with or sense of inappropriateness in the assigned gender role. Some individuals are so convinced they were born the wrong gender that they become preoccupied with methods to eliminate the sex characteristics of the assigned gender, such as requesting opposite gender hormones or surgery to alter sexual characteristics.

Diagnosis/Outcome Identification

Sadock and Sadock (2003) report that intervention with adolescents and adults with gender identity disorder is difficult. Adolescents commonly act out and rarely have the motivation required to alter their cross-gender roles. Adults generally seek therapy to learn how to cope with their altered sexual identity, not to correct it. Becker and Johnson (2003) state:

> Treatment of gender identity disorder in the child is offered in an attempt to help the child avoid peer ostracism and humiliation, be comfortable with his or her own sex, and avoid the possible development of adult gender dysphoria. (p. 749)

Most of the treatment of children with this disorder has been in outpatient clinics. Nurses working in these settings may encounter these clients from time to time,

although the disorder is not common. One-to-one nursing intervention may be provided by a master's-prepared psychiatric clinical nurse specialist.

Based on the data collected during the nursing assessment, possible nursing diagnoses for the client with gender identity disorder in children may include:

Disturbed personal identity related to parenting patterns that encourage culturally unacceptable behaviors for assigned gender.
Impaired social interaction related to socially and culturally unacceptable behaviors.
Low self-esteem related to rejection by peers.

The following criteria may be used for measurement of outcomes in the care of the client with gender identity disorder in children.

The client:

1. Demonstrates trust in a therapist of the same gender.
2. Demonstrates development of a close relationship with the parent of the same gender.
3. Demonstrates interruption in the excessively close relationship with the parent of the opposite gender.
4. Demonstrates behaviors that are culturally appropriate for assigned gender.
5. Verbalizes and demonstrates comfort in, and satisfaction with, assigned gender role.
6. Interacts appropriately with others demonstrating culturally acceptable behaviors.
7. Verbalizes and demonstrates self-satisfaction with assigned gender role.

Planning/Implementation

Table 33–5 provides a plan of care for the client with gender identity disorder in children. Nursing diagnoses are presented, along with outcome criteria, appropriate nursing interventions, and rationales.

Evaluation

The final step of the nursing process is to determine if the nursing interventions have been effective in achieving the intended outcomes. This evaluation process requires that the nurse reassess the client's behaviors and determine if the changes at which the interventions had been directed have occurred. For the child with gender identity disorder, this may be accomplished by using the following types of questions:

1. Does the client demonstrate use of behaviors that are culturally accepted for his or her assigned gender?
2. Does the client perceive that a problem existed that requires a change in behavior for resolution?
3. Can the client use these culturally accepted behaviors in interactions with others?

TABLE 33–5 Care Plan for the Child with Gender Identity Disorder

NURSING DIAGNOSIS: DISTURBED PERSONAL IDENTITY

RELATED TO: Parenting patterns that encourage culturally unacceptable behaviors for assigned gender

EVIDENCED BY: Statements of desiring to be of the opposite gender; exhibiting behaviors culturally associated with the opposite gender

OUTCOME CRITERIA	NURSING INTERVENTIONS	RATIONALE
Client will verbalize knowledge of and demonstrate behaviors that are appropriate and culturally acceptable for assigned gender.	1. Spend time with client and show positive regard.	1. Trust and unconditional acceptance are essential to the establishment of a therapeutic nurse-client relationship.
	2. Be aware of own feelings and attitudes toward this client and his or her behavior.	2. Attitudes influence behavior. The nurse must not allow negative attitudes to interfere with the effectiveness of interventions.
	3. Allow client to describe his or her perception of the problem.	3. It is important to know how the client perceives the problem before attempting to correct misperceptions.
	4. Discuss with client the types of behaviors that are more culturally acceptable. Practice these behaviors through role-playing or with play therapy strategies (e.g., male and female dolls). Positive reinforcement or social attention may be given for use of appropriate behaviors. No response is given for opposite-gender-stereotype behaviors.	4. The goal is to enhance culturally appropriate same-gender behaviors, but not necessarily to extinguish all coexisting opposite-gender behaviors.

NURSING DIAGNOSIS: IMPAIRED SOCIAL INTERACTION

RELATED TO: Social and culturally unacceptable behaviors

EVIDENCED BY: Peer rejection and identification with members of the opposite gender

OUTCOME CRITERIA	NURSING INTERVENTIONS	RATIONALE
Client will interact with others using culturally acceptable behaviors.	1. Once client feels comfortable with the new behaviors in role-playing or one-to-one nurse-client interactions, they may be tried in group situations. If possible, remain with client during interactions with others. Observe client behaviors and the responses he or she elicits from others. Give social attention (e.g., smile, nod) to desired behaviors. Follow up these "practice" sessions with one-to-one processing of the interaction. Give positive reinforcement for efforts. Offer support if client is feeling hurt from peer ridicule. Matter-of-factly discuss the behaviors that elicited the ridicule. Offer no personal reaction to the behavior.	1. The goal is to create a trusting, non-threatening atmosphere for the client in an attempt to change behavior and improve social interactions. Long-term studies have not yet revealed the significance of therapy with these children or psychosexual relationship development in adolescence or adulthood. One variable that must be considered is the evidence of psychopathology within the families of many of these children.

NURSING DIAGNOSIS: LOW SELF-ESTEEM

RELATED TO: Rejection by peers

EVIDENCED BY: Difficulty accepting positive reinforcement; self-negating verbalizations; inability to form close personal relationships

OUTCOME CRITERIA	NURSING INTERVENTIONS	RATIONALE
Client will verbalize positive statements about self, including past accomplishments and future prospects.	1. Encourage child to engage in activities in which he or she is likely to achieve success. Help the child to focus on aspects of his or her life for which positive feelings exist. Discourage rumination about situations that are perceived as failures or over which client has no control. Give positive reinforcement for these behaviors.	1. Success and positive feedback enhance self-esteem.

(Continued on opposite page)

OUTCOME CRITERIA	NURSING INTERVENTIONS	RATIONALE
	2. Help client identify behaviors or aspects of life he or she would like to change. If realistic, assist child in problem solving to find ways to bring about the change.	2. Having some control over his or her life may decrease feelings of powerlessness and increase feelings of self-worth.
	3. Offer to be available for support when the child is feeling rejected by peers.	3. Having an available support person who does not judge the child's behavior and who provides unconditional acceptance assists the child to progress toward acceptance of self as a worthwhile person.

4. Is the client accepted by peers when same-gender behaviors are used?
5. If the client is refusing to change behaviors, what is peer reaction?
6. What is the client's response to negative peer reaction?
7. Can the client verbalize positive statements about self?
8. Can the client discuss past accomplishments without dwelling on the perceived failures?
9. Has the client shown progress toward accepting self as a worthwhile person regardless of others' responses to his or her behavior?

VARIATIONS IN SEXUAL ORIENTATION

Homosexuality

Homosexual activity occurs under some circumstances in probably all known human cultures and all mammalian species for which it has been studied. The term **homosexuality** is derived from the Greek root *homo* meaning "same" and refers to sexual preference for individuals of the same gender. It may be applied in a general way to homosexuals of both genders but is often used to specifically denote male homosexuality. The term **lesbianism**, used to identify female homosexuality, is traced to the Greek poet Sappho who lived on the island of Lesbos and is famous for the love poems she wrote to other women. Most homosexuals prefer the term "gay" because it is less derogatory in its lack of emphasis on the sexual aspects of the orientation. A heterosexual individual is referred to as "straight."

The psychiatric community in general does not consider consensual homosexuality to be a mental disturbance (Sadock & Sadock, 2003). The concept of homosexuality as a disturbance in sexual orientation no longer appears in the *DSM*. Instead, the *DSM-IV-TR* (APA, 2000) is concerned only with the individual who experiences "persistent and marked distress about his or her sexual orientation."

Many members of the American culture disapprove of homosexuality. In a *USA Today*/CNN/GALLUP poll conducted in July 2003, 49 percent of Americans opposed homosexuality as an "acceptable alternative lifestyle" (*USA Today*, 2003). Some experts believe that many Americans' attitudes toward homosexuals can best be described as homophobic. *Homophobia* is defined as a negative attitude toward or fear of homosexuality or homosexuals (Sadock & Sadock, 2003). It may be indicative of a deep-seated insecurity about one's own gender identity. Homophobic behaviors include extreme prejudice against, abhorrence of, and discomfort around homosexuals. These behaviors are usually rationalized by religious, moral, or legal considerations.

Relationship patterns are as varied among homosexuals as they are among heterosexuals. Some homosexuals may remain with one partner for an extended period of time, even for a lifetime, whereas others prefer not to make a commitment, and "play the field" instead.

No one knows for sure why people become homosexual or heterosexual. Various theories have been proposed regarding the issue, but no single etiological factor has consistently emerged. Many contributing factors likely influence the development of sexual orientation.

Predisposing Factors

Biological Theories

A study by Bailey and Pillard (1991) revealed a 52 percent concordance for homosexual orientation in monozygotic twins and 22 percent in dizygotic twins. These data were significant to suggest a possible heritable trait. Sadock and Sadock (2003) state:

Gay men show a familial distribution; they have more brothers who are gay than do heterosexual men. One study found that 33 out of 40 pairs of gay brothers shared a genetic marker on the bottom half of the X chromosome. (p. 698)

A number of studies have been conducted to determine whether or not there is a hormonal influence in the etiology of homosexuality. It has been hypothesized that levels of testosterone may be lower and levels of estrogen higher in homosexual men than in heterosexual men. Results have been inconsistent. It has also been suggested that exposure to inappropriate levels of androgens during the critical fetal period of sexual differentiation may contribute to homosexual orientation. This hypothesis lacks definitive evidence, and conclusions regarding its validity remain tentative.

Psychosocial Theories

Freud (1930) believed that all humans are inherently bisexual, with the capacity for both heterosexual and homosexual behavior. He theorized all individuals go through a homoerotic phase as children. Thus, if homosexuality occurs later in life it is due to arrest of normal psychosexual development. He also believed homosexuality could occur as a result of pathological family relationships in which the child adopts a negative Oedipal position; that is, there is sexualized attachment to the parent of the same gender and identification with the parent of the opposite gender.

Some theories suggest that a dysfunctional family pattern may have an etiological influence in the development of homosexuality. These "nurture" theories focus on the parent–child relationship, and most specifically, the relationship with the same-gender parent. Gay men often have a dominant, supportive mother and a weak, remote, or hostile father (Johnson, 2003). Lesbians may have had a dysfunctional mother–daughter relationship. Both subsequently try to meet their unmet same-gender needs through sexual relationships.

These theories of family dynamics have been disputed by some clinicians who believe that parents have very little influence on the outcome of their children's sexual-partner orientation. Others suggest there may not be one single answer—that sexual orientation may result from a complex interaction between environmental, cognitive, and anatomical factors, shaping the individual at an early age (Johnson, 2003).

Special Concerns

People with homosexual preferences have problems that are similar to those of their heterosexual counterparts. Considerations of attractiveness, finding a partner, and concerns about sexual adequacy are common to both. STDs are epidemic among sexually active individuals of all sexual orientations. Of particular concern is acquired immunodeficiency syndrome (AIDS), which was considered a "gay disease" for the first few years of the epidemic (see Chapter 39). AIDS is a fatal viral illness that, initially in the Western world, was indeed largely transmitted by male homosexual activity. Although AIDS is now known to spread through contaminated blood products, the sharing of needles by intravenous drug users, and heterosexual contact, some individuals still believe AIDS is

God's way of punishing homosexuals. These societal attitudes are considered by many homosexuals to be their greatest burden.

Some homosexuals live in fear of the discovery of their sexual orientation; they fear being rejected by parents and significant others. They experience a great deal of cognitive dissonance related to the disparity between their overt behavior and their inner feelings. Social sanctions still exist in some areas for homosexuals in regard to employment, housing, and public accommodations. The Human Rights Commission protects homosexuals; however, discrimination is still widespread.

Nurses must examine their personal attitudes and feelings about homosexuality. They must be able to recognize when negative feelings are compromising the care they give. Increasing numbers of homosexuals are being honest about their sexual orientation. Health care workers must ensure that these individuals receive care with dignity, which is the right of all human beings. Nurses who have come to terms with their own feelings about homosexuality are better able to separate the person from the behavior. Unconditional acceptance of each individual is an essential component of compassionate nursing.

Transsexualism

Transsexualism is a disorder of gender identity or gender dysphoria (unhappiness or dissatisfaction with one's gender) of the most extreme variety. An individual, despite having the anatomical characteristics of a given gender, has the self-perception of being of the opposite gender. The disorder is relatively rare, with an estimated prevalence of 1 in 30,000 for men and 1 in 100,000 for women (Sadock & Sadock, 2003).

The *DSM-IV-TR* does not identify transsexualism as a specific disorder, choosing instead to discuss the broader category of *gender identity disorder*; however, transsexualism is included in the 10th revision of the *International Classification of Diseases (ICD-10)*.

Individuals with this disorder do not feel comfortable wearing the clothes of their assigned gender and often engage in cross-dressing. They may find their own genitals repugnant and may repeatedly submit requests to the health care system for hormonal and surgical gender reassignment. Depression and anxiety are common and are often attributed by the individual to his or her inability to live in the desired gender role.

Predisposing Factors

Biological Theories

Several studies have been conducted to determine if sex hormone levels are abnormal in individuals with gender dysphoria. In some studies, decreased levels of testosterone were found in male transsexuals, and abnormally high levels of testosterone were found in female transsexuals, but the results have been inconsistent (Becker & Johnson, 2003).

As with homosexuality, there has been some speculation that gender-disordered individuals may be exposed to inappropriate hormones during the prenatal period, which can result in a genetic woman or a genetic man possessing the qualities and perception of the opposite gender. However, evidence that prenatal exposure to these hormones predisposes to transsexualism remains inconclusive.

Psychosocial Theories

It is generally accepted that transsexualism has physiological origins. However, some clinicians believe that the etiology is based on a combination of biological and environmental factors, particularly family dynamics. Some of these theories were previously discussed in the section on gender identity disorder.

Special Concerns

Treatment of the transsexual individual is a complex process. The true transsexual intensely desires to have the genitalia and physical appearance of the assigned gender changed to conform to his or her gender identity. This change requires a great deal more than surgical alteration of physical features. In most cases, the individual must undergo extensive psychological testing and counseling, as well as live in the role of the desired gender for up to 2 years before surgery.

Hormonal treatment is initiated during this period. Male clients receive estrogen, which results in a redistribution of body fat in a more "feminine" pattern, enlargement of the breasts, a softening of the skin, and reduction in body hair. Women receive testosterone, which also causes a redistribution of body fat, growth of facial and body hair, enlargement of the clitoris, and deepening of the voice (Becker & Johnson, 2003). Amenorrhea occurs within a few months.

Surgical treatment for the male-to-female transsexual involves removal of the penis and testes and creation of an artificial vagina. Care is taken to preserve sensory nerves in the area so that the individual may continue to experience sexual stimulation.

Surgical treatment for the female-to-male transsexual is more complex. A mastectomy and sometimes a hysterectomy are preformed. A penis and scrotum are constructed from tissues in the genital and abdominal area, and the vaginal orifice is closed. A penile implant is used to attain erection.

Both men and women continue to receive maintenance hormone therapy following surgery. Satisfaction with the results is high, and most consider the pain

and discomfort worthwhile. Sadock and Sadock (2003) state:

> Outcome studies are highly variable in terms of how success is defined and measured (for example, successful intercourse and body image satisfaction). About 70 percent of male-to-female and 80 percent of female-to-male reassignment surgery patients report satisfactory results. (p. 737)

Nursing care of the post-sex-reassignment surgical client is similar to that of most other postsurgical clients. Particular attention is given to maintaining comfort, preventing infection, preserving integrity of the surgical site, maintaining elimination, and meeting nutritional needs. Psychosocial needs may have to do with body image, fears and insecurities about relating to others, and being accepted in the new gender role. Meeting these needs can begin with nursing in a nonthreatening, nonjudgmental healing atmosphere.

Bisexuality

A bisexual person is not exclusively heterosexual or homosexual; he or she engages in sexual activity with members of both genders. Bisexuals are also sometimes referred to as ambisexual.

Bisexuality is more common than exclusive homosexuality. Statistics suggest that approximately 75 percent of all men are exclusively heterosexual and only 2 percent are exclusively homosexual, leaving a relatively large percentage who have engaged in sexual activity with both men and women.

A diversity of sexual preferences exists among bisexuals. Some individuals prefer men and women equally, whereas others have a preference for one gender but also accept sexual activity with the other gender. Some bisexuals may alternate between homosexual and heterosexual activity for long periods; others may have both a male and a female lover at the same time. Whereas some individuals maintain their bisexual orientation throughout their lives, others may become exclusively homosexual or heterosexual.

Predisposing Factors

Little research exists on the etiology of bisexuality. As previously stated, Freud (1930) believed that all humans are inherently bisexual; that is, he believed that all individuals have the capacity for both heterosexual and homosexual interactions.

Much research on the development of homosexuality rests on the assumption that it is somehow determined by pathological conditions in childhood. Many heterosexual individuals, however, have their first homosexual encounter later in life. It is unlikely that an initial homosexual encounter that occurs in the 30s or 40s was determined by a pathological condition that occurred when the individual was 3 or 4 years old. Some encounters, too, are based solely on the situation, such as the heterosexual man who engages in homosexual behavior while in prison and then returns to heterosexuality following his release. This behavior most likely was determined by circumstances rather than a pathological process that occurred in childhood.

Gender identity (determining whether one is male or female) is usually established by the age of 2 to 3 years. Sexual identity (determining whether one is heterosexual or homosexual or both) may continue to evolve throughout one's lifetime.

SEXUALLY TRANSMITTED DISEASES

Sexually transmitted diseases (STDs) refer to infections that are contracted primarily through sexual activities or intimate contact with the genitals, mouth, or rectum of another individual (Cook, 2003). They may be transmitted from one person to another through heterosexual or homosexual contact, and external genital evidence of pathology may or may not be manifested.

STDs are at epidemic levels in the United States. Individuals are beginning an active sex life at an earlier age. More women are sexually active than ever before. The social changes that may have contributed to the increase in STDs are sometimes referred to as the three Ps: permissiveness, promiscuity, and the pill. The widespread knowledge that antibiotics were available to cure infections and the availability of the pill to prevent pregnancy resulted in significant increases in promiscuity and the subsequent exposure to and spread of STDs.

A primary nursing responsibility in STD control is education that is aimed at prevention of the disease. Nurses must know which diseases are most prevalent, how they are transmitted, their signs and symptoms, available treatment, and consequences of avoiding treatment (Table 33–6). They must teach this information to clients in hospitals and clinics and take an active role in programs of education in the community. Early education is important to decrease the spread of STDs.

STDs have a particularly emotive significance because they can be transmitted between sexual partners. Consequently, STDs carry strong connotations of illicit sex and considerable social stigma, as well as potentially disastrous medical consequences. Feelings of guilt in clients with STDs can be overwhelming. These individuals need strong support to overcome not only the physical difficulties but also the social and emotional ones associated with having this type of illness.

Prevention of STDs is the ideal goal, but early detection and appropriate treatment continue to be considered a realistic objective. Nurses are in an excellent position to provide the education required for prevention, as well as the physical treatment and social and emotional support to assist clients with STDs regain and maintain optimal wellness.

SUMMARY

This chapter has provided information related to the development of sexuality throughout the life cycle. Normal sexual response patterns were described in an effort to provide background information for the recognition and treatment of sexual and gender identity disorders.

The *DSM-IV-TR* identifies two major categories of sexual disorders (paraphilias and sexual dysfunctions) and two categories of gender identity disorders (those occurring in children and those occurring in adolescents and adults).

Paraphilias are a group of behaviors involving sexual activity with nonhuman objects or with nonconsenting partners or that involve suffering to others. Types of paraphilias include exhibitionism, fetishism, frotteurism, pedophilia, sexual masochism or sadism, and voyeurism.

Sexual dysfunctions are disturbances that occur in any of the phases of the normal human sexual response cycle. They include sexual desire disorders, sexual arousal disorders, orgasmic disorders, and sexual pain disorders.

Gender identity disorders occur when there is an incongruence between anatomical sex and the assigned gender role. Individuals experience extreme discomfort in the assigned gender and desire to be, or insist that they are, the opposite gender. Cross-dressing is common, and some individuals pursue hormonal therapy or surgery to alter physical characteristics to match cognitive self-perception.

Predisposing factors and symptomatology for each of these disorders were presented as background assessment data. A content outline for obtaining a sexual history was included. The delivery of nursing care was described in the context of the nursing process.

A description of current medical treatment modalities for each of the disorders was presented. Variations in sexual orientation, including homosexuality, transsexualism, and bisexuality, were discussed. Finally, information on the transmission, signs and symptoms, treatment, and potential complications of the most prevalent STDs was suggested as material for use in programs of education targeted for decreasing the spread of sexually transmitted diseases.

Human sexuality influences all aspects of physical and mental health. Clients are becoming more open to discussing matters pertaining to sexuality, and it is therefore important for nurses to integrate information on sexuality into the care they give. This can be done by focusing on preventive, therapeutic, and educational interventions to assist individuals to attain, regain, or maintain sexual wellness.

TABLE 33–6   **Sexually Transmitted Diseases**

DISEASE	ORGANISM OF TRANSMISSION	METHOD OF TRANSMISSION	SIGNS AND SYMPTOMS	TREATMENT	POTENTIAL COMPLICATIONS
Gonorrhea	*Neisseria gonorrhoeae (bacterium)*	Vaginal sex; anal sex; genital-oral sex; via hand moistened with infected secretions and placed in contact with mucous membranes (e.g., the eyes)	Males: urethritis; dysuria, purulent discharge from urethra; proctitis; pharyngitis. Females: initially asymptomatic. Progress to infection of cervix, urethra, and fallopian tubes.	Ceftriaxone, cefixime, ciprofloxacin, ofloxacin	Men: Sterility from orchitis or epididymitis. Women: Chronic pelvic inflammatory disease; infertility; ectopic pregnancy; blindness from gonococcal conjunctivitis.
Syphilis	*Treponema pallidum (spirochete)*	Vaginal sex; anal sex; genital-oral sex; via contact of infected secretions with intact mucous membranes or abraded skin.	Primary stage: painless chancre on penis, vulva, vagina, mouth, anus, or other point of contact with mucous membranes or abraded skin. Secondary stage: rash, headache, anorexia, weight loss, fever, sore throat, body aches, anemia.	Long-acting penicillin G; tetracycline; erythromycin; ceftriaxone	Latent stage: lasts many years; no symptoms but can be passed on to fetus. Tertiary stage: blindness, heart disease, insanity, ulcerated lesions on skin, mucous membranes, or internal organs.
Chlamydial infection	*Chlamydia trachomatis* (intracellular bacterium)	Vaginal sex; anal sex; via hand moistened with infected secretions and placed in contact with mucous membranes.	Women: cervicitis (either asymptomatic or may have discharge, dysuria, soreness, bleeding) Men: urethral discharge and dysuria.	Tetracycline; erythromycin; azithromycin	Scarring in the fallopian tubes; ectopic pregnancy; infertility.
Genital herpes	Herpes simplex virus, type 1 or type 2	Vaginal sex; anal sex; genital-oral sex; skin-to-skin contact with infected areas; to newborn through vaginal delivery.	Blistery lesions in the genital area causing pain, itching, burning. Also vaginal or urethral discharge, fever, headache, malaise, and myalgias.	There is no cure. Treatment is palliative with acyclovir, valacyclovir, or famciclovir	Recurrences are possible. Potential complications include: meningitis, encephalitis, urethral strictures. Possible risk of cervical cancer.
Genital warts	*Condyloma acuminatum* (human papilloma virus)	Vaginal sex; anal sex; skin-to-skin contact with infected areas.	Cauliflowerlike warts that appear on penis or scrotum in men, and labia, vaginal walls or cervix in women. Mild itching may occur.	Application of fluorouracil (5-FU) or podophyllin; cryotherapy; electrocautery; surgical removal.	Recurrences are possible. Possible increased risk of cervical cancer.
Hepatitis B	Hepatitis B virus	Vaginal sex; anal sex; genital-oral sex; contact with infectious blood or blood products; contact of infectious secretions with mucous membranes or abrased skin.	Malaise, anorexia, nausea/vomiting, fever, headache, mild pain in right upper quadrant of abdomen, jaundice.	No cure. Treatment involves supportive care; bedrest for extended period. Medications generally have not been found to be useful.	Complications include chronic hepatitis; cirrhosis; liver cancer.
AIDS	Human immunodeficiency virus (HIV)	Exchange of body fluids via: anal sex; vaginal sex; genital-oral sex; shared use of needles during drug use. Skin-to-skin contact when there are open sores on the skin. Transfusion with contaminated blood. Perinatal transmission: during delivery and through breast milk.	May be asymptomatic for as long as 10 years following infection with HIV. Early signs of AIDS include severe weight loss, diarrhea, fever, night sweats or the presence of a persistent opportunistic infection (e.g., herpes or candidiasis).	No cure. Antiretroviral medication used to slow growth of the virus. Other medications given for symptomatic relief and to treat opportunistic infections.	Regardless of treatment, AIDS is eventually fatal.

REVIEW QUESTIONS

SELF-EXAMINATION/LEARNING EXERCISE

Select the answer that is *most* appropriate for each of the following questions.

1. Janice, age 24, and her husband are seeking treatment at the sex therapy clinic. They have been married for 3 weeks and have never had sexual intercourse together. Pain and vaginal tightness prevent penile entry. Sexual history reveals Janice was raped when she was 15 years old. The physician would most likely assign which of the following diagnoses to Janice?
   a. Dyspareunia
   b. Vaginismus
   c. Anorgasmia
   d. Sexual aversion disorder

2. The most appropriate nursing diagnosis for Janice would be:
   a. Pain related to vaginal constriction.
   b. Altered sexuality patterns related to inability to have vaginal intercourse.
   c. Sexual dysfunction related to history of sexual trauma.
   d. Dysfunctional grieving related to loss of self-esteem because of rape.

3. The first phase of treatment may be initiated by the nurse. It would include which of the following?
   a. Sensate focus exercises
   b. Tense and relaxation exercises
   c. Systematic desensitization
   d. Education about the disorder

4. The second phase of treatment includes which of the following?
   a. Gradual dilation of the vagina
   b. Sensate focus exercises
   c. Hypnotherapy
   d. Administration of minor tranquilizers

5. Statistically, the outcome of therapy for Janice and her husband is likely to:
   a. Be unsuccessful.
   b. Be very successful.
   c. Be of very long duration.
   d. Result in their getting a divorce.

Match each of the paraphilias listed on the left with its correct behavioral description from the column on the right.

_____ 6. Exhibitionism

_____ 7. Transvestic fetishism

_____ 8. Voyeurism

_____ 9. Frotteurism

_____ 10. Pedophilia

a. Tom watches his neighbor through her window each night as she undresses for bed. Later he fantasizes about having sex with her.

b. Frank drives his car up to a strange woman, stops, and asks her for directions. As she is explaining, he reveals his erect penis to her.

c. Tim, age 17, babysits for his 11-year-old neighbor, Jeff. Six months ago, Tim began fondling Jeff's genitals. They now engage in mutual masturbation each time they are together.

d. John is 32 years old. He buys women's clothing at the thrift shop. Sometimes he dresses as a woman and goes to a singles' bar. He becomes sexually excited as he fantasizes about men being attracted to him as a women.

e. Fred rides a crowded subway every day. He stands beside a woman he views as very attractive. Just as the subway is about to stop, he places his hand on her breast and rubs his genitals against her buttocks. As the door opens, he dashes out and away. Later he fantasizes she is in love with him.

TEST YOUR CRITICAL THINKING SKILLS

Sarah was hospitalized on the psychiatric unit for depression. During her nursing assessment interview, she stated, "According to my husband, I can't do anything right—not even have sex." When asked to explain further, Sarah said she and her husband had been married for 17 years. She said that in the beginning, they had experienced a mutually satisfying sexual relationship and "made love" two or three times a week. Their daughter was born after they had been married 2 years, followed 2 years later by the birth of their son. They now have two teenagers (ages 15 and 13) who, by Sarah's admission, require a great deal of her time and energy. She says, "I'm too tired for sex. And, besides, the kids might hear. I would be so embarrassed if they did. I walked in on my parents having sex

once when I was a teenager, and I thought I would die! And my parents never mentioned it. It was just like it never happened! It was so awful! But sex is just so important to my husband, though, and we haven't had sex in months. We argue all the time about it. I'm afraid it's going to break us up."

Answer the following questions related to Sarah:

1. What would be the primary nursing diagnosis for Sarah?
2. What interventions might the nurse include in the treatment plan for Sarah?
3. What would be a realistic goal for which Sarah might strive?

 INTERNET REFERENCES

Additional information about sexual disorders may be located at the following Web sites:

- http://www.sexualhealth.com/
- http://www-hsl.mcmaster.ca/tomflem/sexual.html
- http://www.priory.com/sex.htm

Additional information about gender identity disorders may be located at the following Web sites:

- http://www.avitale.com/
- http://eserver.org/gender/

Additional information about sexually transmitted diseases may be located at the following Web sites:

- http://www.cdc.gov/std/
- http://www.niaid.nih.gov/factsheets/stdinfo.htm

IMPLICATIONS OF RESEARCH FOR EVIDENCE-BASED PRACTICE

Bacon, C.G., Mittleman, M.A., Kawachi, I., Glovannucci, E., Glasser, D.B., & Rimm, E.B. (2003). Sexual function in men older than 50 years of age: Results from the health professionals follow-up study. *Annals of Internal Medicine, 139*, 161–168.

Description of the Study: The purpose of the Health Professionals Follow-up Study was to describe the association between age and several aspects of sexual functioning in men older than 50 years of age. Participants included 31,742 male dentists, optometrists, osteopaths, podiatrists, pharmacists, and veterinarians in the United States. The participants were mailed questionnaires every 2 years between 1986 and 2000. Age range of participants was 53 to 90 years. Measures of sexual function included ability to have and maintain an erection adequate for intercourse, sexual desire, and ability to reach orgasm. Independent modifiable health behaviors included physical activity, smoking, obesity, alcohol consumption, and sedentary lifestyle (measured by hours of TV viewing).

Results of the Study: The results of this study reinforced those of previous studies that linked sexual dysfunction to increasing age, certain disease processes (e.g., diabetes, cancer, stroke, and hypertension), and medications (e.g., antidepressants; beta-blockers). This study also addressed more specifically the correlation between sexual dysfunction and independent, modifiable risk factors. A higher risk for sexual dysfunction was associated with obesity, sedentary lifestyle, smoking, and excess alcohol consumption. Regular physical exercise (>32 metabolic equivalent hours per week), leanness, moderate alcohol consumption, and not smoking were statistically significant with decreased risk.

Implications for Nursing Practice: This study has strong implications for nursing in terms of educating men older than age 50 about contributing factors to sexual dysfunction. Establishing and conducting classes for weight reduction (including programs of regular exercise) and smoking cessation are well within the scope of nursing practice. Nurses can intervene to assist clients with behavior modification to achieve and/or maintain sexual wellness.

REFERENCES

Abel, G.G., Rouleau, J.L., & Osborn, C.A. (1994). Sexual disorders. In G. Winokur, & P.J. Clayton (Eds.). *The medical basis of psychiatry* (2nd ed.). Philadelphia: W.B. Saunders.

Administration on Aging. (2003). *A profile of older Americans: 2003.* Washington, DC: U.S. Department of Health and Human Services.

Altman, A., & Hanfling, S. (2003). *Sexuality in midlife and beyond.* Boston, MA: Harvard Health Publications.

American Psychiatric Association (APA). (2000). *Diagnostic and statistical manual of mental disorders* (4th ed.) *Text Revision.* Washington, DC: American Psychiatric Association.

Atwood, J.D., & Schwartz, L. (2002). Cyber-sex: The new affair treatment considerations. *Couple & Relationship Therapy, 1*(3), 37–56.

Bailey, J.M., & Pillard, R.C. (1991). A genetic study of male sexual orientation. *Archives of General Psychiatry, 48*, 1089–1096.

Becker, J.V., & Johnson, B.R. (2003). Sexual and gender identity disorders. In R.E. Hales & S.C. Yudofsky (Eds.). *Textbook of clinical psychiatry* (4th ed.) Washington, DC: American Psychiatric Publishing.

Bell, R. (1998). *Changing bodies, changing lives* (3rd ed.). New York: Random House.

Berman, J., & Berman, L. (2001). *For women only: A revolutionary guide to overcoming sexual dysfunction and reclaiming your sex life.* New York: Henry Holt.

Brosman, S.A., & Leslie, S.W. (2004). Erectile dysfunction. Retrieved April 27, 2005 from the World Wide Web at http://www.emedicine.com/med/topic3023.htm

Clayton, A.H. (2002). Sexual dysfunction. In S.G. Kornstein & A H. Clayton (Eds.). *Women's mental health.* New York: The Guilford Press.

Cook, L.H. (2003). Nursing care of patients with sexually transmitted diseases. In L.S. Williams & P.D. Hopper (Eds.). *Understanding medical surgical nursing* (2nd ed.). Philadelphia: F.A. Davis.

Dreyfus, E.A. (1998). *Sexuality and sex therapy: When there is sexual dysfunction.* Retrieved March 22, 2002 from the World Wide Web at http://www.shpm.com/articles/sex/sexther2.html

Johnson, R.D. (2003). Homosexuality: Nature or nurture. *AllPsych Journal.* Retrieved April 28, 2005 from the World Wide Web at http://allpsych.com/journal/homosexuality.html

Leiblum, S.R. (1999). Sexual problems and dysfunction: Epidemiology, classification, and risk factors. *The Journal of Gender-Specific Medicine, 2*(5), 41–45.

Masters, W.H., Johnson, V.E., & Kolodny, R.C. (1995). *Human sexuality* (5th ed.). New York: Addison-Wesley Longman.

Meston, C.M., & Frohlich, P.F. (2002). The psychobiology of sexual and gender identity disorders. In H. D'haenen, J.A. denBoer, & P. Willner (Eds.). *Biological psychiatry* (3rd ed.). London: John Wiley & Sons.

Murray, R.B., & Zentner, J.P. (2001). *Health promotion strategies through the life span* (7th ed.). Upper Saddle River, NJ: Prentice-Hall.

Nappi, R., Salonia, A., Traish, A.M., vanLunsen, R.H.W., Vardi, Y., Kodiglu, A., & Goldstein, I. (2005). Clinical biologic pathophysiologies of women's sexual dysfunction. *Journal of Sexual Medicine, 2*(1), 4–25.

Noviasky, J.A., Masood, A., & Lo, V. (2004, July 15). Tadalafil for erectile dysfunction. *American Family Physician, 70*(2), 359.

Phillips, N.A. (2000, July 1). Female sexual dysfunction: Evaluation and treatment. *American Family Physician, 62*(1), 127–136, 141–142.

Rhodes, J.C., Kjerulff, K.H., Langenberg, P.W., & Guzinski, G.M. (1999). Hysterectomy and sexual functioning. *Journal of the American Medical Association, 282*(20), 1934–1941.

Robins, L.N., Helzer, J.E., Weissman, M.M., Orvaschel, H., Gruenberg, E., Burke, J.D. Jr., & Regier, D.A. (1984). Lifetime prevalence of specific psychiatric disorders in three sites. *Archives of General Psychiatry, 41*, 949–958.

Sadock, B.J., & Sadock, V.A. (2003). *Synopsis of psychiatry: Behavioral sciences/clinical psychiatry* (9th ed.). Philadelphia: Lippincott Williams & Wilkins.

Shenenberger, D., & Knee, T. (2004). Hyperprolactinemia. Retrieved April 27, 2005 from the World Wide Web at http://www.emedicine.com/med/topic1098.htm

Sinclair Intimacy Institute. (2002). Sexual dysfunction in the United States. Retrieved March 20, 2002 from the World Wide Web at http://www.intimacyinstitute.com/about/research/

Spear, J. (2001). Changing attitudes towards sex. *Gale Encyclopedia of Psychology* (2nd ed.). Retrieved April 26, 2005 from the World Wide Web at http://www.findarticles.com/p/articles/mi_g2699/is_0003/ai_2699000313

USA Today. (2003). *Poll shows backlash on gay issues.* Retrieved April 28, 2005 from the World Wide Web at http://www.usatoday.com/news/washington/2003-07–28-poll_x.htm

Zhou, J., Horman, M.A., Gooren, L.J., & Swaab, D.F. (1995). A sex difference in the human brain and its relation to transsexuality. *Nature, 378*, 68–70.

CLASSICAL REFERENCES

Freud, S. (1930). *Three contributions to the theory of sex* (4th ed.). New York: Nervous and Mental Disease Publishing.

Masters, W.H., & Johnson, V.E. (1966). *Human sexual response.* Boston: Little, Brown.

Masters, W.H., & Johnson, V.E. (1970). *Human sexual inadequacy.* Boston: Little, Brown.

EATING DISORDERS

CHAPTER OUTLINE

OBJECTIVES

EPIDEMIOLOGICAL FACTORS

APPLICATION OF THE NURSING PROCESS

TREATMENT MODALITIES

SUMMARY

REVIEW QUESTIONS

KEY TERMS

amenorrhea
anorexia nervosa
anorexiants
binging

bulimia nervosa
emaciated
obesity
purging

CORE CONCEPTS

anorexia
body image
bulimia

OBJECTIVES

After reading this chapter, the student will be able to:

1. Identify and differentiate among the various eating disorders.
2. Discuss epidemiological statistics related to eating disorders.
3. Describe symptomatology associated with anorexia nervosa, bulimia nervosa, and obesity, and use the information in client assessment.
4. Identify predisposing factors in the development of eating disorders.

5. Formulate nursing diagnoses and outcomes of care for clients with eating disorders.
6. Describe appropriate interventions for behaviors associated with eating disorders.
7. Identify topics for client and family teaching relevant to eating disorders.
8. Evaluate the nursing care of clients with eating disorders.
9. Discuss various modalities relevant to treatment of eating disorders.

Nutrition is required to sustain life, and most individuals acquire nutrients from eating food; however, nutrition and life sustenance are not the only reasons most people eat food. Indeed, in an affluent culture, life sustenance may not even be a consideration. It is sometimes difficult to remember that many people within this affluent American culture, as well as all over the world, are starving from lack of food.

The hypothalamus contains the appetite regulation center within the brain. This complex neural system regulates the body's ability to recognize when it is hungry and when it has been sated. Halmi (2003) states:

Eating behavior is now known to reflect an interaction between an organism's physiological state and environmental conditions. Salient physiological variables include the balance of various neuropeptides and neurotransmitters, metabolic state, metabolic rate, condition of the gastrointestinal tract, amount of storage tissue, and sensory receptors for taste and smell. Environmental conditions include features of the food such as taste, texture, novelty, accessibility, and nutritional composition, and other external conditions such as ambient temperature, presence of other people, and stress. (p. 1001)

Society and culture have a great deal of influence on eating behaviors. Eating is a social activity; seldom does an event of any social significance occur without the presence of food. Yet, society and culture also influence how people (and in particular, women) must look. History reveals a regularity of fluctuation in what society has considered desirable in the human female body. Archives and historical paintings reveal the fashionableness and desirability of the plump, full-figured women of the 16th and 17th centuries. In the Victorian era beauty was characterized by a slender, wan appearance that continued through the flapper era of the 1920s. During the Depression era and World War II, the full-bodied woman was again admired, only to be superseded in the late 1960s by the image of the super-thin models propagated by the media, which remains the ideal of today. As it has been said, "A woman can't be too rich or too thin." Eating disorders, as we know them, can dispute this quote.

This chapter explores the disorders associated with undereating and overeating. Because psychological or behavioral factors play a potential role in the presentation of these disorders, they fall well within the realm of psychiatry and psychiatric nursing. Epidemiological statistics are presented along with predisposing factors that have been implicated in the etiology of anorexia nervosa, bulimia nervosa, and obesity. An explanation of the symptomatology is presented as background knowledge for assessing the client with an eating disorder. Nursing care is described in the context of the nursing process. Various treatment modalities are explored.

EPIDEMIOLOGICAL FACTORS

The incidence of **anorexia nervosa** has increased in the past 30 years both in the United States and in Western Europe (Halmi, 2003). Studies indicate a prevalence rate among young women in the United States of approximately 0.5 to 1 percent (Sadock & Sadock, 2003). Anorexia nervosa occurs predominantly in females aged 12 to 30 years. Fewer than 10 percent of the cases occur in males (American Psychiatric Association [APA], 2000). Anorexia nervosa was once believed to be more prevalent in the higher socioeconomic classes, but evidence is lacking to support this hypothesis.

Bulimia nervosa is more prevalent than anorexia nervosa. Estimates of the disorder range from 1 to 3 percent of young women (Sadock & Sadock, 2003). Onset of bulimia nervosa occurs in late adolescence or early adulthood. Cross-cultural research suggests that bulimia nervosa occurs primarily in societies that place emphasis on thinness as the model of attractiveness for women and where an abundance of food is available (Bryant-Waugh & Lask, 2004).

Obesity has been defined as a body mass index (BMI) (weight/height^2) of 30 or greater. In 2002, among adults 20 years of age or older, 65 percent were overweight, with 31 percent of these in the obese range (National Center for Health Statistics [NCHS], 2005). Obesity is more common in black women than in white women and more common in white men than in black men. The

prevalence among lower socioeconomic classes is six times that in upper socioeconomic classes, and there is an inverse relationship between obesity and level of education (American Obesity Association [AOA], 2005a). In 2002, 4.7 percent of the U.S. adult population was categorized as "morbidly" obese, which is defined by the National Institutes of Health as a BMI greater than 40 (AOA, 2005b).

APPLICATION OF THE NURSING PROCESS

Background Assessment Data (Symptomatology)

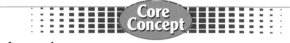

Anorexia
Prolonged loss of appetite.

Body Image
A subjective concept of one's physical appearance based on the personal perceptions of self and the reactions of others.

Anorexia Nervosa

Anorexia nervosa is characterized by a morbid fear of obesity. Symptoms include gross distortion of **body image**, preoccupation with food, and refusal to eat. The term *anorexia* is actually a misnomer. It was initially believed that anorexics did not experience sensations of hunger. However, research indicates that they do indeed suffer from pangs of hunger, and it is only with food intake of less than 200 calories per day that hunger sensations actually cease.

The distortion in body image is manifested by the individual's perception of being "fat" when he or she is obviously underweight or even **emaciated**. Weight loss is usually accomplished by reduction in food intake and often extensive exercising. Self-induced vomiting and the abuse of laxatives or diuretics may also occur.

Weight loss is marked. For example, the individual may present for health care services weighing less than 85 percent of expected weight. Other symptoms include hypothermia, bradycardia, hypotension, edema, lanugo, and a variety of metabolic changes. **Amenorrhea** usually follows weight loss but in some instances may precede it (APA, 2000).

There may be an obsession with food. For example, these individuals may hoard or conceal food, talk about food and recipes at great length, or prepare elaborate meals for others, only to restrict themselves to a limited amount of low-calorie food intake. Compulsive behaviors, such as hand washing, may also be present.

Age at onset is usually early to late adolescence. It is estimated to occur in approximately 0.5 to 1 percent of adolescent females, and is 10 to 20 times more common in females than in males (Sadock & Sadock, 2003). Psychosexual development is generally delayed.

Feelings of depression and anxiety often accompany this disorder. In fact, some studies have suggested a possible interrelationship between eating disorders and affective disorders. Table 34–1 outlines the *DSM-IV-TR* (APA, 2000) diagnostic criteria for anorexia nervosa.

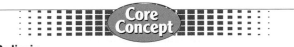

Bulimia
Excessive, insatiable appetite.

Bulimia Nervosa

Bulimia nervosa is an episodic, uncontrolled, compulsive, rapid ingestion of large quantities of food over a short period of time (**binging**), followed by inappropriate compensatory behaviors to rid the body of the excess calories. The food consumed during a binge often has a high caloric content, a sweet taste, and a soft or smooth texture that can be eaten rapidly, sometimes even without

being chewed (Sadock & Sadock, 2003). The binging episodes often occur in secret and are usually only terminated by abdominal discomfort, sleep, social interruption, or self-induced vomiting. Although the eating binges may bring pleasure while they are occurring, self-degradation and depressed mood commonly follow.

To rid the body of the excessive calories, the individual may engage in **purging** behaviors (self-induced vomiting, or the misuse of laxatives, diuretics, or enemas) or other inappropriate compensatory behaviors, such as fasting or excessive exercise. There is a persistent overconcern with personal appearance, particularly regarding how they believe others perceive them. Weight fluctuations are common because of the alternating binges and fasts. However, most individuals with bulimia are within a normal weight range—some slightly underweight, some slightly overweight.

Excessive vomiting and laxative/diuretic abuse may lead to problems with dehydration and electrolyte imbalance. Gastric acid in the vomitus also contributes to the erosion of tooth enamel. In rare instances, the individual may experience tears in the gastric or esophageal mucosa.

Some people with this disorder are subject to mood disorders, anxiety disorders, or substance abuse or dependence, most frequently involving amphetamines or alcohol (APA, 2000). Diagnostic criteria for bulimia nervosa are presented in Table 34–2.

TABLE 34–1   Diagnostic Criteria for Anorexia Nervosa

A. Refusal to maintain body weight at or above a minimally normal weight for age and height (e.g., weight loss leading to maintenance of body weight less than 85% of that expected; or failure to make expected weight gain during period of growth, leading to body weight less than 85% of that expected).
B. Intense fear of gaining weight or becoming fat, even though underweight.
C. Disturbance in the way in which one's body weight or shape is experienced, undue influence of body weight or shape on self-evaluation, or denial of the seriousness of the current low body weight.
D. In postmenarchal females, amenorrhea; i.e., the absence of at least three consecutive menstrual cycles. (A woman is considered to have amenorrhea if her periods occur only following hormone, e.g., estrogen, administration.)
Specify type:
Restricting Type: During the current episode of anorexia nervosa, the person has not regularly engaged in binge-eating or purging behavior (i.e., self-induced vomiting or the misuse of laxatives, diuretics, or enemas).
Binge-Eating/Purging Type: During the current episode of anorexia nervosa, the person has regularly engaged in binge eating or purging behavior (i.e., self-induced vomiting or the misuse of laxatives, diuretics, or enemas).

SOURCE: American Psychiatric Association (2000), with permission.

TABLE 34–2   Diagnostic Criteria for Bulimia Nervosa

A. Recurrent episodes of binge eating. An episode of binge eating is characterized by both of the following:
   1. Eating, in a discrete period of time (e.g., within any 2-hour period) an amount of food that is definitely larger than most people would eat during a similar period of time and under similar circumstances.
   2. A sense of lack of control over eating during the episode (e.g., a feeling that one cannot stop eating or control what or how much one is eating).
B. Recurrent inappropriate compensatory behavior in order to prevent weight gain, such as self-induced vomiting; misuse of laxatives, diuretics, enemas, or other medications; fasting; or excessive exercise.
C. The binge eating and inappropriate compensatory behaviors both occur, on average, at least twice a week for 3 months.
D. Self-evaluation is unduly influenced by body shape and weight.
E. The disturbance does not occur exclusively during episodes of anorexia nervosa.
Specify type:
Purging Type: During the current episode of bulimia nervosa, the person has regularly engaged in self-induced vomiting or the misuse of laxatives, diuretics, or enemas.
Nonpurging Type: During the current episode of bulimia nervosa, the person has used other inappropriate compensatory behaviors, such as fasting or excessive exercise, but has not regularly engaged in self-induced vomiting or the misuse of laxatives, diuretics, or enemas.

SOURCE: American Psychiatric Association (2000), with permission.

Predisposing Factors to Anorexia Nervosa and Bulimia Nervosa

Biological Influences

Genetics. A hereditary predisposition to eating disorders has been hypothesized on the basis of family histories and an apparent association with other disorders for which the likelihood of genetic influences exists. Anorexia nervosa is more common among sisters and mothers of those with the disorder than among the general population. Several studies have reported a higher than expected frequency of mood disorders among first-degree biological relatives of people with anorexia nervosa and bulimia nervosa and of substance abuse and dependence in relatives of individuals with bulimia nervosa (APA, 2000).

Neuroendocrine Abnormalities. Some speculation has occurred regarding a primary hypothalamic dysfunction in anorexia nervosa. Studies consistent with this theory have revealed elevated cerebrospinal fluid cortisol levels and a possible impairment of dopaminergic regulation in individuals with anorexia (Halmi, 2003). Additional evidence in the etiological implication of hypothalamic dysfunction is gathered from the fact that many people with anorexia experience amenorrhea before the onset of starvation and significant weight loss.

Neurochemical Influences. Neurochemical influences in bulimia may be associated with the neurotransmitters serotonin and norepinephrine. This hypothesis has been supported by the positive response these individuals have shown to therapy with the selective serotonin reuptake inhibitors (SSRIs). Some studies have found high levels of endogenous opioids in the spinal fluid of clients with anorexia, promoting the speculation that these chemicals may contribute to denial of hunger (Sadock & Sadock, 2003). Some of these individuals have been shown to gain weight when given naloxone, an opioid antagonist.

Psychodynamic Influences

Psychodynamic theories suggest that eating disorders result from very early and profound disturbances in mother–infant interactions. The result is retarded ego development in the child and an unfulfilled sense of separation–individuation. This problem is compounded when the mother responds to the child's physical and emotional needs with food. Manifestations include a disturbance in body identity and a distortion in body image. When events occur that threaten the vulnerable ego, feelings emerge of lack of control over one's body (self). Behaviors associated with food and eating serve to provide feelings of control over one's life.

Family Influences

Conflict Avoidance. In the theory of the family as a system, psychosomatic symptoms, including anorexia nervosa, are reinforced in an effort to avoid spousal conflict.

Parents are able to deny marital conflict by defining the sick child as the family problem. In these families, there is an unhealthy involvement between the members (enmeshment); the members strive at all costs to maintain "appearances"; and the parents endeavor to retain the child in the dependent position. Conflict avoidance may be a strong factor in the interpersonal dynamics of some families in which children develop eating disorders.

Elements of Power and Control. The issue of control may become the overriding factor in the family of the client with an eating disorder. These families often consist of a passive father, a domineering mother, and an overly dependent child. A high value is placed on perfectionism in this family, and the child feels he or she must satisfy these standards. Parental criticism promotes an increase in obsessive and perfectionistic behavior on the part of the child, who continues to seek love, approval, and recognition. The child eventually begins to feel helpless and ambivalent toward the parents. In adolescence, these distorted eating patterns may represent a rebellion against the parents, viewed by the child as a means of gaining and remaining in control. The symptoms are often triggered by a stressor that the adolescent perceives as a loss of control in some aspect of his or her life.

Obesity

Obesity is not classified as a psychiatric disorder in the *DSM-IV-TR*, but because of the strong emotional factors associated with the condition, it may be considered under "Psychological Factors Affecting Medical Condition."

A third category of eating disorder is also being considered by the American Psychiatric Association. Research criteria for binge eating disorder (BED) are presented in the *DSM-IV-TR* (see Table 34–3). Obesity is a factor in BED because the individual binges on large amounts of food but does not engage in behaviors to rid the body of the excess calories. The following formula is used to determine degree of obesity in an individual:

$$\text{Body mass index} = \frac{\text{Weight (kg)}}{\text{Height (m)}^2}$$

The BMI range for normal weight is 20 to 24.9. Studies by the National Center for Health Statistics indicate that *overweight* is defined as a BMI of 25.0 to 29.9 (based on U.S. Dietary Guidelines for Americans). Based on criteria of the World Health Organization, *obesity* is defined as a BMI of 30.0 or greater. These guidelines, which were released by the National Heart, Lung, and Blood Institute in July 1998, markedly increased the number of Americans considered to be overweight. The average American woman has a BMI of 26, and fashion models typically have BMIs of 18 (Priesnitz, 2005). Table 34–4 presents an example of some BMIs based on weight (in pounds) and height (in inches).

Table 34–3   Research Criteria for Binge-Eating Disorder

A. Recurrent episodes of binge eating. An episode of binge eating is characterized by both of the following:
  (1) Eating, in a discrete period of time (e.g., within any 2-hour period), an amount of food that is definitely larger than most people would eat in a similar period of time under similar circumstances
  (2) A sense of lack of control over eating during the episode (e.g., a feeling that one cannot stop eating or control what or how much one is eating)
B. The binge-eating episodes are associated with three (or more) of the following:
  (1) Eating much more rapidly than normal
  (2) Eating until feeling uncomfortably full
  (3) Eating large amounts of food when not feeling physically hungry
  (4) Eating alone because of being embarrassed by how much one is eating
  (5) Feeling disgusted with oneself, depressed, or very guilty after overeating
C. Marked distress regarding binge eating is present.
D. The binge eating occurs, on average, at least 2 days a week for 6 months.
  NOTE: The method of determining frequency differs from that used for Bulimia Nervosa; future research should address whether the preferred method of setting a frequency threshold is counting the number of days on which binges occur or counting the number of episodes of binge eating.
E. The binge eating is not associated with the regular use of inappropriate compensatory behaviors (e.g., purging, fasting, excessive exercise) and does not occur exclusively during the course of anorexia nervosa or bulimia nervosa.

SOURCE: American Psychiatric Association (2000), with permission.

Obese people often present with hyperlipidemia, particularly elevated triglyceride and cholesterol levels. They commonly have hyperglycemia and are at risk for developing diabetes mellitus. Osteoarthritis may be evident owing to trauma to weight-bearing joints. Work load on the heart and lungs is increased, often leading to symptoms of angina or respiratory insufficiency (National Heart, Lung, and Blood Institute, 2005).

Predisposing Factors to Obesity

Biological Influences

Genetics. Genetics have been implicated in the development of obesity in that 80 percent of offspring of two obese parents are obese (Halmi, 2003). Studies of twins and adoptees reared by normal and overweight parents have also supported this implication of heredity as a predisposing factor to obesity.

Physiological Factors. Lesions in the appetite and satiety centers in the hypothalamus may contribute to overeating and lead to obesity. Hypothyroidism is a problem that interferes with basal metabolism and may lead to weight gain. Weight gain can also occur in response to the decreased insulin production of diabetes mellitus and the increased cortisone production of Cushing's disease.

Lifestyle Factors. On an elementary level, obesity can be viewed as an ingestion of a greater number of calories than are expended. Weight gain occurs when caloric intake exceeds caloric output in terms of basal metabolism and physical activity. Many overweight individuals lead sedentary lifestyles, making it very difficult to burn off calories.

Psychosocial Influences

The psychoanalytical view of obesity proposes that obese individuals have unresolved dependency needs and are

Table 34–4   Body Mass Index (BMI) Chart

BMI	19	20	21	22	23	24	25	26	27	28	29	30	31	32	33	34	35	36	37	38	39	40
HEIGHT (INCHES)										**BODY WEIGHT (POUNDS)**											
58	91	96	100	105	110	115	119	124	129	134	138	143	148	153	158	162	167	172	177	181	186	191
59	94	99	104	109	114	119	124	128	133	138	143	148	153	158	163	168	173	178	183	188	193	198
60	97	102	107	112	118	123	128	133	138	143	148	153	158	163	168	174	179	184	189	194	199	204
61	100	106	111	116	122	127	132	137	143	148	153	158	164	169	174	180	185	190	195	201	206	211
62	104	109	115	120	126	131	136	142	147	153	158	164	169	175	180	186	191	196	202	207	213	218
63	107	113	118	124	130	135	141	146	152	158	163	169	175	180	186	191	197	203	208	214	220	225
64	110	116	122	128	134	140	145	151	157	163	169	174	180	186	192	197	204	209	215	221	227	232
65	114	120	126	132	138	144	150	156	162	168	174	180	186	192	198	204	210	216	222	228	234	240
66	118	124	130	136	142	148	155	161	167	173	179	186	192	198	204	210	216	223	229	235	241	247
67	121	127	134	140	146	153	159	166	172	178	185	191	198	204	211	217	223	230	236	242	249	255
68	125	131	138	144	151	158	164	171	177	184	190	197	203	210	216	223	230	236	243	249	256	262
69	128	135	142	149	155	162	169	176	182	189	196	203	209	216	223	230	236	243	250	257	263	270
70	132	139	146	153	160	167	174	181	188	195	202	209	216	222	229	236	243	250	257	264	271	278
71	136	143	150	157	165	172	179	186	193	200	208	215	222	229	236	243	250	257	265	272	279	286
72	140	147	154	162	169	177	184	191	199	206	213	221	228	235	242	250	258	265	272	279	287	294
73	144	151	159	166	174	182	189	197	204	212	219	227	235	242	250	257	265	272	280	288	295	302
74	148	155	163	171	179	186	194	202	210	218	225	233	241	249	256	264	272	280	287	295	303	311
75	152	160	168	176	184	192	200	208	216	224	232	240	248	256	264	272	279	287	295	303	311	319
76	156	164	172	180	189	197	205	213	221	230	238	246	254	263	271	279	287	295	304	312	320	328

SOURCE: National Heart, Lung, and Blood Institute of the National Institutes of Health (2005).

fixed in the oral stage of psychosexual development. The symptoms of obesity are viewed as depressive equivalents, attempts to regain "lost" or frustrated nurturance and care.

Sadock and Sadock (2003) state:

Although psychological factors are evidently crucial to the development of obesity, how such psychological factors result in obesity is not known. Overweight persons may suffer from every conceivable psychiatric disorder and come from a variety of disturbed backgrounds. Many obese patients are emotionally disturbed persons who, because of the availability of the overeating mechanism in their environments, have learned to use hyperphagia as a means of coping with psychological problems. Some patients may show signs of serious mental disorder when they attain normal weight because they no longer have that coping mechanism. (pp. 752–753)

Transactional Model of Stress/Adaptation

The etiology of eating disorders is most likely influenced by multiple factors. In Figure 34–1, a graphic depiction of this theory of multiple causation is presented in the transactional model of stress/adaptation.

Diagnosis/Outcome Identification

Based on the data collected during the nursing assessment, possible nursing diagnoses for the client with eating disorders include:

Imbalanced nutrition: Less than body requirements related to refusal to eat

Deficient fluid volume (risk for or actual) related to decreased fluid intake; self-induced vomiting; laxative and/or diuretic abuse.

Ineffective denial related to retarded ego development and fear of losing the only aspect of life over which he or she perceives some control (eating).

Imbalanced nutrition: More than body requirements related to compulsive overeating.

Disturbed body image/low self-esteem related to retarded ego development, dysfunctional family system, or feelings of dissatisfaction with body appearance.

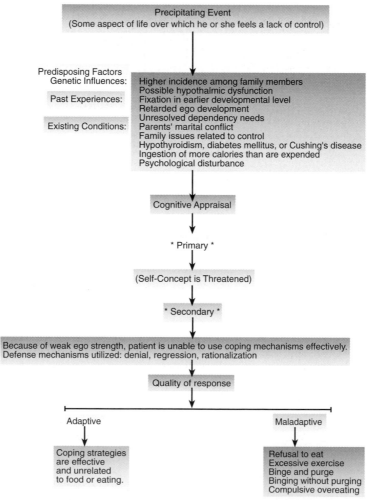

FIGURE 34–1 The dynamics of eating disorders using the transactional model of stress/adaptation.

Anxiety (moderate to severe) related to feelings of help-lessness and lack of control over life events.

The following criteria may be used for measurement of outcomes in the care of the client with eating disorders.

The client:

1. Has achieved and maintained at least 80 percent of expected body weight.
2. Has vital signs, blood pressure, and laboratory serum studies within normal limits.
3. Verbalizes importance of adequate nutrition.
4. Verbalizes knowledge regarding consequences of fluid loss caused by self-induced vomiting (or laxative/diuretic abuse) and importance of adequate fluid intake.
5. Verbalizes events that precipitate anxiety and demon-strates techniques for its reduction.
6. Verbalizes ways in which he or she may gain more control of the environment and thereby reduce feel-ings of helplessness.
7. Expresses interest in welfare of others and less preoc-cupation with own appearance.
8. Verbalizes that image of body as "fat" was mispercep-

tion and demonstrates ability to take control of own life without resorting to maladaptive eating behav-iors (anorexia nervosa).
9. Has established a healthy pattern of eating for weight control, and weight loss toward a desired goal is progressing.
10. Verbalizes plans for future maintenance of weight control.

Planning/Implementation

Tables 34–5 and 34–6 provide plans of care for clients with eating disorders. Nursing diagnoses are presented, along with outcome criteria, appropriate nursing inter-ventions, and rationales.

Some institutions are using a case management model to coordinate care (see Chapter 9 for a more detailed explanation). In case management models, the plan of care may take the form of a critical pathway. Table 34–7 depicts an example of a critical pathway of care for a client with anorexia nervosa.

The concept map care plan is an innovative approach to planning and organizing nursing care (see Chapter 9).

TABLE 34–5   Care Plan for Client with Eating Disorders: Anorexia Nervosa and Bulimia Nervosa

NURSING DIAGNOSES: IMBALANCED NUTRITION: LESS THAN BODY REQUIREMENTS. DEFICIENT FLUID VOLUME (RISK FOR OR ACTUAL)

RELATED TO: Refusal to eat/drink; self-induced vomiting; abuse of laxatives/diuretics

EVIDENCED BY: Loss of weight; poor muscle tone and skin turgor; lanugo; bradycardia; hypotension; cardiac arrhythmias; pale, dry mucous membranes

OUTCOME CRITERIA	NURSING INTERVENTIONS	RATIONALE
Client will achieve 80% of body weight and be free of signs and symptoms of malnutrition/dehydration.	1. Dietitian will determine number of calories required to provide adequate nutrition and realistic weight gain.	1. Adequate calories are required to allow a weight gain of 2–3 pounds per week.
	2. Explain to the client that privileges and restrictions will be based on compliance with treatment and direct weight gain. Do not focus on food and eating.	2. The real issues have little to do with food or eating patterns. Focus on the control issues that have precipitated these behaviors.
	3. Weigh client daily, immediately upon aris-ing and following first voiding. Always use same scale, if possible. Keep strict record of intake and output. Assess skin turgor and integrity regularly. Assess moistness and color of oral mucous membranes.	3. These assessments are important measurements of nutritional status and provide guidelines for treatment.
	4. Stay with client during established time for meals (usually 30 min) and for at least 1 hour following meals.	4. Lengthy mealtimes put excessive focus on food and eating and provide client with attention and reinforcement. The hour following meals may be used to discard food stashed from tray or to engage in self-induced vomiting.
	5. If weight loss occurs, use restrictions. Client must understand that if nutritional status deteriorates, tube feedings will be initiated. This is implemented in a matter-of-fact, nonpunitive way.	5. Restrictions and limits must be estab-lished and carried out consistently to avoid power struggles, to encourage client compliance with therapy, and to ensure client safety.

(Continued on following page)

| TABLE 34–5 | Care Plan for Client with Eating Disorders: Anorexia Nervosa and Bulimia Nervosa (Continued) |

NURSING DIAGNOSIS: INEFFECTIVE DENIAL

RELATED TO: Retarded ego development and fear of losing the only aspect of life over which client perceives some control (eating)

EVIDENCED BY: Inability to admit the impact of maladaptive eating behaviors on life pattern

OUTCOME CRITERIA	NURSING INTERVENTIONS	RATIONALE
Client will verbalize understanding that eating behaviors are maladaptive and demonstrate the ability to cope with issues of control in a more adaptive manner.	1. Develop a trusting relationship. Convey positive regard. 2. Avoid arguing or bargaining with the client who is resistant to treatment. State matter-of-factly which behaviors are unacceptable and how privileges will be restricted for noncompliance. 3. Encourage client to verbalize feelings regarding role within the family and issues related to dependence/independence, the intense need for achievement, and sexuality. Help client recognize ways in which he or she can gain control over these problematic areas of life.	1. Trust and unconditional acceptance promote dignity and self-worth and provide a strong foundation for a therapeutic relationship. 2. The person who is denying a problem and who also has a weak ego will use manipulation to achieve control. Consistency and firmness by staff will decrease use of these behaviors. 3. When client feels control over major life issues, the need to gain control through maladaptive eating behaviors will diminish.

NURSING DIAGNOSIS: DISTURBED BODY IMAGE/LOW SELF-ESTEEM

RELATED TO: Retarded ego development and dysfunctional family system

EVIDENCED BY: Distorted body image, difficulty accepting positive reinforcement, depressed mood and self-deprecating thoughts

OUTCOME CRITERIA	NURSING INTERVENTIONS	RATIONALE
Client will acknowledge misperception of body image as "fat" and verbalize positive self-attributes.	1. Help client to develop a realistic perception of body image and relationship with food. Compare specific measurement of the client's body with the client's perceived calculations. 2. Promote feelings of control within the environment through participation and independent decision making. Through positive feedback, help client learn to accept self as is, including weaknesses as well as strengths. 3. Help client realize that perfection is unrealistic, and explore this need with him or her.	1. There may be a large discrepancy between the actual body size and the client's perception of his or her body size. Client needs to recognize that the misperception of body image is unhealthy and that maintaining control through maladaptive eating behaviors is dangerous—even life threatening. 2. Client must come to understand that he or she is a capable, autonomous individual who can perform outside the family unit and who is not expected to be perfect. Control of his or her life must be achieved in other ways besides dieting and weight loss. 3. As client begins to feel better about self, identifies positive self-attributes, and develops the ability to accept certain personal inadequacies, the need for unrealistic achievement should diminish.

It is a diagrammatic teaching and learning strategy that allows visualization of interrelationships between medical diagnoses, nursing diagnoses, assessment data, and treatments. Examples of concept map care plans for clients with eating disorders are presented in Figures 34–2 and 34–3.

Client/Family Education

The role of client teacher is important in the psychiatric area, as it is in all areas of nursing. A list of topics for client/family education relevant to eating disorders is presented in Table 34–8.

TABLE 34–6   **Care Plan for the Client with an Eating Disorder: Obesity**

NURSING DIAGNOSIS: IMBALANCED NUTRITION: MORE THAN BODY REQUIREMENTS
RELATED TO: Compulsive Overeating
EVIDENCED BY: Weight of more than 20% over expected body weight for age and height; BMI ≥ 30

OUTCOME CRITERIA	NURSING INTERVENTIONS	RATIONALE
Client will demonstrate change in eating patterns resulting in a steady weight loss.	1. Encourage the client to keep a diary of food intake.	1. A food diary provides the opportunity for client to gain a realistic picture of the amount of food ingested and provides a database on which to tailor the dietary program.
	2. Discuss feelings and emotions associated with eating.	2. This helps to identify when client is eating to satisfy an emotional need rather than a physiological one.
	3. With input from the client, formulate an eating plan that includes food from the required food groups with emphasis on low-fat intake. It is helpful to keep the plan as similar to client's usual eating pattern as possible.	3. Diet must eliminate calories while maintaining adequate nutrition. Client is more likely to stay on the eating plan if he or she is able to participate in its creation and it deviates as little as possible from usual types of foods.
	4. Identify realistic increment goals for weekly weight loss.	4. Reasonable weight loss (1–2 pounds per week) results in more lasting effects. Excessive, rapid weight loss may result in fatigue and irritability and ultimately lead to failure in meeting goals for weight loss. Motivation is more easily sustained by meeting "stair-step" goals.
	5. Plan progressive exercise program tailored to individual goals and choice.	5. Exercise may enhance weight loss by burning calories and reducing appetite, increasing energy, toning muscles, and enhancing sense of well-being and accomplishment. Walking is an excellent choice for overweight individuals.
	6. Discuss the probability of reaching plateaus when weight remains stable for extended periods.	6. Client should know this is likely to happen as changes in metabolism occur. Plateaus cause frustration, and client may need additional support during these times to remain on the weight-loss program.
	7. Provide instruction about medications to assist with weight loss if ordered by physician.	7. Appetite-suppressant drugs (e.g., sibutramine) and others that have weight loss as a side effect (e.g., fluoxetine) may be helpful to someone who is severely overweight. They should be used for this purpose for only a short period while the individual attempts to adjust to the new pattern of eating.

NURSING DIAGNOSIS: DISTURBED BODY IMAGE/LOW SELF-ESTEEM
RELATED TO: Dissatisfaction with appearance
EVIDENCED BY: Verbalization of negative feelings about the way he or she looks and desire to lose weight

OUTCOME CRITERIA	NURSING INTERVENTIONS	RATIONALE
Client will begin to accept self based on self-attributes rather than on appearance, while actively pursuing weight loss as desired.	1. Assess client's feelings and attitudes about being obese.	1. Obesity and compulsive eating behaviors may have deep-rooted psychological implications, such as compensation for lack of love and nurturing or a defense against intimacy.

(Continued on following page)

OUTCOME CRITERIA	NURSING INTERVENTIONS	RATIONALE
	2. Ensure that the client has privacy during self-care activities.	2. The obese individual may be sensitive or self-conscious about his or her body.
	3. Have client recall coping patterns related to food in family of origin and explore how these may affect current situation.	3. Parents are role models for their children. Maladaptive eating behaviors are learned within the family system and are supported through positive reinforcement. Food may be substituted by the parent for affection and love, and eating is associated with a feeling of satisfaction, becoming the primary defense.
	4. Determine client's motivation for weight loss and set goals.	4. The individual may harbor repressed feelings of hostility, which may be expressed inward on the self. Because of a poor self-concept, the person often has difficulty with relationships. When the motivation is to lose weight for someone else, successful weight loss is less likely to occur.
	5. Help client identify positive self-attributes. Focus on strengths and past accomplishments unrelated to physical appearance.	5. It is important that self-esteem not be tied solely to size of the body. Client needs to recognize that obesity need not interfere with positive feelings regarding self-concept and self-worth.
	6. Refer client to support or therapy group.	6. Support groups can provide companionship, increase motivation, decrease loneliness and social ostracism, and give practical solutions to common problems. Group therapy can be helpful in dealing with underlying psychological concerns.

TABLE 34-7   Critical Pathway of Care for a Client with Anorexia Nervosa

Estimated Length of Stay: 28 Days*

Variations from Designated Pathway Should Be Documented in Progress Notes

Nursing Diagnoses and Categories of Care	Time Dimension	Goals and/or Actions	Time Dimension	Goals and/or Actions	Time Dimension	Discharge Outcome
Imbalanced nutrition: Less than body requirements. Risk for deficient fluid volume.	Ongoing	Client will gain 3 lb/wk and maintain adequate state of hydration			Day 28	Client will exhibit no signs or symptoms of malnutrition or dehydration
Referrals	Day 1 and ongoing	Consult dietitian	Days 2–28	Fulfill nutritional needs. Client consumes 75% of food provided and at least 1000 ml fluid/day.		
Diagnostic studies	Day 1	Electrolytes Electrocardiogram Blood urea nitrogen/creatinine Urinalysis Complete blood count Thyroid function	Day 14	Repeat of selected diagnostic studies.	Day 28	All laboratory values are within normal limits.
Additional assessments	Daily; q shift	Vital signs	Days 7–28	Vital signs within normal limits	Days 22–28	Client is able to refrain from self–induced vomiting.
	Daily; q shift	Intake & output	Days 7–28	Appropriate balance is achieved.		
	Day 1	Weight	Days 2–28	Client gains approximately $1/2$ lb/day.		
	Day 1	Monitor for purging following meals.	Days 1–21	Client bathroom is locked for 1 hr following meals.		

(Continued on opposite page)

Nursing Diagnoses and Categories of Care	Time Dimension	Goals and/or Actions	Time Dimension	Goals and/or Actions	Time Dimension	Discharge Outcome
Client education	Day 1	Unit orientation; behavior modification plan	Days 7–14	Principles of nutrition; foods for maintenance of wellness	Days 15–18	Client demonstrates ability to select appropriate foods for healthy diet.
Ineffective denial	Day 1	Client will cooperate with orientation to unit and explanation of behavior modification plan.	Days 2–28	Client cooperates with therapy to restore nutritional status	Days 18–28	Client accepts that eating behaviors are maladaptive and demonstrates ability to cope more adaptively.
Referrals	Day 7 (or when physical condition is stable)	Psychologist; social worker; psychodramatist	Days 8–28	Client attends group psychotherapies daily.	Day 28	Client verbalizes ways to gain control in life situation.
Additional assessments	Days 1–17	Assess client's ability to trust; use of manipulation to achieve control.	Day 14	Client has developed trusting relationship with at least one staff member on each shift.	Day 28	Client no longer manipulates others to achieve control.
Client education	Day 1 and ongoing as required	Describe privileges and responsibilities of behavior modification program. Explain consequences of noncompliance.	Day 21	Discuss role of support groups for individuals with eating disorders.	Day 28	Client and family verbalize intention to attend community support group.
Disturbed body image; low self-esteem	Day 7	Client acknowledges that attention will not be given to the discussion of body image and food.	Day 21	Client acknowledges misperception of body image as fat and verbalizes positive self-attributes.	Day 28	Client perceives body image correctly, is not obsessed with food, and has given up the need for perfection.
Referrals	Day 1 (or when condition is stable)	Occupational therapy; recreational therapy; music therapy; art therapy.	Days 2–28	Client attends therapy sessions on a daily basis.	Day 28	Through self-expression, client has gained self-awareness and verbalizes positive attributes of self.
Additional assessments	Day 7	Compare specific measurements of client's body with client's perceived calculations. Clarify discrepancies.	Days 8-28	Discuss strengths and weaknesses. Client should strive to achieve self-acceptance.	Day 28	Client verbalizes acceptance of self, including "imperfections"
Medications	At physician's discretion	For associated symptoms: Antidepressant (e.g., SSRI) and/or antianxiety (e.g.,benzodiazepine)			Day 28	Discharge with medications as required.
Client education	Days 14–28	Discuss alternative coping strategies for dealing with feelings. Have client keep diary of feelings, particularly when thinking about food. Discuss action and side effects of medications.			Day 28	Client demonstrates adaptive coping strategies unrelated to eating behaviors for dealing with feelings. Client verbalizes understanding of need for and side effects of medications.

*Length of stay and type of treatment (in-patient, outpatient, or partial hospitalization) is determined by severity of client's illness and the level of intensity of care required.

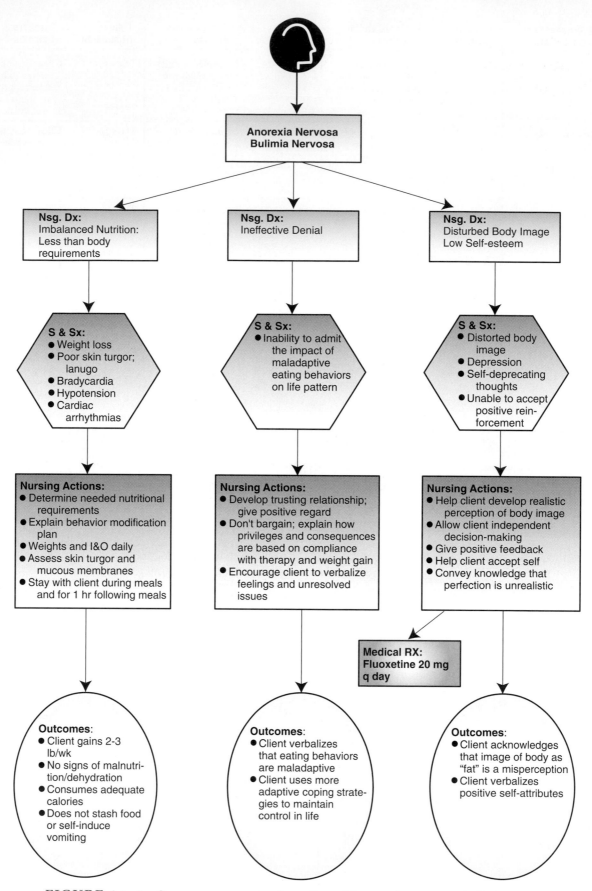

FIGURE 34–2 Concept map care plan for a client with anorexia nervosa or bulimia nervosa.

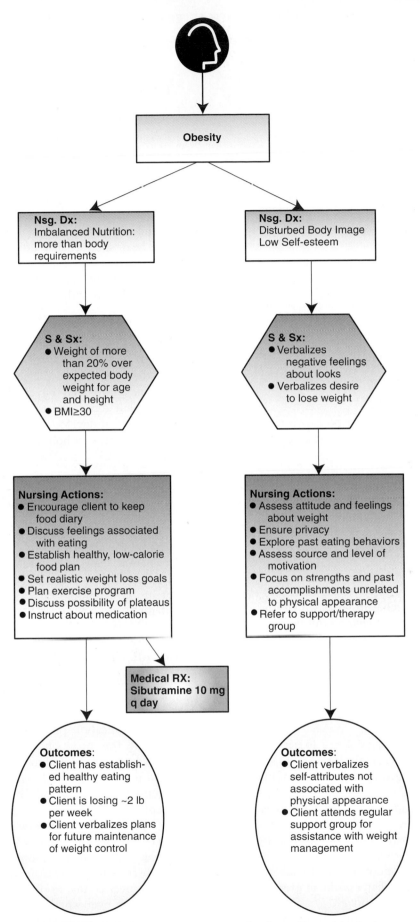

FIGURE 34–3 Concept map care plan for a client with obesity.

TABLE 34–8   Topics for Client/Family Education Related to Eating Disorders

Nature of the Illness
1. Symptoms of anorexia nervosa
2. Symptoms of bulimia nervosa
3. What constitutes obesity
4. Causes of eating disorders
5. Effects of the illness or condition on the body

Management of the Illness
1. Principles of nutrition (foods for maintenance of wellness)
2. Ways client may feel in control of life (aside from eating)
3. Importance of expressing fears and feelings, rather than holding them inside.
4. Alternative coping strategies (to maladaptive eating behaviors)
5. For the obese client:
   a. How to plan a reduced-calorie, nutritious diet
   b. How to read food content labels
   c. How to establish a realistic weight loss plan
   d. How to establish a planned program of physical activity
6. Correct administration of prescribed medications (e.g., antidepressants, anorexigenics)
7. Indication for and side effects of prescribed medications
8. Relaxation techniques
9. Problem-solving skills

Support Services
1. Weight Watchers International
2. Overeaters Anonymous
3. National Association of Anorexia Nervosa and Associated Disorders (ANAD)
   P.O. Box 7
   Highland Park, IL 60035
   (847) 831–3438
4. The American Anorexia/Bulimia Association, Inc.
   165 W. 46th St., Suite 1108
   New York, NY 10036
   (212) 575–6200

Evaluation

Evaluation of the client with an eating disorder requires a reassessment of the behaviors for which the client sought treatment. Behavioral change will be required on both the part of the client and family members. The following types of questions may provide assistance in gathering data required for evaluating whether the nursing interventions have been effective in achieving the goals of therapy.

For anorexia or bulimia:

1. Has the client steadily gained 2 to 3 lb per week to at least 80 percent of body weight for age and size?
2. Is the client free of signs and symptoms of malnutrition and dehydration?
3. Does the client consume adequate calories as determined by the dietitian?
4. Have there been any attempts to stash food from the tray to discard later?
5. Have there been any attempts to self-induce vomiting?
6. Has the client admitted that a problem exists and that eating behaviors are maladaptive?
7. Have behaviors aimed at manipulating the environment been discontinued?

8. Is the client willing to discuss the real issues concerning family roles, sexuality, dependence/independence, and the need for achievement?
9. Does the client understand how he or she has used maladaptive eating behaviors in an effort to achieve a feeling of some control over life events?
10. Has the client acknowledged that perception of body image as "fat" is incorrect?

For obesity:

1. Has the client shown a steady weight loss since starting the new eating plan?
2. Does he or she verbalize a plan to help stay on the new eating plan?
3. Does the client verbalize positive self-attributes not associated with body size or appearance?

For anorexia, bulimia, and obesity:

1. Has the client been able to develop a more realistic perception of body image?
2. Has the client acknowledged that past self-expectations may have been unrealistic?
3. Does client accept self as less than perfect?
4. Has the client developed adaptive coping strategies to deal with stress without resorting to maladaptive eating behaviors?

TREATMENT MODALITIES

The immediate aim of treatment in eating disorders is to restore the client's nutritional status. Complications of emaciation, dehydration, and electrolyte imbalance can lead to death. Once the physical condition is no longer life threatening, other treatment modalities may be initiated.

Behavior Modification

Efforts to change the maladaptive eating behaviors of clients with anorexia or bulimia have become the widely accepted treatment. The importance of instituting a behavior modification program with these clients is to ensure that the program does not "control" them. Issues of control are central to the etiology of these disorders, and in order for the program to be successful, the client must perceive that he or she is in control of the treatment.

Successes have been observed when the client with anorexia is allowed to contract for privileges based on weight gain. The client has input into the care plan and can clearly see what the treatment choices are. The client has control over eating, over the amount of exercise pursued, and even over whether or not to induce vomiting. Goals of therapy, along with the responsibilities of each for goal achievement, are agreed on by client and staff.

Staff and client also agree on a system of rewards and privileges that can be earned by the client, who is given ultimate control. He or she has a choice of whether or not to abide by the contract—a choice of whether or not to gain weight—a choice of whether or not to earn the desired privilege.

Individual Therapy

Although individual psychotherapy is not the therapy of choice for eating disorders, it can be helpful when underlying psychological problems are contributing to the maladaptive behaviors. In supportive psychotherapy, the therapist encourages the client to explore unresolved conflicts and to recognize the maladaptive eating behaviors as defense mechanisms used to ease the emotional pain. The goals are to resolve the personal issues and establish more adaptive coping strategies for dealing with stressful situations.

Family Therapy

Kirkpatrick and Caldwell (2001) state:

Eating disorders have a profound effect on families. While these disorders can help bring families together, they always cause some level of distress. Stresses can cause a breakdown of the whole family unit if there isn't some form of intervention. Family therapy aims at finding solutions to help the healing process for everyone in the family. (p. 159)

In many instances, eating disorders may be considered *family* disorders, and resolution cannot be achieved until dynamics within the family have improved. Family therapy deals with education of the members about the disorder's manifestations, possible etiology, and prescribed treatment. Support is given to family members as they deal with feelings of guilt associated with the perception that they may have contributed to the onset of the disorder. Support is also given as they deal with the social stigma of having a family member with emotional problems.

In some instances when the dysfunctional family dynamics are related to conflict avoidance, the family may be noncompliant with therapy, as they attempt to maintain equilibrium by keeping a member in the sick role. When this occurs, it is essential to focus on the functional operations within the family and to help them manage conflict and create change.

Referrals are made to local support groups for families of individuals with eating disorders. Resolution and growth can sometimes be achieved through interaction with others who are experiencing, or have experienced, the numerous problems of living with a family member with an eating disorder.

Psychopharmacology

There are no medications specifically indicated for eating disorders. Various medications have been prescribed for associated symptoms such as anxiety and depression. Halmi (2003) reports on success with fluoxetine (Prozac) and clomipramine (Anafranil) in clients with anorexia nervosa, and particularly those with depression or obsessive–compulsive symptoms. Cyproheptadine (Periactin), in its unlabeled use as an appetite stimulant, and the antipsychotic chlorpromazine (Thorazine) have also been used to treat this disorder in selected clients. Recent success was reported in an open trial of olanzapine (Zyprexa) with anorexic clients (Barbarich et al., 2004).

Fluoxetine (Prozac) has been found to be useful in the treatment of bulimia nervosa (Walsh et al., 2000). A dosage of 60 mg/day (triple the usual antidepressant dosage) was found to be most effective with bulimic clients. It is possible that fluoxetine, a selective serotonin reuptake inhibitor, may decrease the craving for carbohydrates, thereby decreasing the incidence of binge eating, which is often associated with consumption of large amounts of carbohydrates. Other antidepressants, such as imipramine (Tofranil), desipramine (Norpramin), amitriptyline (Elavil), nortriptyline (Aventyl), and phenelzine (Nardil), also have been shown to be effective in controlled treatment studies (Halmi, 2003). Fluoxetine has also been successful in treating clients who are overweight, possibly for the same reason that was explained for clients with bulimia. The effective dosage for promoting weight loss is 60 mg/day.

A recent study was conducted with topiramate (Topamax), a novel anticonvulsant, in the long-term treatment of binge-eating disorder with obesity (McElroy et al., 2004). The median dose was 250 mg/day. Participants experienced a significant decline in mean weekly binge frequency and significant reduction in body weight.

Sadock and Sadock (2003) state:

Sympathomimetics are used in the treatment of obesity because of their anorexia-inducing effects. Because tolerance develops for the anorectic effects and because of the drugs' high abuse potential, their use for this indication is limited. (p. 1118)

Withdrawal from **anorexiants** may result in a rebound weight gain and, in some clients, a concomitant lethargy and depression. Two anorexiants that were once widely used, fenfluramine and dexfenfluramine, have been removed from the market because of their association with serious heart and lung disease.

A medication for treating obesity, called sibutramine (Meridia), was approved by the U.S. Food and Drug Administration (FDA) in 1998. It has been suggested only for individuals who have a significant amount of weight to lose. The mechanism of action in the control of appetite appears to occur by inhibiting the neurotransmitters serotonin and norepinephrine. Common side effects include headache, dry mouth, constipation, and insomnia. More troublesome side effects include increased blood pressure, rapid heart rate, and seizures. Some concern has recently been expressed about possible cardiac disease associated with the use of sibutramine. Several individuals have claimed cardiovascular-related deaths in association with use of the drug. This claim as yet is unsubstantiated. Caution must be taken in prescribing this medication for an individual with a history of cardiac disease.

SUMMARY

The incidence of eating disorders has continued to increase over the past 30 years. Individuals with anorexia nervosa, a disorder that is characterized by a morbid fear of obesity and a gross distortion of body image, literally can starve themselves to death. The individual believes he or she is fat even when emaciated. The disorder is commonly accompanied by depression and anxiety.

Bulimia nervosa is an eating disorder characterized by the consumption of huge amounts of food, usually in a short period of time, and often in secret. Tension is relieved and pleasure felt during the time of the binge, but is soon followed by feelings of guilt and depression. Individuals with this disorder "purge" themselves of the excessive intake with self-induced vomiting or the misuse of laxatives, diuretics, or enemas. They also are subject to mood and anxiety disorders.

Compulsive eating can result in obesity, which is defined by the NIH as a BMI of 30. Obesity predisposes the individual to many health concerns, and at the morbid level (a BMI of 40), the weight alone can contribute to increases in morbidity and mortality.

This chapter explored the predisposing factors to these three eating disorders. Symptomatology was identified as background assessment data. Nursing care was presented in the context of the six steps of the nursing process. Care plans for anorexia/bulimia and obesity and a critical pathway of care for the client with anorexia nervosa were included. The treatment modalities of behavior modification, individual psychotherapy, family therapy, and psychopharmacology were discussed.

REVIEW QUESTIONS

SELF-EXAMINATION/LEARNING EXERCISE

Select the answer that is *most* appropriate for each of the following questions.

1. Some obese individuals take amphetamines to suppress appetite and help them lose weight. Which of the following is an adverse effect associated with use of amphetamines that makes this practice undesirable?
   a. Bradycardia
   b. Amenorrhea
   c. Tolerance
   d. Convulsions

2. Psychoanalytically, the theory of obesity relates to the individual's unconscious equation of food with:
   a. Nurturance and caring.
   b. Power and control.
   c. Autonomy and emotional growth.
   d. Strength and endurance.

3. From a physiological point of view, the *most common* cause of obesity is probably:
   a. Lack of nutritional education.
   b. More calories consumed than expended.
   c. Impaired endocrine functioning.
   d. Low basal metabolic rate.

4. Nancy, age 14, has just been admitted to the psychiatric unit for anorexia nervosa. She is emaciated and refusing to eat. What is the primary nursing diagnosis for Nancy?
   a. Dysfunctional grieving
   b. Imbalanced nutrition: Less than body requirements.
   c. Interrupted family processes
   d. Anxiety (severe)

5. Which of the following physical manifestations would you expect to assess in Nancy?
   a. Tachycardia, hypertension, hyperthermia
   b. Bradycardia, hypertension, hyperthermia
   c. Bradycardia, hypotension, hypothermia
   d. Tachycardia, hypotension, hypothermia

6. Nancy continues to refuse to eat. What is the most appropriate response by the nurse?
   a. "You know that if you don't eat, you will die."
   b. "If you continue to refuse to take food orally, you will be fed through a nasogastric tube."
   c. "You might as well leave if you are not going to follow your therapy regimen."
   d. "You don't have to eat if you don't want to. It is your choice."

7. Which medication might you expect the physician to prescribe for Nancy?
   a. Sibutramine (Meridia)
   b. Diazepam (Valium)
   c. Fluoxetine (Prozac)
   d. Carbamazepine (Tegretol)

8. Jane is hospitalized on the psychiatric unit. She has a history and current diagnosis of bulimia nervosa. Which of the following symptoms would be congruent with Jane's diagnosis?
   a. Binging, purging, obesity, hyperkalemia
   b. Binging, purging, normal weight, hypokalemia
   c. Binging, laxative abuse, amenorrhea, severe weight loss
   d. Binging, purging, severe weight loss, hyperkalemia

9. Jane has stopped vomiting in the hospital and tells the nurse she is afraid she is going to gain weight. Which is the most appropriate response by the nurse?
   a. "Don't worry. The dietitian will ensure you don't get too many calories in your diet."
   b. "Don't worry about your weight. We are going to work on other problems while you are in the hospital."
   c. "I understand that you are concerned about your weight and we will talk about good nutrition; but now I want you to tell me about your recent invitation to join the National Honor Society. That's quite an accomplishment."
   d. "You are not fat, and the staff will ensure that you do not gain weight while you are in the hospital, because we know that is important to you."

10. The binging episode is thought to involve:
    a. A release of tension, followed by feelings of depression.
    b. Feelings of fear, followed by feelings of relief.
    c. Unmet dependency needs and a way to gain attention.
    d. Feelings of euphoria, excitement, and self-gratification.

TEST YOUR CRITICAL THINKING SKILLS

Janice, a high school sophomore, wanted desperately to become a cheerleader. She practiced endlessly before try-outs, but she was not selected. A week later, her boyfriend, Roy, broke up with her to date another girl. Janice, who was 5'3" tall and weighed 110 pounds, decided it was because she was too fat. She began to exercise at every possible moment. She skipped meals, and tried to keep her daily consumption to no more than 300 calories. She lost a great deal of weight but became very weak. She felt cold all of the time and wore sweaters in the warm weather. She collapsed during her physical edu-cation class at school and was rushed to the emergency department. On admission, she weighed 90 pounds. She was emaciated and anemic. The physician admitted her with a diagnosis of anorexia nervosa.

Answer the following questions about Janice:

1. What will be the *primary* consideration in her care?
2. How will treatment be directed toward helping her gain weight?
3. How will the nurse know if Janice is using self-induced vomiting to rid herself of food consumed at meals?

IMPLICATIONS OF RESEARCH FOR EVIDENCE-BASED PRACTICE

Long, J.D., & Stevens, K.R. (2004). Using technology to promote self-efficacy for healthy eating in adolescents. *Journal of Nursing Scholarship, 36*(2), 134–139.

Description of the Study: Obesity and overweight have reached epidemic proportions and they are risk factors for the development of chronic disease. The purpose of this study was to test the effects of a classroom and World Wide Web (WWW) educational intervention on self-efficacy for healthy eating. The sample consisted of 63 adolescents in the participant group and 58 in the control group. The age range was between 12 and 16 years. The participant group received the intervention that consisted of 10 hours of classroom and 5 hours of Web-based nutrition education endorsed by the American Cancer Society and the National Cancer Institute. Information is included to encourage healthy eating behaviors that reduce the risk of cancer, obesity, heart disease, and diabetes. Participants in the control group received the nutrition education integrated in the health, science, and home economics curriculum. All participants completed six questionnaires to measure dietary knowledge and eating behaviors. Pre- and post-tests were administered to both groups.

Results of the Study: Although no difference was found between groups in food consumption during the month of intervention, the participant group had significantly higher scores related to knowledge of good nutrition and healthy eating behaviors. The study was limited to individual adolescents and did not attempt to initiate change in the home or school environment

Implications for Nursing Practice: Nurses, and especially school nurses, can become actively involved in nutrition education for children and adolescents. The authors report that 9 million young people are overweight—a number that more than doubled in the last 20 years. This has serious implications for nursing to assist in the educational process needed to reverse this unhealthy trend.

IMPLICATIONS OF RESEARCH FOR EVIDENCE-BASED PRACTICE

McIntosh, V.V.W., Jordan, J., Carter, F.A., Luty, S.E., McKenzie, J.M., Bulik, C.M., Frampton, C.M.A., & Joyce, P.R. (2005). **Three psychotherapies for anorexia nervosa: A randomized, controlled trial.** *American Journal of Psychiatry 162*, 741–747.

Description of the Study: The objective of this study was to examine the efficacy of three types of therapies in treatment of anorexia nervosa. Fifty-six women (age range: 17 to 40 years) with anorexia nervosa were randomly assigned to one of three treatments. Two were specialized psychotherapies: cognitive behavior therapy (CBT) and interpersonal psychotherapy (IPT). The third (the intervention) included treatment combining clinical management and supportive psychotherapy (called nonspecific supportive clinical management). They participated in 20 therapy sessions over a minimum of 20 weeks. The intervention consisted of education, care, and support, fostering a therapeutic relationship that promotes adherence to treatment. Emphasis was placed on resumption of normal eating and restoration of weight. Information on weight maintenance strategies, energy requirements, and relearning to eat normally were included. Outcomes were measured on a global anorexia nervosa measure using a 4-point ordinal scale:

4 = meets full criteria for the anorexia nervosa spectrum
3 = not full anorexia nervosa, but having a number of features of eating disorders

2 = few features of eating disorders
1 = no significant features of eating disorders

Results of the Study: Fifty-six percent of the participants who received nonspecific supportive clinical management received a score of 1 or 2 on the final outcome measure, compared with 32 percent and 10 percent of those receiving CBT and IPT, respectively. They suggest that IPT may not have been as successful because of the lack of symptom focus and relatively long time taken to decide on the problem area. They hypothesize that the CBT may have been less effective because of the large amount of psychoeducational material and extensive skills acquisition associated with this therapy, and the difficulty of anorexia clients to generate alternatives due to cognitive rigidity. These results were in direct opposition to the original hypothesis generated by the researchers in the beginning of the study.

Implications for Nursing Practice: Nurses in advanced practice are usually trained to provide CBT and IPT. Often, generalist nurses do not have the theoretical background to perform these therapies. The interventions associated with nonspecific supportive clinical management are within the scope of nursing practice, and the results of this study indicate that they are superior to CBT and IPT in the treatment of anorexia nervosa. Nurses could become instrumental in establishing programs based on this type of treatment for individuals with this type of eating disorder.

 INTERNET REFERENCES

Additional information about anorexia nervosa and bulimia nervosa may be located at the following Web sites:

* http://www.aabainc.org
* http://www.psych.org/public_info/eatingdisorders52201.cfm
* http://www.mentalhealth.com/dis/p20-et01.html
* http://www.anred.com/
* http://www.mentalhealth.com/dis/p20-et02.html

* http://www.nimh.nih.gov/publicat/eatingdisorders.cfm
* http://medlineplus.nlm.nih.gov/medlineplus/eatingdisorders.html

Additional information about obesity may be located at the following Web sites:

* http://www.shapeup.org/
* http://www.obesity.org/
* http://medlineplus.nlm.nih.gov/medlineplus/obesity.html
* http://www.asbp.org/
* http://win.niddk.nih.gov/publications/binge.htm

REFERENCES

American Obesity Association (AOA). (2005a). *Obesity in the U.S.* Retrieved April 30, 2005 from the World Wide Web at http://www.obesity.org/subs/fastfacts/obesity_US.shtml

American Obesity Association (AOA). (2005b). *Morbid obesity.* Retrieved April 30, 2005 from the World Wide Web at http://www.obesity.org/subs/fastfacts/morbidobesity.shtml

American Psychiatric Association (APA) (2000). *Diagnostic and statistical manual of mental disorders* (4th ed.) *Text Revision.* Washington, DC: American Psychiatric Association.

Barbarich, N.C., McConaha, C.W., Gaskill, J., LaVia, M., Frank, G.K., Achenbach, S., Plotnicov, K.H., & Kaye, W.H. (2004). An open trial of olanzapine in anorexia nervosa. *Journal of Clinical Psychiatry, 65*(11), 1480–1482.

Bryant-Waugh, R., & Lask, B. (2004). *Eating disorders.* New York: Brunner-Routledge.

Halmi, K.A. (2003). Eating disorders: Anorexia nervosa, bulimia nervosa, and obesity. In R.E. Hales & S.C. Yudofsky (Eds.). *Textbook of clinical psychiatry* (4th ed.). Washington, DC: American Psychiatric Publishing.

Kirkpatrick, J., & Caldwell, P. (2001). *Eating disorders: Everything you need to know.* Buffalo, NY: Firefly Books.

McElroy, S.L., Shapira, N.A., Arnold, L.M., Keck, P.E., Rosenthal, N.R., Wu, S.C., Capece, J.A., Fazzio, L., & Hudson, J.I. (2004). Topiramate in the long-term treatment of binge-eating disorder associated with obesity. *Journal of Clinical Psychiatry, 65*(11), 1463–1469.

National Center for Health Statistics (NCHS). (2005). *Prevalence of overweight and obesity among adults: United States, 1999–2002.* Retrieved April 30, 2005 from the World Wide Web at http://www.cdc.gov/nchs/products/pubs/pubd/hestats/obese/obse99.htm

National Heart, Lung, and Blood Institute. (2005). Clinical guidelines on the identification, evaluation, and treatment of overweight and obesity in adults. Retrieved April 30, 2005 from the World Wide Web at http://www.nhlbi.nih.gov/guidelines/obesity

Priesnitz, W. (2005). Are you dying to lose weight? *Natural Life Magazine, 84*(2). Retrieved April 30, 2005 from the World Wide Web at http://www.life.ca/nl/84/weight.html

Sadock, B.J., & Sadock, V.A. (2003). *Synopsis of psychiatry: Behavioral sciences/clinical psychiatry* (9th ed.). Philadelphia: Lippincott Williams & Wilkins.

Walsh, T., Agras, W.S., Devlin, M.J., Fairburn, C.G., Wilson, G..T., Kahn, C., & Chally, M.K. (2000, August). Fluoxetine for bulimia nervosa following poor response to psychotherapy. *The American Journal of Psychiatry, 157,* 1332–1334.

ADJUSTMENT AND IMPULSE CONTROL DISORDERS

CHAPTER OUTLINE

OBJECTIVES

HISTORICAL AND EPIDEMIOLOGICAL FACTORS

APPLICATION OF THE NURSING PROCESS

TREATMENT MODALITIES

SUMMARY

REVIEW QUESTIONS

KEY TERMS

adjustment disorder
Gamblers Anonymous
kleptomania

pathological gambling
pyromania
trichotillomania

CORE CONCEPTS

adjustment
impulsive

OBJECTIVES

After reading this chapter, the student will be able to:

1. Discuss historical aspects and epidemiological statistics related to adjustment and impulse control disorders.
2. Describe various types of adjustment and impulse control disorders and identify symptomatology associated with each; use this information in client assessment.
3. Identify predisposing factors in the development of adjustment and impulse control disorders.
4. Formulate nursing diagnoses and goals of

care for clients with adjustment and impulse control disorders.
5. Describe appropriate nursing interventions for behaviors associated with adjustment and impulse control disorders.
6. Identify topics for client and family teaching relevant to adjustment and impulse control disorders.
7. Evaluate nursing care of clients with adjustment and impulse control disorders.
8. Discuss various modalities relevant to treatment of adjustment and impulse control disorders.

lthough **adjustment disorder** and impulse control disorders are two separate diagnostic categories in the *DSM-IV-TR* (American Psychiatric Association [APA], 2000), they do share some common characteristics. It is likely that they are precipitated by a type of psychosocial stress, the sever-

ity of which may or may not directly affect the individual response. Conversely, adjustment disorders are quite common, and impulse control disorders are relatively rare.

This chapter focuses on disorders that occur in response to stressful situations with which the individual cannot cope. The behavior may include:

1. Impairment in an individual's usual social and occupational functioning.
2. Compulsive acts that may be harmful to the person or others.

Historical and epidemiological statistics are presented. Predisposing factors that have been implicated in the etiology of adjustment and impulse control disorders provide a framework for studying the dynamics of these pathological conditions.

An explanation of the symptomatology is presented as background knowledge for assessing the client with an adjustment or impulse control disorder. Nursing care is described in the context of the nursing process. Various medical treatment modalities are explored.

HISTORICAL AND EPIDEMIOLOGICAL FACTORS

Historically, clients with symptoms identified by adjustment or impulse control disorders were classified as having personality disturbances. Problems with these diagnostic categories began after World War II, when, as a result of the lack of a standardized diagnostic system, psychiatrists began to experience difficulties formulating diagnoses for behaviors attributed to combat stress.

The concept of impulse disorders dates back to the 19th century and was identified by the term *instinctive monomania*. The original monomanias included alcoholism, firesetting, homicide, and kleptomania.

A number of studies have indicated that adjustment disorders are probably quite common. Sadock and Sadock (2003) report:

> Adjustment disorders are one of the most common psychiatric diagnoses for disorders of patients hospitalized for medical and surgical problems. In one study, 5 percent of people admitted to a hospital over a 3-year period were classified as having an adjustment disorder. (p. 795)

Adjustment disorder is more common in women than in men by about 2 to 1 (APA, 2000).

The *DSM-IV-TR* (APA, 2000) identifies five specific categories of impulse control disorders: intermittent explosive disorder, **kleptomania, pathological gambling, pyromania**, and **trichotillomania**. Apparently these disorders are quite rare. Various sources place the prevalence range at from less than 1 percent to 5 percent of the adult population, with kleptomania being at the higher end of the range. Intermittent explosive disorder, pathological gambling, and pyromania are more common among men, whereas kleptomania and trichotillomania are diagnosed more often in women (APA, 2000).

APPLICATION OF THE NURSING PROCESS

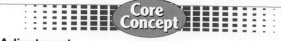

Adjustment
The process of modifying one's behavior in changed circumstances or an altered environment in order to fulfill psychological, physiological, and social needs.

Adjustment Disorders

Classifications of Adjustment Disorder: Background Assessment Data

An adjustment disorder is characterized by a maladaptive reaction to an identifiable psychosocial stressor or stressors that results in the development of clinically significant emotional or behavioral symptoms (APA, 2000). The response occurs within 3 months after onset of the stressor and persists for no longer than 6 months. An exception to the 6 months' criterion is a situation in which the symptoms occur in response to a chronic stressor, such as a chronic, disabling physical illness.

The individual shows impairment in social and occupational functioning or exhibits symptoms that are in excess of an expected reaction to the stressor. The symptoms are expected to remit soon after the stressor is relieved, or if the stressor persists, when a new level of adaptation is achieved. The *DSM-IV-TR* diagnostic criteria for adjustment disorders are presented in Table 35–1.

The stressor itself can be almost anything, but an individual's response to any particular stressor cannot be predicted. If an individual is highly predisposed or vulnerable to maladaptive response, a severe form of the

TABLE 35–1   Diagnostic Criteria for Adjustment Disorders

A. The development of emotional or behavioral symptoms in response to an identifiable stressor(s) occurring within 3 months of the onset of the stressor(s).
B. These symptoms or behaviors are clinically significant as evidenced by either of the following:
   1. Marked distress that is in excess of what would be expected from exposure to the stressor.
   2. Significant impairment in social or occupational (academic) functioning.
C. The stress-related disturbance does not meet the criteria for another specific axis I disorder and is not merely an exacerbation of a preexisting axis I or axis II disorder.
D. The symptoms do not represent bereavement.
E. Once the stressor (or its consequences) has terminated, the symptoms do not persist for more than an additional 6 months.
Specify if:
Acute: If the disturbance lasts less than 6 months.
Chronic: If the disturbance lasts for 6 months or longer.

SOURCE: American Psychiatric Association (2000), with permission.

disorder may follow what most people would consider only a mild or moderate stressor. On the other hand, a less vulnerable individual may develop only a mild form of the disorder in response to what others might consider a severe stressor.

A number of clinical presentations are associated with adjustment disorders. The following categories, identified by the *DSM-IV-TR*, are distinguished by the predominant features of the maladaptive response.

Adjustment Disorder with Anxiety

This category denotes a maladaptive response to a psychosocial stressor in which the predominant manifestation is anxiety. For example, the symptoms may reveal nervousness, worry, and jitteriness. The clinician must differentiate this diagnosis from those of anxiety disorders.

Adjustment Disorder with Depressed Mood

This category is the most commonly diagnosed adjustment disorder. The clinical presentation is one of predominant mood disturbance, although less pronounced than that of major depression. The symptoms, such as depressed mood, tearfulness, and feelings of hopelessness, exceed what is an expected or normative response to an identified psychosocial stressor.

Adjustment Disorder with Disturbance of Conduct

This category is characterized by conduct in which there is violation of the rights of others or of major age-appropriate societal norms and rules. Examples include truancy, vandalism, reckless driving, fighting, and defaulting on legal responsibilities. Differential diagnosis must be made from conduct disorder or antisocial personality disorder.

Adjustment Disorder with Mixed Disturbance of Emotions and Conduct

The predominant features of this category include emotional disturbances (e.g., anxiety or depression) as well as disturbances of conduct in which there is violation of the rights of others or of major age-appropriate societal norms and rules (e.g., truancy, vandalism, fighting).

Adjustment Disorder Unspecified

This subtype is used when the maladaptive reaction is not consistent with any of the other categories. Manifestations may include physical complaints, social withdrawal, or work or academic inhibition, without significant depressed or anxious mood (APA, 2000).

Predisposing Factors to Adjustment Disorders

Biological Theory

Chronic disorders, such as cognitive disorders or mental retardation, are thought to impair the ability of an individual to adapt to stress, causing increased vulnerability to adjustment disorder. Sadock and Sadock (2003) suggest that genetic factors also may influence individual risks for maladaptive response to stress.

Psychosocial Theories

Some proponents of psychoanalytical theory view adjustment disorder as a maladaptive response to stress that is caused by early childhood trauma, increased dependency, and retarded ego development. Other psychoanalysts put considerable weight on the constitutional factor, or birth characteristics that contribute to the manner in which individuals respond to stress. In many instances, adjustment disorder is precipitated by a specific meaningful stressor having found a point of vulnerability in an individual of otherwise adequate ego strength.

Some studies relate a predisposition to adjustment disorder to factors such as developmental stage, timing of the stressor, and available support systems. When a stressor occurs, and the individual does not have the developmental maturity, available support systems, or adequate coping strategies to adapt, normal functioning is disrupted, resulting in psychological or somatic symptoms. The disorder also may be related to a dysfunctional grieving process. The individual may remain in the denial or anger stage, with inadequate defense mechanisms to complete the grieving process.

Transactional Model of Stress/Adaptation

Why are some individuals able to confront stressful situations adaptively and even gain strength from the experience, whereas others not only fail to cope adaptively, but may even encounter psychopathological dysfunction? The transactional model of stress/adaptation takes into consideration the interaction between the individual and the environment.

The type of stressor that one experiences may influence one's adaptation. Sudden-shock stressors occur without warning, and continuous stressors are those that an individual is exposed to over an extended period. Although many studies have been directed to individuals' responses to sudden-shock stressors, it has been found that continuous stressors were more commonly cited than sudden-shock stressors as precipitants to maladaptive functioning.

Both situational and intrapersonal factors most likely contribute to an individual's stress response. Situational factors include personal and general economic conditions; occupational and recreational opportunities; the availability of social supports such as family, friends, neighbors, and cultural or religious support groups.

Intrapersonal factors such as constitutional vulnerability have also been implicated in the predisposition to adjustment disorder. Some studies have indicated that a child with a difficult temperament (defined as one who cries loudly and often; adapts to changes slowly; and has irregular patterns of hunger, sleep, and elimination) is at greater risk of developing a behavior disorder. Freud

(1964) theorized that traumatic childhood experiences created points of fixation to which the individual, during times of stress, would be likely to regress. This might also apply to other unresolved conflicts or developmental issues. Other intrapersonal factors that might influence one's ability to adjust to a painful life change include social skills, coping strategies, the presence of psychiatric illness, degree of flexibility, and level of intelligence.

The etiology of adjustment disorder is most likely influenced by multiple factors. A graphic depiction of this theory of multiple causation is presented in Figure 35–1.

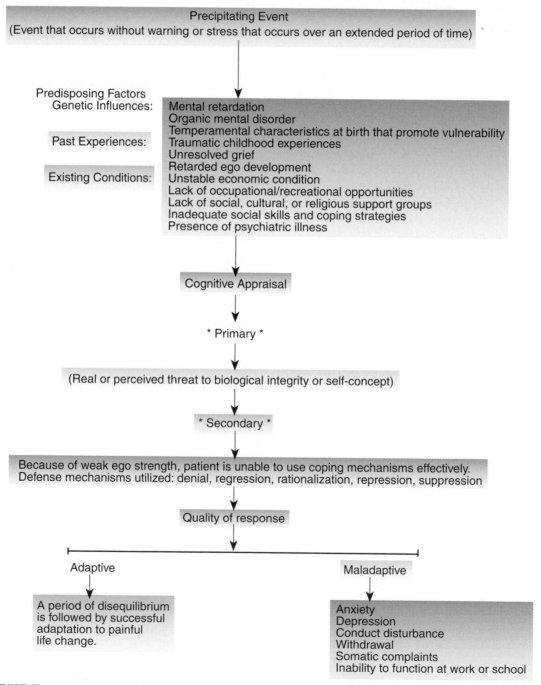

FIGURE 35–1 The dynamics of adjustment disorder using the transactional model of stress/adaptation.

Diagnosis/Outcome Identification

Nursing diagnoses are formulated from the data gathered during the assessment phase and with background knowledge regarding predisposing factors to the disorder. Nursing diagnoses may be used for the client with an adjustment disorder include:

Dysfunctional grieving related to real or perceived loss of any concept of value to the individual, evidenced by interference with life functioning, developmental regression, or somatic complaints.

Impaired adjustment related to change in health status requiring modification in lifestyle (e.g., chronic illness, physical disability), evidenced by inability to problem-solve or set realistic goals for the future.
   NOTE: According to the NANDA International definition, this diagnosis would be appropriate for the person with adjustment disorder only if the precipitating stressor was a change in health status.

The following criteria may be used for measurement of outcomes in the care of the client with an adjustment disorder.

   The client:

1. Verbalizes acceptable behaviors associated with each stage of the grief process.
2. Demonstrates a reinvestment in the environment.
3. Accomplishes activities of daily living independently.
4. Demonstrates ability for adequate occupational and social functioning.
5. Verbalizes awareness of change in health status and the effect it will have on lifestyle.
6. Solves problems and sets realistic goals for the future.
7. Demonstrates ability to cope effectively with change in lifestyle.

Planning/Implementation

Table 35–2 provides a plan of care for the client with adjustment disorder. Nursing diagnoses are presented, along with outcome criteria, appropriate nursing interventions, and rationales.

   The concept map care plan is an innovative approach to planning and organizing nursing care (see Chapter 9). It is a diagrammatic teaching and learning strategy that allows visualization of interrelationships between medical diagnoses, nursing diagnoses, assessment data, and treatments. An example of a concept map care plan for a client with an adjustment disorder is presented in Figure 35–2.

TABLE 35–2	Care Plan for the Client with Adjustment Disorder

NURSING DIAGNOSIS: DYSFUNCTIONAL GRIEVING
RELATED TO: Real or perceived loss of any concept of value to the individual
EVIDENCED BY: Interference with life functioning, developmental regression, or somatic complaints

OUTCOME CRITERIA	NURSING INTERVENTIONS	RATIONALE
Client will be able to function adequately at age-appropriate level with evidence of progression toward resolution of grief.	1. Determine stage of grief in which client is fixed. Identify behaviors associated with this stage.	1. Accurate baseline assessment data are necessary to plan effective care for the grieving client.
	2. Develop trusting relationship with the client. Show empathy and caring. Be honest and keep all promises.	2. Trust is the basis for a therapeutic relationship.
	3. Convey an accepting attitude so that the client is not afraid to express feelings openly.	3. An accepting attitude conveys to the client that you believe he or she is a worthwhile person. Trust is enhanced.
	4. Allow client to express anger. Do not become defensive if initial expression of anger is displaced on the nurse. Assist client to explore angry feelings so that they may be directed toward the intended object or person.	4. Verbalization of feelings in a non-threatening environment may help client come to terms with unresolved issues.
	5. Assist client to discharge pent-up anger through participation in large motor activities (e.g., brisk walks, jogging, volleyball, punching bag, exercise bike).	5. Physical exercise provides a safe and effective method for discharging pent-up tension.
	6. Explain to the client the normal stages of grief and the behaviors associated with each stage. Help client to understand that feelings such as guilt and anger toward the lost concept are appropriate and acceptable during the grief process.	6. Knowledge of the availability of the feelings associated with normal grieving may help to relieve some of the guilt that these responses generate.

(Continued on following page)

OUTCOME CRITERIA	NURSING INTERVENTIONS	RATIONALE
	7. Encourage client to review personal perception of the loss or change. With support and sensitivity, point out reality of the situation in areas where misrepresentations are expressed.	7. Client must give up idealized perception and be able to accept both positive and negative aspects about the painful life change before the grief process is complete.
	8. Communicate to client that crying is acceptable. Use of touch is generally therapeutic, although specific knowledge about the client is important before using it.	8. Use of touch is considered inappropriate in some cultures.
	9. Assist client in solving problems as he or she attempts to determine methods for more adaptive coping with the stressor. Provide positive feedback for strategies identified and decisions made.	9. Positive reinforcement enhances self-esteem and encourages repetition of desirable behaviors.
	10. Encourage client to reach out for spiritual support during this time in whatever form is desirable. Assess client's spiritual needs and assist as necessary in their fulfillment.	10. Spiritual support can enhance successful adaptation to painful life experiences.

NURSING DIAGNOSIS: IMPAIRED ADJUSTMENT

RELATED TO: Change in health status requiring modification in lifestyle

EVIDENCED BY: Inability to problem solve or set realistic goals for the future

OUTCOME CRITERIA	NURSING INTERVENTIONS	RATIONALE
Client will willingly demonstrate competence to function independently to his or her optimal level of ability, considering change in health status.	1. Encourage client to talk about lifestyle prior to the change in health status. Discuss coping mechanisms that were used at stressful times in the past.	1. Identify the client's strengths so that they may be used to facilitate adaptation to the change in health status.
	2. Encourage client to discuss the health change and particularly to express anger associated with it.	2. Anger is a normal stage in the grieving process and if not released in an appropriate manner, may be turned inward on the self, leading to pathological depression.
	3. Encourage client to express fears associated with the change or alteration in lifestyle that the change has created.	3. Change often creates a feeling of disequilibrium, and the individual may respond with fears that are irrational or unfounded. He or she may benefit from feedback that corrects misperceptions about how life will be with the change in health status.
	4. Provide assistance with activities of daily living as required, but encourage independence to the limit that client's ability will allow. Give positive feedback for activities accomplished independently.	4. Independent accomplishments and positive feedback enhance self-esteem and encourage repetition of desired behaviors. Successes also provide hope that adaptive functioning is possible and decrease feelings of powerlessness.
	5. Help client with decision making regarding incorporation of change into lifestyle. Identify problems the change is likely to create. Discuss alternative solutions, weighing potential benefits and consequences of each alternative. Support client's decision in the selection of an alternative.	5. The high degree of anxiety that usually accompanies a major lifestyle change often interferes with an individual's ability to solve problems and to make appropriate decisions. Client may need assistance with this process in an effort to progress toward successful adaptation.
	6. Use role-play to practice stressful situations that might occur in relation to the health status change.	6. This type of anticipatory guidance arms the client with a measure of security and serves to decrease anxiety.
	7. Ensure that client and family are fully knowledgeable regarding the physiology of the change in health status and its necessity for optimal wellness. Encourage them to ask questions, and provide printed material explaining the change to which they may refer. Ensure that client can identify resources within the community from which he or she may seek assistance in adapting to the change in health status.	7. Increased knowledge enhances successful adaptation.

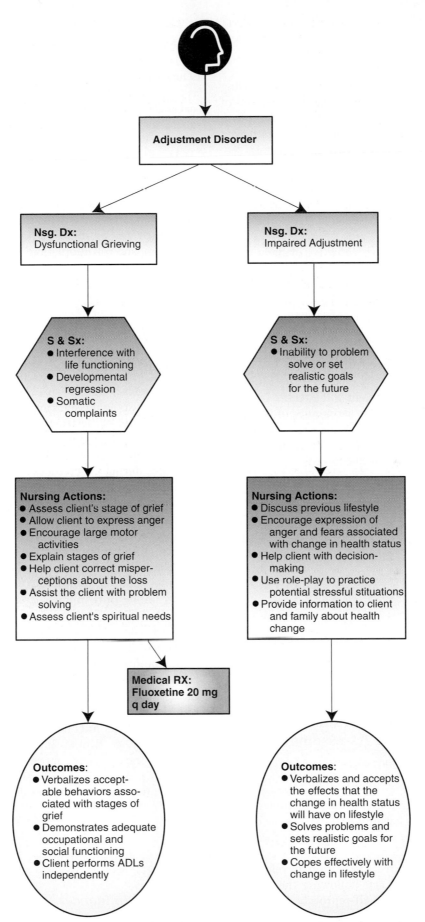

FIGURE 35–2 Concept map care plan for client with adjustment disorder.

Evaluation

Reassessment is conducted to determine if the nursing actions have been successful in achieving the objectives of care. Evaluation of the nursing actions for the client with adjustment disorder may be facilitated by gathering information using the following types of questions:

1. Does the client verbalize understanding of the grief process and his or her position in the process?
2. Does the client recognize his or her adaptive and maladaptive behaviors associated with the grief response?
3. Can the client accomplish activities of daily living independently?
4. If assistance is required, can he or she verbalize resources from whom help may be sought?
5. Does the client demonstrate evidence of progression along the grief response?
6. Does the client demonstrate the ability to perform occupational and social activities adequately?
7. Does the client discuss the change in health status and modification of lifestyle it will effect?
8. Does the client demonstrate acceptance of the modification?
9. Can the client participate in decision making and problem solving for his or her future?
10. Does the client set realistic goals for the future?
11. Does the client demonstrate new adaptive coping strategies for dealing with the change in lifestyle?
12. Can the client verbalize available resources to whom he or she may go for support or assistance should it be necessary?

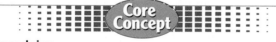

Core Concept

Impulsive
The urge or inclination to act without consideration to the possible consequences of one's behavior.

Impulse Control Disorders

Classifications of Impulse Control Disorders: Background Assessment Data

The *DSM-IV-TR* (APA, 2000) describes the essential features of impulse control disorders as follows:

1. Failure to resist an impulse, drive, or temptation to perform an act that is harmful to the person or others.
2. An increasing sense of tension or arousal before committing the act.
3. An experience of pleasure, gratification, or relief at the time of committing the act. Following the act there may or may not be regret, self-reproach, or guilt.

Individuals who suffer from impulse control disorders follow their impulses to behave in a certain manner without regard to the consequences of their behavior. They seldom know why they do what they do or why it is pleasurable. These behaviors have been likened to sexual excitement and orgasmic release. Some authors have noted that many of the behaviors have adverse or even destructive consequences for the person.

Many people with impulse control disorders function fairly well in other areas of their lives. They are merely unable to contain their behavior in the moment when tension builds, and immediate gratification prevails. Some researchers have associated other behaviors, such as substance abuse, obsessive–compulsive behaviors, and self-mutilation, with disorders of impulse control.

A description of the five categories of impulse control disorders identified by the *DSM-IV-TR* (APA, 2000) follows.

Intermittent Explosive Disorder

This disorder is characterized by discrete episodes of failure to resist aggressive impulses resulting in serious assaultive acts or destruction of property (APA, 2000). The individual is not normally an aggressive person between episodes, and the degree of aggressiveness expressed during the episodes is grossly out of proportion to any precipitating psychosocial stressor.

The symptoms appear suddenly, without any apparent provocation, and the violence is usually the result of an irresistible impulse to lash out. Some clients report sensorium changes, such as confusion during episodes or amnesia for events that occurred during episodes (Sadock & Sadock, 2003). Symptoms terminate abruptly, commonly lasting only minutes or at most a few hours, and are followed by feelings of genuine remorse and self-reproach about the inability to control and the consequences of the aggressive behavior.

Symptoms of the disorder most often begin in adolescence or young adulthood and gradually disappear as the individual approaches middle age. Clients often have histories of learning disabilities, hyperkinesis, and proneness to accidents in childhood (Sadock & Sadock, 2003; Scott, Hilty, & Brook, 2003). The disorder, which is relatively rare, occurs more often in males than in females (APA, 2000). The *DSM-IV-TR* diagnostic criteria for intermittent explosive disorder are presented in Table 35–3.

Predisposing Factors to Intermittent Explosive Disorder

Biological Influences

1. **Genetic.** Some studies have suggested that the disorder is more common in first-degree biological relatives

TABLE 35–3 Diagnostic Criteria for Intermittent Explosive Disorder
A. Several discrete episodes of failure to resist aggressive impulses that result in serious assaultive acts or destruction of property.
B. The degree of aggressiveness expressed during the episodes is grossly out of proportion to any precipitating psychosocial stressors.
C. The aggressive episodes are not better accounted for by another mental disorder (e.g., antisocial personality disorder, borderline personality disorder, a psychotic disorder, a manic episode, conduct disorder, or attention-deficit/hyperactivity disorder) and are not due to the direct physiological effects of a substance (e.g., a drug of abuse, a medication) or a general medical condition (e.g., head trauma, Alzheimer's disease).

SOURCE: American Psychiatric Association (2000), with permission.

of people with the disorder than in the general population.

2. **Physiological**. Any central nervous system insult may predispose an individual to the syndrome. Predisposing factors in childhood are thought to include perinatal trauma, infantile seizures, head trauma, encephalitis, minimal brain dysfunction, and hyperactivity (Sadock & Sadock, 2003). Strain and Newcorn (2003) report:

Patients with episodic violent behavior frequently have abnormal neurological examination results (65%), abnormal neuropsychological test results (58%), [and] abnormal electroencephalogram (EEG) results (55%). (p. 783)

Psychosocial Influences

1. **Family Dynamics**. Individuals with intermittent explosive disorder often have strong identifications with assaultive parental figures. The typical history includes a chaotic and violent early family milieu with heavy drinking by one or both parents, parental hostility, child abuse, threats to life, and the emotional or physical unavailability of a father figure. The individual often has childhood memories of parental inconsistencies and unpredictability.

Kleptomania

The *DSM-IV-TR* describes kleptomania as "the recurrent failure to resist impulses to steal items even though the items are not needed for personal use or for their monetary value." The stolen items are either given away, discarded, returned surreptitiously, or kept and hidden (Sadock & Sadock, 2003). The individual usually has enough money to pay for the stolen objects.

The individual with kleptomania steals purely for the sake of stealing and for the sense of relief and gratification that follows an episode. The impulsive stealing is in response to increasing tension, and even though the

individual almost always knows that the act is wrong, he or she cannot resist the force of mounting tension and the pursuit of pleasure and relief that follows. Seldom is attention given to the possibility or consequences of being apprehended.

The individual, who usually steals without assistance or collaboration from others, may feel shame or remorse following the incident. Others never experience guilt or regret for their behavior. Symptoms of depression and anxiety have been associated with the disorder.

Onset of the disorder is usually in adolescence. It tends to be chronic, with periods of waxing and waning throughout the course of the disorder. The condition is rare but is thought to be more common among women than men. Fewer than 5 percent of arrested shoplifters give a history that is consistent with kleptomania (APA, 2000).

The *DSM-IV-TR* diagnostic criteria for kleptomania are presented in Table 35–4.

Predisposing Factors to Kleptomania

Biological Influences

As with other disorders of impulse control, brain disease and mental retardation have been associated with kleptomania (Sadock & Sadock, 2003). Disinhibition and poor impulse control have been linked with cortical atrophy in the frontal region and enlargement of the lateral ventricles of the brain.

Psychosocial Influences

Cupchick (2002), a Toronto psychologist who has studied and treated theft offenders for almost 30 years, states that most individuals who steal compulsively do so in response to some personal crisis. He states, "Most often what we found is that these people had experienced some unfair, personally devastating loss, and they responded by causing someone else an unfair loss—like a retail store." In the results of two separate studies, he found that almost 75 percent of the cases could be linked to a

TABLE 35–4 Diagnostic Criteria for Kleptomania
A. Recurrent failure to resist impulses to steal objects not needed for personal use or for their monetary value.
B. Increasing sense of tension immediately before committing the theft.
C. Pleasure, gratification, or relief at the time of committing the theft.
D. The stealing is not committed to express anger or vengeance and is not in response to a delusion or a hallucination.
E. The stealing is not better accounted for by conduct disorder, a manic episode, or antisocial personality disorder.

SOURCE: American Psychiatric Association (2000), with permission.

personal crisis, such as a life-threatening diagnosis or the death of a loved one.

Pathological Gambling

This disorder is defined by the *DSM-IV-TR* as persistent and recurrent maladaptive gambling behavior (APA, 2000). The preoccupation with and impulse to gamble intensifies when the individual is under stress. Many impulsive gamblers describe a physical sensation of restlessness and anticipation that can be relieved only by placing a bet. Blume (2002) states:

> In some cases the initial change in gambling behavior leading to pathological gambling begins with a "big win," bringing a rapid development of preoccupation, tolerance, and loss of control. Winning brings feelings of special status, power, and omnipotence. The gambler increasingly depends on this activity to cope with disappointments, problems, and negative emotional states, pulling away from emotional attachment to family and friends.

As the need to gamble increases, the individual is forced to obtain money by any means available. This may include borrowing money from illegal sources or pawning personal items (or items that belong to others). As gambling debts accrue, or out of a need to continue gambling, the individual may desperately resort to forgery, theft, or even embezzlement. Family relationships are disrupted, and impairment in occupational functioning may occur because of absences from work in order to gamble.

Gambling behavior usually begins in adolescence; however, compulsive behaviors rarely occur before young adulthood. The disorder generally runs a chronic course, with periods of waxing and waning, largely dependent on periods of psychosocial stress. Lifetime prevalence rates of pathological gambling range from 0.4 to 3.4 percent in adults and 2.8 to 8 percent among adolescents and college students (APA, 2000). It is more common among men than women.

Various personality traits have been attributed to pathological gamblers. Unwin, Davis, and Leeuw (2000) state:

> Evidence points to the common existence of narcissistic personality characteristics and impulse control problems in pathologic gamblers. High rates of personality disorders (e.g., obsessive-compulsive, avoidant, schizotypal and paranoid) are noted in several studies. Personality profiles of persons who are alcoholics and pathologic gamblers are also similar in some studies. Some experts view pathologic gambling as an addictive disorder, citing as evidence the tolerance and withdrawal symptoms exhibited by pathologic gamblers because of debt escalation behaviors. However, no physical or biochemical markers exist to help physicians make the diagnosis.

The *DSM-IV-TR* diagnostic criteria for pathological gambling are presented in Table 35–5.

TABLE 35–5 Diagnostic Criteria for Pathological Gambling

A. Persistent and recurrent maladaptive gambling behavior as indicated by five (or more) of the following:
  1. Is preoccupied with gambling (e.g., preoccupied with reliving past gambling experiences, handicapping or planning the next venture, or thinking of ways to get money with which to gamble).
  2. Needs to gamble with increasing amounts of money in order to achieve the desired excitement.
  3. Has repeated unsuccessful efforts to control, cut back, or stop gambling.
  4. Is restless or irritable when attempting to cut down or stop gambling.
  5. Gambles as a way of escaping from problems or of relieving a dysphoric mood (e.g., feelings of helplessness, guilt, anxiety, depression).
  6. After losing money gambling, often returns another day to get even ("chasing" one's losses).
  7. Lies to family members, therapist, or others to conceal the extent of involvement with gambling.
  8. Has committed illegal acts such as forgery, fraud, theft, or embezzlement to finance gambling.
  9. Has jeopardized or lost a significant relationship, job, or educational or career opportunity because of gambling.
  10. Relies on others to provide money to relieve a desperate financial situation caused by gambling.
B. The gambling behavior is not better accounted for by a manic episode.

SOURCE: American Psychiatric Association (2000), with permission.

Predisposing Factors to Pathological Gambling

Biological Influences

1. **Genetic.** The fathers of men with the disorder and the mothers of women with the disorder are more likely to have the disorder than is the population at large (Sadock & Sadock, 2003). The *DSM-IV-TR* reports that both pathological gambling and alcohol dependence are more common among the parents of individuals of pathological gambling than in the general population (APA, 2000).
2. **Physiological.** Moreyra and associates (2000) suggest that links may exist between pathological gambling and abnormalities in the serotonergic and noradrenergic receptor systems. Studies have also suggested a possible connection to dysfunction in the dopaminergic system. Other studies have indicated alterations in the ectroencephalographic patterns of pathologic gamblers (Regard et al., 2003).

Psychosocial Influences

Sadock and Sadock (2003) report that the following may be predisposing factors to the development of pathological gambling: loss of a parent by death, separation, divorce, or desertion before the child is 15 years of age; inappropriate parental discipline (absence, inconsistency, or harshness); exposure to and availability of gambling activities for the adolescent; a family emphasis on material and financial symbols; and a lack of family emphasis on saving, planning, and budgeting.

The early psychoanalytical view attempted to explain compulsive gambling in terms of psychosexual maturation. In this theory, the gambling is compared to masturbation; both of these activities derive motive force from a build-up of tension that is released through repetitive actions or the anticipation of them. Another view suggests a masochistic component to pathological gambling and the gambler's inherent need for punishment, which is then achieved through losing (Moreyra et al., 2000).

Pyromania

Pyromania is the inability to resist the impulse to set fires. The act of starting the fire is preceded by tension or affective arousal. The individual experiences intense pleasure, gratification, or relief when setting the fires, witnessing their effects, or participating in their aftermath (APA, 2000). The sole motive for setting the fire is self-gratification, not revenge, insurance collection, or sabotage. They may take precautions to avoid apprehension; however, many individuals with pyromania are totally indifferent to the consequences of their behavior.

The onset of symptoms is usually in childhood. Many individuals with pyromania report early fascination with fire and excitement associated with firefighting equipment and activities. The disorder is relatively rare and is much more common in men than in women. Features associated with pyromania include low intelligence, learning disabilities, alcoholism, psychosexual dysfunction, chronic personal frustrations, resentment of authority figures, and the occurrence of sexual arousal secondary to fires (Sadock & Sadock, 2003).

The *DSM-IV-TR* diagnostic criteria for pyromania are presented in Table 35–6.

TABLE 35–6	**Diagnostic Criteria for Pyromania**

A. Deliberate and purposeful fire setting on more than one occasion.
B. Tension or affective arousal before the act.
C. Fascination with, interest in, curiosity about, or attraction to fire and its situational contexts (e.g., paraphernalia, uses, consequences).
D. Pleasure, gratification, or relief when setting fires, or when witnessing or participating in their aftermath.
E. The fire setting is not done for monetary gain, as an expression of sociopolitical ideology, to conceal criminal activity, to express anger or vengeance, to improve one's living circumstances, in response to a delusion or hallucination, or as a result of impaired judgment (e.g., in dementia, mental retardation, substance intoxication).
F. The fire setting is not better accounted for by conduct disorder, a manic episode, or antisocial personality disorder.

SOURCE: American Psychiatric Association (2000), with permission.

Predisposing Factors to Pyromania

Biological Influences

Mild mental retardation and learning disabilities have been associated with firesetting. A biochemical influence has been suggested based on evidence of significantly low cerebrospinal fluid levels of 5-hydroxyindole acetic acid (5-HIAA) and 3-methoxy-4-hydroxyphenylglycol (MHPG) found in a study of individuals with pyromania (Scott, Hilty, & Brook, 2003). The same study showed a possible hypoglycemic tendency in these individuals.

Psychosocial Influences

Three major psychoanalytical issues that have been associated with impulsive firesetting include: (1) an association between firesetting and sexual gratification, (2) a feeling of impotence and powerlessness, and (3) poor social skills. This is consistent with Freud's (1964) view of fire as a symbol of sexuality. He suggested that the warmth radiated by fire can be compared to the sensation that accompanies a state of sexual excitation. Several authors have described clients who have masturbated after setting fires and describe the gratification they experience as "orgasmic." Other psychoanalytical writers have suggested that fire may symbolize activities deriving from various levels of libidinal and aggressive development. They view the act of firesetting as a means of relieving accumulated rage over the frustration caused by a sense of social, physical, and sexual inferiority (Sadock & Sadock, 2003).

Trichotillomania

The *DSM-IV-TR* defines this disorder as the recurrent pulling out of one's own hair that results in noticeable hair loss (APA, 2000). The impulse is preceded by an increasing sense of tension and results in a sense of release or gratification from pulling out the hair. The most common sites for hair pulling are the scalp, eyebrows, and eyelashes but may occur in any area of the body on which hair grows. These areas of hair loss are more likely found on the opposite side of the body from the dominant hand (Scott, Hilty, & Brook, 2003). Pain is seldom reported to accompany the hairpulling, although tingling and pruritus in the area are not uncommon.

The disorder usually begins in childhood and may be accompanied by nail biting, head banging, scratching, biting, or other acts of self-mutilation. This relatively rare phenomenon occurs more often in women than in men.

The *DSM-IV-TR* diagnostic criteria for trichotillomania are presented in Table 35–7.

TABLE 35–7   Diagnostic Criteria for Trichotillomania

A. Recurrent pulling out of one's hair resulting in noticeable hair loss.
B. An increasing sense of tension immediately before pulling out the hair or when attempting to resist the behavior.
C. Pleasure, gratification, or relief when pulling out the hair.
D. The disturbance is not better accounted for by another mental disorder and is not due to a general medical condition (e.g., a dermatological condition).
E. The disturbance causes clinically significant distress or impairment in social, occupational, or other important areas of functioning.

SOURCE: American Psychiatric Association (2000), with permission.

Predisposing Factors to Trichotillomania

Biological Influences

Trichotillomania may be present as a major symptom in mental retardation, obsessive–compulsive disorder, schizophrenia, borderline personality disorder, and depression (Scott, Hilty, & Brook, 2003). Sadock and Sadock (2003) state:

Trichotillomania is increasingly being viewed as having a biologically determined substrate that may reflect inappropriately released motor activity or excessive grooming behaviors. (p. 790)

Psychosocial Influences

The onset of trichotillomania can be related to stressful situations in more than one quarter of cases. Additional factors that have been implicated include disturbances in mother–child relationships, fear of abandonment, and recent object loss. Studies also have shown a possible correlation between trichotillomania and a history of childhood abuse (e.g., physical, emotional, or sexual) or emotional neglect (Lochner et al., 2002).

Transactional Model of Stress/Adaptation

The etiology of impulse control disorders is most likely influenced by multiple factors. In Figure 35–3 a graphic depiction of this theory of multiple causation is presented in the transactional model of stress/adaptation.

Diagnosis/Outcome Identification

Nursing diagnoses are formulated from the data gathered during the assessment phase and with background knowledge regarding predisposing factors to the disorder. The following nursing diagnoses may be used for the client with impulse control disorder:

Risk for other-directed violence related to dysfunctional family system; possible genetic or physiological influ-

ences evidenced by episodes of violent, aggressive, or assaultive behavior.

Ineffective coping related to possible hereditary factors, physiological alterations, dysfunctional family, or unresolved developmental issues evidenced by inability to control impulse to gamble, steal, set fires, or pull out own hair.

The following criteria may be used for measurement of outcomes in the care of the client with impulse control disorder.

The client:

1. Has not caused harm to self or others.
2. Is able to inhibit the impulse for violence and aggression.
3. Verbalizes the symptoms of increasing tension.
4. Verbalizes strategies to avoid becoming violent.
5. Verbalizes actual object at which anger is directed.
6. Continues to work on increasing frustration tolerance.
7. Verbalizes more adaptive strategies for coping with stressful situations.
8. Demonstrates the ability to delay gratification.
9. Verbalizes understanding that behavior is unacceptable and accepts responsibility for own behavior.

Planning/Implementation

Table 35–8 provides a plan of care for the client with an impulse control disorder. Nursing diagnoses are presented, along with outcome criteria, appropriate nursing interventions, and rationales.

Evaluation

Reassessment is conducted in order to determine if the nursing actions have been successful in achieving the objectives of care. Evaluation of the nursing actions for the client with an impulse control disorder may be facilitated by gathering information using the following types of questions:

1. Has violence, aggression, or assaultive behavior been avoided?
2. Have the client and others escaped harm?
3. Does the client verbalize understanding of the unacceptability of his or her behavior?
4. Can the client verbalize and demonstrate more adaptive strategies for coping with stress?
5. Can the client demonstrate the ability to delay gratification?
6. Can the client verbalize the symptoms of tension that precede unacceptable behavior?
7. Can the client demonstrate ways to intervene that inhibit the compulsion for maladaptive behavior when tension rises?

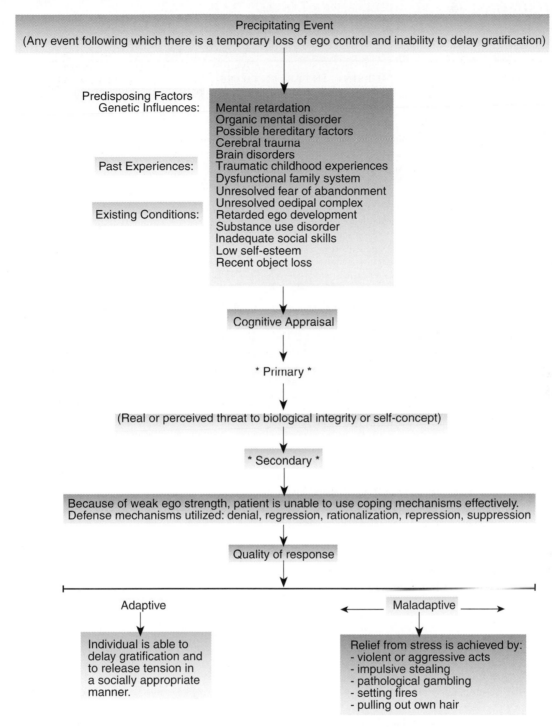

FIGURE 35–3 The dynamics of impulse control disorders using the transactional model of stress/adaptation.

8. Can the client verbalize the types of stress that create the tension?
9. Can the client verbalize a plan to deal with the stress in the future without resorting to behaviors that are socially unacceptable?

Table 35–9 provides topics for client and family education related to adjustment and impulse control disorders.

TREATMENT MODALITIES

Adjustment Disorders

Various treatments are used for clients with adjustment disorder. Strain and Newcorn (2003) cite the following as major goals of therapy for these individuals:

TABLE 35–8	Care Plan for the Client with an Impulse Control Disorder

NURSING DIAGNOSIS: RISK FOR OTHER-DIRECTED VIOLENCE

RELATED TO: Dysfunctional family system; possible genetic or physiological influences

EVIDENCED BY: Episodes of violent, aggressive, or assaultive behavior

OUTCOME CRITERIA	NURSING INTERVENTIONS	RATIONALE
Client will not harm others or the property of others.	1. Convey an accepting attitude toward this client. Feelings of rejection are undoubtedly familiar to him or her. Work on development of trust. Be honest, keep all promises, and convey the message that it is not him or her but the behavior that is unacceptable.	1. An attitude of acceptance promotes feelings of self-worth. Trust is the basis of a therapeutic relationship.
	2. Maintain low level of stimuli in client's environment (low lighting, few people, simple decor, low noise level).	2. A stimulating environment may increase agitation and promote aggressive behavior.
	3. Remove all potentially dangerous objects from the client's environment. Help client identify the true object of his or her hostility.	3. Client safety is a nursing priority. Because of weak ego development, client may be unable to use ego defense mechanisms correctly. Helping him or her recognize this in a non-threatening manner may help reveal unresolved issues so that they may be confronted.
	4. Staff should maintain and convey a calm attitude.	4. Anxiety is contagious and can be transferred from staff to client. A calm attitude provides client with a feeling of safety and security.
	5. Help client recognize the signs that tension is increasing and ways in which violence can be averted.	5. Activities that require physical exertion are helpful in relieving pent-up tension.
	6. Explain to client that should explosive behavior occur, staff will intervene in whatever way is required (e.g., tranquilizing medication, restraints, isolation) to protect client and others.	6. This conveys to the client evidence of control over the situation and provides a feeling of safety and security.

NURSING DIAGNOSIS: INEFFECTIVE COPING

RELATED TO: Possible hereditary factors, physiological alterations, dysfunctional family, or unresolved developmental issues

EVIDENCED BY: Inability to control impulse to gamble, steal, set fires, or pull out own hair

OUTCOME CRITERIA	NURSING INTERVENTIONS	RATIONALE
Client will be able to delay gratification and use adaptive coping strategies in response to stress.	1. Help client gain insight into his or her own behaviors. Often these individuals rationalize to such an extent that they deny that what they have done is wrong.	1. Client must come to understand that certain behaviors will not be tolerated within the society and that severe consequences will be imposed upon those individuals who refuse to comply. Client must *want* to become a productive member of society before he or she can be helped.
	2. Talk about past behaviors with client. Discuss behaviors that are acceptable by societal norms and those that are not. Help client identify ways in which he or she has exploited others. Encourage client to explore how he or she would feel if the circumstances were reversed.	2. An attempt may be made to enlighten the client to the sensitivity of others by promoting self-awareness in an effort to assist the client to gain insight into his or her own behavior.

(Continued on opposite page)

OUTCOME CRITERIA	NURSING INTERVENTIONS	RATIONALE
	3. Throughout relationship with client, maintain attitude of "It is not you, but your behavior, that is unacceptable."	3. An attitude of acceptance promotes feelings of dignity and self-worth.
	4. Work with client to increase the ability to delay gratification. Reward desirable behaviors and provide immediate positive feedback.	4. Rewards and positive feedback enhance self-esteem and encourage repetition of desirable behaviors.
	5. Help client identify and practice more adaptive strategies for coping with stressful life situations.	5. The impulse to perform the maladaptive behavior may be so great that the client is unable to see any other alternatives to relieve stress.

TABLE 35–9 Topics for Client/Family Education Related to Adjustment and Impulse Control Disorders

Nature of the Illness
1. Define adjustment disorder.
2. Describe types and symptoms of adjustment disorder.
3. Describe types and symptoms of impulse control disorders.
4. Discuss possible causes of the disorders.

Management of the Illness
1. Adjustment disorder
   a. Discuss possible need for lifestyle changes.
   b. Discuss ways to identify onset of escalating anxiety.
   c. Discuss problem-solving techniques.
   d. Teach assertive and relaxation techniques.
   e. Ways to increase feelings of control and decrease feelings of powerlessness.
   f. Pharmacology: Antianxiety agents and antidepressants. If these medications are given for associated symptoms, teach client about what to expect and possible adverse effects that may occur.
2. Impulse control disorder
   a. Discuss ways to identify onset of escalating anxiety and methods to prevent maladaptive responses.
   b. Discuss alternative adaptive coping strategies.
   c. Teach assertive and relaxation techniques.
   d. Teach ways to increase feelings of control and decrease feelings of powerlessness.
   e. Pharmacology. The following drugs may be prescribed for impulse control disorders. Ensure that client and family have sufficient knowledge about the medication prior to its administration.
      (1) Intermittent explosive disorder: lithium, anticonvulsants, serotonin-modulating drugs, beta blockers, antipsychotics
      (2) Kleptomania: SSRIs, tricyclic antidepressants, trazodone, lithium, valproate, and naltrexone
      (3) Pathological gambling: clomipramine, SSRIs, lithium, carbamazepine, and naltrexone
      (4) Trichotillomania: chlorpromazine, amitriptyline, lithium, SSRIs/pimozide

Support Services
1. Support groups:
   Gamblers Anonymous
   P.O. Box 17173
   Los Angeles, CA 90017
   (213) 386–8789
   www.gamblersanonymous.org

   National Council on
   Problem Gambling
   208 G Street, N.E.
   Washington, D.C. 20002
   1–800–522–4700
   www.npcgambling.org
2. Individual psychotherapy
3. Crisis intervention
4. Behavior therapy
5. Family therapy

1. To relieve symptoms associated with a stressor
2. To enhance coping with stressors that cannot be reduced or removed
3. To establish support systems that maximize adaptation

Individual Psychotherapy

Individual psychotherapy is the most common treatment for adjustment disorder. Individual psychotherapy allows the client to examine the stressor that is causing the problem, possibly assign personal meaning to the stressor, and confront unresolved issues that may be exacerbating this crisis. Treatment works to remove these blocks to adaptation so that normal developmental progression can resume. Techniques are used to clarify links between the current stressor and past experiences, and to assist with the development of more adaptive coping strategies.

Family Therapy

The focus of treatment is shifted from the individual to the system of relationships in which the individual is involved. The maladaptive response of the identified client is viewed as symptomatic of a dysfunctional family system. All family members are included in the therapy, and treatment serves to improve the functioning within the family network. Emphasis is placed on communication, family rules, and interaction patterns among the family members.

Behavioral Therapy

The goal of behavioral therapy is to replace ineffective response patterns with more adaptive ones. The situations that promote ineffective responses are identified, and carefully designed reinforcement schedules, along with role modeling and coaching, are used to alter the maladaptive response patterns. This type of treatment is very effective when implemented in an inpatient setting where the client's behavior and its consequences may be more readily controlled.

Self-Help Groups

Group experiences with or without a professional facilitator provide an arena in which members may consider and compare their responses to individuals with similar life experiences. Members benefit from learning that they are not alone in their painful experiences. Hope is derived from knowing that others have survived and even grown from similar experiences. Members of the group exchange advice, share coping strategies, and provide support and encouragement for each other.

Crisis Intervention

In crisis intervention the therapist, or other intervener, becomes a part of the individual's life situation. Because of increased anxiety, the individual is unable to problem solve, so he or she requires guidance and support from another to help mobilize the resources needed to resolve the crisis. Crisis intervention is short term and relies heavily on orderly problem-solving techniques and structured activities that are focused on change. The ultimate goal of crisis intervention in the treatment of adjustment disorder is to resolve the immediate crisis, restore adaptive functioning, and promote personal growth.

Psychopharmacology

Adjustment disorder is not commonly treated with medications, for the following reasons: (1) their effect may be temporary and only mask the real problem, interfering with the possibility of finding a more permanent solution and (2) psychoactive drugs carry the potential for physiological and psychological dependence.

When the client with adjustment disorder has symptoms of anxiety or depression, the physician may prescribe antianxiety or antidepressant medication. These medications are considered only adjuncts to psychotherapy and should not be given as the primary therapy. In these instances they are given to alleviate symptoms so that the individual may more effectively cope while attempting to adapt to the stressful situation.

Impulse Control Disorders

Intermittent Explosive Disorder

Individual psychotherapy with intermittent explosive disorder has not been successful. Group therapy, with its elements of group loyalty, peer pressure, expectation, and

confrontation, may be more useful. Family therapy may be helpful when the client is an adolescent or young adult (Sadock & Sadock, 2003).

Clients with intermittent explosive disorder are commonly treated with psychopharmacological agents. A variety of agents have been tried, including mood stabilizers (e.g., lithium), anticonvulsants (e.g., carbamazepine, gabapentin, phenytoin, valproate), serotonin-modulating drugs (e.g., selective serotonin reuptake inhibitors [SSRIs], buspirone, clomipramine, trazodone), and beta-blockers (e.g., propranolol) (Scott, Hilty, & Brook, 2003). Although antipsychotics have been used in the past for aggressive behavior, this practice has been reevaluated because of adverse side effects. The newer atypical antipsychotics, with a more acceptable side effect profile, may prove to be a better choice.

Kleptomania

Insight-oriented psychodynamic psychotherapy has been successful in the treatment of kleptomania. It has been most helpful with those individuals who experience guilt and shame and are thus motivated to change their behavior.

Sadock and Sadock (2003) report the following behavioral therapy methods as useful in the treatment of kleptomania: systematic desensitization, aversive conditioning, and a combination of aversive conditioning and altered social contingencies.

Success in the treatment of kleptomania has been achieved with some medications, including the SSRIs, tricyclic antidepressants, trazodone, lithium, and valproate. One recent study reported effective results in the treatment of kleptomania with naltrexone (Grant & Kim, 2002). The authors state:

> As the treatment progressed, many patients expressed that their struggle to resist the urges to steal and thoughts associated with stealing were reduced or abolished altogether. In addition to reducing urges, naltrexone seemed to reduce the subjective experience of pleasure if they engaged in stealing. (p. 355)

Electroconvulsive therapy has also shown to be effective in some cases.

Pathological Gambling

Because most pathological gamblers deny that they have a problem, treatment is difficult. In fact, most gamblers seek treatment only because of legal difficulties, family pressures, or other psychiatric complaints. Behavioral therapy, cognitive therapy, and psychoanalysis have been used with pathological gambling, with various degrees of success (Moreyra et al., 2000).

Some medications have been used with effective results in the treatment of pathological gambling. The SSRIs and clomipramine have been used successfully in the treatment of pathological gambling as a form of obsessive–compulsive disorder (Moreyra et al., 2000). Lithium, carbamazepine, and naltrexone have also been shown to be effective.

Possibly the most effective treatment of pathological gambling is participation by the individual in **Gamblers Anonymous** (GA). This organization of inspirational group therapy is modeled after Alcoholics Anonymous. The only requirement for GA membership is an expressed desire to stop gambling. Treatment is based on peer pressure, public confession, and the availability of other reformed gamblers to help individuals resist the urge to gamble. Gam-Anon (for family and spouses of compulsive gamblers) and Gam-a-Teen (for adolescent children of compulsive gamblers) are also important sources of treatment.

Pyromania

Treatment of individuals with pyromania has been difficult because of the lack of motivation for change. Denial of problems, refusal to take responsibility for their behavior, and often the existence of alcoholism interfere with improvement in this disorder. Sadock and Sadock (2003) state, "Incarceration may be the only method of preventing a recurrence. Behavior therapy can then be administered in the institution."

Trichotillomania

Behavior modification has been used to treat trichotillomania. Various techniques have been tried, including covert desensitization and habit-reversal practices. These include a system of rewards and punishment that are applied in an effort to modify the hair-pulling behaviors.

Psychodynamic intervention has been used in children with trichotillomania. Exploration is conducted into areas of parent–child relationships or other areas of potential conflict that may provide some enlightenment about the problem.

Various psychopharmacological agents, including chlorpromazine, amitriptyline, and lithium carbonate, have been tried in the treatment of trichotillomania, with moderate results. Recent success with SSRIs augmented with pimozide has been reported.

SUMMARY

This chapter has focused on disorders that occur in response to stressful situations with which the individual cannot cope. The behavior may include:

1. Impairment in an individual's usual social and occupational functioning.
2. Compulsive acts that may be harmful to the person or others.

Adjustment disorders are relatively common. In fact, some studies indicate it is the most commonly ascribed psychiatric diagnosis. Clinical symptoms include inability to function socially or occupationally in response to a psychosocial stressor. The disorder is distinguished by the predominant features of the maladaptive response. These include anxiety, depression, disturbance of conduct, and mixed disturbance of emotions and conduct.

Of the two types of stressors discussed (i.e., sudden-shock and continuous), more individuals respond with maladaptive behaviors to long-term continuous stressors. Treatment modalities for adjustment disorders include individual psychotherapy, family therapy, behavior therapy, self-help groups, and psychopharmacology.

Impulse control disorders are quite rare but involve compulsive acts that may be harmful to the individual or to others. Individuals with impulse control disorders experience increased tension, followed by the inability to resist committing a specific act, after which the individual feels a sense of release and gratification.

Impulse control disorders include:

1. **Intermittent Explosive Disorder:** violent or aggressive behavior that culminates in serious assaultive acts or the destruction of property.
2. **Kleptomania:** inability to resist the impulse to steal.
3. **Pathological Gambling:** inability to resist the impulse to gamble.
4. **Pyromania:** inability to resist the impulse to set fires.
5. **Trichotillomania:** inability to resist the impulse to pull out one's own hair.

Nursing care of individuals with adjustment and impulse control disorders is accomplished using the steps of the nursing process. Background assessment data were presented, along with nursing diagnoses common to each disorder. Interventions appropriate to each nursing diagnosis and relevant outcome criteria for each were included. An overview of current medical treatment modalities was discussed.

INTERNET REFERENCES

Additional information about adjustment disorder may be located at the following Web sites:

- http://www.mentalhealth.com/rx/p23-aj01.html
- http://www.findarticles.com/cf_dls/g2601/0000/2601000025/p1/article.jhtml
- http://www.athealth.com/Consumer/disorders/Adjustment.html
- http://www.mentalhealth.com/dis/p20-aj01.html

Additional information about impulse control disorders may be located at the following Web sites:

- http://www.ncpgambling.org/
- http://www.gamblersanonymous.org/
- http://www.crescentlife.com/disorders/pyromania.htm
- http://www.biopsychiatry.com/klepto.htm
- http://www.psychdirect.com/forensic/Criminology/impulse/explosive.htm
- http://healthgate.partners.org/browsing/browseContent.asp?fileName=11723.xml&title=Kleptomania

IMPLICATIONS OF RESEARCH FOR EVIDENCE-BASED PRACTICE

Petry, N.M., & Tawfik, Z. (2001). Comparison of problem-gambling and non-problem-gambling youths seeking treatment for marijuana abuse. *Journal of the American Academy of Child and Adolescent Psychiatry, 40* **(11), 1324–1331.**

Description of the Study: The objective of this study was to evaluate the prevalence and parallels of problem gambling in marijuana-abusing adolescents. Data was collected from 255 adolescents entering treatment for marijuana abuse in Philadelphia, PA, and Hartford, CT, between 1998 and 2000. A retrospective analysis was conducted.

Results of the Study: Twenty-two percent of the 255 participants experienced gambling problems. Comparisons were made between the problem-gamblers (PGs) and the non-problem-gamblers (NPGs) with the following results. PGs were more likely than NPGs to be male, of African-American ethnicity, and to live in single-parent homes. Other differences emerged between the two groups as well. PGs showed a greater severity of drug and alcohol use than NPGs. PGs were involved in more illegal activity and experienced a higher number of somatization and anxiety symptoms. PGs also reported more recent sexual partners and human immunodeficiency virus risk behaviors.

Implications for Nursing Practice: The authors suggest that these data support the need for early identification and treatment of problem gambling in substance-abusing adolescents. This has particularly important implications for nurses who work in the area of substance abuse and addictions. Information about problem gambling should become a routine part of the nursing assessment in these areas.

REVIEW QUESTIONS

SELF-EXAMINATION/LEARNING EXERCISE

Select the answer that is most appropriate for the questions that follow the situation.

Situation: Linda has been admitted to the psychiatric unit with a diagnosis of adjustment disorder with depressed mood. She recently left her husband after 10 years of a very stormy marriage. She did not want to leave but decided that the move was best for herself and her two children (who are living with her). Linda was very dependent on her husband and is having difficulty living an independent lifestyle.

1. The *priority* nursing diagnosis for Linda would be:
   a. Impaired adjustment related to breakup of marriage.
   b. Dysfunctional grieving related to breakup of marriage.
   c. Ineffective coping related to problems with dependency.
   d. Social isolation related to depressed mood.

2. Linda says to the nurse, "I feel so bad. I thought I would feel better once I left, but I feel worse!" Which is the *best* response by the nurse?
   a. "Cheer up, Linda. You have a lot to be happy about."
   b. "You are grieving for the marriage you did not have. It's natural for you to feel badly."
   c. "Try not to dwell on how you feel. If you don't think about it, you'll feel better."
   d. "You did the right thing, Linda. Knowing that should make you feel better."

3. The physician orders sertraline (Zoloft) for Linda. This medication is intended to:
   a. Increase energy and elevate mood.
   b. Stimulate the central nervous system.
   c. Prevent psychotic symptoms.
   d. Produce a calming effect.

4. Which of the following is true regarding adjustment disorder?
   a. Linda will require long-term psychotherapy to achieve relief.
   b. Linda likely inherited a genetic tendency for the disorder.
   c. Linda's symptoms will likely remit once she has accepted the change in her life.
   d. Linda probably would not have experienced adjustment disorder if she had a higher level of intelligence.

5. The category of adjustment disorder with depressed mood identifies the individual who:
   a. Violates the rights of others to feel better.
   b. Expresses symptoms that reveal a high level of anxiety.
   c. Exhibits severe social isolation and withdrawal.
   d. Is experiencing a dysfunctional grieving process.

Match the behavior on the right to the appropriate diagnosis on the left.

_____ 6. Kleptomania.

a. Tony has been fascinated by fire for as long as he can remember. He played with matches as a child. As an adult, he has set numerous fires, always feeling exhilarated and even sexually stimulated afterward.

_____ 7. Intermittent explosive disorder.

b. Janet received a great deal of money and property in a divorce settlement. Shortly after the divorce, she experienced an impulse to enter a large department store and steal some inexpensive costume jewelry. Although she had been apprehended twice for shoplifting, she was indifferent to being discovered at this time.

_____ 8. Pathological gambling

c. Frankie, a 16-year-old boy, had had temper tantrums since age 2. As he matured, the "tantrums" intensified, with explosions of rage, usually without identifiable provocation. He had attempted to molest his 12-year-old sister and went after his father with a butcher knife. He has an abnormal electroencephalogram.

_____ 9. Pyromania

d. Callie, a 10-year-old girl, has been pulling her hair out of the crown of her head for several years. She has been referred to psychiatry from the dermatology clinic. Her mother reports the hair pulling usually occurs at night when Callie is tired. Further history reveals Callie's father left her mother when Callie was 4 years old and has never been heard from since. Callie tells the psychiatrist he left because she was a bad girl.

_____ 10. Trichotillomania

e. Harold has borrowed a great deal of money from an illegal source in an effort to pay back a gambling debt. He has continued to gamble so that he can pay back the loan with his winnings. Last night, the loan sharks threatened harm if he did not pay soon. He withdraws all the money from his joint account with his wife and heads for the racetrack.

TEST YOUR CRITICAL THINKING SKILLS

Alice, age 48, underwent a mastectomy of the right breast after her mammogram revealed a lump that proved to be malignant when biopsied. Since her surgery 6 weeks ago, Alice has refused to see any of her friends. She stays in her bedroom, speaks to her husband only when he speaks first, is having difficulty sleeping, and eats very little. She refuses to look at the mastectomy scar and has refused to see the Reach to Recovery representative who has tried several times to help fit her with a prosthesis. Her husband has become very worried about her and spoke to the family doctor, who recommended a psychiatrist. She has been admitted to the psychiatric unit with a diagnosis of adjustment disorder with depressed mood.

Answer the following questions about Alice:

1. What would be the primary nursing diagnosis for Alice?
2. Describe a short-term goal and a long-term goal for Alice.
3. Discuss a priority nursing intervention in working with Alice.

REFERENCES

American Psychiatric Association. (2000). *Diagnostic and statistical manual of mental disorders* (4th ed.) *Text revision.* Washington, DC: American Psychiatric Association.

Blume, S.G. (2002). *Pathological gambling: Recognition and intervention.* Retrieved on May 3, 2005 from the World Wide Web at http://www.iupui.edu/~flip/reading4.html

Grant, J.E., & Kim, S.W. (2002). An open-label study of naltrexone in the treatment of kleptomania. *Journal of Clinical Psychiatry, 63*(4), 349–356.

Lochner, C., duToit, P.L., Zungu-Dirwayi, N., Marais, A., vanKradenburg, J., Curr, B., Seedat, S., Niehaus, D.J.H., & Stein, D.J. (2002). Childhood trauma in obsessive-compulsive disorder, trichotillomania, and controls. *Depression and Anxiety, 15,* 66–68.

Moreyra, P., Ibanez, A., Saiz-Ruiz, J., Nissenson, K., & Blanco, C. (2000). Review of the phenomenology, etiology and treatment of pathological gambling. *German Journal of Psychiatry, 3,* 37–52.

Regard, M., Knoch, D., Gutling, E., & Landis, T. (2003). Brain damage and addictive behavior: A neuropsychological and electroencephalogram investigation with pathologic gamblers. *Cognitive and Behavioral Neurology, 16*(1), 47–53.

Sadock, B.J., & Sadock, V.A. (2003). *Synopsis of psychiatry: Behavioral sciences/clinical psychiatry* (9th ed.). Philadelphia: Lippincott Williams & Wilkins.

Scott, C.L., Hilty, D.M., & Brook, M. (2003). Impulse-control disorders not elsewhere classified. In R.E. Hales & S.C. Yudofsky (Eds.). *Textbook of clinical psychiatry* (4th ed.). Washington, DC: American Psychiatric Publishing.

Strain, J.J., & Newcorn, J. (2003). Adjustment disorders. In R.E. Hales & S.C. Yudofsky (Eds.). *Textbook of clinical psychiatry* (4th ed.). Washington, DC: American Psychiatric Publishing.

Unwin, B.K., Davis, M.K., & Leeuw, J.B. (2000). Pathologic gambling. *American Family Physician, 61*(3), 741–749.

CLASSICAL REFERENCE

Freud, S. (1964). New introductory lectures on psychoanalysis and other works. In *The standard edition of the complete psychological works of Sigmund Freud* (Vol. 22). London: Hogarth Press.

PSYCHOLOGICAL FACTORS AFFECTING MEDICAL CONDITIONS

CHAPTER OUTLINE

OBJECTIVES

HISTORICAL ASPECTS

APPLICATION OF THE NURSING PROCESS

TREATMENT MODALITIES

SUMMARY

REVIEW QUESTIONS

KEY TERMS

autoimmune

cachexia

carcinogens

essential hypertension

migraine personality

type A personality

type B personality

type C personality

type D personality

CORE CONCEPT

psychophysiological

OBJECTIVES

After reading this chapter, the student will be able to:

1. Differentiate between somatoform and psychophysiological disorders.
2. Identify various types of psychophysiological disorders.
3. Discuss historical and epidemiological statistics related to various psychophysiological disorders.
4. Describe symptomatology associated with various psychophysiological disorders and use these data in client assessment.
5. Identify various predisposing factors to psychophysiological disorders.
6. Formulate nursing diagnoses and outcomes for clients with various psychophysiological disorders.
7. Describe appropriate nursing interventions for behaviors associated with various psychophysiological disorders.
8. Identify topics for client and family teaching relevant to psychophysiological disorders.
9. Evaluate the nursing care of clients with psychophysiological disorders.
10. Discuss various modalities relevant to treatment of psychophysiological disorders.

*P*sychophysiological responses differ from somatoform disorders in that there is evidence of either demonstrable organic pathology or a known pathophysiological process involved. No such organic involvement can be identified in somatoform disorders.

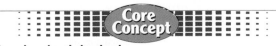

Psychophysiological

A condition that is identified as such because psychological factors have been identified as contributing to the initiation or exacerbation of the symptoms.

The *DSM-IV-TR* (American Psychiatric Association [APA], 2000) states:

> Psychological factors can influence the course of the general medical condition, which can be inferred by a close temporal association between the factors and the development or exacerbation of, or delayed recovery from, the medical condition. (p. 731)

Several types of psychological factors are implicated by the *DSM-IV-TR* as those that can affect the general medical condition. They include:

1. Mental disorders (e.g., axis I disorders, such as major depression).
2. Psychological symptoms (e.g., depressed mood or anxiety).
3. Personality traits or coping style (e.g., denial of the need for medical care).
4. Maladaptive health behaviors (e.g., smoking or overeating).
5. Stress-related physiological responses (e.g., tension headaches).
6. Other or unspecified psychological factors (e.g., interpersonal or cultural factors).

The *DSM-IV-TR* diagnostic criteria for psychological factors affecting medical condition are presented in Table 36–1.

Virtually any organic disorder can be considered psychophysiological. Sadock and Sadock (2003) state,

TABLE 36–1 Psychological Factors (Specify) Affecting Medical Condition

A. A general medical condition (coded on Axis III) is present.
B. Psychological factors adversely affect the general medical condition in one of the following ways:
1. The factors have influenced the course of the general medical condition as shown by a close temporal association between the psychological factors and the development or exacerbation of, or delayed recovery from, the general medical condition.
2. The factors interfere with the treatment of the general medical condition.
3. The factors constitute additional health risks for the individual.
4. Stress-related physiological responses precipitate or exacerbate symptoms of the general medical condition.

Specify type of psychological factor:
Mental disorder (e.g., axis I disorder such as major depressive disorder delaying recovery from a myocardial infarction).
Psychological symptoms (e.g., depressive symptoms delaying recovery from surgery; anxiety exacerbating asthma).
Personality traits or coping style (e.g, pathological denial of the need for surgery in a patient with cancer; hostile, pressured behavior contributing to cardiovascular disease).
Maladaptive health behaviors (e.g., overeating, lack of exercise, unsafe sex).
Stress-related physiological response (e.g., stress-related exacerbations of ulcer, hypertension, arrhythmia, or tension headache).
Other or unspecified psychological factors (e.g., interpersonal, cultural, or religious factors).

SOURCE: American Psychiatric Association (2000), with permission.

TABLE 36–2 Examples of Psychophysiological Disorders

Acne	Immune disease (e.g., multiple sclerosis, systemic lupus erythematosus)
Amenorrhea	
Angina pectoris	Impotence
Asthma	Irritable bowel syndrome
Cancer	Migraine headache
Cardiospasm	Nausea and vomiting
Coronary heart disease	Neurodermatitis
Duodenal ulcer	Obesity
Dysmenorrhea	Pylorospasm
Enuresis	Regional enteritis
Essential hypertension	Rheumatoid arthritis
Gastric ulcer	Sacroiliac pain
Herpes	Skin disease (e.g., psoriasis)
Hyperglycemia	Tension headache
Hyperthyroidism	Tuberculosis
Hypoglycemia	Ulcerative colitis

SOURCES: Modified from American Psychiatric Association (2000), Kaplan & Sadock (1998), and Pelletier (1992).

"…psychological or behavioral factors play a role in almost every medical condition." A list of some (although certainly not all) psychophysiological disorders is presented in Table 36–2.

The following psychophysiological disorders are discussed in this chapter:

Asthma
Cancer
Coronary heart disease
Peptic ulcer
Migraine headache
Hypertension
Rheumatoid arthritis
Ulcerative colitis

Historical and epidemiological statistics are presented. Predisposing factors that have been implicated in the etiology of each psychophysiological disorder provide a framework for study. An explanation of the symptomatology is presented as background knowledge for assessing the client with a psychophysiological disorder. Nursing care is described in the context of the nursing process. Various medical treatment modalities are explored.

HISTORICAL ASPECTS

For more than a century, physicians have agreed that in some disorders an interaction exists between emotional and physical factors. Four general types of reaction to stress have been identified, and they parallel Peplau's (1963) four levels of anxiety (see Chapter 2). These reactions are:

1. *The normal reaction* (mild anxiety), in which there is increased alertness and a mobilization of defenses for action.
2. *The psychophysiological reaction* (moderate anxiety), in

which the defenses fail and the response is translated into somatic symptoms.

3. *The neurotic reaction* (severe anxiety), in which the anxiety is so great that the defense becomes ineffective and neurotic symptoms develop.
4. *The psychotic reaction* (panic anxiety), in which loss of control results in misperception of the environment.

Hans Selye (1976) studied the physiological response of a biological system to change imposed on it. He found that regardless of the stressor, the biological entity responded with a syndrome of symptoms that he called the *general adaptation syndrome*. (This syndrome of symptoms is described in Chapter 1.) In this aroused state, the individual garners the strength to face the stress and mobilize the defenses to resolve it. If the defenses fail and the stressor is not quickly resolved, however, the body remains in this aroused state indefinitely, becoming susceptible to psychophysiological illness.

Historically, mind and body have been viewed as two distinct entities, each subject to different laws of causality. Indeed, in many instances—particularly in highly specialized areas of medicine—the biological and psychological components of disease remain separate. However, medical research shows that a change is occurring. Research associated with biological functioning is being expanded to include the psychological and social determinants of health and disease. This psychobiological approach to illness reflects a more holistic perspective and one that promotes concern for helping clients achieve optimal functioning.

APPLICATION OF THE NURSING PROCESS

Background Assessment Data: Types of Psychophysiological Disorders

Asthma

Definition and Epidemiological Statistics. Asthma is a disorder of the bronchial airways characterized by inflammation of the mucosal lining of the bronchial tree and spasm of the bronchial smooth muscles, which causes narrowed airways and air trapping (Hopper, 2003). It affects 18 million Americans, including approximately 6 million children younger than age 18 (Centers for Disease Control [CDC], 2005). Asthma may occur at any age, although it is more common in individuals younger than age 40.

Signs and Symptoms. Asthma is characterized by episodes of bronchial constriction resulting in dyspnea, wheezing, productive cough, restlessness, and eosinophilia. Expiration is prolonged and breathing reflects use of accessory muscles. Tachypnea and nasal flaring are common. The individual is usually diaphoretic and quite apprehensive, with total attention focused on his or her breathing.

Predisposing Factors

Biological Influences. Hereditary factors may play a role in the etiology of asthma. People who have a family history of asthma have an increased risk of developing the disease. Asthma also appears to be more common in families that have individuals with hay fever or eczema.

Allergies play a major role in precipitating the attacks associated with asthma. Allergic asthma is triggered by allergens such as pollen, foods, medications, animal dander, air pollution, molds, or dust mites (Hopper, 2003). Other factors known to stimulate bronchoconstriction include exercise, cold air, smoking, and respiratory infection.

Psychosocial Influences. Asthma has long been recognized as a "typical" psychophysiological response with evidence of symptoms being induced by emotional stress. Individuals with asthma are characterized as having excessive dependency needs, although no specific personality type has been identified (Sadock & Sadock, 2003). Individuals with asthma have been associated with certain personality characteristics, including fears, emotional lability, increased anxiety, and depression (Levenson, 2003; Sadock & Sadock, 2003).

Cancer

Definition and Epidemiological Statistics. Cancer is a malignant neoplasm in which the basic structure and activity of the cells have become deranged, usually because of changes in the DNA. These mutated cells grow wildly and rapidly and lose their similarity to the original cells. The malignant cells spread to other areas by invading surrounding tissues and by entering the blood and lymphatic system. If left untreated, the malignant neoplasms usually result in death.

Cancer is the second leading cause of death in the United States. However, 5-year survival rates have increased as a result of early diagnosis and treatment and the improvement of treatment modalities for most cancers. The largest number of deaths from cancer in both men and women is attributed to cancer of the lung (American Cancer Society [ACS], 2005).

The incidence and mortality rates for cancer are higher for African Americans than for whites, and lower for Latino Americans than for both blacks and whites (ACS, 2005). Cancer has been called a "disease of the aging," as the likelihood of developing cancer increases with age.

Signs and Symptoms. Significant changes that may occur as early warning signs of cancer have been identified (National Cancer Institute, 2005). They include:

- Thickening or lump in the breast or any other part of the body
- Obvious change in a wart or mole
- A sore that does not heal
- Nagging cough or hoarseness

● Changes in bowel or bladder habits
● Indigestion or difficulty swallowing
● Unexplained changes in weight
● Unusual bleeding or discharge

Specific effects are determined by site. Malignant tumors can also create effects at sites distant to the primary site. Late-stage cancer symptoms may include anemias, infections, thrombocytopenia, **cachexia**, weakness, weight loss, dyspnea, ascites, and pleural effusion.

Predisposing Factors

Biological Influences. Certain cancers, such as those of the stomach, breast, colon, kidney, uterus, and lung tend to occur in a familial pattern. Whether this indicates an inherited susceptibility or common exposure to an etiological factor is unknown.

Continuous irritation also may predispose individuals to certain types of cancer. For example, chronic exposure to the sun is thought to predispose to melanoma, and prolonged alcohol consumption may be related to the development of esophageal cancer.

Exposure to occupational or environmental **carcinogens** may lead to specific cancers. Examples include cigarette smoke, aniline dye, radium, asphalt, arsenic, chromate, uranium, and asbestos. Various drugs have been implicated in the onset of cancer. They include immunosuppressive agents, diethylstilbestrol, oral contraceptives, cytotoxic agents, and radioisotopes.

Certain viruses have been isolated and identified as the causative factor of cancer in some animals. However, the role that viruses play in the etiology of cancer in humans has not been definitely established.

Psychosocial Influences. Karren and associates (2002) report on a number of research studies dealing with personality characteristics that have been associated with individuals who develop cancer. The term **type C personality** has been coined to describe these characteristics. Cancer has sometimes been called the "nice guy's disease." Common characteristics that were found to be associated with type C personality include repression of negative emotions, passivity, and a tendency to be apologetic and overly cooperative.

Other researchers who have studied these characteristics identify the following profile for the type C personality:

● Suppresses anger and hostility to an extreme (experiences these emotions but does not express them).
● Exhibits a calm, placid exterior.
● Commonly feels depressed and in despair.
● Has low self-esteem, low self-worth.
● Puts others' needs before his or her own.
● Has a tendency toward self-pity (acts as the martyr).
● Sets unrealistic standards and is inflexible in the enforcement of these standards.

● Resents others for perceived "wrongs," although others are never aware of these feelings.

Levenson (2003) reports on a number of studies that provide support, as well as a lack of support, for several psychological factors associated with the onset and progression of cancer. Depression has been linked to a higher-than-normal risk of developing cancer, as well as death from the disease. The ability to express one's emotions rather than repress them has been shown to have an association with a more positive cancer prognosis. A lack of closeness with parents and less than satisfactory interpersonal relationships have been linked to later development of cancer. Variables of positive relationships have been associated with increased survival rates.

Some studies have been conducted in an effort to determine if there is a link between psychosocial stress and the onset of cancer symptoms. Results suggest a positive correlation between the effects of stress and the induction and growth of neoplastic tumors in extensive work with experimental animals and in more limited studies with humans. Biopsychosocial events appear to reduce immunological competence at a critical time and may allow a mutant cell to thrive and grow (Pelletier, 1992).

Coronary Heart Disease

Definition and Epidemiological Statistics. Coronary heart disease (CHD) is also called *coronary artery disease* or *ischemic heart disease*. It is defined as myocardial impairment caused by a decrease in blood supply to the heart muscle (Tazbir & Keresztes, 2005). It is the leading cause of death in the United States. Five million people have CHD. It is more prevalent in men than in women, although the number of women with CHD is increasing, probably as a result of greater social and economic pressures on women and changes in their lifestyles. The incidence of CHD is higher in older individuals and those in the lower socioeconomic groups (Mensah et al., 2005).

Signs and Symptoms. Atherosclerosis, or changes in the lining of the coronary arteries that affect lumen size, is the basic underlying problem associated with coronary heart disease. Size of the lumen is decreased because of an accumulation of cells, lipids, and connective tissue that adheres to the intima of the artery. This results in decreased oxygenated blood flow to the myocardium and possible myocardial ischemia. Myocardial ischemia may be asymptomatic or may cause discomfort in the chest.

Angina pectoris can occur spontaneously or in relation to increased myocardial oxygen demand. Common descriptions of pain associated with angina include squeezing, burning, pressing, choking, aching, or bursting pressure (Tazbir & Keresztes, 2005). The discomfort of angina usually lasts from 2 to 5 minutes, sometimes as long as 15 minutes, and rarely as long as 30 minutes.

Pain associated with myocardial infarction (MI) is

similar to that experienced in angina but lasts longer than 15 to 30 minutes. Symptoms may also include indigestion, nausea and vomiting, diaphoresis, syncope, palpitations, or dyspnea. Up to one third of people experiencing MI will not experience chest pain (Canto et al., 2000). This phenomenon is more prevalent among the elderly population, in women, and in clients with diabetes.

Predisposing Factors

Biological Influences. A number of risk factors have been identified as predisposing factors to the development of CHD. A family history of CHD increases an individual's risk of developing atherosclerosis. Other possible hereditary risk factors for CHD include high serum lipoprotein levels, particularly cholesterol and triglycerides, hypertension, and diabetes mellitus. It is not known whether there is a direct genetic link or if the risk is related more to environmental lifestyle patterns.

Various lifestyle habits have been implicated. The association between cigarette smoking and CHD has now been clearly established. Obesity, defined as body mass index (weight/height^2) of 30 or greater, has been associated with increased risk of developing CHD. It is unclear whether the increased risk is associated with the obesity itself or to other factors that frequently accompany obesity, such as high blood pressure or diabetes.

Sedentary lifestyle has also been implicated. It is thought that physical exercise offers some protection by helping to maintain a lower blood pressure, keeping the body at a healthy weight, and correcting dyslipidemias (McKechnie & Mosca, 2003).

Psychosocial Influences. Friedman and Rosenman (1974) have completed the most comprehensive research to date in the area of personality and CHD. They developed a detailed profile of the CHD-prone individual, which they identified as **type A personality**. They also studied personality characteristics of individuals who experienced stress in a different manner and seemed less prone to CHD. This personality profile was designated **type B personality**.

Friedman and Rosenman identified two character traits that when occurring together automatically classify an individual as type A personality. These two traits are excessive competitive drive and a chronic, continual sense of time urgency. Additional type A characteristics include:

- Having easily aroused hostility that is usually kept under control but flares up unexpectedly, often when others would consider it unwarranted.
- Being very aggressive, very ambitious, concentrating almost exclusively on his or her career.
- Having no time for hobbies, and during any leisure time, feeling guilty just relaxing as if wasting time.
- Seldom feeling satisfied with accomplishments; always feeling must do more.

- Measuring achievements in numbers produced and dollars earned.
- Continually struggling to achieve and feeling there is never enough time (time becomes the enemy of the person with type A personality).
- Appearing to be very extroverted and social; often dominating conversation; having an outgoing personality but often concealing a deep-seated insecurity about his or her own worth.
- Experiencing driving ambition and the need to win (leads the person with type A personality to undertake all activities with the same competitive drive, with even recreational activities becoming aggressive when the individual puts undue pressure on himself or herself to compete).

People with type B personalities are not the opposite of those with type A, only different. Those with type B personality are no less successful than those with type A. They may perform just as well on their jobs—maybe better. Those with type B do not feel the constant sense of time urgency that those with type A feel. They can function under time pressure when it is required, but it is not a pervasive part of their lives as it is with those type A individuals. Ambition of individuals with type B personalities probably is based on goals that have been well thought out. There is not the constant need for competition and comparison with peers. Self-worth often comes from goals other than material and social success. Individuals with type B personality recognize and accept both strengths and limitations. They view leisure time as a time to relax, and they do so without feeling guilty. They take the time to consider alternatives and to think things through before deciding or acting. These characteristics often result in more creative output by people with type B personality. Those with type A are prone to making more errors because of their impulsivity (i.e., acting before thinking things through).

Rosenman and colleagues (1975) reported the results of an 8$\frac{1}{2}$-year follow-up study for predicting CHD in men between the ages of 39 and 59. In this study, the incidence of CHD was significantly associated with parental history, diabetes, education, smoking, blood pressure, and serum cholesterol levels. The study also concluded that type A behavior was a strong factor and that "this association could not be explained by association of behavior pattern with any single predictive risk factor or any combination of them" (Rosenman et al., 1975). Type A behavior risk factor was clearly a contributing factor in itself.

The most recent research associated with CHD personality characteristics has revealed a behavior pattern being termed ***type D personality*** (the *distressed* personality) (Denollet, 1997). Individuals with type D personality have a tendency to experience negative emotions and the inability to express feelings in social situations. Karren and associates (2002) state:

[It was found] that certain negative emotions, such as anger, anxiety, depression, worry, and hopelessness all increased the risk of coronary artery disease. The problem did not occur from the *occasional* experiencing of these negative emotions, but from the tendency to experience these negative emotions across time and a variety of situations and the tendency to suppress negative emotions. (p. 151)

In a review of current research on type D personality in the context of CHD, Pedersen and Denollet (2003) concluded that accumulating evidence indicates that cardiac patients with type D personality are at increased risk for cardiovascular morbidity and mortality, independent of standard cardiac risk factors, and that they appeared to benefit less from medical and invasive treatment. Karren and associates (2002) report on research suggesting that the presence of either negative emotions or social inhibition without the other does not necessarily increase the risk of CHD, but that it takes a combination of the two. A study by Denollet and Brutsaert (1998) showed that type D personality:

● Increases the risk of cardiac death, especially among patients with established coronary heart disease.
● Causes increased risk of subsequent heart attack among myocardial infarction patients.
● Increases the risk of death by four times among coronary artery disease patients.

The researchers believe that this knowledge about type D personality may help identify individuals at risk for CHD. However, some clinicians have suggested that personality traits such as those identified as type D—social inhibition and negative feelings—are much harder to change than some other characteristics identified with type A personality. Continued research is needed to substantiate conclusions in the long term.

Peptic Ulcer

Definition and Epidemiological Statistics. Peptic ulcers are an erosion of the mucosal wall in the esophagus, stomach, duodenum, or jejunum. Deeper lesions may penetrate the mucosal layer and extend into the muscular layers of the intestinal wall (Dawson, 2003).

Peptic ulcers occur four times more frequently in men than in women. The disease occurs in approximately 10 percent of the population, and peak ages have been identified as 40 to 60 years (Murphy-Blake & Hawks, 2005). Hospitalization, surgery, and mortality related to peptic ulcer disease place an economic burden on this country in the billions of dollars annually.

Signs and Symptoms. Pain is the characteristic clinical manifestation of peptic ulcer disease. It is usually experienced in the upper abdomen near the midline, and may radiate to the back, sternum, or lower abdomen. Pain is usually worse when the stomach is empty and gastric secretions are high. Food or antacid medication often relieves the pain.

Predisposing Factors

Biological Influences. Approximately 80 percent of ulcers are thought to be caused by infection of the digestive tract with the bacterium *Helicobacter pylori*. It is unknown how the infection spreads, but it may be transmitted orally or through contaminated food or water. Not all people who are infected with *H. pylori* develop ulcers. Ulcers form when an upset in the balance between the damaging effects of gastric acids and the body's natural protective mechanisms occurs, making the lining of the digestive tract susceptible to erosion. It is thought that *H. pylori* contributes to this weakening of protective mechanisms. A vaccine against *H. pylori* is currently being developed.

Several environmental factors have been associated with peptic ulcer disease. Cigarette smoking and regular use of aspirin have been strongly implicated. Other agents such as alcohol, steroids, and nonsteroidal anti-inflammatory drugs are also ulcerogenic in that they can cause damage to the gastric mucosal barrier. There also appears to be a familial predisposition to peptic ulcer disease.

Psychosocial Influences. Studies have observed increased gastric secretion and motility in the presence of hostility, resentment, and frustration (Karren et al., 2002). The link between ulcers and stress has been related by some psychodynamic investigators to an unfulfilled dependency need in ulcer-prone individuals. These individuals tend to have an unhealthy attachment to others, and although they are dependent by nature, they perceive that they have few people on whom they can depend in times of crisis. They are excessive worriers, and seem to have more times of crises than most people, possibly because they are such pessimists and always seem to expect the worst from a situation (Karren et al., 2002). Anxiety and depression are common among ulcer-prone individuals.

Essential Hypertension

Definition and Epidemiological Statistics. **Essential hypertension** is the persistent elevation of blood pressure for which there is no apparent cause or associated underlying disease (Fanning & Lewis, 2003). It is a major cause of cerebrovascular accident (stroke), cardiac disease, and renal failure.

Approximately 30 percent of the adult population in the United States are hypertensive, a condition characterized by a blood pressure of 140/90 mm Hg or higher (American Heart Association, 2005). Because hypertension is often asymptomatic, it is estimated that 30 percent of persons with hypertension do not know they have it.

The disorder is more common in men than in women and is twice as prevalent in the African-American population as it is in the white population.

Signs and Symptoms. Most commonly, hypertension produces no symptoms, particularly in the early stages. When symptoms do occur, they may include headache, vertigo, flushed face, spontaneous nosebleed, or blurred vision. Chronic, progressive hypertension may reveal signs and symptoms associated with specific organ system damage. For example, dyspnea, chest pain, or cardiac hypertrophy may indicate cardiovascular damage; confusion and parasthesia may suggest cerebrovascular damage; and elevated serum creatinine or blood urea nitrogen may signal kidney damage.

Predisposing Factors

Biological Influences. Individuals who have a positive family history of hypertension are at greater risk of developing the disorder than those who do not.

Physiological influences that have been hypothesized include an imbalance of circulating vasoconstrictors (e.g., angiotensin) and vasodilators (e.g., prostaglandins), increased sympathetic nervous system activity resulting in increased vasoconstriction, and impairment of sodium and water excretion (DeMartinis, 2005). Other conditions that may contribute to hypertension are obesity and cigarette smoking.

Psychosocial Influences. Karren and associates (2002) report on studies that suggest there is a correlation between suppressed anger and hypertension. Some psychoanalysts believe this may be associated with childhood rearing that forbade expression of angry feelings. Several studies showed consistent results of a significant relationship between suppressed anger and elevated blood pressure. One study measured blood pressure in three groups of men with three different types of anger management: expression, suppression, and "cool reflection." Karren and associates (2002) report on the results of that study:

> The men with the lowest blood pressure were those who kept their cool, who acknowledged their anger but were not openly hostile, either verbally or physically. That may be because they were managing their anger appropriately. Those with the highest blood pressure were the ones who either bottled up their anger or became openly hostile. (pp. 206–207)

Migraine Headache

Definition and Epidemiological Statistics. The word *migraine* comes from the Greek word *hemikranion* (meaning "half of the cranium"). In migraine headache, pain usually affects one side of the head. Pain most commonly originates in the muscles of the face, neck, and head; the blood vessels; and the dura mater. The blood vessels dilate and become congested with blood. Pain results from the exertion of pressure on nerves that lie in or around these congested blood vessels.

Migraine headaches can occur at any age but commonly begin in persons between ages 16 and 30 years. They are more common in women than in men and often are associated with various phases of the menstrual cycle. Approximately 5 percent of the general population suffers from migraine headaches.

Signs and Symptoms. The "classic" migraine headache occurs in two distinctive phases. In the prodromal phase, which may begin from minutes to days before the actual pain of the headache, the individual may experience visual disturbances, weakness and numbness on one side of the body, mental confusion, irritability, fatigue, sweating, and dizziness. The headache phase usually consists of pain on one side of the head. As it intensifies, the pain may spread to the other side as well. The ache is frequently dull, deep, and throbbing, and often begins in the forehead, ear, jaw, or in or around an eye or temple. Nausea, vomiting, mental cloudiness, total body achiness, abdominal pain, chills, and cold hands and feet commonly accompany the headache. Pain from a migraine headache lasts from 4 to 72 hours, after which sore muscles, total body exhaustion, and a continued mild mental cloudiness may persist for days.

The most common form of migraine headache is a variation of the classic version. Many of the symptoms are similar, but in common migraine the distinctive phases of the classic migraine do not occur. Photophobia (sensitivity to light) and hyperacusis (sensitivity to sound) may be present in both types.

Predisposing Factors

Biological Influences. A number of biological influences have been identified as triggers for headache-prone individuals. Periods of hormonal change have been implicated, such as during menstruation, during ovulation, during menopause, and at the beginning or just following pregnancy.

Heredity appears to play an important role in the etiology of migraine headaches. It is common for individuals from several generations within the same family to experience the disorder. Occasionally members of one or two generations are spared, but it is not uncommon to track a history of headaches in aunts, uncles, cousins, or grandparents.

Some foods, beverages, and drugs can precipitate migraine in certain individuals. These substances include caffeine, chocolate, aged cheese, vinegar, organ meats, alcoholic beverages, sour cream, yogurt, aspartame, citrus fruits, bananas, raisins, avocados, onions, smoked meats, monosodium glutamate, and products preserved with nitrites. Drugs that lower blood pressure, in particular reserpine and hydralazine, have also been known to trigger migraine headaches.

Some people experience attacks only during or after physical exertion. This may be caused by the chemical or blood vessel changes that occur during physical exercise.

Various other factors that have been implicated in the development of migraine headaches include cigarette smoking, bright lights, changes in the weather, high elevations, oral contraceptives, altered sleep patterns, and skipping meals.

Psychosocial Influences. Certain characteristics have been identified as "the **migraine personality**." Migraine sufferers have been described as perfectionistic, overly conscientious, and somewhat inflexible. They may be meticulously neat and tidy, compulsive, and often very hard workers. They are usually quite intelligent, exacting, and place a very high premium on success, setting high (sometimes unrealistic) expectations on themselves and others. Delegation of responsibility is difficult, as they feel no one can perform the task as well as they can. Classically, there is repressed or suppressed anger. The individual experiences hostility and anger but cannot express these feelings openly. Some researchers have identified the "migraine personality" as a clone of the Type A personality (Karren et al., 2002).

Emotions play a critical role in the precipitation of migraine headaches. An individual experiencing emotional stress may develop a migraine headache in response to the secondary gains one receives from assuming the sick role. Migraine headaches therefore may provide a means of escape for dealing with the stressful situation. Other individuals experience migraine attacks only *after* the emotionally distressing event has passed or lessened. This has been called "let-down" headache and can be one of the influential factors in provoking the weekend or holiday migraine, when the anxiety has been relieved and the individual finally relaxes.

Rheumatoid Arthritis

Definition and Epidemiological Statistics. Rheumatoid arthritis is a disease characterized by chronic musculoskeletal pain arising from inflammation of the joints (Sadock & Sadock, 2003). It is a *systemic* disease and may also be manifested by lesions of the major organs of the body. Rheumatoid arthritis is more prevalent in women than in men by a ratio of 2:1 or 3:1. It affects approximately 1 to 3 percent of the population of the United States, with an estimated 200,000 cases diagnosed annually. The disease is characterized by periods of remission and exacerbation.

Signs and Symptoms. Onset of the disease is usually insidious, with joint inflammation preceding the systemic symptoms of fatigue, malaise, anorexia, weight loss, low-grade fever, myalgias, and paresthesias (Kebicz & Ignatavicius, 2003). Some individuals recover from a first attack of the disorder and never suffer a recurrence, whereas others tend to be chronic and progressive. Joint involvement is usually characterized by swelling, pain, redness, warmth, and tenderness. Joints of the hands and feet are often affected early. As the disease progresses, any freely movable joint may be involved.

About one out of every five rheumatoid arthritis clients develop systemic manifestations, which can occur in virtually any body system. Cardiac, pulmonary, and renal involvement are the most serious consequences of rheumatoid arthritis.

Predisposing Factors

Biological Influences. Heredity appears to be influential in the predisposition to rheumatoid arthritis. The serum protein rheumatoid factor is found in at least half of people with rheumatoid arthritis and frequently in their close relatives. Rheumatoid arthritis affects people with a family history of the disease two to three times more often than the rest of the population (Kebicz & Ignatavicius, 2003). Although the rheumatoid factor is present in clients with other diseases, it is rare in the population at large.

An additional theory postulates that rheumatoid arthritis may be the result of a dysfunctional immune mechanism initiated by an infectious process, although the causative agent is yet to be identified. In such an instance, antibodies that form in keeping with a normal reaction to infection become directed instead against the self in an **autoimmune** response that results in tissue damage.

Psychosocial Influences. Rheumatoid arthritis clients are postulated to be self-sacrificing, anxious, unassertive, inhibited, and perfectionistic, with an inherent inability to express anger (Karren et al., 2002). Female rheumatoid clients are described as nervous, tense, worried, moody, and depressed, and typically had mothers whom they felt rejected them and fathers who were unduly strict (Pelletier, 1992).

Some evidence suggests that emotionally traumatic life events, such as the loss of a key person by death or separation, often precede the first symptoms of rheumatoid arthritis and precipitate its onset in some individuals. Thus, emotional decompensation in predisposed individuals may result in the onset or exacerbation of rheumatoid arthritis.

Ulcerative Colitis

Definition and Epidemiological Statistics. Ulcerative colitis is a chronic inflammatory ulcerative disease of the colon, usually associated with bloody diarrhea (Sadock & Sadock, 2003). The prevalence rate in the United States is estimated at 70 to 150 per 100,000 population. It can occur at any age, but is most prevalent between the ages of 15 and 35 years. Ulcerative colitis affects males and females equally. The disease is more common in Caucasians than in African Americans and Asian Americans. There is a higher incidence of ulcerative colitis in the Jewish population (Al-Ataie & Shenoy, 2005).

Signs and Symptoms. The mucosa of the colon and rectum become inflamed, with diffuse areas of bleeding. Diarrhea is the predominant symptom of ulcerative colitis. There may be as many as 15 to 20 liquid stools a day containing blood, mucus, and pus (Rogers, 2005). Abdominal cramping may or may not precede the bowel movement. Generalized manifestations include fever, anorexia, weight loss, nausea, and vomiting. During exacerbation of the illness, anemia and elevated white cell count are common.

As the disease progresses, the inflammation advances up the colon and the bleeding points enlarge and become ulcerated. The ulcers may bleed or perforate, forming scar tissue as it heals. The scar tissue causes the colon to thicken and become rigid, and normal elasticity and absorptive capability are diminished. Changes in the mucosa may cause the formation of pseudopolyps that can become cancerous.

Predisposing Factors

Biological Influences. A genetic factor may be involved in the development because individuals who have a family member with ulcerative colitis are at greater risk than the general population. This theory is supported by sibling and twin studies, although no genetic marker has been identified.

The possibility that ulcerative colitis may be an autoimmune disease has generated a great deal of research interest. High rates of anticolon antibodies are found in relatives of ulcerative colitis clients. Serum and mucosal autoantibodies against intestinal epithelial cells may be involved. Individuals with ulcerative colitis are often found to have p-antineutrophil cytoplasmic antibodies (Al-Ataie & Shenoy, 2005).

Psychosocial Influences. Regarding personality characteristics associated with individuals who have ulcerative colitis, Sadock and Sadock (2003) state, "Studies of patients with ulcerative colitis have shown a predominance of obsessive–compulsive traits. They are neat, orderly, punctual, and have difficulty expressing anger." A pathological mother–child relationship resulting in feelings of helplessness and hopelessness has also been implicated.

Onset or exacerbation of ulcerative colitis has been associated with stressful life events or psychological trauma. The altered immune status that accompanies psychological stress may be an influencing factor in predisposed individuals.

Transactional Model of Stress/Adaptation

The etiology of psychophysiological disorders is most likely influenced by multiple factors. In Figure 36–1, a graphic depiction of this theory of multiple causation is presented in the transactional model of stress/adaptation.

Diagnosis/Outcome Identification

Nursing diagnoses are formulated from the data gathered during the assessment phase and with background knowledge regarding predisposing factors to the disorder. Some common nursing diagnoses for clients with specific psychophysiological disorders include:

ASTHMA
Ineffective airway clearance
Activity intolerance
Anxiety (severe)

CANCER
Fear
Anticipatory grieving
Disturbed body image

CORONARY HEART DISEASE
Pain
Fear
Activity intolerance

PEPTIC ULCER DISEASE
Pain
Impaired tissue integrity

HYPERTENSION
Risk for ineffective tissue perfusion
Risk for sexual dysfunction

MIGRAINE HEADACHE
Pain
Ineffective role performance

RHEUMATOID ARTHRITIS
Pain
Self-care deficit
Activity intolerance

ULCERATIVE COLITIS
Pain
Diarrhea
Risk for imbalanced nutrition: less than body requirements

Some nursing diagnoses common to the general category of psychological factors affecting medical condition include:

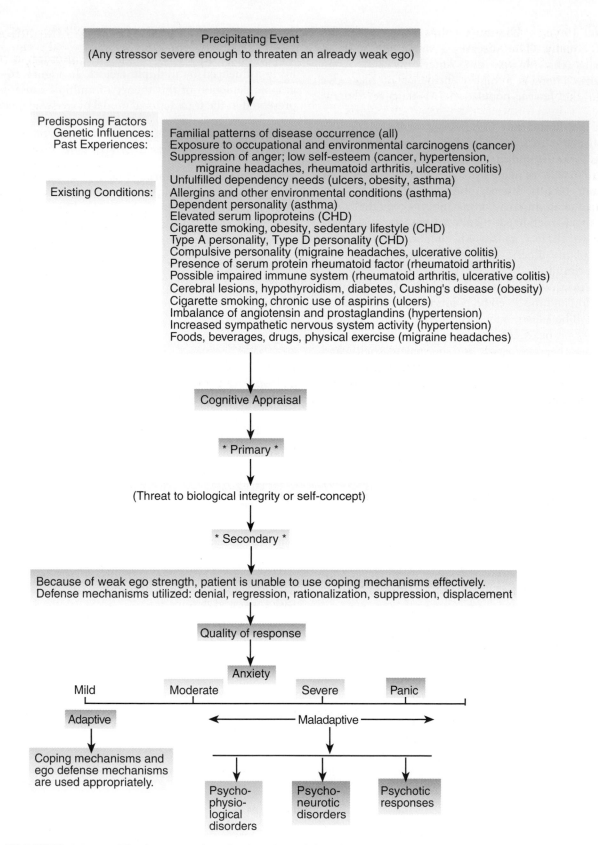

FIGURE 36–1   The dynamics of psychophysiological disorders using the transactional model of stress/adaptation.

Ineffective coping related to repressed anxiety and inadequate coping methods, evidenced by initiation or exacerbation of physical illness.

Deficient knowledge related to psychological factors affecting medical condition, evidenced by statements such as "I don't know why the doctor put me on the psychiatric unit. I have a physical problem."

Low self-esteem related to unmet dependency needs, evidenced by self-negating verbalizations and demanding sick-role behaviors.

Ineffective role performance related to physical illness accompanied by real or perceived disabling symptoms, evidenced by changes in usual patterns of responsibility.

The following criteria may be used for measurement of outcomes in the care of the client with a psychophysiological disorder:

The client:

1. Denies pain or other physical complaint.
2. Demonstrates the ability to perform more adaptive coping strategies in the face of stressful situations.
3. Verbalizes stressful situations that have led to or worsened physical symptoms in the past.

4. Verbalizes a plan to cope with stressful situations in an effort to prevent exacerbation of physical symptoms.
5. Performs activities of daily living independently.

Planning/Implementation

In Table 36–3, selected nursing diagnoses common to the general category are presented in a plan of care. Nursing diagnoses are included, along with outcome criteria, appropriate nursing interventions, and rationales.

The concept map care plan is an innovative approach to planning and organizing nursing care (see Chapter 9). It is a diagrammatic teaching and learning strategy that allows visualization of interrelationships between medical diagnoses, nursing diagnoses, assessment data, and treatments. An example of a concept map care plan for a client with a psychophysiological disorder is presented in Figure 36–2.

Client/Family Education

The role of client teacher is important in the psychiatric area, as it is in all areas of nursing. A list of topics for

---

TABLE 36–3	Care Plan for the Client with a Psychophysiological Disorder

NURSING DIAGNOSIS: INEFFECTIVE COPING
RELATED TO: Repressed anxiety and inadequate coping methods
EVIDENCED BY: Initiation or exacerbation of physical illness

OUTCOME CRITERIA	NURSING INTERVENTIONS	RATIONALE
Client will achieve physical wellness and demonstrate the ability to prevent exacerbation of physical symptoms as a coping mechanism in response to stress.	1. Perform thorough physical assessment.	1. Physical assessment is necessary to determine specific care required for client's physical condition.
	2. Monitor laboratory values, vital signs, intake and output, and other assessments.	2. This is necessary to maintain an accurate ongoing appraisal.
	3. Together with the client, identify goals of care and ways in which client believes he or she can best achieve those goals. Client may need assistance with problem solving.	3. Personal involvement in his or her own care provides a feeling of control and increases chances for positive outcomes.
	4. Encourage client to discuss current life situations that he or she perceives as stressful and the feelings associated with each.	4. Verbalization of true feelings in a nonthreatening environment may help client come to terms with unresolved issues.
	5. During client's discussion, note times during which a sense of powerlessness or loss of control over life situations emerges. Focus on these times and discuss ways in which the client may maintain a feeling of control.	5. A sense of self-worth develops and is maintained when an individual feels power over his or her own life situations.
	6. As client becomes able to discuss feelings more openly, assist him or her in a nonthreatening manner to relate certain feelings to the appearance of physical symptoms.	6. Client may be unaware of the relationship between physical symptoms and emotional problems.

(Continued on following page)

OUTCOME CRITERIA	NURSING INTERVENTIONS	RATIONALE
	7. Discuss stressful times when physical symptoms did not appear and the adaptive coping strategies that were used during those situations. Therapy is facilitated by considering areas of strength and using them to the client's benefit. Provide positive reinforcement for adaptive coping mechanisms identified or used. Suggest alternative coping strategies but allow client to determine which can most appropriately be incorporated into his or her lifestyle.	7. Positive reinforcement enhances self-esteem and encourages repetition of desired behaviors. Client may require assistance with problem solving but must be allowed and encouraged to make decisions independently.
	8. Help client to identify a resource within the community (friend, significant other, group) to use as a support system for the expression of feelings.	8. A positive support system may help to prevent maladaptive coping through physical illness.

NURSING DIAGNOSIS: KNOWLEDGE DEFICIT

RELATED TO: Psychological factors affecting medical condition

EVIDENCED BY: Statements such as "I don't know why the doctor put me on the psychiatric unit. I have a physical problem."

OUTCOME CRITERIA	NURSING INTERVENTIONS	RATIONALE
Client will be able to verbalize psychological factors affecting his or her physical condition.	1. Assess client's level of knowledge regarding effects of psychological problems on the body.	1. An adequate database is necessary for the development of an effective teaching plan.
	2. Assess client's level of anxiety and readiness to learn.	2. Learning does not occur beyond the moderate level of anxiety.
	3. Discuss physical examinations and laboratory tests that have been conducted. Explain purpose and results of each.	3. Client has the right to know about and accept or refuse any medical treatment.
	4. Explore feelings and fears held by client. Go slowly. These feelings may have been suppressed/repressed for so long that their disclosure may be a very painful experience. Be supportive.	4. Expression of feelings in the presence of a trusted individual and in a nonthreatening environment may encourage the individual to confront unresolved feelings.
	5. Have client keep a diary of appearance, duration, and intensity of physical symptoms. A separate record of situations that the client finds especially stressful should also be kept.	5. Comparison of these records may provide objective data from which to observe the relationship between physical symptoms and stress.
	6. Help client identify needs that are being met through the sick role. Together, formulate more adaptive means for fulfilling these needs. Practice by role-playing.	6. Repetition through practice serves to reduce discomfort in the actual situation.
	7. Provide instruction in assertiveness techniques, especially the ability to recognize the differences among passive, assertive, and aggressive behaviors and the importance of respecting the rights of others while protecting one's own basic rights.	7. These skills will preserve client's self-esteem while also improving his or her ability to form satisfactory interpersonal relationships.
	8. Discuss adaptive methods of stress management, such as relaxation techniques, physical exercise, meditation, breathing exercises, and autogenics.	8. Use of these adaptive techniques may decrease appearance of physical symptoms in response to stress.

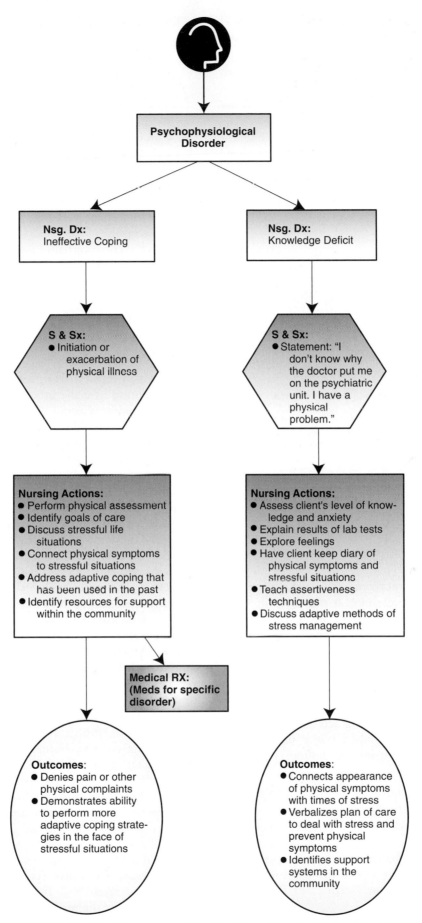

FIGURE 36–2 Concept map care plan for client with a psychophysiological disorder.

TABLE 36–4   Topics for Client/Family Education Related to Psychological Factors Affecting Medical Condition

Nature of the Illness

1. Provide information to the client about specific disease process:
   a. Asthma
   b. Cancer
   c. Coronary heart disease
   d. Peptic ulcer
   e. Essential hypertension
   f. Migraine headache
   g. Rheumatoid arthritis
   h. Ulcerative colitis
   i. Other
2. Discuss psychological implications of exacerbation or delayed healing

Management of the Illness

1. Discuss ways to identify onset of escalating anxiety.
2. Discuss ways to interrupt escalating anxiety:
   a. Assertive techniques
   b. Relaxation techniques
   c. Physical activities
   d. Talking with trusted individual
   e. Meditation
3. Discuss pain management.
4. Discuss how family can prevent reinforcing the illness.
5. Pharmacology
   a. Discuss why physician has prescribed certain medications.
   b. Discuss possible side effects of medications.
   c. Provide printed information about what symptoms to report to physician.
6. Discuss medical treatment modalities of the illness.
7. Discuss possible lifestyle changes related to the illness.

Support Services

1. Support groups
2. Individual psychotherapy
3. Biofeedback

---

client and family education relevant to psychological factors that affect medical condition is presented in Table 36–4.

Evaluation

Reassessment is conducted to determine if the nursing actions have been successful in achieving the objectives of care. Evaluation of the nursing actions for the client with a psychophysiological disorder may be facilitated by gathering information using the following types of questions.

1. Does the client complain of pain or other physical symptoms?
2. Are the physical symptoms interfering with role responsibilities?
3. Does the client verbalize that physical symptoms have been relieved?
4. Can the client carry out activities of daily living independently?
5. Can the client verbalize alternative coping strategies for dealing with stress?

6. Can the client demonstrate the ability to utilize these more adaptive coping strategies in the face of stress?
7. Does the client recognize which types of stressful situations or maladaptive health behaviors exacerbate physical symptoms?
8. Can the client correlate the appearance of the physical symptoms with a stressful situation or maladaptive health behavior?
9. Can the client verbalize unfulfilled needs for which the sick role may be compensating?
10. Can the client verbalize alternative ways to fulfill these needs?
11. Can the client verbalize resources to whom he or she may go when feeling the need for assistance in times of stress?

TREATMENT MODALITIES

Asthma

The goals of medical treatment for clients with asthma are prevention of acute attacks and promotion of normal functioning (Cronin & Miracle, 2005). The most commonly prescribed medications for asthma are bronchodilators and corticosteroids, usually from a metered-dose inhaler. Bronchodilators increase the airway diameter and corticosteroids reduce the inflammatory response.

The most commonly used bronchodilators are the beta-adrenergic agonists (e.g., metaproterenol, albuterol). Theophylline and other methylxanthines are also used, but, because they are usually given orally, they may produce greater side effects than those administered by inhaler.

Corticosteroids, such as fluticasone and beclomethasone, may be used in inhalant form for the prophylactic treatment of asthma. Other medications prescribed for asthma include leukotriene receptor antagonists, which inhibit bronchoconstriction by blocking the leukotriene receptor, and mast cell stabilizers, which occupy a position on the mast cell and prevent release of the chemicals that stimulate bronchospasm and promote inflammation.

Some clients with asthma may be candidates for short-term or long-term psychotherapy. The internist or family physician maintains care of the physical component of the client's illness, whereas the psychotherapist focuses on attitudes and emotions and helping the client to progress with the separation–individuation process. The psychological aspects are kept separate from the physical aspects of the illness so that the therapeutic relationship is not destroyed if the client suffers an asthmatic attack during psychotherapy. Exacerbations during the treatment offer both the therapist and the client an opportunity to become aware of the psychological context in which they occur. They then may be able to understand the emotional factors involved and, hopefully, to modify them.

Cancer

Surgery is perhaps the oldest method used to control or cure cancer. Surgical procedures can be used to diagnose malignancy (e.g., biopsy), to cure malignancies (e.g., mastectomy, hysterectomy), for rehabilitation measures (e.g., breast reconstruction), and for various other purposes of improving quality of life for cancer clients when a cure is impossible (e.g., palliative and supportive measures).

Radiation therapy is the use of high-energy ionizing emissions from a radioactive source to destroy malignant cells with as little damage to normal tissues as possible (Meier, 2005). It can be used singly or in combination with other forms of treatment to achieve maximum tumor control. It is also used as a palliative measure to control the pain of bone metastasis in clients with advanced neoplastic disease.

Chemotherapy is the administration of antineoplastic drugs, in a systemic or regional manner, to cure or control a malignancy by destroying tumor cells without excessive destruction of normal cells (Meier, 2005). These drugs can effect a cure in about 10 percent of all cancers. When a cure is not possible, they may be given for palliative measures, to control symptoms, or to extend the client's useful life. They are often given in combination with other therapies, such as surgery or radiation therapy. Most chemotherapeutic agents have significant adverse effects (e.g., bone marrow depression, severe nausea and vomiting, alopecia), which should be measured against the potential benefits when outlining a course of treatment for a cancer client.

With respect to the psychosomatic dimensions of cancer, the classic work of Simonton and Simonton (1975) must be considered. They have reported positive results with autogenic relaxation and mental imagery in the role of adjunct therapy for clients with malignant disease. Once relaxation has been achieved, the individual is taught to visualize the malignancy within his or her body. Then the person visualizes a killer attack (from his or her own fantasy) on the malignant cells, followed by a visualization of the army of white cells transporting the dead cancer cells out of the body. The Simontons have had convincing results with this technique, particularly in clients who maintain a positive attitude about therapy. They strongly emphasize a high correlation between positive response to treatment and positive attitudes, both to the disease and to life in a more general sense. They also emphasize that the application of relaxation and visualization techniques is an *adjunct* to traditional treatment, not an *alternative*.

Psychotherapy may help those possibly cancer-prone individuals with type C personality characteristics. The individual must learn to express the feelings and emotions that have been suppressed. Overcoming some of the characteristics associated with type C personality may have the potential of diminishing the risk of developing cancer and facilitating recovery from the disease. It is thought that immune responses are enhanced when the individual perceives a greater feeling of well being through the attainment of a more positive sense of self-control (Karren et al., 2002).

Coronary Heart Disease

Surgical intervention with coronary artery bypass grafting (CABG) is indicated for clients with significant obstruction of the major coronary arteries. It provides symptomatic relief in 80 to 90 percent of cases (Tazbir & Keresztes, 2005).

Percutaneous transluminal coronary angioplasty (PTCA) is a technique that does not alter the general disease process but is an alternative approach to CABG. PTCA attempts to restore patency of the arterial lumen by compressing atheromatous plaques against the wall of the artery. This procedure reduces the symptoms of CHD, but the underlying progression of atherosclerosis continues.

Chemotherapeutic agents used in the treatment of CHD include:

1. Vasodilators: to increase coronary tissue perfusion (e.g., nitroglycerin, isosorbide).
2. Beta-adrenergic blocking agents: to treat angina and hypertension (e.g., propranolol, atenolol).
3. Calcium antagonists: to treat angina and hypertension (e.g., verapamil, nifedipine, diltiazem).
4. Antihyperlipidemic agents: to lower serum cholesterol and triglyceride levels (e.g., simvastatin, atorvastatin, gemfibrozil).

Various techniques, such as progressive relaxation, autohypnosis, meditation, biofeedback, and group therapy, have been tried (with mixed results) in an attempt to modify the type A behavior pattern associated with CHD. Positive outcomes in the reduction of type A behaviors have been observed with combinations of education, interpersonal counseling, and behavior modification therapy. Karren and associates (2002) report that eight controlled studies have now shown that the toxic, hostile parts of type A (and even the excessive busyness) can indeed be transformed into safer behaviors.

Peptic Ulcer

The focus of treatment for peptic ulcer disease is to alleviate symptoms, promote healing, and prevent complications and recurrence.

Pharmacological interventions include:

1. Antacids: to neutralize gastric acid (e.g., calcium carbonate, magnesium/aluminum salts).
2. Antisecretory agents: to inhibit secretion of hydrochloric acid (HCl) in the stomach.

    a. Histamine H_2 antagonists (e.g., cimetidine, ranitidine).

    b. Proton pump inhibitors (e.g., omeprazole, esomeprazole, lansoprazole)

    c. Anticholinergics (e.g., atropine, belladonna, propantheline).

3. Cytoprotective agents: to coat ulcerated mucosal tissue and inhibit pepsin activity (e.g., sucralfate).

4. Antibiotics and anti-infectives: treatment of *H. pylori* infection (e.g., amoxicillin; tetracycline; metronidazole).

The selection of foods in dietary intervention is determined by client tolerance. The traditional bland diet with emphasis on dairy products has become controversial. Spicy foods do, however, cause dyspepsia in some individuals. A reduction or elimination of caffeine and alcohol is recommended. Smoking and the intake of aspirin should be avoided.

Surgical intervention may be necessary if medical management does not result in symptomatic relief, when serious, life-threatening complications occur, or when there is possible malignancy. The most common types of surgical intervention include gastrectomy (removal of a portion of the stomach), vagotomy (severing the vagus nerve to reduce vagally stimulated HCl), and pyloroplasty (repairing or reopening of the pylorus to enhance gastric emptying).

Psychotherapy has been beneficial with ulcer clients whose personality characteristics, ego strength, and coping mechanisms favor increased vulnerability to stress. Troublesome conflicts that have been associated with peptic ulcer disease, such as passivity, dependency, aggression, anger, and frustration, need to be evaluated and properly addressed in treatment, respecting the client's defensive structure and need for support and reassurance. In studies with peptic ulcer clients, a combination of medication with psychotherapy has been more beneficial than treatment with medication alone. Levenson (2003) states:

> Patients with peptic ulcer whose condition is refractory to treatment should be screened for high state and trait anxiety characteristics. Cognitive-behavioral therapy can help patients feel a greater sense of mastery over feared calamities and less helpless and overwhelmed. Clinicians also should identify depression, overuse of NSAIDs, alcohol abuse, smoking, job stress, and other psychosocial factors that may aggravate peptic ulcer for appropriate therapeutic intervention. (p. 646)

Essential Hypertension

The treatment of clients with hypertension is directed toward lowering blood pressure in an attempt to halt or reverse progressive organ damage. Some individuals can lower their blood pressure by altering their lifestyle. If the individual is unable or unwilling to do so, pharmacological therapy is recommended. Many individuals are treated with a combination of both approaches.

Dietary Modifications

Two effective nonpharmacological modalities for the reduction of elevated blood pressure include weight reduction and sodium restriction. It may be necessary for the individual who is on diuretic therapy to ensure that there is a sufficient intake of potassium, either through diet or with supplements. It is also important for the individual with high blood pressure to decrease intake of caffeine, alcohol, and saturated fats.

Environmental Factors

Individuals with hypertension should not smoke.

Physical Exercise

Increased physical activity (e.g., 30 to 45 minutes of brisk walking three to five times a week) has been shown to lower blood pressure in some hypertensive individuals. Exercise helps prevent and control hypertension by reducing weight, decreasing peripheral resistance, and decreasing body fat (Fanning & Lewis, 2003). Caution with isotonic exercises, such as weight lifting, is advised for hypertensive individuals, as an acute rise in blood pressure can occur.

Pharmacotherapy

Physicians commonly take a "stepped-care" approach to prescribing antihypertensive medications. If weight control, dietary restrictions, and physical exercise are not sufficient to maintain a lowered pressure, the first step of pharmacological intervention is usually with a low dose of a diuretic, beta-blocker, calcium channel blocker, or angiotensin-converting enzyme inhibitor. If these medications are not successful in lowering the pressure, either the dosage is increased or a second drug of a different classification is substituted or added (DeMartinis, 2005). This continues until the desired blood pressure is achieved, side effects become intolerable, or the maximum amount of each drug has been reached.

Relaxation Techniques

Relaxation techniques, such as meditation, yoga, hypnosis, and biofeedback reduce blood pressure in some individuals. They are especially useful for individuals with higher initial pressures and as adjunctive therapy to pharmacological treatment. Supportive psychotherapy, during which the individual is encouraged to express honest feelings, particularly anger, may also be helpful.

Migraine Headache

Pharmacological intervention for migraine headache is directed toward prevention with drugs such as propranolol, amitriptyline, fluoxetine, verapamil, venlafaxine, topiramate, or divalproex sodium. Once a migraine attack has begun, some physicians will administer an injection of a narcotic, such as meperidine or codeine, which blocks the pain and allows the individual to sleep until the attack subsides. A newer class of drugs, the serotonin receptor agonists (sumatriptan, naratriptan, zolmitriptan, almotriptan, eletriptan, frovatriptan, and rizatriptan), which are available in oral, injectable, and inhalant forms, has been shown to be effective in interrupting migraine attacks.

Other treatments during a migraine attack that may provide some relief include cold compresses to the head and neck; bedrest in a quiet, darkened room; application of pressure to the temples; and perhaps heat to neck and shoulder muscles that have contracted in response to headache pain.

Some medications are prescribed to be taken at the first sign of onset of a migraine attack. If taken in the prodromal phase at the very first sign, ergotamine tartrate may prevent the vasodilation that creates the pain of migraine. It is ineffective once the attack has begun. Ergotamine is available in combination with other drugs, such as caffeine, sedatives, and antiemetics, and is marketed in various forms, including tablets, suppositories, inhalants, and sublinguals. Ergotamine can safely be taken only once or twice a week at the most, so it is not appropriate for individuals who have headaches more often than this. It can be very harmful because of its vasoconstrictive properties and potential for preventing adequate tissue perfusion.

A number of nonpharmacological interventions associated with migraine management and prevention have been suggested:

1. Reduce or eliminate aggravating factors. This can be accomplished by keeping a headache diary for a time, recording the time of day the headache occurs and circumstances (including food/medication/beverage intake) that may have triggered the attack.
2. Regularly participate in enjoyable hobbies and relaxing activities. Practice regular relaxation exercises.
3. Regular physical exercise is advisable, unless it has been known to provoke migraine attacks.
4. Try to obtain the same amount of sleep each night. Do not oversleep or go without sleep.
5. Biofeedback, behavior modification, yoga, or meditation appear to be worthwhile in some cases of migraine.
6. Migraine may be related to repressed or suppressed anger, hostility, and guilt. Honest expression of these feelings may remove some of the emotional predisposition to the disorder. Psychotherapy may be necessary in some instances, both to help relieve unresolved anger and to help modify some of the characteristics associated with "migraine personality."
7. Some individuals report relief from migraines after they quit smoking. It is possible that the products of combustion may play a role in dilating arteries.

Rheumatoid Arthritis

The goals of therapy for rheumatoid arthritis are to relieve discomfort and achieve remission. Treatment depends on the extent of the disability, psychosocial variables, and the results of laboratory examinations.

Pharmacological Treatment

Medications used in the treatment of rheumatoid arthritis include the following:

1. Nonsteroidal anti-inflammatory agents (NSAIDs). Examples include ibuprofen, naproxen, ketoprofen, indomethacin, fenoprofen, and piroxicam. This category also includes the selective Cox-2 inhibitors (e.g., celecoxib and valdecoxib). However, these medications have recently come under a great deal of controversy. One drug within this classification, rofecoxib, was removed from the worldwide market because of safety concerns associated with an increased risk of cardiovascular events (including heart attack and stroke).
2. Disease-modifying antirheumatic drugs (DMARDs). These drugs refer to a second line of defense, when NSAIDs are deemed ineffective. DMARDs include hydroxychloroquine, gold salts, penicillamine, methotrexate, azathioprine, sulfasalazine, cyclosporine, leflunomide, etanercept, adalimumab, and infliximab (MacDonald, 2005).
3. Corticosteroids. Low-dose prednisone is used as a bridge, to carry clients from unsuccessful NSAID therapy until they experience the benefits of the slower-acting DMARDs (MacDonald, 2005).

Surgical Treatment

Various surgical treatments are available for clients with rheumatoid arthritis. Synovectomy is performed to relieve pain and maintain muscle and joint balance. Joint fusion may provide stability to a joint and decrease deformity. Spinal fusion may be necessary to treat subluxation. Total joint replacement is performed to restore motion to a joint and function to the muscles, ligaments, and other soft tissue structures that control a joint (MacDonald, 2005).

Psychological Treatment

Psychotherapy and prompt recognition and treatment of psychiatric morbidity may help clients cope and adapt to this condition. A client's initial reaction to the diagnosis of rheumatoid arthritis depends on the degree of incapacity at the time and the immediate threat to his or her lifestyle. Denial of the illness is a common initial response, followed progressively by other responses associated with the grieving response. Clients may blame themselves or believe that the disease is the result of past behaviors. Depression may need to be treated separately. Clients should be encouraged to function as independently as possible. The focus on cure should be deflected to a focus on control of the disease and prevention of disability.

Ulcerative Colitis

The goals of care for the client with ulcerative colitis are to relieve discomfort and promote and maintain remission of the disease. This is accomplished through nutritional therapy, pharmacological treatment, surgical intervention if necessary, and psychological support.

Nutritional Therapy

There are no general restrictions on diet. Clients should avoid foods that they identify as irritating. Usually a low-residue diet is initiated and advanced as tolerated with one food added at a time. Milk may be a problem for some clients. When the disease is severe or extensive, and absorption problems have resulted in dehydration and cachexia, total parenteral nutrition may be necessary.

Pharmacological Treatment

Pharmacological treatment may include sulfasalazine, which appears to have both anti-inflammatory and antimicrobial properties. Severe forms of the disease are treated with corticosteroids (e.g., hydrocortisone, prednisone, prednisolone). Corticosteroids provide relief through suppression of inflammation but do not cure ulcerative colitis. To provide symptomatic relief, antidiarrheals (e.g., loperamide, diphenoxylate) and antispasmodics (e.g., propantheline) may be prescribed. Antibiotics (e.g., metronidazole, ciprofloxacin) may be administered when an infectious process is present.

Surgical Treatment

Surgery is indicated for the client with ulcerative colitis intractable to medical management or to treat complications such as perforation, hemorrhage, obstruction, or toxic megacolon (Rogers, 2005). Types of surgery that may be performed include proctocolectomy with permanent or continent ileostomy, total colectomy with ileorectal anastomosis, or total colectomy with ileoanal reservoir. Surgery is considered curative, and recurrences rarely occur.

Psychological Support

Ulcerative colitis can be a lifetime illness with periods of exacerbation and remission that can disrupt the person's life situation. Because emotions and stress have been known to play a role in exacerbation of the illness, psychological support may help to decrease the frequency of these attacks by helping the individual to recognize the stressors that precipitate exacerbations and identify more adaptive ways of coping. The person with ulcerative colitis often feels a lack of control over his or her life. Psychological support may help the client cope with feelings of insecurity, dependency, and depression. It is extremely important that the individual express feelings of repressed or suppressed anger and hostility.

Fears and anxieties associated with possible sexual dysfunction need to be explored. The individual who has undergone surgical intervention for ulcerative colitis may be experiencing a disturbed body image that could interfere with sexual functioning. The person must be given the opportunity to discuss these sexual concerns. He or she may require assistance in communicating these concerns to the sexual partner. Alternate ways of meeting sexuality needs can be explored.

SUMMARY

Psychophysiological disorders are those in which psychological factors contribute to the initiation or exacerbation of the physical condition. There is evidence of either demonstrable organic pathology or involvement of a known pathophysiological process. The *DSM-IV-TR* (APA, 2000) identifies this category as "psychological factors affecting medical condition." Types of psychological factors identified by the *DSM-IV-TR* include mental disorders, psychological symptoms, personality traits or coping styles, maladaptive health behaviors, stress-related physiological responses, and others.

Virtually any organic disorder can be considered psychophysiological. The following disorders were discussed in this chapter:

- Asthma
- Cancer
- Coronary heart disease
- Peptic ulcer disease
- Essential hypertension
- Migraine headache

● Rheumatoid arthritis
● Ulcerative colitis

Psychophysiological disorders are thought to occur when the body remains in a prolonged state of moderate-to-severe anxiety. This prolonged period of arousal may contribute to the initiation or exacerbation of the physical symptoms in otherwise predisposed individuals.

Predisposing factors to the development of psychophysiological disorders include heredity, allergies, environmental conditions, viruses, elevated serum lipoproteins, cigarette smoking, alcohol abuse, specific foods, and dysfunctional immune system. The following personality characteristics have also been implicated in the predisposition to psychophysiological disorders:

● Asthma: unfulfilled dependency needs
● Cancer: repressed anger and low self-esteem (type C personality)
● Coronary heart disease: competitive drive and continual sense of time urgency (type A personality)
● Peptic ulcer: unfulfilled dependency needs

● Hypertension: suppressed anger
● Migraine headache: repressed or suppressed anger, perfectionism
● Rheumatoid arthritis: repressed anger, self-sacrificing traits
● Ulcerative colitis: repressed anger, obsessive–compulsive traits

Nursing care of the client with psychophysiological disorders is accomplished using the steps of the nursing process. Background assessment data were presented, along with nursing diagnoses common to each disorder and to the general psychophysiological condition. Interventions appropriate to each general nursing diagnosis and relevant outcome criteria for each were included. An overview of current medical treatment modalities for each disorder was discussed.

Nurses in all areas of clinical practice should be aware of client potential for psychophysiological responses and the possible psychosocial influences associated with these disorders. Nurses will most likely (at least initially) encounter these clients in areas other than psychiatry.

REVIEW QUESTIONS

SELF-EXAMINATION/LEARNING EXERCISE

Match the following psychophysiological disorders to the psychosocial profile with which it has been associated:

_____ 1. Asthma

_____ 2. Cancer

_____ 3. Coronary heart disease

_____ 4. Peptic ulcer disease

_____ 5. Essential hypertension

_____ 6. Migraine headache

_____ 7. Rheumatoid arthritis

_____ 8. Ulcerative colitis

a. Competitive; aggressive; ambitious; no time for leisure; never satisfied with accomplishments; easily aroused hostility.

b. Obsessive–compulsive by nature; anxious; rigid; excessively neat; repressed anger; depression is common.

c. Unfulfilled dependency needs; anxiety and depression are common; fearful and emotionally labile

d. Self-sacrificing; inhibited; perfectionistic; repressed anger; depression is common.

e. Unfulfilled dependency needs; suppressed anxiety; resentment and frustration resulting in increased gastric secretion.

f. Perfectionistic; somewhat rigid; compulsive; sets unrealistic expectations; suppresses or represses anger.

g. "The nice guy"; suppresses anger; low self-esteem; depression is common; feelings of hopelessness.

h. Suppresses anger; may stem from not being able to express anger as a child

9. Which of the following is the primary nursing diagnosis for clients in the general category of psychophysiological disorders?
   a. Pain, evidenced by classic pain behaviors
   b. Ineffective coping, evidenced by exacerbation of physical symptoms
   c. Ineffective role performance, evidenced by inability to perform usual responsibilities
   d. Activity intolerance, evidenced by inability to participate in activities

10. The difference between somatoform disorders and psychophysiological disorders can be explained by which of the following statements?
    a. Somatoform disorders occur at the panic level of anxiety and psychophysiological disorders do not.
    b. Psychophysiological disorders occur at the panic level of anxiety and somatoform disorders do not.
    c. Organic pathology is evident in somatoform disorders but not in psychophysiological disorders.
    d. Organic pathology is evident in psychophysiological disorders but not in somatoform disorders.

37

PERSONALITY DISORDERS

C H A P T E R   O U T L I N E

OBJECTIVES

HISTORICAL ASPECTS

TYPES OF PERSONALITY DISORDERS

APPLICATION OF THE NURSING PROCESS

TREATMENT MODALITIES

SUMMARY

REVIEW QUESTIONS

K E Y   T E R M S

histrionic
narcissism
object constancy
passive–aggressive

schizoid
schizotypal
splitting

C O R E   C O N C E P T

personality

O B J E C T I V E S

After reading this chapter, the student will be able to:

1. Define *personality*.
2. Compare stages of personality development according to Sullivan, Erikson, and Mahler.
3. Identify various types of personality disorders.
4. Discuss historical and epidemiological statistics related to various personality disorders.
5. Describe symptomatology associated with borderline personality disorder and antisocial personality disorder, and use these data in client assessment.
6. Identify predisposing factors for borderline personality disorder and antisocial personality disorder.

7. Formulate nursing diagnoses and goals of care for clients with borderline personality disorder and antisocial personality disorder.
8. Describe appropriate nursing interventions for behaviors associated with borderline personality disorder and antisocial personality disorder.
9. Evaluate nursing care of clients with borderline personality disorder and antisocial personality disorder.
10. Discuss various modalities relevant to treatment of personality disorder.

 he word **personality** is derived from the Greek term *persona*. It was used originally to describe the theatrical mask worn by some dramatic actors at the time. Over the years, it lost its connotation of pretense and illusion and came to represent the person behind the mask—the "real" person.

The *DSM-IV-TR* (American Psychiatric Association [APA], 2000) defines personality *traits* as "enduring

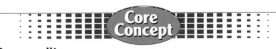

Personality
The totality of emotional and behavioral characteristics that are particular to a specific person and that remain somewhat stable and predictable over time.

715

patterns of perceiving, relating to, and thinking about the environment and oneself that are exhibited in a wide range of social and personal contexts." Personality *disorders* occur when these traits become inflexible and maladaptive and cause either significant functional impairment or subjective distress. These disorders are coded on axis II of the multiaxial diagnostic system used by the APA (see Chapter 2 for an explanation of this system). Virtually all individuals exhibit some behaviors associated with the various personality disorders from time to time. It is only when significant functional impairment occurs in response to these personality characteristics that the individual is thought to have a personality disorder.

Personality development occurs in response to a number of biological and psychological influences. These variables include (but are not limited to) heredity, temperament, experiential learning, and social interaction. A number of theorists have attempted to provide information about personality development. Most suggest that it occurs in an orderly, stepwise fashion. These stages overlap, however, as maturation occurs at different rates in different individuals. The theories of Sullivan (1953),

Erikson (1963), and Mahler (Mahler, Pine, & Bergman, 1975) were presented at length in Chapter 3. The stages of personality development according to these three theorists are compared in Table 37–1. The nurse should understand "normal" personality development before learning about what is considered maladaptive.

Historical and epidemiological aspects of personality disorders are discussed in this chapter. Predisposing factors that have been implicated in the etiology of personality disorders are presented. Symptomatology is explained to provide background knowledge for assessing clients with personality disorders.

Individuals with personality disorders are not often treated in acute care settings for the personality disorder as their primary psychiatric diagnosis. However, many clients with other psychiatric and medical diagnoses manifest symptoms of personality disorders. Nurses are likely to encounter clients with these personality characteristics frequently in all health care settings.

Nurses working in psychiatric settings may often encounter clients with borderline and antisocial personality characteristics. The behavior of borderline clients is very unstable, and hospitalization is often required as a

| ■ TABLE 37–1   Comparison of Personality Development—Sullivan, Erikson, and Mahler |

MAJOR DEVELOPMENTAL TASKS AND DESIGNATED AGES		
SULLIVAN	**ERIKSON**	**MAHLER**
Birth to 18 months: Relief from anxiety through oral gratification of needs.	Birth to 18 months: To develop a basic trust in the mothering figure and be able to generalize it to others.	Birth to 1 month: Fulfillment of basic needs for survival and comfort
18 months to 6 years: Learning to experience a delay in personal gratification without undue anxiety.	18 months to 3 years: To gain some self-control and independence within the environment.	1 to 5 months: Developing awareness of external source of need fulfillment.
6 to 9 years: Learning to form satisfactory peer relationships.	3 to 6 years: To develop a sense of purpose and the ability to initiate and direct own activities.	5 to 10 months: Commencement of a primary recognition of separateness from the mothering figure.
9 to 12 years: Learning to form satisfactory relationships with persons of the same sex; the initiation of feelings of affection for another person.	6 to 12 years: To achieve a sense of self-confidence by learning, competing, performing successfully, and receiving recognition from significant others, peers, and acquaintances.	10 to 16 months: Increased independence through locomotor functioning; increased sense of separateness of self.
12 to 14 years: Learning to form satisfactory relationships with persons of the opposite sex; developing a sense of identity.	12 to 20 years: To integrate the tasks mastered in the previous stages into a secure sense of self.	16 to 24 months: Acute awareness of separateness of self; learning to seek "emotional refueling" from mothering figure to maintain feeling of security.
14 to 21 years: Establishing self-identity; experiences satisfying relationships; working to develop a lasting, intimate opposite-sex relationship.	20 to 30 years: To form an intense, lasting relationship or a commitment to another person, a cause, an institution, or a creative effort.	24 to 36 months: Sense of separateness established; on the way to object constancy: able to internalize a sustained image of loved object/person when it is out of sight; resolution of separation anxiety.
	30 to 65 years: To achieve the life goals established for oneself, while also considering the welfare of future generations.	
	65 years to death: To review one's life and derive meaning from both positive and negative events, while achieving a positive sense of self-worth.	

result of attempts at self-injury. The client with antisocial personality disorder may enter the psychiatric arena as a result of judicially ordered evaluation. Psychiatric intervention may be an alternative to imprisonment for antisocial behavior if it is deemed potentially helpful.

Nursing care of clients with borderline personality disorder or antisocial personality disorder is presented in this chapter in the context of the nursing process. Various medical treatment modalities for personality disorders are explored.

HISTORICAL ASPECTS

The concept of a personality disorder has been described for thousands of years (Phillips, Yen, & Gunderson, 2003). In the 4th century B.C., Hippocrates concluded that all disease stemmed from an excess of or imbalance among four bodily humors: yellow bile, black bile, blood, and phlegm. Hippocrates identified four fundamental personality styles that he concluded stemmed from excesses in the four humors: the irritable and hostile choleric (yellow bile); the pessimistic melancholic (black bile); the overly optimistic and extraverted sanguine (blood); and the apathetic phlegmatic (phlegm).

Within the profession of medicine, the first recognition that personality disorders, apart from psychosis, were cause for their own special concern was in 1801, with the awareness that an individual can behave irrationally even when the powers of intellect are intact. Nineteenth-century psychiatrists embraced the term *moral insanity*, the concept of which defines what we know today as personality disorders.

A major difficulty for psychiatrists has been the establishment of a classification of personality disorders. The *DSM-IV-TR* provides specific criteria for diagnosing these disorders. The *DSM-IV-TR* groups the personality disorders into three clusters. These clusters, and the disorders classified under each, are described as follows:

1. Cluster A: behaviors described as odd or eccentric
   a. Paranoid personality disorder
   b. Schizoid personality disorder
   c. Schizotypal personality disorder
2. Cluster B: behaviors described as dramatic, emotional, or erratic
   a. Antisocial personality disorder
   b. Borderline personality disorder
   c. Histrionic personality disorder
   d. Narcissistic personality disorder
3. Cluster C: behaviors described as anxious or fearful
   a. Avoidant personality disorder
   b. Dependent personality disorder
   c. Obsessive–compulsive personality disorder
      NOTE: The third edition of the *DSM* included passive–aggressive personality disorder in cluster C.

In the *DSM-IV-TR*, this disorder has been included in the section on *Criteria Provided for Further Study*. For purposes of this text, passive–aggressive personality disorder will be described with the cluster C disorders.

Historically, individuals with personality disorders have been labeled as "bad" or "immoral" and as deviants in the range of normal personality dimensions. The events and sequences that result in pathology of the personality are complicated and difficult to unravel. Continued study is needed to facilitate understanding of this complex behavioral phenomenon.

TYPES OF PERSONALITY DISORDERS

Paranoid Personality Disorder

Definition and Epidemiological Statistics

The *DSM-IV-TR* defines paranoid personality disorder as "a pervasive distrust and suspiciousness of others such that their motives are interpreted as malevolent, beginning by early adulthood and present in a variety of contexts" (APA, 2000). Sadock and Sadock (2003) identify the characteristic feature as a long-standing suspiciousness and mistrust of people in general. Prevalence is difficult to establish because individuals with the disorder seldom seek assistance for their problem or require hospitalization. When they present for treatment at the insistence of others, they may be able to pull themselves together sufficiently so that their behavior does not appear maladaptive. The disorder is more commonly diagnosed in men than in women.

Clinical Picture

Individuals with paranoid personality disorder are constantly on guard, hypervigilant, and ready for any real or imagined threat. They appear tense and irritable. They have developed a hard exterior and become immune or insensitive to the feelings of others. They avoid interactions with other people, lest they be forced to relinquish some of their own power. They always feel that others are there to take advantage of them.

They are extremely oversensitive and tend to misinterpret even minute cues within the environment, magnifying and distorting them into thoughts of trickery and deception. Because they trust no one, they are constantly "testing" the honesty of others. Their intimidating manner provokes almost everyone with whom they come in contact into exasperation and anger.

Individuals who are paranoid maintain their self-esteem by attributing their shortcomings to others. They do not accept responsibility for their own behaviors and feelings and project this responsibility on to others. They are envious and hostile toward others who are highly successful and believe the only reason they are not as successful is because they have been treated unfairly. People who are paranoid are extremely vulnerable and constantly on the defensive. Any real or imagined threat can release hostility and anger that is fueled by animosities from the past. The desire for reprisal and vindication is so intense that a possible loss of control can result in aggression and violence. These outbursts are usually brief, and the paranoid person soon regains the external control, rationalizes the behavior, and reconstructs the defenses central to his or her personality pattern.

The *DSM-IV-TR* diagnostic criteria for paranoid personality disorder are presented in Table 37–2.

Predisposing Factors

Research has indicated a possible hereditary link in paranoid personality disorder. Studies have revealed a higher incidence of paranoid personality disorder among relatives of clients with schizophrenia than among control subjects (Sadock & Sadock, 2003).

Psychosocially, people with paranoid personality disorder may have been subjected to parental antagonism and harassment. They likely served as scapegoats for displaced parental aggression and gradually relinquished all hope of affection and approval. They learned to perceive the world as harsh and unkind, a place calling for protective vigilance and mistrust. They entered the world with a "chip-on-the-shoulder" attitude and were met with many rebuffs and rejections from others. Anticipating

humiliation and betrayal by others, the paranoid person learned to attack first.

Schizoid Personality Disorder

Definition and Epidemiological Statistics

Schizoid personality disorder is characterized primarily by a profound defect in the ability to form personal relationships or to respond to others in any meaningful, emotional way (Phillips, Yen, & Gunderson, 2003). These individuals display a lifelong pattern of social withdrawal, and their discomfort with human interaction is very apparent. The prevalence of schizoid personality disorder within the general population has been estimated at between 3 and 7.5 percent. Significant numbers of people with the disorder are never observed in a clinical setting. The gender ratio of the disorder is unknown, although it is diagnosed more frequently in men.

Clinical Picture

People with schizoid personality disorder appear cold, aloof, and indifferent to others. They prefer to work in isolation and are unsociable, with little need or desire for emotional ties. They are able to invest enormous affective energy in intellectual pursuits.

In the presence of others they appear shy, anxious, or uneasy. They are inappropriately serious about everything and have difficulty acting in a lighthearted manner. Their behavior and conversation exhibit little or no spontaneity. Typically they are unable to experience pleasure, and their affect is commonly bland and constricted.

The *DSM-IV-TR* diagnostic criteria for schizoid personality disorder are presented in Table 37–3.

TABLE 37–2 Diagnostic Criteria for Paranoid Personality Disorder

A. A pervasive distrust and suspiciousness of others such that their motives are interpreted as malevolent, beginning by early adulthood and present in a variety of contexts, as indicated by four (or more) of the following:
1. Suspects, without sufficient basis, that others are exploiting, harming, or deceiving him or her.
2. Is preoccupied with unjustified doubts about the loyalty or trustworthiness of friends or associates.
3. Is reluctant to confide in others because of unwarranted fear that the information will be used maliciously against him or her.
4. Reads hidden demeaning or threatening meanings into benign remarks or events.
5. Persistently bears grudges, (i.e., is unforgiving of insults, injuries, or slights).
6. Perceives attacks on his or her character or reputation that are not apparent to others and is quick to react angrily or to counterattack.
7. Has recurrent suspicions, without justification, regarding fidelity of spouse or sexual partner.
B. Does not occur exclusively during the course of schizophrenia, a mood disorder with psychotic features, or another psychotic disorder and is not due to the direct physiological effects of a general medical condition.

SOURCE: American Psychiatric Association (2000), with permission.

TABLE 37–3 Diagnostic Criteria for Schizoid Personality Disorder

A. A pervasive pattern of detachment from social relationships and a restricted range of expression of emotions in interpersonal settings, beginning by early adulthood and present in a variety of contexts, as indicated by four (or more) of the following:
1. Neither desires nor enjoys close relationships, including being part of a family.
2. Almost always chooses solitary activities.
3. Has little, if any, interest in having sexual experiences with another person.
4. Takes pleasure in few, if any, activities.
5. Lacks close friends or confidants other than first-degree relatives.
6. Appears indifferent to the praise or criticism of others.
7. Shows emotional coldness, detachment, or flattened affectivity.
B. Does not occur exclusively during the course of schizophrenia, a mood disorder with psychotic features, another psychotic disorder, or a pervasive development disorder and is not due to the direct physiological effects of a general medical condition.

SOURCE: American Psychiatric Association (2000), with permission.

Predisposing Factors

Although the role of heredity in the etiology of schizoid personality disorder is unclear, the feature of introversion appears to be a highly inheritable characteristic (Phillips, Yen, & Gunderson, 2003). Further studies are required before definitive statements can be made.

Psychosocially, the development of schizoid personality is probably influenced by early interactional patterns that the person found to be cold and unsatisfying. The childhoods of these individuals have often been characterized as bleak, cold, unempathic, and notably lacking in nurturing. A child brought up with this type of parenting may become a schizoid adult if that child possesses a temperamental disposition that is shy, anxious, and introverted. Phillips, Yen, and Gunderson (2003) state:

> Clinicians have noted that schizoid personality disorder occurs in adults who experienced cold, neglectful, and ungratifying relationships in early childhood, which leads these persons to assume that relationships are not valuable or worth pursuing. (pp. 812–813)

Schizotypal Personality Disorder

Definition and Epidemiological Statistics

Individuals with **schizotypal** personality disorder were once described as "latent schizophrenics." Their behavior is odd and eccentric but does not decompensate to the level of schizophrenia. Schizotypal personality is a graver form of the pathologically less severe schizoid personality pattern. Recent studies indicate that approximately 3 percent of the population has this disorder (APA, 200).

Clinical Picture

Individuals with schizotypal personality disorder are aloof and isolated and behave in a bland and apathetic manner. Magical thinking, ideas of reference, illusions, and depersonalization are part of their everyday world. Examples include superstitiousness, belief in clairvoyance, telepathy, or "sixth sense," or beliefs that "others can feel my feelings" (APA, 2000).

The speech pattern is sometimes bizarre. People with this disorder often cannot orient their thoughts logically and become lost in personal irrelevancies and in tangential asides that seem vague, digressive, and not pertinent to the topic at hand. This feature of their personality only further alienates them from others.

Under stress, these individuals may decompensate and demonstrate psychotic symptoms, such as delusional thoughts, hallucinations, or bizarre behaviors, but they are usually of brief duration (Sadock & Sadock, 2003). They often talk or gesture to themselves, as if "living in their own world." Affect is bland or inappropriate, such

TABLE 37–4 Diagnostic Criteria for Schizotypal Personality Disorder

A. A pervasive pattern of social and interpersonal deficits marked by acute discomfort with, and reduced capacity for, close relationships as well as by cognitive or perceptual distortions and eccentricities of behavior, beginning by early adulthood and present in a variety of contexts, as indicated by five (or more) of the following:
  1. Ideas of reference (excluding delusions of reference)
  2. Odd beliefs or magical thinking that influences behavior and is inconsistent with subcultural norms (e.g., superstitiousness, belief in clairvoyance, telepathy, or "sixth sense"; in children and adolescents, bizarre fantasies or preoccupations)
  3. Unusual perceptual experiences, including bodily illusions
  4. Odd thinking and speech (e.g., vague, circumstantial, metaphorical, overelaborate, or stereotyped)
  5. Suspiciousness or paranoid ideation
  6. Inappropriate or constricted affect
  7. Behavior or appearance that is odd, eccentric, or peculiar
  8. Excessive social anxiety that does not diminish with familiarity and tends to be associated with paranoid fears rather than negative judgments about self
B. Does not occur exclusively during the course of schizophrenia, a mood disorder with psychotic features, another psychotic disorder, or a pervasive developmental disorder.

SOURCE: American Psychiatric Association (2000), with permission.

as laughing at their own problems or at a situation that most people would consider sad.

The *DSM-IV-TR* diagnostic criteria for schizotypal personality disorder are presented in Table 37–4.

Predisposing Factors

Some evidence suggests that schizotypal personality disorder is more common among the first-degree biological relatives of people with schizophrenia than among the general population, indicating a possible hereditary factor (APA, 2000). Although speculative, other biogenic factors that may contribute to the development of this disorder include anatomical deficits or neurochemical dysfunctions resulting in diminished activation, minimal pleasure–pain sensibilities, and impaired cognitive functions. These possible biological etiological factors support the close link between schizotypal personality disorder and schizophrenia and are considered in classifying schizotypal personality disorder with schizophrenia rather than with the personality disorders in the *International Classification of Diseases (ICD-10)* (Phillips, Yen, & Gunderson, 2003).

The early family dynamics of the individual with schizotypal personality disorder may have been characterized by indifference, impassivity, or formality, leading to a pattern of discomfort with personal affection and closeness. Early on, affective deficits made them unattractive and unrewarding social companions. They were likely shunned, overlooked, rejected, and disgraced by others, resulting in feelings of low self-esteem and a marked distrust of interpersonal relations. Having failed repeatedly to cope with these adversities, they began to withdraw and reduce contact with individuals and situations that evoked sadness and humiliation. Their new inner world provided them with a more significant and potentially rewarding existence than the one experienced in reality.

Antisocial Personality Disorder

Definition and Epidemiological Statistics

Antisocial personality disorder is a pattern of socially irresponsible, exploitative, and guiltless behavior that reflects a disregard for the rights of others (Phillips, Yen, & Gunderson, 2003). These individuals exploit and manipulate others for personal gain and have a general disregard for the law. They have difficulty sustaining consistent employment and in developing stable relationships. It is one of the oldest and best researched of the personality disorders and has been included in all editions of the *Diagnostic and Statistical Manual of Mental Disorders*. In the United States, prevalence estimates range from 3 percent in men to about 1 percent in women (APA, 2000). The disorder is more common among the lower socioeconomic classes, and particularly so among highly mobile residents of impoverished urban areas (Sadock & Sadock, 2003). The *ICD-10* identifies this disorder as *dissocial personality disorder*.

> **NOTE:** The clinical picture, predisposing factors, nursing diagnoses, and interventions for care of clients with antisocial personality disorder are presented later in this chapter.

Borderline Personality Disorder

Definition and Epidemiological Statistics

Borderline personality disorder is characterized by a pattern of intense and chaotic relationships, with affective instability and fluctuating attitudes toward other people. These individuals are impulsive, are directly and indirectly self-destructive, and lack a clear sense of identity. Prevalence estimates of borderline personality range from 2 to 3 percent of the population. It is the most common form of personality disorder, occurring in every culture (Phillips, Yen, & Gunderson, 2003). It is more common in women than in men, with female-to-male ratios being estimated as high as 4 to 1 (Finley-Belgrad & Davies, 2004). The *ICD-10* identifies this disorder as *emotionally unstable personality disorder*.

> **NOTE:** The clinical picture, predisposing factors, nursing diagnoses, and interventions for care of clients with borderline personality disorder are presented later in this chapter.

Histrionic Personality Disorder

Definition and Epidemiological Statistics

This disorder is characterized by colorful, dramatic, and extroverted behavior in excitable, emotional people. They have difficulty maintaining long-lasting relationships, although they require constant affirmation of approval and acceptance from others. The prevalence of the disorder is thought to be about 2 to 3 percent, and it is more common in women than in men.

Clinical Picture

People with histrionic personality disorder have a tendency to be self-dramatizing, attention seeking, overly gregarious, and seductive. They use manipulative and exhibitionistic behaviors in their demands to be the center of attention. People with histrionic personality disorder often demonstrate, in mild pathological form, what our society tends to foster and admire in its members: to be well liked, successful, popular, extroverted, attractive, and sociable. However, beneath these surface characteristics is a driven quality—an all-consuming need for approval and a desperate striving to be conspicuous and to evoke affection or attract attention at all costs. Failure to evoke the attention and approval they seek often results in feelings of dejection and anxiety.

Individuals with this disorder are highly distractible and flighty by nature. They have difficulty paying attention to detail. They can portray themselves as carefree and sophisticated on the one hand and as inhibited and naive on the other. They tend to be highly suggestible, impressionable, and rather easily influenced by others. They are strongly dependent.

Interpersonal relationships are fleeting and superficial. The person with histrionic personality disorder, having failed throughout life to develop the richness of inner feelings and lacking resources from which to draw, lacks the ability to provide another with genuinely sustained affection. Somatic complaints are not uncommon in these individuals, and fleeting episodes of psychosis may occur during periods of extreme stress.

The *DSM-IV-TR* diagnostic criteria for histrionic personality disorder are presented in Table 37–5.

Predisposing Factors

Neurobiological correlates have been proposed in the predisposition to histrionic personality disorder. Coccaro and Siever (2000) relate the characteristics of enhanced sensitivity and reactivity to environmental stimuli to heightened noradrenergic activity in the individual with histrionic personality disorder. They suggested that the trait of impulsivity may be associated with decreased serotonergic activity.

TABLE 37–5 Diagnostic Criteria for Histrionic Personality Disorder
A pervasive pattern of excessive emotionality and attention seeking, beginning by early adulthood and present in a variety of contexts, as indicated by five (or more) of the following: 1. Is uncomfortable in situations in which he or she is not the center of attention.   2. Interaction with others is often characterized by inappropriate sexually seductive or provocative behavior.   3. Displays rapidly shifting and shallow expression of emotions.   4. Consistently uses physical appearance to draw attention to self.   5. Has a style of speech that is excessively impressionistic and lacking in detail.   6. Shows self-dramatization, theatricality, and exaggerated expression of emotion.   7. Is suggestible, i.e., easily influenced by others or circumstances.   8. Considers relationships to be more intimate than they actually are.

SOURCE: American Psychiatric Association (2000), with permission.

Heredity also may be a factor because the disorder is apparently more common among first-degree biological relatives of people with the disorder than in the general population. Phillips, Yen, and Gunderson (2003) report on research that suggests that the behavioral characteristics of histrionic personality disorder may be associated with a biogenetically determined temperament. From this perspective, histrionic personality disorder would arise out of "an extreme variation of temperamental disposition."

From a psychosocial perspective, learning experiences may contribute to the development of histrionic personality disorder. The child may have come to learn that positive reinforcement was contingent on the ability to perform parentally approved and admired behaviors. It is likely that the child rarely received either positive or negative feedback. Parental acceptance and approval came inconsistently and only when the behaviors met parental expectations. Hannig (2005) states:

> The root causes [of histrionic personality disorder] surround an unbonded mother relationship and an abusive paternal relationship. When a child is not the center of a parent's attention, neglect, lack of bonding, and deprivation leaves one starving for attention, approval, praise, and reassurance.

Narcissistic Personality Disorder

Definition and Epidemiological Statistics

Persons with narcissistic personality disorder have an exaggerated sense of self-worth. They lack empathy, and are hypersensitive to the evaluation of others. They believe that they have the inalienable right to receive special consideration and that their desire is justification for possessing whatever they seek.

This diagnosis appeared for the first time in the third edition of the *Diagnostic and Statistical Manual of Mental Disorders*. However, the concept of **narcissism** has its roots in the 19th century. It was viewed by early psychoanalysts as a normal phase of psychosexual development. The *DSM-IV-TR* (APA, 2000) estimates that the disorder occurs in 2 to 16 percent of the clinical population and less than 1 percent of the general population. It is diagnosed more often in men than in women.

Clinical Picture

Individuals with narcissistic disorder appear to lack humility, being overly self-centered and exploiting others to fulfill their own desires. They often do not conceive of their behavior as being inappropriate or objectionable. Because they view themselves as "superior" beings, they believe they are entitled to special rights and privileges.

Although often grounded in grandiose distortions of reality, their mood is usually optimistic, relaxed, cheerful, and carefree. This mood can easily change, however, because of their fragile self-esteem. If they do not meet self-expectations, do not receive the positive feedback they expect from others, or draw criticism from others, they may respond with rage, shame, humiliation, or dejection. They may turn inward and fantasize rationalizations that convince them of their continued stature and perfection.

The exploitation of others for self-gratification results in impaired interpersonal relationships. In selecting a mate, narcissistic individuals frequently choose a person who will provide them with the praise and positive feedback that they require and who will not ask much from his or her partner in return.

The *DSM-IV-TR* diagnostic criteria for narcissistic personality disorder are presented in Table 37–6.

Predisposing Factors

Several psychodynamic theories exist regarding the predisposition to narcissistic personality disorder. Phillips, Yen, and Gunderson (2003) suggest that, as children, these individuals had their fears, failures, or dependency needs responded to with criticism, disdain, or neglect. They grow up with contempt for these behaviors in themselves and others and are unable to view others as sources of comfort and support. They project an image of invulnerability and self-sufficiency that conceals their true sense of emptiness and contributes to their inability to feel deeply.

Mark (2002) suggests that the parents of individuals with narcissistic personality disorder were often narcissistic themselves. The parents were demanding, perfectionistic, and critical, and they placed unrealistic expectations on the child. Children model their parents'

46

TABLE 37–6 Diagnostic Criteria for Narcissistic Personality Disorder

A pervasive pattern of grandiosity (in fantasy or behavior), need for admiration, and lack of empathy, beginning by early adulthood and present in a variety of contexts, as indicated by five (or more) of the following:
1. Has a grandiose sense of self-importance (e.g., exaggerates achievements and talents, expects to be recognized as superior without commensurate achievements).
2. Is preoccupied with fantasies of unlimited success, power, brilliance, beauty, or ideal love.
3. Believes that he or she is "special" and unique and can be understood only by, or should associate with, other special or high-status people (or institutions).
4. Requires excessive admiration.
5. Has a sense of entitlement (i.e., unreasonable expectations of especially favorable treatment or automatic compliance with his or her expectations).
6. Is interpersonally exploitative (i.e., takes advantage of others to achieve his or her own ends).
7. Lacks empathy: is unwilling to recognize or identify with the feelings and needs of others.
8. Is often envious of others or believes that others are envious of him or her.
9. Shows arrogant, haughty behaviors or attitudes.

SOURCE: American Psychiatric Association (2000), with permission.

behavior, giving way to the adult narcissist. Mark (2002) also suggests that the parents may have subjected the child to physical or emotional abuse or neglect.

Narcissism may also develop from an environment in which parents attempt to live their lives vicariously through their child. They expect the child to achieve the things they did not achieve, possess that which they did not possess, and have life better and easier than they did. The child is not subjected to the requirements and restrictions that may have dominated the parents' lives, and thereby grows up believing he or she is above that which is required for everyone else. Mark (2002) states:

[Some] researchers believe that parents who over-indulge their children or who provide indiscriminate praise and those who do not set limits as to what is appropriate in their children's behavior can also produce adults who will suffer from narcissistic personality disorder. The message here appears to be inconsistency – inconsistency in parenting – the child does not know where to turn or how to behave appropriately; they do not know what is reality and what is fantasy. This of course is a major aspect of the symptoms of narcissistic personality disorder – sufferers tend to shun reality.

Avoidant Personality Disorder

Definition and Epidemiological Statistics

The individual with avoidant personality disorder is extremely sensitive to rejection and because of this may lead a very socially withdrawn life. It is not that he or she is asocial; in fact, there may be a strong desire for companionship. The extreme shyness and fear of rejection, however, create needs for unusually strong guarantees of uncritical acceptance (Sadock & Sadock, 2003). Prevalence of the disorder in the general population is between 0.5 and 1 percent, and it appears to be equally common in men and women (APA, 2000).

Clinical Picture

Individuals with this disorder are awkward and uncomfortable in social situations. From a distance, others may perceive them as timid, withdrawn, or perhaps cold and strange. Those who have closer relationships with them, however, soon learn of their sensitivities, touchiness, evasiveness, and mistrustful qualities.

Their speech is usually slow and constrained, with frequent hesitations, fragmentary thought sequences, and occasional confused and irrelevant digressions. They are often lonely, and express feelings of being unwanted. They view others as critical, betraying, and humiliating. They desire to have close relationships but avoid them because of their fear of being rejected. Depression, anxiety, and anger at oneself for failing to develop social relations are commonly experienced.

The *DSM-IV-TR* diagnostic criteria for avoidant personality disorder are presented in Table 37–7.

Predisposing Factors

It is possible that there is a hereditary influence with avoidant personality disorder because it seems to occur more frequently in certain families (Rettew & Jellinek, 2004). Some infants who exhibit traits of hyperirritabil-

TABLE 37–7 Diagnostic Criteria for Avoidant Personality Disorder

A pervasive pattern of social inhibition, feelings of inadequacy, and hypersensitivity to negative evaluation, beginning by early adulthood and present in a variety of contexts, as indicated by four (or more) of the following:
1. Avoids occupational activities that involve significant interpersonal contact, because of fears of criticism, disapproval, or rejection.
2. Is unwilling to get involved with people unless certain of being liked.
3. Shows restraint within intimate relationships because of the fear of being shamed or ridiculed.
4. Is preoccupied with being criticized or rejected in social situations.
5. Is inhibited in new interpersonal situations because of feelings of inadequacy.
6. Views self as socially inept, personally unappealing, or inferior to others.
7. Is unusually reluctant to take personal risks or to engage in any new activities because they may prove embarrassing.

SOURCE: American Psychiatric Association (2000), with permission.

ity, crankiness, tension, and withdrawal behaviors may possess a temperamental disposition toward an avoidant pattern.

The primary psychosocial predisposing influence to avoidant personality disorder is parental rejection and censure, which if often reinforced by peers (Phillips, Yen, & Gunderson, 2003). These children are often reared in a family in which they are belittled, abandoned, and criticized, such that any natural optimism is extinguished and replaced with feelings of low self-worth and social alienation. They learn to be suspicious and to view the world as hostile and dangerous.

Dependent Personality Disorder

Definition and Epidemiological Statistics

Dependent personality disorder is characterized by "a pervasive and excessive need to be taken care of that leads to submissive and clinging behavior and fears of separation" (APA, 2000). These characteristics are evident in the tendency to allow others to make decisions, to feel helpless when alone, to act submissively, to subordinate needs to others, to tolerate mistreatment by others, to demean oneself to gain acceptance, and to fail to function adequately in situations that require assertive or dominant behavior.

The disorder is relatively common. Sadock and Sadock (2003) discuss the results of one study of personality disorders in which 2.5 percent of the sample were diagnosed with dependent personality disorder. It is more common in women than in men and more common in the youngest children of a family.

Clinical Picture

Individuals with dependent personality disorder have a notable lack of self-confidence that is often apparent in their posture, voice, and mannerisms. They are typically passive and acquiescent to the desires of others. They are overly generous and thoughtful and underplay their own attractiveness and achievements. They may appear to others to "see the world through rose-colored glasses," but when alone, they may feel pessimistic, discouraged, and dejected. Others are not made aware of these feelings; their "suffering" is done in silence.

Individuals with dependent personality disorder assume the passive and submissive role in relationships. They are willing to let others make their important decisions. Should the dependent relationship end, they feel helpless and fearful because they feel incapable of caring for themselves (Phillips, Yen, & Gunderson, 2003). They may hastily and indiscriminately attempt to establish another relationship with someone they

TABLE 37–8 Diagnostic Criteria for Dependent Personality Disorder
A pervasive and excessive need to be taken care of that leads to submissive and clinging behavior and fears of separation, beginning by early adulthood and present in a variety of contexts, as indicated by five (or more) of the following: 1. Has difficulty making everyday decisions without an excessive amount of advice and reassurance from others. 2. Needs others to assume responsibility for most major areas of his or her life. 3. Has difficulty expressing disagreement with others because of fear of loss of support or approval.   **NOTE:** Do not include realistic fears of retribution. 4. Has difficulty initiating projects or doing things on his or her own (because of a lack of self-confidence in judgment or abilities rather than a lack of motivation or energy). 5. Goes to excessive lengths to obtain nurturance and support from others, to the point of volunteering to do things that are unpleasant. 6. Feels uncomfortable or helpless when alone because of exaggerated fears of being unable to care for himself or herself. 7. Urgently seeks another relationship as a source of care and support when a close relationship ends. 8. Is unrealistically preoccupied with fears of being left to take care of himself or herself.

SOURCE: American Psychiatric Association (2000), with permission.

believe can provide them with the nurturance and guidance they need.

They avoid positions of responsibility and become anxious when forced into them. They have feelings of low self-worth and are easily hurt by criticism and disapproval. They will do almost anything, even if it is unpleasant or demeaning, to earn the acceptance of others.

The *DSM-IV-TR* diagnostic criteria for dependent personality disorder are presented in Table 37–8.

Predisposing Factors

An infant may be genetically predisposed to a dependent temperament. Twin studies measuring submissiveness have shown a higher correlation between identical twins than fraternal twins.

Psychosocially, dependency is fostered in infancy when stimulation and nurturance are experienced exclusively from one source. The infant becomes attached to one source to the exclusion of all others. If this exclusive attachment continues as the child grows, the dependency is nurtured. A problem may arise when parents become overprotective and discourage independent behaviors on the part of the child. Parents who make new experiences unnecessarily easy for the child and refuse to allow him or her to learn by experience encourage their child to give up efforts at achieving autonomy. Dependent behaviors may be subtly rewarded in this environment, and the child may come to fear a loss of love or attachment from the parental figure if independent behaviors are attempted.

Obsessive–Compulsive Personality Disorder

Definition and Epidemiological Statistics

Individuals with obsessive–compulsive personality disorder are very serious and formal and have difficulty expressing emotions. They are overly disciplined, perfectionistic, and preoccupied with rules. They are inflexible about the way in which things must be done and have a devotion to productivity to the exclusion of personal pleasure. An intense fear of making mistakes leads to difficulty with decision-making. The disorder is relatively common and occurs more often in men than in women. Within the family constellation, it appears to be most common in oldest children.

Clinical Picture

Individuals with obsessive–compulsive personality disorder are inflexible and lack spontaneity. They are meticulous and work diligently and patiently at tasks that require accuracy and discipline. They are especially concerned with matters of organization and efficiency and tend to be rigid and unbending about rules and procedures.

Social behavior tends to be polite and formal. They are very "rank conscious," a characteristic that is reflected in their contrasting behaviors with "superiors" as opposed to "inferiors." They can be very solicitous to and ingratiating with authority figures. However, with subordinates the compulsive person is quite autocratic and condemnatory, often appearing pompous and self-righteous.

People with obsessive–compulsive personality disorder typify the "bureaucratic personality," the so-called company man. They see themselves as conscientious, loyal, dependable and responsible and are contemptuous of people whose behavior they consider frivolous and impulsive. Emotional behavior is considered immature and irresponsible.

Although on the surface these individuals appear to be calm and controlled, underneath this exterior lies a great deal of ambivalence, conflict, and hostility. Individuals with this disorder commonly use the defense mechanism of reaction formation. Not daring to expose their true feelings of defiance and anger, they withhold these feelings so strongly that the opposite feelings come forth. The defenses of isolation, intellectualization, rationalization, reaction formation, and undoing are also commonly evident (Phillips, Yen, & Gunderson, 2003).

The *DSM-IV-TR* diagnostic criteria for obsessive–compulsive personality disorder are presented in Table 37–9.

TABLE 37–9   Diagnostic Criteria for Obsessive–Compulsive Personality Disorder

A pervasive pattern of preoccupation with orderliness, perfectionism, and mental and interpersonal control, at the expense of flexibility, openness, and efficiency, beginning by early adulthood and present in a variety of contexts, as indicated by four (or more) of the following:

1. Is preoccupied with details, rules, lists, order, organization, or schedules to the extent that the major point of the activity is lost.
2. Shows perfectionism that interferes with task completion (e.g., is unable to complete a project because his or her own overly strict standards are not met).
3. Is excessively devoted to work and productivity to the exclusion of leisure activities and friendships (not accounted for by obvious economic necessity).
4. Is overconscientious, scrupulous, and inflexible about matters of morality, ethics, or values (not accounted for by cultural or religious identification).
5. Is unable to discard worn-out or worthless objects even when they have no sentimental value.
6. Is reluctant to delegate tasks or to work with others unless they submit to exactly his or her way of doing things.
7. Adopts a miserly spending style toward both self and others; money is viewed as something to be hoarded for future catastrophes.
8. Shows rigidity and stubbornness.

SOURCE: American Psychiatric Association (2000), with permission.

Predisposing Factors

In the psychoanalytical view, the parenting style in which the individual with obsessive–compulsive personality disorder was reared is one of over-control. These parents expect their children to live up to their imposed standards of conduct and condemn them if they do not. Praise for positive behaviors is bestowed on the child with much less frequency than punishment for undesirable behaviors. In this environment, individuals become experts in learning what they must *not* do to avoid punishment and condemnation rather than what they *can* do to achieve attention and praise. They learn to heed rigid restrictions and rules. Positive achievements are expected, taken for granted, and only occasionally acknowledged by their parents, whose comments and judgments are limited to pointing out transgressions and infractions of rules.

Passive–Aggressive Personality Disorder

Definition and Epidemiological Statistics

The *DSM-IV-TR* defines this disorder as a pervasive pattern of negativistic attitudes and passive resistance to demands for adequate performance in social and occupational situations that begins by early adulthood and occurs in a variety of contexts. The name of the disorder is based on the assumption that such people are passively expressing covert aggression. Passive–aggressive disorder has been included in all editions of the *Diagnostic and*

Statistical Manual of Mental Disorders, and although no statistics exist that speak to its prevalence, the syndrome appears to be relatively common.

Clinical Picture

Passive–aggressive individuals feel cheated and unappreciated. They believe that life has been unkind to them, and they express envy and resentment over the "easy life" that they perceive others having. When they feel another person has wronged them, they may go to great lengths to seek retribution, or "get even," but always in a subtle and passive manner rather than discussing their feelings with the offending individual. They demonstrate passive resistance and general obstructiveness in response to the expectations of others. As a tactic of interpersonal behavior, passive–aggressive individuals commonly switch among the roles of the martyr, the affronted, the aggrieved, the misunderstood, the contrite, the guilt-ridden, the sickly, and the overworked. In this way, they are able to vent their anger and resentment subtly, while gaining the attention, reassurance, and dependency they crave.

The *DSM-IV-TR* research criteria for passive–aggressive personality disorder are presented in Table 37–10.

Predisposing Factors

Contradictory parental attitudes and behavior are implicated in the predisposition to passive–aggressive personality disorder. In the nuclear family dynamics, at any moment and without provocation, these children may receive the kindness and support they crave or hostility and rejection. Parental responses are inconsistent and unpredictable, and these children internalize the conflicting attitudes toward themselves and others. For example, they do not know whether to think of themselves as competent or incompetent and are unsure as to whether they love or hate those on whom they depend. Double-bind communication may also be exhibited in these families. Expressions of concern and affection may be verbalized, only to be negated and undone through subtle and devious behavioral manifestations. This *approach-avoidance* pattern is modeled by the children, who then become equally equivocal and ambivalent in their own thinking and actions.

Through this type of environment, children learn to control their anger for fear of provoking parental withdrawal and not receiving love and support—-even on an inconsistent basis. Overtly the child appears polite and undemanding; hostility and inefficiency are manifested only covertly and indirectly.

APPLICATION OF THE NURSING PROCESS

Borderline Personality Disorder

Background Assessment Data

Historically, there have been a group of clients who did not classically conform to the standard categories of neuroses or psychoses. The designation "borderline" was introduced to identify these clients who seemed to fall on the border between the two categories. Other terminology that has been used in an attempt to identify this disorder includes *ambulatory schizophrenia*, *pseudoneurotic schizophrenia*, and *emotionally unstable personality*. When the term *borderline* was first proposed for inclusion in the third edition of the *DSM*, some psychiatrists feared it might be used as a "wastebasket" diagnosis for difficult-to-treat clients. However, a specific set of criteria has been established for diagnosing what has been described as "a consistent and stable course of unstable behavior" (Table 37–11).

Clinical Picture

Individuals with borderline personality always seem to be in a state of crisis. Their affect is one of extreme intensity and their behavior reflects frequent changeability. These changes can occur within days, hours, or even minutes. Often these individuals exhibit a single, dominant affective tone, such as depression, which may give way periodically to anxious agitation or inappropriate outbursts of anger.

Chronic Depression. Depression is so common in clients with this disorder that before the inclusion of borderline personality disorder in the *DSM*, many of these clients were diagnosed as depressed. Depression occurs in response to feelings of abandonment by the mother in early childhood (see "Predisposing Factors"). Underlying the depression is a sense of rage that is sporadically

TABLE 37–10   Research Criteria for Passive–Aggressive Personality Disorder
A. A pervasive pattern of negativistic attitudes and passive resistance to demands for adequate performance, beginning by early adulthood and present in a variety of contexts, as indicated by four (or more) of the following:
1. Passively resists fulfilling routine social and occupational tasks.
2. Complains of being misunderstood and unappreciated by others.
3. Is sullen and argumentative.
4. Unreasonably criticizes and scorns authority.
5. Expresses envy and resentment toward those apparently more fortunate.
6. Voices exaggerated and persistent complaints of personal misfortune.
7. Alternates between hostile defiance and contrition.
B. Does not occur exclusively during major depressive episodes and is not better accounted for by dysthymic disorder.

SOURCE: American Psychiatric Association (2000), with permission.

TABLE 37–11   Diagnostic Criteria for Borderline Personality Disorder

A pervasive pattern of instability of interpersonal relationships, self-image, and affects, and marked impulsivity beginning by early adulthood and present in a variety of contexts, as indicated by five (or more) of the following:
  1. Frantic efforts to avoid real or imagined abandonment.
     NOTE: Does not include suicidal or self-mutilating behavior covered in criterion 5.
  2. A pattern of unstable and intense interpersonal relationships characterized by alternating between extremes of idealization and devaluation.
  3. Identity disturbance: markedly and persistently unstable self-image or sense of self.
  4. Impulsivity in at least two areas that are potentially self-damaging (e.g., spending, sex, substance abuse, reckless driving, binge eating).
     NOTE: Do not include suicidal or self-mutilating behavior covered in criterion 5.
  5. Recurrent suicidal behavior, gestures, or threats, or self-mutilating behavior.
  6. Affective instability due to marked reactivity of mood (e.g., intense episodic dysphoria, irritability, or anxiety, usually lasting a few hours and only rarely more than a few days).
  7. Chronic feelings of emptiness.
  8. Inappropriate, intense anger or difficulty controlling anger (e.g., frequent displays of temper, constant anger, recurrent physical fights).
  9. Transient, stress-related paranoid ideation or severe dissociative symptoms.

SOURCE: American Psychiatric Association (2000), with permission.

turned inward on the self and externally on the environment. Seldom is the individual aware of the true source of these feelings until well into long-term therapy.

Inability to Be Alone. Because of this chronic fear of abandonment, clients with borderline personality disorder have little tolerance for being alone. They prefer a frantic search for companionship, no matter how unsatisfactory, to sitting with feelings of loneliness, emptiness, and boredom (Sadock & Sadock, 2003).

Patterns of Interaction

Clinging and Distancing. The client with borderline personality disorder commonly exhibits a pattern of interaction with others that is characterized by clinging and distancing behaviors. When clients are clinging to another individual, they may exhibit helpless, dependent, or even childlike behaviors. They overidealize a single individual with whom they want to spend all their time, with whom they express a frequent need to talk, or from whom they seek constant reassurance. Acting-out behaviors, even self-mutilation, may result when they cannot be with this chosen individual. Distancing behaviors are characterized by hostility, anger, and devaluation of others, arising from a feeling of discomfort with closeness. Distancing behaviors also occur in response to separations, confrontations, or attempts to limit certain behaviors. Devaluation of others is manifested by discrediting or undermining their strengths and personal significance.

Splitting. Splitting is a primitive ego defense mechanism that is common in people with borderline personality disorder. It arises from their lack of achievement of **object constancy** and is manifested by an inability to integrate and accept both positive and negative feelings. In their view, people—including themselves—and life situations are either all good or all bad. For example, if a caregiver is nurturing and supportive, he or she is lovingly idealized. Should the nurturing relationship be threatened in any way (e.g., the caregiver must move because of his or her job), suddenly the individual is devalued, and the idealized image changes from beneficent caregiver to one of hateful and cruel persecutor.

Manipulation. In their efforts to prevent the separation they so desperately fear, clients with this disorder become masters of manipulation. Virtually any behavior becomes an acceptable means of achieving the desired result: relief from separation anxiety. Playing one individual against another is a common ploy to allay these fears of abandonment.

Self-Destructive Behaviors. Repetitive, self-mutilative behaviors are classic manifestations of borderline personality disorder. Although these acts can be fatal, most commonly they are manipulative gestures designed to elicit a rescue response from significant others. Suicide attempts are not uncommon and result from feelings of abandonment following separation from a significant other. The endeavor is often attempted, however, incorporating a measure of "safety" into the plan (e.g., swallowing pills in an area where the person will surely be discovered by others; or swallowing pills and making a phone call to report the deed to someone).

Other types of destructive behaviors include cutting, scratching, and burning. Various theories abound regarding why these individuals are able to inflict pain on themselves. One hypothesis suggests they may have higher levels of endorphins in their bodies than most people, thereby increasing their threshold for pain. Another theory relates to the individual's personal identity disturbance. It proposes that since much of the self-mutilating behaviors take place when the individual is in a state of depersonalization and derealization, he or she does not initially feel the pain. They continue the mutilation until the pain is felt in an effort to counteract the feelings of unreality. Some clients with borderline personality disorder have reported that "… to feel pain is better than to feel nothing." Pain validates their existence.

Impulsivity. Individuals with borderline personality disorder have poor impulse control based on primary process functioning. Impulsive behaviors associated with borderline personality disorder include substance abuse, gambling, promiscuity, reckless driving, and binging and purging (APA, 2000). Many times these acting-out behaviors occur in response to real or perceived feelings of abandonment.

Predisposing Factors

Biological Influences

Biochemical. Cummings and Mega (2003) have suggested a possible serotonergic defect in clients with borderline personality disorder. In positron emission tomography using α-[^{11}C]methyl-L-tryptophan (α-[^{11}C]MTrp), which reflects serotonergic synthesis capability, clients with borderline personality demonstrated significantly decreased α-[^{11}C]MTrp in medial frontal, superior temporal, and striatal regions of the brain. Cummings and Mega (2003) state:

> These functional imaging studies support a medial and orbitofrontal abnormality that may promote the impulsive aggression demonstrated by patients with the borderline personality disorder. (p. 230)

Genetic. The decrease in serotonin may also have genetic implications for borderline personality disorder. Sadock and Sadock (2003) report that depression is common in the family backgrounds of clients with borderline personality disorder. They state:

> These patients have more relatives with mood disorders than do control groups, and persons with borderline personality disorder often have mood disorder as well. (p. 800)

Psychosocial Influences

Childhood Trauma. Studies have shown that many individuals with borderline personality disorder were reared in families with chaotic environments. Finley-Belgrad and Davies (2004) state, "Risk factors [for borderline personality disorder] include family environments characterized by trauma, neglect, and/or separation; exposure to sexual and physical abuse; and serious parental psychopathology such as substance abuse and antisocial personality disorder." Forty to 71 percent of borderline personality disorder clients report having been sexually abused, usually by a non-caregiver (National Institute of Mental Health [NIMH], 2001). In some instances, this disorder has been likened to posttraumatic stress disorder in response to childhood trauma and abuse. Oldham and associates (2002) state:

> Even when full criteria for comorbid PTSD are not present, patients with borderline personality disorder may experience PTSD-like symptoms. For example, symptoms such as intrusion, avoidance, and hyperarousal may emerge during psychotherapy. Awareness of the trauma-related nature of these symptoms can facilitate both psychotherapeutic and pharmacological efforts in symptom relief. (p. 804)

Developmental Factors. According to Mahler's theory of object relations (Mahler, Pine, & Bergman, 1975), the infant passes through six phases from birth to 36 months, when a sense of separateness from the parenting figure is finally established. These phases include the following:

Phase 1 (Birth to 1 Month), Autistic Phase. During this period, the baby spends most of his or her time in a half-waking, half-sleeping state. The main goal is fulfillment of needs for survival and comfort.

Phase 2 (1 to 5 Months), Symbiotic Phase. At this time, there is a type of psychic fusion of mother and child. The child views the self as an extension of the parenting figure, although there is a developing awareness of external sources of need fulfillment.

Phase 3 (5 to 10 Months), Differentiation Phase. The child is beginning to recognize that there is a separateness between the self and the parenting figure.

Phase 4 (10 to 16 Months), Practicing Phase. This phase is characterized by increased locomotor functioning and the ability to explore the environment independently. A sense of separateness of the self is increased.

Phase 5 (16 to 24 Months), Rapprochement Phase. Awareness of separateness of the self becomes acute. This is frightening to the child, who wants to regain some lost closeness but not return to symbiosis. The child wants the mother there as needed for "emotional refueling" and to maintain feelings of security.

Phase 6 (24 to 36 Months), On the Way to Object Constancy Phase. In this phase, the child completes the individuation process and learns to relate to objects in an effective, constant manner. A sense of separateness is established, and the child is able to internalize a sustained image of the loved object or person when out of sight. Separation anxiety is resolved.

The individual with borderline personality disorder becomes fixed in the rapprochement phase of development. This occurs when the child shows increasing separation and autonomy. The mother, who feels secure in the relationship as long as the child is dependent, begins to feel threatened by the child's increasing independence. The mother may indeed be experiencing her own fears of abandonment. In response to separation behaviors, the mother withdraws the emotional support or "refueling" that is so vitally needed during this phase for the child to feel secure. Instead, the mother rewards clinging, dependent behaviors, and punishes (withholding emotional support) independent behaviors. With his or her sense of emotional survival at stake, the child learns to behave in a manner that satisfies the parental wishes. An internal conflict develops within the child, based on fear of abandonment. He or she wants to achieve independence common to this stage of development, but fears that mother will withdraw emotional support as a result. This unresolved fear of abandonment remains with the child into adulthood. Unresolved grief for the nurturing they failed to receive results in internalized rage that manifests itself in the depression so common in people with borderline personality disorder.

Diagnosis/Outcome Identification

Nursing diagnoses are formulated from the data gathered during the assessment phase and with background knowledge regarding etiological implications for the disorder. Some common nursing diagnoses for the client with borderline personality disorder include:

Risk for self-mutilation related to parental emotional deprivation (unresolved fears of abandonment).

Dysfunctional grieving related to maternal deprivation during rapprochement phase of development (internalized as a loss, with fixation in anger stage of grieving process), evidenced by depressed mood, acting-out behaviors.

Impaired social interaction related to extreme fears of abandonment and engulfment evidenced by alternating clinging and distancing behaviors.

Disturbed personal identity related to underdeveloped ego evidenced by feelings of depersonalization and derealization.

Anxiety (severe to panic) related to unconscious conflicts based on fear of abandonment evidenced by transient psychotic symptoms (disorganized thinking; misinterpretation of the environment).

Chronic low self-esteem related to lack of positive feedback evidenced by manipulation of others and inability to tolerate being alone.

The following criteria may be used for measurement of outcomes in the care of clients with borderline personality disorder.

The client:

1. Has not harmed self.
2. Seeks out staff when desire for self-mutilation is strong.
3. Is able to identify true source of anger.
4. Expresses anger appropriately.
5. Relates to more than one staff member.
6. Completes activities of daily living independently.
7. Does not manipulate one staff member against the other in order to fulfill own desires.

Planning/Implementation

In Table 37–12, selected nursing diagnoses common to the client with borderline personality disorder are presented in a plan of care. Outcome criteria along with appropriate nursing interventions and rationales are included for each.

The concept map care plan is an innovative approach to planning and organizing nursing care (see Chapter 9). It is a diagrammatic teaching and learning strategy that allows visualization of interrelationships between medical diagnoses, nursing diagnoses, assessment data, and treatments. An example of a concept map care plan for a client with borderline personality disorder is presented in Figure 37–1.

Evaluation

Reassessment is conducted to determine if the nursing actions have been successful in achieving the objectives of care. Evaluation of the nursing actions for the client with borderline personality disorder may be facilitated by gathering information using the following types of questions:

1. Has the client been able to seek out staff when feeling the desire for self-harm?
2. Has the client avoided self-harm?
3. Can the client correlate times of desire for self-harm to times of elevation in level of anxiety?
4. Can the client discuss feelings with staff (particularly feelings of depression and anger)?
5. Can the client identify the true source toward which the anger is directed?
6. Can the client verbalize understanding of the basis for his or her anger?
7. Can the client express anger appropriately?
8. Can the client function independently?
9. Can the client relate to more than one staff member?
10. Can the client verbalize the knowledge that the staff members will return and are not abandoning the client when leaving for the day?
11. Can the client separate from the staff in an appropriate manner?
12. Can the client delay gratification and refrain from manipulating others in order to fulfill own desires?
13. Can the client verbalize resources within the community from whom he or she may seek assistance in times of extreme stress?

Antisocial Personality Disorder

Background Assessment Data

In the *DSM-I*, antisocial behavior was categorized as a "sociopathic or psychopathic" reaction that was symptomatic of any of several underlying personality disorders. The *DSM-II* represented it as a distinct personality type, a distinction that has been retained in subsequent editions. The *DSM-IV-TR* diagnostic criteria for antisocial personality disorder are presented in Table 37–13.

Individuals with antisocial personality disorder are not seen often in most clinical settings, and when they are, it is commonly a way to avoid legal consequences. Sometimes they are admitted to the healthcare system by court order for psychological evaluation. Most frequently, however, these individuals may be encountered in prisons, jails, and rehabilitation services.

NURSING DIAGNOSIS: RISK FOR SELF-MUTILATION

RELATED TO: Parental emotional deprivation (unresolved fears of abandonment)

OUTCOME CRITERIA	NURSING INTERVENTIONS	RATIONALE
Client will not harm self.	1. Observe client's behavior frequently. Do this through routine activities and interactions; avoid appearing watchful and suspicious.	1. Close observation is required so that intervention can occur if required to ensure client's (and others') safety.
	2. Secure a verbal contract from client that he or she will seek out staff member when urge for self-mutilation is felt.	2. Discussing feelings of self-harm with a trusted individual provides a degree of relief to the client. A contract gets the subject out in the open and places some of the responsibility for his or her safety with the client. An attitude of acceptance of the client as a worthwhile individual is conveyed.
	3. If self-mutilation occurs, care for client's wounds in a matter-of-fact manner. Do not give positive reinforcement to this behavior by offering sympathy or additional attention.	3. Lack of attention to the maladaptive behavior may decrease repetition of its use.
	4. Encourage client to talk about feelings he or she was having just before this behavior occurred.	4. To problem solve the situation with the client, knowledge of the precipitating factors is important.
	5. Act as a role model for appropriate expression of angry feelings, and give positive reinforcement to client when attempts to conform are made.	5. It is vital that the client expresses angry feelings because suicide and other self-destructive behaviors are often viewed as a result of anger turned inward on the self.
	6. Remove all dangerous objects from client's environment.	6. Client safety is a nursing priority.
	7. If warranted by high acuity of the situation, staff may need to be assigned on a one-to-one basis.	7. Because of their extreme fear of abandonment, clients with this disorder should not be left alone at a stressful time as it may cause an acute rise in anxiety and agitation levels.

NURSING DIAGNOSIS: DYSFUNCTIONAL GRIEVING

RELATED TO: Maternal deprivation during rapprochement phase of development (internalized as a loss, with fixation in anger stage of grieving process)

EVIDENCED BY: Depressed mood, acting-out behaviors

OUTCOME CRITERIA	NURSING INTERVENTIONS	RATIONALE
Client will be able to identify true source of anger, accept ownership of the feelings, and express them in a socially acceptable manner in an effort to initiate progression through the grief process.	1. Convey an accepting attitude—one that creates a nonthreatening environment for the client to express feelings. Be honest and keep all promises.	1. An accepting attitude conveys to the client that you believe he or she is a worthwhile person. Trust is enhanced.
	2. Identify the function that anger, frustration, and rage serve for the client. Allow him or her to express these feelings within reason.	2. Verbalization of feelings in a nonthreatening environment may help client come to terms with unresolved issues.
	3. Encourage client to discharge pent-up anger through participation in large motor activities (e.g., brisk walks, jogging, physical exercises, volleyball, punching bag, exercise bike).	3. Physical exercise provides a safe and effective method for discharging pent-up tension.
	4. Explore with client the true source of the anger. This is a painful therapy that often leads to regression as the client deals with the feelings of early abandonment.	4. Reconciliation of the feelings associated with this stage is necessary before progression through the grieving process can continue.

(Continued on following page)

OUTCOME CRITERIA	NURSING INTERVENTIONS	RATIONALE
	5. As anger is displaced onto the nurse or therapist, caution must be taken to guard against the negative effects of counter-transference (see Chapter 7). These are very difficult clients who have the capacity for eliciting a whole array of negative feelings from the therapist.	5. The existence of negative feelings by the nurse or therapist must be acknowledged, but they must not be allowed to interfere with the therapeutic process.
	6. Explain the behaviors associated with the normal grieving process. Help the client recognize his or her position in this process.	6. Knowledge of the acceptability of the feelings associated with normal grieving may help to relieve some of the guilt that these responses generate.
	7. Help client to understand appropriate ways to express anger. Give positive reinforcement for behaviors used to express anger appropriately. Act as a role model.	7. Positive reinforcement enhances self-esteem and encourages repetition of desirable behaviors.
	8. Set limits on acting-out behaviors and explain consequences of violation of those limits. Be supportive, yet consistent and firm in caring for this client.	8. Client lacks sufficient self-control to limit maladaptive behaviors, so assistance is required from staff. Without consistency on the part of all staff members working with this client, however, a positive outcome will not be achieved.

NURSING DIAGNOSIS: IMPAIRED SOCIAL INTERACTION

RELATED TO: Extreme fears of abandonment and engulfment

EVIDENCED BY: Alternating clinging and distancing behaviors and staff splitting

OUTCOME CRITERIA	NURSING INTERVENTIONS	RATIONALE
Client will exhibit no evidence of splitting or clinging and distancing behaviors in relationships with staff and/or peers.	1. Encourage client to examine these behaviors (to recognize that they are occurring).	1. Client may be unaware of splitting or of clinging and distancing pattern of interaction with others. Recognition must occur before change can occur.
	2. Help client realize that you will be available, without reinforcing dependent behaviors.	2. Knowledge of your availability may provide needed security for the client.
	3. Give positive reinforcement for independent behaviors.	3. Positive reinforcement enhances self-esteem and encourages repetition of desirable behaviors.
	4. Rotate staff members who work with the client to avoid client's developing dependence on particular individuals.	4. Client must learn to relate to more than one staff member in an effort to decrease use of splitting, and diminish fears of abandonment.
	5. Explore feelings that relate to fears of abandonment and engulfment with client. Help client understand that clinging and distancing behaviors are engendered by these fears.	5. Exploration of feelings with a trusted individual may help client come to terms with unresolved issues.
	6. Help client understand how these behaviors interfere with satisfactory relationships.	6. Client may be unaware of others' perception of him or her and why these behaviors are not acceptable to others.
	7. Assist client to work toward achievement of object constancy. Be available, without promoting dependency.	7. This may help client resolve fears of abandonment and develop the ability to establish satisfactory intimate relationships.

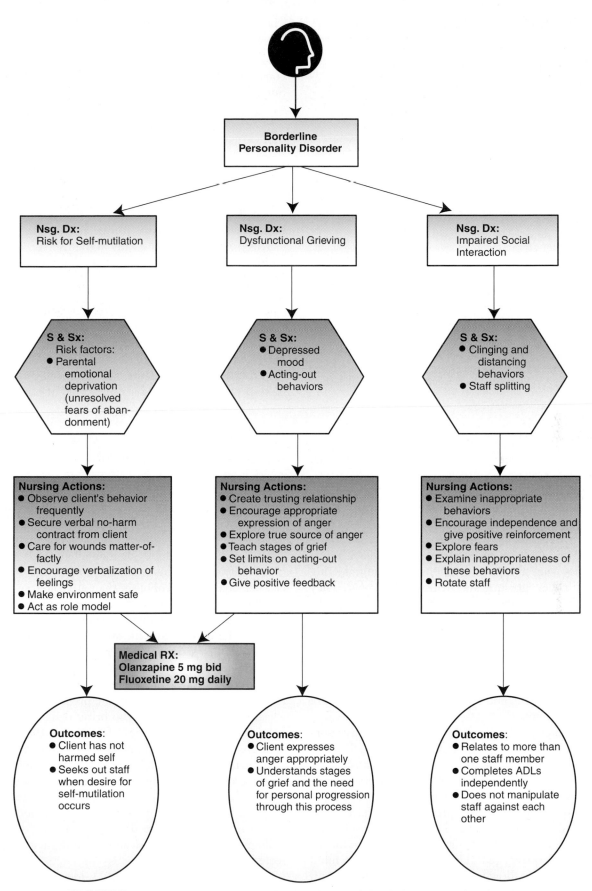

FIGURE 37–1 Concept map care plan for client with borderline personality disorder.

TABLE 37–13   Diagnostic Criteria for Antisocial Personality Disorder

A. There is a pervasive pattern of disregard for and violation of the rights of others occurring since age 15 years, as indicated by three (or more) of the following:
  1. Failure to conform to social norms with respect to lawful behaviors as indicated by repeatedly performing acts that are grounds for arrest.
  2. Deceitfulness, as indicated by repeated lying, use of aliases, or conning others for personal profit or pleasure.
  3. Impulsivity or failure to plan ahead.
  4. Irritability and aggressiveness, as indicated by repeated physical fights or assaults.
  5. Reckless disregard for safety of self or others.
  6. Consistent irresponsibility, as indicated by repeated failure to sustain consistent work behavior or honor financial obligations.
  7. Lack of remorse, as indicated by being indifferent to or rationalizing having hurt, mistreated, or stolen from another.
B. Individual is at least 18 years old.
C. There is evidence of conduct disorder with onset before age 15 years.
D. The occurrence of antisocial behavior is not exclusively during the course of schizophrenia or a manic episode.

SOURCE: American Psychiatric Association (2000), with permission.

Clinical Picture

Phillips, Yen, and Gunderson (2003) describe antisocial personality disorder as a pattern of socially irresponsible, exploitative, and guiltless behavior that reflects a disregard for the rights of others. These individuals exploit and manipulate others for personal gain and have a general disregard for the law. They have difficulty sustaining consistent employment and in developing stable relationships. They appear cold and callous, often intimidating others with their brusque and belligerent manner. They tend to be argumentative and, at times, cruel and malicious. They lack warmth and compassion and are often suspicious of these qualities in others.

Individuals with antisocial personality have a very low tolerance for frustration, act impetuously, and are unable to delay gratification. They are restless and easily bored, often taking chances and seeking thrills, as if they were immune to danger.

When things go their way, individuals with this disorder act cheerful, even gracious and charming. Because of their low tolerance for frustration, this pleasant exterior can change very quickly. When what they desire at the moment is challenged, they are likely to become furious and vindictive. Easily provoked to attack, their first inclination is to demean and dominate. They believe that "good guys come in last," and show contempt for the weak and underprivileged. They exploit others to fulfill their own desires, showing no trace of shame or guilt for their behavior.

Individuals with antisocial personalities see themselves as victims, using projection as the primary ego defense mechanism. They do not accept responsibility for the consequences of their behavior. Gorman, Raines, and Sultan (2002) state:

> Manipulative individuals have come to suspect that any person or institution may try to control them, rendering them powerless and vulnerable to attack. (p. 168)

In their own minds, this perception justifies their malicious behavior, lest they be the recipient of unjust persecution and hostility from others.

Satisfying interpersonal relationships are not possible because individuals with antisocial personalities have learned to place their trust only in themselves. They have a philosophy that "everyone is out to 'help number one' and that one should stop at nothing to avoid being pushed around" (APA, 2000).

One of the most distinctive characteristics of antisocial personalities is their tendency to ignore conventional authority and rules. They act as though established social norms and guidelines for self-discipline and cooperative behavior do not apply to them. They are flagrant in their disrespect for the law and for the rights of others.

Predisposing Factors

Biological Influences. The *DSM-IV-TR* reports that antisocial personality is more common among first-degree biological relatives of those with the disorder than among the general population (APA, 2000). Twin and adoptive studies have implicated the role of genetics in antisocial personality disorder (Phillips, Yen, & Gunderson, 2003). These studies of families of individuals with antisocial personality show higher numbers of relatives with antisocial personality or alcoholism than are found in the general population. The studies have also shown that children of parents with antisocial behavior are more likely to be diagnosed with antisocial personality, even when they are separated at birth from their biological parents and reared by individuals without the disorder.

Characteristics associated with temperament in the newborn may be significant in the predisposition to antisocial personality. Parents who bring their children with behavior disorders to clinics often report that the child displayed temper tantrums from infancy and would become furious when awaiting a bottle or a diaper change. As these children mature, they commonly develop a bullying attitude toward other children. Parents report that they are undaunted by punishment and generally quite unmanageable. They are daring and foolhardy in their willingness to chance physical harm and, they seem unaffected by pain.

Fischer and associates (2002) identified attention-deficit hyperactivity disorder and conduct disorder during childhood and adolescence as predisposing factors to antisocial personality disorder.

Although these biogenetic influences may describe some familial pattern to the development of antisocial personality disorder, no basic pathology process has yet been determined as an etiological factor. Bienenfeld (2004) states:

Low levels of behavioral inhibition may be mediated by serotonergic dysregulation in the septohippocampal system. There may also be developmental or acquired abnormalities in the prefrontal brain systems and reduced autonomic activity in antisocial personality disorder. This may underlie the low arousal, poor fear conditioning, and decision-making deficits described in antisocial personality disorder.

Family Dynamics. Antisocial personality disorder frequently arises from a chaotic home environment. Parental deprivation during the first 5 years of life appears to be a critical predisposing factor in the development of antisocial personality disorder. Separation due to parental delinquency appears to be more highly correlated with the disorder than is parental loss from other causes. The presence or intermittent appearance of inconsistent impulsive parents, not the loss of a consistent parent, is environmentally *most* damaging.

Studies have shown that individuals with antisocial personality disorder often have been severely physically abused in childhood. The abuse contributes to the development of antisocial behavior in several ways. First, it provides a model for behavior. Second, it may result in injury to the child's central nervous system, thereby impairing the child's ability to function appropriately. Finally, it engenders rage in the victimized child, which is then displaced onto others in the environment.

A number of factors associated with disordered family functioning have been implicated in the development of antisocial personality (Hill, 2003; Phillips, Yen, & Gunderson, 2003; Ramsland, 2005). The following circumstances may influence the predisposition to antisocial personality disorder:

1. Absence of parental discipline
2. Extreme poverty
3. Removal from the home
4. Growing up without parental figures of both sexes
5. Erratic and inconsistent methods of discipline
6. Being "rescued" each time they are in trouble (never having to suffer the consequences of one's own behavior)
7. Maternal deprivation

Diagnosis/Outcome Identification

Nursing diagnoses are formulated from the data gathered during the assessment phase and with background knowledge regarding predisposing factors to the disorder. Some common nursing diagnoses for the client with antisocial personality disorder include:

Risk for other-directed violence related to rage reactions, negative role-modeling, inability to tolerate frustration.

Defensive coping related to dysfunctional family system, evidenced by disregard for societal norms and laws, absence of guilty feelings, or inability to delay gratification.

Chronic low self-esteem related to repeated negative feedback resulting in diminished self-worth, evidenced by manipulation of others to fulfill own desires or inability to form close, personal relationships.

Impaired social interaction related to negative role modeling and low self-esteem, evidenced by inability to develop a satisfactory, enduring, intimate relationship with another.

Deficient knowledge (self-care activities to achieve and maintain optimal wellness) related to lack of interest in learning and denial of need for information, evidenced by demonstration of inability to take responsibility for meeting basic health practices.

The following criteria may be used to measure outcomes in the care of the client with antisocial personality disorder:

The client:

1. Discusses angry feelings with staff and in group sessions.
2. Has not harmed self or others.
3. Can rechannel hostility into socially acceptable behaviors.
4. Follows rules and regulations of the therapy environment.
5. Can verbalize which of his or her behaviors are not acceptable.
6. Shows regard for the rights of others by delaying gratification of own desires when appropriate.
7. Does not manipulate others in an attempt to increase feelings of self-worth.
8. Verbalizes understanding of knowledge required to maintain basic health needs.

Planning/Implementation

Table 37–14 presents a care plan of selected nursing diagnoses common to the client with antisocial personality disorder. Outcome criteria, appropriate nursing interventions, and rationales are included for each.

The concept map care plan is an innovative approach to planning and organizing nursing care (see Chapter 9). It is a diagrammatic teaching and learning strategy that allows visualization of interrelationships between medical diagnoses, nursing diagnoses, assessment data, and treatments. An example of a concept map care plan for a client with antisocial personality disorder is presented in Figure 37–2.

NURSING DIAGNOSIS: RISK FOR OTHER-DIRECTED VIOLENCE
RELATED TO: Rage reactions, negative role-modeling, inability to tolerate frustration

OUTCOME CRITERIA	NURSING INTERVENTIONS	RATIONALE
Client will not harm self or others.	1. Convey an accepting attitude toward this client. Feelings of rejection are undoubtedly familiar to him or her. Work on development of trust. Be honest, keep all promises, and convey the message that it is not *him* or *her* but the *behavior* that is unacceptable.	1. An attitude of acceptance promotes feelings of self-worth. Trust is the basis on which a therapeutic relationship is established.
	2. Maintain low level of stimuli in client's environment (low lighting, few people, simple decor, low noise level).	2. A stimulating environment may increase agitation and promote aggressive behavior.
	3. Observe client's behavior frequently during routine activities and interactions; avoid appearing watchful and suspicious.	3. Close observation is required so that intervention can occur if required to ensure client's (and others') safety.
	4. Remove all dangerous objects from client's environment.	4. Client safety is a nursing priority.
	5. Help client identify the true object of his or her hostility.	5. Because of weak ego development, client may be misusing the defense mechanism of displacement. Helping him or her recognize this in a nonthreatening manner may help reveal unresolved issues so that they may be confronted.
	6. Encourage client to verbalize hostile feelings gradually.	6. Verbalization of feelings in a nonthreatening environment may help client come to terms with unresolved issues.
	7. Explore with client alternative ways of handling frustration (e.g., large motor skills that channel hostile energy into socially acceptable behaviors).	7. Physically demanding activities help to relieve pent-up tension.
	8. Staff should maintain and convey a calm attitude.	8. Anxiety is contagious and can be transferred from staff to client. A calm attitude provides client with a feeling of safety and security.
	9. Have sufficient staff available to present a show of strength to client if necessary.	9. This conveys to client evidence of control over the situation and provides some physical security for staff.
	10. Administer tranquilizing medications as ordered by physician or obtain an order if necessary. Monitor for effectiveness and for adverse side effects.	10. Antianxiety agents (e.g., diazepam, chlordiazepoxide, oxazepam) produce a calming effect and may help to allay hostile behaviors (**Note:** Medications are not often prescribed for clients with this disorder because of these individuals' strong susceptibility to addictions.)
	11. If client is not calmed by "talking down" or by medication, use of mechanical restraints may be necessary. Be sure to have sufficient staff available to assist. Follow protocol established by the institution in executing this intervention. The Joint Commission on Accreditation of Healthcare Organizations (JCAHO) requires that the physician reevaluate and issue a new order for restraints every 4 hr for adults age 18 and older. If the client has previously refused medication, administer it after restraints have been applied. Most states consider this intervention appropriate in emergency situations or in the event that a client is likely to harm self or others. Never use restraints as a punitive measure; they should be used as a protective measure for a client who is out of control. Observe the client in restraints every 15 min (or according to	11. Client safety is a nursing priority.

(Continued on opposite page)

| | institutional policy). Ensure that circulation to extremities is not compromised (check temperature, color, pulses). Assist client with needs related to nutrition, hydration, and elimination. Position client so that comfort is facilitated and aspiration can be prevented. | |
| | 12. As agitation decreases, assess client's readiness for restraint removal or reduction. Remove one restraint at a time, while assessing client's response. | 12. This minimizes risk of injury to client and staff. |

NURSING DIAGNOSIS: DEFENSIVE COPING
RELATED TO: Dysfunctional family system
EVIDENCED BY: Disregard for societal norms and laws; absence of guilty feelings; inability to delay gratification

OUTCOME CRITERIA	NURSING INTERVENTIONS	RATIONALE
Client will be able to follow rules and delay personal gratification.	1. From the onset, client should be made aware of which behaviors are acceptable and which are not. Explain consequences of violation of the limits. A consequence must involve something of value to the client. All staff must be consistent in enforcing these limits. Consequences should be administered in a matter-of-fact manner immediately following the infraction.	1. Because client cannot (or will not) impose own limits on maladaptive behaviors, they must be delineated and enforced by staff. Undesirable consequences may help to decrease repetition of these behaviors.
	2. Do not attempt to coax or convince client to do the "right thing." Do not use the words "You should (or shouldn't)…"; instead, use "You will be expected to…" The ideal would be for client to eventually internalize societal norms, beginning with this step-by-step, "either/or" approach (*either* you do [don't do] this, *or* this will occur).	2. Explanations must be concise, concrete, and clear, with little or no capacity for misinterpretation.
	3. Provide positive feedback or reward for acceptable behaviors.	3. Positive reinforcement enhances self-esteem and encourages repetition of desirable behaviors.
	4. Begin to increase the length of time requirement for acceptable behavior in order to achieve the reward. For example, 2 hr of acceptable behavior may be exchanged for a phone call, 4 hr for 2 hr of television; 1 day of acceptable behavior for a recreational therapy bowling activity, 5 days for a weekend pass.	4. This type of intervention may assist the client in learning to delay gratification.
	5. A milieu unit provides the appropriate environment for the client with antisocial personality.	5. The democratic approach, with specific rules and regulations, community meetings, and group therapy sessions emulates the type of societal situation in which the client must learn to live. Feedback from peers is often more effective than confrontation from an authority figure. The client learns to follow the rules of the group as a positive step in the progression toward internalizing the rules of society.
	6. Help client to gain insight into his or her own behaviors. Often these individuals rationalize to such an extent that they deny that what they have done is wrong (e.g., "The owner of this store has so much money, he'll never miss the little bit I take. He has everything, and I have nothing. It's no fair! I deserve to have some of what he has.")	6. Client must come to understand that certain behaviors will not be tolerated within the society and that severe consequences will be imposed on those individuals who refuse to comply. Client must *want* to become a productive member of society before he or she can be helped.

(Continued on following page)

TABLE 37–14	**Care Plan for the Client with Antisocial Personality Disorder** *(Continued)*	
OUTCOME CRITERIA	**NURSING INTERVENTIONS**	**RATIONALE**
	7. Talk about past behaviors with client. Discuss behaviors that are acceptable by society and those which are not. Help client identify ways in which he or she has exploited others. Encourage client to explore how he or she would feel if the circumstances were reversed.	7. An attempt may be made to enlighten the client to the sensitivity of others by promoting self-awareness in an effort to help the client gain insight into his or her own behavior.
	8. Throughout relationship with client, maintain attitude of "It is not *you*, but your *behavior*, that is unacceptable."	8. An attitude of acceptance promotes feelings of dignity and self-worth.

Evaluation

Reassessment is conducted to determine if the nursing actions have been successful in achieving the objectives of care. Evaluation of the nursing actions for the client with antisocial personality disorder may be facilitated by gathering information using the following types of questions:

1. Does the client recognize when anger is getting out of control?
2. Can the client seek out staff instead of expressing anger in an inappropriate manner?
3. Can the client use other sources for rechanneling anger (e.g., physical activities)?
4. Has harm to others been avoided?
5. Can the client follow rules and regulations of the therapeutic milieu with little or no reminding?
6. Can the client verbalize which behaviors are appropriate and which are not?
7. Does the client express a desire to change?
8. Can the client delay gratifying own desires in deference to those of others when appropriate?
9. Does the client refrain from manipulating others to fulfill own desires?
10. Does the client fulfill activities of daily living willingly and independently?
11. Can the client verbalize methods of achieving and maintaining optimal wellness?
12. Can the client verbalize community resources from which he or she can seek assistance with daily living and healthcare needs when required?

TREATMENT MODALITIES

Few would argue that treatment of individuals with personality disorders is difficult and, in some instances, may even seem impossible. Personality characteristics are learned very early in life and perhaps may even be genetic. It is not surprising, then, that these enduring patterns of behavior may take years to change, if change occurs. Phillips, Yen, and Gunderson (2003) state:

Because personality disorders consist of deeply ingrained attitudes and behavior patterns that consolidate during development and have endured since early adulthood, they have always been believed to be very resistant to change. Moreover, treatment efforts are further confounded by the degree to which patients with a personality disorder do not recognize their maladaptive personality traits as undesirable or needing to be changed. (p. 809)

Most clinicians believe it best to strive for lessening the inflexibility of the maladaptive traits and reducing their interference with everyday functioning and meaningful relationships. Little research exists to guide the decision of which therapy is most appropriate in the treatment of personality disorders. Selection of intervention is generally based on the area of greatest dysfunction, such as cognition, affect, behavior, or interpersonal relations. Following is a brief description of various types of therapies and the disorders to which they are customarily suited.

Interpersonal Psychotherapy

Depending on the therapeutic goals, interpersonal psychotherapy with personality disorders is brief and time limited, or it may involve long-term exploratory psychotherapy. Interpersonal psychotherapy may be particularly appropriate because personality disorders largely reflect problems in interpersonal style.

Long-term psychotherapy attempts to understand and modify the maladjusted behaviors, cognition, and affects of clients with personality disorders that dominate their personal lives and relationships. The core element of treatment is the establishment of an empathic therapist–client relationship, based on collaboration and guided discovery in which the therapist functions as a role model for the client.

Interpersonal psychotherapy is suggested for clients with paranoid, schizoid, schizotypal, borderline, dependent, narcissistic, and obsessive–compulsive personality disorders.

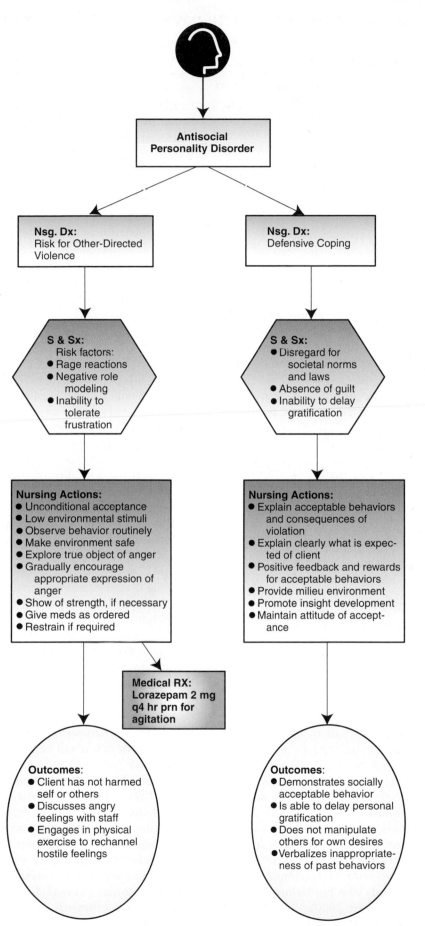

FIGURE 37–2 Concept map care plan for client with antisocial personality disorder.

Psychoanalytical Psychotherapy

The treatment of choice for individuals with histrionic personality disorder has been psychoanalytical psychotherapy (Phillips, Yen, & Gunderson, 2003). Treatment focuses on the unconscious motivation for seeking total satisfaction from others and for being unable to commit oneself to a stable, meaningful relationship.

Milieu or Group Therapy

This treatment is especially appropriate for individuals with antisocial personality disorder, who respond more adaptively to support and feedback from peers. In milieu or group therapy, feedback from peers is more effective than in one-to-one interaction with a therapist. Group therapy—particularly homogeneous supportive groups that emphasize the development of social skills—may be helpful in overcoming social anxiety and developing interpersonal trust and rapport in clients with avoidant personality disorder (Phillips, Yen, & Gunderson, 2003). Feminist consciousness-raising groups can be useful in helping dependent clients struggling with social-role stereotypes.

Cognitive/Behavioral Therapy

Behavioral strategies offer reinforcement for positive change. Social skills training and assertiveness training teach alternative ways to deal with frustration. Cognitive strategies help the client recognize and correct inaccurate internal mental schemata. This type of therapy may be useful for clients with obsessive–compulsive, passive–aggressive, antisocial, and avoidant personality disorders.

Psychopharmacology

Psychopharmacology may be helpful in some instances. Although these drugs have no effect in the direct treatment of the disorder itself, some symptomatic relief can be achieved. Antipsychotic medications are helpful in the treatment of psychotic decompensations experienced by clients with paranoid, schizotypal, and borderline personality disorders (Coccaro & Siever, 2000).

A variety of pharmacological interventions have been used with borderline personality disorder. The selective serotonin reuptake inhibitors (SSRIs) and monoamine oxidase inhibitors (MAOIs) have been successful in decreasing impulsivity and self-destructive acts in these clients (Phillips, Yen, & Gunderson, 2003). SSRIs also have been successful in reducing anger, impulsiveness, and mood instability in clients with borderline personality disorder (Coccaro & Siever, 2000). Antipsychotics

have resulted in improvement in illusions, ideas of reference, paranoid thinking, anxiety, and hostility in some clients.

Lithium carbonate and propranolol (Inderal) may be useful for the violent episodes observed in clients with antisocial personality disorder (Coccaro & Siever, 2000). Caution must be given to prescribing medications outside the structured setting because of the high risk for substance abuse by these individuals.

For the client with avoidant personality disorder, anxiolytics are sometimes helpful whenever previously avoided behavior is being attempted. The mere possession of the medication may be reassurance enough to help the client through the stressful period. Antidepressants, such as sertraline (Zoloft) and paroxetine (Paxil), may be useful with these clients if panic disorder develops.

SUMMARY

Clients with personality disorders are undoubtedly some of the most difficult ones health care workers are likely to encounter. Personality characteristics are formed very early in life and are difficult, if not impossible, to change. In fact, some clinicians believe the therapeutic approach is not to try to change the characteristics but rather to decrease the inflexibility of the maladaptive traits and reduce their interference with everyday functioning and meaningful relationships.

This chapter presents a review of the development of personality according to Sullivan, Erikson, and Mahler. The stages identified by these theorists represent the "normal" progression and establish a foundation for studying dysfunctional patterns.

The concept of a personality disorder has been present throughout the history of medicine. Problems have arisen in the attempt to establish a classification system for these disorders. The *DSM-IV-TR* groups them into three clusters. Cluster A (behaviors described as odd or eccentric) includes paranoid, schizoid, and schizotypal personality disorders. Cluster B (behaviors described as dramatic, emotional, or erratic) includes antisocial, borderline, histrionic, and narcissistic personality disorders. Cluster C (behaviors described as anxious or fearful) includes avoidant, dependent, and obsessive–compulsive disorders. Passive–aggressive personality disorder, which the *DSM-IV-TR* includes in "Criteria Provided for Further Study," was included with the cluster C disorders.

Nursing care of the client with a personality disorder is accomplished using the steps of the nursing process. Background assessment data were presented, along with information regarding possible etiological implications for each disorder. An overview of current medical treatment modalities for each disorder was presented.

Care of clients with borderline personality disorder and antisocial personality disorder was described at length. Individuals with borderline personality disorder may enter the health care system because of their instability and frequent attempts at self-destructive behavior. The individual with antisocial personality disorder may become part of the health care system to avoid legal consequences or because of a court order for psychological evaluation. Nursing diagnoses common to each disorder were presented along with appropriate interventions and relevant outcome criteria for each.

Nurses who work in all types of clinical settings should be familiar with the characteristics associated with personality-disordered individuals. Nurses working in psychiatry must be knowledgeable about appropriate intervention with these clients, for it is unlikely that they will encounter a greater professional challenge than these clients present.

REVIEW QUESTIONS

SELF-EXAMINATION/LEARNING EXERCISE

Select the answer that is *most* appropriate for each of the following questions:

1. Kim has a diagnosis of borderline personality disorder. She often exhibits alternating clinging and distancing behaviors. The most appropriate nursing intervention with this type of behavior would be to:
   a. Encourage Kim to establish trust in one staff person, with whom all therapeutic interaction should take place.
   b. Secure a verbal contract from Kim that she will discontinue these behaviors.
   c. Withdraw attention if these behaviors continue.
   d. Rotate staff members who work with Kim so that she will learn to relate to more than one person.

2. Kim manipulates the staff in an effort to fulfill her own desires. All of the following may be examples of manipulative behaviors in the borderline client except:
   a. Refusal to stay in room alone, stating, "It's so lonely."
   b. Asking Nurse Jones for cigarettes after 30 minutes, knowing the assigned nurse has explained she must wait 1 hour.
   c. Stating to Nurse Jones, "I really like having you for my nurse. You're the best one around here."
   d. Cutting arms with razor blade after discussing dismissal plans with physician.

3. "Splitting" by the client with borderline personality disorder denotes:
   a. Evidence of precocious development.
   b. A primitive defense mechanism in which the client sees objects as all good or all bad.
   c. A brief psychotic episode in which the client loses contact with reality.
   d. Two distinct personalities within the borderline client.

4. According to Margaret Mahler, predisposition to borderline personality disorder occurs when developmental tasks go unfulfilled in which of the following phases?
   a. Autistic phase, during which the child's needs for security and comfort go unfulfilled
   b. Symbiotic phase, during which the child fails to bond with the mother
   c. Differentiation phase, during which the child fails to recognize a separateness between self and mother
   d. Rapprochement phase, during which the mother withdraws emotional support in response to the child's increasing independence

Situation: Jack was arrested for breaking into a jewelry store and stealing thousands of dollars worth of diamonds. At his arraignment, the judge ordered a psychological evaluation. He has just been admitted by court order to the locked unit. Based on a long history of maladaptive behavior, he has been given the diagnosis of antisocial personality disorder.

5. Which of the following characteristics would you expect to assess in Jack?
   a. Lack of guilt for wrongdoing
   b. Insight into his own behavior
   c. Ability to learn from past experiences
   d. Compliance with authority

6. Milieu therapy is a good choice for clients with antisocial personality disorder because it:
   a. Provides a system of punishment and rewards for behavior modification.
   b. Emulates a social community in which the client may learn to live harmoniously with others.
   c. Provides mostly one-to-one interaction between the client and therapist.
   d. Provides a very structured setting in which the clients have very little input into the planning of their care.

7. In evaluating Jack's progress, which of the following behaviors would be considered the most significant indication of positive change?
   a. Jack got angry only once in group this week.
   b. Jack was able to wait a whole hour for a cigarette without verbally abusing the staff.
   c. On his own initiative, Jack sent a note of apology to a man he had injured in a recent fight.
   d. Jack stated that he would no longer start any more fights.

8. Donna and Katie work in the secretarial pool of a large organization. It is 30 minutes until quitting time when a supervisor hands Katie a job that will take an hour and says he wants it before she leaves. She then says to Donna, "I can't stay over! I'm meeting Bill at 5 o'clock! Be a doll, Donna. Do this job for me!" Donna agrees, although silently she is furious at Katie because this is the third time this has happened in 2 weeks. Katie leaves and Donna says to herself, "This is crazy. I'm not finishing this job for her. Let's see how she likes getting in trouble for a change." Donna leaves without finishing the job. This is an example of which type of personality characteristic?
   a. Antisocial
   b. Paranoid
   c. Passive–aggressive
   d. Obsessive–compulsive

9. Carol is a new nursing graduate being oriented on a medical/surgical unit by the head nurse, Mrs. Carey. When Carol describes a new technique she has learned for positioning immobile clients, Mrs. Carey states, "What are you trying to do … tell me how to do my job? We have always done it this way on this unit, and we will continue to do it this way until I say differently!" This is an example of which type of personality characteristic?
   a. Antisocial
   b. Paranoid
   c. Passive–aggressive
   d. Obsessive–compulsive

10. Which of the following behavioral patterns is characteristic of individuals with histrionic personality disorder?
   a. Belittling themselves and their abilities
   b. Overreacting inappropriately to minor stimuli
   c. Suspicious and mistrustful of others
   d. A lifelong pattern of social withdrawal

TEST YOUR CRITICAL THINKING SKILLS

Lana, age 32, was diagnosed with borderline personality disorder when she was 26 years old. Her husband took her to the emergency department when he walked into the bathroom and found her cutting her legs with a razor blade. At that time, assessment revealed that Lana had a long history of self-mutilation, which she had carefully hidden from her husband and others. Lana began long-term psychoanalytical psychotherapy on an outpatient basis. Therapy revealed that Lana had been physically and sexually abused as a child by both her mother and her father, both now deceased. She admitted to having chronic depression, and her husband related episodes of rage reactions. Lana has been hospitalized on the psychiatric unit for a week because of suicidal ideations. After making a no-suicide contract with the staff, she is allowed to leave the unit on pass to keep a dental appointment that she made a number of weeks ago. She has just returned to the unit and says to her nurse, "I just took 20 Desyrel while I was sitting in my car in the parking lot."

Answer the following questions related to Lana:

1. The nurse is well acquainted with Lana and believes this is a manipulative gesture. How should the nurse handle this situation?
2. What is the priority nursing diagnosis for Lana?
3. Lana likes to "split" the staff into "good guys" and "bad guys." What is the most important intervention for splitting by a person with borderline personality disorder?

IMPLICATIONS OF RESEARCH FOR EVIDENCE-BASED PRACTICE

Zanarini, M.C., & Frankenburg, F.R. (2001). Olanzapine treatment of female borderline personality disorder patients: A double-blind, placebocontrolled pilot study. *Journal of Clinical Psychiatry*, 62(11), 849–854.

Description of the Study: The intent of this study was to compare the efficacy and safety of olanzapine versus placebo in the treatment of women meeting the criteria for borderline personality disorder (BPD). Subjects included 28 women meeting the Revised Diagnostic Interview for Borderlines and the *DSM-IV* criteria for BPD. The subjects were randomly assigned, 19 to olanzapine and 9 to placebo. Treatment duration was 6 months. Outcomes were self-reported on the Symptom Checklist-90, which measured changes in anxiety, depression, paranoia, anger/hostility, and interpersonal sensitivity.

Results of the Study: Olanzapine was associated with a significantly greater rate of improvement over time than placebo in all of the symptom areas studied except depression. Weight gain was modest but higher in the olanzapine group than in the placebo group. No serious movement disorders were noted.

Implications for Nursing Practice: Olanzapine appears to be a safe and effective agent in the treatment of women meeting the criteria for BPD. Nurses who work with individuals who have BPD should be familiar with this medication and understand the nursing implications associated with its administration. The implications of this study are particularly significant for nurses who have prescriptive authority and treat clients with BPD.

IMPLICATIONS OF RESEARCH FOR EVIDENCE-BASED PRACTICE

Dekovic, M., Janssens, J.A.M., & VanAs, N.M.C. (2003). Family predictors of antisocial behavior in adolescence. *Family Process*, 42(2), 223–235.

Description of the Study: The objective of this study was to examine the combined and unique ability of different aspects of family functioning to predict involvement in antisocial behavior in a large community (nonclinical) sample of adolescents. The aspects of family functioning that were measured included:

1. *Proximal factors*: parental childrearing behaviors and the quality of the parent-adolescent relationship.
2. *Distal factors:* parental characteristics (e.g., depression; parental confidence in his or her competence as a parent)
3. *Contextual factors:* family characteristics (e.g., family cohesion, quality of the marital relationship; involvement between members)
4. *Global factors:* family socioeconomic status; family composition (e.g., single-parent family)

The researchers hypothesized that proximal factors would play a stronger role in future antisocial behavior than the other three variables. The sample included 508 families with an adolescent between 12 and 18 years. There were 254 females and 254 males. The parent sample consisted of 969 parents (502 mothers and 467 fathers). Ninety-one percent of the families were intact families, 7 percent of the parents were divorced or separated, and 2 percent were widowed. There was a wide range of socioeconomic and educational backgrounds, although the parents with low educational and occupational levels were slightly underrepresented. Data were gathered in the subjects' homes through a battery of questionnaires administered individually to adolescents, mothers, and fathers.

Results of the Study: Results showed that proximal factors were significant predictors of antisocial behavior, independent of their shared variance with other factors. Also consistent with the hypothesized model, the effects of distal and contextual factors appear to be mostly indirect: after their association with proximal factors was taken into account, these factors were no longer significantly related to antisocial behavior. Global indicators of family functioning (socioeconomic status and family composition) were unrelated to adolescent antisocial behavior. This study showed that supportive parents, parents who use more subtle means of guidance (i.e., supervision rather than punitive strategies) and parents who are consistent in their behavior toward adolescents, have a lower risk that their child would become involved in antisocial behavior. Adolescents who are exposed to coercive and hostile parenting probably adopt this aggressive style of interacting with others. The parent-adolescent relationship that was characterized by elevated levels of conflict and a lack of closeness and acceptance emerged as a risk factor for involvement in antisocial behavior. Parental depression, conflict in the marital dyad, and lack of cohesion between members were also found to influence adolescent antisocial behavior, but less directly than the proximal factors.

Implications for Nursing Practice: Nurses must use this information to design and implement effective parenting programs. Nurses can become actively involved in teaching parents, in inpatient, outpatient, and community education programs. The researchers state, "The findings of this study suggest that, when designing interventions that focus on family factors, in addition to teaching parents adequate child-rearing skills, more attention should be given to finding methods to improve the general *quality* of the parent-adolescent relationship."

INTERNET REFERENCES

Additional information about personality disorders may be located at the following Web sites:

- http://www.mentalhealth.com/dis/p20-pe04.html
- http://www.mentalhealth.com/dis/p20-pe08.html
- http://www.mentalhealth.com/dis/p20-pe05.html
- http://www.mentalhealth.com/dis/p20-pe09.html
- http://www.mentalhealth.com/dis/p20-pe06.html
- http://www.mentalhealth.com/dis/p20-pe07.html
- http://www.mentalhealth.com/dis/p20-pe10.html
- http://www.mentalhealth.com/dis/p20-pe01.html
- http://www.mentalhealth.com/dis/p20-pe02.html
- http://www.mentalhealth.com/dis/p20-pe03.html
- http://www.mentalhealth.com/p13.html#Per

REFERENCES

American Psychiatric Association. (2000). *Diagnostic and statistical manual of mental disorders.* (4th ed.) *Text revision.* Washington, DC: American Psychiatric Association.

Bienenfeld, D. (2004). Personality disorders. Retrieved May 11, 2005 from the World Wide Web at http://www.emedicine.com/med/topic3472.htm

Coccaro, E.F., & Siever, L.J. (2000). The neuropsychopharmacology of personality disorders. *Psychopharmacology: The fourth generation of progress.* The American College of Neuropsychopharmacology. Retrieved May 10, 2005 from the World Wide Web at http://www.acnp.org/G4/GN401000152/CH148.html

Cummings, J.L., & Mega, M.S. (2003). *Neuropsychiatry and behavioral neuroscience.* New York: Oxford University Press.

Finley-Belgrad, E.A., & Davies, J.A. (2004). Personality disorder: Borderline. Retrieved May 10, 2005 from the World Wide Web at http://www.emedicine.com/ped/topic270.htm

Fischer, M., Barkley, R.A., Smallish, L., & Fletcher, K. (2002). Young adult follow-up of hyperactive children: Self-reported psychiatric disorders, comorbidity, and the role of childhood conduct problems and teen CD. *Journal of Abnormal Child Psychology, 30*(5), 463–475.

Gorman, L., Raines, M.L., & Sultan, D.F. (2002). *Psychosocial nursing for general patient care* (2nd ed.). Philadelphia: F.A. Davis.

Hannig, P.J. (2005). *Histrionic personality disorder.* Retrieved May 10, 2005 from the World Wide Web http://www.nvo.com/psych_help/histrionicpersonalitydisorder

Hill, J. (2003). Early identification of individuals at risk for antisocial personality disorder. *British Journal of Psychiatry, 182* (Suppl. 44), s11–s14.

Mark, R. (2002). *How to deal with narcissistic personality disorder.* Retrieved May 10, 2005 from the World Wide Web at http://wiwi.essortment.com/narcissisticp_rwmn.htm

National Institute of Mental Health (NIMH). (2001). Borderline personality disorder: Raising questions, finding answers. Retrieved May 10, 2005 from the World Wide Web at http://www.nimh.nih.gov/publicat/bpd.cfm

Oldham, J.M., Gabbard, G.O., Goin, M.K., Gunderson, J., Soloff, P., Spiegel, D., Stone, M., & Phillips, K.A. (2002). Practice guideline for the treatment of patients with borderline personality disorder. In *The American Psychiatric Association Practice Guidelines for the Treatment of Psychiatric Disorders, Compendium 2002.* Washington, DC: American Psychiatric Publishing.

Phillips, K.A., Yen, S., & Gunderson, J.G. (2003). Personality Disorders. In R.E. Hales & S.C. Yudofsky (Eds.). *Textbook of clinical psychiatry* (4th ed.). Washington, DC: American Psychiatric Publishing.

Ramsland, K. (2005). *Born or made? Theories of psychopathy.* Retrieved May 11, 2005 from the World Wide Web at http://www.crimelibrary.com/criminal_mind/psychology/psychopath/2.html?sect=4

Rettew, D.C., & Jellinek, M.S. (2004). *Personality disorder: Avoidant personality.* Retrieved May 10, 2005 from the World Wide Web at http://www.emedicine.com/ped/topic189.htm

Sadock, B.J., & Sadock, V.A. (2003). *Synopsis of psychiatry: Behavioral sciences/clinical psychiatry* (9th ed.). Philadelphia: Lippincott Williams & Wilkins.

Tyrer, P., & Stein, G. (1993). *Personality disorder reviewed.* London: Royal College of Psychiatrists.

CLASSICAL REFERENCES

Erikson, E. (1963). *Childhood and society* (2nd ed.). New York: W.W. Norton.

Mahler, M., Pine, F., & Bergman, A. (1975). *The psychological birth of the human infant.* New York: Basic Books.

Sullivan, H.S. (1953). *The interpersonal theory of psychiatry.* New York: W.W. Norton.

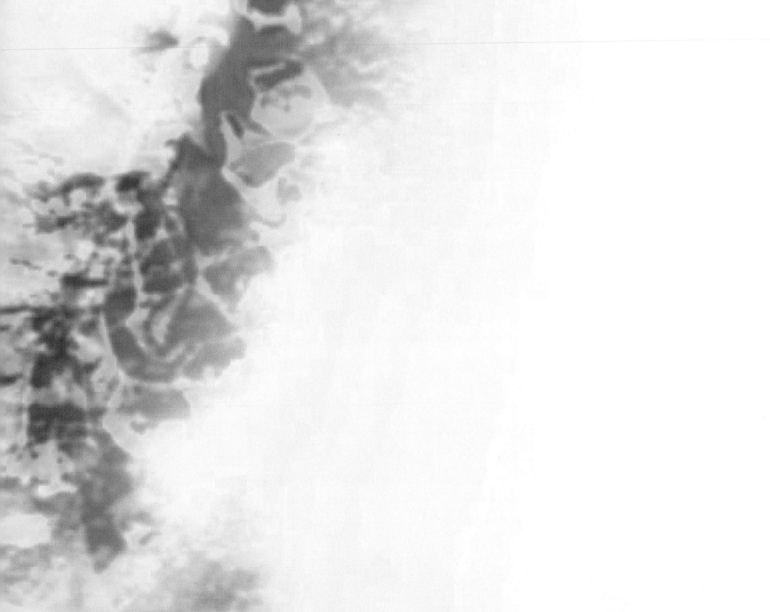

UNIT FIVE

PSYCHIATRIC/MENTAL HEALTH NURSING OF SPECIAL POPULATIONS

THE AGING INDIVIDUAL

CHAPTER OUTLINE

OBJECTIVES

HOW OLD IS *OLD*?

EPIDEMIOLOGICAL STATISTICS

THEORIES OF AGING

THE NORMAL AGING PROCESS

SPECIAL CONCERNS OF THE ELDERLY

APPLICATION OF THE NURSING PROCESS

SUMMARY

REVIEW QUESTIONS

KEY TERMS

attachment theory
bereavement overload
disengagement theory
geriatrics
gerontology

geropsychiatry
"granny-bashing"
"granny-dumping"
long-term memory
Medicaid

Medicare
menopause
osteoporosis
reminiscence therapy
short-term memory

OBJECTIVES

After reading this chapter, the student will be able to:

1. Discuss societal perspectives on aging.
2. Describe an epidemiological profile of aging in the United States.
3. Discuss various theories of aging.
4. Describe biological, psychological, sociocultural, and sexual aspects of the normal aging process.
5. Discuss retirement as a special concern to the aging individual.
6. Explain personal and sociological perspec-

tives of long-term care of the aging individual.
7. Describe the problem of elder abuse as it exists in today's society.
8. Discuss the implications of the increasing number of suicides among the elderly population.
9. Apply the steps of the nursing process to the care of aging individuals.

hat is it like to grow old? It is not likely that many people in the American culture would state that it is something they want to do. Most would agree, however, that it is "better than the alternative."

Roberts (1991) tells the following often-told tale of Supreme Court Justice Oliver Wendell Holmes, Jr. In the year before he retired at age 91 as the oldest justice ever to sit on the Supreme Court of the United States, Holmes and his close friend Justice Louis Brandeis, then a mere 74 years old, were out for one of their frequent walks on Washington's Capitol Hill. On this particular day, the justices spotted a very attractive young woman approaching them. As she passed, Holmes paused, sighed, and said to Brandeis, "Oh, to be 70 again!" Obviously, old age is relative to the individual experiencing it.

Growing old has not been popular among the youth-oriented American culture. However, with 66 million "baby-boomers" reaching their 65th birthdays by the year 2030, greater emphasis is being placed on the needs of an aging population. The disciplines of **gerontology** (the study of the aging process), **geriatrics** (the branch of clinical medicine specializing in problems of the elderly), and **geropsychiatry** (the branch of clinical medicine specializing in psychopathology of the elderly population) are expanding rapidly in response to this predictable demand.

Growing old in a society that has been obsessed with youth may have a critical impact on the mental health of many people. This situation has serious implications for psychiatric nursing.

What is it like to grow old? More and more people will be able to answer this question as the 21st century progresses. Perhaps they will also be asking the question that Roberts (1991) asks: "How did I get here so fast?"

This chapter focuses on physical and psychological changes associated with the aging process, as well as special concerns of the elderly population, such as retirement, long-term care, elder abuse, and rising suicide rates. The nursing process is presented as the vehicle for delivery of nursing care to elderly individuals.

HOW OLD IS *OLD*?

The concept of "old" has changed drastically over the years. Our prehistoric ancestors probably had a life span of 40 years, with the average individual living around 18 years. As civilization developed, mortality rates remained high as a result of periodic famine and frequent malnutrition. An improvement in the standard of living was not truly evident until about the middle of the 17th century. Since that time, assured food supply, changes in food production, better housing conditions, and more progressive medical and sanitation facilities have contributed to population growth, declining mortality rates, and substantial increases in longevity.

In 1900, the average life expectancy in the United States was 47 years, and only 4 percent of the population was age 65 or over. By 2003, the average life expectancy at birth was 74.8 years for men and 80.1 years for women (National Center for Health Statistics [NCHS], 2005).

The U.S. Census Bureau has created a system for classification of older Americans:

Older:	55 through 64 years
Elderly:	65 through 74 years
Aged:	75 through 84 years
Very old:	85 years and older

Some gerontologists have elected to used a simpler classification system:

Young old:	60 through 74 years
Middle old:	75 through 84 years
Old old:	85 years and older

So how old is *old*? Obviously the term cannot be defined by a number. Myths and stereotypes of aging have long obscured our understanding of the aged and the process of aging. Ideas that all elderly individuals are sick, depressed, obsessed with death, senile, and incapable of change affect the way elderly people are treated. They even shape the pattern of aging of the people who believe them. They can become self-fulfilling prophecies—people start to believe they should behave in certain ways and, therefore, act according to those beliefs. Generalized assumptions can be demeaning and interfere with the quality of life for older individuals.

Just as there are many differences in individual adaptation at earlier stages of development, so it is in the elderly person. Erikson (1963) has suggested that the mentally healthy older person possesses a sense of ego integrity and self-acceptance that will help in adapting to the ambiguities of the future with a sense of security and optimism.

Murray and Zentner (2001) state:

> Having accomplished the earlier [developmental] tasks, the person accepts life as his or her own and as the only life for the self. He or she would wish for none other and would defend the meaning and the dignity of the lifestyle. The person has further refined the characteristics of maturity described for the middle-aged adult, achieving both wisdom and an enriched perspective about life and people. (p. 800)

Everyone, particularly health care workers, should see aging people as individuals, each with specific needs and abilities, rather than as a stereotypical group. Some individuals may seem "old" at 40, whereas others may not seem "old" at 70. Variables such as attitude, mental health, physical health, and degree of independence strongly influence how an individual perceives himself or herself. Surely, in the final analysis, whether one is considered "old" must be self-determined.

EPIDEMIOLOGICAL STATISTICS

The Population

In 1980, Americans 65 years of age or older numbered 25.5 million. By 2003, these numbers had increased to approximately 36 million, representing just over 12 percent of the population (NCHS, 2004). This trend is expected to continue, with a projection for 2030 at about 71.5 million, or 20 percent of the population.

Marital Status

In 2003, of individuals age 65 and older, 74.4 percent of men and 43.4 percent of women were married (NCHS, 2004). Forty-four percent of all women in this age group were widowed. There were over three times as many widows as widowers because women live longer than men and tend to marry men older than themselves.

Living Arrangements

The majority of individuals age 65 or older live alone, with a spouse, or with relatives (NCHS, 2004). At any one time, fewer than 5 percent of people in this age group live in institutions. This percentage increases dramatically with age, ranging from 1.1 percent for persons 65 to 74 years, to 4.3 percent for persons 75 to 84 years, and 18.3 percent for persons 85 and older. See Figure 38–1 for a distribution of living arrangements.

Economic Status

Approximately 3.6 million persons age 65 or older were below the poverty level in 2002 (AoA, 2003). Older women had a higher poverty rate than older men, and older Hispanic women living alone had the highest poverty rate. Poor people who have worked all their lives can expect to become poorer in old age, and others will become poor only after becoming old. However, there are still a substantial number of affluent and middle-income older persons who enjoy a high quality of life.

Of individuals in this age group, 80 percent owned their own homes in 2003 (U.S. Census Bureau, 2005). However, the housing of this population of Americans is usually older and less adequate than that of the younger population; therefore, a higher percentage of income must be spent on maintenance and repairs.

Employment

With the passage of the Age Discrimination in Employment Act in 1967, forced retirement has been virtually eliminated in the workplace. Evidence suggests that involvement in purposeful activity is vital to successful adaptation and perhaps even to survival. Individuals age 65 or older constituted 3.3 percent of the U.S. labor force in 2004 (Bureau of Labor Statistics, 2005).

Health Status

The number of days in which usual activities are restricted because of illness or injury increases with age. The American Geriatrics Society (2005) reports that 82 percent of individuals 65 and older have at least one chronic condition, and two-thirds have more than one chronic condition. The most commonly occurring conditions among the elderly population are hypertension, arthritis, heart disease, cancer, sinusitis, and diabetes (AoA, 2003).

Emotional and mental illnesses increase over the life cycle. Depression is particularly prevalent and suicide is increasing among elderly Americans. Organic mental disease increases dramatically in old age.

THEORIES OF AGING*

A number of theories related to the aging process have been described. These theories are grouped into two broad categories: biological and psychosocial.

Biological Theories

Biological theories attempt to explain the physical process of aging, including molecular and cellular changes in the major organ systems and the body's ability to function adequately and resist disease. They also attempt to explain why people age differently and what factors affect longevity and the body's ability to resist disease.

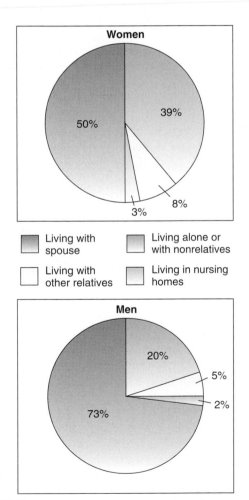

FIGURE 38–1 Living arrangements of persons age 65 and older (NCHS, 2004).

---

*This section was adapted from Stanley, M., Blair, K.A., & Beare, P.G. (2005). *Gerontological nursing: Promoting successful aging with older adults* (3rd ed.). Philadelphia: F.A. Davis, with permission.

Genetic Theory

According to genetic theory, aging is an involuntarily inherited process that operates over time to alter cellular or tissue structures. This theory suggests that life span and longevity changes are predetermined. Stanley, Blair, and Beare (2005) state,

> [Genetic] theories posit that the replication process at the cellular level becomes deranged by inappropriate information provided from the cell nucleus. The DNA molecule becomes cross-linked with another substance that alters the genetic information. This cross-linking results in errors at the cellular level that eventually cause the body's organs and systems to fail. (p. 12)

The development of free radicals, collagen, and lipofuscin in the aging body, and of an increased frequency in the occurrence of cancer and autoimmune disorders, provide some evidence for this theory and the proposition that error or mutation occurs at the molecular and cellular level.

Wear-and-Tear Theory

Proponents of this theory believe that the body wears out on a scheduled basis. Free radicals, which are the waste products of metabolism, accumulate and cause damage to important biological structures. Free radicals are molecules with unpaired electrons that exist normally in the body; they also are produced by ionizing radiation, ozone, and chemical toxins. According to this theory, these free radicals cause DNA damage, cross-linkage of collagen, and the accumulation of age pigments.

Environmental Theory

According to this theory, factors in the environment (e.g., industrial carcinogens, sunlight, trauma, and infection) bring about changes in the aging process. Although these factors are known to accelerate aging, the impact of the environment is a secondary rather than a primary factor in aging. Science is only beginning to uncover the many environmental factors that affect aging.

Immunity Theory

The immunity theory describes an age-related decline in the immune system. As people age, their ability to defend against foreign organisms decreases, resulting in susceptibility to diseases such as cancer and infection. Along with the diminished immune function, a rise in the body's autoimmune response occurs, leading to the development of autoimmune diseases such as rheumatoid arthritis and allergies to food and environmental agents.

Neuroendocrine Theory

This theory proposes that aging occurs because of a slowing of the secretion of certain hormones that have an impact on reactions regulated by the nervous system. This is most clearly demonstrated in the pituitary gland, thyroid, adrenals, and the glands of reproduction. Although research has given some credence to a predictable biological clock that controls fertility, there is much more to be learned from the study of the neuroendocrine system in relation to a systemic aging process that is controlled by a "clock."

Psychosocial Theories

Psychosocial theories focus on social and psychological changes that accompany advancing age, as opposed to the biological implications of anatomic deterioration. Several theories have attempted to describe how attitudes and behavior in the early phases of life affect people's reactions during the late phase. This work is called the process of "successful aging."

Personality Theory

Personality theories address aspects of psychological growth without delineating specific tasks or expectations of older adults. Murray and Zentner (2001) state, "Evidence supports the general hypothesis that personality characteristics in old age are highly correlated with early life characteristics." In extreme old age, however, people show greater similarity in certain characteristics, probably because of similar declines in biological functioning and societal opportunities.

In a classic study by Reichard, Livson, and Peterson (1962), the personalities of older men were classified into five major categories according to their patterns of adjustment to aging. According to this study:

1. *Mature men* are considered well-balanced persons who maintain close personal relationships. They accept both the strengths and weaknesses of their age, finding little to regret about retirement and approaching most problems in a relaxed or convivial manner without continually having to assess blame.
2. *"Rocking chair" personalities* are found in passive-dependent individuals who are content to lean on others for support, to disengage, and to let most of life's activities pass them by.
3. *Armored men* have well-integrated defense mechanisms, which serve as adequate protection. Rigid and stable, they present a strong silent front and often rely on activity as an expression of their continuing independence.
4. *Angry men* are bitter about life, themselves, and other people. Aggressiveness is common, as is suspicion of

others, especially of minorities or women. With little tolerance for ambiguity or frustration, they have always shown some instability in work and their personal lives, and now feel extremely threatened by old age.

5. *Self-haters* are similar to angry men, except that most of their animosity is turned inward on themselves. Seeing themselves as dismal failures, being old only depresses them all the more.

The investigators identified the mature, "rocking chair," or armored categories as characteristic of healthy, adjusted individuals and the angry and self-hater categories as less successful agers. In all cases, the evidence suggested that the personalities of the subjects, although distinguished by age-specific criteria, had not changed appreciably throughout most of adulthood.

In a more recent study of personality traits, Srivastava and associates (2003) examined the "big five" personality trait dimensions in a large sample to determine how personality changes over the life span. Age range of the subjects was from 21 to 60. The personality traits tested included conscientiousness, agreeableness, neuroticism, openness, and extraversion. They found that conscientiousness (being organized, planful, and disciplined) increased throughout the age range studied, with the biggest increases during the 20s. Agreeableness (being warm, generous, and helpful) increased most during a person's 30s. Neuroticism (being anxious and emotionally labile) declined with age for women, but did not decline for men. Openness (being acceptable to new experiences) showed small declines with age for both men and women. Extraversion (being outwardly expressive and interested in the environment) declined for women but did not show changes in men. This study contradicts the view that personality traits tend to stop changing in early adulthood. These researchers suggest that personality traits change gradually but systematically throughout the life span.

Developmental Task Theory

Developmental tasks are the activities and challenges that one must accomplish at specific stages in life to achieve successful aging. Erikson (1963) described the primary task of old age as being able to see one's life as having been lived with integrity. In the absence of achieving that sense of having lived well, the older adult is at risk for becoming preoccupied with feelings of regret or despair.

Disengagement Theory

Disengagement theory describes the process of withdrawal by older adults from societal roles and responsibilities. According to the theory, this withdrawal process is predictable, systematic, inevitable, and necessary for the proper functioning of a growing society. Older adults were said to be happy when social contacts diminished and responsibilities were assumed by a younger generation. The benefit to the older adult is thought to be in providing time for reflecting on life's accomplishments and for coming to terms with unfulfilled expectations. The benefit to society is thought to be an orderly transfer of power from old to young.

There have been many critics of this theory, and the postulates have been challenged. For many healthy and productive older individuals, the prospect of a slower pace and fewer responsibilities is undesirable.

Activity Theory

In direct opposition to the disengagement theory is the activity theory of aging, which holds that the way to age successfully is to stay active. Multiple studies have validated the positive relationship between maintaining meaningful interaction with others and physical and mental well-being.

Sadock and Sadock (2003) suggest that social integration is the prime factor in determining psychosocial adaptation in later life. Social integration refers to how the aging individual is included and takes part in the life and activities of his or her society. This theory holds that the maintenance of activities is important to most people as a basis for deriving and sustaining satisfaction, self-esteem, and health.

Continuity Theory

This theory, also known as the developmental theory, is a follow-up to the disengagement and activity theories. It emphasizes the individual's previously established coping abilities and personal character traits as a basis for predicting how the person will adjust to the changes of aging. Basic lifestyle characteristics are likely to remain stable in old age, barring physical or other types of complications that necessitate change. A person who has enjoyed the company of others and an active social life will continue to enjoy this lifestyle into old age. One who has preferred solitude and a limited number of activities will probably find satisfaction in a continuation of this lifestyle.

Maintenance of internal continuity is motivated by the need for preservation of self-esteem, ego integrity, cognitive function, and social support. As they age, individuals maintain their self-concept by reinterpreting their current experiences so that old values can take on new meanings in keeping with present circumstances. Internal self-concepts and beliefs are not readily vulnerable to environmental change; and external continuity in skills, activities, roles, and relationships can remain remarkably stable into the 70s. Physical illness or death of friends and loved ones may preclude continued social interaction (Sadock & Sadock, 2003).

THE NORMAL AGING PROCESS

Biological Aspects of Aging

Individuals are unique in their physical and psychological aging processes, as influenced by their predisposition or resistance to illness; the effects of their external environment and behaviors; their exposure to trauma, infections, and past diseases; and the health and illness practices they have adopted during their life span. As the individual ages, there is a quantitative loss of cells and changes in many of the enzymatic activities within cells, resulting in a diminished responsiveness to biological demands made on the body. Age-related changes occur at different rates for different individuals, although in actuality, when growth stops aging begins. This section presents a brief overview of the normal biological changes that occur with the aging process.

Skin

One of the most dramatic changes that occurs in aging is the loss of elastin in the skin. This effect, as well as changes in collagen, causes aged skin to wrinkle and sag. Excessive exposure to sunlight compounds these changes and increases the risk of developing skin cancer.

Fat redistribution results in a loss of the subcutaneous cushion of adipose tissue. Thus, older people lose "insulation" and are more sensitive to extremes of ambient temperature than are younger people (Stanley, Blair, & Beare, 2005). Fewer blood vessels to the skin result in a slower rate of healing.

Cardiovascular System

The age-related decline in the cardiovascular system is thought to be the major determinant of decreased tolerance for exercise and loss of conditioning and the overall decline in energy reserve. The aging heart is characterized by modest hypertrophy with reduced ventricular compliance and diminished cardiac output (Murray & Zentner, 2001; Sadock & Sadock, 2003). This results in a decrease in response to work demands and some diminishment of blood flow to the brain, kidneys, liver, and muscles. Heart rate also slows with time. If arteriosclerosis is present, cardiac function is further compromised.

Respiratory System

Thoracic expansion is diminished by an increase in fibrous tissue and loss of elastin. Pulmonary vital capacity decreases, and the amount of residual air increases. Scattered areas of fibrosis in the alveolar septa interfere with exchange of oxygen and carbon dioxide. These changes are accelerated by the use of cigarettes or other inhaled substances. Cough and laryngeal reflexes are re- duced, causing decreased ability to defend the airway. Decreased pulmonary blood flow and diffusion ability result in reduced efficiency in responding to sudden respiratory demands.

Musculoskeletal System

Skeletal aging involving the bones, muscles, ligaments, and tendons probably generates the most frequent limitations on activities of daily living experienced by aging individuals. Loss of muscle mass is significant, although this occurs more slowly in men than in women. Demineralization of the bones occurs at a rate of about 1 percent per year throughout the life span in both men and women. However, this increases to approximately 10 percent in women around **menopause**, making them particularly vulnerable to **osteoporosis**.

Individual muscle fibers become thinner and less elastic with age. Muscles become less flexible following disuse. There is diminished storage of muscle glycogen, resulting in loss of energy reserve for increased activity. These changes are accelerated by nutritional deficiencies and inactivity.

Gastrointestinal System

In the oral cavity, the teeth show a reduction in dentine production, shrinkage and fibrosis of root pulp, gingival retraction, and loss of bone density in the alveolar ridges. There is some loss of peristalsis in the stomach and intestines, and gastric acid production decreases. Levels of intrinsic factor may also decrease, resulting in vitamin B_{12} malabsorption in some aging individuals. A significant decrease in absorptive surface area of the small intestine may be associated with some decline in nutrient absorption. Motility slowdown of the large intestine, combined with poor dietary habits, dehydration, lack of exercise, and some medications, may give rise to problems with constipation.

There is a modest decrease in size and weight of the liver resulting in losses in enzyme activity required to deactivate certain medications by the liver. These age-related changes can influence the metabolism and excretion of these medications. These changes, along with the pharmacokinetics of the drug, must be considered when giving medications to aging individuals.

Endocrine System

A decreased level of thyroid hormones causes a lowered basal metabolic rate. Decreased amounts of adrenocorticotropic hormone may result in less efficient stress response.

Impairments in glucose tolerance are evident in aging individuals (Pietraniec-Shannon, 2003). Studies of glucose challenges show that insulin levels are equivalent to or slightly higher than those from younger challenged individuals, although peripheral insulin resistance appears to play a significant role in carbohydrate intolerance. The observed glucose clearance abnormalities and insulin resistance in older people may be related to many factors other than biological aging (e.g., obesity, family history of diabetes) and may be influenced substantially by diet or exercise.

Genitourinary System

Age-related declines in renal function occur because of a steady attrition of nephrons and sclerosis within the glomeruli over time (Stanley, Blair, & Beare, 2005). Vascular changes affect blood flow to the kidneys and results in reduced glomerular filtration and tubular function (Murray & Zentner, 2001). Elderly people are prone to develop the syndrome of inappropriate antidiuretic hormone secretion, and levels of blood urea nitrogen and creatinine may be elevated slightly. The overall decline in renal functioning has serious implications for physicians in prescribing medications for elderly individuals.

In men, enlargement of the prostate gland is common as aging occurs. Prostatic hypertrophy is associated with an increased risk for urinary retention and may also be a cause of urinary incontinence (Beers & Jones, 2004). Loss of muscle and sphincter control, as well as the use of some medications, may cause urinary incontinence in women. Not only is this problem a cause of social stigma, but also, if left untreated, it increases the risk of urinary tract infection and local skin irritation. Normal changes in the genitalia are discussed in the section on "Sexual Aspects of Aging."

Immune System

Aging results in changes in both cell-mediated and antibody-mediated immune responses. The size of the thymus gland declines continuously from just beyond puberty to about 15 percent of its original size at age 50. The consequences of these changes include a greater susceptibility to infections and a diminished inflammatory response that results in delayed healing. There is also evidence of an increase in various autoantibodies (e.g., rheumatoid factor) as a person ages, increasing the risk of autoimmune disorders (Beers & Jones, 2004).

Because of the overall decrease in efficiency of the immune system, the proliferation of abnormal cells is facilitated in the elderly individual. Cancer is the best example of aberrant cells allowed to proliferate due to the ineffectiveness of the immune system.

Nervous System

With aging, there is an absolute loss of neurons, which correlates with decreases in brain weight of about 10 percent by age 90 (Murray & Zentner, 2001). Gross morphological examination reveals gyral atrophy in the frontal, temporal, and parietal lobes; widening of the sulci; and ventricular enlargement. However, it must be remembered that these changes have been identified in careful study of adults with normal intellectual function.

The brain has enormous reserve, and little cerebral function is lost over time, although greater functional decline is noted in the periphery (Stanley, Blair, & Beare, 2005). There appears to be a disproportionately greater loss of cells in the cerebellum, the locus ceruleus, the substantia nigra, and olfactory bulbs, accounting for some of the more characteristic aging behaviors such as mild gait disturbances, sleep disruptions, and decreased smell and taste perception.

Some of the age-related changes within the nervous system may be due to alterations in neurotransmitter release, uptake, turnover, catabolism, or receptor functions (Beers & Jones, 2004). A great deal of attention is being given to brain biochemistry and in particular to the neurotransmitters acetylcholine, dopamine, norepinephrine, and epinephrine. These biochemical changes may be responsible for the altered responses of many older persons to stressful events and some biological treatments.

Sensory Systems

Vision. Visual acuity begins to decrease in mid-life. Presbyopia (blurred near vision) is the standard marker of aging of the eye. It is caused by a loss of elasticity of the crystalline lens, and results in compromised accommodation.

Cataract development is inevitable if the individual lives long enough for the changes to occur. Cataracts occur when the lens of the eye becomes less resilient (due to compression of fibers) and increasingly opaque (as proteins lump together), ultimately resulting in a loss of visual acuity.

The color in the iris may fade, and the pupil may become irregular in shape. A decrease in production of secretions by the lacrimal glands may cause dryness and result in increased irritation and infection. The pupil may become constricted, requiring an increase in the amount of light needed for reading.

Hearing. Hearing changes significantly with the aging process. Gradually over time, the ear loses its sensitivity to discriminate sounds because of damage to the hair cells of the cochlea. The most dramatic decline appears to be in perception of high-frequency sounds.

Although hearing loss is significant in all aging individuals, the decline is more dramatic in men than in women. Men are twice as likely as women to have hearing loss (Murray & Zentner, 2001).

Taste and Smell. Taste sensitivity decreases over the life span. Taste discrimination decreases, and bitter taste sensations predominate. Sensitivity to sweet and salty tastes is diminished.

The deterioration of the olfactory bulbs is accompanied by loss of smell acuity. The aromatic component of taste perception diminishes.

Touch and Pain. Organized sensory nerve receptors on the skin continue to decrease throughout the life span; thus, the touch threshold increases with age (Pietraniec-Shannon, 2003). The ability to feel pain also decreases in response to these changes, and the ability to perceive and interpret painful stimuli changes. These changes have critical implications for the elderly in their potential lack of ability to use sensory warnings for escaping serious injury.

Psychological Aspects of Aging

Memory Functioning

Age-related memory deficiencies have been extensively reported in the literature. Although **short-term memory** seems to deteriorate with age, perhaps because of poorer sorting strategies, **long-term memory** does not show similar changes. However, in nearly every instance, well-educated, mentally active people do not exhibit the same decline in memory functioning as their age peers who lack similar opportunities to flex their minds. Nevertheless, with few exceptions, the time required for memory scanning is longer for both recent and remote recall among older people. This can sometimes be attributed to social or health factors (e.g., stress, fatigue, illness), but it can also occur because of certain normal physical changes associated with aging (e.g., decreased blood flow to the brain).

Intellectual Functioning

There appears to be a high degree of regularity in intellectual functioning across the adult age span. Crystallized abilities, or knowledge acquired in the course of the socialization process, tend to remain stable over the adult life span. Fluid abilities, or abilities involved in solving novel problems, tend to decline gradually from young to old adulthood. In other words, intellectual abilities of older people do not decline but do become obsolete. The age of their formal educational experiences is reflected in their intelligence scoring.

Learning Ability

The ability to learn is not diminished by age. Studies, however, have shown that some aspects of learning do change with age. The ordinary slowing of reaction time with age for nearly all tasks or the over-arousal of the central nervous system may account for lower performance levels on tests requiring rapid responses. Under

conditions that allow for self-pacing by the participant, differences in accuracy of performance diminish. Ability to learn continues throughout life, although strongly influenced by interests, activity, motivation, health, and experience. Adjustments do need to be made in teaching methodology and time allowed for learning.

Adaptation to the Tasks of Aging

Loss and Grief. Individuals experience losses from the very beginning of life. By the time individuals reach their 60s and 70s, they have experienced numerous losses, and mourning has become a life-long process. Unfortunately, with the aging process comes a convergence of losses, the timing of which makes it impossible for the aging individual to complete the grief process in response to one loss before another occurs. Because grief is cumulative, this can result in **bereavement overload**, which has been implicated in the predisposition to depression in the elderly.

Attachment to Others. Many studies have confirmed the importance of interpersonal relationships at all stages in the life cycle. Murray and Zentner (2001) state:

[Social networks] contribute to well-being of the senior by promoting socialization and companionship, elevating morale and life satisfaction, buffering the effects of stressful events, providing a confident, and facilitating coping skills and mastery.

This need for **attachment** is consistent with the activity theory of aging that correlates the importance of social integration with successful adaptation in later life.

Maintenance of Self-Identity. Self-concept and self-image appear to remain stable over time. Factors that have been shown to favor good psychosocial adjustment in later life are sustained family relationships, maturity of ego defenses, absence of alcoholism, and absence of depressive disorder (Vaillant, 2003). Studies show that the elderly have a strong need for and remarkable capability of retaining a persistent self-concept in the face of the many changes that contribute to instability in later life.

Dealing with Death. Death anxiety among the aging is apparently more of a myth than a reality. Studies have not supported the negative view of death as an overriding psychological factor in the aging process. Various investigators who have worked with dying persons report that it is not death itself, but abandonment, pain, and confusion that is feared. What many desire most is someone to talk with, to show them their life's meaning is not shattered merely because they are about to die (Kübler-Ross, 1969; Murray & Zentner, 2001).

Psychiatric Disorders in Later Life. The later years constitute a time of especially high risk for emotional distress. Sadock and Sadock, (2003) state:

Several psychosocial risk factors predispose older people to mental disorders. These risk factors include loss of social roles, loss of autonomy, the deaths of friends and relatives, declining health, increased isolation, financial constraints, and decreased cognitive functioning. (p. 1320)

Dementing disorders are the most common causes of psychopathology in the elderly (Sadock & Sadock, 2003). About half of these disorders are of the Alzheimer's type, which is characterized by an insidious onset and a gradually progressive course of cognitive impairment. No curative treatment is currently available. Symptomatic treatments, including pharmacological interventions, attention to the environment, and family support, can help to maximize the client's level of functioning.

Delirium is one of the most common and important forms of psychopathology in later life. A number of factors have been identified that predispose elderly people to delirium, including structural brain disease, reduced capacity for homeostatic regulation, impaired vision and hearing, a high prevalence of chronic disease, reduced resistance to acute stress, and age-related changes in the pharmacokinetic and pharmacodynamics of drugs. Delirium needs to be recognized and the underlying condition treated as soon as possible. A high mortality is associated with this condition.

Depressive disorders are the most common affective illnesses occurring after the middle years. The incidence of increased depression among elderly people is influenced by the variables of physical illness, functional disability, cognitive impairment, and loss of a spouse (Stanley, Blair, & Beare, 2005). Hypochondriacal symptoms are common in the depressed elderly. Symptomatology often mimics that of dementia, a condition that is referred to as pseudodementia. (See Table 26–3 for a comparison of the symptoms of dementia and pseudodementia.) Suicide is more prevalent in the elderly, with declining health and decreased economic status being considered important influencing factors. Treatment of depression in the elderly individual is with psychotropic medications or electroconvulsive therapy.

Schizophrenia and delusional disorders may continue into old age or may manifest themselves for the first time only during senescence (Blazer, 2003). In most instances, individuals who manifest psychotic disorders early in life show a decline in psychopathology as they age. Late-onset schizophrenia (after age 60) is not common, but when it does occur, it often is characterized by delusions or hallucinations of a persecutory nature. The course is chronic, and treatment is with neuroleptics and supportive psychotherapy.

Most anxiety disorders begin in early to middle adulthood, but some appear for the first time after age 60. Sadock and Sadock (2003) state:

The fragility of the autonomic nervous system in older persons may account for the development of anxiety after a major stressor. Because of concurrent physical disability, older persons react more severely to posttraumatic stress disorder than younger persons. (p. 1325)

In older adults, symptoms of anxiety and depression often accompany each other, making it difficult to determine which disorder is dominant. Personality disorders are uncommon in the elderly population. The incidence of personality disorders among individuals over age 65 is less than 5 percent. Most elderly people with personality disorder have likely manifested the symptomatology for many years.

Sleep disorders are very common in the aging individual. Sleep disturbances affect 50 percent of people age 65 and older who live at home and 66 percent of those who live in long-term care facilities (Stanley, Blair, & Beare, 2005). Some common causes of sleep disturbances among elderly people include age-dependent decreases in the ability to sleep ("sleep decay"); increased prevalence of sleep apnea; depression; dementia; anxiety; pain; impaired mobility; medications; and psychosocial factors such as loneliness, inactivity, and boredom. Sedative-hypnotics, along with non-pharmacological approaches, are often used as sleep aids with the elderly. Changes in aging associated with metabolism and elimination must be considered when maintenance medications are administered for chronic insomnia in the aging client.

Sociocultural Aspects of Aging

Old age brings many important socially induced changes, some of which have the potential for negative effect on both the physical and mental well-being of older persons. In American society, old age is arbitrarily defined as being 65 years or older because that is the age when most people have been able to retire with full Social Security and other pension benefits. Recent legislation has increased the age beyond 65 years for full Social Security benefits.

Elderly people in virtually all cultures share some basic needs and interests. There is little doubt that most individuals choose to live the most satisfying life possible until their demise. They want protection from hazards and release from the weariness of everyday tasks. They want to be treated with the respect and dignity that is deserving of individuals who have reached this pinnacle in life; and they want to die with the same respect and dignity.

From the beginning of human culture, the aged have had a special status in society. Even today, in some cultures the aged are the most powerful, the most engaged, and the most respected members of the society. This has not been the case in the modern industrial societies, although trends in the status of the aged differ widely between one industrialized country and another. For example, the status and integration of the aged in Japan have remained relatively high when compared with the other industrialized nations. The aged are awarded a position of honor in cultures that place emphasis on family cohesiveness. In these cultures, the aged are revered for their knowledge and wisdom gained through their years of life experiences (Giger & Davidhizar, 2004).

Many negative stereotypes color the perspective on aging in the United States. Ideas that elderly individuals are always tired or sick, slow and forgetful, isolated and lonely, unproductive, and angry determine the way younger individuals relate to the elderly in this society. Increasing disregard for the elderly has resulted in a type of segregation, as aging individuals voluntarily seek out or are involuntarily placed in special residences for the aged.

Assisted living centers, retirement apartment complexes, and even entire retirement communities intended solely for individuals over age 50, are becoming more and more common. In 2002, about half (52 percent) of persons age 65 and older lived in nine states, with the majority in California, Florida, and New York (AoA, 2003). It is important for elderly individuals to feel part of an integrated group, and they are migrating to these areas in an effort to achieve this integration. This phenomenon provides additional corroboration for the activity theory of aging, and the importance of attachment to others.

Employment is another area in which the elderly experience discrimination. Although compulsory retirement has been virtually eliminated, discrimination still exists in hiring and promotion practices. Many employers are not eager to retain or hire older workers. It is difficult to determine how much of the failure to hire and promote results from discrimination based on age alone and how much of it is related to a realistic and fair appraisal of the aged employee's ability and efficiency. It is true that some elderly individuals are no longer capable of doing as good a job as a younger worker; however, there are many who likely can do a *better* job than their younger counterparts, if given the opportunity. Nevertheless, surveys have shown that some employers accept the negative stereotypes about elderly individuals and believe that older workers are hard to please, set in their ways, less productive, frequently absent, and involved in more accidents.

The status of the elderly may improve with time and as their numbers increase with the aging of the "baby boomers." As older individuals gain political power, the benefits and privileges designed for the elderly will increase. There is power in numbers, and the 21st century promises power for individuals ages 65 and older.

Sexual Aspects of Aging

Sexuality and the sexual needs of elderly people are frequently misunderstood, condemned, stereotyped, ridiculed, repressed, and ignored. Americans have grown up in a society that has liberated sexual expression for all other age groups, but still retains certain Victorian standards regarding sexual expression by the elderly. Negative stereotyped notions concerning sexual interest and activity of the elderly are common. Some of these include ideas that older people have no sexual interests or desires; that they are sexually undesirable; or that they are all too fragile or too ill to engage in sexual activity. Some people even believe it is disgusting or comical to consider elderly individuals as sexual beings.

These cultural stereotypes undoubtedly play a large part in the misperception many people hold regarding sexuality of the aged, and they may be reinforced by the common tendency of the young to deny the inevitability of aging. With reasonably good health and an interesting and interested partner, there is no inherent reason why individuals should not enjoy an active sexual life well into late adulthood (Altman & Hanfling, 2003).

Physical Changes Associated with Sexuality

Many of the changes in sexuality that occur in later years are related to the physical changes that are taking place at that time of life.

Changes in the Female. Menopause may begin anytime during the 40s or early 50s. During this time there is a gradual decline in the functioning of the ovaries and the subsequent production of estrogen, which results in a number of changes. The walls of the vagina become thin and inelastic, the vagina itself shrinks in both width and length, and the amount of vaginal lubrication decreases noticeably. Orgastic uterine contractions may become spastic. All of these changes can result in painful penetration, vaginal burning, pelvic aching, or irritation on urination. In some women, the discomfort may be severe enough to result in an avoidance of intercourse. Paradoxically, these symptoms are more likely to occur with infrequent intercourse of only one time a month or less. Regular and more frequent sexual activity results in a greater capacity for sexual performance (King, 2005). Other symptoms that are associated with menopause in some women include hot flashes, night sweats, sleeplessness, irritability, mood swings, migraine headaches, urinary incontinence, and weight gain.

Some menopausal women elect to take hormone replacement therapy for relief of these changes and symptoms. With estrogen therapy, the symptoms of menopause are minimized or do not occur at all. However, some women choose not to take the hormone because of an increased risk of breast cancer, and when given alone, an increased risk of endometrial cancer. To combat this latter effect, most women also take a second hormone, progesterone. Taken for 7 to 10 days during the month, progesterone decreases the risk of estrogen-induced endometrial cancer. Some physicians are electing to prescribe a low dose of progesterone that is taken, along with estrogen, for the entire month. A combination pill, taken in this manner, is also available.

Results of the Women's Health Initiative (WHI), as reported in the *Journal of the American Medical Association*, indicate that the combination pill is associated with an increased risk of cardiovascular disease and breast cancer (Rossouw et al., 2002). Benefits related to decreased risk of colon cancer and osteoporosis were reported; however, investigators stopped this arm of the study and suggested discontinuation of this type of therapy.

Changes in the Male. Testosterone production declines gradually over the years, beginning between ages 40 and 60. A major change resulting from this hormone reduction is that erections occur more slowly and require more direct genital stimulation to achieve. There may also be a modest decrease in the firmness of the erection in men older than age 60. The refractory period lengthens with age, increasing the amount of time following orgasm before the man may achieve another erection. The volume of ejaculate gradually decreases, and the force of ejaculation lessens. The testes become somewhat smaller, but most men continue to produce viable sperm well into old age. Prolonged control over ejaculation in middle-aged

and elderly men may bring increased sexual satisfaction for both partners.

Sexual Behavior in the Elderly

Coital frequency in early marriage and the overall quantity of sexual activity between age 20 and 40 correlate significantly with frequency patterns of sexual activity during aging (Masters, Johnson, & Kolodny, 1995). Although sexual interest and behavior do appear to decline somewhat with age, studies show that significant numbers of elderly men and women have active and satisfying sex lives well into their 80s. A survey commissioned by the American Association of Retired Persons (AARP) and *Modern Maturity* magazine provided some revealing information regarding the sexual attitudes and behavior of senior citizens. Some statistics from the survey are summarized in Table 38–1. The information from this survey clearly indicates that sexual activity can

---

TABLE 38–1   **AARP/Modern Maturity Survey on Sexual Attitudes and Behavior (A survey of Americans ages 45 and older)**

	AGES	MEN	WOMEN	BOTH
Have sex at least once a week:	45—59			~ 50 %
	60—74	30%	24%	
Have sex at least once a month:	45 and older			> 70%
Extremely or very satisfied with their physical relationships:	All	67%	61%	
Very satisfied with emotional relationship:	All	70%	62%	
Report sexual activity is important to their overall quality of life:	All	60%	35%	
Believe non-marital sex is okay:	< 60		66%	
	60–74		50%	
	≥ 75		33%	
	All	A majority of men of all ages believe non-marital sex is okay.		
Report having a chronic health problem affecting sex life:	All			20%
Report taking hormone replacement therapy:	45–59		36%	
	≥ 75		10%	
Report having taken antidepressant therapy:	45–59		14%	
	60–74		8%	
Report prostate problems interfere with sex life:	All	18%		
Report being treated for prostate problems:	All	50%		
Report being impotent:	< 60	2.5%		
	60–74	16%		
	≥ 75	37%		
Report using a medicine, hormone, or other treatment for impotence:	All	10%		
Describe their partners as physically attractive:	45–59	59%	52%	
	≥ 75	63%	57%	
What would most improve your sex life?	45–59			Less stress/more free time
	≥ 60	Better health		
	60–74		Better health for partner	
	≥ 75		Finding a partner	

SOURCE: Adapted from Jacoby (1999).

and does continue well past the 70s for healthy active individuals who have regular opportunities for sexual expression. King (2005) states: "For healthy men and women with healthy partners, sexual activity will probably continue throughout life if they had a positive attitude about sex when they were younger."

SPECIAL CONCERNS OF THE ELDERLY

Retirement

Statistics reflect that a larger percentage of Americans of both sexes are living longer and that many of them are retiring earlier. Reasons often given for the increasing pattern of early retirement include health problems, Social Security and other pension benefits, attractive "early out" packages offered by companies, and long-held plans (e.g., turning a hobby into a money-making situation). Even eliminating the mandatory retirement age and the possibility of delaying the age of eligibility for Social Security benefits from 65 to 67 by the year 2027 is not expected to have a significant effect on the trend toward earlier retirement.

Sadock and Sadock (2003) report that of those people who voluntarily retire, most reenter the work force within 2 years. The reasons they give for doing this include negative reactions to being retired, feelings of being unproductive, economic hardship, and loneliness.

About 4.4 million older Americans were in the labor force (working or actively seeking work) in 2004. These included 2.5 million men and 1.9 million women, and constituted 3.3 percent of the U.S. labor force (Bureau of Labor Statistics, 2005).

Retirement has both social and economical implications for elderly individuals. The role is fraught with a great deal of ambiguity and is one that requires many adaptations on the part of those involved.

Social Implications

Retirement is often anticipated as an achievement in principle, but met with a great deal of ambiguity when it actually occurs. Our society places a great deal of importance on productivity, making as much money as possible, and doing it at as young an age as possible. These types of values contribute to the ambiguity associated with retirement. Although leisure has been acknowledged as a legitimate reward for workers, leisure during retirement historically has lacked the same social value. Adjustment to this life cycle event becomes more difficult in the face of societal values that are in direct conflict with the new lifestyle.

Historically, many women have derived a good deal of their self-esteem from their families—birthing them, rearing them, and being a "good mother." Likewise,

many men have achieved self-esteem through work-related activities—creativity, productivity, and earning money. With the termination of these activities may come a loss of self-worth, resulting in depression in some individuals who are unable to adapt satisfactorily. Murray and Zentner (2001) list four developmental tasks related to successful adaptation in retirement:

● Remaining actively involved and having a sense of belonging unrelated to work
● Reevaluating life satisfaction related to family and social relations and spiritual life rather than to work
● Reevaluating the world's outlook, keeping a view of the world that is coherent and meaningful and a view that one's own world is meaningful
● Maintaining a sense of health, integrating mind and body to avoid complaints or illness when work is no longer the focus (p. 811)

American society often identifies an individual by his or her occupation. This is reflected in the conversation of people who are meeting each other for the first time. Undoubtedly, most everyone has either asked or been asked at some point in time, "What do you do?" or "Where do you work?" Occupation determines status, and retirement represents a significant change in status. The basic ambiguity of retirement occurs in an individual's or society's definition of this change. Is it undertaken voluntarily or involuntarily? Is it desirable or undesirable? Is one's status made better or worse by the change?

In looking at the trend of the past two decades, we may presume that retirement is becoming, and will continue to become, more accepted by societal standards. With more and more individuals retiring earlier and living longer, the growing number of aging people will spend a significantly longer time in retirement. At present, retirement has become more of an institutionalized expectation and there appears to be increasing acceptance of it as a social status.

Economical Implications

Because retirement is generally associated with 20 to 40 percent reduction in personal income, the standard of living after retirement may be adversely affected. Most older adults derive postretirement income from a combination of Social Security benefits, public and private pensions, and income from savings or investments.

In 2002, the median income in households containing families headed by persons 65 or over was $33,802 and 3.6 million elderly were below the poverty level (AoA, 2003). The rate of those living in poverty was higher among women than men and higher among African Americans and Latino Americans than whites.

The Social Security Act of 1935 promised assistance with financial security for the elderly. Since then, the original legislation has been modified, yet the basic philosophy remains intact. Its effectiveness, however, is now being questioned. Faced with deficits, the program is forced to pay benefits to those currently retired from both the reserve funds and monies being collected at present. There is genuine concern about future generations, when there may be no reserve funds from which to draw. Because many of the programs that benefit older adults depend on contributions from the younger population, the growing ratio of older Americans to younger people may affect society's ability to supply the goods and services necessary to meet this expanding demand.

Medicare and **Medicaid** were established by the government to provide medical care benefits for elderly and indigent Americans. Medicaid funds are matched by the states, and coverage varies significantly from state to state. Medicare covers only a percentage of health care costs; therefore, to reduce risk related to out-of-pocket expenditures, many older adults purchase private "medigap" policies designed to cover charges in excess of those approved by Medicare.

The magnitude of retirement earnings depends almost entirely on pre-retirement income. The poor will remain poor and the wealthy are unlikely to lower their status during retirement; however, for many in the middle classes, the relatively fixed income sources may be inadequate, possibly forcing them to face financial hardship for the first time in their lives.

Long-Term Care

The concept of long-term care covers a broad spectrum of comprehensive health care that addresses both illness and wellness and the support services necessary to provide the physical, psychological, social, spiritual, and economic needs of persons with chronic illnesses, including disabilities (Stanley, Blair, & Beare, 2005). Long-term care facilities are defined by the level of care they provide. They may be skilled nursing facilities, intermediate care facilities, or a combination of the two. Some institutions provide convalescent care for individuals recovering from acute illness or injury, some provide long-term care for individuals with chronic illness or disabilities, and still others provide both types of assistance.

Most elderly individuals prefer to remain in their own homes or in the homes of family members for as long as this can meet their needs without deterioration of family or social patterns. Many elderly individuals are placed in institutions as a last resort only after heroic efforts have been made to keep them in their own or a relative's home. The increasing emphasis on home health care has extended the period of independence for aging individuals.

In 2002, approximately 5 percent of the population aged 65 and older lived in nursing homes (NCHS, 2004).

The percentage increases dramatically with age, ranging from 1.1 percent for persons aged 65 to 74, 4.3 percent for persons aged 75 to 84, to 18.3 percent for persons aged 85 and older. A profile of the "typical" elderly nursing home resident is about 80 years of age, white, female, widowed, with multiple chronic health conditions.

In determining who in our society will need long-term care, several factors have been identified that appear to place people at risk. The following risk factors are taken into consideration to predict potential need for services and to estimate future costs.

Age. Because people grow older in very different ways, and the range of differences becomes greater with the passage of time, age is becoming a less relevant characteristic than it was historically. However, because of the high prevalence of chronic health conditions and disabilities, as well as the greater chance of diminishing social supports associated with advancing age, the 65-and-older population is often viewed as an important long-term care target group.

Health. Level of functioning, as determined by ability to perform various behaviors or activities—such as bathing, eating, mobility, meal preparation, handling finances, judgment, and memory—is a measurable risk factor. The need for ongoing assistance from another person is critical in determining the need for long-term care.

Mental Health Status. Mental health problems are risk factors in assessing need for long-term care. Many of the symptoms associated with certain mental disorders (especially the dementias) such as memory loss, impaired judgment, impaired intellect, and disorientation would render the individual incapable of meeting the demands of daily living independently.

Socioeconomic and Demographic Factors. Low income generally is associated with greater physical and mental health problems among the elderly. Because many elderly individuals have limited finances, they are less able to purchase care resources available outside of institutions (e.g., home healthcare), although Medicare and Medicaid now contribute a limited amount to this type of noninstitutionalized care.

Women are at greater risk of being institutionalized than men, not because they are less healthy but because they tend to live longer and, thus, reach the age at which more functional and cognitive impairments occur. They are also more likely to be widowed. Whites have a higher rate of institutionalization than nonwhites. This may be related to cultural and financial influences.

Marital Status, Living Arrangement, and the Informal Support Network. Individuals who are married and live with a spouse are the least likely of all disabled people to be institutionalized. Those who live alone without resources for home care and with few or no relatives living nearby to provide informal care are at higher risk for institutionalization.

Attitudinal Factors

Many people dread the thought of even visiting a nursing home, let alone moving to one or placing a relative in one. The media picture and subsequent reputation of nursing homes has not been positive. Stories of substandard care and patient abuse have scarred the industry, making it difficult for those facilities that are clean, well-managed, and provide innovative, quality care to their residents to rise above the stigma.

State and national licensing boards perform periodic inspections to ensure that standards set forth by the federal government are being met. These standards address quality of patient care as well as adequacy of the nursing home facility. Yet, many elderly individuals and their families perceive nursing homes as a place to go to die, and the fact that many of these institutions are poorly equipped, understaffed, and disorganized keeps this societal perception alive. There are, however, many excellent nursing homes that strive to go beyond the minimum federal regulations for Medicaid and Medicare reimbursement. In addition to medical, nursing, rehabilitation, and dental services, social and recreational services are provided to increase the quality of life for elderly people living in nursing homes. These activities include playing cards, bingo, and other games; parties; church activities; books; television; movies; and arts, crafts, and other classes. Some nursing homes provide occupational and professional counseling. These facilities strive to enhance opportunities for improving quality of life and for becoming "places to live," rather than "places to die."

Elder Abuse

Abuse of elderly individuals, which at times has been referred to in the media as "**granny-bashing**," is a prevalent and serious form of family violence. Sadock and Sadock (2003) estimate that 10 percent of individuals older than age 65 are the victims of abuse or neglect. The abuser is often a relative who lives with the elderly person and may be the assigned caregiver. Typical caregivers who are likely to be abusers of the elderly were described by Murray and Zentner (2001) as being under economic stress, substance abusers, themselves the victims of previous family violence, and exhausted and frustrated by the caregiver role. Identified risk factors for victims of abuse included being a white female age 70 and older, being mentally or physically impaired, being unable to meet daily self-care needs, and having care needs that exceeded the caretaker's ability.

Abuse of elderly individuals may be psychological, physical, or financial. Neglect may be intentional or unintentional. Psychological abuse includes yelling, insulting, harsh commands, threats, silence, and social isolation. Physical abuse is described as striking, shoving, beating, or restraint. Financial abuse refers to misuse or theft of finances, property, or material possessions. Neglect implies failure to do the obviously necessary things that a person cannot do independently. Unintentional neglect is inadvertent, whereas intentional neglect is deliberate. In addition, elderly individuals may be the victims of sexual abuse, which is sexual intimacy between two persons that occurs without the consent of one of the persons involved. Another type of abuse, which has been called "**granny-dumping**" by the media, involves abandoning elderly individuals at emergency departments, nursing homes, or other facilities—literally leaving them in the hands of others when the strain of caregiving becomes intolerable. Types of elder abuse are summarized in Table 38–2.

Elder victims often minimize the abuse or deny that it has occurred. The elderly person may be unwilling to disclose information because of fear of retaliation, embarrassment about the existence of abuse in the family, protectiveness toward a family member, or unwillingness to institute legal action. Adding to this unwillingness to report is the fact that infirm elders are often isolated so their mistreatment is less likely to be noticed by those who might be alert to symptoms of abuse. For these reasons, detection of abuse in the elderly is difficult at best.

TABLE 38–2	Examples of Elder Abuse

Physical Abuse
Striking, hitting, beating
Shoving
Bruising
Cutting
Restraining

Psychological Abuse
Yelling
Insulting, name-calling
Harsh commands
Threats
Ignoring, silence, social isolation
Withholding of affection

Neglect (intentional or unintentional)
Withholding food and water
Inadequate heating
Unclean clothes and bedding
Lack of needed medication
Lack of eyeglasses, hearing aids, false teeth

Financial Abuse or Exploitation
Misuse of the elderly person's income by the caregiver
Forcing the elderly person to sign over financial affairs to another person against his or her will or without sufficient knowledge about the transaction

Sexual Abuse
Sexual molestation; rape
Any type of sexual intimacy against the elderly person's will

SOURCE: Adapted from Sadock & Sadock (2003) and Murray & Zentner (2001).

Factors that Contribute to Abuse

A number of contributing factors have been implicated in the abuse of elderly individuals.

Longer Life. The 65-and-older age group has become the fastest growing segment of the population. Within this segment, the number of elderly older than age 75 has increased most rapidly. This trend is expected to continue well into the 21st century. The 75 and older age group is the one most likely to be physically or mentally impaired, requiring assistance and care from family members. This group also is the most vulnerable to abuse from caregivers.

Dependency. Dependency appears to be the most common precondition in domestic abuse. Changes associated with normal aging or induced by chronic illness often result in loss of self-sufficiency in the elderly person, requiring that they become dependent on another for assistance with daily functioning. Long life may also consume finances to the point that the elderly individual becomes financially dependent on another as well. This dependence increases the elderly person's vulnerability to abuse.

Stress. The stress inherent in the caregiver role is a factor in most abuse cases. Some clinicians believe that elder abuse results from individual or family psychopathology. Others suggest that even psychologically healthy family members can become abusive as the result of the exhaustion and acute stress caused by overwhelming caregiving responsibilities. This is compounded in an age group that has been dubbed the "sandwich generation"—those individuals who elected to delay childbearing so that they are now at a point in their lives when they are "sandwiched" between providing care for their children and providing care for their aging parents.

Learned Violence. Children who have been abused or witnessed abusive and violent parents are more likely to evolve into abusive adults. Stanley, Blair, and Beare (2005) state:

> Violence is a learned behavior that is passed down from generation to generation in some families because violence has been modeled as an acceptable coping behavior, with no substantial penalties for the behavior. This model suggests that a child who grows up in a violent family will also become violent. Some believe that elder mistreatment may be related to retribution on the part of an adult offspring who was abused as a child. (p. 290)

Identifying Elder Abuse

Because so many elderly individuals are reluctant to report personal abuse, health care workers need to be able to detect signs of mistreatment when they are in a position to do so. Table 38–2 listed a number of *types* of elder abuse. The following *manifestations* of the various categories of abuse have been identified (Murray & Zentner, 2001; Stanley, Blair, & Beare, 2005):

- Indicators of psychological abuse include a broad range of behaviors such as the symptoms associated with depression, withdrawal, anxiety, sleep disorders, and increased confusion or agitation.
- Indicators of physical abuse may include bruises, welts, lacerations, burns, punctures, evidence of hair pulling, and skeletal dislocations and fractures.
- Neglect may be manifested as consistent hunger, poor hygiene, inappropriate dress, consistent lack of supervision, consistent fatigue or listlessness, unattended physical problems or medical needs, or abandonment.
- Sexual abuse may be suspected when the elderly person is presented with pain or itching in the genital area, bruises or bleeding in external genitalia, vaginal, or anal areas, or unexplained sexually transmitted disease.
- Financial abuse may be occurring when there is an obvious disparity between assets and satisfactory living conditions or when the elderly person complains of a sudden lack of sufficient funds for daily living expenses.

Health care workers often feel intimidated when confronted with cases of elder abuse. In these instances, referral to an individual experienced in management of victims of such abuse may be the most effective approach to evaluation and intervention. Health care workers are responsible for reporting any suspicions of elder abuse. An investigation is then conducted by regulatory agencies, whose job it is to determine if the suspicions are corroborated. Every effort must be made to ensure the client's safety, but it must be kept in mind that a competent elderly person has the right to choose his or her health care options. As inappropriate as it may seem, some elderly individuals choose to return to the abusive situation. In this instance, he or she should be provided with names and phone numbers to call for assistance if needed. A follow-up visit by an adult protective service representative should be conducted.

Increased efforts need to be made to ensure that health care providers have comprehensive training in the detection of and intervention in elder abuse. More research is needed to increase knowledge and understanding of the phenomenon of elder abuse and ultimately to effect more sophisticated strategies for prevention, intervention, and treatment.

Suicide

Although persons older than age 65 comprise only 12 percent of the population, they represent a disproportionately high percentage of individuals who commit suicide. Of all suicides, 20 percent are committed by this age group, and suicide is the 15th leading cause of death among the elderly (Charbonneau, 2003). The group especially at risk appears to be white men. Predisposing factors include loneliness, financial problems, physical illness, loss, and depression (Sadock & Sadock, 2003).

Although the rate of suicide among the elderly remains high, the numbers of suicides among this age group dropped steadily from 1930 to 1980. Investigators who study these trends surmise that this decline was due to increases in services for older people and an understanding of their problems in society. However, from 1980 to 1986 the number of suicides among people age 65 and older increased by 25 percent, which suggests that other factors are contributing to the problem. It has been suggested that increased social isolation may be a contributing factor to suicide among the elderly. The number of elderly individuals who are divorced, widowed, or otherwise living alone has increased. Among men aged 75 years and older, the suicide rate for divorced men is 3.4 times, and the rate for widowed men is 2.6 times, that for married men. In the same age group, the suicide rate for divorced women is 2.8 times, and for widowed women is 1.9 times, the rate for married women (Merck Institute of Aging & Health, 2005).

The National Institute of Mental Health [NIMH] (2003) suggests that major depression is a significant predictor of suicide in older adults. Unfortunately, it is widely under-recognized and under-treated by the medical community. The NIMH (2003) states:

> Several studies have found that many older adults who die by suicide—up to 75 percent—have visited a primary care physician within a month of their suicide. These findings point to the urgency of enhancing both the detection and the adequate treatment of depression as a means of reducing suicide risk among older persons.

Many elderly individuals express symptoms associated with depression that are never recognized as such. Any sign of helplessness or hopelessness should elicit a supportive intervening response. In assessing suicide intention, direct questions should be asked, but concern and compassion should be used:

● Have you thought life is not worth living?
● Have you considered harming yourself?
● Do you have a plan for hurting yourself?
● Have you ever acted on that plan?
● Have you ever attempted suicide? (Stanley, Blair, & Beare, 2005)

Components of intervention with a suicidal elderly person should include demonstrations of genuine concern, interest, and caring; indications of empathy for their fears and concerns; and help in identifying, clarifying, and formulating a plan of action to deal with the unresolved issue. If the elderly person's behavior seems particularly lethal, additional family or staff coverage and contact should be arranged to prevent isolation.

APPLICATION OF THE NURSING PROCESS

Assessment

Assessment of the elderly individual may follow the same framework used for all adults, but with consideration of the possible biological, psychological, sociocultural, and sexual changes that occur in the normal aging process described previously in this chapter. In no other area of nursing is it more important for nurses to practice holistic nursing than with the elderly. Older adults are likely to have multiple physical problems that contribute to problems in other areas of their lives. Obviously, these components cannot be addressed as separate entities. Nursing the elderly is a multifaceted, challenging process because of the multiple changes occurring at this time in the life cycle and the way in which each change affects every aspect of the individual.

Several considerations are unique to assessment of the elderly. Assessment of the older person's thought processes is a primary responsibility. Knowledge about the presence and extent of disorientation or confusion will influence the way in which the nurse approaches elder care.

Information about sensory capabilities is also extremely important. Because hearing loss is common, the nurse should lower the pitch and loudness of his or her voice when addressing the older person. Looking directly into the face of the older person when talking facilitates communication. Questions that require a declarative sentence in response should be asked; in this way, the nurse is able to assess the client's ability to use words correctly. Visual acuity can be determined by assessing adaptation to the dark, color matching, and the perception of color contrast. Knowledge about these aspects of sensory functioning is essential in the development of an effective care plan.

The nurse should be familiar with the normal physical changes associated with the aging process. Examples of some of these changes include:

● Less effective response to changes in environmental temperature, resulting in hypothermia.
● Decreases in oxygen use and the amount of blood pumped by the heart, resulting in cerebral anoxia or hypoxia.
● Skeletal muscle wasting and weakness, resulting in difficulty in physical mobility.
● Limited cough and laryngeal reflexes, resulting in risk of aspiration.
● Demineralization of bones, resulting in spontaneous fracturing.
● Decrease in gastrointestinal motility, resulting in constipation.
● Decrease in the ability to interpret painful stimuli, resulting in risk of injury.

Common psychosocial changes associated with aging include:

● Prolonged and exaggerated grief, resulting in depression.
● Physical changes, resulting in disturbed body image.
● Changes in status, resulting in loss of self-worth.

This list is by no means exhaustive. The nurse should consider many other alterations in his or her assessment of the client. Knowledge of the client's functional capabilities is essential for determining the physiological, psychological, and sociological needs of the elderly individual. Age alone does not preclude the occurrence of all these changes. The aging process progresses at a wide range of variance, and each client must be assessed as a unique individual.

Diagnosis/Outcome Identification

Virtually any nursing diagnosis may be applicable to the aging client, depending on individual needs for assistance. Based on normal changes that occur in the elderly, the following nursing diagnoses may be considered:

Physiologically Related Diagnoses

Risk for trauma related to confusion, disorientation, muscular weakness, spontaneous fractures, falls.

Hypothermia related to loss of adipose tissue under the skin, evidenced by increased sensitivity to cold and body temperature below 98.6 degrees.

Decreased cardiac output related to decreased myocardial efficiency secondary to age-related changes, evidenced by decreased tolerance for activity and decline in energy reserve.

Ineffective breathing pattern related to increase in fibrous tissue and loss of elasticity in lung tissue, evidenced by dyspnea and activity intolerance.

Risk for aspiration related to diminished cough and laryngeal reflexes.

Impaired physical mobility related to muscular wasting and weakness, evidenced by need for assistance in ambulation.

Imbalanced nutrition, less than body requirements, related to inefficient absorption from gastrointestinal tract, difficulty chewing and swallowing, anorexia, difficulty in feeding self, evidenced by wasting syndrome, anemia, weight loss.

Constipation related to decreased motility; inadequate diet; insufficient activity or exercise, evidenced by decreased bowel sounds; hard, formed stools; or straining at stool.

Stress incontinence related to degenerative changes in pelvic muscles and structural supports associated with increased age, evidenced by reported or observed dribbling with increased abdominal pressure or urinary frequency.

Urinary retention related to prostatic enlargement, evidenced by bladder distention, frequent voiding of small amounts, dribbling, or overflow incontinence.

Disturbed sensory perception related to age-related alterations in sensory transmission, evidenced by decreased visual acuity, hearing loss, diminished sensitivity to taste and smell, or increased touch threshold.

Disturbed sleep pattern related to age-related decrease in ability to sleep ("sleep decay"), dementia, or medications, evidenced by interrupted sleep, early awakening, or falling asleep during the day.

Pain related to degenerative changes in joints, evidenced by verbalization of pain or hesitation to use weight-bearing joints.

Self-care deficit (specify) related to weakness, confusion, or disorientation, evidenced by inability to feed self, maintain hygiene, dress/groom self, or toilet self without assistance.

Risk for impaired skin integrity related to alterations in nutritional state, circulation, sensation, or mobility.

Psychosocially Related Diagnoses

Disturbed thought processes related to age-related changes that result in cerebral anoxia, evidenced by short-term memory loss, confusion, or disorientation.

Dysfunctional grieving related to bereavement overload, evidenced by symptoms of depression.

Risk for suicide related to depressed mood and feelings of low self-worth.

Powerlessness related to lifestyle of helplessness and dependency on others, evidenced by depressed mood, apathy, or verbal expressions of having no control or influence over life situation.

Low self-esteem related to loss of pre-retirement status, evidenced by verbalization of negative feelings about self and life.

Fear related to nursing home placement, evidenced by symptoms of severe anxiety and statements such as, "Nursing homes are places to go to die."

Disturbed body image related to age-related changes in skin, hair, fat distribution, evidenced by verbalization of negative feelings about body.

Ineffective sexuality patterns related to dyspareunia, evidenced by reported dissatisfaction with decrease in frequency of sexual intercourse.

Sexual dysfunction related to medications (e.g., antihypertensives) evidenced by inability to achieve an erection.

Social isolation related to total dependence on others, evidenced by expression of inadequacy in or absence of significant purpose in life.

Risk for trauma (elder abuse) related to caregiver role strain.

Caregiver role strain related to severity and duration of the care receiver's illness; lack of respite and recreation for the caregiver, evidenced by feelings of stress in relationship with care receiver; feelings of depression and anger; or family conflict around issues of providing care.

The following criteria may be used for measurement of outcomes in the care of the elderly client.

The client:

1. Has not experienced injury.
2. Maintains reality orientation consistent with cognitive level of functioning.
3. Manages own self-care with assistance.
4. Expresses positive feelings about self, past accomplishments, and hope for the future.

5. Compensates adaptively for diminished sensory perception.

Caregivers:

1. Can problem-solve effectively regarding care of elderly client.
2. Demonstrate adaptive coping strategies for dealing with stress of caregiver role.
3. Openly express feelings.
4. Express desire to join support group of other caregivers.

Planning/Implementation

In Table 38–3, selected nursing diagnoses are presented for the elderly client. Outcome criteria are included,

TABLE 38–3 Care Plan for the Elderly Client

NURSING DIAGNOSIS: RISK FOR TRAUMA
RELATED TO: Confusion, disorientation, muscular weakness, spontaneous fractures, falls

OUTCOME CRITERIA	NURSING INTERVENTIONS	RATIONALE

Client will not experience injury.	1. The following measures may be instituted:
	  a. Arrange furniture and other items in the room to accommodate client's disabilities.
	  b. Store frequently used items within easy access.
	  c. Keep bed in unelevated position. Pad siderails and headboard if client has history of seizures. Keep bedrails up when client is in bed (if permitted by institutional policy).
	  d. Assign room near nurses' station; observe frequently.
	  e. Assist client with ambulation.
	  f. Keep a dim light on at night.
	  g. If client is a smoker, cigarettes and lighter or matches should be kept at the nurses' station and dispensed only when someone is available to stay with client while he or she is smoking.
	  h. Frequently orient client to place, time, and situation.
	  i. Soft restraints may be required if client is very disoriented and hyperactive.
		1. To ensure client safety.

NURSING DIAGNOSIS: DISTURBED THOUGHT PROCESSES
RELATED TO: Age-related changes that result in cerebral anoxia
EVIDENCED BY: Short-term memory loss, confusion, or disorientation

OUTCOME CRITERIA	NURSING INTERVENTIONS	RATIONALE
Client will interpret the environment accurately and maintain reality orientation to the best of his or her cognitive ability.	1. Frequently orient client to reality. Use clocks and calendars with large numbers that are easy to read. Notes and large, bold signs may be useful as reminders. Allow client to have personal belongings.	1. To help maintain orientation and aid in memory and recognition.

(Continued on opposite page)

OUTCOME CRITERIA	NURSING INTERVENTIONS	RATIONALE
	2. Keep explanations simple. Use face-to-face interaction. Speak slowly and do not shout.	2. To facilitate comprehension. Shouting may create discomfort, and in some instances, may provoke anger.
	3. Discourage rumination of delusional thinking. Talk about real events and real people.	3. Rumination promotes disorientation. Reality orientation increases sense of self-worth and personal dignity.
	4. Monitor for medication side effects.	4. Physiological changes in the elderly can alter the body's response to certain medications. Toxic effects may intensify altered thought processes.

NURSING DIAGNOSIS: SELF-CARE DEFICIT (SPECIFY)
RELATED TO: Weakness, disorientation, confusion, or memory deficits
EVIDENCED BY: Inability to fulfill activities of daily living

OUTCOME CRITERIA	NURSING INTERVENTIONS	RATIONALE
Client will accomplish activities of daily living to the best of his or her ability. Unfulfilled needs will be met by caregivers.	1. Provide a simple, structured environment: a. Identify self-care deficits and provide assistance as required. Promote independent actions as able. b. Allow plenty of time for client to perform tasks. c. Provide guidance and support for independent actions by talking the client through the task one step at a time. d. Provide a structured schedule of activities that do not change from day to day. e. Activities of daily living should follow home routine as closely as possible. f. Allow consistency in assignment of daily caregivers.	1. To minimize confusion.

NURSING DIAGNOSIS: CAREGIVER ROLE STRAIN
RELATED TO: Severity and duration of the care receiver's illness; lack of respite and recreation for the caregiver
EVIDENCED BY: Feelings of stress in relationship with care receiver; feelings of depression and anger; family conflict around issues of providing care

OUTCOME CRITERIA	NURSING INTERVENTIONS	RATIONALE
Caregivers will achieve effective problem-solving skills and develop adaptive coping mechanisms to regain equilibrium.	1. Assess prospective caregivers' ability to anticipate and fulfill client's unmet needs. Provide information to assist caregivers with this responsibility. Ensure that caregivers are aware of available community support systems from which they can seek assistance when required. Examples include adult day-care centers, housekeeping and homemaker services, respite care services, or a local chapter of the Alzheimer's Disease and Related Disorders Association. This organization sponsors a nationwide 24-hour hotline to provide information and link families who need assistance with nearby chapters and affiliates. The hotline number is 800-621-0379.	1. Caregivers require relief from the pressures and strain of providing 24-hour care for their loved one. Studies have shown that elder abuse arises out of caregiving situations that place overwhelming stress on the caregivers.

(Continued on following page)

TABLE 38–3   Care Plan for the Elderly Client *(Continued)*

OUTCOME CRITERIA	NURSING INTERVENTIONS	RATIONALE
	2. Encourage caregivers to express feelings, particularly anger.	2. Release of these emotions can serve to prevent psychopathology, such as depression or psychophysiological disorders, from occurring.
	3. Encourage participation in support groups composed of members with similar life situations.	3. Hearing others who are experiencing the same problems discuss ways in which they have coped may help caregiver adopt more adaptive strategies. Individuals who are experiencing similar life situations provide empathy and support for each other.

NURSING DIAGNOSIS: LOW SELF-ESTEEM

RELATED TO: Loss of pre-retirement status

EVIDENCED BY: Verbalization of negative feelings about self and life

OUTCOME CRITERIA	NURSING INTERVENTIONS	RATIONALE
Client will demonstrate increased feelings of self-worth by expressing positive aspects of self and past accomplishments.	1. Encourage client to express honest feelings in relation to loss of prior status. Acknowledge pain of loss. Support client through process of grieving.	1. Client may be fixed in anger stage of grieving process, which is turned inward on the self, resulting in diminished self-esteem.
	2. If lapses in memory are occurring, devise methods for assisting client with memory deficit. Examples: a. Name sign on door identifying client's room. b. Identifying sign on outside of dining room door. c. Identifying sign on outside of restroom door. d. Large clock, with oversized numbers and hands, appropriately placed. e. Large calendar, indicating one day at a time, with month, day, and year in bold print. f. Printed, structured daily schedule, with one copy for client and one posted on unit wall. g. "News board" on unit wall where current news of national and local interest may be posted.	2. These aids may assist client to function more independently, thereby increasing self-esteem.
	3. Encourage client's attempts to communicate. If verbalizations are not understandable, express to client what you think he or she intended to say. It may be necessary to reorient client frequently.	3. The ability to communicate effectively with others may enhance self-esteem.
	4. Encourage reminiscence and discussion of life review (see Table 38–4). Also discuss present-day events. Sharing picture albums, if possible, is especially good.	4. Reminiscence and life review help client resume progression through the grief process associated with disappointing life events and increase self-esteem as successes are reviewed.
	5. Encourage participation in group activities. May need to accompany client at first, until he or she feels secure that the group members will be accepting, regardless of limitations in verbal communication.	5. Positive feedback from group members will increase self-esteem.
	6. Encourage client to be as independent as possible in self-care activities. Provide written schedule of tasks to be performed. Intervene in areas where client requires assistance.	6. The ability to perform independently preserves self-esteem.

(Continued on opposite page)

NURSING DIAGNOSIS: DISTURBED SENSORY PERCEPTION
RELATED TO: Age-related alterations in sensory transmission
EVIDENCED BY: Decreased visual acuity, hearing loss, diminished sensitivity to taste and smell, and increased touch threshold

OUTCOME CRITERIA	NURSING INTERVENTIONS*	RATIONALE
Client will attain optimal level of sensory stimulation. Client will not experience injury due to diminished sensory-perception.	1. The following nursing strategies are indicated: a. Provide meaningful sensory stimulation to all special senses through conversation, touch, music, or pleasant smells. b. Encourage wearing of glasses, hearing aids, prostheses, and other adaptive devices. c. Use bright, contrasting colors in the environment. d. Provide large-print reading materials, such as books, clocks, calendars, and educational materials. e. Maintain room lighting that distinguishes day from night and that is free of shadows and glare. f. Teach client to scan the environment to locate objects. g. Help client to locate food on plate using "clock" system, and describe food if client is unable to visualize; assist with feeding as needed. h. Arrange physical environment to maximize functional vision. i. Place personal items and call light within client's field of vision. j. Teach client to watch the person who is speaking. k. Reinforce wearing of hearing aid; if client does not have an aid, may consider a communication device (e.g., amplifier). l. Communicate clearly, distinctly, and slowly, using a low-pitched voice and facing client; avoid overarticulation. m. Remove as much unnecessary background noise as possible. n. Do not use slang or extraneous words. o. As speaker, position self at eye level and no farther than 6 feet away. p. Get the client's attention before speaking. q. Avoid speaking directly into the client's ear. r. If the client does not understand what is being said, rephrase the statement rather than simply repeating it. s. Help client select foods from the menu that will ensure a discrimination between various tastes and smells. t. Ensure that food has been properly cooled so that client with diminished pain threshold is not burned. u. Ensure that bath or shower water is appropriate temperature. v. Use backrubs and massage as therapeutic touch to stimulate sensory receptors.	1. To assist client with diminished sensory perception and because client safety is a nursing priority.

*The interventions for this nursing diagnosis were adapted from Rogers-Seidl (1997).

767

along with appropriate nursing interventions and rationale for each.

Reminiscence therapy is especially helpful with elderly clients. This therapeutic intervention is highlighted in Table 38–4.

Evaluation

Reassessment is conducted to determine if the nursing actions have been successful in achieving the objectives of care. Evaluation of the nursing actions for the elderly client may be facilitated by gathering information using the following types of questions:

1. Has the client escaped injury from falls, burns, or other means to which he or she is vulnerable because of age?
2. Can caregivers verbalize means of providing a safe environment for the client?
3. Does the client maintain reality orientation at an optimum for his or her cognitive functioning?
4. Can the client distinguish between reality-based and non-reality-based thinking?
5. Can caregivers verbalize ways in which to orient client to reality, as needed?
6. Is the client able to accomplish self-care activities independently to his or her optimum level of functioning?
7. Does the client seek assistance for aspects of self-care that he or she is unable to perform independently?
8. Does the client express positive feelings about himself or herself?
9. Does the client reminisce about accomplishments that have occurred in his or her life?
10. Does the client express some hope for the future?
11. Does the client wear eyeglasses or a hearing aid, if needed, to compensate for sensory deficits?
12. Does the client consistently look at others in the face to facilitate hearing when they are talking to him or her?
13. Does the client use helpful aids, such as signs identifying various rooms, to help maintain orientation?
14. Can the caregivers work through problems and make decisions regarding care of the elderly client?
15. Do the caregivers include the elderly client in the decision-making process, if appropriate?
16. Can the caregivers demonstrate adaptive coping strategies for dealing with the strain of long-term caregiving?
17. Are the caregivers open and honest in expression of feelings?
18. Can the caregivers verbalize community resources to which they can go for assistance with their caregiving responsibilities?
19. Have the caregivers joined a support group?

Table 38–4	**Reminiscence Therapy and Life Review with the Elderly**

Stanley, Blair, and Beare (2005) state:

> Stimulation of life memories helps older adults to work through their losses and maintain self-esteem. Life review provides older adults with an opportunity to come to grips with guilt and regrets and to emerge feeling good about themselves. (p. 268)

Studies have indicated that *reminiscence*, or thinking about the past and reflecting on it, may promote better mental health in old age. *Life review* is related to reminiscence, but differs from it in that it is a more guided or directed cognitive process that constructs a history or story in an autobiographical way (Murray & Zentner, 2001).

Elderly individuals who spend time thinking about the past experience an increase in self-esteem and are less likely to suffer depression. Some psychologists believe that life review may help some people adjust to memories of an unhappy past. Others view reminiscence and life review as ways to bolster feelings of well-being, particularly in older people who can no longer remain active.

Reminiscence therapy can take place on a one-to-one basis or in a group setting. In reminiscence groups, elderly individuals share significant past events with peers. The nurse leader facilitates the discussion of topics that deal with specific life transitions, such as childhood, adolescence, marriage, childbearing, grandparenthood, and retirement. Members share both positive and negative aspects, including personal feelings, about these life cycle events.

Reminiscence on a one-to-one basis can provide a way for elderly individuals to work through unresolved issues from the past. Painful issues may be too difficult to discuss in the group setting. As the individual reviews his or her life process, the nurse can validate feelings and help the elderly client come to terms with painful issues that may have been long suppressed. This process is necessary if the elderly individual is to maintain (or attain) a sense of positive identity and self-esteem and ultimately achieve the goal of ego integrity as described by Erikson (1963).

A number of creative measures can be used to facilitate life review with the elderly individual. Having the client keep a journal for sharing may be a way to stimulate discussion (as well as providing a permanent record of past events for significant others). Pets, music, and special foods have a way of provoking memories from the client's past. Photographs of family members and past significant events are an excellent way of guiding the elderly client through his or her autobiographical review.

Care must be taken in the life review to assist clients to work through unresolved issues. Anxiety, guilt, depression, and despair may result if the individual is unable to work through the problems and accept them. Life review can work in a negative way if the individual comes to believe that his or her life was meaningless. However, it can be a very positive experience for the person who can take pride in past accomplishments and feel satisfied with his or her life, resulting in a sense of serenity and inner peace in the older adult.

SUMMARY

Care of the aging individual presents one of the greatest challenges for nursing. The growing population of individuals aged 65 and older suggests that the challenge will progress well into the 21st century.

America is a youth-oriented society. It is not desirable to be old; in fact, to some it is repugnant. Most, however, if faced with a choice, would choose growing old to the alternative—death. In some cultures, the elderly are revered and hold a special place of honor within the society, but in highly industrialized countries such as the United States, status declines with the decrease in productivity and participation in the mainstream of society.

Individuals experience many changes as they age. Physical changes occur in virtually every body system. Psychologically, there may be age-related memory deficiencies, particularly for recent events. Intellectual functioning does not decline with age, but length of time required for learning increases.

Aging individuals experience many losses, potentially leading to bereavement overload. They are vulnerable to depression and to feelings of low self-worth. The elderly population represents a disproportionately high percentage of individuals who commit suicide. Dementing disorders are the most frequent causes of psychopathology in the elderly. Sleep disorders are very common.

The need for sexual expression by the elderly is often misunderstood within our society. Although many physical changes occur at this time of life that alter an individual's sexuality, if he or she has reasonably good health and a willing partner, sexual activity can continue well past the 70s for most people.

Retirement has both social and economical implications for elderly individuals. Society often equates an individual's status with occupation, and loss of employment may result in the need for adjustment in the standard of living because retirement income may be reduced by 20 to 40 percent of pre-retirement earnings.

Less than 5 percent of the population aged 65 and older live in nursing homes. A profile of the typical elderly nursing home resident is a white woman about 78 years old, widowed, with multiple chronic health conditions. Much stigma is attached to what some still call "rest homes" or "old age homes," and many elderly people still equate them with a place "to go to die."

The strain of the caregiver role has become a major dilemma in our society. Elder abuse is sometimes inflicted by caregivers for whom the role has become overwhelming and intolerable. There is an intense need to find assistance for these people, who must provide care for their loved ones on a 24-hour basis. Home health care, respite care, support groups, and financial assistance are needed to ease the burden of this role strain.

Nursing of the elderly individual is accomplished through the six steps of the nursing process. Assessment requires that changes occurring in the normal aging process—biological, psychological, sociocultural, and sexual—be taken into consideration before an accurate plan of care can be formulated.

Nursing of elderly individuals requires a special kind of inner strength and compassion. The following poem, which has become familiar over the years, is excellent in eliciting empathy for what the elderly must feel. I thank the anonymous author for sharing. It conveys a powerful message.

WHAT DO YOU SEE, NURSE?

What do you see, nurse, what do you see?
What are you thinking when you look at me?
A crabbed old woman, not very wise.
Uncertain of habit, with faraway eyes.
Who dribbles her food and makes no reply
When you say in a loud voice, "I do wish you'd try."
Who seems not to notice the things that you do
And forever is losing a stocking or shoe.
Who unresisting or not, lets you do as you will
With bathing and feeding, the long day to fill.
Is that what you're thinking, is that what you see?
Then open your eyes, you're not looking at me.
I'll tell you who I am as I sit there so still.
As I move at your bidding, as I eat at your will.
I'm a small child of ten with a father and mother,
Brothers and sisters who love one another.
A young girl at sixteen with wings on her feet
Dreaming that soon now a lover she'll meet.
A bride soon at twenty—my heart gives a leap
Remembering the vows that I promised to keep.
At twenty-five, now, I have young of my own
Who need me to build a secure happy home.
A woman of thirty, my young now grow fast
Bound to each other with ties that should last.
At forty my young now will soon be gone,
But my man stays beside me to see I don't mourn.
At fifty once more babies play round my knee.
Again we know children, my loved one and me.
Dark days are upon me, my husband is dead.
I look at the future, I shudder with dread.
For my young are all busy rearing young of their own.
And I think of the years and the love I have known.
I'm an old woman now and nature is cruel.
Tis her jest to make old age look like a fool.
The body it crumbles, grace and vigor depart.
There is now just a stone where I once had a heart.
But inside this old carcass a young girl still dwells.
And now and again my battered heart swells.
I remember the joys, I remember the pain.
And I'm loving and living life all over again.
I think of the years all too few—gone so fast.
And accept the stark fact that nothing can last.
So open your eyes, nurse, open and see.
Not a crabbed old woman—look closer—SEE ME.

Author unknown.

REVIEW QUESTIONS

SELF-EXAMINATION/LEARNING EXERCISE

Select the answer that is *most* appropriate for each of the following questions.

Situation: Stanley, a 72-year-old widower, was brought to the hospital by his son, who reports that Stanley has become increasingly withdrawn. He has periods of confusion and forgetfulness, but most of the time his thought processes are intact. He eats very little and has lost some weight. His wife died 5 years ago and the son reports, "He did very well, didn't even cry." Stanley attended the funeral of his best friend 1 month ago, after which these symptoms began. Stanley has been admitted for testing and evaluation.

1. In her admission assessment, the nurse notices an open sore on Stanley's arm. When she questions him about it he says, "I scraped it on the fence 2 weeks ago. It's smaller than it was." How might the nurse analyze these data?
   a. Stanley was trying to commit suicide.
   b. The delay in healing may indicate that Stanley has developed skin cancer.
   c. A diminished inflammatory response in the elderly increases healing time.
   d. Age-related skin changes and distribution of adipose tissue delay healing in the elderly.

2. Stanley is deaf on his right side. Which is the most appropriate nursing intervention for communicating with Stanley?
   a. Speak loudly into his left ear.
   b. Speak to him from a position on his left side.
   c. Speak face-to-face in a high-pitched voice.
   d. Speak face-to-face in a low-pitched voice.

3. Why is it important to have the nurse check the temperature of the water before Stanley takes a shower?
   a. Stanley may catch cold if the water temperature is too low.
   b. Stanley may burn himself because of a higher pain threshold.
   c. Stanley has difficulty discriminating between hot and cold.
   d. The water must be exactly 98.6° F.

4. From the information provided in the situation, which would be the priority nursing diagnosis for Stanley?
   a. Dysfunctional grieving
   b. Imbalanced nutrition: less than body requirements
   c. Social isolation
   d. Risk for injury

5. The physician diagnoses Stanley with major depression. A suicide assessment is conducted. Why is Stanley at high risk for suicide?
   a. All depressed people are at high risk for suicide.
   b. Stanley is in the age group in which the highest percentage of suicides occur.
   c. Stanley is a white man, recently bereaved, living alone.
   d. His son reports that Stanley owns a gun.

6. Which of the following would be a *priority* nursing intervention with Stanley?
   a. Take blood pressure once each shift.
   b. Ensure that Stanley attends group activities.
   c. Encourage Stanley to eat all of the food on his food tray.
   d. Encourage Stanley to talk about his wife's death.

7. In group exercise, Stanley becomes tired and short of breath very quickly. This is most likely due to:
   a. Age-related changes in the cardiovascular system.
   b. Stanley's sedentary lifestyle.
   c. The effects of pathological depression.
   d. Medication the physician has prescribed for depression.

8. Stanley says to the nurse, "I'm all alone now. My wife is gone. My best friend is gone. My son is busy with his work and family. I might as well just go, too." Which is the best response by the nurse?
   a. "Are you thinking that you want to die, Stanley?"
   b. "You have lots to live for, Stanley."
   c. "Cheer up, Stanley. It's almost time for activity therapy."
   d. "Tell me about your family, Stanley."

9. Stanley says to the nurse, "I don't want to go to that crafts class. I'm too old to learn anything." Based on knowledge of the aging process, which of the following is a true statement?
   a. Memory functioning in the elderly most likely reflects loss of long-term memories of remote events.
   b. Intellectual functioning declines with advancing age.
   c. Learning ability remains intact, but time required for learning increases with age.
   d. Cognitive functioning is rarely affected in aging individuals.

10. According to the literature, which of the following is most important for Stanley to maintain a healthy, adaptive old age?
    a. To remain socially interactive.
    b. To disengage slowly in preparation of the last stage of life.
    c. To move in with his son and family.
    d. To maintain total independence and accept no help from anyone.

TEST YOUR CRITICAL THINKING SKILLS

Mrs. M., age 76, is seeing her primary physician for her regular 6-month physical exam. Mrs. M.'s husband died 2 years ago, at which time she sold her home in Kansas and came to live in California with her only child, a daughter. The daughter is married and has 3 children (one in college and two teenagers at home). The daughter reports that her mother is becoming increasingly withdrawn, stays in her room, and eats very little. She has lost 13 pounds since her last 6-month visit. The primary physician refers Mrs. M. to a psychiatrist who hospitalizes her for evaluation. He diagnoses Mrs. M. with Major Depression.

Mrs. M. tells the nurse, "I didn't want to leave my home, but my daughter insisted. I would have been all right. I miss my friends and my church. Back home I drove my car everywhere. But there's too much traffic out here. They sold my car and I have to depend on my daughter or grandkids to take me places. I hate being so dependent! I miss my husband so much. I just sit and think about him and our past life all the time. I don't have any interest in meeting new people. I want to go home!!"

Mrs. M. admits to having some thoughts of dying, although she denies feeling suicidal. She denies having a plan or means for taking her life. "I really don't want to die, but I just can't see much reason for living. My daughter and her family are so busy with their own lives. They don't need me—or even have time for me!"

Answer the following questions about Mrs. M.:

1. What would be the *primary* nursing diagnosis for Mrs. M.?
2. Formulate a short-term goal for Mrs. M.
3. From the assessment data, identify the major problem that may be a long-term focus of care for Mrs. M.

IMPLICATIONS OF RESEARCH FOR EVIDENCE-BASED PRACTICE

Turvey, C.L., Conwell, Y., Jones, M.P., Phillips, C., Simonsick, E., Pearson, J.L., & Wallace, R. (2002). Risk factors for late-life suicide: A prospective, community-based study. *American Journal of Geriatric Psychiatry*, *10*(4), 398–406.

Description of the study: Studies have suggested that a negative or depressive mental outlook, being widowed or divorced, sleeping more than 9 hours per day, and drinking more than three alcoholic beverages per day were risk factors for late-life suicide. The primary aim of this study was to examine the relationship between completed suicide in late life and physical health, disability, and social support. The participants were 14,456 individuals selected from a general population of elderly subjects age 65 and older. Control subjects were a group of 420 individuals who were matched by age and sex. It was a 10-year longitudinal study beginning in 1981. Variables were assessed at baseline, year 3, and year 6, with a 10-year mortality follow-up. Baseline variables included sleep quality, social support, alcohol use, medical illness, physical impairment, cognitive impairment, and depressive symptoms.

Results of the Study: The 10-year mortality follow-up indicated that 75 percent of the control subjects had died, but none had died from suicide. Twenty-one of the 14,456 participants committed suicide within the follow-up period. Twenty of the 21 suicide victims were male. Average age was 78.6 years, with a range from 67 to 90 years. The most common means was gunshot. Other means included hanging, cutting, overdose, drowning, carbon monoxide inhalation, and one participant jumped to his death. In this study, presence of friends or relatives to confide in was negatively associated with suicide. Likewise, regular church attendance was more common in control subjects than the participant sample, indicating an even wider range of community support. Those who committed suicide had reported more depressive symptoms than those who did not, but they did not consume more alcohol (inconsistent with previous studies). Poor sleep quality was positively correlated with suicide in this study, but no specific physical illness was identified as a predisposition. The authors identify the small suicide sample as a limitation of this study.

Implications for Nursing Practice: This study identified depression, poor sleep quality, and limited social support as important variables in the potential for elderly suicide. Sleep disturbance may be an important indicator of depression, whereas limited social support may be a contributing factor. The study provides reinforcement for the U.S. Department of Health and Human Services (USDHHS) recommendation in their *National Strategy for Suicide Prevention: Goals and Objectives for Action* (2001). The USDHHS recommends detection and treatment of depression as a strategy to prevent late-life suicide. The authors state, "Because both depression and social support are amenable to intervention, this study provides further evidence for the possible effectiveness of such strategies to reduce suicides among older adults." Nurses can become actively involved in assessing for these risk factors, as well as planning, implementing, and evaluating the effectiveness of strategies for preventing suicide in the elderly population.

INTERNET REFERENCES

Additional sources related to aging may be located at the following Web sites:

- http://www.4woman.org/Menopause
- http://www.aarp.org/
- http://www.oaktrees.org/elder/
- http://www.acjnet.org/docs/eldabpfv.html

- http://www.ssa.gov/
- http://www.nih.gov/nia/
- http://www.medicare.gov/
- http://www.seniorlaw.com/
- http://www.growthhouse.org/cesp.html
- http://www.agenet.com/
- http://www.aoa.dhhs.gov/
- http://www.nsclc.org/

REFERENCES

Administration on Aging (AoA). (2003). *A profile of older Americans: 2003*. Washington, DC: U.S. Department of Health and Human Services.

Altman, A. & Hanfling, S. (2003). *Sexuality in midlife and beyond*. Boston, MA: Harvard Health Publications.

American Geriatrics Society. (2005). Summary of Geriatric and Chronic Care Management Act of 2005 (S. 40/H.R. 467). Retrieved May 13, 2005 from the World Wide Web at http://www.american-geriatrics.org/policy/summ_gerchroniccaremgmt05PF.shtml

Beers, M.H., & Jones, T.V. (Eds.). (2004). *The Merck manual of health & aging*. Whitehouse Station, NJ: Merck Research Laboratories.

Blazer, D. (2003). Geriatric psychiatric. In R.E. Hales & S.C. Yudofsky (Eds.). *Textbook of clinical psychiatry* (4th ed.). Washington, DC: American Psychiatric Publishing.

Bureau of Labor Statistics. (2005). *Employment status by race, age, sex, and Hispanic or Latino ethnicity, 2004 annual averages*. Retrieved May 15, 2005 from the World Wide Web at http://www.bls.gov/cps/wlf-table3-2005.pdf

Charbonneau, A. (2003). Elderly suicide prevention. Regions VII/VIII Suicide Prevention Planning Meeting. Kansas City, KS: University of Kansas Medical Center, October 29, 2003.

Giger, J.N., & Davidhizar, R.E. (2004). *Transcultural nursing: Assessment and intervention* (4th ed.). St. Louis: C.V. Mosby.

Jacoby, S. (1999). Great sex: What's age got to do with it? *Modern Maturity, 42W*(5), 40–45.

King, B.M. (2005). *Human sexuality today* (5th ed.). Upper Saddle River, NJ: Pearson Prentice-Hall.

Masters, W.H., Johnson, V.E., & Kolodny, R.C. (1995). *Human sexuality* (5th ed.). New York: Addison-Wesley Longman.

Merck Institute of Aging & Health. (2005). *Suicide in older adults: We can all help to prevent it.* Retrieved May 16, 2005 from the World Wide Web at http://www.miahonline.org/resources/nursesnotes/articles/02_17_05.suicide.html

Murray, R.B., & Zentner, J.P. (2001). *Health promotion strategies through the life span* (7th ed.). Upper Saddle River, NJ: Prentice-Hall.

National Center for Health Statistics (NCHS). (2004). *Older Americans 2004: Key indicators of well-being.* Federal Interagency Forum on Aging-Related Statistics. Washington, DC: U.S. Government Printing Office.

National Center for Health Statistics (NCHS). (2005). National Vital Statistics Report, Vol. 53, No. 15, February 28, 2005. Retrieved May 13, 2005 from the World Wide Web at http://www.cdc.gov/nchs/

National Institute of Mental Health [NIMH]. (2003). *Older adults: Depression and suicide facts.* Retrieved May 16, 2005 from the World Wide Web at http://www.nimh.nih.gov/publicat/elderlydepsuicide.cfm

Pietraniec-Shannon, M. (2003). Nursing care of elderly patients. In L.S. Williams & P.D. Hopper (Eds.). *Understanding medical-surgical nursing* (2nd ed.). Philadelphia: F.A. Davis.

Roberts, C.M. (1991). *How did I get here so fast?* New York: Warner Books.

Rogers-Seidl, F.F. (1997). *Geriatric nursing care plans* (2nd ed.). St. Louis: Mosby Year Book.

Rossouw, J.E., Anderson, G.L., Prentice, R.L., LaCroix, A.Z., Kooperberg, C., Stefanick, M.L., Jackson, R.D., Beresford, S.A., Howard, B.V., Johnson, K.C., Kotchen, J.M., Ockene, J., & Writing Group for the Women's Health Initiative Investigators. (2002). Risks and benefits of estrogen plus progestin in healthy postmenopausal women: Principal results from the Women's Health Initiative randomized controlled trial. *Journal of the American Medical Association, 288*(3), 321–333, 366–368.

Sadock, B.J., & Sadock, V.A. (2003). *Synopsis of psychiatry: Behavioral sciences/clinical psychiatry* (9th ed.). Philadelphia: Lippincott Williams & Wilkins.

Srivastava, S., John, O.P., Gosling, S.D., & Potter, J. (2003). Development of personality in early and middle adulthood: Set like plaster or persistent change? *Journal of Personality and Social Psychology, 84*(5), 1041–1053.

Stanley, M., Blair, K.A., & Beare, P.G. (2005). *Gerontological nursing: Promoting successful aging with older adults* (3rd ed.). Philadelphia: F.A. Davis.

U.S. Census Bureau. (2005). Public Information Office. Retrieved May 13, 2005 from the World Wide Web at http://www.census.gov/PressRelease/www/releases/archives/facts_for_features_special_editions/004210.html

Vaillant, G.E. (2003). *Aging Well: Surprising guideposts to a happier life from the landmark Harvard study of adult development.* New York: Little, Brown.

CLASSICAL REFERENCES

Erikson, E.H. (1963). *Childhood and society* (2nd ed.). New York: W.W. Norton.

Kübler-Ross, E. (1969). *On death and dying.* New York: Macmillan.

Reichard, S., Livson, F., & Peterson, P.G. (1962). *Aging and personality.* New York: John Wiley & Sons.

39
C H A P T E R

THE INDIVIDUAL WITH HIV DISEASE

C H A P T E R   O U T L I N E

OBJECTIVES

PATHOPHYSIOLOGY INCURRED
BY INFECTION WITH THE HIV

HISTORICAL ASPECTS

EPIDEMIOLOGICAL STATISTICS

PREDISPOSING FACTORS

APPLICATION OF THE NURSING PROCESS

TREATMENT MODALITIES

SUMMARY

REVIEW QUESTIONS

K E Y   T E R M S

HIV-associated
  dementia
HIV wasting
  syndrome
hospice
Kaposi's sarcoma
opportunistic
  infection

persistent generalized
  lymphadenopathy
Pneumocystis
  pneumonia
seroconversion
Standard Precautions
Transmission-Based
  Precautions

C O R E   C O N C E P T S

acquired immuno-
  deficiency syndrome
human immuno-
  deficiency virus
lymphocytes

O B J E C T I V E S

After reading this chapter, the student will be able to:

1. Discuss the human immunodeficiency virus (HIV) as the causative agent in the development of acquired immunodeficiency syndrome (AIDS).
2. Describe the pathophysiology incurred by HIV.
3. Discuss historical perspectives associated with HIV disease.
4. Relate epidemiological statistics associated with HIV disease.
5. Identify predisposing factors to HIV disease.
6. Describe symptomatology associated with HIV infection and AIDS and use this data in client assessment.
7. Formulate nursing diagnoses and goals of care for clients with HIV disease.
8. Describe appropriate nursing interventions for clients with HIV disease.
9. Identify topics for client and family teaching relevant to HIV disease.
10. Evaluate nursing care of clients with HIV disease.
11. Discuss various modalities relevant to treatment of clients with HIV disease.

774

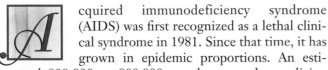

cquired immunodeficiency syndrome (AIDS) was first recognized as a lethal clinical syndrome in 1981. Since that time, it has grown in epidemic proportions. An estimated 800,000 to 900,000 people currently are living with HIV disease in the United States, with approximately 40,000 new infections occurring each year (Kaiser Family Foundation, 2004). Much research is now focused on HIV infection as a possible means of altering the course of the epidemic.

Core Concept

Acquired Immunodeficiency syndrome (AIDS)
A disease of the human immune system caused by the human immunodeficiency virus (HIV) that is characterized by a T4 cell count less than 200, thereby rendering the individual highly vulnerable to life-threatening conditions.

Core Concept

Human Immunodeficiency Virus (HIV)
The etiological agent that produces the immunosuppression resulting in AIDS.

Individuals are diagnosed as having HIV infection when the virus is directly identified in host tissues by virus isolation or indirectly identified by the presence of HIV antibodies in body fluid using laboratory immunoassay testing. Many individuals with HIV infection remain asymptomatic for years. Left untreated, the disease progresses over a period of 10 or more years to the late stage—AIDS. The availability of potent combinations of drugs that specifically block HIV replication has dramatically improved the prognosis for HIV-infected individuals.

In 1993, the Centers for Disease Control defined HIV disease as "a specific group of diseases or conditions which are indicative of severe immunosuppression related to infection with the human immunodeficiency virus (HIV)." HIV disease identifies a full spectrum of conditions caused by HIV infection, including asymptomatic HIV infection, symptomatic infection, and AIDS. The individual with HIV infection is considered to have "CDC-defined AIDS" when the T4 lymphocyte count falls to less than $200/mm^3$, or there is evidence of an **opportunistic infection** associated with advanced HIV disease.

This chapter presents physical and psychological manifestations of HIV disease. Delivery of nursing care is described in terms of the nursing process. Various medical treatment modalities are discussed.

PATHOPHYSIOLOGY INCURRED BY INFECTION WITH THE HIV

Core Concept

Lymphocyte
Lymphocytes are white blood cells responsible for much of the body's immune protection. T4 lymphocytes (also called CD4 lymphocytes and T4 helper cells) are the targets of the HIV.

The Normal Immune Response

Cells responsible for nonspecific immune reactions include neutrophils, monocytes, and macrophages. They work to destroy the invasive organism and initiate and facilitate damaged tissue. If these cells are not effective in accomplishing a satisfactory healing response, specific immune mechanisms take over.

Specific immune mechanisms are divided into two major types: the cellular response and the humoral response. The controlling elements of the cellular response are the T lymphocytes (T cells), and those of the humoral response are called B lymphocytes (B cells). When the body is invaded by a specific antigen, the T cells—and particularly the T4 lymphocytes (also called T helper cells)—become sensitized to and specific for the foreign antigen. These antigen-specific T4 cells divide many times, producing antigen-specific T4 cells with other functions. One of these, the T killer cell, destroys viruses that reproduce inside other cells by puncturing the cell membrane of the host cell and allowing the contents of the cell, including viruses, to spill out into the bloodstream, where they can be engulfed by macrophages. Another cell produced through division of the T4 cells is the suppressor T cell, which serves to stop the immune response once the foreign antigen has been destroyed (Scanlon & Sanders, 2003).

The humoral response is activated when antigen-specific T4 cells communicate with B cells in the spleen and lymph nodes. These B cells in turn produce the antibodies specific to the foreign antigen. Antibodies attach themselves to foreign antigens so that they are unable to invade body cells. These invader cells are then destroyed without being able to multiply.

The Immune Response to HIV

HIV infection results in a profound depletion of T4 lymphocytes. The HIV infects the T4 lymphocyte, thereby destroying the very cell the body needs to direct an attack on the virus.

An individual with a healthy immune system may present with a T4 count between $600/mm^3$ and $1200/mm^3$. The individual with HIV infection may experience a drop at the time of acute infection, with a subsequent increase when the acute stage subsides. Typically, the T-cell count is about 500 to 600 when the individual begins to develop **chronic persistent generalized lymphadenopathy** (PGL). Opportunistic infections are common when the T-cell count reaches 200. T4 cell counts in individuals with advanced HIV disease drop dramatically, in some cases down to zero (New Mexico AIDS InfoNet, 2005).

When an individual is infected with HIV, T4 lymphocytes become the main target of attack by the virus. The T4 cells that escape assault seem to lose the ability to function at full capacity and are therefore unable to initiate responses by various other components of the immune system. Because of this, the B cells demonstrate a decreased ability to mount an antibody response to a *new* antigen (Fondere et al., 2003).

The HIV continues to infiltrate new T4 cells, reproducing until they burst out of the cell membrane and begin to float freely in the blood, infecting other T4 cells, of which the body has a limited supply. B cells are stimulated by free-floating HIVs to start producing antibodies. Unfortunately, by the time enough antibodies to HIV are produced to mount an effective attack, the viruses have invaded other cells where they are safe from the attacking antibodies. Protection by monocytes and macrophages is also compromised as a result of lack of stimulation by T4 cells and additionally because some monocytes and macrophages are directly infected by HIV.

Investigators and clinicians require a great deal more knowledge about the effects of HIV on the immune system. Currently, researchers are actively trying to develop a vaccine against HIV that could prevent infection or clinical progression. Until there is a greater understanding of what type of immunity will provide a protective response to HIV, development of a vaccine remains in the future.

HISTORICAL ASPECTS

The first description of what was to later be called AIDS appeared in the CDC's *Morbidity and Mortality Weekly Report* (MMWR) of June 5, 1981. The report described unusual outbreaks of *Pneumocystis carinii* pneumonia (PCP) and Kaposi's sarcoma (KS) among specific groups of young homosexual men in California and New York. Appearance of these syndromes was considered unusual because of the frequency with which they were occurring and the population being affected. Historically, these conditions were seen infrequently and generally only in severely immunosuppressed individuals.

Because these first cases were identified only in homosexual and bisexual men, investigators assumed that the immune deficiency was etiologically related to the gay lifestyle. The disease was even referred to at that time as

gay-related immune deficiency (Kanabus & Fredriksson, 2005).

Numbers of reported cases were mounting rapidly. Within a brief period, AIDS cases began appearing in other special populations: heterosexual intravenous (IV) drug users and hemophiliacs. Soon after, the first AIDS cases associated with blood transfusions were suspected. These individuals were found to have a history of receiving blood transfusions within the preceding 3 to 5 years.

By 1983, independent laboratories were reporting isolation of a newly recognized retrovirus from patients with or at risk for AIDS (Hare, 2004). Initially, different names were assigned to the new retrovirus, including lymphadenopathy-associated virus (LAV), AIDS-associated retrovirus (ARV), and human T-lymphotropic virus III (HTLV-III) (Kanabus & Fredriksson, 2005). In 1986, the retrovirus came to be known as "human immunodeficiency virus."

Subsequently, a second, closely related retrovirus was identified. This second virus was endemic to West Africa and had similar modes of transmission and associated clinical syndromes (Noble, 2004). To distinguish between these two viruses, the initially discovered retrovirus that is now associated with most of the world's HIV disease is called human immunodeficiency virus type 1 (HIV-1) and the second virus, isolated in West Africa, is called human immunodeficiency virus type 2 (HIV-2). The term "HIV" commonly refers to HIV-1, because HIV-2 is rare in most parts of the world (Noble, 2004).

Once the retrovirus had been isolated, a test for identifying HIV antibodies in the blood was developed, making it possible to determine if individuals had been infected by HIV. Screening of blood and blood products also became possible, curbing transmission of the virus through blood transfusion.

The HTLV-III may have originated in Africa with a virus called simian T-cell leukemia virus (STLV) found in more than 30 species of monkeys and apes. Spread of the virus progressed from subprimate to African humans. The virus then reportedly moved at elevated rates to the Caribbean and northern South America and at lower rates to North America and Europe.

The AIDS epidemic has assumed major proportions, with the numbers of cases continuing to grow internationally. Virtually every major country in the world is confronting what has become the major health crisis of modern times. If progression is not curtailed, it will undoubtedly come to be ranked among history's greatest killers.

EPIDEMIOLOGICAL STATISTICS

Estimates by the United Nations Joint Programme on HIV/AIDS (UNAIDS) and the World Health Organization (WHO), a cosponsor of the Joint Programme, indicate that as of the end of 2004, approximately 40 million people were infected with HIV. During 2004, an estimated 3 million people lost their lives to the disease (UNAIDS/WHO, 2004). The largest number of infections (approximately 64 percent) are concentrated in Sub-Saharan Africa.

Almost 930,000 cases of AIDS were diagnosed in the United States through 2003 (Centers for Disease Control and Prevention [CDC], 2004). In the United States, HIV disease has now been reported in all 50 states and the District of Columbia. Geographical distribution shows the highest number of cases in New York, California, and Florida and the lowest in North Dakota and Wyoming (CDC, 2004).

The number of estimated deaths among persons with AIDS has declined steadily since 1995, and may have stabilized (CDC, 2004). This is due in part to the widespread introduction of highly active antiretroviral therapy (HAART). These highly effective medications delay the disease progression among HIV-infected persons who are receiving treatment.

Behavioral changes have resulted in a decline in the number of cases among homosexual men. However, the number of cases transmitted through heterosexual contact and IV drug use have increased, accounting for about one third of new diagnoses in 2003 (CDC, 2004).

Nursing care of clients with HIV disease is moving away from the acute care hospitals. Length of acute care hospital stays is decreasing, and a greater focus is being placed on alternative services, such as expanded outpatient clinics, day care facilities, chronic care facilities, home care programs, and hospice programs.

The epidemiology of HIV disease changes rapidly, and current information becomes outdated almost before it is published. Nurses must maintain awareness of the latest available information about the disease and the issues that affect provision and outcome of nursing care of clients with HIV disease.

PREDISPOSING FACTORS

The etiological agent associated with AIDS is HIV. It is currently known to have two subtypes, which have been called type 1 and type 2 (HIV-1 and HIV-2). Most of the cases of AIDS worldwide are linked to HIV-1 with the exception of Africa, where HIV-2 is prevalent. HIV-1 and HIV-2 are clinically similar, except that HIV-2 appears to be less easily transmitted, and the period between initial infection and illness is longer with HIV-2 (Noble, 2004). Several new strains have been discovered, and the HIV-1 has subsequently been classified into three groups, with a number of genetically distinct subtypes (Noble, 2004). Classification is a complex issue and subject to change as new discoveries are made.

The major routes for transmission of HIV are sexual, bloodborne, and perinatal transmission. There has been a shift in the identification of at-risk populations from that of merely belonging to a specific group to identifying characteristic behaviors that place individuals at risk. The risk for HIV infection is having sex with someone who is infected or being exposed to blood that is infected. The risk is not being a member of any particular group.

Sexual Transmission

It is now clear that both homosexual and heterosexual activity play major roles in the transmission of HIV infection worldwide. In the United States and Europe, the largest percentage of AIDS cases are among homosexual men; in Africa, however, most cases result from heterosexual transmission of HIV (Hare, 2004).

Heterosexual Transmission

The virus is found in greater concentration in semen than in vaginal secretions, which more readily facilitates transmission from men to women than from women to men. Male-to-female transmission has been reported in cases of HIV-positive female partners of hemophiliacs, bisexual men, and male IV drug users, and in women artificially inseminated by specimens from men who are infected with HIV.

HIV may be transmitted from an infected man to his female sexual partner by vaginal or anal intercourse. The possibility of oral transmission through sexual practices such as fellatio seems to be relatively low, although clear cases have occurred (Hare, 2004). Data on female-to-male transmission in the United States have been limited; however, this mode of transmission is biologically plausible because HIV has been isolated in vaginal secretions, and cases of female-to-male transmission have been documented (Hare, 2004).

Homosexual Transmission

The most significant risk factors for homosexual transmission of HIV are receptive anal intercourse and the number of male sexual partners. Other behaviors that may injure rectal mucosa increase the risk of viral invasion. The lining of the anal canal is delicate and prone to tearing and bleeding, making anal intercourse an easy way for infections to be passed from one person to another. The presence of concomitant infections with other diseases such as hepatitis, herpes, and other sexually transmitted diseases increases the risk of infection with HIV because of antigenic overload in the host, resulting in acceleration of pathogenesis of immunodeficiency.

Bloodborne Transmission

Transfusion with Blood Products

HIV transmission through transfusion of blood and blood products has been greatly diminished. Only 219 cases were reported in 2003 (CDC, 2004). Although laboratory tests are more than 99 percent sensitive, screening problems may occur when donations are received from individuals recently infected with HIV-1 who have not yet developed antibodies or from persistently antibody-negative donors who are infected with HIV. In March, 1996, the American Red Cross (ARC) implemented the HIV-1 p24 antigen test. This test, when used in combination with the HIV antibody test, further improves the safety of the blood supply for transfusions. The ARC reports that the risk of HIV infection through transfusion is now one in 676,000 units.

Individuals at highest risk for HIV infection from blood transfusion are hemophiliacs, simply because of their massive requirements for blood products. Other individuals who require blood because of temporary illness or surgery also may be at risk.

Transmission by Needles Infected with HIV-1

The highest number of cases occurring via this route are among IV drug users who share needles and other equipment contaminated with HIV-1-infected blood. In some areas of the country, this is the most prevalent mode of transmission. IV drug abusers are also at higher risk because of the immunosuppressive factors associated with many of the drugs of abuse and the common underlying existence of malnutrition. Some regions (e.g., New York City) have established programs to provide drug users with clean needles in an effort to diminish the spread of HIV.

A second bloodborne mode of transmission of HIV with contaminated needles is through accidental needle sticks by health care workers, as well as by other means and with other contaminated equipment used for therapeutic purposes. Some examples include:

● Needle sticks caused by recapping needles and by improper disposal of syringes.
● Coming in contact with blood or other body fluids during treatments without wearing gloves and while having chapped hands or cuts on the hands.
● Having blood or other body fluids splashed on face during treatments, causing entry through ocular, nasal, or oral mucous membranes.
● Being cut with a sharp object that has been contaminated with the blood of a client who is HIV positive
● Dressing open wounds without wearing gloves.

Perinatal Transmission

Worldwide, approximately 500,000 infants are perinatally infected with HIV each year, most of whom are born in developing countries (Kanabus & Pennington, 2005). Modes of transmission include transplacental, through exposure to maternal blood and vaginal secretions during delivery, and through breast milk. Delivery by cesarean section may provide somewhat less risk than vaginal delivery (American Academy of Family Physicians [AAFP], 2001). Because breast milk has been implicated as a mode of transmission, women should be counseled to use other forms of infant feeding when possible.

The risk of perinatal transmission has been significantly reduced in recent years with the advent of free or low-cost prenatal care, provision of access to anti-HIV medication during pregnancy, and education about the dangers of breastfeeding. The use of zidovudine during pregnancy can reduce the rate of passing HIV from mother to baby by about two thirds (AAFP, 2001).

Other Possible Modes of Transmission

To date, HIV has been isolated from blood, semen, vaginal secretions, saliva, tears, breast milk, cerebrospinal fluid, and amniotic fluid. However, only blood, semen, vaginal secretions, and breast milk have been epidemiologically linked to transmission of the virus (CDC, 2003a).

The risk of being infected with HIV through casual, nonsexual contact is so low as to be virtually nonexistent. Even in those isolated cases that have been reported, most consistently exhibit additional risk factors that may account for the infection.

APPLICATION OF THE NURSING PROCESS

Background Assessment Data

The CDC now identifies HIV infection as a continuous and progressive process. In 1993, the CDC revised the classification system for HIV infection and expanded the surveillance case definition for AIDS among adolescents and adults. These categories are identified by T4 cell count and presence of symptomatic conditions or opportunistic infections. The information is categorized here according to early-, middle-, and late-stage HIV disease and is summarized in Table 39–1.

Early-Stage (Category 1) HIV Disease (≥500 T4 Cells/mm³)

Acute (Primary) HIV Infection. The acute HIV infection is identified by a characteristic syndrome of symptoms that occurs from 6 days to 6 weeks after exposure to the virus.

TABLE 39-1	Stages and Symptoms of HIV Disease
STAGE (T4 CELLS/MM³)	CONDITION/SYMPTOMS
Early Stage (≥500)	**Acute HIV Infection** Fever, malaise, sore throat, lymphadenopathy, anorexia, nausea and vomiting, headaches, skin rash, diarrhea **Seroconversion** HIV antibodies are detected in the blood (most often occurs from 6 weeks to 6 months after exposure) **Asymptomatic Infection** No manifestations of illness. Slow deterioration of immune system with decline in T4 cell count
Middle Stage (499–200)	**Persistent Generalized Lymphadenopathy** Lymph nodes of the neck, armpit, and groin swell and remain swollen for months. **Systemic Complaints** Fever, night sweats, chronic diarrhea, fatigue, minor oral infections, headaches, weight loss
Late Stage (≤200)	**HIV Wasting Syndrome** Severe weight loss; large-volume diarrhea; fever and weakness **Opportunistic Infections** *Pneumocystis carinii* pneumonia (fever, dyspnea, cough) Cryptosporidiosis (profuse watery diarrhea) Toxoplasmosis (neurological abnormalities) Candidiasis (lesions in oral cavity, esophagus, vagina) Cryptococcosis (meningitis) Cytomegalovirus (retinitis, enteritis, pneumonitis, cerebral disease, hepatitis, adrenal necrosis, and others) Herpes simplex (watery blisters orally and on genitals) Herpes zoster (painful, blistery lesions on skin along nerve track; disseminated disease may involve lungs and CNS) *Mycobacterium avium* (HIV wasting syndrome) *Mycobacterium tuberculosis* (tuberculosis) Others **AIDS-Related Malignancies** Kaposi's sarcoma (pigmented lesions that transform into tumors form on the body and in any organ system) Non-Hodgkin's lymphoma Hodgkin's disease Malignant melanoma Testicular cancers Primary hepatocellular carcinoma Invasive cervical cancer **Altered Mental States** Delirium (fluctuating consciousness, abnormal vital signs, and psychotic phenomena) Dementia (cognitive, motor, and behavioral changes)

The symptoms have an abrupt onset, are somewhat vague, and are similar to those sometimes seen in mononucleosis. Symptoms of acute HIV infection include fever, myalgia, malaise, lymphadenopathy, sore throat, anorexia, nausea and vomiting, headaches, skin rash, and diarrhea (Blair, 2005). Most symptoms resolve themselves in 1 to 3 weeks, with the exception of fever, myalgia, lymphadenopathy, and malaise, which may continue for several months.

Seroconversion, the detectability of HIV antibodies in the blood, most often is detected between 6 and 12 weeks (Sadock & Sadock, 2003). Most people show positive for HIV by 3 months after infection. In some individuals it may take up to 6 months. The time between infection and seroconversion is called the *window period*.

Asymptomatic Infection. The acute infection progresses to an asymptomatic stage. Probably the largest number of HIV-infected individuals fall within this group. Individuals may remain in this asymptomatic stage for 10 or more years. The progression of the illness is much faster in infants and children than it is in adults.

During this asymptomatic period, there is slow deterioration of the immune system with a decline in the T4 cell count. The length of this stage correlates with the level of HIV replication and individual genetic differences in strength of immune function.

Middle-Stage (Category 2) HIV Disease (499 to 200 T4 Cells/mm³)

Persistent Generalized Lymphadenopathy. Following the asymptomatic period, clients with HIV infection may develop a generalized lymphadenopathy, in which lymph nodes in at least two different locations in the body swell and remain swollen for months, with no other signs of a related infectious disease. The lymph nodes that are most frequently affected are those in the areas of the neck, jaw, groin, and armpits. This syndrome often occurs within a few months of seroconversion for HIV antibody.

Other Symptoms of Middle-Stage HIV Disease

Fever. Fever is common during this stage, even in the absence of any specific **opportunistic infection**. Management is frequently through intermittent or long-term use of nonsteroidal anti-inflammatory drugs.

Night Sweats. The most common description of this symptom is severe drenching night sweats that occur repeatedly over a prolonged period (Viera, Bond, & Yates, 2003). They are often associated with the fever and may be controlled through the regular use of antipyretic agents.

Chronic Diarrhea. In middle-stage HIV disease, diarrhea can be induced by infection of the gastrointestinal tract with the HIV or another microbial organism. The diarrhea can be severe enough to result in dehydration and general debilitation. At this stage, it is treated symptomatically and effectively with common antidiarrheal medications. In late-stage HIV disease, diarrhea is usually associated with opportunistic GI pathogens.

Fatigue. This symptom can range from mild limitations in a usually active lifestyle to severe debilitation. At this stage, the client should be evaluated for depression, of which fatigue is a common symptom, and which is quite treatable in individuals with HIV disease. In late-stage HIV disease, fatigue may be associated with endocrine malfunction.

Minor Oral Infections. Oral infections with *Candida albicans* are common in early symptomatic HIV disease. Various topical and oral agents are successful in treating the symptom, although a high rate of recurrence is common.

Headache. Headaches are a common symptom in all stages of the illness. These may be quite severe and are often identified as bifrontal or occipital. Treatment is symptomatic, and nonsteroidal anti-inflammatory agents are preferred over narcotics because of the chronicity of this complaint.

Late-Stage (Category 3) HIV Disease (<200 T4 Cells/mm³)

HIV Wasting Syndrome. **HIV wasting syndrome**, involving diarrhea and weight loss, occur in most individuals with advanced HIV disease. Symptoms are associated with nutrient malabsorption, or enterocolitis or intestinal injury related to an opportunistic pathogen. Involuntary weight loss of more than 10 percent of baseline body weight is common. Large-volume diarrhea, fever, and weakness accompany the syndrome. A low-fat, lactose-free diet supplemented with medium-chain triglycerides may be beneficial. Parenteral nutrition may be used in refractory cases.

Opportunistic Infections. Opportunistic infections have long been a defining characteristic of AIDS. Common ones are defined here.

***Pneumocystis carinii* pneumonia.** The most common opportunistic infection seen in clients with AIDS is **pneumocystis pneumonia** (Smith, 2003). Symptoms include fever, exertional dyspnea, and nonproductive cough.

Cryptosporidiosis. This parasitic infection may cause chronic profuse watery diarrhea in AIDS clients. Other symptoms include abdominal cramping and pain, anorexia, nausea, vomiting, profound weight loss, fever, fatigue, myalgia, and electrolyte imbalance (Blair, 2005).

Toxoplasmosis. This protozoan infection frequently causes central nervous system (CNS) disease in AIDS clients. Common presenting symptoms include headache, impaired cognition, hemiparesis, aphasia, ataxia, vision loss, cranial nerve palsies, motor problems, and seizures (Blair, 2005). Infection can also involve other organ systems, such as the heart, lungs, skin, stomach, abdomen, and testes.

Candidiasis. Most commonly caused by the fungus *Candida albicans*, this infection usually occurs in the oral cavity and esophagus of the HIV-infected individual. Vaginal and anal infections are seen less frequently. Oral candidiasis, commonly called thrush, is characterized by white plaques on the oral mucosa. Esophageal candidiasis presents with painful lesions in the esophagus, making swallowing difficult.

Cryptococcosis. This yeast infection, caused by *Cryptococcus neoformans*, most commonly causes lung and brain infection in AIDS clients (Blair, 2005). Infection in the CNS produces symptoms of low-grade fever, fatigue, headaches, nausea, vomiting, and altered mental status. Pulmonary manifestations include cough, dyspnea, and pleuritic chest pain (Blair, 2005).

Cytomegalovirus. Cytomegalovirus (CMV) is common in most human populations. In most instances, it is latent and asymptomatic. Immunosuppression by HIV reactivates the virus. CMV causes retinitis (and possible blindness), enteritis (manifested by profuse watery diarrhea), pneumonitis, cerebral disease, myelitis, pericarditis, endometritis, glomerulitis, epididymitis, hepatitis, and adrenal necrosis.

Herpes Simplex. Herpes simplex virus (HSV) infections are found in the oral, genital, or rectal area of people with AIDS. Symptoms include blisterlike lesions that rupture and leave ulcerations, fever, pain, or bleeding (Smith, 2003). HSV can also cause encephalitis, esophagitis, bronchitis, keratitis, pericarditis, and hand infection (Blair, 2005).

Herpes Zoster. Herpes zoster has been found to cause both dermatomal (shingles) and disseminated disease in clients with HIV infection. After initial infection (usually in childhood), herpes zoster lies latent in the dorsal root ganglia of the peripheral nerves. Reactivation results in painful lesions on the skin area supplied by the affected nerve. Dissemination to the lung or CNS can result in pneumonia or encephalitis. Ophthalmic nerve involvement can cause blindness.

Mycobacteria. *Mycobacterium avium-intracellulare* complex (MAC) and *M. tuberculosis* occur with great frequency among clients with HIV disease. MAC may contribute to the HIV wasting syndrome, with symptoms of diarrhea and malabsorption. Other symptoms include fever, chills, weight loss, night sweats, lymphadenopathy, and fatigue. *M. tuberculosis* is associated with the development of tuberculosis in clients with HIV disease. The primary manifestation is pulmonary lesions. Extrapulmonary lesions may involve bones, joints, liver, spleen, CNS, skin, gastrointestinal tract, urine, and blood (Blair, 2005).

AIDS-Related Malignancies. A number of malignant neoplasms have been associated with HIV disease. Common ones are described here.

Kaposi's Sarcoma. Kaposi's sarcoma (KS) is caused by a virus called Kaposi's sarcoma herpes virus (KSHV), or herpes virus type 8. KS is unrelated to low T4 cell counts and can occur early in HIV infection (Blair, 2005). Lesions associated with KS may appear on any body surface or in the viscera. KS lesions usually manifest as flat, "patchy," spots that look like a bruise. In light-skinned people, they appear reddish to purple in color, whereas in dark skinned people, they are generally dark brown to black. The initial lesions become elevated and develop into papules or plaques. Eventually the plaques enlarge, coalesce, and form tumor nodules. Krown (2003) describes the following characteristics of plaque formation:

Distinctive cutaneous lesion distributions may occur, such as on the nose, on or behind the ears, or involving the periorbital tissues; on the lower legs or feet (with large plaques on the soles of the feet in some patients); large clusters of lesions in the upper medial thighs or the suprapubic and genital areas; and widespread and scattered over the trunk, but sparing the face and extremities. Lesions may be symmetric and linear, and distributed around skin folds. The factors that predispose to these varied distributions are unknown.

Virtually any organ system, including the heart and lungs, may be affected. GI involvement is common and may result in pain, obstruction, and bleeding. Clients with pulmonary KS may present with symptoms similar to those of pneumonia, thereby creating some difficulty with differential diagnosis. KS rarely involves the CNS. Lymphedema from lymphatic obstruction may occur with KS. Occasionally, massive nodal enlargement may occur, and lymph nodes may be replaced by KS (Krown, 2003). KS is not viewed as a metastatic disease, but rather

one with multifocal origin. A poor prognosis is associated with visceral involvement.

The number of cases of KS has declined in the U.S. in recent years. This decline is attributed to the increased effectiveness of antiretroviral medication and safer sex practices among homosexual men, who historically have had the highest incidence of KS (Krown, 2003).

Other Malignancies. Individuals with HIV disease are at increased risk for developing non-Hodgkin's lymphomas, a group of neoplasms that includes primary central nervous system lymphomas, systemic lymphomas, and primary effusion lymphomas (Kaplan, 1998). Extranodal sites, including the CNS and bone marrow, are frequently involved. Major primary extranodal sites have been identified as the brain, anus, rectum, head, neck, lung, and liver (Kaplan, 1998). Clinical features are consistent with regional involvement. Hodgkin's disease, squamous-cell carcinomas, malignant melanoma, testicular cancers, and primary hepatocellular carcinoma also have been reported in association with HIV disease.

Altered Mental States

Delirium. Delirium is one of the most common cognitive disorders seen in AIDS clients. Clinical manifestations may include a fluctuating level of consciousness, reversal of sleep-wake cycle, abnormal vital signs, and psychotic phenomena (e.g., hallucinations). Contributing factors to the development of delirium include CNS infections, CNS neoplastic disease, side effects of various chemotherapeutic agents, hypoxemia from respiratory compromise, electrolyte imbalance, and sensory deprivation. In some clients, delirium may be superimposed on, or evolve into, dementia.

Depressive Syndromes. Depression is the most common psychiatric disorder observed among HIV-positive clients (Remien & Rabkin, 2001). Anticipatory or actual grief is an important cause of depressive symptoms in clients with HIV disease. Transient suicidal ideation on learning of HIV positivity is quite common, although the incidence of serious suicidal behavior is low. Depression in AIDS clients may be related to receiving a new diagnosis of HIV positivity or AIDS, perceiving rejection by loved ones, experiencing multiple losses of friends to the disease, having an inadequate social and financial support system, and presence of an early cognitive disorder.

HIV-Associated Dementia. HIV-associated dementia (HAD) is a neuropathological syndrome experienced by 7 to 27 percent of people with HIV infection, usually in the late stages (Sahai-Srivastava & Jones, 2004). Incidence rates of the disorder continue to show decline, especially following the introduction of HAART, although the actual number of cases may continue to rise as survival rates for individuals with advanced HIV infection lengthen (McArthur, 2002). Sadock and Sadock (2003)

TABLE 39–2	Signs and Symptoms of HIV-Associated Dementia
EARLY	**LATE**
Cognitive	**Cognitive**
Forgetfulness	Severe cognitive deficits
Loss of concentration	Mutism
Confusion	
Slowness of thought	
Motor	**Motor**
Loss of balance	Psychomotor retardation
Leg weakness	Ataxia
Deterioration in handwriting	Hypertonia
	Paralysis
	Tremors
	Vegetative state
Behavioral	**Behavioral**
Apathy	Organic psychosis—
Social withdrawal	persistent
Dysphoric mood	Vacant staring
Organic psychosis	Lethargy
Regressed behavior	Hypersomnolence
Other	**Other**
Headache	Bowel and bladder
Seizures	incontinence
	Myoclonus
	Seizures

SOURCE: Adapted from Blair (2005); Yahya, Garewal, & Thomas (2005); and Sahai-Srivastava & Jones (2004).

suggest that possible etiologies of the dementia include "HIV encephalopathy, CNS infections, CNS neoplasms, CNS abnormalities caused by systemic disorders and endocrinopathies, and adverse CNS responses to drugs." Early clinical manifestations include subtle cognitive, behavioral, and motor symptoms, which become more severe with progression of the disease (Table 39–2).

Psychosocial Implications of HIV/AIDS

The psychosocial problems that confront a person with HIV disease can be overwhelming. Health care workers still face a number of unknowns related to the disease, thereby setting clients with HIV disease apart from individuals with other life-threatening illnesses. Persons with HIV disease are often the victims of discrimination because of fear of contagion, prejudices, and stigmatization surrounding the illness. Fredriksson and Kanabus (2004) identify the following aspects that have contributed to the psychosocial problems experienced by individuals with HIV disease:

1. HIV disease is a life-threatening disease.
2. People are afraid of contracting the disease from a person who is HIV positive.
3. The disease is associated with behaviors (e.g., sex

between men and IV drug use) that are already stigmatized in many societies.
4. Religious or moral beliefs lead some people to believe that having HIV disease is the result of amoral behavior (e.g., promiscuity or "deviant sex") that deserves to be punished.

The individual with newly diagnosed HIV seropositivity commonly responds with shock and disbelief, followed by guilt, anger, and depression. In some instances, a symptom complex similar to posttraumatic stress disorder is common in the first few weeks after a person receives notification of his or her HIV positivity. The person may become extremely anxious and hypervigilant about physical symptoms, exhibiting marked dependence on health care workers. Feelings of guilt prevail over previous life activities and self-blame for becoming infected. Depressive thoughts are common, and acute suicidal crises may occur. Some individuals may become socially isolated. They may fear that they will infect others or be rejected by others. Crisis intervention with newly diagnosed HIV-positive persons is aimed at restoring a positive psychological equilibrium and providing education for making the necessary lifestyle behavioral changes to protect self and others.

Denial is a common defense mechanism among individuals with high-risk behaviors. Denial prevents individuals from undergoing HIV testing; it delays some HIV-positive individuals from seeking early medical care; and it prevents some HIV-positive individuals from changing their behavior to prevent HIV transmission.

Significant others of clients with HIV disease face many stresses associated with the client's illness. Initially they may experience emotions typical of the grief response. The reality of the situation is felt when the person begins to accept the immense responsibility for the physical and emotional care of his or her loved one. The significant other may experience financial concerns and lack of social support.

When the significant other is a gay lover, guilt over having infected the partner or fear of having been infected by the partner may be felt. The gay lover may be rejected by the client's family members, who themselves may be experiencing unique stresses associated with learning for the first time of their relative's lifestyle. Parents may blame themselves and their childrearing practices. The family may experience a lack of social support owing to the stigma attached to the illness. Grief responses by family members are common.

Psychiatric Disorders Common in Clients with HIV Infections

Mood disorders, substance use disorders, and cognitive impairment are the most commonly observed neuropsychiatric disorders in clients with HIV disease (Remien & Rabkin, 2001). Other psychiatric disorders common to individuals with HIV disease include anxiety disorders, psychotic disorders, adjustment disorders, and sleep disorders (McDaniel et al., 2002).

Anxiety Disorders. Individuals with HIV infection express fears about the illness and uncertainty about their future. Symptoms of intense anxiety may remit when a crisis can be temporarily resolved. However, persistence of anxiety symptoms for weeks to months can become a diagnosable anxiety disorder requiring evaluation and treatment. McDaniel and associates (2002) state:

> For persons infected with HIV, there are numerous points at various stages of the illness when anxiety about the future, physical symptoms, or clinical decisions can become overwhelming. Psychotherapeutic approaches to situational anxiety can help patients work through intense affects and provide a structure within which sound decisions can be made. [Because of adverse interactions between anxiolytics and antiretroviral medications] psychiatrists may need to adjust medication doses and consider medical setbacks when treating patients with prominent anxiety symptoms. Psychotherapy may be effective in managing anxiety while reducing the need for medications. (p. 174)

Major Depression. Symptoms associated with the diagnosis of major depression in individuals with HIV disease include depressed mood, dysphoria, low self-esteem, hopelessness, worthlessness, guilt, helplessness, and suicidal ideation. Physical signs, such as fatigue, anorexia, insomnia, weakness, and diminished libido, which are often used to diagnose major depression in healthy individuals, may be related to the disease process or to medications in individuals with HIV disease.

Other symptoms, such as apathy, withdrawal, mental slowing, and avoidance of complex tasks, which are considered common symptoms of major depression, may be related to early symptoms of cognitive impairment of HIV-associated dementia. Taking a careful history and making a clinical examination are required for a differential diagnosis. The management of major depression in HIV-infected individuals entails (1) supportive psychotherapy; (2) the control of distressing physical symptoms, especially pain; (3) adjunctive measures such as behavioral interventions; and (4) psychopharmacological measures (Remien & Rabkin, 2001).

AIDS is associated with an increased frequency of suicidal ideation, suicide attempts, and suicides than in the general population. Feelings of hopelessness, guilt about past behavior, multiple bereavements, absent or inadequate social supports, and isolation from family and friends have been identified as common predisposing factors. McDaniel and associates (2002) state:

> Recent evidence has shown that patients with greater levels of "fighting spirit," a specific pattern of adjustment to life-threatening illnesses, tend to have lower levels of suicidal ideation. Evaluation of suicide risk and other violent acts is an integral part of a comprehensive evaluation for HIV/AIDS patients. Psychiatric treatments that promote greater adaptation to living with HIV infection may lower the risk of suicide for many patients. (p. 180)

Mania. Mania in individuals with HIV disease may be secondary to AIDS-associated brain infections, neoplasms, or treatment with medications (McDaniel et al., 2002). AIDS-related mania that occurs late in the course of the disease may be associated with the direct effects of the HIV on the central nervous system. Research shows that mania in AIDS carries a poor prognosis. It is often associated with cognitive impairments and occurs in patients with more advanced immunosuppression (N.Y. State Department of Health AIDS Institute, 2005).

Dementia and Delirium. HAD was discussed previously in this chapter. It is not uncommon for delirium to be superimposed on HAD and to occur with greater frequency in advanced disease due to adverse effects of specific diseases associated with HIV disease. Examples include hypoxemia due to *Pneumocystis carinii* pneumonia, uremia due to HIV nephropathy, or elevated ammonia levels due to cirrhosis (McDaniel et al., 2002). Delirium can also be an adverse reaction to medications, such as high-dose corticosteroids. Symptoms of delirium include fluctuating level of consciousness, misperceptions, delusions, loss of sleep–wake cycle, and agitation or withdrawal. General treatment measures include judicious use of appropriate medications to treat agitation, maintain orientation, and restore the sleep–wake cycle.

Diagnosis/Outcome Identification

Nursing diagnoses are formulated from the data gathered during the assessment phase and with background knowledge regarding predisposing factors to the disorder. The following nursing diagnoses may be used for the client with HIV disease:

Ineffective protection related to compromised immune status secondary to diagnosis of HIV disease evidenced by laboratory values indicating decreased numbers of T4 cells and presence of opportunistic infections manifested by fever, night sweats, copious watery diarrhea, weight loss, fatigue, malaise, swollen lymph glands, cough, dyspnea, rash, skin lesions, white patches in mouth, headache, ataxia, anorexia, bleeding, bruising, and various neurological effects.

Interrupted family processes related to crisis associated with having a family member diagnosed with HIV disease evidenced by difficulty making decisions that affect all family members; inability to meet physical, emotional, spiritual, and security needs of its members.

Deficient knowledge (prevention of transmission and protection of the client) related to lack of exposure to accurate information evidenced by inaccurate statements by client and family.

Disturbed thought processes related to primary HIV infection, opportunistic infections that invade the CNS, and/or adverse effects of therapy evidenced by confusion, disorientation, memory deficits, and inappropriate non-reality-based thinking. (Refer to Table 26–4, Care Plan for Client with a Cognitive Disorder.)

Risk for suicide related to new diagnosis of HIV infection, evidenced by statements of wishing to take own life and preferring dying rather than facing future with AIDS. (Refer to Table 18–4, Care Plan for the Suicidal Client.)

Impaired adjustment related to change in health status requiring modification in lifestyle, evidenced by elevated level of anxiety and fear of the future. (Refer to Table 35–2, Care Plan for the Client with Adjustment Disorder.)

The following criteria may be used for measurement of outcomes in the care of the client with HIV/AIDS.

The client:

1. Shows no new signs or symptoms of infection.
2. Does not experience respiratory distress.
3. Maintains optimal nutrition and hydration.
4. Has experienced no further weight loss.
5. Maintains integrity of skin and mucous membranes.
6. Manifests evidence of wound healing.
7. Attains and maintains normal fluid and electrolyte balance.
8. Has fewer bowel movements, with increased stool consistency.
9. Explores feelings about self and illness.
10. Verbalizes understanding about disease process, modes of transmission, and prevention of infection.

The family/significant others:

1. Discuss feelings regarding client's diagnosis and prognosis.
2. Can make rational decisions regarding care of their loved one and the effect on family function.
3. Can verbalize precautions for preventing transmission of HIV to themselves and others and infection of the client.
4. Verbalize knowledge of resources within the community from which they may seek support and assistance.

Planning/Implementation

Table 39–3 provides a plan of care for the client with HIV/AIDS. Nursing diagnoses are presented, along with outcome criteria, appropriate nursing interventions, and rationales.

TABLE 39–3   **Care Plan for the Client with HIV Disease***

NURSING DIAGNOSIS: INEFFECTIVE PROTECTION

RELATED TO: Compromised immune status secondary to diagnosis of HIV disease

EVIDENCED BY: Laboratory values indicating decreased numbers of T4 cells and presence of opportunistic infections manifested by fever, night sweats, diarrhea, weight loss, fatigue, malaise, swollen lymph glands, cough, dyspnea, rash, skin lesions, white patches in mouth, headache, ataxia, anorexia, bleeding, bruising, and various neurological effects

OUTCOME CRITERIA	NURSING INTERVENTIONS	RATIONALE
Client safety and comfort will be maximized.	1. Implement universal blood and body fluid precautions.	1–8. To prevent infection in an immunocompromised individual.
	2. Wash hands with antibacterial soap before entering and on leaving client's room.	
	3. Monitor vital signs at regular intervals.	
	4. Monitor complete blood counts (CBCs) for leukopenia/neutropenia.	
	5. Monitor for signs and symptoms of specific opportunistic infections.	
	6. Protect client from individuals with infections.	
	7. Maintain meticulous sterile technique for dressing changes and any invasive procedure.	
	8. Administer antibiotics as ordered.	
	9. Provide low-residue, high-protein, high-calorie, soft, bland diet. Maintain hydration with adequate fluid intake.	9–16. To restore nutritional status and decrease nausea/vomiting and diarrhea.

(Continued on opposite page)

10. Obtain daily weight and record intake and output.
11. Monitor serum electrolytes and CBCs.
12. If client is unable to eat, provide isotonic tube feedings as tolerated. Check for gastric residual frequently.
13. If client is unable to tolerate oral intake/tube feedings, consult physician regarding possibility of parenteral hyperalimentation. Observe hyperalimentation administration site for signs of infection.
14. Administer antidiarrheals and antiemetics as ordered.
15. Perform frequent oral care. Promote prevention and healing of lesions in the mouth.
16. Have the client eat small, frequent meals with high-calorie snacks rather than three large meals per day.
17. Monitor skin condition for signs of redness and breakdown.
18. Reposition client every 1 to 2 hours.
19. Encourage ambulation and chair activity as tolerated.
20. Use "egg crate" mattress or air mattress on bed.
21. Wash skin daily with soap and rinse well with water.
22. Apply lotion to skin to maintain skin softness.
23. Provide wound care as ordered for existing pressure sores or lesions.
24. Cleanse skin exposed to diarrhea thoroughly and protect rectal area with ointment.
25. Apply artificial tears to eyes as appropriate.
26. Perform frequent oral care; apply ointment to lips.
27. Assess respiratory status frequently:
    a. Monitor depth, rate, and rhythm of respirations.
    b. Auscultate lung fields every 2 hr and p.r.n.
    c. Monitor arterial blood gases.
    d. Check color of skin, nail beds, and sclerae.
    e. Assess sputum for color, odor, and viscosity.
28. Encourage coughing and deep-breathing exercises.
29. Provide humidified oxygen as ordered.
30. Suction as needed using sterile technique.
31. Space nursing care to allow client adequate rest periods between procedures.
32. Administer analgesics or sedatives judiciously to prevent respiratory depression.
33. Administer bronchodilators and antibiotics as ordered.
34. Follow protocol for maintenance of skin integrity.
35. Provide safe environment to minimize falling or bumping into objects.
36. Provide soft toothbrush or "toothette" swabs for cleaning teeth and gums.
37. Ensure that client does not take aspirin or other medications that increase the potential for bleeding.
38. Clean up areas contaminated by client's blood with household bleach diluted 1:10 with water.
39. Provide frequent tepid water sponge baths.
40. Provide antipyretic as ordered by physician (avoid aspirin).
41. Place client in cool room, with minimal clothing and bed covers.
42. Encourage intake of cool liquids (if not contraindicated).

17–26. To promote improvement of skin and mucous membrane integrity.

27–33. To maximize oxygen consumption and minimize respiratory distress.

34–38. To minimize the potential for easy bleeding caused by HIV-induced thrombocytopenia.

39–42. To maintain near-normal body temperature.

(Continued on following page)

NURSING DIAGNOSIS: INTERRUPTED FAMILY PROCESSES

RELATED TO: Crisis associated with having a family member diagnosed with HIV disease

EVIDENCED BY: Difficulty making decisions that affect all family members; inability to meet physical, emotional, spiritual, and security needs of its members

OUTCOME CRITERIA	NURSING INTERVENTIONS	RATIONALE
Family will verbalize areas of dysfunction and demonstrate ability to cope more effectively. Family members will express feelings regarding loved one's diagnosis and prognosis.	1. Create an environment that is comfortable, supportive, private, and promotes trust. 2. Encourage each individual member to express feelings regarding loved one's diagnosis and prognosis. 3. If the client is homosexual, and this is family's first awareness, help them deal with guilt and shame they may experience. Help parents to understand they are not responsible, and their child is still the same individual they have always loved. 4. Serve as facilitator between client's family and homosexual partner. The family may have difficulty accepting the partner as a person who is as significant as a spouse. Clarify roles and responsibilities of family and partner. Do this by bringing both parties together to define and distribute the tasks involved in the client's care. 5. Encourage use of stress management techniques (e.g., relaxation exercises, guided imagery, attendance at support group meetings for significant others of AIDS clients). 6. Provide educational information about AIDS and opportunity to ask questions and express concerns. 7. Make family referrals to community organizations that provide supportive help or financial assistance to clients with HIV disease	1. Basic needs of the family must be met before crisis resolution can be attempted. 2. Each individual is unique and must feel that his or her private needs can be met within the family constellation. 3. Resolving guilt and shame enables family members to respond adaptively to the crisis. Their response can affect the client's remaining future and the family's future as well. 4. By minimizing the lack of legally defined roles, and by focusing on the need for making realistic decisions about the client's care, communication and resolution of conflict is enhanced. 5. Reduction of stress and support from others who share similar experiences enables individuals to begin to think more clearly and develop new behaviors to cope with this situational crisis. 6. Many misconceptions about the disease abound within the public domain. Clarification may calm some of the family's fears and facilitate interaction with the client. 7. Extended care can place a financial burden on client and family members. Respite care may provide family members with occasional much-needed relief away from the stress of physical and emotional caregiving responsibilities.

NURSING DIAGNOSIS: DEFICIENT KNOWLEDGE (PREVENTION OF TRANSMISSION AND PROTECTION OF THE CLIENT)

RELATED TO: Lack of exposure to accurate information

EVIDENCED BY: Inaccurate statements by client and family

OUTCOME CRITERIA	NURSING INTERVENTIONS	RATIONALE

Client and family will be able to verbalize accurate information regarding transmission of HIV and protection of the immunodeficient client.	1. Teach that HIV cannot be contracted from:
	  a. Casual or household contact with an individual with HIV infection.
	  b. Shaking hands, hugging, social (dry) kissing, holding hands, or other nonsexual physical contact.
	  c. Touching unsoiled linens or clothing, money, furniture, or other inanimate objects.
	  d. Being near someone who has HIV disease at work, school, stores, restaurants, elevators.
	  e. Toilet seats, bathtubs, towels, showers, or swimming pools.
		All of this information may be given to client and significant others in an effort to clarify misconceptions, calm fears, and support an environment of appropriate interventions for care of the client with HIV disease.

(Continued on opposite page)

f. Dishes, silverware, or food handled by a person with HIV disease.
g. Animals (pets may transmit opportunistic organisms).
h. (Very unlikely spread by) coughing, sneezing, spitting, kissing, tears, saliva.
2. HIV dies quickly outside the body because it requires living tissue to survive. It is readily killed by soap, cleansers, hot water, and disinfectants.
3. Teach client to protect self from infections by taking the following precautions:
  a. Avoid unpasteurized milk or milk products.
  b. Cook all raw vegetables and fruits before eating.
  c. Cook all meals well before eating.
  d. Avoid direct contact with persons with known contagious illnesses.
  e. Consult physician before getting a pet.
  f. Avoid touching animal feces, urine, emesis, litter boxes, aquariums, or bird cages. Always wear mask and gloves when cleaning up after a pet.
  g. Avoid traveling in countries with poor sanitation.
  h. Avoid vaccines or vaccinations that contain live organisms.
 	
  i. Exercise regularly.
  j. Control stress factors. A counselor or support group may be helpful.
  k. Stop smoking.
 	
  l. Maintain good personal hygiene.
4. Teach client/significant others about prevention of transmission:
  a. Do not donate blood, plasma, body organs, tissues, or semen.
  b. Inform physician, dentists, and anyone providing care that you have HIV disease.
  c. Do not share needles or syringes.
  d. Do not share personal items, such as toothbrushes, razors, or other implements that may be contaminated with blood or body fluids.
  e. Do not eat or drink from the same dinnerware and utensils without washing them between uses.
  f. Avoid becoming pregnant if at risk for HIV infection.
  g. Engage in only "safer" sexual practices (those *not* involving exchange of body fluids).
  h. Avoid sexual practices medically classified as "unsafe," such as anal or vaginal intercourse and oral sex.
  i. Avoid the use of recreational drugs because of their immunosuppressive effects.
5. Teach the home caregiver(s) to protect self from HIV infection by taking the following precautions:
  a. Wash hands thoroughly with liquid antibiotic soap before and after each client contact. Use moisturizing lotion afterward to prevent dry, cracking skin.
  b. Wear gloves when in contact with blood or body fluids (e.g., open wounds, suctioning, feces). Gown or aprons may be worn if soiling is likely.
  c. Wear a mask:
    (1) When client has a productive cough and tuberculosis has not been ruled out.
    (2) To protect client if caregiver has a cold.
    (3) During suctioning.
	
	Raw or improperly washed foods may transmit microbes.
	
	Pets require extra infection control precautions because of the opportunistic organisms carried by animals.
	
	Vaccination with live organisms may be fatal to severely immunosuppressed persons.
	
	Smoking predisposes to respiratory infections.

(Continued on following page)

TABLE 39–3	Care Plan for the Client with HIV Disease* *(Continued)*	
OUTCOME CRITERIA	**NURSING INTERVENTIONS**	**RATIONALE**
	d. Bag disposable gloves and masks with client's trash.	
	e. Dispose of the following in the toilet:	
	(1) Organic material on clothes or linen before laundering.	
	(2) Blood or body fluids.	
	(3) Soiled tissue or toilet paper.	
	(4) Cleaners or disinfectants used to clean contaminated articles.	
	(5) Solutions contaminated with blood or body fluids.	
	f. Double-bag client's trash and soiled dressings in an impenetrable, plastic bag. *Tie* the bag shut and discard with household trash.	
	g. Do not recap needles, syringes, and other sharp items. Use puncture-proof covered containers for disposal (e.g., coffee cans, jars).	
	h. Place soiled linen and clothing in a plastic bag and tie shut until washed. Launder these separately from other laundry. Use bleach or other disinfectant in hot water.	
	i. When house cleaning, all equipment used in care of the client, as well as bathroom and kitchen surfaces, should be cleaned with a 1:10 dilute bleach solution.	
	j. Mops, sponges, and other items used for cleaning should be reserved specifically for that purpose.	

*The interventions for this care plan have been adapted from "Nursing Care Plan for the AIDS Patient," written by the nursing staff of Hospice, Inc., Wichita, KS.

Client/Family Education

The role of client teacher is important in the psychiatric area, as it is in all areas of nursing. A list of topics for client and family education relevant to HIV disease is presented in Table 39–4.

Evaluation

Reassessment is conducted in order to determine if the nursing actions have been successful in achieving the objectives of care. Evaluation of the nursing actions for clients with HIV/AIDS may be facilitated by gathering information using the following types of questions:

1. Have precautions been successful in preventing new infection of the client?
2. Have fever and night sweats been controlled?
3. Has there been a decrease in frequency and increase in consistency of stools?
4. Have weight and nutritional status stabilized?
5. Are fluid and electrolyte values within normal limits?
6. Does the client experience respiratory distress?
7. Have bleeding and bruising been avoided?
8. Are skin and mucous membranes intact?
9. Do family members/significant others verbalize feelings (including anger) regarding the client's diagnosis and prognosis?
10. Can members identify areas of dysfunction within the family?
11. If the client has a homosexual lover, has any conflict been resolved?
12. Have caregiving responsibilities been defined and distributed in a manner acceptable to all?
13. Have the parents worked through feelings of guilt and shame?
14. Are the client and family/significant other(s) able to verbalize educational information presented regarding ways in which HIV can and cannot be transmitted, ways to protect the client from infections, and ways to prevent transmission to caregivers and others?
15. Can the client and family/significant other(s) identify resources within the community from which they may seek support and assistance (e.g., AIDS support groups, home care, respite care, hospice, financial support)?

TABLE 39–4	Topics for Client/Family Education Related to HIV Disease

Nature of the Illness

1. What is HIV infection?
2. What is AIDS?
3. How can you find out if you have it?
4. Discuss usual progression of the illness:
   a. Time dimensions
   b. Symptoms associated with various stages
   c. Associated medical conditions

Management of the Illness

1. Discuss methods of transmission:
   a. Sexually
   b. Bloodborne
   c. Perinatal
   d. Ways to prevent transmission of the virus to others:
      (1) Safer sex
      (2) Don't share needles.
      (3) Prevent pregnancy.
      (4) Don't breastfeed.
2. Dispel myths regarding transmission.
3. Provide guidelines to caregivers for preventing transmission of HIV during home care.
4. Discuss ways to prevent transmission of infections to the individual with HIV infection.
5. Provide guidelines for when to seek medical assistance.
6. Discuss opportunistic infections.
7. Discuss treatment modalities and medication:
   a. Reverse transcriptase inhibitors
   b. Protease inhibitors
   c. Medications for opportunistic infections
   d. Antianxiety agents
   e. Antidepressants
   f. Mood stabilizing agents
   g. Antipsychotics
8. Discuss legal issues.
9. Discuss financial issues.
10. Discuss psychological and social issues.

Support Services

1. Support groups
2. Individual psychotherapy
3. CDC AIDS hotline number: 1-800-342-AIDS
4. HIV-Associated Dementia Hotline: Project Inform: 1-800-822-7422

TREATMENT MODALITIES

Pharmacology

Antiretroviral Therapy

The first antiretroviral agent approved by the FDA in the treatment of HIV infection was zidovudine (azidothymidine [AZT]). Marketed under the trade name of Retrovir, it was initially prescribed for clients with severe symptomatic HIV disease (<200 T4 cells). More recent data, however, justify treating clients who have fewer than 500 T4 cells. Zidovudine belongs to the classification of drugs known as *nucleoside reverse transcriptase inhibitors* (NRTIs).

Since the approval of zidovudine by the FDA, a number of other NRTIs have been approved in the treatment of HIV infection. Some of these include didanosine [ddI] (Videx), lamivudine [3TC] (Epivir), stavudine [d4T] (Zerit), and abacavir [ABC] (Ziagen).

A second classification of antiretroviral drugs is the *non-nucleoside reverse transcriptase inhibitors* (NNRTIs). Examples of NNRTIs include delavirdine [DLV] (Rescriptor), nevirapine [NVP] (Viramune), and efavirenz [EFP] (Sustiva). Both NRTIs and NNRTIs work (albeit in different ways) by disabling the HIV reproductive enzyme called *reverse transcriptase*. In doing so, viral replication inside the host cell is inhibited.

Another class of antiretrovirals, called *protease inhibitors* (PIs), are also being used by some individuals with HIV disease. Protease inhibitors, examples of which include saquinavir (Fortovase), indinavir (Crixivan), nelfinavir (Viracept), ritonavir (Norvir), and amprenavir (Agenerase), prevent or slow down the action of an HIV enzyme, called *protease*, which is needed by the HIV to break down proteins for replication. Protease inhibitors have been very effective in increasing T4 cell counts and decreasing viral load within the blood.

For individuals who have become resistant to NRTIs, NNRTIs, and PIs, there is an additional classification called entry inhibitors. Entry inhibitors work by preventing HIV from entering healthy T cells in the body. Only one entry inhibitor, enfuvirtide (Fuzeon), has currently been approved by the FDA. Enfuvirtide is a fusion inhibitor that attaches to the gp41 protein on the HIV surface preventing viral entry into the host cell. Other entry inhibitors that target proteins on host cells are currently under investigation.

Single drug therapy is no longer the treatment of choice. Triple drug therapy with two nucleosides and one protease inhibitor is the most potent antiretroviral treatment available (Sadock & Sadock, 2003). The term *highly active antiretroviral therapy* (HAART) is used to describe a combination of three or more antiretroviral medications used to treat HIV. Resistance readily develops to monotherapy, but it has been found that if two or more antiretrovirals are taken together, the rate at which resistance develops is vastly reduced.

When to initiate antiretroviral therapy remains controversial. Available data continue to support the practice of not starting therapy for asymptomatic individuals who have T4 cell counts above 350 mm³, and consideration for initiating antiretroviral therapy below this point, but before the count drops to 200 mm³ (Saag, 2004). Initiation of therapy is considered earlier when symptoms are apparent. Considerations in delaying treatment are related to long-term toxicity of the drugs and client quality of life.

Other Chemotherapeutic Agents

Various other drugs are used in individuals with HIV to treat the opportunistic infections and malignancies associated with the disease. Some examples include antibiotics, antifungal agents, antiviral agents, and antineoplastic agents. Hare (2004) states:

Many commonly encountered opportunistic infections may be prevented by administering prophylactic antibiotics to those at risk. In general, secondary prophylaxis (treatment to prevent recurrence of an opportunistic infection) should be provided as long as immune impairment persists. Among individuals who experience reconstitution of immunologic function with antiretroviral therapy, as assessed by sustained increases in T4 count to levels above those associated with opportunistic infections, discontinuation of primary prophylaxis or secondary prophylaxis has been shown to be safe.

The U.S. Food and Drug Administration has approved a number of medications for the prophylaxis and treatment of AIDS-related illnesses. Some of these include fluconazole (treatment of candidiasis and cryptococcal meningitis); foscarnet (treatment of cytomegalovirus retinitis); rifabutin (prophylaxis for *Mycobacterium avium* complex); trimethoprim/sulfamethoxazole (prophylaxis for *Pneumocystis carinii* pneumonia); and famvir (treatment of herpes simplex infections). Some studies have indicated that zidovudine may be helpful in slowing or preventing the symptoms of HIV-associated dementia (McDaniel et al., 2002; Sadock & Sadock, 2003).

Psychotropic Medications

Antianxiety Agents. Benzodiazepines, such as alprazolam, oxazepam or lorazepam, are often prescribed for relief of anxiety in clients with HIV disease. Interaction of the benzodiazepines with antiretroviral agents may require adjustment in dosage. Buspirone (BuSpar) may be useful in the management of chronic anxiety symptoms, although it takes from 2 to 3 weeks for it to become effective as an anxiolytic. No reports of HIV-related drug-drug interactions with buspirone have been noted (McDaniel, 2002).

Antidepressants. The tricyclic antidepressants and selective serotonin reuptake inhibitors (SSRIs) may be used for relief of depression in clients with HIV disease. The SSRIs may be selected because of their minimal anticholinergic side effects, a benefit for HIV clients who suffer from excessive dryness of the mouth. They are also less sedating than the tricyclics. Their main disadvantages are that initially they may produce a stimulant effect that may aggravate anxiety in HIV clients and that they tend to cause sexual dysfunction. Drug-drug interaction with the protease inhibitors needs to be considered when prescribing these antidepressants for individuals with HIV disease.

Monoamine oxidase inhibitors (MAOIs), although highly effective antidepressants, may be a risky choice for HIV-infected clients with cognitive defects because of the diet and concomitant medication restrictions required with administration of these drugs. Stimulants, such as methylphenidate (Ritalin) and amphetamine, may also be useful in HIV clients with neurocognitive impairment, fatigue, and to a lesser extent, in some clients with depression (McDaniel et al., 2002). They are generally considered safe with no reports of interactions with antiretroviral agents, but should be avoided or used with caution in clients with a history of amphetamine abuse.

Mood Stabilizers. Lithium has been the drug of choice for manic symptoms. However, lithium therapy poses potential problems for clients with HIV disease. Lithium toxicity is particularly risky with these clients because of altered renal function, dehydration, vomiting, and diarrhea. If the manic behavior can be attributable to a medication being administered to the client, the medication should be decreased or stopped as soon as is medically feasible. Carbamazepine (Tegretol) and valproic acid (Depakote) have been used successfully to stabilize mood in clients with HIV-associated mania.

Antipsychotics. Psychotic symptoms are often seen in the client with HIV disease who experiences delirium. Certain medications administered for HIV-related problems may also result in psychosis. McDaniel and associates (2002) state:

> For all antipsychotic agents, the possibility of drug-drug interactions must be considered for those patients also taking antiretroviral medication. Antipsychotic dosage adjustment may be required to minimize side effects such as extrapyramidal side effects. Because of the rare dose-related side effect of agranulocytosis among patients taking clozapine, this particular agent should be monitored closely if given to any HIV patient. Likewise, clinicians should monitor for risk of seizures if clozapine is administered with ritonavir, since ritonavir inhibits the cytochrome P450 isoenzyme 2D6, clozapine's primary metabolic pathway. Depot antipsychotic medication should be avoided in advanced HIV disease. (p. 197)

Universal Isolation Precautions*

In January 1996, the Centers for Disease Control and Prevention (CDC) issued new guidelines for isolation precautions in hospitals. The guidelines, based on the latest epidemiologic information on transmission of infection in hospitals, are intended primarily for use in acute-care hospitals, although some of the recommendations may be applicable to subacute-care or extended-care facilities. The recommendations are not intended for use in day care, well care, or domiciliary care programs.

The revised guidelines contain two tiers of precautions. In the first tier are those precautions designed for the care of all patients in hospitals regardless of their diagnosis or presumed infection status. Implementation of these "Standard Precautions" is the primary strategy for successful nosocomial infection control. In the second tier are precautions designed only for the care of specified patients. These additional "Transmission-Based

---

*This section is reprinted from *Taber's Cyclopedic Medical Dictionary* (20th ed.). (2005). Philadelphia: F.A. Davis. With permission.

Precautions" are used for patients known or suspected to be infected or colonized with epidemiologically important pathogens that can be transmitted by airborne or droplet transmission or by contact with dry skin or contaminated surfaces.

Standard Precautions synthesize the major features of Universal (Blood and Body Fluid) Precaution (designed to reduce the risk of transmission of pathogens from moist body substances). Standard Precautions apply to (1) blood; (2) all body fluids, secretions, and excretions *except sweat*, regardless of whether they contain visible blood; (3) nonintact skin; and (4) mucous membranes. Standard Precautions are designed to reduce the risk of transmission of both recognized and unrecognized sources of infection in hospitals.

Transmission-Based Precautions are designed for patients documented or suspected to be infected or colonized with highly transmissible or epidemiologically important pathogens for which additional precautions beyond Standard Precautions are needed to interrupt transmission in hospitals. There are three types of Transmission-Based Precautions: *Airborne Precautions, Droplet Precautions, and Contact Precautions.* They may be combined for diseases that have multiple routes of transmission. When used either singly or in combination, they are to be used in addition to Standard Precautions. (**Author's Note:** Knowledge of Transmission-Based Precautions is important in caring for clients with opportunistic infections associated with HIV disease.)

Standard Precautions

The following Standard Precautions, or the equivalent, should be used for the care of all patients.

● **Handwashing**
1. Wash hands after touching blood, body fluids, secretions, excretions, and contaminated items, whether or not gloves are worn. Wash hands immediately after gloves are removed, between patient contacts, and when otherwise indicated to avoid transfer of microorganisms to other patients or environments. It may be necessary to wash hands between tasks and procedures on the same patient to prevent cross-contamination of different body sites.
2. Use a plain (nonantimicrobial) soap for routine handwashing.
3. Use an antimicrobial agent or a waterless antiseptic agent for specific circumstances (e.g., control of outbreaks or hyperendemic infections), as defined by the infection control program.

● **Gloves:** Wear gloves (clean, nonsterile gloves are adequate) when touching blood, body fluids, secretions, excretions, and contaminated items. Put on clean gloves just before touching mucous membranes and

nonintact skin. Change gloves between tasks and procedures on the same patient after contact with material that may contain a high concentration of microorganisms. Remove gloves promptly after use, before touching noncontaminated items and environmental surfaces, and before going to another patient, and wash hands immediately to avoid transfer of microorganisms to other patients or environments.

● **Mask, Eye Protection, Face Shield:** Wear a mask and eye protection or a face shield to protect mucous membranes of the eyes, nose, and mouth during procedures and patient-care activities that are likely to generate splashes or sprays of blood, body fluids, secretions, and excretions.

● **Gown:** Wear a gown (a clean, nonsterile gown is adequate) to protect skin and to prevent soiling of clothing during procedures and patient-care activities that are likely to generate splashes or sprays of blood, body fluids, secretions, or excretions. Select a gown that is appropriate for the activity and amount of fluid likely to be encountered. Remove a soiled gown as promptly as possible, and wash hands to avoid transfer of microorganisms to other patients or environments.

● **Patient-Care Equipment:** Handle used patient-care equipment soiled with blood, body fluids, secretions, and excretions in a manner that prevents skin and mucous membrane exposures, contamination of clothing, and transfer of microorganisms to other patients and environments. Ensure that reusable equipment is not used for the care of another patient until it has been cleaned and reprocessed appropriately. Ensure that single-use items are discarded properly.

● **Environmental Control:** Ensure that the hospital has adequate procedures for the routine care, cleaning, and disinfection of environmental surfaces, beds, bedrails, bedside equipment, and other frequently touched surfaces, and ensure that these procedures are being followed.

● **Linen:** Handle, transport and process used linen soiled with blood, body fluids, secretions, and excretions in a manner that prevents skin and mucous membrane exposures and contamination of clothing, and that avoids transfer of microorganisms to other patients and environments.

● **Occupational Health and Bloodborne Pathogens:**
1. Take care to prevent injuries when using needles, scalpels, and other sharp instruments or devices; when handling sharp instruments after procedures; when cleaning used instruments; and when disposing of used needles. Never recap used needles, or otherwise manipulate them using both hands, or use any other technique that involves directing the point of a needle toward any part of the body; rather, use either a one-handed "scoop" technique or a mechanical device designed for holding the needle sheath. Do not remove used needles from

disposable syringes by hand, and do not bend, break, or otherwise manipulate used needle by hand. Place used disposable syringes and needles, scalpel blades, and other sharp items in appropriate puncture-resistant containers, which are located as close as practical to the area in which the items were used, and place reusable syringes and needles in a puncture-resistant container for transport to the reprocessing area.

2. Use mouthpieces, resuscitation bags, or other ventilation devices as an alternative to mouth-to-mouth resuscitation methods in areas where the need for resuscitation is predictable.

● **Patient Placement:** Place a patient who contaminates the environment or who does not (or cannot be expected to) assist in maintaining appropriate hygiene or environmental control in a private room. If a private room is not available, consult with infection control professionals regarding patient placement or other alternatives.

Hospice Care

Hospice is a program that provides palliative and supportive care to meet the special needs of people who are dying and their families. Hospice care provides physical, psychological, spiritual, and social care for the person for whom aggressive treatment is no longer appropriate or desired. Various models of hospice exist, including freestanding institutions that provide both inpatient and home care; those affiliated with hospitals in which hospice services are provided within the hospital setting; and hospice organizations that provide home care only. Historically, the hospice movement in the United States has evolved mainly as a system of home-based care.

Hospice helps clients achieve physical and emotional comfort so that they can concentrate on living life as fully as possible. Clients are urged to stay active for as long as they are able—to take part in activities they enjoy, and to focus on the quality of life. (Please see Chapter 45 for a detailed description of hospice care.)

Incorporating HIV Prevention in the Medical Care of Persons Living with HIV

Indications are that the optimism caused by effective AIDS drugs may be eroding safer sex practices and leading to increased sexual risk-taking by some individuals (Shewmaker, 2004). In 2003, the CDC provided guidelines for health care professionals to help HIV-positive individuals practice safer sex behaviors consistently. The recommendations were developed by using an evidence-based approach and are categorized into three major

components: (1) risk screening, (2) behavioral interventions, and (3) partner counseling and referral services, including partner notification (CDC, 2003b).

Risk Screening

This step involves assessment of HIV-positive clients' behavioral risk factors for HIV transmission, and testing for the presence of other STDs. The CDC suggests that this assessment can be achieved with a self-administered questionnaire; a computer-, audio-, or video-assisted questionnaire; or a brief interview with the clinician. Any indication of high-risk behavior from this initial assessment should launch a more in-depth discussion of the risks associated with HIV transmission. Initial screening for pregnancy should be accomplished in this stage, as well.

Laboratory testing and assessment of physical signs and symptoms associated with other STDs should be performed. Compliance with state reporting requirements must be considered.

Behavioral Interventions

Behavioral interventions are strategies designed to change knowledge, attitudes, behaviors, or practices to reduce personal health risks or the risk of transmitting HIV to others (CDC, 2003b). Health care environments can be structured to support and enhance prevention. Providing information about HIV transmission risks and how to prevent transmission of HIV and other STDs should be a basic part of this approach. Condoms could be made readily accessible at the health care site, along with education about the importance of their use.

Discussion should include information about the client's responsibility for disclosure of HIV serostatus to sex and needle-sharing partners. Education about HIV transmission with specific sexual behaviors and the effect of antiretroviral therapy on HIV transmission should be included. These prevention messages should be ongoing and reinforced at all clinical visits. Referrals for other types of services identified in the needs assessment should be made.

Partner Counseling and Referral Services, Including Partner Notification

This part of the prevention service involves informing current partners (and past partners who may have been exposed) that a person who is HIV infected has identified them as a sex or needle-sharing partner and advising them to have HIV counseling and testing (CDC, 2003b). Some states have laws requiring health care workers to report to individuals known to be at risk for HIV transmission from clients known to be infected (i.e., duty to warn). Partners can be informed of their exposure by health department staff, clinicians in the private sector, or the individual with HIV disease (CDC, 2003b).

Incorporating these guidelines into practice could contribute significantly toward reducing risk behaviors associated with HIV transmission. Nurses in the hospital and in the community are in a prime position for initiating these interventions into clinical practice.

SUMMARY

AIDS is likely to be one of this century's major killers. The disease is the terminal end of a continuum of syndromes identified by HIV infection. The continuum begins with the acute response that occurs when the individual is initially infected with the virus, and progresses to a period of asymptomatic infection that may last for as long as 10 years. Advanced stages of the disease present with lymphadenopathy, neurological involvement, opportunistic infections, HIV wasting syndrome, malignancies, and finally death.

The HIV invades the T4 cells (normal range 600/mm^3 to 1200/mm^3) until in the very advanced stage of the disease the individual may be almost depleted of these protective cells. Examples of opportunistic infections that attack the body of an individual with AIDS include *Pneumocystis carinii* pneumonia (PCP), candidiasis, cytomegalovirus (CMV), herpes, *M. tuberculosis*, and toxoplasmosis. Many of these were rarely observed before the AIDS epidemic. Common malignancies associated with AIDS include Kaposi's sarcoma (KS) and non-Hodgkin's lymphoma. Any infectious or other disease process can prove fatal to an individual with AIDS whose immune system is severely depressed.

Approximately 20 to 30 percent of AIDS clients develop HIV-associated dementia, which is thought to be the most common CNS complication of HIV infection. Cognitive, motor, and behavioral processes are affected to a point when the individual may become totally vegetative. Psychiatric syndromes commonly associated with HIV infection include depression, anxiety, mania, and psychosis.

Transmission of HIV infection is via three major routes: sexual, bloodborne, and perinatal. Sexual transmission can occur through any activity in which there is an exchange of body fluids with an infected individual. Although most sexual transmission in the past has occurred within the homosexual population, increasing numbers of cases are occurring from heterosexual contact. Bloodborne transmission can occur when an individual is transfused with blood or blood products that have been contaminated with HIV. Other modes of bloodborne transmission include the sharing of contaminated needles by IV drug users and accidental sticks with contaminated needles by health care workers. Perinatal transmission occurs in infants born to HIV-infected women through exposure to maternal blood and vaginal secretions during delivery. It can also occur transplacentally and through infant feeding with breast milk.

This chapter discussed delivery of care to the client with HIV disease via the steps of the nursing process. Background assessment data included a description of the predisposing factors as well as symptomatology associated with various aspects of the disease. Nursing diagnoses and a plan of care for the client with HIV disease were presented, along with outcome criteria and guidelines for evaluation of nursing care. Other treatment modalities including pharmacology, universal isolation precautions, hospice care, and guidelines for prevention of transmission were discussed.

REVIEW QUESTIONS

SELF-EXAMINATION/LEARNING EXERCISE

Select the answer that is *most* appropriate for the questions that follow this situation.

Situation: Joe is a 34-year-old homosexual man. He and his partner were both tested and found to be HIV positive 8 years ago. His partner died 2 years ago. Joe had taken care of him until his death. Joe has seen his primary physician, who is admitting him to the hospital with a loss of 15 pounds in the past 2 weeks, fever, night sweats, persistent diarrhea, and enlarged cervical, axillary, and inguinal lymph nodes. His laboratory T4 count is 400/mm^3. Oral candidiasis (thrush) is evident upon examination. This is his third hospitalization in 15 months. He previously had a diagnosis of persistent generalized lymphadenopathy.

1. During the initial nursing assessment, Joe says to the nurse, "I didn't mention it to my doctor, but I found this spot on my foot yesterday that I hadn't noticed before. It doesn't hurt or anything." Upon inspection, the nurse observes a small, bluish spot that is slightly raised on the sole of Joe's foot. Taking note of this symptom, of what might the nurse be concerned?
   a. Herpes simplex
   b. Candidiasis
   c. Herpes zoster
   d. Kaposi's sarcoma

2. Oral candidiasis presents with which of the following symptoms?
   a. Bleeding gums
   b. Dry, cracking lips
   c. White patches on the oral mucosa
   d. Blisters on the tongue

3. What type of organism is *Candida*?
   a. Fungus
   b. Protozoan
   c. Bacterium
   d. Virus

4. Joe's physician prescribed the antiviral agent zidovudine for him 5 years ago. What is the rationale behind administration of this medication?
   a. It cures HIV infection.
   b. It prevents the HIV-infected person from getting other viruses.
   c. It slows down the progression from HIV infection to full-blown AIDS.
   d. It prevents entry of HIV into the CNS.

5. In providing nursing care for Joe, which of the following interventions would be most appropriate for preventing transmission to the caregiver?
   a. Wear a gown to carry in Joe's food tray.
   b. Do not recap Joe's medication injection needles.
   c. Wear a mask when changing the linen on Joe's bed.
   d. Wear gloves to change the bag on Joe's continuous IV fluids.

6. Which of the following interventions would be most appropriate for prevention of infection to Joe?
   a. Allow only one staff person to provide care for Joe.
   b. Place Joe in protective isolation.
   c. Put a "no visitors" sign on Joe's door.
   d. Wash hands before entering Joe's room.

7. Joe is discharged from the hospital after 2 weeks. Which of the following would be appropriate to teach Joe and his caregivers?
   a. Joe should cook all vegetables and fruits before eating them.
   b. Joe should abstain from all sexual activities.
   c. Joe should refrain from exercising because of weakness and fatigue.
   d. Joe should not kiss anyone on the mouth.

8. Fourteen months later Joe is readmitted. He has lost a great deal more weight. He is unable to take nourishment by mouth and has apparent difficulty breathing. He has a dry, nonproductive cough, and a fever of 101.2°F. The physician diagnoses PCP. PCP is an example of:
   a. An opportunistic infection.
   b. A hospital-acquired infection.
   c. An infection acquired due to lack of immunization.
   d. A hypersensitivity reaction to a medication Joe has been taking for his AIDS.

9. Joe's condition continues to deteriorate and he is transferred to hospice care. The primary goal of hospice care is:
   a. To assist with legal and financial problems of long-term care and dying.
   b. To provide quality of life for the terminally ill person until death occurs.
   c. To assist family and significant others through their loved one's dying process.
   d. To fulfill the emotional and spiritual needs of the client and family and/or significant others.

10. Which of the following medications might be helpful in slowing down the progression of symptoms in HIV-associated dementia?
    a. Haloperidol
    b. Zidovudine
    c. Carbamazepine
    d. Alprazolam

TEST YOUR CRITICAL THINKING SKILLS

George, a 37-year-old man, presents himself to his physician complaining of fever, sore throat, anorexia, and fatigue. These symptoms have persisted for about 3 weeks. George says, "I've had these flu symptoms, but they just don't seem to go away."

George is a professional writer and has had two of his novels published. He is gay and has been in a monogamous relationship for 9 years. He and his partner, Steve, both were found to be negative for HIV in tests they took 6 years ago. George confides to the physician that one night about 2 months ago after an argument with Steve, he left the apartment angry, went to a bar, and met a man with whom he had an unprotected sexual encounter. The next day, he and Steve resumed their relationship and he never saw the man from the bar again.

A lab test reveals that George is HIV-positive. The acute symptoms disappear, and George has no further symptoms of the illness. However, George is devastated by the diagnosis and begins experiencing symptoms of anxiety and depression. He becomes preoccupied with dying. He cannot sleep without having nightmares about dying. He cannot eat, and continues to lose weight. He cannot write, and refuses to see anyone.

Steve tests negative for HIV at this time. George has moved out of their apartment and has rented a room for himself. Steve goes to see him every day. George is obsessed with reading everything he can find about AIDS, but panics when he hears about people he knows dying of the disease. He has become nonfunctional and just sits and stares out his window. Steve talks him into seeing a psychiatrist who hospitalizes George with a diagnosis of Adjustment Disorder with Mixed Anxiety and Depressed Mood.

Answer the following questions related to George:

1. Describe priority information the nurse must gather during the intake assessment interview.
2. List the two priority nursing diagnoses for George.
3. Identify three important nursing interventions in working with George.

IMPLICATIONS OF RESEARCH FOR EVIDENCE-BASED PRACTICE

Brown, E.J., & Jemmott, L.S. (2000). HIV among people with mental illness: Contributing factors, prevention needs, barriers, and strategies. *Journal of Psychosocial Nursing, 38*(4), 14–19.

Description of the Study: The purpose of this study was to improve the understanding of HIV-related contributing factors, prevention needs, barriers to prevention, and prevention strategies among people with mental illness (PWMI) by conducting an extensive review of the literature and by interviewing key informants. Database searches were conducted revealing 28 articles pertaining to HIV/AIDS among PWMI. These articles were analyzed by examining 4 content areas: contributing factors associated with the development of HIV; HIV prevention needs; HIV prevention intervention strategies; and barriers to the implementation of HIV prevention intervention strategies for PWMI. Key informants were interviewed and asked the following questions: "What factors contribute to PWMI acquiring HIV?", "What are the HIV prevention needs of PWMI?", "Which HIV prevention strategies could be used with PWMI to help meet the needs that you identified?", and "What barriers prevent the implementation of these strategies in your agency or similar agencies?"

Results of the Study: Several factors were found to contribute to the incidence and prevalence of HIV among PWMI: PWMI are sexually active, although they are often perceived by mental health professionals as not sexually active; women with chronic mental illness were found to be more sexually active than their male counterparts; knowledge deficits among PWMI concerning risk of HIV/AIDS and measures to prevent contracting HIV. Cognitive deficits, lack of impulse control, co-morbid alcohol and drug abuse, and increased vulnerability to sexual abuse were also seen as risk factors. Information from key informants supported findings from the literature. Identified prevention needs of PWMI included HIV prevention intervention programs, HIV testing and counseling, and STD prevention screening and treatment services. Barriers to these programs that were identified included the lack of cognitive ability among PWMI to integrate HIV prevention information into their behavior because of their impaired psychosocial functioning. Other barriers identified included mental health care professionals' denial of sexual activity on the part of PWMI and inadequate integration of HIV intervention services into mental health programs.

Implications for Nursing Practice: The following nursing strategies for prevention of HIV in PWMI were suggested: (1) health education and risk reduction strategies for prevention, skill building activity, negotiation, counseling, and support, with information related to sexual coercion and provision of condoms; (2) institutionally based health education and risk reduction strategies within partial day programs, residential programs, long term acute care, etc.; (3) HIV counseling and testing, including personal risk assessment, education about prevention strategies and transmission of HIV, and encouragement for future testing if risk behavior continues; (4) prevention case management for those PWMI who are not connected to comprehensive programs and services; and (5) education of mental health care professionals regarding the susceptibility of PWMI to acquisition and transmission of HIV. Mental health professionals need to be sensitized to the specialized needs of PWMI so that appropriate HIV preventive strategies can be provided. The authors suggest that "nurses, due to their close interaction with PWMI, are in key positions to document HIV risk-related behaviors and to advocate for integrating HIV risk reduction strategies into the therapeutic milieu."

 INTERNET REFERENCES

Additional information about HIV/AIDS may be located at the following Web sites:

- http://www.avert.org/
- http://www.aegis.com/main/
- http://www.critpath.org/
- http://www.HIVpositive.com/index.html
- http://research.med.umkc.edu/teams/cml/AIDS.html
- http://www.cdc.gov/hiv
- http://hivinsite.ucsf.edu/InSite?page=KB
- http://www.cdc.gov/mmwr/preview/mmwrhtml/rr5212a1.htm

REFERENCES

American Academy of Family Physicians (AAFP). (2001). *HIV, pregnancy, and AZT.* Retrieved April 19, 2002 from http://familydoctor.org/handouts/093.html

Blair, M. (2005). Management of clients with acquired immunodeficiency syndrome. In J.M. Black & J.H. Hawks (Eds.). *Medical-surgical nursing: Clinical management for positive outcomes* (7th ed.). St. Louis: W.B. Saunders.

Centers for Disease Control and Prevention (CDC). (2003a). *HIV and its transmission.* Retrieved May 18, 2005 from the World Wide Web at http://www.cdc.gov/hiv/pubs/facts/transmission.htm

Centers for Disease Control and Prevention (CDC). (2003b). Incorporating HIV prevention into the medical care of persons living with HIV. *Morbidity and Mortality Weekly Report, 52*(12), 1–24.

Centers for Disease Control and Prevention (CDC). (2004). *HIV/AIDS surveillance report* (Vol. 15). Atlanta, GA: CDC.

Fondere, J., Huguet, M., Yssel, H., Baillat, V., Reynes, J., van de Perre, P., & Vendrell, J. (2003). Detection of peripheral HIV-1-specific memory B cells in patients untreated or receiving highly active antiretroviral therapy. *AIDS, 17*(16), 2323–2330.

Fredriksson, J., & Kanabus, A. (2004). HIV & AIDS: Stigma and discrimination. Retrieved May 19, 2005 from the World Wide Web at http://www.avert.org/aidsstigma.htm

Hare, C.B. (2004). Clinical overview of HIV disease. HIV InSite knowledge base chapter. Retrieved May 17, 2005 from http://hivinsite.ucsf.edu/InSite.jsp?page=kb-03-01-01

Kaiser Family Foundation. (2004). *The HIV/AIDS epidemic in the*

United States. Retrieved May 17, 2005 from the World Wide Web at http://www.kff.org

Kanabus, A., & Fredriksson, J. (2005). *The history of AIDS: 1981–1986.* AVERT. Retrieved May 17, 2005 from the World Wide Web at http://www.avert.org/his81_86.htm

Kanabus, A., & Pennington, J. (2005). *Preventing mother-to-child transmission of HIV.* Retrieved May 18, 2005 from the World Wide Web at http://www.avert.org/motherchild.htm

Kaplan, L.D. (1998). *Clinical presentation and management of HIV-associated lymphoma.* University of California San Francisco. Retrieved April 19, 2002 from http://hivinsite.ucsf.edu/InSite.jsp?page=kb-06&doc=kb-06-03-02

Krown, S.E. (2003). *Clinical characteristics of Kaposi's sarcoma.* University of California at San Francisco. Retrieved May 19, 2005 from http://hivinsite.ucsf.edu/InSite.jsp?page=kb-06-02-03

McArthur, J. (2002). *The Geneva Report: Update on neurology.* The Johns Hopkins University, Division of Infectious Diseases and AIDS Service. Retrieved April 19, 2002 from the World Wide Web at http://www.hopkins-aids.edu/geneva/hilites_mcar_dem.html

McDaniel, J.S., Brown, L., Cournos, F., Forstein, M., Goodkin, K., Lyketsos, C., & Chung, J.Y. (2002). Practice guideline for the treatment of patients with HIV/AIDS. In *American Psychiatric Association practice guidelines for the treatment of psychiatric disorders: Compendium 2002.* Washington, DC: American Psychiatric Publishing.

New Mexico AIDS InfoNet. (2005). *T-cell tests.* Retrieved May 17, 2005 from the World Wide Web at http://www.aidsinfonet.org

Noble, R. (2004). *Introduction to HIV types, groups, and subtypes.*

AVERT. Retrieved May 17, 2005 from the World Wide Web at http://www.avert.org/hivtypes.htm

Remien, R.H., & Rabkin, J.G. (2001). Psychological aspects of living with HIV disease. *Western Journal of Medicine, 175*(5), 332–335.

Saag, M.S. (2004). Initiation of antiretroviral therapy: Implications of recent findings. *Topics in HIV Medicine, 12*(3), 83–88.

Sadock, B.J., & Sadock, V.A. (2003). *Synopsis of psychiatry: Behavioral sciences/clinical psychiatry* (9th ed.). Philadelphia: Lippincott Williams & Wilkins.

Sahai-Srivastava, S., & Jones, B. (2004). *Dementia due to HIV disease.* Retrieved May 19, 2005 from the World Wide Web at http://www.emedicine.com/med/topic3151.htm

Scanlon, V.C., & Sanders, T. (2003). *Essentials of anatomy and physiology* (4th ed.). Philadelphia: F.A. Davis.

Shewmaker, S.Z. (2004, November/December). A new prescription for HIV prevention. *The American Nurse, 36*(6), 15.

Smith, G.B. (2003). Nursing care of patients with HIV disease and AIDS. In L.S. Williams & P.D. Hopper (Eds.). *Understanding medical surgical nursing* (2nd ed.). Philadelphia: F.A. Davis.

Yahya, S., Garewal, M., & Thomas, F.P. (2005). HIV-1 encephalopathy and AIDS dementia complex. Retrieved May 19, 2005 from the World Wide Web at http://www.emedicine.com/NEURO/topic447.htm

United Nations Joint Programme on HIV/AIDS (UNAIDS) and World Health Organization (WHO). (2004). *AIDS epidemic update—December 2004.* Retrieved May 17, 2005 from the World Wide Web at http://www.unaids.org/wad2004/report_pdf.html

Viera, A.J., Bond, M.M., & Yates, S.W. (2003). Diagnosing night sweats. *American Family Physician, 67*(5), 1019–1024.

40
CHAPTER

PROBLEMS RELATED TO ABUSE OR NEGLECT

CHAPTER OUTLINE

OBJECTIVES
HISTORICAL PERSPECTIVES
PREDISPOSING FACTORS
APPLICATION OF THE NURSING PROCESS

TREATMENT MODALITIES
SUMMARY
REVIEW QUESTIONS

KEY TERMS

child sexual abuse
compounded rape
    reaction
controlled response
    pattern
cycle of battering
date rape
emotional abuse
emotional neglect

expressed response
    pattern
marital rape
physical neglect
safe house or shelter
sexual exploitation
    of a child
silent rape reaction
statutory rape

CORE CONCEPTS

abuse
battering
incest
neglect
rape

OBJECTIVES

After reading this chapter, the student will be able to:

1. Discuss historical perspectives associated with intimate partner abuse, child abuse, and sexual assault.
2. Describe epidemiological statistics associated with intimate partner abuse, child abuse, and sexual assault.
3. Discuss characteristics of victims and victimizers.
4. Identify predisposing factors to abusive behaviors.
5. Describe physical and psychological effects

on the victims of intimate partner abuse, child abuse, and sexual assault.
6. Identify nursing diagnoses, goals of care, and appropriate nursing interventions for care of victims of intimate partner abuse, child abuse, and sexual assault.
7. Evaluate nursing care of victims of intimate partner abuse, child abuse, and sexual assault.
8. Discuss various modalities relevant to treatment of victims of abuse.

 buse is on the rise in this society. Books, newspapers, movies, and television inundate their readers and viewers with stories of "man's inhumanity to man" (no gender bias intended).

Nearly 5.3 million intimate partner victimizations occur each year among United States women ages 18 and older (Centers for Disease Control and Prevention [CDC], 2003). More injuries are attributed to intimate partner violence than to all rapes, muggings, and auto-

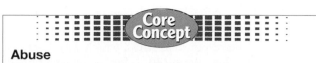

Core Concept

Abuse
The maltreatment of one person by another.

mobile accidents combined. Rape is vastly underreported in the United States. Because many of these attacks occurring daily go unreported and unrecognized, sexual assault can be considered a silent-violent epidemic in the United States today.

An increase in the incidence of child abuse and related fatalities has also been documented. In 2003, an estimated 2.9 million cases of possible child abuse or neglect were reported to child protective services, and about 906,000 of these cases were substantiated (U.S. Department of Health and Human Services [USDHHS], 2005). About 1,500 children died from causes related to abuse or neglect in 2003.

Abuse affects all populations equally. It occurs among all races, religions, economic classes, ages, and educational backgrounds. The phenomenon is cyclical in that many abusers were themselves victims of abuse as children.

This chapter discusses intimate partner violence, child abuse (including neglect), and sexual assault. Elder abuse is discussed in Chapter 38. Factors that predispose individuals to commit acts of abuse against others, as well as the physical and psychological effects on the victims, are examined.

Nursing of individuals who have experienced abusive behavior from others is presented within the context of the nursing process. Various treatment modalities are described.

HISTORICAL PERSPECTIVES

Family violence is not a new problem; in fact, it is probably as old as humankind and has been documented as far back as Biblical times. In the United States, spouse and child abuse arrived with the Puritans; however, it was not until 1973 that public outrage initiated an active movement against the practice. Child abuse became a mandatory reportable occurrence in the United States in 1968. Responsibility for the protection of elders from abuse rests primarily with the states. In 1987, Congress passed amendments to the Older Americans Act of 1965 that provide for state Area Agencies on Aging to assess the need for elder abuse prevention services. These events have made it possible for individuals who once felt powerless to stop the abuse against them, to come forward and seek advice, support, and protection.

Historically, violence against female partners (whether in a married or an unmarried intimate relationship) has not been considered a social problem but rather a fact of

life. Some individuals have been socialized within their cultural context to accept violence against women in relationships (American Nurses Association [ANA], 1998).

From Roman times until the beginning of the 20th century, women were considered the personal property of men. Very early on in Roman times, women were purchased as brides, and their status, as well as that of their children, was closely akin to that of slaves. Violent beatings and even death occurred if women acted contrary to their husbands' wishes or to the social code of the time.

Women historically have been socialized to view themselves as sexual objects. In early Biblical times, women were expected to subjugate themselves to the will of men, and those who refused were often severely punished. Rape is largely a crime against women, although men and children also fall victim to this heinous act. Rape is the extreme manifestation of the domination of one individual over another. Rape is viewed as a ritual of power.

During the Puritan era, "spare the rod and spoil the child" was a theme supported by the Bible. Children were considered the property of their parents and could be treated accordingly. Harsh treatment by parents was justified by the belief that severe physical punishment was necessary to maintain discipline, transmit educational decisions, and expel evil spirits. Change began in the mid-19th and early 20th centuries with the child welfare movement and the passage of laws for the protection of children.

Historical examination reveals an inclination toward violence among human beings from very early in civilization. Little has changed, for violence permeates every aspect of today's society, the victims of which are inundating the health care system. Aside from the personal physical, psychological, and social devastation that violence incurs, there are economic implications as well. The World Health Organization (WHO) reports that in the United States alone, costs related to interpersonal violence reach 3.3 percent of the gross domestic product (WHO, 2005).

PREDISPOSING FACTORS

What predisposes individuals to be abusive? Although no one really knows for sure, several theories have been espoused. A brief discussion of ideas associated with biological, psychological, and sociocultural views is presented here.

Biological Theories

Neurophysiological Influences

Various components of the neurological system in both humans and animals have been implicated in both the facilitation and inhibition of aggressive impulses. Areas of the brain that may be involved include the temporal lobe, the limbic system, and the amygdaloid nucleus (Tardiff, 2003).

Biochemical Influences

Studies show that various neurotransmitters—in particular norepinephrine, dopamine, and serotonin—may play a role in the facilitation and inhibition of aggressive

impulses (Siever, 2002). This theory is consistent with the "fight or flight" arousal described by Selye (1956) in his theory of the response to stress, which was described in Chapter 1. (See Figure 40–1 for an explanation of these biochemical influences on violent behavior.)

Genetic Influences

Various genetic components related to aggressive behavior have been investigated. Some studies have linked

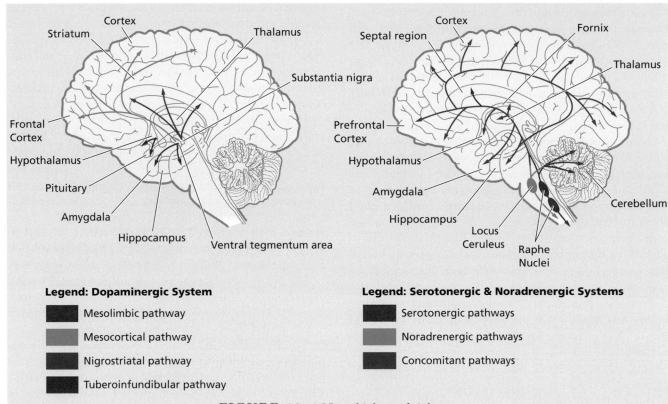

FIGURE 40–1 Neurobiology of violence.

Neurotransmitters
Neurotransmitters that have been implicated in the etiology of aggression and violence include decreases in serotonin, and increases in norepinephrine and dopamine (Siever, 2002; Tardiff, 2003).

Associated Areas of the Brain

- Limbic structures: Emotional alterations
- Prefrontal & frontal cortices: Modulation of social judgment
- Amygdala: Anxiety, rage, fear
- Hypothalamus: Stimulates sympathetic nervous system in "fight-or-flight" response
- Hippocampus: Learning and memory

Medications used to Modulate Aggression

1. Studies have suggested that selective serotonin reuptake inhibitors (SSRIs) may reduce irritability and aggression consistent with the hypothesis of reduced serotonergic activity in aggression.
2. Mood stabilizers that dampen limbic irritability may be important in reducing the susceptibility to react to provocation or threatening stimuli by overactivation of limbic system structures such as the amygdala (Siever, 2002). Carbamazepine (Tegretol), phenytoin (Dilantin), and divalproex sodium (Depakote) have yielded positive results. Lithium has also been used effectively in violent individuals (Tardiff, 2003).
3. Anti-adrenergic agents such as β-blockers (e.g., propranolol) have been shown to reduce aggression in some individuals, presumably by dampening excessive noradrenergic activity (Siever, 2002).
4. In their ability to modulate excessive dopaminergic activity, antipsychotics—both typical and atypical—have been helpful in the control of aggression and violence, particularly in individuals with co-morbid psychosis.

increased aggressiveness with selective inbreeding in mice, suggesting the possibility of a direct genetic link. Another genetic characteristic that was once thought to have some implication for aggressive behavior was the genetic karyotype XYY. The XYY syndrome has been found to contribute to aggressive behavior in a small percentage of cases (Sadock & Sadock, 2003). The evidence linking this chromosomal aberration to aggressive and deviant behavior has not yet been firmly established.

Disorders of the Brain

Organic brain syndromes associated with various cerebral disorders have been implicated in the predisposition to aggressive and violent behavior (Cummings & Mega, 2003; Sadock & Sadock, 2003; Tardiff, 2003). Brain tumors, particularly in the areas of the limbic system and the temporal lobes; trauma to the brain, resulting in cerebral changes; and diseases, such as encephalitis (or medications that may effect this syndrome) and epilepsy, particularly temporal lobe epilepsy, have all been implicated.

Psychological Theories

Psychodynamic Theory

The psychodynamic theorists imply that unmet needs for satisfaction and security result in an underdeveloped ego and a weak superego. It is thought that when frustration occurs, aggression and violence supply this individual with a dose of power and prestige that boosts the self-image and validates a significance to his or her life that is lacking. The immature ego cannot prevent dominant id behaviors from occurring, and the weak superego is unable to produce feelings of guilt.

Learning Theory

Children learn to behave by imitating their role models, which are usually their parents. Models are more likely to be imitated when they are perceived as prestigious or influential, or when the behavior is followed by positive reinforcement. Children may have an idealistic perception of their parents during the very early developmental stages but, as they mature, may begin to imitate the behavior patterns of their teachers, friends, and others. Individuals who were abused as children or whose parents disciplined with physical punishment are more likely to behave in an abusive manner as adults (Tardiff, 2003).

Adults and children alike model many of their behaviors after individuals they observe on television and in movies. Unfortunately, modeling can result in maladaptive as well as adaptive behavior, particularly when children view heroes triumphing over villains by using violence. It is also possible that individuals who have a biological predisposition toward aggressive behavior may be more susceptible to negative role modeling.

Sociocultural Theories

Societal Influences

Although they agree that perhaps some biological and psychological aspects are influential, social scientists believe that aggressive behavior is primarily a product of one's culture and social structure.

American society essentially was founded on a general acceptance of violence as a means of solving problems. The concept of relative deprivation has been shown to have a profound effect on collective violence within a society. Kennedy and associates (1998) have stated:

> Studies have shown that poverty and income are powerful predictors of homicide and violent crime. The effect of the growing gap between the rich and poor is mediated through an undermining of social cohesion, or social capital, and decreased social capital is in turn associated with increased firearm homicide and violent crime.

Indeed, the United States was populated by the violent actions of one group of people over another. Since that time, much has been said and written, and laws have been passed, regarding the civil rights of all people. However, to this day many people would agree that the statement "All men are created equal" is hypocritical in our society.

Societal influences may also contribute to violence when individuals realize that their needs and desires are not being met relative to other people (Tardiff, 2003). When poor and oppressed people find that they have limited access through legitimate channels, they are more likely to resort to delinquent behaviors in an effort to obtain desired ends. This lack of opportunity and subsequent delinquency may even contribute to a subculture of violence within a society.

APPLICATION OF THE NURSING PROCESS

Background Assessment Data

Intimate Partner Abuse

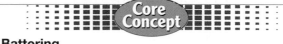

Battering
A pattern of coercive control founded on and supported by physical and/or sexual violence or threat of violence of an intimate partner.

The National Coalition Against Domestic Violence (2002a) states:

> Battering is a pattern of behavior used to establish power and control over another person through fear and intimidation, often including the threat or use of violence. Battering happens when one person believes they are entitled to control another.

The American Medical Association (2005) defines domestic violence as:

> An ongoing, debilitating experience of physical, psychological, and/or sexual abuse in the home, associated with increased isolation from the outside world and limited personal freedom and accessibility to resources.

Physical abuse between domestic partners may be known as spouse abuse, domestic or family violence, wife or husband battering, or intimate partner or relationship abuse. United States Bureau of Justice (2003) statistics for 2001 reflected the following: (1) approximately 85 percent of victims of intimate violence were women, (2) women ages 16 to 24 experienced the highest per capita rates of intimate violence, and (3) intimate partners committed 3 percent of the nonfatal violence against men. In the same study, approximately 60 percent of women and 50 percent of men reported the victimizations to the police. The most common reason for not reporting among women was "fear of reprisal." Among men, the most common reason for not reporting was because it was a "private or personal matter."

Profile of the Victim

Battered women represent all age, racial, religious, cultural, educational, and socioeconomic groups. They may be married or single, housewives or business executives. Many women who are battered have low self-esteem, commonly adhere to feminine sex-role stereotypes, and often accept the blame for the batterer's actions. Feelings of guilt, anger, fear, and shame are common. They may be isolated from family and support systems.

Some women who are in violent relationships grew up in abusive homes and may have left those homes, even gotten married, at a very young age in order to escape the abuse. The battered woman views her relationship as male dominant, and as the battering continues, her ability to see the options available to her and to make decisions concerning her life (and possibly those of her children) decreases. The phenomenon of *learned helplessness* may be applied to the woman's progressing inability to act on her own behalf. Learned helplessness occurs when an individual comes to understand that regardless of his or her behavior, the outcome is unpredictable and usually undesirable.

Profile of the Victimizer

Men who batter usually are characterized as persons with low self-esteem. Pathologically jealous, they present a "dual personality," one to the partner and one to the rest of the world (Meskill & Conner, 2003). They are often under a great deal of stress, but have limited ability to cope with the stress. The typical abuser is very possessive and perceives his spouse as a possession. He becomes threatened when she shows any sign of independence or attempts to share herself and her time with others. Small children are often ignored by the abuser; however, they also become the targets of abuse as they grow older, particularly if they attempt to protect their mother from abuse. The abuser also may use threats of taking the children away as a tactic of emotional abuse.

The abusing man typically wages a continuous campaign of degradation against his female partner. He insults and humiliates her and everything she does at every opportunity. He strives to keep her isolated from others and totally dependent on him. He demands to know where she is at every moment, and when she tells him he challenges her honesty. He achieves power and control through intimidation.

The Cycle of Battering

In her classic studies of battered women and their relationships, Walker (1979) identified a cycle of predictable behaviors that are repeated over time. The behaviors can be divided into three distinct phases that vary in time and intensity both within the same relationship and among different couples. Figure 40–2 depicts a graphic representation of the **cycle of battering**.

Phase I. The Tension-Building Phase. During this phase, the woman senses that the man's tolerance for frustration is declining. He becomes angry with little provocation but, after lashing out at her, may be quick to apologize. The woman may become very nurturing and compliant, anticipating his every whim in an effort to prevent his anger from escalating. She may just try to stay out of his way.

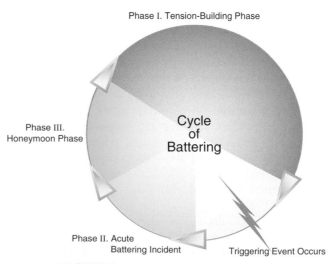

FIGURE 40–2 The cycle of battering.

Minor battering incidents may occur during this phase, and in a desperate effort to avoid more serious confrontations, the woman accepts the abuse as legitimately directed toward her. She denies her anger and rationalizes his behavior (e.g., "I need to do better"; "He's under so much stress at work"; "It's the alcohol. If only he didn't drink"). She assumes the guilt for the abuse, even reasoning that perhaps she *did* deserve the abuse, just as her aggressor suggests.

The minor battering incidents continue and the tension mounts, as the woman waits for the impending explosion. The abuser begins to fear that his partner will leave him. His jealousy and possessiveness increase, and he uses threats and brutality to keep her in his captivity. Battering incidents become more intense, after which the woman becomes less and less psychologically capable of restoring equilibrium. She withdraws from him, which he misinterprets as rejection, further escalating his anger toward her. Phase I may last from a few weeks to many months or even years.

Phase II. The Acute Battering Incident. This phase is the most violent and the shortest, usually lasting up to 24 hours. It most often begins with the batterer justifying his behavior to himself. By the end of the incident, however, he cannot understand what has happened, only that in his rage he has lost control over his behavior.

This incident may begin with the batterer wanting to "just teach her a lesson." In some instances, the woman may intentionally provoke the behavior. Having come to a point in phase I in which the tension is unbearable, long-term battered women know that once the acute phase is behind them, things will be better.

During phase II, women feel their only option is to find a safe place to hide from the batterer. The beating is severe, and many women can describe the violence in great detail, almost as if dissociation from their bodies had occurred. The batterer generally minimizes the severity of the abuse. Help is usually sought only in the event of severe injury or if the woman fears for her life or those of her children.

Phase III. Calm, Loving, Respite ("Honeymoon") Phase. In this phase, the batterer becomes extremely loving, kind, and contrite. He promises that the abuse will never recur and begs her forgiveness. He is afraid she will leave him and uses every bit of charm he can muster to ensure this does not happen. He believes he now can control his behavior, and because now he has "taught her a lesson," he believes she will not "act up" again.

He plays on her feelings of guilt, and she desperately wants to believe him. She wants to believe that he *can* change, and that she will no longer have to suffer abuse. During this phase the woman relives her original dream of ideal love and chooses to believe that *this* is what her partner is *really* like.

This loving phase becomes the focus of the woman's perception of the relationship. She bases her reason for remaining in the relationship on this "magical" ideal phase and hopes against hope that the previous phases will not be repeated. This hope is evident even in those women who have lived through a number of horrendous cycles.

Although phase III usually lasts somewhere between the lengths of time associated with phases I and II, it can be so short as to almost pass undetected. In most instances, the cycle soon begins again with renewed tensions and minor battering incidents. In an effort to "steal" a few precious moments of the phase III kind of loving, the battered woman becomes a collaborator in her own abusive lifestyle. Victim and batterer become locked together in an intense, symbiotic relationship.

Why Does She Stay?

Probably the most common response that battered women give for staying is that they fear for their life and/or the lives of their children. As the battering progresses, the man gains power and control through intimidation and instilling fear with threats such as, "I'll kill you and the kids if you try to leave." Challenged by these threats, and compounded by her low self-esteem and sense of powerlessness, the woman sees no way out. In fact, she may try to leave only to return when confronted by her partner and the psychological power he holds over her.

Women have been known to stay in an abusive relationship for many reasons, some of which include the following (Family Violence Law Center, 2003; National Coalition Against Domestic Violence, 2002b):

1. For the children: She may fear losing custody of the children if she leaves.
2. For financial reasons: She may have no financial resources, access to the resources, or job skills.
3. Fear of retaliation: Her partner may have told her that if she leaves he will find her and kill her and the children.
4. Lack of a support network: She may be under pressure from family members to stay in the marriage and try to work things out.
5. Religious reasons: She may have religious beliefs against divorce. Some clergy strive only to help save the marriage at all costs (rather than to focus on stopping the violence).
6. Hopefulness: She remembers good times and love in the relationship and has hope that her partner will change his behavior and they can have good times again.

Child Abuse

Erik Erikson (1963) stated, "The worst sin is the mutilation of a child's spirit." Children are vulnerable and relatively powerless, and the effects of maltreatment are infinitely deep and long lasting. Child maltreatment typically includes physical or emotional injury, physical or emotional neglect, or sexual acts inflicted upon a child by a caregiver. The Child Abuse Prevention and Treatment Act (CAPTA), as amended and reauthorized in October 1996, identifies a minimum set of acts or behaviors that characterize maltreatment (National Clearinghouse on Child Abuse and Neglect [NCCAN]) (2004). States may use these as foundations on which to establish state legislation.

Physical Abuse

Physical abuse of a child includes "any physical injury as a result of punching, beating, kicking, biting, burning, shaking, throwing, stabbing, choking, hitting (with a hand, stick, strap, or other object), burning, or otherwise harming a child" (NCCAN, 2004). Maltreatment is considered whether or not the caretaker intended to cause harm, or even if the injury resulted from over-discipline or physical punishment. The most obvious way to detect it is by outward physical signs. However, behavioral indicators also may be evident.

Signs of Physical Abuse. Indicators of physical abuse may include any of the following (NCCAN, 2003).
The child:

1. Has unexplained burns, bites, bruises, broken bones, or black eyes.
2. Has fading bruises or other marks noticeable after an absence from school.
3. Seems frightened of the parents and protests or cries when it is time to go home.
4. Shrinks at the approach of adults
5. Reports injury by a parent or another adult caregiver.

Physical abuse may be suspected when the parent or other adult caregiver (NCCAN, 2003):

1. Offers conflicting, unconvincing, or no explanation for the child's injury.
2. Describes the child as "evil," or in some other very negative way.
3. Uses harsh physical discipline with the child.
4. Has a history of abuse as a child.

Emotional Abuse

Emotional abuse involves a pattern of behavior on the part of the parent or caretaker that results in serious impairment of the child's social, emotional, or intellectual functioning. Examples of emotional injury include belittling or rejecting the child, ignoring the child, blaming the child for things over which he or she has no control, isolating the child from normal social experiences, and using harsh and inconsistent discipline. Behavioral indicators of emotional injury may include (NCCAN, 2003):

1. Shows extremes in behavior, such as overly compliant or demanding behavior, extreme passivity, or aggression.
2. Is either inappropriately adult (e.g., parenting other children) or inappropriately infantile (e.g., frequently rocking or head-banging)
3. Is delayed in physical or emotional development
4. Has attempted suicide
5. Reports a lack of attachment to the parent

Emotional abuse may be suspected when the parent or other adult caregiver (NCCAN, 2003):

1. Constantly blames, belittles, or berates the child.
2. Is unconcerned about the child and refuses to consider offers of help for the child's problems.
3. Overtly rejects the child.

Physical and Emotional Neglect

> **Core Concept**
>
> **Neglect**
> *Physical neglect* of a child includes refusal of or delay in seeking health care, abandonment, expulsion from the home or refusal to allow a runaway to return home, and inadequate supervision. *Emotional neglect* refers to a chronic failure by the parent or caretaker to provide the child with the hope, love, and support necessary for the development of a sound, healthy personality.

Indicators of Neglect. The possibility of neglect may be considered when the child (NCCAN, 2003):

1. Is frequently absent from school.
2. Begs or steals food or money.
3. Lacks needed medical or dental care, immunizations, or glasses.
4. Is consistently dirty and has severe body odor.
5. Lacks sufficient clothing for the weather.
6. Abuses alcohol or other drugs.
7. States that there is no one at home to provide care.

The possibility of neglect may be considered when the parent or other adult caregiver (NCCAN, 2003):

1. Appears to be indifferent to the child.
2. Seems apathetic or depressed.
3. Behaves irrationally or in a bizarre manner.
4. Is abusing alcohol or other drugs.

Sexual Abuse of a Child

Various definitions of **child sexual abuse** are available in the literature. CAPTA defines sexual abuse as:

Employment, use, persuasion, inducement, enticement, or coercion of any child to engage in, or assist any other person to engage in, any sexually explicit conduct or any simulation of such conduct for the purpose of producing any visual depiction of such conduct; or the rape, and in cases of caretaker or inter-familial relationships, statutory rape, molestation, prostitution, or other form of sexual exploitation of children, or incest with children. (NCCAN, 2004).

Included in the definition is **sexual exploitation of a child**, in which a child is induced or coerced into engaging in sexually explicit conduct for the purpose of promoting any performance, and child sexual abuse, in which a child is being used for the sexual pleasure of an adult (parent or caretaker) or any other person.

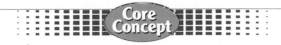

Incest

Incest is the occurrence of sexual contacts or interaction between, or sexual exploitation of, close relatives, or between participants who are related to each other by a kinship bond that is regarded as a prohibition to sexual relations (e.g., caretakers, stepparents, stepsiblings) (Sadock & Sadock, 2003).

Indicators of Sexual Abuse. Child abuse may be considered a possibility when the child (NCCAN, 2003):

1. Has difficulty walking or sitting.
2. Suddenly refuses to change for gym or to participate in physical activities.
3. Reports nightmares or bedwetting.
4. Experiences a sudden change in appetite.
5. Demonstrates bizarre, sophisticated, or unusual sexual knowledge or behavior.
6. Becomes pregnant or contracts a venereal disease, particularly if under age 14.
7. Runs away.
8. Reports sexual abuse by a parent or another adult caregiver.

Sexual abuse may be considered a possibility when the parent or other adult caregiver (NCCAN, 2003):

1. Is unduly protective of the child or severely limits the child's contact with other children, especially of the opposite sex.
2. Is secretive and isolated.
3. Is jealous or controlling with family members.

Characteristics of the Abuser

A number of factors have been associated with adults who abuse or neglect their children. Sadock and Sadock (2003) report that 90 percent of parents who abuse their children were severely physically abused by their own mothers or fathers. Murray and Zentner (2001) identify the following as additional characteristics that may be associated with abusive parents:

- Experiencing a stressful life situation (e.g., unemployment; poverty)
- Having few, if any, support systems; commonly isolated from others
- Lacking understanding of child development or care needs
- Lacking adaptive coping strategies; angers easily; has difficulty trusting others
- Expecting the child to be perfect; may exaggerate any mild difference the child manifests from the "usual"

The Incestuous Relationship

A great deal of attention has been given to the study of father–daughter incest. In these cases there is usually an impaired sexual relationship between the parents. Communication between the parents is ineffective, which prevents them from correcting their problems. Typically, the father is domineering, impulsive, and physically abusing; whereas the mother is passive and submissive, and denigrates her role as wife and mother. She is often aware of, or at least strongly suspects, the incestuous behavior between the father and daughter but may believe in or fear her husband's absolute authority over the family. She may deny that her daughter is being harmed and may actually be grateful that her husband's sexual demands are being met by someone other than herself.

Onset of the incestuous relationship typically occurs when the daughter is 8 to 10 years of age and commonly begins with genital touching and fondling. In the beginning, the child may accept the sexual advances from her father as signs of affection. As the incestuous behavior continues and progresses, the daughter usually becomes more bewildered, confused, and frightened, never knowing whether her father will be paternal or sexual in his interactions with her (Sadock & Sadock, 2003).

The relationship may become a love–hate situation on the part of the daughter. She continues to strive for the ideal father–daughter relationship but is fearful and hateful of the sexual demands he places on her. The mother may be alternately caring and competitive as she witnesses her husband's possessiveness and affections directed toward her daughter. Out of fear that his daughter may expose their relationship, the father may attempt to interfere with her normal peer relationships (Sadock & Sadock, 2003).

It has been suggested that some fathers who participate in incestuous relationships may have unconscious homosexual tendencies and have difficulty achieving a stable heterosexual orientation. On the other hand, some men have frequent sex with their wives and several of their own children but are unwilling to seek sexual partners outside the nuclear family because of a need to maintain the public facade of a stable and competent patriarch. Although the oldest daughter in a family is most vulnerable to becoming a participant in father–daughter incest, some fathers form sequential relationships with several daughters. If incest has been reported with one daughter, it should be suspected with all of the other daughters (Murray & Zentner, 2001).

The Adult Survivor of Incest

Several common characteristics have been identified in adults who have experienced incest as children. Basic to these characteristics is a fundamental lack of trust resulting from an unsatisfactory parent–child relationship, which causes low self-esteem and a poor sense of identity. Children of incest often feel trapped, for they have been admonished not to talk about the experience and may be afraid, or even fear for their lives, if they are exposed. If they do muster the courage to report the incest, particularly to the mother, they frequently are not believed. This is confusing to the child, who is then left with a sense of self-doubt and the inability to trust his or her own feelings. The child develops feelings of guilt with the realization over the years that the parents are using him or her in an attempt to solve their own problems.

Childhood sexual abuse is likely to distort the development of a normal association of pleasure with sexual activity (Reeves, 2003). Peer relationships are often delayed, altered, inhibited, or perverted. In some instances, individuals who were sexually abused as children completely retreat from sexual activity and avoid all close interpersonal relationships throughout life. Other adult manifestations of childhood sexual abuse in women include diminished libido, vaginismus, nymphomania, and promiscuity. In male survivors of childhood sexual abuse, impotence, premature ejaculation, exhibitionism, and compulsive sexual conquests may occur. Lerner (2005) suggests that adult survivors of incest are at risk for experiencing symptoms of posttraumatic stress disorder, sexual dysfunction, somatization disorders, compulsive sexual behaviors, depression, anxiety, eating disorders, substance disorders, and intolerance of or constant search for intimacy.

The conflicts associated with pain (either physical or emotional) and sexual pleasure experienced by children who are sexually abused are commonly manifested symbolically in adult relationships. Women who were abused as children commonly enter into relationships with men who abuse them physically, sexually, or emotionally (Bensley, VanEenwyk, & Wynkoop, 2003).

Adult survivors of incest who decide to come forward with their stories usually are estranged from nuclear family members. They are blamed by family members for disclosing the "family secret" and often accused of overreacting to the incest. Frequently the estrangement becomes permanent when family members continue to deny the behavior and the individual is accused of lying. In recent years, a number of celebrities have come forward with stories of their childhood sexual abuse. Some have chosen to make the disclosure only after the death of their parents. Revelation of these past activities can be one way of contributing to the healing process for which incest survivors so desperately strive.

Sexual Assault

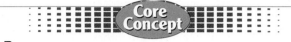

Rape

Rape is the expression of power and dominance by means of sexual violence, most commonly by men over women, although men may also be rape victims.

Sexual assault is viewed as any type of sexual act in which an individual is threatened or coerced, or forced to submit against his or her will. Rape, a type of sexual assault, occurs over a broad spectrum of experiences ranging from the surprise attack by a stranger to insistence on sexual intercourse by an acquaintance or spouse. Regardless of the defining source, one common theme always emerges: Rape is an act of aggression, not one of passion.

Date rape is a term applied to situations in which the rapist is known to the victim (Sadock & Sadock, 2003). They may be out on a first date, may have been dating for a number of months, or merely may be acquaintances or schoolmates. College campuses are the location for a staggering number of these types of rapes, a great many of which go unreported. An increasing number of colleges and universities are establishing programs for rape prevention and counseling for victims of rape.

Marital rape, which has been recognized only in recent years as a legal category, is the case in which a spouse may be held liable for sexual abuse directed at a marital partner against that person's will. Historically, with societal acceptance of the concept of women as marital property, the legal definition of rape held an exemption within the marriage relationship. In 1993, marital rape became a crime in all 50 U.S. states, under at least one section of the sexual offenses code. In 17 states and the District of Columbia, there are no exemptions from rape prosecution granted to husbands. However, in 33 states, there are still some exemptions given to husbands from rape prosecution.

Statutory rape is defined as unlawful intercourse between a man older than 16 years of age and a woman under the age of consent (Sadock & Sadock, 2003). The age of consent varies from state to state, ranging from age 14 to 21. A man who has intercourse with a woman under the age of consent can be arrested for statutory rape, although the interaction may have occurred between consenting individuals. The charges, when they occur, usually are brought by the young woman's parents.

Profile of the Victimizer

Older profiles of the individual who rapes were described by Abrahamsen (1960) and Macdonald (1971), who identified the rapist's childhood as "mother-dominated" and the mother as "seductive but rejecting." The behavior of the mother toward the son was described as overbearing, with seductive undertones. Mother and son shared little secrets, and she rescued him when his delinquent acts created problems with others. However, she was quick to withdraw her love and attention when he went against her wishes, a rejection that was powerful and unyielding. She was domineering and possessive of the son, a dominance that often continued into his adult life. Macdonald (1971) stated:

> The seductive mother arouses overwhelming anxiety in her son with great anger, which may be expressed directly toward her but more often is displaced onto other women. When this seductive behavior is combined with parental encouragement of assaultive behavior, the setting is provided for personality development in the child which may result in sadistic, homicidal sexual attacks on women in adolescence or adult life.

Many rapists report growing up in abusive homes (McCormack, 2002). Even when the parental brutality is discharged by the father, the anger may be directed toward the mother who did not protect her child from physical assault. More recent feminist theories suggest that the rapist displaces this anger on the rape victim because he cannot directly express it toward other men (Sadock & Sadock, 2003).

Statistics show that the greatest number of rapists are between the ages of 25 and 44. Of rapists, 51 percent are white, 47 percent are African American, and the remaining 2 percent come from all other races (Sadock & Sadock, 2003). Many are either married or cohabiting at the time of their offenses. For those with previous criminal activity, the majority of their convictions are for crimes against property rather than against people. Most rapists do not have histories of mental illness.

The Victim

Rape can occur at any age. Although victims have been reported as young as 15 months old and as old as 82 years, the high-risk age group appears to be 16 to 24 years (Sadock & Sadock, 2003). Of rape victims, 70 to 75 percent are single women, and the attack frequently occurs in or close to the victim's own neighborhood.

Scully (1994), in a study of a prison sample of rapists, found that in "stranger rapes," victims were not chosen for any reason having to do with appearance or behavior, but simply because the individual happened to be in a certain place at a certain time. Scully states:

> The most striking and consistent factor in all the stranger rapes, whether committed by a lone assailant or a group, is the unfortunate fact that the victim was "just there" in a location unlikely to draw the attention of a passerby. Almost every one of these men said exactly the same thing, "It could have been any woman," and a few added that because it was dark, they could not even see what their victim looked like very well. (p. 175)

In her study, Scully found that 62 percent of the rapists used a weapon, most frequently a knife. Most suggested that they used the weapon to terrorize and subdue the victim but not to inflict serious injury. The presence of a weapon (real or perceived) appears to be the principal measure of the degree to which a woman resists her attacker.

Rape victims who present themselves for care shortly after the crime has occurred likely may be experiencing an overwhelming sense of violation and helplessness that began with the powerlessness and intimidation experienced during the rape. Burgess (2004) identified two emotional patterns of response that may occur within hours after a rape and with which health care workers may be confronted in the emergency department or rape crisis center. In the **expressed response pattern**, the victim expresses feelings of fear, anger, and anxiety through such behaviors as crying, sobbing, smiling, restlessness, and tension. In the **controlled response pattern**, the feelings are masked or hidden, and a calm, composed, or subdued affect is seen.

The following manifestations may be evident in the days and weeks after the attack (Burgess, 2004):

1. Contusions and abrasions about various parts of the body
2. Headaches, fatigue, sleep pattern disturbances
3. Stomach pains, nausea and vomiting
4. Vaginal discharge and itching, burning upon urination, rectal bleeding and pain
5. Rage, humiliation, embarrassment, desire for revenge, and self-blame
6. Fear of physical violence and death

The long-term effects of sexual assault depend largely on the individual's ego strength, social support system, and the way he or she was treated as a victim (Burgess, 2004). Various long-term effects include increased restlessness, dreams and nightmares, and phobias (particularly those having to do with sexual interaction). Some women report that it takes years to get over the experience; they describe a sense of vulnerability and a loss of control over their own lives during this period. They feel defiled and unable to wash themselves clean, and some women are unable to remain living alone in their home or apartment.

Some victims develop a **compounded rape reaction**, in which additional symptoms such as depression and suicide, substance abuse, and even psychotic behaviors may be noted (Burgess, 2004). Another variation has been called the **silent rape reaction**, in which the victim tells no one about the assault. Anxiety is suppressed and the emotional burden may become overwhelming. The unresolved sexual trauma may not be revealed until the woman is forced to face another sexual crisis in her life that reactivates the previously unresolved feelings.

Diagnosis/Outcome Identification

Nursing diagnoses are formulated from the data gathered during the assessment phase and with background knowledge regarding predisposing factors to the situation. Some common nursing diagnoses for victims of abuse include:

Rape-trauma syndrome related to sexual assault evidenced by verbalizations of the attack; bruises and lacerations over areas of body; severe anxiety.

Powerlessness related to cycle of battering evidenced by verbalizations of abuse; bruises and lacerations over areas of body; fear for her safety and that of her children; verbalizations of no way to get out of the relationship.

Delayed growth and development related to abusive family situation evidenced by sudden onset of enuresis, thumb sucking, nightmares, inability to perform self-care activities appropriate for age.

The following criteria may be used to measure outcomes in the care of abuse victims:

The client who has been sexually assaulted:

1. Is no longer experiencing panic anxiety.
2. Demonstrates a degree of trust in the primary nurse.
3. Has received immediate attention to physical injuries.
4. Has initiated behaviors consistent with the grief response.

The client who has been physically battered:

1. Has received immediate attention to physical injuries.
2. Verbalizes assurance of his or her immediate safety.
3. Discusses life situation with primary nurse.
4. Can verbalize choices from which he or she may receive assistance.

The child who has been abused:

1. Has received immediate attention to physical injuries.
2. Demonstrates trust in primary nurse by discussing abuse through the use of play therapy.
3. Is demonstrating a decrease in regressive behaviors.

Planning/Implementation

Table 40–1 provides a plan of care for the client who has been a victim of abuse. Nursing diagnoses are presented,

along with outcome criteria, appropriate nursing interventions, and rationales for each.

Evaluation

Evaluation of nursing actions to assist victims of abuse must be considered on both a short- and a long-term basis.

Short-term evaluation may be facilitated by gathering information using the following types of questions:

1. Has the individual been reassured of his or her safety?
2. Is this evidenced by a decrease in panic anxiety?
3. Have wounds been properly cared for and provision made for follow-up care?
4. Have emotional needs been attended to?
5. Has trust been established with at least one person to whom the client feels comfortable relating the abusive incident?
6. Have available support systems been identified and notified?
7. Have options for immediate circumstances been presented?

Long-term evaluation may be conducted by health care workers who have contact with the individual long after the immediate crisis has passed.

1. Is the individual able to conduct activities of daily living satisfactorily?
2. Have physical wounds healed properly?
3. Is the client appropriately progressing through the behaviors of grieving?
4. Is the client free of sleep disturbances (nightmares, insomnia); psychosomatic symptoms (headaches, stomach pains, nausea/vomiting); regressive behaviors (enuresis, thumb sucking, phobias); and psychosexual disturbances?
5. Is the individual free from problems with interpersonal relationships?
6. Has the individual considered the alternatives for change in his or her personal life?
7. Has a decision been made relative to the choices available?
8. Is he or she satisfied with the decision that has been made?

TREATMENT MODALITIES

Crisis Intervention

The focus of the initial interview and follow-up with the client who has been sexually assaulted is on the rape incident alone. Problems identified but unassociated with the rape are not dealt with at this time. The goal of crisis intervention is to help victims return to their previous lifestyle as quickly as possible.

TABLE 40–1	Care Plan for Victims of Abuse

NURSING DIAGNOSIS: RAPE-TRAUMA SYNDROME
RELATED TO: Sexual assault
EVIDENCED BY: Verbalizations of the attack; bruises and lacerations over areas of body; severe anxiety

OUTCOME CRITERIA	NURSING INTERVENTIONS	RATIONALE
Client will begin a healthy grief resolution, initiating the process of healing (both physically and psychologically).	1. It is important to communicate the following to the victim of sexual assault: • You are safe here. • I'm sorry that it happened. • I'm glad you survived. • It's not your fault. No one deserves to be treated this way. • You did the best that you could.	1. The woman who has been sexually assaulted fears for her life and must be reassured of her safety. She may also be overwhelmed with self-doubt and self-blame, and these statements instill trust and validate self-worth.
	2. Explain every assessment procedure that will be conducted and why it is being conducted. Ensure that data collection is conducted in a caring, nonjudgmental manner.	2. This may serve to decrease fear/anxiety and increase trust.
	3. Ensure that the client has adequate privacy for all immediate post-crisis interventions. Try to have as few people as possible providing the immediate care or collecting immediate evidence.	3. The post-trauma client is extremely vulnerable. Additional people in the environment increase this feeling of vulnerability and serve to escalate anxiety.
	4. Encourage the client to give an account of the assault. Listen, but do not probe.	4. Nonjudgmental listening provides an avenue for catharsis that the client needs to begin healing. A detailed account may be required for legal follow-up, and a caring nurse, as client advocate, may help to lessen the trauma of evidence collection.
	5. Discuss with the client whom to call for support or assistance. Provide information about referrals for aftercare.	5. Because of severe anxiety and fear, the client may need assistance from others during this immediate post-crisis period. Provide referral information in writing for later reference (e.g., psychotherapist, mental health clinic, community advocacy group).

NURSING DIAGNOSIS: POWERLESSNESS
RELATED TO: Cycle of battering
EVIDENCED BY: Verbalizations of abuse; bruises and lacerations over areas of body; fear for own safety and that of children; verbalizations of no way to get out of the relationship

OUTCOME CRITERIA	NURSING INTERVENTIONS	RATIONALE
Client will recognize and verbalize choices available, thereby perceiving some control over life situation.	1. In collaboration with physician, ensure that all physical wounds, fractures, and burns receive immediate attention. Take photographs if the victim will permit.	1. Client safety is a nursing priority. Photographs may be called in as evidence if charges are filed.
	2. Take the woman to a private area to do the interview.	2. If the client is accompanied by the man who did the battering, she is not likely to be truthful about her injuries.
	3. If she has come alone or with her children, assure her of her safety. Encourage her to discuss the battering incident. Ask questions about whether this has happened before, whether the abuser takes drugs, whether the woman has a safe place to go, and whether she is interested in pressing charges.	3. Some women will attempt to keep secret how their injuries occurred in an effort to protect the partner or because they are fearful that the partner will kill them if they tell.

(Continued on following page)

TABLE 40–1 Care Plan for Victims of Abuse *(Continued)*

OUTCOME CRITERIA	NURSING INTERVENTIONS	RATIONALE
	4. Ensure that "rescue" efforts are not attempted by the nurse. Offer support, but remember that the final decision must be made by the client.	4. Making her own decision will give the client a sense of control over her life situation. Imposing judgments and giving advice are nontherapeutic.
	5. Stress to the victim the importance of safety. She must be made aware of the variety of resources that are available to her. These may include crisis hotlines, community groups for women who have been abused, shelters, counseling services, and information regarding the victim's rights in the civil and criminal justice system. Following a discussion of these available resources, the woman may choose for herself. If her decision is to return to the marriage and home, this choice also must be respected.	5. Knowledge of available choices decreases the victim's sense of powerlessness, but true empowerment comes only when she chooses to use that knowledge for her own benefit.

NURSING DIAGNOSIS: DELAYED GROWTH AND DEVELOPMENT

RELATED TO: Abusive family situation

EVIDENCED BY: Sudden onset of enuresis, thumb sucking, nightmares, inability to perform self-care activities appropriate for age

OUTCOME CRITERIA	NURSING INTERVENTIONS	RATIONALE
Client will develop trusting relationship with nurse and report how evident injuries were sustained. Negative regressive behaviors (enuresis, thumb sucking, nightmares) will diminish.	1. Perform complete physical assessment of the child. Take particular note of bruises (in various stages of healing), lacerations, and client complaints of pain in specific areas. Do not overlook or discount the possibility of sexual abuse. Assess for nonverbal signs of abuse: aggressive conduct, excessive fears, extreme hyperactivity, apathy, withdrawal, age-inappropriate behaviors.	1. An accurate and thorough physical assessment is required to provide appropriate care for the client.
	2. Conduct an in-depth interview with the parent or adult who accompanies the child. Consider: If the injury is being reported as an accident, is the explanation reasonable? Is the injury consistent with the explanation? Is the injury consistent with the child's developmental capabilities?	2. Fear of imprisonment or loss of child custody may place the abusive parent on the defensive. Discrepancies may be evident in the description of the incident, and lying to cover up involvement is a common defense that may be detectable in an in-depth interview.
	3. Use games or play therapy to gain child's trust. Use these techniques to assist in describing his or her side of the story.	3. Establishing a trusting relationship with an abused child is extremely difficult. He or she may not even want to be touched. These types of play activities can provide a nonthreatening environment that may enhance the child's attempt to discuss these painful issues.
	4. Determine whether the nature of the injuries warrants reporting to authorities. Specific state statutes must enter into the decision of whether to report suspected child abuse. Individual state statutes regarding what constitutes child abuse and neglect may be found at http://nccanch.acf.hhs.gov/general/legal/statutes/index.cfm	4. A report is commonly made if there is reason to suspect that a child has been injured as a result of physical, mental, emotional, or sexual abuse. "Reason to suspect" exists when there is evidence of a discrepancy or inconsistency in explaining a child's injury. Most states require that the following individuals report cases of suspected child abuse: all health care workers, all mental health therapists, teachers, child-care providers, firefighters, emergency medical personnel, and law enforcement personnel. Reports are made to the Department of Health and Human Services or a law enforcement agency.

The client should be involved in the intervention from the beginning. This promotes a sense of competency, control, and decision-making. Because an overwhelming sense of powerlessness accompanies the rape experience, active involvement by the victim is both a validation of personal worth and the beginning of the recovery process. Crisis intervention is time limited—usually 6 to 8 weeks. If problems resurface beyond this time, the victim is referred for assistance from other agencies (e.g., long-term psychotherapy from a psychiatrist or mental health clinic).

During the crisis period, attention is given to coping strategies for dealing with the symptoms common to the posttrauma client. Initially the individual undergoes a period of disorganization during which there is difficulty making decisions, extreme or irrational fears, and general mistrust. Observable manifestations may range from stark hysteria to expression of anger and rage to silence and withdrawal. Guilt and feelings of responsibility for the rape, as well as numerous physical manifestations, are common. The crisis counselor will attempt to help the victim draw upon previous successful coping strategies to regain control over his or her life.

If the client is a victim of battering, the counselor ensures that various resources and options are made known to the victim so that she may make a personal decision regarding what she wishes to do with her life. Support groups provide a valuable forum for reducing isolation and learning new strategies for coping with the aftermath of physical or sexual abuse. Particularly for the rape victim, the peer support group provides a therapeutic forum for reducing the sense of isolation she may feel in the aftermath of predictable social and interpersonal responses to her experience.

Sadock and Sadock (2003) state:

Few women emerge from the assault completely unscathed. The manifestations and the degree of damage depend on the violence of the attack itself, the vulnerability of the woman, and the support system available to her immediately after the attack. A rape victim fares best when she receives immediate support and can ventilate her fear and rage to loving family members, sympathetic physicians, and law enforcement officials. Knowing that she has socially acceptable means of recourse, such as the arrest and conviction of the rapist, can help a rape victim. (p. 892)

The Safe House or Shelter

Most major cities in the United States now have **safe houses or shelters** where women can go to be assured of protection for them and their children. These shelters provide a variety of services, and the women receive emotional support from staff and each other. Most shelters provide individual and group counseling; help with bureaucratic institutions such as the police, legal representation, and social services; child care and children's programming; and aid for the woman in making future plans, such as employment counseling and linkages with housing authorities.

The shelters are usually run by a combination of professional and volunteer staff, including nurses, psychologists, lawyers, and others. Women who themselves have been previously abused are often among the volunteer staff members.

Group work is an important part of the service of shelters. Women in residence range from those in the immediate crisis phase to those who have progressed through a variety of phases of the grief process. Those newer members can learn a great deal from the women who have successfully resolved similar problems. Length of stay varies a great deal from individual to individual, depending on a number of factors, such as outside support network, financial situation, and personal resources.

The shelter provides a haven of physical safety for the battered woman and promotes expression of the intense emotions she may be experiencing regarding her situation. A woman often exhibits depression, extreme fear, or even violent expressions of anger and rage. In the shelter, she learns that these feelings are normal and that others also have experienced these same emotions in similar situations. She is allowed to grieve for what has been lost and for what was expected but not achieved. Help is provided in overcoming the tremendous guilt associated with self-blame. This is a difficult step for someone who has accepted responsibility for another's behavior over a long period.

New arrivals at the shelter are given time to experience the relief from the safety and security provided. Making decisions is discouraged during the period of immediate crisis and disorganization. Once the woman's emotions have become more stable, planning for the future begins. Through information from staff and peers, she learns what resources are available to her within the community. Feedback is provided, but the woman makes her own decision about "where she wants to go from here." She is accepted and supported in whatever she chooses to do.

Family Therapy

The focus of therapy with families who use violence is to help them develop democratic ways of solving problems. Studies show that the more a family uses the democratic means of conflict resolution, the less likely they are to engage in physical violence. Families need to learn to deal with problems in ways that can produce mutual benefits for all concerned, rather than engaging in power struggles among family members.

Parents also need to learn more effective methods of disciplining children, aside from physical punishment. Methods that emphasize the importance of positive reinforcement for acceptable behavior can be very effective. Family members must be committed to consistent use of this behavior modification technique for it to be successful.

Teaching parents about expectations for various developmental levels may alleviate some of the stress that accompanies these changes. Knowing what to expect from individuals at various stages of development may provide needed anticipatory guidance to deal with the crises commonly associated with these stages.

Therapy sessions with all family members together may focus on problems with family communication. Members are encouraged to express honest feelings in a manner that is nonthreatening to other family members. Active listening, assertiveness techniques, and respecting the rights of others are taught and encouraged. Barriers to effective communication are identified and resolved.

Referrals to agencies that promote effective parenting skills (e.g., parent effectiveness training) may be made. Alternative agencies that may relieve the stress of parenting (e.g., "Mom's Day Out" programs, sitter-sharing organizations, and day care institutions) also may be considered. Support groups for abusive parents may also be helpful, and assistance in locating or initiating such a group may be provided.

SUMMARY

This chapter provided a discussion of abuse—the maltreatment of one person by another. Intimate partner abuse, child abuse, and sexual assault are all on the rise in this country, and all populations are equally affected.

Abuse of women and children began early in the development of this country when these individuals were considered the property of their husbands and fathers; this physical abuse was considered acceptable. Many women came to believe that they deserved any physical or sexual abuse they encountered.

Various factors have been theorized as influential in the predisposition to violent behavior. Physiological and biochemical influences within the brain have been suggested, as has the possibility of a direct genetic link. Organic brain syndromes associated with various cerebral disorders have been implicated in the predisposition to aggressive and violent behavior.

Psychoanalytical theorists relate the predisposition to violent behavior to underdeveloped ego and a poor self-concept. Learning theorists suggest that children imitate the abusive behavior of their parents. This theory has been substantiated by studies that show that individuals who were abused as children or whose parents disciplined them with physical punishment are more likely to be abusive as adults. Societal influences, such as general acceptance of violence as a means of solving problems, also have been implicated.

Women who are battered usually take blame for their situation. They were often reared in abusive families and have come to expect this type of behavior. Battered women often see no way out of their present situation and may be encouraged by their social support network (family, friends, clergy) to remain in the abusive relationship.

Child abuse includes physical and emotional abuse, physical and emotional neglect, and sexual abuse of a child. A child may experience many years of abuse without reporting it because of fear of retaliation by the abuser. Some children report incest experiences to their mothers, only to be rebuffed by her and told to remain secretive about the abuse. Adult survivors of incest often experience a number of physical and emotional manifestations relating back to the incestuous relationship.

Sexual assault is identified as an act of aggression, not passion. Many rapists report growing up in abusive homes, and some theorists relate the predisposition to rape to a "seductive, but rejecting, mother." Rape is a crisis situation; many women experience flashbacks, nightmares, rage, physical symptoms, depression, and thoughts of suicide for many years after the occurrence.

Nursing implementation with victims of abuse was discussed in the context of the nursing process. Assessment data, nursing diagnoses, outcome criteria, appropriate nursing interventions with rationale, and standards for evaluation were presented. Additional treatment modalities were described, including crisis intervention with the sexual assault victim, safe shelter for battered women, and therapy for families who use violence.

Problems related to abuse and neglect are becoming a national crisis in the United States. Nurses are in a unique position to intervene at the primary, secondary, and tertiary levels of prevention with the victims of these problematic behaviors.

REVIEW QUESTIONS

SELF-EXAMINATION/LEARNING EXERCISE

Select the answer that is *most* appropriate for each of the following questions:

Situation: Sharon is a 32-year-old woman who arrives at the emergency department with her three small children. She has multiple bruises around her face and neck. Her right eye is swollen shut.

1. Sharon says to the nurse, "I didn't want to come. I'm really okay. He only does this when he has too much to drink. I just shouldn't have yelled at him." The best response by the nurse is:
   a. "How often does he drink too much?"
   b. "It is not your fault. You did the right thing by coming here."
   c. "How many times has he done this to you?"
   d. "He is not a good husband. You have to leave him before he kills you."

2. In the interview, Sharon tells the nurse, "He's been getting more and more violent lately. He's been under a lot of stress at work the last few weeks, so he drinks a lot when he gets home. He always gets mean when he drinks. I was getting scared. So I just finally told him I was going to take the kids and leave. He got furious when I said that and began beating me with his fists." With knowledge about the cycle of battering, what does this situation represent?
   a. Phase I. Sharon was desperately trying to stay out of his way and keep everything calm.
   b. Phase I. A minor battering incident for which Sharon assumes all the blame
   c. Phase II. The acute battering incident that Sharon provoked with her threat to leave
   d. Phase III. The honeymoon phase in which the husband believes that he has "taught her a lesson and she won't act up again."

3. The *priority* nursing intervention for Sharon in the emergency department is:
   a. Tending to the immediate care of her wounds.
   b. Providing her with information about a safe place to stay.
   c. Administering the prn tranquilizer ordered by the physician.
   d. Explaining how she may go about bringing charges against her husband.

4. Sharon goes with her children to stay at a women's shelter. She participates in group therapy and receives emotional support from staff and peers. She is made aware of the alternatives open to her. Nevertheless, she decides to return to her home and marriage. The best response by the nurse upon Sharon's departure is:
   a. "I just can't believe you have decided to go back to that horrible man."
   b. "I'm just afraid he will kill you or the children when you go back."
   c. "What makes you think things have changed with him?"
   d. "I hope you have made the right decision. Call this number if you need help."

Situation: Carol is a school nurse. Five-year-old Jana has been sent to her office complaining of nausea. She lies down on the office cot, but eventually vomits and soils her blouse. When Carol removes Jana's blouse to clean it, she notices that Jana has a number of bruises on her arms and torso. Some are bluish in color; others are various shades of green and yellow. She also notices some small scars. Jana's abdomen protrudes on her small, thin frame.

5. From the objective physical assessment, the nurse suspects that:
   a. Jana is experiencing physical and sexual abuse.
   b. Jana is experiencing physical abuse and neglect.
   c. Jana is experiencing emotional neglect.
   d. Jana is experiencing sexual and emotional abuse.

6. Carol tries to talk to Jana about her bruises and scars, but Jana refuses to say how she received them. Another way in which Carol can get information from Jana is to:
   a. Have her evaluated by the school psychologist.
   b. Tell her she may select a "treat" from the treat box (e.g., sucker, balloon, junk jewelry) if she answers the nurse's questions.
   c. Explain to her that if she answers the questions, she may stay in the nurse's office and not have to go back to class.
   d. Use a "family" of dolls to role-play Jana's family with her.

7. Carol strongly suspects that Jana is being abused. What would be the best way for Carol to proceed with this information?
   a. As a healthcare worker, report the suspicion to the Department of Health and Human Services.
   b. Check Jana again in a week and see if there are any new bruises.
   c. Meet with Jana's parents and ask them how Jana got the bruises.
   d. Initiate paperwork to have Jana placed in foster care.

Situation Lana is an 18-year-old freshman at the state university. She was extremely flattered when Don, a senior star football player, invited her to a party. On the way home, he parked the car in a secluded area by the lake. He became angry when she refused his sexual advances. He began to beat her and finally raped her. She tried to fight him, but his physical strength overpowered her. He dumped her in the dorm parking lot and left. The dorm supervisor rushed Lana to the emergency department.

8. Lana says to the nurse, "It's all my fault. I shouldn't have allowed him to stop at the lake." The nurse's best response is:
   a. "Yes, you're right. You put yourself in a very vulnerable position when you allowed him to stop at the lake."
   b. "You are not to blame for his behavior. You obviously made some right decisions, because you survived the attack."
   c. "There's no sense looking back now. Just look forward, and make sure you don't put yourself in the same situation again."
   d. "You'll just have to see that he is arrested so he won't do this to anyone else."

9. The *priority* nursing intervention with Lana would be:
   a. Help her to bathe and clean herself up.
   b. Provide physical and emotional support during evidence collection.
   c. Provide her with a written list of community resources for rape victims.
   d. Discuss the importance of a follow-up visit to evaluate for sexually transmitted diseases.

10. Lana is referred to a support group for rape victims. She has been attending regularly for 6 months. From this group, she has learned that the most likely reason Don raped her was:
    a. He had had too much to drink at the party and was not in control of his actions.
    b. He had not had sexual relations with a girl in many months.
    c. He was predisposed to become a rapist by virtue of the poverty conditions under which he was reared.
    d. He was expressing power and dominance by means of sexual aggression and violence.

TEST YOUR CRITICAL THINKING SKILLS

Sandy is a psychiatric RN who works at the Safe House for battered women. Lisa has just been admitted with her two small children after she was treated in the emergency department. She had been beaten severely by her husband while he was intoxicated last night. She escaped with her children after he passed out in their bedroom.

In her initial assessment, Sandy learns from Lisa that she has been battered by her husband for 5 years, beginning shortly after their marriage. She explained that she "knew he drank quite a lot before we were married, but thought he would stop after we had kids." Instead, the drinking has increased. Sometimes he doesn't even get home from work until 11 o'clock or midnight, after stopping to drink at the bar with his buddies.

Lately, he has begun to express jealousy and a lack of trust in Lisa, accusing her of numerous infidelities and indiscretions, none of which is true. Lisa says, "If only he wasn't under so much stress on his job, then maybe he wouldn't drink so much. Maybe if I tried harder to make everything perfect for him at home—I don't know. What do you think I should do to keep him from acting this way?"

Answer the following questions related to Lisa:

1. What is an appropriate response to Lisa's question?
2. Identify the priority psychosocial nursing diagnosis for Lisa.
3. What must the nurse ensure that Lisa learns from this experience?

IMPLICATIONS OF RESEARCH FOR EVIDENCE-BASED PRACTICE

Sachs, B., Hall, L.A., Lutenbacher, M., & Rayens, M.K. (1999). Potential for abusive parenting by rural mothers with low-birth-weight children. *Image: Journal of Nursing Scholarship, 31*(1), 21–25.

Description of the Study: The purpose of this study was to describe factors influencing the potential for abusive parenting by rural mothers of low-birth-weight (LBW) children. The convenience sample in this study included 48 mothers of LBW children, ranging in age from 18 to 39 years, all living in a rural area of the state, and all living with their LBW infant at the time of the study. Average length of the children's hospitalization after birth was 6 weeks, and the average age at time of the study was 9 months. In-home interviews were conducted using structured questionnaires to assess the mothers' everyday stressors, depressive symptoms, functional social support, quality of family relationships, and child abuse potential.

Results of the Study: According to the questionnaires used for measurement, 54 percent of the mothers indicated a high level of depressive symptoms and 63 percent indicated a high potential for physical child abuse. No significant differences were noted in depressive symptoms and potential for child abuse by birth weight, health status of the child, or time since hospital discharge. Mothers with high child abuse potential reported more everyday stressors and depressive symptoms, less functional social support, and poorer family functioning. Because in this study everyday stressors and the two social support systems (functional social support and quality of family relationships) were examined as predictors of depressive symptoms, it is suggested that everyday stressors exerts both a direct and an indirect effect on mothers' potential for child abuse. The strongest predictor of child abuse potential was mothers' depressive symptoms.

Implications for Nursing Practice: The researchers conclude that rural mothers of LBW children are at risk for abusive parenting. This study demonstrated the adverse effects of everyday stressors, minimal social resources, and depressive symptoms on mothers' potential for abusive parenting. Nurses should provide attention to the mental health of mothers living in isolated, rural areas. Information should be made available to these mothers regarding community resources that offer social support and childcare assistance. Nurses could establish and conduct educational programs to improve parenting skills and promote more positive child health outcomes.

 INTERNET REFERENCES

Additional information related to child abuse may be located at the following Web sites:

- http://nccanch.acf.hhs.gov/
- http://www.childabuse.org/
- http://endabuse.org/
- http://www.child-abuse.com

Additional information related to sexual assault may be located at the following Web sites:

- http://www.vaw.umn.edu/Vawnet/mrape.htm
- http://www.ncweb.com/org/rapecrisis
- http://www.nlm.nih.gov/medlineplus/rape.html

Additional information related to domestic violence may be located at the following Web sites:

- http://www.ndvh.org/
- http://www.cpsdv.org/
- http://home.cybergrrl.com/dv/book/toc.html
- http://crisis-support.org/
- http://www.ama-assn.org/ama/pub/category/3242.html

REFERENCES

American Medical Association (AMA). (2005). *Diagnostic and treatment guidelines on domestic violence*. Retrieved May 21, 2005 from the World Wide Web at http://www.ama-assn.org/ama/pub/category/3548.html

American Nurses Association (ANA). (1998). *Culturally competent assessment for family violence*. Washington, DC: American Nurses Publishing.

Bensley, L., VanEenwyk, J., & Wynkoop, K.S. (2003). Childhood family violence history and women's risk for intimate partner violence and poor health. *American Journal of Preventive Medicine, 25*(1), 38–44.

Burgess, A. (2004). Rape violence. *Nurse Spectrum/Nurseweek CE: Course 25*. Retrieved May 23, 2005 from the World Wide Web at http://www.nursingspectrum.com

Centers for Disease Control and Prevention (CDC). *Intimate partner violence: Fact sheet*. Retrieved May 21, 2005 from the World Wide Web at http://www.cdc.gov/ncipc/factsheets/ipvfacts.htm

Cummings, J.L., & Mega, M.S. (2003). *Neuropsychiatry and behavioral neuroscience*. New York: Oxford University Press.

Family Violence Law Center. (2003). *Why do women stay in violent relationships?* Retrieved May 22, 2005 from the World Wide Web at http://www.fvlc.org

Kennedy, B.P., Kawachi, I., Prothrow, S.D., Lochner, K., & Gupta, V. (1998). Social capital, income inequality, and firearm violent crime. *Social Science and Medicine, 47*(1), 7–17.

Lerner, M. (2005). *Adult manifestations of childhood sexual abuse*. New York: The American Academy of Experts in Traumatic Stress.

McCormack, J. (2002, May). Sexual offenders' perceptions of their early interpersonal relationships: An attachment perspective. *Journal of Sex Research, 39*(2), 85–93.

Meskill, J., & Conner, M. (2003). *Understanding and dealing with domestic violence against women*. Retrieved May 22, 2005 from the World Wide Web at http://www.oregoncounseling.org/

Murray, R.B., & Zentner, J.P. (2001). *Health promotion strategies through the life span* (7th ed.). Upper Saddle River, NJ: Prentice-Hall.

National Clearinghouse on Child Abuse and Neglect (NCCAN). (2004). *What is child abuse and neglect?* Retrieved May 22, 2005 from http://nccanch.acf.hhs.gov/pubs/factsheets/whatiscan.cfm

National Clearinghouse on Child Abuse and Neglect (NCCAN). (2003). *Recognizing child abuse and neglect: Signs and symptoms.* Retrieved May 22, 2005 from http://nccanch.acf.hhs.gov/pubs/factsheets/signs.cfm

National Coalition Against Domestic Violence. (2002a). *What is battering?* Retrieved May 3, 2002 from the World Wide Web at http://www.ncadv.org/problem/what.htm

National Coalition Against Domestic Violence. (2002b). *Why do women stay?* Retrieved May 3, 2002 from the World Wide Web at http://www.ncadv.org/problem/why2.htm

Reeves, C.R. (2003). *Childhood: It should not hurt.* Huntersville, NC: LTI Publishing.

Sadock, B.J., & Sadock, V.A. (2003). *Synopsis of psychiatry: Behavioral sciences/clinical psychiatry* (9th ed.). Philadelphia: Lippincott Williams & Wilkins.

Scully, D. (1994). *Understanding sexual violence: A study of convicted rapists.* New York: Routledge.

Siever, L.J. (2002, August). Neurobiology of impulsive-aggressive personality disordered patients. *Psychiatric Times, 19*(8): Online.

Tardiff, K.J. (2003). Violence. In R.E. Hales & S.C. Yudofsky (Eds.). *Textbook of clinical psychiatry* (4th ed.). Washington, DC: The American Psychiatric Publishing.

United States Bureau of Justice. (2003). *Intimate partner violence, 1993–2001.* Washington, DC: U.S. Department of Justice.

World Health Organization (WHO). (2005). The economic dimensions of interpersonal violence. Geneva, Switzerland: WHO.

CLASSICAL REFERENCES

Abrahamsen, D. (1960). *The psychology of crime.* New York: John Wiley & Sons.

Erikson, E.H. (1963). *Childhood and society* (2nd ed.). New York: W.W. Norton & Co.

Macdonald, J.M. (1971). *Rape: Offenders and their victims.* Springfield, IL: Charles C. Thomas.

Selye, H. (1956). *The stress of life.* New York: McGraw-Hill.

Walker, L.E. (1979). *The battered woman.* New York: Harper & Row.

MEN'S AND WOMEN'S HEALTH ISSUES

CHAPTER OUTLINE

OBJECTIVES
MEN'S HEALTH ISSUES
WOMEN'S HEALTH ISSUES

SUMMARY
REVIEW QUESTIONS

KEY TERMS

andropause
eclampsia
homocysteine

hormone replacement
   therapy (HRT)
menopause

osteoporosis
prostate-specific antigen
   (PSA)

OBJECTIVES

After reading this chapter, the student will be able to:

1. Identify the leading causes of death in men and women.
2. Discuss epidemiological statistics related to common physiological and psychological problems of men and women.
3. Describe risk factors for common physiological and psychological problems of men and women.
4. Discuss various modalities relevant to treatment of common physiological and psychological problems of men and women.
5. Identify gender differences as they pertain to common disorders of men and women.
6. Describe gender differences in the pharmacokinetics of medications.

Author's note: When my daughter came home from 5th grade health class with a note inviting mothers to view a film on menstruation with their daughters, an intense discussion ensued. "What is this word *menstruation*?" she asked. "It's the same thing that we sometimes call a *period*," I responded. She was satisfied for a few moments, then thoughtfully replied, "Hmmmm, menstruation. That's a funny name for it. Seems like it ought to be *women*struation!"

Indeed.

 nly until recently have women been included in clinical research trials. The results of studies on men were presumed to apply also to women. We are now learning, however, that there are differences in the way women and men respond to certain illnesses and also to the treatments. Research has shown that male and female brains develop somewhat differently after a certain point in fetal life, apparently leading to some differences in thinking and behavior.

It is true that physical and mental health issues are *human* issues. Throughout life, however, men and women face different developmental challenges. Men and women are socialized from the time of birth to respond to these challenges differently. Although they share many of the same health issues, the differences in gender responses are significant enough to warrant separate attention to each.

This chapter focuses on salient health issues specific to both genders. Physiological and psychosocial influences related to specific developmental stages are addressed. A number of treatment modalities are discussed.

MEN'S HEALTH ISSUES

Physiological Problems

Cardiovascular Disease

Cardiovascular disease is the leading cause of death among men of all ages and races in the United States (Centers for Disease Control [CDCa], 2005). Its prevalence increases with age, and it is most common in men ages 65 and older. Types of cardiovascular disease include coronary artery disease, myocardial infarction, valvular disease, cardiac dysrhythmias, congestive heart failure, angina pectoris, and hypertension.

Coronary Artery Disease

Coronary artery disease (CAD) affects about 13 million Americans (American Heart Association [AHA], 2005a). This disease occurs when the coronary arteries that feed the heart become narrowed by plaque and other fatty substances, blocking sufficient blood flow to the cardiac muscle. The arteries may be narrowed further by blood clots formed through platelet aggregation. When blood flow through the coronary arteries is insufficient, oxygen supply to the cardiac muscle is compromised. This may result in **angina pectoris**.

Angina Pectoris. Pain from angina pectoris has been described as a heaviness, pressure, squeezing, or burning type of pain. It is often mistaken for indigestion. The pain is usually felt in the chest, but may also occur in the left shoulder, arms, neck, throat, jaw, or back. It is commonly triggered by one of the "four E's": exertion, eating, excitement, or exposure to cold. Weakness, dizziness, nausea, shortness of breath, and palpitations may also be present. Duration is short (from 3 to 30 minutes), and relief usually occurs with rest or medication (Massie & Granger, 2005). Attacks lasting more than 30 minutes may suggest an alternative diagnosis, such as **myocardial infarction**.

Myocardial Infarction. Myocardial infarction (MI) results from prolonged (generally 30 minutes or longer) myocardial ischemia (Massie & Granger, 2005). The pain is similar to that of angina pectoris, but is more severe and is not relieved by rest or oral medications. Dyspnea, nausea and vomiting, arrhythmia, weakness, and extreme anxiety may be present. The goal of treatment is to provide rapid intervention and minimize heart muscle damage.

Risk Factors for Coronary Artery Disease

Risk factors for CAD may be categorized as modifiable (those that can be changed) and nonmodifiable (those that cannot be changed).

NONMODIFIABLE RISK FACTORS

- Family history. CAD occurring in parents or siblings predisposes an individual to the disease.
- Male gender. CAD is more common in men than in women, except after **menopause**.
- Age. The incidence of CAD increases with age.
- Race. African Americans have a greater risk for hypertension than whites, which may play a role in coronary artery disease.

MODIFIABLE RISK FACTORS

- Hyperlipidemia. Elevated levels of cholesterol and triglycerides are thought to predispose individuals to CAD. A low-fat diet or medications to decrease these levels may be prescribed.
- Smoking. Cigarette smoking as a single factor increases the risk of CAD. Acting with other factors, it increases the risk greatly. Smoking increases blood pressure, decreases exercise tolerance, and increases the tendency for blood to clot (AHA, 2005b).
- Hypertension. High blood pressure can cause damage to the lining of the coronary arteries and lead to CAD.
- Obesity. Obesity may be an indirect link to CAD in that it predisposes people to hypertension, diabetes, and hyperlipidemias.
- Carbohydrate intolerance. Individuals with diabetes mellitus often have increased lipid levels, obesity, and hypertension (Masharani, 2005). Control of hyperglycemia (linked to progression of CAD) through diet, exercise, and medications is vital in individuals with diabetes mellitus.
- Homocysteine. Elevated levels of homocysteine have been linked to increased risk of cardiovascular disease (Warren, 2002). Supplements of folic acid, vitamin B_{12}, and vitamin B_6 should be taken by individuals with hyper-homocysteinemia.
- Type A personality. Time management and relaxation exercises may be helpful for individuals with a predisposition to CAD. (See Chapter 36.)
- Depression. Research over the past two decades has shown that people with heart disease are more likely to suffer from depression than otherwise healthy people, and conversely, that people with depression are at greater risk for developing heart disease (National Institute of Mental Health [NIMH], 2002). People with heart disease who are depressed have an increased risk of death after a heart attack compared to those who are not depressed. Treatment for depression helps people manage both diseases, thus enhancing survival and quality of life.

To prevent or reduce the progression of CAD, strategies that target the modifiable risk factors are of prime importance. Examples include: (1) following a diet that is low in fat and high in foods such as fruits, vegetables, and whole-grain products that are naturally low in fat and high in complex carbohydrates and fiber and (2) cessation of smoking or never starting; the risk of heart disease decreases rapidly after quitting and almost returns to that of baseline in 2 to 3 years (Cundiff, 2002). Cessation of smoking is also important in the control of high blood pressure. Additional factors in the control of hypertension include limiting salt intake, keeping weight at an appropriate level, exercising regularly, reducing excessive alcohol consumption, and practicing relaxation techniques. The physician may determine that some individuals require medication to lower serum lipid levels or to maintain blood pressure within normal limits. An antidepressant may be helpful for those individuals who experience chronic depression. A daily dose of aspirin, which has been shown to be beneficial for some individuals in reducing the risk of CAD, is sometimes prescribed for men over 50.

Neoplastic Disease

The second leading cause of death in men is neoplastic disease. Ranked according to type of cancer, lung, prostate, and colon are first through third, respectively (National Cancer Institute [NCI], 2005a).

Signs and symptoms of lung cancer may be insidious and are often related to location of the tumor. Common warning signals include persistent cough, blood in the sputum; unexplained weight loss; fatigue; chest, shoulder, back, or arm pain; or any change in respiratory patterns (York, 2005). Shortness of breath and a unilateral wheeze are common. The primary risk factor for this type of cancer is cigarette smoking, particularly for 20 years or more. Exposure to substances such as arsenic, asbestos, and certain organic chemicals has also been implicated. Treatment of lung cancer consists of surgery, chemotherapy, or radiation, alone or in combination.

African American men have a higher rate of prostate cancer than white men. It is uncommon before age 50, but the incidence increases steadily thereafter (Stoller & Carroll, 2005). Often no signs or symptoms associated with the disease appear until late in its progression, when problems with voiding may occur. Risk factors for the disease are unconfirmed, but determinants such as high-fat diet, hormonal changes, viral infections, and industrial exposure to cadmium have been implicated. Regular screening examinations and a blood test called **prostatic-specific antigen (PSA)** are important for early detection. Treatment of prostate cancer consists of hormonal therapy, radiation therapy (either by external beam or by implant), or surgical resection of the prostate gland. Radical prostatectomy in which perineal nerves are severed generally leaves the client impotent. Nerve-sparing procedures, using a retropubic approach, may be used in cases in which the nerves are not involved. When these procedures are used, erec-

tile capability may be interrupted, but the majority of men regain potency within a few months (Chuang et al., 2005).

Testicular cancer, although not common, is on the increase. It is more common in white men than in African Americans. Two to three men per 100,000 have testicular cancer (NCI, 2005a). Testicular cancer generally appears as a painless nodule. Symptoms such as back pain, cough, or weight loss only occur with advanced disease, which presents a poor prognosis. Risk factors are unknown, although testicular cancer is more common in men who live in rural than in urban areas and in men born with undescended testes. Regular monthly self-examinations of the testes are extremely important for early detection of this disease. If detected and treated early, there is a 90 to 100 percent chance of cure. In early stages, treatment consists of surgical removal of the testicle and nearby lymph nodes. Removal of only one testicle maintains fertility and erectile capability. In later stages of the disease, radiation, chemotherapy, or both also may be administered.

Erectile Dysfunction

Erectile dysfunction (ED), also called *impotence*, can be a total inability to achieve erection, an inconsistent ability to do so, an inability to maintain erections, or the inability to control ejaculation (Perry & Schacht, 2001). This condition affects about 30 million men in the United States. The incidence of ED increases with age, affecting about 35 percent of men older than 65 years of age. It is not necessarily a consequence of aging, however. ED may be caused by vascular changes, including atherosclerosis, high blood pressure, and elevated cholesterol levels; nervous system conditions, such as multiple sclerosis and Alzheimer's disease; endocrine and hormone imbalances, such as diabetes, thyroid disease, or a low level of testosterone; spinal cord injuries and prostate surgeries; smoking; and certain medications, such as antihypertensives and antidepressants (Sisson, 2004). Psychological problems, such as stress, anxiety, guilt, low self-esteem, depression and unsatisfactory relationships, can also be contributing factors. Following initial episodes of ED, fear of sexual failure can have a compounding effect on the problem.

Treatments for ED may include counseling or sex therapy for any emotional problems that may be contributing to the condition. Oral medications, such as the phosphodiesterase type 5 inhibitors (e.g., sildenafil [Viagra], tadalafil [Cialis], and vardenafil [Levitra]) and yohimbine; hormone therapy with testosterone; and injectable medications, such as papaverine or prostaglandin, are effective for some men. For those individuals who are refractory to these medical treatments, surgery to implant a penile prosthesis is available.

Andropause

Is there really a *male menopause*? Most clinicians would respond that there is. Whether it is referred to as male menopause, male climacteric, or the newer term **andropause**, the phenomenon describes the effects of age-related androgen decrease.

Levels of testosterone fall gradually from middle age, and decrease by as much as 50 percent between the ages of 25 and 75 years (Gould, Petty, & Jacobs, 2000). In women, menopause comes on fairly rapidly, around age 45 or 50. It is clearly linked to the cessation of ovulation and a precipitous fall in estrogen concentration.

In addition to aging, several other factors may be associated with diminished testosterone levels (hypotestosteronemia). These include a history of orchitis, testicular trauma, chemotherapy, radiation therapy, malnutrition, physical and psychological stress, alcohol abuse, and obesity (Gould, Petty, & Jacobs, 2000; Vetrosky & Aliabadi, 2002).

Signs and symptoms of andropause vary and are related to the variances in testosterone levels among men. Some common signs and symptoms are listed in Table 41–1. Diamond (2002) states:

As a result of [testosterone] decline, erections take longer to occur and are not quite as firm as they once were. The urge to ejaculate is not as insistent as it once was, and the force of ejaculation is weaker. Men also experience a decline in lean muscle mass and a tendency to put on weight. Aches and pains become more pervasive. Some men complain of anxiety or insomnia. Full-blown depression often occurs, although feelings of anger and frustration are more common. Men report that "everything seems to bother them," while their wives complain that their husbands "used to be loving and gentle, but now there's no pleasing" them. (pp. 7–8)

Symptomatic andropause is treated with testosterone replacement therapy (TRT). About 5 percent of men in the United States receive this therapy (Vetrosky & Aliabdi, 2002). TRT appears to restore libido and sexual functioning and improves bone mass, muscle mass, and strength in older men (Rhoden & Morgentaler, 2004). It is available in oral, intramuscular, gel, and transdermal patch preparations. TRT is not without adverse effects. It has been associated with benign prostatic hyperplasia,

increased levels of PSA, and growth of prostate cancer, if present. Other potential adverse effects include hepatotoxicity (with oral forms), gynecomastia, infertility, and aggressive behavior (especially when physiologic doses are exceeded) (Vetrosky & Aliabadi, 2002). TRT can be beneficial for some men who are experiencing symptoms of andropause; however, follow-up and regular monitoring of testosterone levels should be considered. Digital rectal exam should be performed every 6 months, PSA levels checked, and treatment efficacy and adverse effects reviewed (Rhoden & Morgentaler, 2004).

Psychosocial Problems

A substantial body of research has revealed gender differences in attitudes toward psychotherapy (Mosher, 2002). Surveys show that women express more positive help-seeking views than men do, and that women report a higher tolerance of the social stigma associated with obtaining psychotherapy than men. Women seek counseling about twice as frequently as men.

Depression

Depression affects nearly 10 percent of the population (National Institute of Mental Health [NIMH], 2001). Only one in three people who suffer from depression actually seek help from the medical profession, and the majority of these are women. Our culture is largely to blame for this phenomenon. Men are reared to believe that expressing emotions is largely a feminine trait, and that to express feelings in a vulnerable manner denotes weakness or unmanliness.

Symptoms of depression in men are hardly recognizable as such. Men may demonstrate feelings of depression with displaced anger, substance abuse, or social withdrawal. Cultural norms teach men that they must remain in control. They are more likely than women to express anger; women are more likely to hold anger in and become depressed.

Even the therapy for depression is often seen as feminine. Talking about problems and expressing emotions is much more common among women than it is among men. Fredric Rabinowitz, a psychologist at the University of Redlands, who leads a men's support group, states (Shaw, 2005):

Men tend to downplay emotional distress. They express depression differently [than women]. They have a long way to go in acknowledging depression. A lot of men come into therapy coerced. A partner says, "If you don't get help, I'm leaving." Or the relationship has already blown up. Typically, it has to get pretty bad for a man to come in on his own.

Men do experience depression, and it is vitally important that health care providers recognize the behaviors

TABLE 41–1	**Signs and Symptoms of Andropause**
Depression	Nervousness
Hot flashes	Night sweats
Decreased libido	Erectile dysfunction
Decreased muscle mass	Decreased strength
Easily fatigued	Lethargy
Increased irritability	Decreased visuospatial ability
Mood swings	Weight gain
Insomnia	Decreased bone density

SOURCES: Diamond (2002); Vetrosky & Aliabadi (2002); and Gould, Petty, & Jacobs (2000).

associated with male depression. A recent study by Johns Hopkins medical students found that depressed men were twice as likely as their nondepressed counterparts to develop heart disease or die suddenly because of heart problems (Mann, 2000). And men with depression commit suicide at much higher rates than women, although more women attempt it. Because relatively few men seek medical assistance for primary depression (the primary problem), it is important for health care providers to screen men for secondary depression. That is, when men seek medical care for a physical condition, the mental status should also be considered. This may be the only means to depression therapy for this large segment of the population.

Suicide

Suicide is the eighth leading cause of death among men of all ages and races in the United States (CDCa, 2005). Women attempt suicide more often than men, but men are four times more likely to die as a result than women (CDC, 2004). This is thought to relate to the type of method used. Men tend to select more lethal methods, such as guns, whereas women choose to swallow pills, a method in which a buffer of time is available for rescue.

In 2002, white men accounted for more than half of all suicides in the United States (National Center for Health Statistics, 2004). In fact, the profile for the highest rate of suicides is a white man, over the age of 85, living alone, who has just experienced a significant loss. Most individuals who kill themselves have a diagnosable mental or substance abuse disorder or both, and the majority have depressive illness (CDC, 2005b).

These statistics are strikingly consistent throughout the world and across cultures. Global distribution statistics provided by the World Health Organization (WHO, 2002) indicates that in all countries suicide is significantly more prevalent among men, and that after age 65, the suicide rate for men increases dramatically.

More than 90 percent of people who kill themselves have a treatable mental disorder, commonly a depressive disorder or a substance abuse disorder (CDC, 2005b). Although effective treatments for depression are readily available, there has not been a significant reduction in the suicide rate in the United States, particularly in men over 65. Andersen and colleagues (2000) report that many individuals who commit suicide have visited a physician within a week or a month of their death, some even on the day of the suicide. Health care practitioners may not be satisfactorily evaluating suicide potential during routine office visits by this high-risk population of older men. Routine screening for depression and suicide potential may be the only means of reaching these individuals, who often resist seeking assistance for this common mental health problem.

Substance Use Disorders

In 2002, men accounted for more than two thirds of the admissions for substance abuse treatment (Office of National Drug Control Policy [ONDCP], 2005). Information from the 2003 National Survey on Drug Use and Health (Substance Abuse and Mental Health Services Administration [SAMHSA], 2005) revealed that men are more likely than women to be users of alcohol. About 6 percent of adults were classified as heavy drinkers, somewhat more men than women. Women were about twice as likely as men to be lifetime abstainers. Current drinking was most prevalent in the 25- to 44-year-old age group of white college educated men. Prevalence declined steadily with age from 45 years on.

A recent research study concluded that longer stays in alcohol and drug treatment lead to better posttreatment results, and that factors leading to a successful stay in treatment differ by gender (Mertens & Weisner, 2000). For women, positive predictors for staying in treatment included being unemployed, being married, having higher incomes, and having lower levels of psychiatric severity relative to those who dropped out. For men, the variables associated with staying in treatment were being older, receiving employer pressure to enter treatment, and having a goal to abstain from drinking and drug use. The results of this study indicate both professional and practical applications. Mertens and Weisner (2000) state:

> Clinicians may be able to identify patients who are at risk of dropping out of treatment. Providers might offer some psychiatric services or psychiatric referrals for women with psychiatric problems or motivational enhancement therapy for men who need to increase their motivation levels. Furthermore, people who are entering treatment, as well as their families and friends, may benefit by becoming aware of those risk factors associated with dropping out and plan accordingly.

Men also have a higher rate of illicit drug use and tobacco use than women (SAMHSA, 2005). This is true in all age groups except for 12- to 17-year-olds, in which the gender differences were smaller.

Men tend to drink more frequently in groups and in public, whereas women more often drink privately and alone. Many people drink moderately with no negative impact on their lives. Research has suggested that for some people a glass of wine a day may even be beneficial in preventing heart disease. When, then, can alcohol use be considered a problem? Following are some standard guidelines:

- Using alcohol or drugs for relief when faced with a problem
- Neglecting responsibilities because of substance use
- Drinking or taking drugs first thing in the morning
- Increasing the amount of substance used to achieve the desired effect

- Feeling guilty about substance use and/or concealing it from others
- Experiencing undesirable physical or psychological effects when attempting to decrease intake or abstain from substance use
- Driving (or being arrested for driving) while under the influence of a substance
- Experiencing memory deficits for a period of time while under the influence of a substance

Any of these behaviors might indicate a need for treatment of a substance abuse problem. As was stated previously, men resist seeking medical treatment. They are more likely than women to deny that they have a medical problem. Nurses and other health care providers can be instrumental in assessing this high-risk population for substance abuse problems and targeting them for programs of treatment and rehabilitation.

WOMEN'S HEALTH ISSUES

Physiological Problems

Cardiovascular Disease

Cardiovascular disease is widely thought of as a disease of men; however, it is the leading cause of death in women and after menopause, the prevalence of cardiovascular disease is similar to that of men (Crandall, 2005). African American women are twice as likely to die from coronary artery disease (CAD) than are European American women. Yet, many women still do not consider cardiovascular disease to be a personal health threat.

Risk factors for cardiovascular disease in women are similar to those for men. They include family history of the disease, diabetes mellitus, hypertension, hyperlipidemia, obesity, and smoking. Some studies indicate that more women than men have diabetes, hypertension, and hyperlipidemia (Hansen, 2002). A sedentary lifestyle is also a contributing factor for CAD in some women. Repressed anger, high-level role stress, and depression also have been identified as contributing factors.

Cardiac symptoms may appear differently in women than in men. Women are more likely than men to complain initially of nonexertional chest pain or pain in the jaw, arms, shoulder, back, or epigastric area. Women are also more likely than men to complain of shortness of breath, palpitations, feelings of faintness, or nausea and fatigue (Hansen, 2002).

Because heart disease often does not occur in women until after menopause, women tend to be on the average about 10 years older than men when these problems arise. Hanson (2002) states, "Her advanced age is considered to be the most significant factor in increased cardiac mortality, decreased efficacy of thrombolytics and aspirin, and a tendency toward the underuse of these

medications in women." Advanced age also may be a factor in higher mortality rates from cardiac disease and surgery in women than in men.

In younger women, a concern may exist regarding the effects of oral contraceptives as a risk factor for cardiac disease. Early on, oral contraceptives contained high doses of estrogen and progesterone, a factor that was considered to promote thrombosis. Currently, most oral contraceptives utilize much lower doses of these hormones, reducing the risk of dangerous blood clot formation. However, the risk still exists in women over the age of 35 who smoke and take high-level estrogen contraceptives (Hanson, 2002).

Hormone replacement therapy (HRT) remains a controversial issue among postmenopausal women. Historically, HRT had been thought to have protective factors for menopausal women against coronary heart disease, dementia, and osteoporosis. Recent research has suggested otherwise. The Women's Health Initiative (WHI) is a long-term study by the National Institutes of Health targeting women ages 50 to 79, and focusing on HRT, dietary and lifestyle modifications, and health and risk factors associated with specific disease outcomes. The study will continue for several more years, but began to close down one arm of the investigation in 2002. The combination hormone pill (estrogen plus progestin) was found be associated with an increased risk of breast cancer, stroke, coronary heart disease, and ovarian cancer (WHI, 2005). The positive results included a decrease in endometrial cancer, an increase in bone density and overall decrease in fractures, and a decrease in risk for colorectal cancer.

Women participating in the study who had undergone hysterectomy and did not take the combination pill, but took estrogen therapy alone, continued the study until 2004, when they, too, were asked to stop the HRT. This arm of the study also showed both positive and negative results. Women on estrogen alone showed an increased risk for stroke and increased risk of thrombosis. Estrogen alone did not appear to offer protection against decline in cognitive functioning or colon cancer. Positively, there appeared to be no increase in the risk of breast cancer, and the results indicated some protection against osteoporosis (WIH, 2005). The study continues until 2010, so additional conclusions will be forthcoming.

Prevention of heart disease in women calls for educational programs to modify those risk factors for the disease. Women must have knowledge about the importance of a low-fat diet, adequate physical exercise, maintaining a healthy weight, and not smoking. They should have sufficient information to make appropriate personal choices about whether to take HRT. Hansen (2002) states:

Greater awareness on the part of both the lay public and health care professionals is needed if professionals are to identify women at risk for developing cardiac disease and to help them make good use of preventative measures. Professionals also need to make efforts to educate and counsel women regarding the risks of cardiac disease. (p. 432)

Neoplastic Disease

The second leading cause of death in women is neoplastic disease (CDC, 2005a). Lung and bronchial cancer are the leading cause of cancer-related death in women in the United States (NCI, 2005a).

Lung Cancer. The primary risk factor for lung cancer in women is cigarette smoking. Dr. David Satcher, past Surgeon General of the United States has stated:

When calling attention to public health problems, we must not misuse the word "epidemic." But there is no better word to describe the 600 percent increase since 1950 in women's death rates for lung cancer, a disease primarily caused by cigarette smoking. Clearly, smoking-related disease among women is a full-blown epidemic. (CDC, 2001)

With the large amount of information being dispersed about the negative effects of cigarette smoking, tobacco use is on the decline. However, women are not quitting in the same numbers as men. Statistics show that 23 percent of women smoked cigarettes in 2003 (SAMHSA, 2005). Prevalence is highest among white women with less than a high school education. In 2003, 22 percent of high school girls were current smokers (American Lung Association [ALA], 2004).

Other risk factors for lung cancer in women include exposure to radon, asbestos, certain industrial substances and organic chemicals, radiation exposure, air pollution, tuberculosis, and secondhand tobacco smoke in non-smokers (Chen & Kunkel, 2002). Treatment for lung cancer consists of surgery, chemotherapy, or radiation, individually or in combination, depending on the stage of the cancer.

Breast Cancer. Breast cancer is the most common form of cancer in women and the second leading cause of cancer-related death (NCI, 2005a). The lifetime risk of contracting breast cancer is 1 in 8, and the risk increases with advancing age (NCI, 2005b).

Meier (2005) identifies the following risk factors for breast cancer:

● Female gender (99 percent of all breast cancers occur in women)
● Age 50 years or older
● Early menarche or late menopause or both
● Being childless or having first child after the age of 30
● Mother or sister having had breast cancer

The incidence of breast cancer has been rising for the past three decades, while mortality from breast cancer has declined steadily (NCI, 2005a). Breast cancer is not a lethal disease for the majority of women. Education about the importance of breast self-examination and screening with mammography have led to increased incidence of early detection and successful treatment for many women.

Early-stage tumors of the breast are usually symptomless and can be detected only by physical examination of the breast or by mammogram. Benign tumors are usually painless, have well-defined margins, and are moveable. Malignant tumors also are usually painless, hard, irregularly shaped, and nonmobile (Craft, 2005). The skin over the malignant area may become "dimpled," and there may be some retraction of the nipple. Differential diagnosis is made by tissue examination obtained through needle biopsy or excisional biopsy.

Treatment of breast cancer consists of chemotherapy, hormonal therapy, radiation therapy, surgery, or a combination. Surgical options include lumpectomy (removal of the tumor and small margin of normal tissue) or mastectomy (removal of the entire breast, axillary lymph nodes, and overlying skin) (Craft, 2005). Other breast-preservation procedures, such as partial mastectomy and wedge resection, also are possible.

A great deal of psychological discomfort is associated with the experience of breast cancer and its treatment. Loss of a breast inevitably initiates a grief response in the individual. Anger, anxiety, depression, and fear of recurrence are common emotional responses. Disturbances in body image sometimes occur, and may result in marital or sexual disruption. Chen and Kunkel (2002) state:

The life stage at which the cancer occurs, previous emotional stability, and the presence of interpersonal supports are key factors in the psychosocial adaptation to [breast cancer]. Studies suggest that patients with breast cancer who use an active problem-solving approach to the stresses of illness and exhibit flexibility in their coping efforts are less distressed and adapt better. (p. 371)

Group interventions have been shown to be helpful to breast cancer patients. Being able to express anger and other emotions in a group of individuals who have experienced the same illness and treatment procedures can be extremely beneficial. Chen and Kunkel (2002) state, "A shared group experience can help minimize the negative impact of illness on recovery and well-being."

Gynecological Issues

The Reproductive Cycle

Menstruation. The average age at menarche, or the initial menstrual period, in the United States is 12.8 years (Carroll, 2005). Most women begin to menstruate by the time they are 16 years old. Menstruation is the physical condition that initiates reproductive preparedness in a woman. During the menstrual cycle, increased levels of estrogen and progesterone serve to build up and thicken the lining of the uterus in preparation for receiving a fertilized ovum from the ovary. If the ovum is fertilized, it is implanted in the lining of the uterus. If fertilization does not occur, hormone levels decrease, and the lining of the uterus is sloughed off during menstruation.

Premenstrual Syndrome (PMS) and Premenstrual Dysphoric Disorder (PMDD). It is estimated that up to 80 percent of all women experience some combination of emotional, physical, or behavioral symptoms in the week prior to menstruation (Burt & Hendrick, 2005). Some of the symptoms of PMS include tension and migraine headaches, irritability, food cravings, breast tenderness, bloating, weight gain, anxiety, diarrhea, feeling overwhelmed by the stresses of everyday life, and sadness.

A somewhat more severe form of the syndrome, which is referred to as premenstrual dysphoric disorder, occurs in 3 to 8 percent of menstruating women (Burt & Hendrick, 2005). The *Diagnostic and Statistical Manual of Mental Disorders* [DSM-IV-TR] (APA, 2000) lists the following symptoms for PMDD: depression, self-deprecating thoughts, anxiety, mood swings, anger or irritability, decreased interest in usual activities, difficulty concentrating, fatigue, appetite changes, food cravings, hypersomnia or insomnia, and other physical symptoms, such as breast tenderness or swelling, headaches, joint or muscle pain, a sensation of "bloating," and weight gain.

An imbalance of the hormones estrogen and progesterone has been implicated in the predisposition to premenstrual dysphoric disorder. It has been postulated that excess estrogen or a high estrogen-to-progesterone ratio during the luteal phase may be associated with the symptoms of PMDD (Burt & Hendrick, 2005; Sadock & Sadock, 2003). Abnormal prostaglandin activity has also been implicated (Sadock & Sadock, 2003).

A number of nutritional alterations have also been indicated in the etiology of premenstrual dysphoric disorder. They include deficiencies in the B vitamins, calcium, magnesium, manganese, vitamin E, and linolenic acid (Frackiewicz & Shiovitz, 2001). Glucose tolerance fluctuations, abnormal fatty acid metabolism, and sensitivity to caffeine and alcohol may also play a role in bringing about the symptoms associated with this disorder.

First-line treatment for PMDD is with lifestyle changes, such as diet modifications (reducing salt, caffeine, and alcohol intake), stress-reduction techniques, exercise, counseling, and education. For those women who do not respond to lifestyle changes, pharmacotherapy with a selective serotonin reuptake inhibitor (SSRI) antidepressant is the treatment of choice. Fluoxetine (Sarafem), paroxetine (Paxil), and sertraline (Zoloft) have been approved by the FDA for treatment of PMDD. Some women have experienced relief from the symptoms of PMS and PMDD with herbal medications. Some of these are listed in Table 41–2.

Pregnancy. Pregnancy is a profoundly personal and social event, significant for the prospective mother and all the people in her life. Many variables enter into whether the pregnancy is a positive or negative experience for the woman. Some of these include: whether the pregnancy was planned or unplanned, the age and health of the mother, and the relationship between the mother and the father.

The pregnancy rate for U.S. women declined during the decade from 1990 to 2000 (Ventura et al., 2004). The teenage pregnancy rate fell 27 percent during this period. Preliminary findings indicate that the pregnancy rate increased in 2003 for those women age 30 and older. From 2002 to 2003, there was an increase of 4 percent for women aged 30 to 34, an increase of 6 percent for ages 35 to 39, and an increase of 5 percent for women ages 40 to 44 years (Hamilton, Martin, & Sutton, 2004).

Among the factors believed to be driving the downturn in teen pregnancies are increases in condom use, the adoption of the effective injectable and implant contraceptives, and the leveling off of teen sexual activity.

TABLE 41–2	**Herbals Used for Symptoms of Premenstrual Syndrome**	
HERBAL	**PRECAUTIONS/ADVERSE EFFECTS**	**CONTRAINDICATIONS**
Black cohosh (*Cimicifuga racemosa*)	May potentiate the effects of antihypertensive medications. Some individuals may experience nausea or headache.	Pregnancy
Bugleweed (*Lycopus virginicus*)	No side effects known. Should not be taken concomitantly with thyroid preparations.	Thyroid disease
Chaste tree (*Vitex agnus-castus*)	Occasional rashes may occur. Should not be taken concomitantly with dopamine-receptor antagonists.	Pregnancy and lactation
Evening primrose (*Oenothera biennis*)	May lower the seizure threshold. Should not be taken concomitantly with other drugs that lower the seizure threshold.	
Potentilla (*Potentilla anserine*)	May cause stomach irritation.	
Shepherd's purse (*Capsella bursa-pastoris*)	No side effects known.	Pregnancy
Valerian (*Valeriana officinalis*)	With long-term use: headache, restless states, sleeplessness, mydriasis, disorders of cardiac function. Should not be taken concomitantly with CNS depressants.	Pregnancy and lactation

SOURCE: *PDR for Herbal Medicines* (2nd ed.), 2000.

Economic opportunities have given women a reason to more highly value education and work. Many women are delaying pregnancies in an effort to attain the educational and occupational goals in a growing economy. Thus, more women in their 30s and 40s are currently having babies.

Pregnant women who are older are at higher risk for certain problems during pregnancy than are younger women. Hypertension is more common in pregnant women over forty. This is commonly managed with diet, salt restriction, and exercise. However, medication may be prescribed if the situation becomes critical.

Preeclampsia, also called *toxemia*, is manifested by hypertension, edema, rapid weight gain, and the spilling of protein in the urine (Crombleholme, 2005). The condition usually occurs during the last 6 weeks of the pregnancy. Preeclampsia can lead to **eclampsia**, which is a more serious condition that is characterized by extremely high blood pressure, blurred vision, severe abdominal pain, headaches, and convulsions. Uncontrolled eclampsia can be fatal (Crombleholme, 2005). Treatment is with bed rest and fetal monitoring. Jeopardy to the fetus or mother may result in early delivery.

Older pregnant women are at higher risk for gestational diabetes, a situational condition that occurs only during pregnancy. Gestational diabetes is usually diagnosed around the beginning of the third trimester. The condition is generally not serious; however, diagnosis and appropriate monitoring of mother and baby is critical. A Cesarean section delivery may need to be performed if the baby is very large. This condition occurs when the increase in placental hormones produced to preserve the pregnancy block the production of insulin by the pancreas. Following delivery, when the placental hormones are removed, gestational diabetes usually disappears (Fain, 2005).

The risk of bearing a child with Down syndrome increases with age. The probability is 1 in 365 for a woman over age 35. Some women choose to have amniocentesis or some other form of genetic testing. With amniocentesis, approximately 80 metabolic diseases can be detected, although unless family history reveals a risk of a specific genetic abnormality, only chromosomal analysis and alpha-fetoprotein measurement will be conducted (Pyeritz, 2005). It is essential that a man and woman prepare in advance for the possible results of amniocentesis. That is, they should have a discussion (with the physician and alone) about continuing the pregnancy based on the results of the test. This anticipatory discussion will help to prepare them emotionally.

The decision to terminate a pregnancy can be a traumatic experience. Parents feel angry, guilty, and grief stricken. It may be the hardest decision a woman or couple are ever forced to make, and they will need a great deal of support from significant others. Burt and Hendrick (2005) state:

> Women should be given ample opportunity to express their feelings. After the decision to abort an abnormal fetus, women may experience mourning for the loss of a wished-for baby, and they often benefit from bereavement counseling. In some cases, guilt for having produced a deformed fetus may require sensitive exploration and resolution. (p. 109)

It is extremely important that the couple be allowed and encouraged to grieve. They have experienced a profound loss and they must deal in a healthy manner with the myriad of feelings that are associated with the grief response. This also relates to individuals who experience spontaneous abortion, or *miscarriage*. The loss of a baby is a tragedy, and its grief must be respected. Burt and Hendrick (2005) state:

> Couples who have sustained a pregnancy loss need to work through their bereavement in a safe place where fears can be discussed, disappointments addressed, and grief experienced. For couples who are feeling isolated and alienated, [psychotherapy] may be able to provide an opportunity for such processes to occur. (p. 112)

Twelve to 24 percent of pregnancies result in miscarriage (Burt & Hendrick, 2005). Women who experience this type of loss are at high risk for anxiety, depression, and somatization in the 6 months following the event. Guilt related to feelings of "having done something to cause" the miscarriage may contribute to these symptoms. In addition, variance in the timing of intense feelings on the part of the couple may result in their becoming alienated from one another. Clinicians must be aware of and sensitive to these possibilities.

Menopause. Menopause is technically defined as the cessation of menses due to the loss of ovarian function (Burt & Hendrick, 2005). *Perimenopause* is the interval between regular menstrual cycles and complete cessation of ovarian function. Perimenopause may last as long as 10 years (Null, 2002). Estrogen levels may begin to decline as early as the mid-30s. Symptoms of perimenopause generally begin sometime in the 40s. Symptoms include irregular menstrual cycles, hot flashes, night sweats, sleep disturbances, vaginal dryness, depression, irritability, and mood swings (Null, 2002). Some women experience a gradual decline in libido during this period. The cause may be hormonal, but can also be due to other life stresses and how the individual views getting older. Burt and Hendrick (2005) state:

> Most women who have been sexually active before menopause remain so during the perimenopausal years. Nevertheless, estrogen decline associated with perimenopause may produce dyspareunia and decreased libido. Other factors that may impair sexual function include diminished sexual desire, chronic health problems, depression, anxiety, medication effects, partner unavailability, relationship conflicts, or sexual dysfunction in the partner. (p. 132)

Bone loss, leading to osteoporosis, and increasing cholesterol and triglyceride levels, putting the woman at risk for heart disease, are two potentially serious problems associated with the menopausal and postmenopausal years. Some women may experience depression during this period, but it is more common in women who have a history of PMS and who have experienced depression prior to menopause (Burt & Hendrick, 2005).

Treatment for relief of menopausal symptoms is determined on an individual basis. HRT has been used (and is still used by many) to relieve the symptoms of perimenopause. The concerns and benefits of this therapy were discussed previously in the section addressing cardiovascular disease. Table 41–3 identifies potential capabilities of HRT. Some general guidelines that may be beneficial in alleviating some of the common symptoms of perimenopause include the following:

For hot flashes: Limit caffeine intake (e.g., coffee, tea, cola drinks, chocolate), alcohol intake, sugar, spicy foods, hot soups, and hot drinks. Large meals may also trigger hot flashes, so it may be helpful to consume several smaller meals instead. Some women find that a daily vitamin B-complex tablet and 400 IU of vitamin E are beneficial. Dressing in layers and sleeping in a cool room also may provide some relief.

For vaginal dryness: In addition to the aging process, some medications, such as antihistamines, may contribute to vaginal dryness. Water-based lubricants, used at the time of intercourse, may be helpful. Some women have found some relief with vitamin E suppositories or low-dose estrogen or testosterone creams.

For loss of bone density: 1000 to 1500 milligrams per day of calcium, consumed in a calcium-rich diet or taken in the form of a supplement, is important to prevent loss of bone density. Weight-bearing (e.g., walking) and strength-building exercises also have been shown to be beneficial. Null (2002) states:

Weight-bearing aerobic exercises such as brisk walking, jogging, stair climbing, and dancing produce mechanical stress on the skeletal system, which drives calcium into the long bones. Non-weight-bearing aerobic exercises such as biking, rowing, and swimming are not as helpful in osteoporosis prevention, but they do promote flexibility, which is useful for people prone to arthritis. (p. 452)

Medication also is now available for the treatment and prevention of osteoporosis in postmenopausal women. These include alendronate (Fosamax), risedronate (Actonel), and raloxifene (Evista).

For hyperlipidemia: Although one's heredity for cardiovascular disease is a nonmodifiable factor, adopting a low-fat, high-fiber diet that is rich in fruits, vegetables, and whole grains may provide some benefit. Antihyperlipidemic medications may be required for more problematic cases.

Depression: Treatment of depression in perimenopausal

TABLE 41–3	Estrogen Therapy for the Menopausal Woman
WHAT ESTROGEN *CAN* DO	WHAT ESTROGEN *CANNOT* DO
Relieve vaginal dryness	Prevent/cure depression
Relieve hot flashes	Prevent weight gain
Reduce bone loss	Delay the aging process
Protect against colorectal cancer	

SOURCE: Women's Health Initiative (2005) and Rossouw & Anderson (2002).

women includes the usual treatment modalities: psychotherapy and pharmacotherapy. The serotonin reuptake inhibitors (SSRIs) are used to treat both the depressive and vasomotor symptoms of perimenopause. Some research has shown that estrogen therapy has been helpful in the treatment of perimenopausal depression. However, it is not recommended as primary treatment for depression, particularly in light of the concerns expressed by the WHI. Burt and Hendrick (2005) state:

The perimenopausal woman should be encouraged to discuss other sources of stress [that may be contributing to depression], including possible interpersonal stress, changing sexuality on her part or that of her partner, new-onset health problems, shifting role expectations, and new responsibilities, such as caring for aging and ill parents. In addition to individual psychotherapy, important aspects of treatment include referrals to caregiver support groups, assistance with obtaining financial support, and attention to chronic medical problems. (p. 140)

Psychosocial Problems

Depression

Depression is about twice as common in women as it is in men (APA, 2000). Hormonal factors related to the reproductive cycle may play a role in women's increased vulnerability to depression (Kornstein & Wojcik, 2002). During the luteal phase of the menstrual cycle, a period associated with dysphoric mood changes, there is a withdrawal of both estrogen and progesterone. Premenstrual dysphoric disorder occurs in about 5 percent of women.

Approximately 80 percent of women experience mild depressive symptoms in the postpartum period. Ten to 15 percent suffer from a more severe postpartum depression, and this is more common in women who have a prior history of mood disorder (Kornstein & Wojcik, 2002). Kornstein and Wojcik (2002) state, "A woman who has experienced a postpartum depression is at risk for future episodes of depression, both in association with and independent of reproductive events. The risk of a subsequent postpartum episode may exceed 50 percent" (p. 149).

The Edinburgh Postnatal Depression Scale (EPDS) was developed to assist primary care health professionals to detect mothers suffering from postpartum depression. The validation study showed that mothers who scored above 92.3 percent were likely to be suffering from a depressive illness of varying severity. The score on this depression scale and a careful clinical assessment can be used to confirm the diagnosis of postpartum depression. The EPDS is presented in Table 41–4.

A number of other factors have been implicated in the vulnerability of women to depression. From very early in life, developmental socialization processes reflect gender differences in coping styles and methods of processing emotional stimuli. Kornstein and Wojcik (2002) state:

> Parents and teachers tend to have different expectations of girls and boys, which may result in girls' becoming more nurturing and more concerned with the evaluations of others, and in boys' developing a greater sense of mastery and independence. Such stereotypical gender socialization is hypothesized to lead to differences in self-concept and vulnerability to depression. (p. 150)

More women than men have a tendency to become depressed following major stressful life events (Harvard Medical School, 2004). Living in poverty, being single

---

TABLE 41–4   The Edinburgh Postnatal Depression Scale (EPDS)

Instructions for users:
1. The mother is asked to underline the response that comes closest to how she has been feeling in the previous 7 days.
2. All ten items must be completed.
3. Care should be taken to avoid the possibility of the mother discussing her answers with others.
4. The mother should complete the scale herself, unless she has limited English or has difficulty with reading.
5. The EPDS may be used at 6-8 weeks to screen postnatal women. The child health clinic, postnatal check-up or a home visit may provide suitable opportunities for its completion.

Name:_____
Address:_____
Baby's Age:_____

As you have recently had a baby, we would like to know how you are feeling. Please UNDERLINE the answer that comes closest to how you have felt IN THE PAST 7 DAYS, not just how you feel today.

1. I have been able to laugh and see the funny side of things.
   • As much as I always could
   • Not quite so much now
   • Definitely not so much now
   • Not at all

2. I have looked forward with enjoyment to things
   • As much as I ever did
   • Rather less than I used to
   • Definitely less than I used to
   • Hardly at all

3. I have blamed myself unnecessarily when things went wrong.*
   • Yes, most of the time
   • Yes, some of the time
   • Not very often
   • No, never

4. I have been anxious or worried for no good reason.
   • No, not at all
   • Hardly ever
   • Yes, sometimes
   • Yes, very often

5. I have felt scared or panicky for a not very good reason.*
   • Yes, quite a lot
   • Yes, sometimes
   • No, not much
   • No, not at all

6. Things have been getting on top of me.*
   • Yes, most of the time I haven't been able to cope at all
   • Yes, sometimes I haven't been coping as well as usual
   • No, most of the time I have coped quite well
   • No, I have been coping as well as ever

7. I have been so unhappy that I have had difficulty sleeping.*
   • Yes, most of the time
   • Yes, sometimes
   • Not very often
   • No, not at all

8. I have felt sad or miserable.*
   • Yes, most of the time
   • Yes, quite often
   • Not very often
   • No, not at all

9. I have been so unhappy that I have been crying.*
   • Yes, most of the time
   • Yes, quite often
   • Only occasionally
   • No, never

10. The thought of harming myself has occurred to me.*
    • Yes, quite often
    • Sometimes
    • Hardly ever
    • Never

Response categories are scored 0, 1, 2, and 3 according to increased severity of the symptoms. Items marked with an asterisk are reverse scored (i.e., 3, 2, 1, and 0). The total score is calculated by adding together the scores for each of the ten items. Scores above 92.3 percent are a possible indication of postpartum depression.

SOURCE: J.L. Cox, J.M. Holden, & R. Sagovsky (June 1987). *British Journal of Psychiatry, 150,* 782-786.
(**NOTE:** The authors give permission to reproduce the scale providing users respect copyright by quoting the names of the authors, the title and the source of the paper in all reproduced copies.)

mothers, experiencing lower educational achievements, and facing fewer opportunities and salary inequities in the workplace have all been implicated in the propensity for depression in women.

Women have more of a tendency to gain weight when they are depressed, whereas men are more likely to lose weight. Women also report higher rates of disturbed sleep, psychomotor retardation, expressed anger, anxiety, and somatization (Kornstein & Wojcik, 2002).

As stated previously, women attempt suicide more often than men, but men are 4 times more likely to die from suicide than women (CDC, 2004). Men choose more lethal means, such as guns, whereas women more often take overdoses of medication. Even in childhood and adolescence, girls express more suicidal ideation than boys (Kornstein & Wojcik, 2002). Among adolescents, depression is a strong predictor of suicidal behavior in both genders; however, suicide rates are higher in girls with comorbid substance use or conduct disorder.

Depressed women are more likely than men to have comorbid phobias, generalized anxiety disorder, panic disorder, or eating disorder; men are more likely to have comorbid substance use disorder (Kornstein & Wojcik, 2002). Recent research has indicated that depression may be a factor in the development of cardiovascular disease in both genders (Lesperance & Jaffe, 2002; NIMH, 2002).

There is a growing body of research showing gender differences in the absorption, metabolism, and excretion of many medications, including antidepressants. Robinson (2002) reports on a number of studies, which indicate that, compared to men, women have slower gastric emptying time, lower gastric acid secretion, higher percentage of body fat, a possible higher level of cerebral blood flow, decreased metabolism of drugs in the liver, and lower renal clearance. In addition, hormonal fluctuations during the menstrual cycle, pregnancy, postpartum, and menopause also affect the pharmacokinetics of medications. These differences may lead to greater bioavailability and slower clearance of drugs compared with men, suggesting that optimal doses for men may be relatively high in women (Robinson, 2002). Another consequence of these phenomena is that women experience side effects of psychotropic medications more often than men.

Gender differences in response to specific antidepressants have been demonstrated (Kornstein & Wojcik, 2000; Kornstein et al., 2000). These studies indicate that men respond more favorably to tricyclic antidepressants, particularly imipramine, whereas women seem to achieve better results with the selective serotonin reuptake inhibitors (SSRIs) and monoamine oxidase inhibitors (MAOIs). Robinson (2002) states:

The clinician should be aware that men and women may respond differently to a given antidepressant, and in women [hormonal] status should be taken into account when choos-

ing an antidepressant. Proper attention to dosage in women is very important to prevent excessive side effects. Women may need lower doses of antidepressants than men as their physiology tends to result in higher serum levels of drug. On the other hand, there may be times during the menstrual cycle, such as premenstrually, when women require more medication.

Much more research is needed to study the specific gender responses to medications. The clinician prescribing psychotropic medications should be aware of the gender differences and the effects of the menstrual cycles, reproductive events, and possible interactions with HRT.

Substance Use Disorders

The prevalence of illicit drug, alcohol, and tobacco use by adults is higher among men than it is in women. However, the gender difference among adolescents is negligible. Women ages 18 to 34 report more drinking-related problems than older women; however, middle-aged women (ages 35 to 49) have a higher incidence of alcohol dependence (Canterbury, 2002).

White women are more likely to drink alcohol than African American women. African American women who do drink are more likely to drink heavily and have more alcohol-related health problems. Hispanic women are more likely to drink infrequently or to abstain. Alcohol use in women is also associated with low household income, lower levels of education, and widowhood (Canterbury, 2002). With regard to binge drinking, college women have a higher likelihood than women of the same age who are not in college.

Women absorb and metabolize alcohol differently than men. Women have less body water than men of similar body weight, so that women achieve higher concentrations of alcohol in the blood after drinking equivalent amounts of alcohol. Women have less dehydrogenase, an enzyme that breaks down alcohol, in their bodies than men. Because of this, women become intoxicated more quickly and remain so longer (Burt & Hendrick, 2005). An increase in estrogen levels increases women's susceptibility to alcohol and results in even faster intoxication. This affects women during their premenstrual periods and women who take oral contraceptives or HRT.

The negative effects of alcohol on the liver appear to be worse in women than in men. Alcohol-induced liver disease appears in women over a shorter period of time and after consuming less alcohol (National Institute on Alcohol Abuse and Alcoholism [NIAAA], 1999). Women also are more likely than men to develop alcoholic hepatitis and to die from cirrhosis.

Alcohol-related medical complications (e.g., peptic ulcer, liver disease, anemia, and cerebral atrophy) develop more quickly in women, and women have higher relative mortality rates from alcoholism than do men (Greenfield et al., 2003). Studies also indicate an increase in the risk for breast cancer with moderate to heavy alcohol consumption (Horn-Ross et al., 2004).

Risk factors that may predispose women to alcohol abuse or dependence include genetic influences, early initiation of drinking, and victimization in childhood (NIAAA, 1999). Genetic factors have been confirmed through twin and adoption studies. Other studies have shown that women who start drinking alcohol before age 16 are most likely to engage in heavy drinking later in life (Pitkanen, Lyyra, & Pulkkinen, 2005). Brems and colleagues (2004) found that women with a history of childhood physical or sexual abuse reported earlier age at onset of drinking and more problems associated with use of alcohol and drugs.

Women who drink alcohol during pregnancy are at risk of delivering babies with fetal alcohol syndrome, a leading cause of mental retardation. Smoking during pregnancy increases the risk of having stillborn or premature infants or infants with low birthweight (Canterbury, 2002). Use of drugs such as heroin, methadone, amphetamines, or cocaine may result in the birth of an infant who is dependent on the drug and may experience drug withdrawal or have other medical problems at birth.

Women who seek treatment for substance dependence are more likely than men to be poor and without insurance (Canterbury, 2002). Many women are hindered in their endeavor to procure treatment by inadequate financial resources, lack of childcare facilities, and fear of losing their children. On the other hand, it is sometimes this fear of losing their children that forces women into a rehabilitation program.

Although men have higher prevalence rates for substance abuse and dependence, the gender gap is closing rapidly. Canterbury (2002) states:

> Changing societal roles and attitudes toward women—especially the increase in women entering the workplace in general, and previously male-dominated sports and professions in particular—may influence not only opportunities to drink, but also drinking culture. (p. 237)

SUMMARY

There are differences in the way women and men respond to certain illnesses and also to the treatments. Men and women face different physical and mental health challenges at various times in their lives.

Cardiovascular disease is the leading cause of death among men of all ages and races in the United States. Its prevalence increases with age, and it is most common in men ages 65 and older. Types of cardiovascular disease discussed in this chapter include coronary artery disease, angina pectoris, and myocardial infarction. Modifiable and nonmodifiable risk factors were described.

Neoplastic disease is the second leading cause of death in men, with lung cancer being the most prevalent type. The primary risk factor for lung cancer is cigarette smoking. Exposure to arsenic, asbestos, and certain organic chemicals has also been implicated. African American men have a higher rate of prostate cancer than white men. The incidence of this type of cancer increases with age and may be related to consumption of a high-fat diet, hormonal changes, viral infections, and industrial exposure to cadmium. Testicular cancer is more common in white men than in African Americans. It is generally detected as a painless nodule and, if detected and treated early, there is a 90 to 100 percent chance of cure.

Erectile dysfunction (ED) affects about 30 million men in the United States. Incidence of the disorder increases with age and may be related to vascular changes, certain nervous system conditions, endocrine and hormone imbalances, spinal cord injuries, prostate surgeries, smoking, and some medications. Psychological problems can also contribute to problems with ED. Medications or hormonal therapy may be effective for some men. Surgical interventions also are available.

Andropause is the term applied to the phenomenon that describes the effects of age-related androgen decrease in men. Some of these symptoms include depression, night sweats, decreased libido, ED, decreased muscle mass, decreased strength, easy fatigability, insomnia, and weight gain. Symptoms of andropause may be treated with testosterone replacement therapy.

Men may demonstrate depression with displaced anger, substance abuse, or social withdrawal. Suicide is the eighth leading cause of death among men of all ages and races in the United States. The profile for the highest rate of suicides is a white man, over the age of 85, living alone, who has just experienced a significant loss. The majority of individuals who commit suicide are suffering from a depressive disorder.

More men than women are diagnosed with substance use disorders. Men have a higher rate of alcohol use, illicit drug use, and tobacco use than women, and they are more likely than women to deny that they have a problem. Often men must receive pressure from an employer before they will enter a treatment program.

Cardiovascular disease is also the leading cause of death in women. African American women are twice as likely to die from CAD than white women. Heart disease often does not occur in women until after menopause.

The second leading cause of death in women is neoplastic disease, with lung cancer being the leading type. The primary risk factor for lung cancer in women is cigarette smoking. Smoking-related disease among women is at epidemic proportions, and women are not quitting in the same numbers as men.

Breast cancer is the most common form of cancer in women and the second leading cause of cancer-related death. The lifetime risk of contracting breast cancer is one in eight, and the risk increases with advancing age. Treatment is with chemotherapy, hormonal therapy, radiation therapy, surgery, or a combination.

PMDD occurs in 2 to 9 percent of menstruating women. An imbalance of the hormones estrogen and progesterone has been implicated in the predisposition to PMDD, resulting in symptoms of depression, mood swings, irritability, fatigue, appetite and sleep changes, difficulty concentrating, headaches, and weight gain. Treatment consists of diet modifications, stress-reduction techniques, and possibly an SSRI antidepressant.

The pregnancy rate for U.S. women fell during the decade from 1990 to 2000. In 2003, there was a sharp increase in the pregnancy rate for women age 30 and older. Many women are delaying pregnancy to pursue education and careers, and more women are becoming pregnant in their 30s and 40s. Older women are at higher risk for certain problems during pregnancy: eclampsia, gestational diabetes, and bearing a child with Down syndrome.

Symptoms of perimenopause usually begin sometime around age 40 and include irregular menstrual cycles, hot flashes, night sweats, sleep problems, vaginal dryness, difficulty concentrating, and mood swings. The risk for osteoporosis and heart disease increases in the post-menopausal years. Treatment for perimenopausal symptoms includes a number of lifestyle factors, and some women may elect to take hormone replacement therapy. Alternative therapies, such as soy products and some herbal preparations are effective for some individuals.

Depression is about twice as common in women as it is in men. Hormones may play a role in the etiology of this disorder in women. Depression is common in a number of women during the luteal phase of the menstrual cycle and also during the postpartum period. Women attempt suicide more often than men, but men are four times more likely to die as a result than women. Research has indicated gender differences in the pharmacokinetics of many medications, including antidepressants, and also gender differences in response to specific antidepressants.

White women are more likely to drink alcohol than African American or Hispanic women. Women absorb and metabolize alcohol differently than men. The negative effects of chronic alcohol use appear to affect women more rapidly than they do men. An increase in the risk of breast cancer has been associated with moderate to heavy alcohol consumption. Risk factors that may predispose women to alcohol abuse or dependence include genetic influences, early initiation of drinking, and victimization in childhood. Many women seek treatment for substance disorders only when they fear losing their children because of their substance use. Changing societal roles and attitudes may be contributing to increased substance use by women.

Health care providers need to become aware of the gender differences associated with various illnesses and their treatments. Only recently have women even been included in clinical research trials. Now the knowledge base is broadening and with increased information, such as the different ways in which men and women present with certain illnesses and respond to certain medications, health care providers can give their clients the best possible health care available.

REVIEW QUESTIONS

SELF-EXAMINATION/LEARNING EXERCISE

Select the answer that is *most* appropriate for each of the following questions.

1. Which of the following is the leading cause of death among men of all ages and races in the United States?
   a. Prostate cancer
   b. Lung cancer
   c. Suicide
   d. Cardiovascular disease

2. Recent research has identified which of the following as a possible risk factor for coronary artery disease?
   a. Depression
   b. Obsessive–compulsive disorder
   c. Panic disorder
   d. Posttraumatic stress disorder

3. The leading cause of death from cancer in men is:
   a. Prostate cancer.
   b. Lung cancer.
   c. Testicular cancer.
   d. Colon cancer.

4. Symptoms of andropause are directly related to:
   a. Increased cholesterol levels.
   b. Increased testosterone levels.
   c. Decreased triglyceride levels.
   d. Decreased testosterone levels.

5. Sam, age 50, complains to his doctor that he can feel his heart beating fast lately. He is afraid he is having a heart attack. His wife tells the doctor that Sam is angry all the time, he has started drinking heavily, and doesn't want to see any of their friends or family. In addition to checking for heart disease in Sam, what might the physician also suspect?
   a. Substance dependence
   b. Depression
   c. Brain cancer
   d. Anxiety disorder

6. The leading cause of death in women is:
   a. Breast cancer.
   b. Lung cancer.
   c. Cardiovascular disease.
   d. Stroke.

7. The most common form of cancer in women is:
   a. Breast cancer.
   b. Lung cancer.
   c. Colon cancer.
   d. Cancer of the uterus.

8. Which of the following is implicated in the predisposition to premenstrual dysphoric disorder?
   a. Deficiencies in vitamin C and potassium
   b. Overwhelming stress
   c. Imbalance of estrogen and progesterone
   d. Increased antidiuretic hormone

9. Which statement is true about postpartum depression?
   a. Once a woman has experienced postpartum depression, she is most likely not to experience it again.
   b. Postpartum depression is most common among women of the lower socioeconomic group.
   c. Postpartum depression is most common among women who have smoked during their pregnancy.
   d. Postpartum depression is more common in women who have a prior history of mood disorder.

10. Gender differences in the pharmacokinetics of medications may lead to which of the following in women?
    a. Higher serum concentrations from the same dosages
    b. Lower serum concentrations from the same dosages
    c. More rapid renal clearance of medications
    d. Wider distribution of most medications

11. Compared to men, women may become intoxicated quicker from drinking alcohol and remain so longer for which of the following reasons?
    a. Less total body water results in higher blood concentrations of alcohol.
    b. Women have less dehydrogenase, an enzyme that breaks down alcohol.
    c. Increased estrogen levels increase women's susceptibility to alcohol.
    d. All of the above.

IMPLICATIONS OF RESEARCH FOR EVIDENCE-BASED PRACTICE

Dunn, A.L., Trivedi, M.H., Kampert, J.B., Clark, C.G., & Chambliss, H.O. (2005). Exercise treatment for depression: Efficacy and dose response. *American Journal of Preventive Medicine, 28*(1), 1–8.

Description of the Study: The purpose of this study was to examine (1) whether exercise is an efficacious treatment for mild to moderate major depressive disorder (MDD), and (2) the dose-response relation of exercise and reduction in depressive symptoms. Subjects included 80 men and women ages 20 to 45 years who had been diagnosed with mild to moderate MDD. Subjects were screened and eliminated from the study if they were 160 percent over ideal weight, consumed more than 21 drinks per week, had attempted suicide in the last 2 years or were assessed as a suicide risk, had been hospitalized for a psychiatric disorder in the last 5 years, were unable to exercise because of a medical condition, or were pregnant or planned to become pregnant. Measurement of depression was determined using the Hamilton Rating Scale for Depression (HRSD) at baseline and after 12 weeks of exercise intervention. Subjects were randomly assigned to 1 of 4 study groups: low-dose (7 kcal/kg per week) exercise 3 times a week (LD/3), public health recommended dose (17.5 kcal/kg per week) exercise 3 times a week (PHD/3), low-dose exercise 5 times a week (LD/5), public health dose exercise 5 times a week (PHD/5), or the control group, which was defined as 3 days per week of stretching flexibility exercise for 15 to 20 minutes per session. The exercise groups received aerobic training on a treadmill or stationary bicycle.

Results of the Study: Forty-six percent of participants in the PHD group had a therapeutic response to treatment, defined as a 50 percent reduction in baseline HRSD score, and 42 percent of the PHD group had remission of symptoms, defined as an HRSD ≤ 7. In contrast, the LD group did not respond any better than the exercise placebo control group, although both groups had reductions in depressive symptoms. The finding of no difference in results for the 3-day/week and the 5-day/week conditions suggests that the determining factor for reduction and remission of symptoms is total energy expenditure. The response and remission rates in the PHD group are comparable to other depression treatments, such as medication or cognitive behavioral therapy.

Implications for Nursing Practice: Aerobic exercise in the amount recommended by consensus public health recommendations was found to be an effective monotherapy in treating mild to moderate MDD. This is important information for nurses who work in all types of practice settings. Many depressed clients do not seek therapy from psychiatric professionals, and many do not want to take antidepressant medication. Nurses can educate clients about the positive effects of exercise for relief from mild to moderate depression.

REFERENCES

American Heart Association (AHA). (2005a). *Heart disease and stroke statistics—2005 update.* Dallas, TX: American Heart Association.

American Heart Association (AHA). (2005b). *Cigarette smoking and cardiovascular diseases.* Retrieved May 24, 2005 from the World Wide Web at http://www.americanheart.org/

American Lung Association (ALA). (2004). *Women and smoking fact sheet.* Retrieved May 27, 2005 from the World Wide Web at http://www.lungusa.org/

American Psychiatric Association (APA). (2000). *Diagnostic and statistical manual of mental disorders* (4th ed.) *Text revision.* Washington, DC: American Psychiatric Association.

Andersen, U.A., Andersen, M., Rosholm, J.U., & Gram, L.F. (2000). Contacts to the health care system prior to suicide: A comprehensive analysis using registers for general and psychiatric hospital admissions, contacts to general practitioners and practicing specialists, and drug prescriptions. *ACTA Psychiatrica Scandinavica, 102,* 126–134.

Brems, C., Johnson, M.E., Neal, D., & Freemon, M. (2004). Childhood abuse history and substance use among men and women receiving detoxification services. *American Journal of Drug and Alcohol Abuse, 30*(4), 799–821.

Burt, V.K., & Hendrick, V.C. (2005). *Clinical manual of women's mental health.* Washington, DC: American Psychiatric Publishing.

Canterbury, R.J. (2002). Alcohol and other substance abuse. In S.G. Kornstein & A.H. Clayton (Eds.). *Women's mental health.* New York: The Guilford Press.

Carroll, R.G. (2005). The reproductive systems. In J.M. Black & J.H. Hawks (Eds.). *Medical-surgical nursing: Clinical management for positive outcomes* (7th ed.). St. Louis: W.B. Saunders.

Centers for Disease Control (CDC). (2001). *Women and smoking: A report of the Surgeon General—2001.* National Center for Chronic Disease Prevention and Health Promotion, Office on Smoking and Health. Atlanta, GA: CDC.

Centers for Disease Control (CDC). (2004). *Leading causes of death, 2002.* Retrieved May 26, 2005 from http://webappa.cdc.gov/sasweb/ncipc/leadcaus.html

Centers for Disease Control (CDC). (2005a). National Center for Health Statistics. *National Vital Statistics Report, 53*(17), 13.

Centers for Disease Control (CDC). (2005b). National Center for Injury Prevention and Control. *Suicide: Fact Sheet.* Retrieved May 26, 2005 from the World Wide Web at http://www.cdc.gov/ncipc/factsheets/suifacts.htm

Chen, E.I., & Kunkel, E.J.S. (2002). Oncology: Women with breast, gynecologic, or lung cancer. In S.G. Kornstein & A.H. Clayton (Eds.). *Women's mental health.* New York: The Guilford Press.

Chuang, M.S., O'Connor, R.C., Laven, B.A., Orvieto, M.A., & Brendler, C.B. (2005). Early release of the neurovascular bundles and optical loupe magnification lead to improved and earlier return of potency following radical retropubic prostatectomy. *The Journal of Urology, 173*(2), 537–539.

Craft, M. (2005). Management of clients with breast disorders. In J.M. Black & J.H. Hawks (Eds.). *Medical-surgical nursing: Clinical management for positive outcomes* (7th ed.). St. Louis: W.B. Saunders.

Crandall, C.J. (2005). *Heart Disease in Women.* Retrieved May 26, 2005 from the World Wide Web at http://www.medicinenet.com

Crombleholme, W.R. (2005). Obstetrics. In L.M. Tierney, S.J. McPhee, & M.A. Papadakis (Eds.). *Current medical diagnosis & treatment* (44th ed.). New York: McGraw-Hill.

Cundiff, D.K. (2002). Coronary artery bypass grafting (CABG): Reassessing efficacy, safety, and cost. *Medscape General Medicine, 4*(2), Online.

Diamond, J. (2002, March). Male menopause? Yes, there really is such a thing. *Bottom Line Tomorrow, 10*(3), 7–8.

Fain, J.A. (2005). Management of clients with diabetes mellitus. In J.M. Black & J.H. Hawks (Eds.). *Medical-surgical nursing: Clinical management for positive outcomes* (7th ed.). St. Louis: W.B. Saunders.

Frackiewicz, E.J., & Shiovitz, T.M. (2001). Evaluation and management of premenstrual syndrome. *Journal of the American Pharmaceutical Association, 41*(3), 437–447.

Gould, D.C., Petty, R., & Jacobs, H.S. (2000, March 25). For and against: The male menopause—does it exist? *British Medical Journal, 320,* 858–861.

Greenfield, S.F., Manwani, S.G., & Nargiso, J.E. (2003). Epidemiology of substance use disorders in women. *Obstetrics and Gynecology Clinics of North America, 30,* 413–446.

Hamilton, B.E., Martin, J.A., & Sutton, P.D. (2004). Births: Preliminary data for 2003. *National Vital Statistics Reports,* Vol. 53, No. 9. Hyattsville, MD: National Center for Health Statistics.

Hansen, S. (2002). Cardiovascular disease. In S.G. Kornstein and A.H. Clayton (Eds.). *Women's mental health.* New York: The Guilford Press.

Harvard Medical School. (2004). Women and depression. *Harvard Mental Health Letter,* Vol. 20, No. 11. Boston, MA: Harvard Health Publications.

Horn-Ross, P.L., Canchola, A.J., West, D.W., Stewart, S.L., Bernstein, L., Deapen, D., Pinder, R., Ross, R.K., Anton-Culver, H., Peel, D., Ziogas, A., Reynolds, P., & Wright, W. (2004). Patterns of alcohol consumption and breast cancer risk in the California Teachers Study cohort. *Cancer Epidemiology Biomarkers & Prevention, 13*(3), 405–411.

Kornstein, S.G., & Wojcik, B.A. (2000). Gender effects in the treatment of depression, *Psychiatric Clinics of North America Annual of Drug Therapy, 7,* 23–57.

Kornstein, S.G., & Wojcik, B.A. (2002). Depression. In S.G. Kornstein & A.H. Clayton (Eds.). *Women's mental health.* New York: The Guilford Press.

Kornstein, S.G., Thase, M.E., McCullough, J.P., Gelenberg, A.J., & Harrison, W.M. (2000). Gender differences in treatment response to sertraline versus imipramine in chronic depression. *American Journal of Psychiatry, 157,* 1445–1452.

Lesperance, F., & Jaffe, A.S. (2002). *Beyond the blues: Understanding the link between coronary artery disease and depression.* Retrieved April 5, 2002 from the World Wide Web at http://www.medscape.com/viewarticle/423461_2

Mann, D. (2000). *Depression affects men differently than women: Cultural expectations may explain why.* Retrieved May 11, 2002 from the World Wide Web at http://my.webmd.com/living_better_content/emo/article/1728.62155

Masharani, U. (2005). Diabetes mellitus and hypoglycemia. In L.M. Tierney, S.J. McPhee, & M.A. Papadakis (Eds.). *Current medical diagnosis and treatment* (44th ed.). New York: McGraw-Hill.

Massie, B.M., & Granger, C.B. (2005). Heart. In L.M. Tierney, S.J. McPhee, & M.A. Papadakis (Eds.). *Current medical diagnosis and treatment* (44th ed.). New York: McGraw-Hill.

Meier, P. (2005). Clients with cancer. In J.M. Black & J.H. Hawks (Eds.). *Medical-surgical nursing: Clinical management for positive outcomes* (7th ed.). St. Louis: W.B. Saunders.

Mertens, J.R., & Weisner, C.M. (2000, October). Predictors of substance abuse treatment retention among women and men in an HMO. *Alcoholism: Clinical & Experimental Research, 24*(10), 1524–1533.

Mosher, C.E. (2002). Impact of gender and problem severity upon intervention selection. *Sex Roles: A Journal of Research, 46*(3-4), 113–119.

National Cancer Institute (NCI). (2005a). *SEER cancer statistics review 1975–2002.* Retrieved May 24, 2005 from http://seer.cancer.gov/csr/1975_2002/

National Cancer Institute (NCI). (2005b). *Lifetime probability of breast cancer in American women.* Retrieved May 27, 2005 from http://cis.nci.nih.gov/fact/5_6.htm

National Center for Health Statistics (NCHS). (2004). *Health, United States 2004.* Hyattsville, MD: NCHS.

National Institute of Mental Health (NIMH). (2001). *Depression in women and men: What's the difference?* Retrieved May 11, 2002 from the World Wide Web at http://www.nimh.nih.gov/research/differencesummary.cfm

National Institute of Mental Health (NIMH). (2002). Depression and heart disease. NIH Publication No. 02-5004. Bethesda, MD: NIMH.

National Institute on Alcohol Abuse and Alcoholism (NIAAA). (1999). Are women more vulnerable to alcohol effects? *Alcohol Alert,* No. 46. Rockville, MD: U.S. Department of Health and Human Services.

Null, G. (2002). *Women's health solutions*. New York: Seven Stories Press.

Office of National Drug Control Policy (ONDCP). (2005). *Drug Facts*. Retrieved May 26, 2005 from the World Wide Web at http://www.whitehousedrugpolicy.gov/drugfact/women

Parry, B.L. (2000). Hormonal basis of mood disorders in women. In E. Frank (Ed.). *Gender and its effects on psychopathology*. Washington, DC: American Psychiatric Press.

Perry, A., & Schacht, M. (2001). *American Medical Association complete guide to men's health*. New York: John Wiley & Sons.

PDR for Herbal Medicines (2nd ed.). (2000). Montvale, NJ: Medical Economics Company.

Pitkanen, T., Lyyra, A.L., & Pulkkinen, L. (2005). Age of onset of drinking and the use of alcohol in adulthood: A follow-up study from age 8-42 for females and males. *Addiction, 100*(5), 652–661.

Pyeritz, R.E. (2005). Medical genetics. In L.M. Tierney, S.J. McPhee, & M.A. Papadakis (Eds.). *Current medical diagnosis & treatment* (44th ed.). New York: McGraw-Hill.

Rhoden, E.L., & Morgentaler, A. (2004). Medical progress: Risks of testosterone replacement therapy and recommendations for monitoring. *New England Journal of Medicine, 350*, 482–492.

Robinson, G.E. (2002). Women and psychopharmacology. *Medscape Women's Health eJournal, 7*(1). Retrieved March 11, 2002 from the World Wide Web at http://www.medscape.com/viewarticle/423938

Sadock, B.J., & Sadock, V.A. (2003). *Synopsis of psychiatry: Behavioral sciences/clinical psychiatry* (9th ed.). Philadelphia: Lippincott Williams & Wilkins.

Shaw, G. (2005). *Men get angry, not sad*. Retrieved May 25, 2005 from http://my.webmd.com/content/pages/7/1663_51924.htm

Sisson, E.M. (2004). *Erectile dysfunction*. Retrieved May 24, 2005 from http://health.discovery.com/diseasesandcond/encyclopedia/3105.html

Stoller, M.L., & Carroll, P.R. (2005). Urology. In L. M. Tierney, S.J. McPhee, & M.A. Papadakis (Eds.). *Current medical diagnosis and treatment* (44th ed.). New York: McGraw-Hill.

Substance Abuse and Mental Health Services Administration (SAMHSA). (2005). *2003 National Survey on Drug Use & Health: Results*. Retrieved May 26, 2005 from the World Wide Web at http://www.oas.samhsa.gov/NHSDA/2k3NSDUH/2k3results.htm

Ventura, S.J., Abma, J.C., Mosher, W.D., & Henshaw, S. (2004). Estimated pregnancy rates for the United States, 1990–2000: An update. *National vital statistics reports*, Vol. 52, No. 23. Hyattsville, MD: National Center for Health Statistics.

Vetrosky, D.T., & Aliabadi, Z. (2002). The andropause debate: Aging process or disease state? *Clinician Reviews, 12*(3), 78–85.

Warren, C.J. (2002). Emergent cardiovascular risk factor. *Progress in Cardiovascular Nursing, 17*(1), 35–41.

Women's Health Initiative (WHI). (2005). *Study findings*. Retrieved May 27, 2005 from the World Wide Web at http://www.whi.org/findings/

World Health Organization (WHO). (2002). *Distribution of suicide rates by gender and age, 2000*. Retrieved May 26, 2005 from the World Wide Web at http://www.who.int/mental_health/en/

York, N.L. (2005). Management of clients with parenchymal and pleural disorders. In J.M. Black & J.H. Hawks (Eds.). *Medical-surgical nursing: Clinical management for positive outcomes* (7th ed.). St. Louis: W.B. Saunders.

COMMUNITY MENTAL HEALTH NURSING

CHAPTER OUTLINE

OBJECTIVES

THE CHANGING FOCUS OF CARE

THE PUBLIC HEALTH MODEL

THE ROLE OF THE NURSE

CASE MANAGEMENT

THE COMMUNITY AS CLIENT

RURAL MENTAL HEALTH NURSING

SUMMARY

REVIEW QUESTIONS

KEY TERMS

case management
case manager
deinstitutionalization
diagnostically related
  groups (DRGs)

managed care
mobile outreach units
prospective payment
shelters
store-front clinics

CORE CONCEPTS

community
primary prevention
secondary prevention
tertiary prevention

OBJECTIVES

After reading this chapter, the student will be able to:

1. Discuss the changing focus of care in the field of mental health.
2. Define the concepts of care associated with the model of public health:
   a. Primary prevention
   b. Secondary prevention
   c. Tertiary prevention
3. Differentiate between the roles of basic level and advanced practice psychiatric/mental health registered nurses.
4. Define the concepts of case management and identify the role of case management in community mental health nursing.
5. Discuss primary prevention of mental illness within the community.
6. Identify populations at risk for mental illness within the community.
7. Discuss nursing intervention in primary prevention of mental illness within the community.

8. Discuss secondary prevention of mental illness within the community.
9. Describe treatment alternatives related to secondary prevention within the community.
10. Discuss tertiary prevention of mental illness within the community as it relates to the chronically and homeless mentally ill.
11. Relate historical and epidemiological factors associated with caring for the chronically and homeless mentally ill within the community.
12. Identify treatment alternatives for care of the chronically and homeless mentally ill within the community.
13. Apply steps of the nursing process to care of the chronically and homeless mentally ill within the community.
14. Describe principal aspects of the role of the mental health nurse in rural settings.

his chapter explores the concepts of primary and secondary prevention of mental illness within communities. Additional focus is placed on tertiary prevention of mental illness: treatment with community resources of those who are chronically mentally ill and homeless persons who are mentally ill. Emphasis is given to the role of the psychiatric nurse in the various treatment alternatives within the community setting.

THE CHANGING FOCUS OF CARE

Before 1840, there was no known treatment for individuals who were mentally ill. Because mental illness was perceived as incurable, the only "reasonable" intervention was thought to be removing these ill persons from the community to a place where they would do no harm to themselves or others.

In 1841, Dorothea Dix, a former schoolteacher, began a personal crusade across the land on behalf of institutionalized mentally ill clients. The efforts of this self-appointed "inspector" resulted in more humane treatment of the mentally ill and the establishment of a number of hospitals for the mentally ill.

After the movement initiated by Dix, the number of hospitals for persons with mental illness increased, although unfortunately not as rapidly as did the population with mental illness. The demand soon outgrew the supply, and hospitals became overcrowded and understaffed, with conditions that would have sorely distressed Dorothea Dix.

The community mental health movement gained impetus in the 1940s. With establishment of the National Mental Health Act of 1946, the U.S. government awarded grants to the states to develop mental health programs outside of state hospitals. Outpatient clinics and psychiatric units in general hospitals were inaugurated. Then, in 1949, as an outgrowth of the National Mental Health Act, the National Institute of Mental Health (NIMH) was established. The U.S. government has charged this agency with the responsibility for mental health in the United States.

In 1955, the Joint Commission on Mental Health and Illness was established by Congress to identify the nation's mental health needs and to make recommendations for improvement in psychiatric care. In 1961, the Joint Commission published a report, *Action for Mental Health*, in which recommendations were made for treatment of clients with mental illness, training for caregivers, and improvements in education and research of mental illness. With consideration given to these recommendations, Congress passed the Mental Retardation Facilities and Community Mental Health Centers Construction Act (often called the Community Mental

Health Centers Act) of 1963. This act called for the construction of comprehensive community health centers, the cost of which would be shared by federal and state governments. The **deinstitutionalization** movement (the closing of state mental hospitals and discharging of individuals with mental illness) had begun.

Unfortunately, many state governments did not have the capability to match the federal funds required for the establishment of these mental health centers. Some communities found it difficult to follow the rigid requirements for services required by the legislation that provided the grant.

In 1980 the Community Mental Health Systems Act, which was to have played a major role in renovation of mental health care, was established. Funding was authorized for community mental health centers, identification and services to high-risk populations, and for rape research and services. Approval was also granted for the appointment of an associate director for minority concerns at NIMH. Before this plan could be enacted, however, the newly inaugurated administration set forth its intention to diminish federal involvement. Budget cuts reduced the number of mandated services, and federal funding for community mental health centers was terminated in 1984.

Meanwhile, costs of care for hospitalized psychiatric clients continued to rise. The problem of the "revolving door" began to intensify. Individuals with chronic mental illness had no place to go when their symptoms exacerbated, except back to the hospital. Individuals without support systems remained in the hospital for extended periods because of lack of appropriate community services. Hospital services were paid for by cost-based, retrospective reimbursement: Medicaid, Medicare, and private health insurance. Retrospective reimbursement encouraged hospital expenditure; the more services provided, the more payment received.

This system of delivery of health care was interrupted in 1983 with the advent of **prospective payment**—the Reagan administration's proposal of cost containment. It was directed at control of Medicare costs by setting forth preestablished amounts that would be reimbursed for specific diagnoses, or **diagnostically related groups (DRGs)**. Since that time, prospective payment has also been integrated by the states (Medicaid) and by some private insurance companies, drastically affecting the amount of reimbursement for health care services.

Mental health services have been influenced by prospective payment. General hospital services to psychiatric clients have been severely restricted. Clients who present with acute symptoms, such as acute psychosis, suicidal ideations or attempts, or manic exacerbations, constitute the largest segment of the psychiatric hospital census. Clients with less serious illnesses (e.g., moderate depression or adjustment disorders) may be hospitalized, but length of stay has been shortened considerably by the reimbursement guidelines. Clients are being discharged from the hospital with a greater need for aftercare than in the past, when hospital stays were longer.

Deinstitutionalization continues to be the changing focus of mental health care in the United States. Care for the client in the hospital has become cost prohibitive, whereas care for the client in the community is cost effective. The reality of the provision of health care services today is often more of a political and funding issue than providers would care to admit. Decisions about how to treat are rarely made without consideration of cost and method of payment.

Provision of outpatient mental health services not only is the wave of the future but also has become a necessity today. We must serve the consumer by providing the essential services to assist with health promotion or prevention, to initiate early intervention, and to ensure rehabilitation or prevention of long-term disability.

THE PUBLIC HEALTH MODEL

The premise of the model of public health is based largely on the concepts set forth by Gerald Caplan (1964) during the initial community mental health movement. They include primary prevention, secondary prevention, and tertiary prevention. These concepts no longer have relevance only to mental health nursing, but also have been widely adapted as guiding principles in many clinical and community settings over a range of medical and nursing specialties.

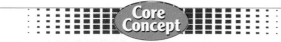

Primary Prevention
Services aimed at reducing the incidence of mental disorders within the population.

Primary prevention targets both individuals and the environment. Emphasis is twofold:

1. Assisting individuals to increase their ability to cope effectively with stress.
2. Targeting and diminishing harmful forces (stressors) within the environment.

Nursing in primary prevention is focused on the targeting of groups at risk and the provision of educational programs. Examples include:

1. Teaching parenting skills and child development to prospective new parents.
2. Teaching physical and psychosocial effects of alcohol/drugs to elementary school students.
3. Teaching techniques of stress management to virtually anyone who desires to learn.

4. Teaching groups of individuals ways to cope with the changes associated with various maturational stages.
5. Teaching concepts of mental health to various groups within the community.
6. Providing education and support to unemployed or homeless individuals.
7. Providing education and support to other individuals in various transitional periods (e.g., widows and widowers, new retirees, and women entering the work force in middle life).

These are only a few examples of the types of services nurses provide in primary prevention. These services can be offered in a variety of settings that are convenient for the public (e.g., churches, schools, colleges, community centers, YMCAs and YWCAs, workplace of employee organizations, meetings of women's groups, or civic or social organizations such as PTAs, health fairs, and community shelters).

Secondary Prevention
Services aimed at reducing the prevalence of psychiatric illness by shortening the course (duration) of the illness (Sadock & Sadock, 2003).

Secondary prevention is accomplished through early identification of problems and prompt initiation of effective treatment. Nursing in secondary prevention focuses on recognition of symptoms and provision of, or referral for, treatment. Examples include:

1. Ongoing assessment of individuals at high risk for illness exacerbation (e.g., during home visits, at day care, in community health centers, or in any setting where screening of high risk individuals might occur).
2. Provision of care for individuals in whom illness symptoms have been assessed (e.g., individual or group counseling, medication administration, education and support during period of increased stress [crisis intervention], staffing rape crisis centers, suicide hotlines, homeless shelters, shelters for abused women, or mobile mental health units).
3. Referral for treatment of individuals in whom illness symptoms have been assessed. Referrals may come from support groups, community mental health centers, emergency services, psychiatrists or psychologists, and day or partial hospitalization. Inpatient therapy on a psychiatric unit of a general hospital or in a private psychiatric hospital may be necessary. Chemotherapy and various adjunct therapies may be initiated as part of the treatment.

Secondary prevention has been addressed extensively in Unit Four of this text. Nursing assessment, diagnosis/

outcome identification, plan/implementation, and evaluation were discussed for many of the mental illnesses identified in the *DSM-IV-TR* (APA, 2000). These concepts may be applied in any setting where nursing is practiced.

Core Concept

Tertiary Prevention
Services aimed at reducing the residual defects that are associated with severe or chronic mental illness.

Tertiary prevention is accomplished in two ways:

1. Preventing complications of the illness.
2. Promoting rehabilitation that is directed toward achievement of each individual's maximum level of functioning.

Sadock and Sadock (2003) suggest that the term *chronic mental illness*, which historically has been associated with long hospitalizations that resulted in loss of social skills and increased dependency, now may also refer to clients from the deinstitutionalized generation. These individuals may never have experienced hospitalization, but they still do not possess adequate skills to live productive lives within the community.

Nursing in tertiary prevention focuses on helping clients learn or relearn socially appropriate behaviors so that they may achieve a satisfying role within the community. Examples include:

1. Consideration of the rehabilitation process at the time of initial diagnosis and treatment planning.
2. Teaching the client daily living skills and encouraging independence to his or her maximum ability.
3. Referring clients for various aftercare services (e.g., support groups, day treatment programs, partial hospitalization programs, psychosocial rehabilitation programs, group home or other transitional housing).
4. Monitoring effectiveness of aftercare services (e.g., through home health visits or follow-up appointments in community mental health centers).
5. Making referrals for support services when required (e.g., some communities have programs linking individuals with chronic mental disorders to volunteers who serve to develop friendships with the individuals and who may assist with household chores, shopping, and other activities of daily living with which the individual is having difficulty, in addition to participating in social activities with the individual).

Nursing care at the tertiary level of prevention can be administered on an individual or group basis and in a variety of settings, such as inpatient hospitalization, day or partial hospitalization, group home or halfway house, shelters, home health care, nursing homes, and community mental health centers.

THE ROLE OF THE NURSE

One emphasis of the National Mental Health Act of 1946 was to increase the supply of mental health professionals. This Act named four major mental health disciplines: psychiatry, clinical psychology, social work, and nursing. To increase the numbers of trained mental health professionals, grants were provided to institutions, and stipends and fellowships were awarded to individuals.

Nurses who work in the field of psychiatry may practice at one of two levels: the psychiatric/mental health registered nurse or the psychiatric/mental health advanced practice registered nurse. These two levels have been differentiated through the efforts of the Coalition of Psychiatric Nursing Organizations, under the leadership of the Executive Committee of the American Nurses Association's (ANA) Council on Psychiatric and Mental Health Nursing.

The Psychiatric/Mental Health Registered Nurse

Definition: A registered nurse (RN) who is educationally prepared in nursing and licensed to practice in his or her individual state (ANA, 2000).

Education: Baccalaureate degree in nursing (BSN), has worked in the field of psychiatric/mental health nursing for a minimum of 2 years, and demonstrates competency in the skills of psychiatric-mental health nursing (ANA, 2000).

Additional credentialing: In addition to professional licensure by the state, psychiatric/mental health RNs may apply to sit for ANA examinations that certify them as basic level psychiatric/mental health nurses.

Employment settings: Inpatient psychiatric hospital unit, day treatment and partial hospitalization programs, community health centers, home health care, long-term care centers.

Professional responsibilities: Health promotion and health maintenance, intake screening and evaluation, case management, provision of a therapeutic environment (e.g., milieu therapy), promotion of self-care activities, administering and monitoring psychobiological treatment regimens (including prescribed psychopharmacological agents and their effects), health teaching, crisis intervention, counseling, complementary interventions, and psychiatric rehabilitation (ANA, 2000).

The Psychiatric/Mental Health Advanced Practice Registered Nurse

Definition: A licensed RN who is educationally prepared either as a clinical nurse specialist or a nurse practitioner at least at the master's degree level in the specialty of psychiatric/mental health nursing (ANA, 2000).

Education: Minimum of a master's degree in psychiatric and mental health nursing. This preparation is distinguished by a depth of knowledge of theory and practice, validated experience in clinical practice, and competence in advanced clinical nursing skills (ANA, 2000).

Additional credentialing: Master's- or doctorate-prepared nurses may sit for ANA examinations that certify them as a psychiatric/mental health clinical nurse specialist or nurse practitioner. In addition, some states have special licensure that may be granted to nurses with advanced education that permits them to practice at a more independent level (Advanced Practice Registered Nurse [APRN]) and that makes them eligible for prescriptive authority, inpatient admission privileges, third-party reimbursement, and other specific privileges (ANA, 2000).

Employment settings: Inpatient psychiatric hospital units; day treatment and partial hospitalization programs, community mental health centers; private mental health facilities; individual private practice; crisis intervention services; or in the capacity of mental health consultant, supervisor, educator, administrator, or researcher.

Professional responsibilities: In addition to those required at the basic RN level, the RN in advanced psychiatric/mental health nursing practice must demonstrate knowledge and expertise related to psychopharmacological interventions, complementary interventions, various forms of psychotherapy, community interventions, case management, consultation-liaison, clinical supervision, and expanded advocacy activities (ANA, 2000).

CASE MANAGEMENT

Because of the rising costs of hospitalization and in keeping with the concept of deinstitutionalization, there has become a need for managing the care of clients (particularly the chronically ill) in an outpatient setting. **Case management** was defined and discussed in Chapter 9 of this text. Case management at the secondary level of prevention strives to organize client care so that specific outcomes are achieved within an allotted time frame. Commonly, this time frame is determined by the established protocols for length of stay as defined by the DRGs.

Ideally, case management incorporates concepts of care at the primary, secondary, and tertiary levels of prevention. Various definitions have emerged and should be clarified.

Managed care is a concept designed to control the balance between cost and quality of client care. In a managed-care program, individuals receive health care based on need, as assessed by coordinators of the provider. Managed care exists in many settings, including (but not limited to):

● Insurance-based programs
● Employer-based medical provider programs
● Social service programs
● The public health sector

Managed care may exist in virtually any setting in which health care provision is a part of the service; that is, in any setting in which an organization (whether it be private or government based) is responsible for payment of health care services for a group of people. Examples of managed care are health maintenance organizations (HMOs) and preferred provider organizations (PPOs).

Case management is the method used to achieve managed care. It is the actual coordination of services required to meet the needs of the client. The Case Management Society of America (CMSA) defines case management as "a collaborative process which assesses, plans, implements, coordinates, monitors, and evaluates options and services to meet an individual's health needs through communication and available resources to promote quality cost-effective outcomes" (CMSA, 2002). Types of clients who benefit from case management include (but are not limited to):

● The frail elderly.
● Those who are developmentally disabled.
● Those who are physically handicapped.
● Those who are mentally handicapped.
● Individuals with long-term medically complex problems that require multifaceted, costly care (e.g., high-risk infants, persons with human immunodeficiency virus or AIDS, and transplant patients).

● Individuals who are severely compromised by an acute episode of illness or an acute exacerbation of a chronic illness (e.g., schizophrenia).

The **case manager** is responsible for negotiating with multiple health care providers to obtain a variety of services for the client. The very nature of nursing that incorporates knowledge about the biological, psychological, and sociocultural aspects related to human functioning makes nurses highly appropriate as case managers. The American Nurse's Credentialing Center (ANCC) now offers national certification by exam for nursing case management. The applicant must hold a current license as a registered nurse with a baccalaureate degree, associate degree, or diploma in nursing. In addition, he or she must have functioned as a nursing case manager for a minimum of 2,000 hours of practice within the last 2 years. Some case management programs prefer master's-prepared clinical nurse specialists who have experience working with the specific populations for whom the case management service will be rendered.

Case management is becoming a recommended method of treatment for individuals with a chronic mental illness. This type of care enhances functioning by increasing the individual's ability to solve problems, improving work and socialization skills, promoting leisure time activities, and endeavoring to diminish dependency on others.

THE COMMUNITY AS CLIENT

Primary Prevention

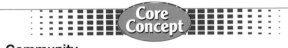

Community
A group, population, or cluster of people with at least one common characteristic, such as geographic location, occupation, ethnicity, or health concern (Langley, 2002).

Primary prevention within communities encompasses the twofold emphasis defined earlier in this chapter. These include:

1. Identifying stressful life events that precipitate crises and targeting the relevant populations at high risk.
2. Intervening with these high-risk populations to prevent or minimize harmful consequences.

Populations at Risk

One way to view populations at risk is to focus on types of crises that individuals experience in their lives. Two broad categories are maturational crises and situational crises.

Maturational Crises

Maturational crises are crucial experiences that are associated with various stages of growth and development. Erikson (1963) described eight stages of the life cycle during which individuals struggle with developmental "tasks." Crises can occur during any of these stages, although several developmental periods and life-cycle events have been recognized as having increased crisis potential: adolescence, marriage, parenthood, midlife, and retirement.

Adolescence. The task for adolescence according to Erikson (1963) is *identity versus role confusion*. This is the time in life when individuals ask questions such as "Who am I?" "Where am I going?" and "What is life all about?"

Adolescence is a transition into young adulthood. It is a very volatile time in most families. Commonly, there is conflict over issues of control. Parents sometimes have difficulty relinquishing even a minimal amount of the control they have had throughout their adolescent's infancy, toddlerhood, and school-age years, at a time when the adolescent is seeking independence. It may seem that the adolescent is 25 years old one day and 5 years old the next. An often-quoted definition of an adolescent, by an anonymous author, is: "A toddler with hormones and wheels."

At this time, adolescents are "trying out their wings," although they possess an essential need to know that the parents (or surrogate parents) are available if support is required. Mahler, Pine, and Bergman (1975) have termed this vital concept "emotional refueling," and although they were referring to toddlers when they coined the term, it is highly applicable to adolescents as well. In fact, it is believed that the most frequent immediate precipitant to adolescent suicide is loss, or threat of loss, or abandonment by parents or closest peer relationship.

Adolescents have many issues to deal with and many choices to make. Some of these include issues that relate to self-esteem and body image (in a body that is undergoing rapid changes), peer relationships (with both genders), education and career selection, establishing a set of values and ideals, sexuality and sexual experimentation (including issues of birth control and prevention of sexually transmitted diseases), drug and alcohol abuse, and physical appearance.

Nursing interventions with adolescents at the primary level of prevention focus on providing adolescents with support and accurate information to ease the difficult transition they are undergoing. Educational offerings can be presented in schools, churches, youth centers, or any location in which groups of teenagers gather. Types of programs may include (but are not limited to):

● Alateen groups for adolescents with alcoholic parent(s).
● Other support groups for teenagers who are in need of

assistance to cope with stressful situations (e.g., children dealing with divorce of their parents, pregnant teenagers, teenagers coping with abortion, adolescents coping with the death of a parent).

● Educational programs that inform about and validate bodily changes and emotional feelings about which there may be some concerns.

● Educational programs that inform about nutritional needs specific for this age group.

● Educational programs that inform about sexuality, pregnancy, contraception, and sexually transmitted diseases.

● Educational programs that inform about the use and abuse of alcohol and other drugs.

Marriage. The "American Dream" of the 1950s—especially that of the American woman—was to marry, have two or three children, buy a house in the suburbs, and drive a station wagon. To not be at least betrothed by their mid-20s caused many women to fear becoming an "old maid." Living together without the benefit of marriage was an unacceptable and rarely considered option.

Times have changed considerably in 50 years. Today's young women are choosing to pursue careers before entering into marriage, to continue their careers after marriage, or to not get married at all. Many couples are deciding to live together without being married, and, as with most trends, the practice now receives more widespread societal acceptance than it once did.

Why is marriage considered one of the most common maturational crises? Sheehy (1976), in her classic volume about life's passages, wrote:

No two people can possibly coordinate all their developmental crises. The timing of outside opportunities will almost never be the same. But more importantly, each one has an inner life structure with its own idiosyncrasies. Depending on what has gone before, each one will alternate differently between times of feeling full of certainty, hope, and heightened potential and times of feeling vulnerable, unfocused, and scared. (p. 138)

Additional conflicts sometimes also arise when the marriage is influenced by crossovers in religion, ethnicity, social status, or race, although these types of differences have become more individually and societally acceptable than they once were.

Nursing interventions at the primary level of prevention with individuals in this stage of development involve education regarding what to expect at various stages in the marriage. Many high schools now offer courses in marriage and family living in which students role-play through anticipatory marriage and family situations. Nurses could offer these kinds of classes within the community to individuals considering marriage. Too many people enter marriage with the notion that, as sure as the depth of their love, their soon-to-be husband or wife will discontinue his or her "undesirable" traits and change

into the perceived ideal spouse. Primary prevention with these individuals involves:

● Encouraging honest communication.
● Determining what each person expects from the relationship.
● Ascertaining whether or not each individual can accept compromise.

This type of intervention can be effective in individual or couple's therapy and in support or educational groups of couples experiencing similar circumstances.

Parenthood. Murray and Zentner (2001) state:

The coming of the child is a crisis, a turning point in the couple's life in which old patterns of living must be changed for new ways of living and new values. With the advent of parenthood, a couple is embarking on a journey from which there is no return. To put it simply, parents cannot quit. The child's birth brings a finality to many highly valued privileges and a permanence of responsibilities. (p. 326)

There is probably no developmental stage that creates an upheaval equal to that of the arrival of a child. Even when the child is desperately wanted and pleasurably anticipated, his or her arrival usually results in some degree of chaos within the family system.

Because the family operates as a system, the addition of a new member influences all parts of the system as a whole. If it is a first child, the relationship between the spouses is likely to be affected by the demands of caring for the infant on a 24-hour basis. If there are older children, they may resent the attention showered on the new arrival and show their resentment in a variety of creative ways.

The concept of having a child (particularly the first one) is often romanticized, with little or no consideration given to the realities and responsibilities that accompany this "bundle of joy." Many young parents are shocked to realize that such a tiny human can create so many changes in so many lives. It is unfortunate that parenting is one of the most important positions an individual will hold in life and one for which he or she is often least prepared.

Nursing intervention at the primary level of prevention with the developmental stage of parenthood must begin long before the child is even born. How do we prepare individuals for parenthood? *Anticipatory guidance* is the term used to describe the interventions used to help new parents know what they might expect. Volumes have been written on the subject, but it is also important for expectant parents to have a support person or network with whom they can talk, express feelings, excitement, and fears. Nurses can provide the following type of information to help ease the transition into parenthood (Mercer, 2000; Murray & Zentner, 2001; Spock, 2004).

1. Prepared childbirth classes: what most likely will happen but with additional information about possible variations from that which is expected.

2. Information about what to expect after the baby arrives:
   a. **Parent–infant bonding**. Expectant parents should know that it is not unusual for parent–infant bonding not to occur immediately. The strong attachment will occur as parent and infant get to know each other.
   b. **Changing husband–wife relationships**. The couple should be encouraged to engage in open honest communication and role playing of typical situations that are likely to arise after the baby becomes a part of the family.
   c. **Clothing and equipment**. Expectant parents need to know what is required to care for a newborn child. Family economics, space available, and lifestyle should be considered.
   d. **Feeding**. Advantages and disadvantages of breast-feeding and formula-feeding should be presented. The couple should be supported in whatever method is chosen. Anticipatory guidance related to technique should be provided for one or both methods, as the expectant parents request.
   e. **Other expectations**. It is important for expectant parents to receive anticipatory guidance about the infant's sleeping and crying patterns, bathing the infant, care of the circumcision and cord, toys that provide stimulation of the newborn's senses, aspects of providing a safe environment, and when to call the physician.
3. Stages of growth and development: It is very important for parents to understand what behaviors should be expected at what stage of development. It is also important to know that their child may not necessarily follow the age guidelines associated with these stages. However, a substantial deviation from these guidelines should be reported to their physician.

Midlife. What is middle age? A colleague once remarked that upon turning 50 years of age she stated, "Now I can say I am officially middle aged … until I began thinking about how few individuals I really knew who were 100!"

Midlife crises are not defined by a specific number. Various sources in the literature identify these conflicts as occurring anytime between age 35 and 65.

What is a midlife crisis? This, too, is very individual, but a number of patterns have been identified within three broad categories:

1. **An alteration in perception of the self**. One's perception of self may occur slowly. One may suddenly become aware of being "old" or "middle aged." Murray and Zentner (2001) state:

   The individual looks in the mirror and sees changes that others may have noticed for sometime. Gray thinning hair and wrinkles, coarsening features, decreased muscular tone, weight gain, varicosities, and capillary breakage

may be the first signs of impending age, and may suddenly become frighteningly apparent to the individual. (p. 699)

Other biological changes that occur naturally with the aging process may also impact on the crises that occur at this time. In women, a gradual decrease in the production of estrogen initiates the menopause, which results in a variety of physical and emotional symptoms. Some physical symptoms include "hot flashes," vaginal dryness, cessation of menstruation, loss of reproductive ability, night sweats, insomnia, headaches, and minor memory disturbances. Emotional symptoms include anxiety, depression, crying for no reason, and temper outbursts.

Although the menopausal period in men is not as evident as it is in women, most clinicians subscribe to the belief that men undergo a climacteric experience related to the gradual decrease in production of testosterone. Although sperm production diminishes with advancing age, there is usually no complete cessation, as there is of ovum production in women at menopause (Scanlon & Sanders, 2003). Some men experience hot flashes, sweating, chills, dizziness, and heart palpitations (Murray & Zentner, 2001), whereas others may experience severe depression and an overall decline in physical vigor (Sadock & Sadock, 2003). An alteration in sexual functioning is not uncommon (see Chapter 38).

2. **An alteration in perception of others**. A change in relationship with adult children requires a sensitive shift in caring. Wright and Leahey (2000) state:

   The family of origin must relinquish the primary roles of parent and child. They must adapt to the new roles of parent and adult child. This involves renegotiation of emotional and financial commitments. The key emotional process during this stage is for family members to deal with a multitude of exits from and entries into the family system. (pp. 112–113)

These experiences are particularly difficult when parents' values conflict with the relationships and types of lifestyles their children choose. An alteration in perception of one's parents also begins to occur during this time. Having always looked to parents for support and comfort, the middle-aged individual may suddenly find that the roles are beginning to reverse. Aging parents may look to their children for assistance with making decisions regarding their everyday lives and for assistance with chores that they have previously accomplished independently. When parents die, middle-aged individuals must come to terms with their own mortality. The process of recognition and resolution of one's own finitude begins in earnest at this time.

3. **An alteration in perception of time**. Middle age has been defined as the end of youth and the beginning of old age. Individuals often experience a sense that time is running out: "I haven't done all I want to do or accomplished all I intended to accomplish!" Depres-

sion and a sense of loss may occur as individuals realize that some of the goals established in their youth may go unmet.

The "empty nest syndrome" has been identified as the adjustment period parents experience when the last child leaves home to establish an independent residence. The crisis is often more profound for the mother who has devoted her life to nurturing her family. As the last child leaves, she may perceive her future as uncertain and meaningless.

Some women who have devoted their lives to rearing their children decide to develop personal interests and pursue personal goals once the children are grown. This occurs at a time when many husbands have begun to decrease what may have been a compulsive drive for occupational security during the earlier years of their lives. This disparity in common goals may create conflict between husband and wife. At a time when she is experiencing more value in herself and her own life, he may begin to feel less valued. This may also relate to a decrease in the amount of time and support from the wife to which the husband has become accustomed. This type of role change will require numerous adaptations on the part of both spouses.

Finally, an alteration in one's perception of time may be related to the societal striving for eternal youth. Murray and Zentner (2001) state:

> Whether a man or a woman, the person who lacks self-confidence and who cannot accept the changing body, has a compulsion to try cosmetics, clothes, hair styles, and the other trappings of youth in the hope that the physical attributes of youth will be attained. The person tries to regain a youthful figure and face, perhaps through surgery; tints the hair to cover signs of gray; and turns to hormone creams to restore the skin. (pp. 731–732)

This yearning for youth may take the form of sexual promiscuity or extramarital affairs with much younger individuals, in an effort to prove that one "still has what it takes." Some individuals reach for the trappings of youth with regressive-type behaviors, such as the middle-aged man who buys a motorcycle and joins a motorcycle gang and the 50-year-old woman who wears miniskirts and flirts with her daughter's boyfriends. These individuals may be denying their own past and experience. With a negative view of self, they strongly desire to relive their youth.

Nursing intervention at the primary level of prevention with the developmental stage of midlife involves providing accurate information regarding changes that occur during this time of life and support for adapting to these changes effectively. These interventions might include:

1. Nutrition classes to inform individuals in this age group about the essentials of diet and exercise. Educational materials on how to avoid obesity or reduce weight can be included, along with the importance of good nutrition.
2. Assistance with ways to improve health (e.g., quit smoking, cease or reduce alcohol consumption, reduce fat intake).
3. Discussions of the importance of having regular physical examinations, including Pap and breast examinations for women and prostate examinations for men. Monthly breast self-examinations should be taught and yearly mammograms encouraged.
4. Classes on menopause should be given. Provide information about what to expect. Myths that abound regarding this topic should be expelled. Support groups for women (and men) undergoing the menopausal experience should be formed.
5. Support and information related to physical changes occurring in the body during this time of life. Assist with the grief response that some individuals will experience in relation to loss of youth, "empty nest," and sense of identity.
6. Support and information related to care of aging parents should be given. Individuals should be referred to community resources for respite and assistance before strain of the caregiver role threatens to disrupt the family system.

Retirement. Retirement, which is often anticipated as an achievement in principle, may be met with a great deal of ambivalence when it actually occurs. Our society places a great deal of importance on productivity and on earning as much money as possible at as young an age as possible. These types of values contribute to the ambivalence associated with retirement. Although leisure has been acknowledged as a legitimate reward for workers, leisure during retirement is generally not accorded the same social value. Adjustment to this life-cycle event becomes more difficult in the face of societal values that are in direct conflict with the new lifestyle.

Historically many women have derived much of their self-esteem from having children, rearing children, and being a "good mother." Likewise, many men have achieved self-esteem through work-related activities—creativity, productivity, and earning money. Termination of these activities may result in a loss of self-worth. Individuals who are unable to adapt satisfactorily may become depressed.

It would appear that retirement is becoming, and will continue to become, more accepted by societal standards. With more and more individuals retiring earlier and living longer, the growing number of aging persons will spend a significantly longer time in retirement. At present, retirement has become more of an institutionalized expectation, and there appears to be increasing acceptance of it as a social status.

Nursing intervention at the primary level of prevention with the developmental task of retirement involves providing information and support to individuals who have retired or are considering retirement. Support can be on a one-to-one basis to assist these individuals to sort out their feelings regarding retirement. Murray and Zentner (2001) state:

> The retiree may be faced with these questions: Can I face loss of job satisfaction? Will I feel the separation from people close to me at work? If I need continued employment on a part-time basis to supplement Social Security payments, will the old organization provide it, or must I adjust to a new job? Shall I remain in my present home or seek a different one because of easier maintenance or reduced cost of upkeep? Might a different climate be better, and if so, will I miss my relatives and neighbors? (p. 812)

Support can also be provided in a group environment. Support groups of individuals undergoing the same types of experiences can be extremely helpful. Nurses can form and lead these types of groups to assist retiring individuals through this critical period. These groups can also serve to provide information about available resources that offer assistance to individuals in or nearing retirement, such as information concerning Medicare, Social Security, and Medicaid; information related to organizations that specialize in hiring retirees; and information regarding ways to use newly acquired free time constructively.

Situational Crises

Situational crises are acute responses that occur as a result of an external circumstantial stressor. The number and types of situational stressors are limitless and may be real or exist only in the perception of the individual. Some types of situational crises that put individuals at risk for mental illness include the following.

Poverty. A number of studies have identified poverty as a direct correlation to emotional illness. This may have to do with the direct consequences of poverty, such as inadequate and crowded living conditions, nutritional deficiencies, medical neglect, unemployment, or being homeless.

High Rate of Life Change Events. Miller and Rahe (1997) found that frequent changes in life patterns due to a large number of significant events occurring in close proximity tend to decrease a person's ability to deal with stress, and physical or emotional illness may be the result. These include life change events such as death of a loved one, divorce, fired from a job, change in living conditions, change in place of employment or residence, physical illness, or change in body image as a result of loss of a body part or function.

Environmental Conditions. Environmental conditions can create situational crises. Tornados, floods, hurricanes, and earthquakes have wreaked devastation on thousands of individuals and families in recent years.

Trauma. Individuals who have encountered traumatic experiences must be considered at risk for emotional illness. These include traumatic experiences usually considered outside the range of usual human experience, such as participating in military combat, being a victim of violent personal assault, undergoing torture, being taken hostage or kidnapped, or being the victim of a natural or manmade disaster (APA, 2000).

Nursing intervention at the primary level of prevention with individuals experiencing situational crises is aimed at maintaining the highest possible level of functioning while offering support and assistance with problem solving during the crisis period. Interventions for nursing of clients in crisis include the following:

1. Use a reality-oriented approach. The focus of the problem is on the here and now.
2. Remain with the individual who is experiencing panic anxiety.
3. Establish a rapid working relationship by showing unconditional acceptance, by active listening, and by attending to immediate needs.
4. Discourage lengthy explanations or rationalizations of the situation; promote an atmosphere for verbalization of true feelings.
5. Set firm limits on aggressive, destructive behaviors. At high levels of anxiety, behavior is likely to be impulsive and regressive. Establish at the outset what is acceptable and what is not, and maintain consistency.
6. Clarify the problem that the individual is facing. The nurse does this by describing his or her perception of the problem and comparing it with the individual's perception of the problem.
7. Help the individual determine what he or she believes precipitated the crisis.
8. Acknowledge feelings of anger, guilt, helplessness, and powerlessness, while taking care not to provide positive feedback for these feelings.
9. Guide the individual through a problem-solving process by which he or she may move in the direction of positive life change:
   a. Help the individual confront the source of the problem that is creating the crisis response.
   b. Encourage the individual to discuss changes he or she would like to make. Jointly determine whether desired changes are realistic.
   c. Encourage exploration of feelings about aspects that cannot be changed, and explore alternative ways of coping more adaptively in these situations.
   d. Discuss alternative strategies for creating changes that are realistically possible.
   e. Weigh benefits and consequences of each alternative.
   f. Assist the individual to select alternative coping strategies that will help alleviate future crisis situations.
10. Identify external support systems and new social networks from whom the individual may seek assistance in times of stress.

Nursing at the level of primary prevention focuses largely on education of the consumer to prevent initiation or exacerbation of mental illness. An example of just one type of teaching plan for use in primary prevention situations is presented in Table 42–1.

Secondary Prevention
Populations at Risk

Secondary prevention within communities relates to using early detection and prompt intervention with indi-

| TABLE 42–1 | Client Education for Primary Prevention: Drugs of Abuse |

CLASS OF DRUGS	EFFECTS	SYMPTOMS OF OVERDOSE	TRADE NAMES	COMMON NAMES	EFFECTS ON THE BODY (CHRONIC OR HIGH-DOSE USE)
CNS Depressants Alcohol	Relaxation, loss of inhibitions, lack of concentration, drowsiness, slurred speech, sleep	Nausea, vomiting; shallow respirations; cold, clammy skin; weak, rapid pulse; coma; possible death.	Ethyl alcohol, beer, gin, rum, vodka, bourbon, whiskey, liqueurs, wine, brandy, sherry, champagne.	Booze, alcohol, liquor, drinks, cocktails, highballs, nightcaps, moonshine, white lightning, firewater.	Peripheral nerve damage, skeletal muscle wasting, encephalopathy, psychosis, cardiomyopathy, gastritis, esophagitis, pancreatitis, hepatitis, cirrhosis of the liver, leukopenia, thrombocytopenia, sexual dysfunction.
Other (barbiturates and non-barbiturates)	Same as alcohol.	Anxiety, fever, agitation, hallucinations, disorientation, tremors, delirium, convulsions, possible death.	Seconal Nembutal Amytal Valium Librium Chloral hydrate Equanil, Miltown	Red birds Yellow birds Blue birds Blues/yellows Green & whites Mickies Downers	Decreased REM sleep, respiratory depression, hypotension, possible kidney or liver damage, sexual dysfunction.
CNS Stimulants Amphetamines and related drugs	Hyperactivity, agitation, euphoria, insomnia, loss of appetite.	Cardiac arrhythmias, headache, convulsions, hypertension, rapid heart rate, coma, possible death.	Dexedrine, Didrex, Tenuate, Preludin, Ritalin, Plegine, Cylert, Ionamin, Sanorex	Uppers, pep pills, wakeups, bennies, eye-openers, speed, black beauties, sweet A's	Aggressive, compulsive behavior; paranoia; hallucinations; hypertension.
Cocaine	Euphoria, hyperactivity, restlessness, talkativeness, increased pulse, dilated pupils.	Hallucinations, convulsions, pulmonary edema, respiratory failure, coma, cardiac arrest, possible death.	Cocaine hydrochloride	Coke, flake, snow, dust, happy dust, gold dust, girl, cecil, C, toot, blow, crack	Pulmonary hemorrhage; myocardial infarction; ventricular fibrillation.
Opioids	Euphoria, lethargy, drowsiness, lack of motivation.	Shallow breathing, slowed pulse, clammy skin, pulmonary edema, respiratory arrest, convulsions, coma, possible death.	Heroin Morphine Codeine Dilaudid Demerol Methadone Percodan Talwin Opium	Snow, stuff, H, Harry, horse M, morph, Miss Emma Schoolboy Lords Doctors Dollies Perkies T's Big O, black stuff	Respiratory depression, constipation, fecal impaction, hypotension, decreased libido, retarded ejaculation, impotence, orgasm failure.
Hallucinogens	Visual hallucinations, disorientation, confusion, paranoid delusions, euphoria, anxiety, panic, increased pulse.	Agitation, extreme hyperactivity, violence, hallucinations, psychosis, convulsions, possible death.	LSD PCP Mescaline DMT STP	Acid, cube, big D Angel dust, Hog, crystal Mesc Businessman's trip Serenity and peace	Panic reaction, acute psychosis, flashbacks.
Cannabinols	Relaxation, talkativeness, lowered inhibitions, euphoria, mood swings.	Fatigue, paranoia, delusions, hallucinations, possible psychosis.	Cannabis Hashish	Marijuana, pot, grass, joint, Mary Jane, MJ Hash, rope, Sweet Lucy	Tachycardia, orthostatic hypotension, chronic bronchitis, problems with infertility, amotivational syndrome.

viduals experiencing mental illness symptoms. The same maturational and situational crises that were presented in the previous section on primary prevention are used to discuss intervention at the secondary level of prevention.

Maturational Crises

Adolescence. The need for intervention at the secondary level of prevention in adolescence occurs when disruptive and age-inappropriate behaviors become the norm, and the family can no longer cope adaptively with the situation. All levels of dysfunction are considered—from dysfunctional family coping to the need for hospitalization of the adolescent.

Nursing intervention with the adolescent at the secondary level of prevention may occur in the community setting at community mental health centers, physician's offices, schools, public health departments, and crisis intervention centers. Nurses may work with families to problem solve and improve coping and communication skills, or they may work on a one-to-one basis with the adolescent in an attempt to modify behavior patterns.

Adolescents may be hospitalized for a variety of reasons. The *DSM-IV-TR* (APA, 2000) identifies a number of problems, the severity of which would determine whether the adolescent required inpatient care. Conduct disorders, adjustment disorders, eating disorders, substance-related disorders, depression, and anxiety disorders are the most common diagnoses for which adolescents are hospitalized. Nursing care of adolescents in the hospital setting focuses on problem identification and stabilizing a crisis situation. Once stability has been achieved, clients are commonly discharged to outpatient care. If an adolescent's home situation has been deemed unsatisfactory, the state may take custody and the child is then discharged to a group or foster home. Care plans for intervention with the adolescent at the secondary level of prevention can be found in Chapter 25.

Marriage. Problems in a marriage are as far-reaching as the individuals who experience them. Problems that are not uncommon to the disruption of a marriage relationship include substance abuse on the part of one or both partners and disagreements on issues of sex, money, children, gender roles, and infidelity, among others. Murray and Zentner (2001) state:

> Staying married to one person and living with the frustrations, conflicts, and boredom that any close and lengthy relationship imposes requires constant work by both parties. (p. 613)

Nursing intervention at the secondary level of prevention with individuals encountering marriage problems may include one or more of the following:

1. Counseling with the couple or with one of the spouses on a one-to-one basis.
2. Referral to a couples' support group.

3. Identification of the problem and possible solutions; support and guidance as changes are undertaken.
4. Referral to a sex therapist.
5. Referral to a financial advisor.
6. Referral to parent effectiveness training.

Murray and Zentner (1997) state:

> When marriage fails and bonds are broken, aloneness, anger, mistrust, hostility, guilt, shame, a sense of betrayal, fear, disappointment, loss of identity, anxiety, and depression, alone or in combination, can appear both in the divorcee and the one initiating the divorce. (p. 677)

In Miller and Rahe's (1997) life change questionnaire, only death of a spouse or other close family member scored higher than divorce in severity of stress experienced. This is an area in which nurses can intervene to help ease the transition and prevent emotional breakdown. In community health settings, nurses can lead support groups for newly divorced individuals. They can also provide one-to-one counseling for individuals experiencing the emotional chaos engendered by the dissolution of a marriage relationship.

Divorce also has an impact on the children involved. Nurses can intervene with the children of divorce in an effort to prevent dysfunctional behaviors associated with the breakup of a marriage.

Parenthood. Intervention at the secondary level of prevention with parents can be required for a number of reasons. A few of these include:

1. Physical, emotional, or sexual abuse of a child.
2. Physical or emotional neglect of a child.
3. Birth of a child with special needs.
4. Diagnosis of a terminal illness in a child.
5. Death of a child.

Nursing intervention at the secondary level of prevention includes being able to recognize the physical and behavioral signs that indicate possible abuse of a child. The child may be cared for in the emergency room or as an inpatient on the pediatric unit or child psychiatric unit of a general hospital.

Nursing intervention with parents may include teaching effective methods of disciplining children, aside from physical punishment. Methods that emphasize the importance of positive reinforcement for acceptable behavior can be very effective. Family members must be committed to consistent use of this behavior modification technique for it to be successful.

Parents should also be informed about behavioral expectations at the various levels of development. Knowledge of what to expect from children at various stages of development may provide needed anticipatory guidance to deal with the crises commonly associated with these various stages.

Therapy sessions with all family members together may focus on problems with family communications.

Members are encouraged to express honest feelings in a manner that is nonthreatening to other family members. Active listening, assertiveness techniques, and respect for the rights of others are taught and encouraged. Barriers to effective communication are identified and resolved.

Referrals to agencies that promote effective parenting skills may be made (e.g., parent effectiveness training). Alternative agencies that may provide relief from the stress of parenting may also be considered (e.g., "Mom's Day Out" programs, sitter-sharing organizations, and day care institutions). Support groups for abusive parents may also be helpful and assistance in locating or initiating such a group may be provided.

The nurse can assist parents who are grieving the loss of a child or the birth of a child with special needs by helping them to express their true feelings associated with the loss. Feelings such as shock, denial, anger, guilt, powerlessness, and hopelessness need to be expressed in order for the parents to progress through the grief response.

Home health care assistance can be provided for the family of a child with special needs. This can be done by making referrals to other professionals, such as speech, physical, and occupational therapists, medical social workers, psychologists, and nutritionists. If the child with special needs is hospitalized, the home health nurse can provide specific information to hospital staff that may be helpful in providing continuity of care for the client and help in the transition for the family.

Nursing intervention also includes providing assistance in the location of and referral to support groups that deal with loss of a child or birth of a child with special needs. Some nurses may serve as leaders of these types of groups in the community.

Midlife. Nursing care at the secondary level of prevention during midlife becomes necessary when the individual is unable to integrate all of the changes that are occurring during this period. An inability to accept the physical and biological changes, the changes in relationships between themselves and their adult children and aging parents, and the loss of the perception of youth may result in depression for which the individual may require help to resolve.

Retirement. Retirement can also result in depression for individuals who are unable to satisfactorily grieve for the loss of this aspect of their lives. This is more likely to occur if the individuals have not planned for retirement and if they have derived most of their self-esteem from their employment.

Nursing intervention at the secondary level of prevention with depressed individuals takes place in both inpatient and outpatient settings. Severely depressed clients with suicidal ideations will need close observation in the hospital setting, whereas those with mild to moderate depression may be treated in the community. A nursing care plan for the client with depression is found in Chapter 29. These concepts apply to the secondary level of prevention and may be used in all nursing care settings.

The physician may elect to use pharmacotherapy with antidepressants. Nurses may intervene by providing information to the client about what to expect from the medication, possible side effects, adverse effects, and how to self-administer the medication.

Situational Crises

Nursing care at the secondary level of prevention with clients undergoing situational crises occurs only if crisis intervention at the primary level failed and the individual is unable to function socially or occupationally. Exacerbation of mental illness symptoms requires intervention at the secondary level of prevention. These disorders were addressed extensively in Unit Four. Nursing assessment, diagnosis and outcome identification, plan and implementation, and evaluation were discussed for many of the mental illnesses identified in the *DSM-IV-TR* (APA, 2000). These skills may be applied in any setting where nursing is practiced.

A case study situation of nursing care at the secondary level of prevention in a community setting is presented in Table 42–2.

Tertiary Prevention

The Chronically Mentally Ill

Historical and Epidemiological Aspects

In 1955, more than half a million individuals resided in public mental hospitals. More recent statistics indicate that approximately 100,000 mentally ill persons inhabit these institutions on a long-term basis (Sadock & Sadock, 2003).

Deinstitutionalization of persons with chronic mental illness began in the 1960s as national policy change and with a strong belief in the individual's right to freedom. Other considerations included the deplorable conditions of some of the state asylums, the introduction of neuroleptic medications, and the cost-effectiveness of caring for these individuals in the community setting.

Deinstitutionalization began to occur rapidly and without sufficient planning for the needs of these individuals as they reentered the community. Those who were fortunate enough to have support systems to provide assistance with living arrangements and sheltered employment experiences most often received the outpatient treatment they required. However, those without adequate support either managed to survive on a meager existence or were forced to join the ranks of the homeless. Some ended up in nursing homes meant to provide care for individuals with physical disabilities.

TABLE 42–2	Secondary Prevention Case Study: Parenthood

The identified patient was a petite, doll-like 4-year-old girl named Tanya. She was the older of two children in a Latino American family. The other child was a boy named Joseph, aged 2. The mother was 5 months pregnant with their third child. The family had been referred to the nurse after Tanya was placed in foster care following a report to the Department of Human Services by her nursery school teacher that the child had marks on her body suspicious of child abuse.

The parents, Paulo and Annette, were in their mid-20s. Paulo had lost his job at an aircraft plant 3 months ago and had been unable to find work since. Annette brought in a few dollars from cleaning houses for other people, but the family was struggling to survive.

Paulo and Annette were angry at having to see the nurse. After all, "Parents have the right to discipline their children." The nurse did not focus on the *intent* of the behavior, but instead looked at factors in the family's life that could be viewed as stressors. This family had multiple stressors: poverty, the father's unemployment, the age and spacing of the children, the mother's chronic fatigue from work at home and in other people's homes, and finally, having a child removed from the home against the parents' wishes.

During therapy with this family, the nurse discussed the behaviors associated with various developmental levels. She also discussed possible deviations from these norms and when they should be reported to the physician. The nurse and the family discussed Tanya's behavior, and how it compared with the norms.

The parents also discussed their own childhoods. They were able to relate some of the same types of behaviors that they observed in Tanya. But they both admitted that they came from families whose main method of discipline was physical punishment. Annette had been the oldest child in her large family and had been expected to "keep the younger ones in line." When she had not done so, she was punished with her father's belt. She expressed anger toward her father, although she had never been allowed to express it at the time.

Paulo's father had died when he was a small boy, and Paulo had been expected to be the "man of the family." From the time he was very young, he worked at odd jobs to bring money into the home. Because of this, he had little time for the usual activities of childhood and adolescence. He held much resentment toward the young men who "had everything and never had to work for it."

Paulo and Annette had high expectations for Tanya. In effect, they expected her to behave in a manner well beyond her developmental level. These expectations were based on the reflections of their own childhoods. They were uncomfortable with the spontaneity and playfulness of childhood because they had had little personal experience with these behaviors. When Tanya balked and expressed the verbal assertions common to early childhood, Paulo and Annette interpreted these behaviors as defiance toward them and retaliated with anger in the manner in which they had been parented.

With the parents, the nurse explored feelings and behaviors from their past so that they were able to understand the correlation to their current behaviors. They learned to negotiate ways to deal with Tanya's age-appropriate behaviors. In combined therapy with Tanya, they learned how to relate to her childishness, and even how to enjoy playing with both of their children.

The parents ceased blaming each other for the family's problems. Annette had spent a good deal of her time deprecating Paulo for his lack of support of his family, and Paulo blamed Annette for being "unable to control her daughter." Communication patterns were clarified, and life in the family became more peaceful.

Without a need to "prove himself" to his wife, Paulo's efforts to find employment met with success because he no longer felt the need to turn down jobs that he knew his wife would perceive to be beneath his capabilities. Annette no longer works outside the home, and both she and Paulo participate in the parenting chores. Tanya and her siblings continue to demonstrate age-appropriate developmental progression.

Certain segments of our population with chronic mental illness problems have been left untreated: the elderly, the "working poor," the homeless, and those individuals previously covered by funds that have been cut by various social reforms. These circumstances have promoted in individuals with chronic mental illness a greater number of crisis-oriented emergency department visits and hospital admissions, and repeated confrontations with law enforcement officials.

In 2002, President George W. Bush established the New Freedom Commission on Mental Health. This commission was charged with the task of conducting a comprehensive study of the United States mental health service delivery system. They were to identify unmet needs and barriers to services and recommend steps for improvement in services and support for individuals with serious mental illness. In July 2003, the commission presented its final report to the President (President's New Freedom Commission on Mental Health, 2003). The Commission identified the following five barriers:

1. **Fragmentation and gaps in care for children.** About 7 to 9 percent of all children (ages 9 to 17) have a serious emotional disturbance (SED). The Commis-

sion found that services for children are even more fragmented than those for adults, with more uncoordinated funding and differing eligibility requirements. Only a fraction of children with SED appear to have access to school-based or school-linked mental health services. Children with SED who are identified for special education services have higher levels of absenteeism, higher drop-out rates, and lower levels of academic achievement than students with other disabilities.

2. **Fragmentation and gaps in care for adults with serious mental illness.** The Commission expresses concern that so many adults with serious mental illness are homeless, dependent on alcohol or drugs, unemployed, and go without treatment. According to the World Health Organization (WHO), mental illness ranks first in terms of causing disability in North America and Western Europe (WHO, 2001). The Commission identifies public attitudes and the stigma associated with mental illness as a major barrier to treatment. Stigma is often internalized by individuals with mental illness, leading to hopelessness, lower self-esteem, and isolation. Stigma deprives these individuals of the support they need to recover.

3. **High unemployment and disability for people with serious mental illness.** Undetected, untreated, and poorly treated mental disorders interrupt careers, leading many individuals into lives of disability, poverty, and long-term dependence. The Commission found a 90 percent unemployment rate among adults with serious mental illness—the worst level of employment of any group of people with disabilities. Some surveys have shown that many individuals with serious mental illness *want* to work, and could, with modest assistance. However, the largest "program" of assistance the United States has for people with mental illness is disability payments. Sadly, societal stigma is also reflected in employment discrimination against people with mental illness.

4. **Older adults with mental illnesses are not receiving care.** The Commission reports that about 5 to 10 percent of older adults have major depression, yet most are not properly recognized and treated. The report states:

   > Older people are reluctant to get care from specialists. They feel more comfortable going to their primary care physician. Still, they are often more sensitive to the stigma of mental illness, and do not readily bring up their sadness and despair. If they acknowledge problems, they are more likely than young people to describe physical symptoms. Primary care doctors may see their suffering as "natural" aging, or treat their reported physical distress instead of the underlying mental disorder. What is often missed is the deep impact of depression on older people's capacity to function in ways that are seemingly effortless for others.

5. **Mental health and suicide prevention are not yet national priorities.** The fact that the United States has failed to prioritize mental health puts many lives at stake. Families struggle to maintain equilibrium while communities strain (and often fail) to provide needed assistance for adults and children who suffer from mental illness. Over 30,000 lives are lost annually to suicide. About 90 percent of those who take their life have a mental disorder. Many individuals who commit suicide have not had the care in the months before their death that would help them to affirm life. Both the American Psychiatric Association and the National Mental Health Association have called on the U.S. Congress to pass parity legislation. Lack of equal access to insurance coverage is conspicuous evidence of the low priority placed on mental health treatment.

The Commission outlined the following goals and recommendations for mental health reform:

Goal 1. Americans will understand that mental health is essential to overall health.
Commission recommendations:

- Advance and implement a national campaign to reduce the stigma of seeking care and a national strategy for suicide prevention.
- Address mental health with the same urgency as physical health.

Goal 2. Mental health care will be consumer and family driven.
Commission recommendations:

- Develop an individualized plan of care for every adult with a serious mental illness and child with a serious emotional disturbance.
- Involve consumers and families fully in orienting the mental health system toward recovery.
- Align relevant federal programs to improve access and accountability for mental health services.
- Create a Comprehensive State Mental Health Plan.
- Protect and enhance the rights of people with mental illness.

Goal 3. Disparities in mental health services will be eliminated.
Commission recommendations:

- Improve access to quality care that is culturally competent.
- Improve access to quality care in rural and geographically remote areas.

Goal 4. Early mental health screening, assessment, and referral to services will be common practice.
Commission recommendations:

- Promote the mental health of young children.
- Improve and expand school mental health programs.
- Screen for co-occurring mental and substance use disorders and link with integrated treatment strategies.
- Screen for mental disorders in primary health care, across the life span, and connect to treatment and supports.

Goal 5. Excellent mental health care will be delivered and research will be accelerated.
Commission recommendations:

- Accelerate research to promote recovery and resilience, and ultimately to cure and prevent mental illnesses.
- Advance evidence-based practices using dissemination and demonstration projects, and create a public-private partnership to guide their implementation.
- Improve and expand the workforce providing evidence-based mental health services and supports.

- Develop the knowledge base in four understudied areas: mental health disparities, long-term effects of medications, trauma, and acute care.

Goal 6. Technology will be used to access mental health care and information.

Commission recommendations:

- Use health technology and telehealth to improve access and coordination of mental health care, especially for Americans in remote areas or in underserved populations.
- Develop and implement integrated electronic health record and personal health information systems.

If these proposals became reality, it would surely mean improvement in the care of chronically mentally ill individuals. Many nurse leaders see this period of health care reform as an opportunity for nurses to expand their roles and assume key positions in education, prevention, assessment, and referral. Nurses are, and will continue to be, in key positions to assist chronically mentally ill clients to remain as independent as possible, to manage their illness within the community setting, and to strive to minimize the number of hospitalizations required.

Treatment Alternatives

Community Mental Health Centers. The goal of community mental health centers in caring for the chronically mentally ill is to improve coping ability and prevent exacerbation of acute symptoms. A major obstacle in meeting this goal has been the lack of advocacy or sponsorship for clients who require services from a variety of sources. This has placed responsibility for health care on a mentally ill individual who is often barely able to cope with everyday life. Case management has become a recommended method of treatment for individuals with a chronic mental illness.

The ANA (1992) has endorsed case management as an effective method of providing care for clients in the community who require long-term assistance:

> Nurses bring broad-based and unique skills and knowledge to case management. The role of the nurse as a coordinator of care has been integral to defining nursing practice for decades. The coordination of services and care is the primary function of case managers. This role is a logical extension of the nursing role. (p. 14)

Bower (1992) has identified five core components and nursing role functions that blend with the steps of the nursing process to form a framework for nursing case management. The core components include:

- **Interaction**. The nurse must develop a trusting relationship with the client, family members, and other

service providers. During an initial screening process the nurse determines if the client is eligible for case management according to preestablished guidelines and, if not, refers the client for appropriate assistance elsewhere.

- **Assessment: Establishment of a Database**. The nurse conducts a comprehensive assessment of the client's physical health status, functional capability, mental status, personal and community support systems, financial resources, and environmental conditions. The data are then analyzed and appropriate nursing diagnoses formulated.
- **Planning**. A service care plan is devised with client participation. The plan should include mutually agreed-on goals, specific actions directed toward goal achievement, and selection of essential resources and services through collaboration among health care professionals, the client, and the family or significant others.
- **Implementation**. In this phase, the client receives the needed services from the appropriate providers. In some instances the nursing case manager is also a provider of care, whereas in others, he or she is only the coordinator of care.
- **Evaluation**. The case manager continuously monitors and evaluates the client's responses to interventions and progress toward preestablished goals. Regular contact is maintained with client, family or significant others, and direct service providers. Ongoing care coordination continues until outcomes have been achieved. The client may then be discharged or assigned to inactive status, as appropriate.

A case study of nursing case management within a community mental health center is presented in Table 42–3.

Assertive Community Treatment (ACT). The National Alliance for the Mentally Ill (NAMI) defines ACT as a service-delivery model that provides comprehensive, locally based treatment to people with serious and persistent mental illnesses (NAMI, 2003). ACT is a type of case-management program that provides highly individualized services directly to consumers. It is a team approach, and includes members from psychiatry, social work, nursing, substance abuse, and vocational rehabilitation. The ACT team provides these services 24 hours a day, seven days a week, 365 days a year.

NAMI (2003) identifies the primary goals of ACT as follows:

- To lessen or eliminate the debilitating symptoms of mental illness each individual client experiences
- To minimize or prevent recurrent acute episodes of the illness
- To meet basic needs and enhance quality of life
- To improve functioning in adult social and employment roles

TABLE 42–3	Nursing Case Management in the Community Mental Health Center: A Case Study

Michael, 73 years old with a history of multiple psychiatric admissions, has lived in various adult foster homes and boarding houses for the past 10 years. He was originally diagnosed as having schizophrenia, but he was recently rediagnosed as having bipolar disorder, mania. His symptoms are well controlled with lithium 300 mg three times a day, which is prescribed by the outpatient psychiatrist.

The nurse practitioner/case manager in the outpatient clinic coordinates Michael's care, advocates for his needs, and counsels him regarding his health problems. She orders routine blood tests to assess his lithium levels. When Michael experienced visual disturbances, she referred him for an emergency eye evaluation. He was found to have a retinal detachment and was sent to a local VA hospital for emergency surgery. After his eye surgery, the nurse practitioner arranged transportation to his follow-up visits with the eye doctor and instructed him about his eye care and instillation of his eye drops. Michael did not like putting eye drops in his eye and tended to neglect doing it. Because he also had glaucoma and required ongoing treatment with pilocarpine and timolol maleate eye drops twice daily, he needed a great deal of education and reassurance to continue using the eye drops.

In addition to routine quarterly visits for ongoing case management, the nurse practitioner also performs his annual health assessment consisting of history, review of systems, mental status exam, and physical assessment. During Michael's last physical exam, the nurse practitioner detected a thyroid mass and referred him for a complete evaluation including thyroid function tests, a thyroid scan, and evaluation by a surgeon and an endocrinologist. She discussed his thyroid problem with the surgeon and the endocrinologist, and they determined that Michael would best benefit from thyroid replacement (i.e., levothyroxine sodium 0.1 mg daily).

Because Michael eats all of his meals in restaurants, the nurse was concerned about his diet. A brief diet review revealed that his diet was low in vitamin C. He was then instructed in which foods and juices he should include in his daily menu. The nurse practitioner discussed ways that Michael could get the best nutrition for the least cost.

Michael currently is living in a boarding house and is totally responsible for taking his own medication, attending to his activities of daily living, and managing his own money. He has very limited income and depends on donations for many of his clothing needs.

Despite his age, he is quite active and alert. He attends many VA-sponsored social activities and does daily volunteer work at the VA, such as pushing wheelchairs, running errands, and escorting other veterans to clinic appointments. His nurse case manager arranged for him to receive free lunches as a reward for some of his volunteer activities.

Nursing case management has helped this elderly gentleman with chronic psychiatric illness and many years of hospitalization to live independently within the community setting.

SOURCE: From Pittman (1989), with permission.

● To enhance an individual's ability to live independently in his or her own community
● To lessen the family's burden of providing care

The ACT team provides treatment, rehabilitation, and support services to individuals with severe and persistent mental illness who are unable on their own to receive treatment from a traditional model of case management. The team is usually able to provide most services with minimal referrals to other mental health programs or providers. Services are provided within community settings, such as a person's home, local restaurants, parks, nearby stores, and any other place that the individual requires assistance with living skills.

Studies have shown that ACT clients spend significantly less time in hospitals and more time in independent living situations, have less time unemployed, earn more income from competitive employment, experience more positive social relationships, express greater satisfaction with life, and are less symptomatic (NAMI, 2003). Only about half of the states currently have ACT programs established or under pilot testing. NAMI (2003) states:

Despite the documented treatment success of ACT, only a fraction of those with the greatest needs have access to this uniquely effective program. In the United States, adults with severe and persistent mental illnesses constitute one-half to one percent of the adult population. It is estimated that 20 to 40 percent of this group could be helped by the ACT model if it were available.

Day/Evening Treatment/Partial Hospitalization Programs. Day or evening treatment programs (also called partial hospitalization) are designed to prevent institutionalization or to ease the transition from inpatient hospitalization to community living. Various types of treatment are offered. Many include therapeutic community (milieu) activities; individual, group, and family therapies; psychoeducation; alcohol and drug education; crisis intervention; therapeutic recreational activities; and occupational therapy. Many programs offer medication administration and monitoring as part of their care. Some programs have established medication clinics for individuals on long-term psychopharmacological therapy. These clinics may include educational classes and support groups for individuals with similar conditions and treatments.

Partial hospitalization programs generally offer a comprehensive treatment plan formulated by an interdisciplinary team of psychiatrists, psychologists, nurses, occupational and recreational therapists, and social workers. Nurses take a leading role in the administration of partial hospitalization programs. They lead groups, provide crisis intervention, conduct individual counseling, act as role models, and make necessary referrals for specialized treatment. Use of the nursing process provides continual evaluation of the program, and modifications can be made as necessary.

Partial hospitalization programs have proven to be an effective method of preventing hospitalization for many individuals with severe and persistent mental illness.

They are a way of transitioning these individuals from the acute care setting back into the mainstream of the community. For some individuals who have been deinstitutionalized, they provide structure, support, opportunities for socialization, and an improvement in their overall quality of life.

Community Residential Facilities. Community residential facilities for persons with chronic mental illness are known by many names: group homes, halfway houses, foster homes, boarding homes, sheltered care facilities, transitional housing, independent living programs, social-rehabilitation residences, and others. These facilities differ by the purpose for which they exist and the activities that they offer.

Some of these facilities provide food, shelter, housekeeping, and minimal supervision and assistance with activities of daily living. Others may also include a variety of therapies and serve as a transition between hospital and independent living. In addition to the basics, services might include individual and group counseling, medical care, job training or employment assistance, and leisure-time activities.

A wide variety of personnel staff these facilities. Some facilities have live-in professionals who are available at all times, some have professional staff who are on call for intervention during crisis situations, and some are staffed by volunteers and individuals with little knowledge or background for understanding and treating persons who are chronically mentally ill.

The concept of transitional housing for individuals who are chronically mentally ill is sound and has proved in many instances to be a successful means of therapeutic support and intervention for maintaining them within the community. However, without guidance and planning, transition to the community can be futile. These individuals may be ridiculed and rejected by the community. They may be targets of unscrupulous individuals who take advantage of their inability to care for themselves satisfactorily. These behaviors may increase maladaptive responses to the demands of community living and exacerbate the mental illness. A period of structured reorientation to the community in a living situation that is supervised and monitored by professionals is more likely to result in a successful transition for the individual with chronic mental illness.

The Homeless Population

Historical and Epidemiological Aspects

In 1992, Dr. Richard Lamb, a recognized expert in the field of severe and persistent mental illness, wrote:

> Alec Guinness, in his memorable role as a British Army colonel in *Bridge on the River Kwai*, exclaims at the end of the film when he finally realizes he has been working to help the enemy, 'What have I done?' As a vocal advocate and spokesman for deinstitutionalization and community treatment of severely mentally ill patients for well over two decades, I often find myself asking that same question.

The number of homeless in the United States has been estimated at somewhere between 250,000 and 4 million. It is difficult to determine the true scope of the problem because even the statisticians who collect the data have difficulty defining homeless persons. They have sometimes been identified as, "those people who sleep in shelters or public spaces." This approach results in underestimates because available shelter services are insufficient to meet the numbers of homeless people (U.S. Conference of Mayors, 2004).

According to the Stewart B. McKinney Act, a person is considered homeless who

> ...lacks a fixed, regular, and adequate night-time residence; and...has a primary night-time residency that is: (A) a supervised publicly or privately operated shelter designed to provide temporary living accommodations, (B) an institution that provides a temporary residence for individuals intended to be institutionalized, or (C) a public or private place not designed for, or ordinarily used as, a regular sleeping accommodation for human beings. (National Coalition for the Homeless [NCH], 2004)

Two methods of counting the homeless are commonly used (NCH, 2002a). The point-in-time method attempts to count all the people who are literally homeless on a given day or during a given week. The second method (called *period prevalence counts*) examines the number of people who are homeless over a given period of time. This second method may result in a more accurate count because the extended time period would allow for including the people who are homeless one day (or week) but find employment and affordable housing later, removing them from the homeless count. At the same time during this extended period, others would lose housing and become homeless.

Who Are the Homeless?

The U.S. Conference of Mayors (2004) reports that during the past year requests for emergency shelter increased in the survey cities by an average of 6 percent. The homeless are increasingly a heterogeneous group. The NCH (2004) provides the following demographics:

Age. Studies have produced a variety of statistics related to age of the homeless: 25 percent are younger than 18 years of age; individuals between the ages of 31 and 50 comprise 51 percent; and persons aged 55 through 60 have been estimated at 2.5 percent to 19.4 percent.

Gender. More men than women are homeless. The U.S. Conference of Mayors (2003) study found that single men comprise 40 percent of the urban homeless population and single women 14 percent.

Families. Families with children are among the fastest growing segments of the homeless population. Families comprise 40 percent of the urban homeless population, but research indicates that this number is likely higher in rural areas, where families, single mothers, and children make up the largest group of homeless people.

Ethnicity. The study by the U.S. Conference of Mayors (2003) found that the homeless population was 49 percent African American, 35 percent Caucasian, 13 percent Hispanic, 2 percent Native American, and 1 percent Asian. The ethnic makeup of homeless populations varies according to geographic location.

Mental Illness and Homelessness

It is thought that approximately 25 to 33 percent of the homeless population suffers from some form of mental illness (Harvard Medical School, 2005). Who are these individuals, and why are they homeless? Some blame the deinstitutionalization movement. Mentally ill persons who were released from state and county mental hospitals and who did not have families with whom they could reside sought residence in board and care homes of varying quality. Halfway houses and supportive group living arrangements were helpful but scarce. Many of those with families returned to their homes, but because families received little if any instruction or support, the consequences of their mentally ill loved one returning to live at home were often turbulent, resulting in the individual frequently leaving home.

Types of Mental Illness Among the Homeless. A number of studies have been conducted, primarily in large, urban areas, which have addressed the most common types of mental illness identified among the homeless. Schizophrenia is frequently described as the most common diagnosis. Other prevalent disorders include bipolar affective disorder, substance abuse and dependence, depression, personality disorders, and organic mental disorders. Many exhibit psychotic symptoms, many are former residents of long-term care institutions for the mentally ill, and many have such a strong desire for independence that they isolate themselves in an effort to avoid being identified as a part of the mental health system. Many of them are clearly a danger to themselves or others, yet they often do not even see themselves as ill.

Contributing Factors to Homelessness Among the Mentally Ill

Deinstitutionalization. As previously stated, deinstitutionalization is frequently implicated as a contributing factor to homelessness among the mentally ill. Deinstitutionalization began out of expressed concern by mental health professionals and others who described the

"deplorable conditions" under which mentally ill individuals were housed.

The advent of psychotropic medications and the community mental health movement began a growing philosophical view that mentally ill individuals receive better and more humanitarian treatment in the community than in state hospitals far removed from their homes. It was believed that commitment and institutionalization in many ways deprived these individuals of their civil rights. Not the least of the motivating factors for deinstitutionalization was the financial burden these clients placed on state governments.

In fact, deinstitutionalization has not failed completely. About 50 percent of the mentally ill population—those who have insight into their illness and need for medication—have done reasonably well. It is the other 50 percent who lack such insight and often stop taking their medication who end up on the streets.

However, because the vast increases in homelessness did not occur until the 1980s, the release of severely mentally ill people from institutions cannot be solely to blame. A number of other factors have been implicated.

Poverty. Cuts in various government entitlement programs have depleted the allotments available for chronically mentally ill individuals living in the community. The job market is prohibitive for individuals whose behavior is incomprehensible or even frightening to many. The stigma and discrimination associated with mental illness may be diminishing slowly, but it is highly visible to those who suffer from its effects.

A Scarcity of Affordable Housing. The National Coalition for the Homeless (NCH, 2002b) states:

> A lack of affordable housing and the limited scale of housing assistance programs have contributed to the current housing crisis and to homelessness. The gap between the number of affordable housing units and the number of people needing them has created a housing crisis for poor people. Between 1970 and 1995, the gap between the number of low-income renters and the amount of affordable housing units skyrocketed from a nonexistent gap to a shortage of 4.4 million affordable housing units—the largest shortfall on record.

In addition, the number of single-room-occupancy (SRO) hotels has diminished drastically. These SRO hotels provided a means of relatively inexpensive housing for chronic psychiatric clients. Although some people believe that these facilities nurtured isolation, they provided adequate shelter from the elements for their occupants. So many individuals currently frequent the shelters of our cities that there is concern that the shelters are becoming mini-institutions for the chronically mentally ill.

Other Factors. Several other factors that may contribute to homelessness have been identified. They include the following:

● **Lack of Affordable Health Care**. For families barely able to scrape together enough money to pay for day-to-day living, a catastrophic illness can create the level of poverty that starts the downward spiral to homelessness.

● **Domestic Violence**. The NCH (2002b) reports on a number of studies that identify domestic violence as a primary cause of homelessness. Battered women are often forced to choose between an abusive relationship and homelessness.

● **Addiction Disorders**. For individuals with alcohol or drug addictions, in the absence of appropriate treatment, the chances increase for being forced into life on the street. The following have been cited as obstacles to addiction treatment for homeless persons: lack of health insurance; lack of documentation; waiting lists; scheduling difficulties; daily contact requirements; lack of transportation; ineffective treatment methods; lack of supportive services; and cultural insensitivity.

Community Resources for the Homeless

Interfering Factors. Among the many issues that complicate service planning for the homeless mentally ill is this population's penchant for mobility. Frequent relocation confounds service delivery and interferes with providers' efforts to ensure appropriate care. Some individuals with chronic mental illness may be affected by homelessness only temporarily or intermittently. These individuals are sometimes called the "episodically homeless." Others move around within neighborhoods or cities as needs change and based on whether or not they can obtain needed services. A large number of the homeless mentally ill population exhibits continuous unbounded movement over wide geographical areas.

Not all of the homeless mentally ill population are mobile. Some studies have indicated that a large percentage remains in the same location over a number of years. Health care workers must identify movement patterns of homeless people in their area to at least try to bring the best care possible to this unique population. This may indeed mean delivering services to those individuals who do not seek out services on their own.

Health Issues. Life as a homeless person can have severe consequences in terms of health. Exposure to the elements, poor diet, sleep deprivation, risk of violence, injuries, and little or no health care lead to a precarious state of health and exacerbate any preexisting illnesses. One of the major afflictions is alcoholism. It has been estimated that about 40 percent of homeless individuals abuse alcohol. Compared to other homeless individuals, those who abuse alcohol are at greater risk for neurolog-

ical impairment, heart disease and hypertension, chronic lung disease, gastrointestinal (GI) disorders, hepatic dysfunction, and trauma.

Thermoregulation is a health problem for all homeless individuals because of their exposure to all kinds of weather. It is a compounded problem for the homeless alcoholic who spends much time in an altered level of consciousness.

It is difficult to determine whether mental illness is a cause or an effect of homelessness. Some behaviors that may seem deviant to some people may in actuality be adaptations to life on the street. It has been suggested that some homeless individuals may even seek hospitalization in psychiatric institutions in an attempt to get off the streets for a while.

Tuberculosis is a growing problem among individuals who are homeless (Raoult, Foucault, & Brouqui, 2001). Crowded shelters provide ideal conditions for spread of respiratory infections among their inhabitants. The risk of acquiring tuberculosis is also increased by the prevalence of alcoholism, drug addiction, HIV infection, and poor nutrition among homeless individuals.

Dietary deficiencies are a continuing problem for homeless individuals. Not only is the homeless person commonly in a poor nutritional state, but the condition itself exacerbates a number of other health problems. Homeless people suffer from higher mortality rates and a greater number of serious disorders than their counterparts in the general population.

Sexually transmitted diseases, such as gonorrhea and syphilis, are a serious problem for the homeless. One of the most serious sexually transmitted diseases prevalent among the homeless is human immunodeficiency virus (HIV) infection. Street life is precarious for individuals whose systems are immunosuppressed by the HIV. Rummaged food scraps are often spoiled, and exposure to the elements is a continuous threat. HIV-infected individuals who stay in shelters often are exposed to the infectious diseases of others, which can be life threatening in their vulnerable condition.

HIV disease is increasing among the homeless population. The NCH (1999) reports that one study revealed a median HIV-positive rate of 2.3 percent for homeless persons under the age of 25. Another suggested that up to 50 percent of persons living with HIV/AIDS are expected to need housing assistance of some kind during their lifetimes.

Homeless children have special health needs. The NCH (2001) reports that children without a home have higher rates of asthma, ear infections, stomach problems, and speech problems than their counterparts who are not homeless. They also experience more mental health problems, such as anxiety, depression, and withdrawal.

They are twice as likely to experience hunger and four times as likely to have delayed development.

Types of Resources Available

Homeless Shelters. The system of shelters for the homeless in the United States varies widely, from converted warehouses that provide cots or floor space on which to sleep overnight to significant operations that provide a multitude of social and health care services. They are run by volunteers and paid professionals and are sponsored by churches, community governments, and a variety of social agencies.

It is impossible, then, to describe a "typical" shelter. One profile may be described as the provision of lodging, food, and clothing to individuals who are in need of these services. Some shelters also provide medical and psychiatric evaluations, first aid and other health care services, and referral for case management services by nurses or social workers.

Individuals who seek services from the shelter are generally assigned a bed or cot, issued a set of clean linen, provided a place to shower, shown laundry facilities, and offered a meal in the shelter kitchen or dining hall. Most shelters attempt to separate dormitory areas for men and women, with various consequences for those who violate the rules.

Shelters cover expenses through private and corporate donations, church sponsorships, and government grants. From the outset, shelters were conceptualized as "temporary" accommodations for individuals who needed a place to spend the night. Realistically, they have become permanent lodging for homeless individuals with little hope for improving their situation. Some individuals use shelters for their mailing address.

In the early 1980s, New York City instituted the Work Experience Program (WEP), which required all employable residents to work 20 hours a week for a $12.50 stipend. Evaluation of the program suggested that WEP kept the residents busy and enhanced their self-esteem, while preventing idleness and depression. Since 1995, under a comprehensive program of welfare reform, more than 250,000 people have moved through the WEP (Human Resources Administration [HRA], 2002).

Shelters provide a safe and supportive environment for homeless individuals who have no other place to go. Some homeless people who inhabit shelters use the resources offered to improve their lot in life, whereas others become hopelessly dependent on the shelter's provisions. To a few, the availability of a shelter may even mean the difference between life and death.

Health Care Centers and Store-Front Clinics. Some communities have established "street clinics" to serve the homeless population. Many of these clinics are operated by nurse practitioners who work in consultation with physicians in the area. In recent years, some of these clinics have provided clinical rotation sites for nursing students in their community health rotation. Some have been staffed by faculties of nursing schools who have established group practices in the community setting.

A wide variety of services are offered at these clinics, including administering medications, assessing vital signs, screening for tuberculosis and other communicable diseases, giving immunizations and flu shots, changing dressings, and administering first aid. Physical and psychosocial assessments, health education, and supportive counseling are also frequent interventions.

Nursing in **store-front clinics** for the homeless provides many special challenges, not the least of which is poor working conditions. These clinics often operate under severe budgetary constraints with insufficient staff, supplies, and equipment, and in high-crime neighborhoods in dilapidated, inadequate facilities. Frustration is often high among nurses who work in these clinics, as they are seldom able to see measurable progress in their homeless clients. Maintenance of health management is virtually impossible for many individuals who have no resources outside the health care setting. When return appointments for preventive care are made, the lack of follow-through is high.

Mobile Outreach Units. Outreach programs literally reach out to the homeless in their own environment in an effort to provide health care. Volunteers and paid professionals form teams to drive or walk around and seek out homeless individuals who are in need of assistance. They offer coffee, sandwiches, and blankets in an effort to show concern and establish trust. If assistance can be provided at the site, it is done so. If not, every effort is made to ensure that the individual is linked with a source that can provide the necessary services.

Mobile outreach units provide assistance to homeless individuals who are in need of physical or psychological care. The emphasis of outreach programs is to accommodate the homeless who refuse to seek treatment elsewhere. Most target the mentally ill segment of the population. When trust has been established, and the individual agrees to come to the team's office, medical and psychiatric treatment is initiated. Involuntary hospitalization is initiated when an individual is deemed harmful to self or others, or otherwise meets the criteria for being considered "gravely disabled."

The Homeless Client and the Nursing Process

The nursing process with the homeless client is demonstrated by the following case study.

CASE STUDY

ASSESSMENT

Joe, age 46, is brought to the Community Health Clinic by two of his peers, who report: "He just had a fit. He needs a drink bad!" Joe is dirty, unkempt, has visible tremors of the upper extremities, and is weak enough to require assistance when ambulating. He is cooperative as the nurse completes the intake assessment. He is coherent, although thought processes are slow. He is disoriented to time and place. He appears somewhat frightened as he scans the unfamiliar surroundings. He is unable to tell the nurse when he had his last drink. He reports no physical injury, and none is observable.

Joe carries a small bag with a few personal items inside, among which is a VA Benefit Card, identifying him as a veteran of the Vietnam war. The nurse finds a cot for Joe to lie down, ensures that his vital signs are stable, and telephones the number on the VA card.

The clinic nurse discovers that Joe is well known to the admissions personnel at the VA. He has a 29-year history of schizophrenia, with numerous hospitalizations. At the time of his last discharge, he was taking fluphenazine (Prolixin) 10 mg twice a day. He told the clinic nurse that he took the medication for a few months after he got out of the hospital but then did not have the prescription refilled. He could not remember when he had last taken fluphenazine.

Joe also has a long history of alcohol-related disorders and has been through the VA substance rehabilitation program three times. He has no home address and receives his VA disability benefit checks at a shelter address. He reports that he has no family. The nurse makes arrangements for VA personnel to drive Joe from the clinic to the VA hospital, where he is admitted for detoxification. She sets up a case management file for Joe and arranges with the hospital to have Joe return to the clinic after discharge.

DIAGNOSIS/OUTCOME IDENTIFICATION

The following nursing diagnosis was formulated for Joe:

Ineffective health maintenance related to ineffective coping skills evidenced by abuse of alcohol, lack of follow-through with neuroleptic medication, and lack of personal hygiene.

Ongoing criteria were selected as outcomes for Joe. They include:

1. Follows the rules of the group home and maintains his residency status.
2. Attends weekly sessions of group therapy at the VA day treatment program.
3. Attends weekly sessions of Alcoholics Anonymous and maintains sobriety.
4. Reports regularly to the health clinic for injections of fluphenazine.
5. Volunteers at the VA hospital 3 days a week.
6. Secures and retains permanent employment.

PLAN/IMPLEMENTATION

During Joe's hospitalization, the clinic nurse remained in contact with his case. Joe received complete physical and dental examinations and treatment during his hospital stay. The clinic nurse attended the treatment team meeting for Joe as his outpatient case manager. It was decided at the meeting to try giving Joe injections of fluphenazine decanoate because of his history of noncompliance with his daily oral medications. The clinic nurse would administer the injection every 4 weeks.

At Joe's follow-up clinic visit the nurse explains to Joe that she has found a group home where he may live with others who have personal circumstances similar to his. At the group home, meals will be provided and the group home manager will ensure that Joe's basic needs are fulfilled. A criterion for remaining at the residence is for Joe to remain alcohol free. Joe is agreeable to these living arrangements.

With Joe's concurrence, the clinic nurse also performs the following interventions:

1. Goes shopping with Joe to purchase some new clothing, allowing Joe to make decisions as independently as possible.
2. Helps Joe move into the group home and introduces him to the manager and residents.
3. Helps Joe change his address from the shelter to the group home so that he may continue to receive his VA benefits.
4. Enrolls Joe in the weekly group therapy sessions of the day treatment facility connected with the VA hospital.
5. Helps Joe locate the nearest Alcoholics Anonymous group and identifies a sponsor who will ensure that Joe gets to the meetings.
6. Sets up a clinic appointment for Joe to return in 4 weeks for his fluphenazine injection; telephones Joe 1 day in advance to remind him of his appointment.
7. Instructs Joe to return to or call the clinic if any of the following symptoms occur: sore throat, fever, nausea and vomiting, severe headache, difficulty urinating, tremors, skin rash, or yellow skin or eyes.
8. Assists Joe in securing transportation to and from appointments.
9. Encourages Joe to set realistic goals for his life and offers recognition for follow-through.
10. When Joe is ready, discusses employment alternatives with him; suggests the possibility of starting with a volunteer job (perhaps as a VA hospital volunteer).

EVALUATION

Evaluation of the nursing process with the homeless mentally ill must be highly individualized. Statistics show that chances for relapse with this population are high. Therefore, it is extremely important that outcome criteria be realistic so as not to set the client up for failure.

RURAL MENTAL HEALTH NURSING

Approximately 20 percent of the U.S. population resides in rural areas (Bushy, 2004). These rural communities make up a type of subculture with their own set of beliefs, attitudes, and values that differ comparatively with the urban population. These differences affect the way in which individuals in the rural areas view mental health and mental illness and the care of individuals with mental illness.

Mental health assistance is much less readily available to rural residents than it is to individuals who reside in urban areas. Not only do fewer general hospitals exist in rural America, but psychiatric services are seldom provided within these institutions. Because of this, rural residents often must travel long distances to procure mental health services. In reality, only about half of rural residents with emotional problems ever seek treatment, and most commonly, the mental health services are provided by a general practitioner, public health nurse, or social service worker. Knowledge of crisis intervention techniques is essential for the rural mental health nurse, as the denial of emotional illness and delay in treatment often necessitates emergency services.

A number of characteristics have been identified in describing the rural population. In comparison to the population in general, rural residents are commonly more religious, conservative, traditional, and family-oriented. These particular values influence not only the way in which rural residents interpret psychopathological behaviors but also the initiative to seek treatment and the type of treatment sought. Some of the barriers to treatment of mental illness by rural residents include stigma, isolation, lack of knowledge, cost of services and medications, and lack of availability of the latest science-based mental health services (Braun, 2005).

The rural mental health nurse must by necessity serve as a generalist. That is, he or she must be able to assess the physical and emotional needs of individuals and make referrals when needed. He or she should also possess the ability to intervene with a variety of skills in a diversity of situations. As a practitioner, the rural mental health nurse may staff a community health center, make home visits, or even serve as primary therapist in crisis intervention, and short- and long-term individual counseling.

Trust may be difficult to establish in the rural community. Because of the stigma attached to mental illness and the ideology that "one takes care of one's own problems," it is less likely that individuals would seek treatment for emotional problems but more likely that they would seek assistance for related physical complaints because these would be more socially acceptable. Personal disclosure is difficult among individuals who "know everyone and everyone's business." Suspicions surrounding confidentiality may interfere with treatment in group situations.

The role of educator is most significant to the rural mental health nurse. Because many individuals who live in rural settings have had little or no health education, the choice of topics is vast. Examples range from basic nutrition and hygiene to information about numerous physical illnesses, how to prevent them, identify symptoms, and treat them. The rural mental health nurse also has an opportunity to decrease stigma surrounding mental illness by increasing knowledge about pathological behaviors and how to prevent and treat them. Information can be dispensed in a variety of ways, including during community health fairs and club meetings, in schools and churches, and in the home or community health clinic.

Change is difficult under the best of circumstances. But the opportunity for change is bountiful, and with enough patience and fortitude the rural mental health nurse can serve as change agent on many levels, including individual, community, state, and even national. Expansion of mental health services in rural areas is sorely needed, and the legislative arena is the most probable source for assistance in generating the resources required to provide these services. A keen opportunity exists for rural mental health nurses to become active in the political process, particularly at this time of volatile health care reform.

Outreach programs have been shown to be effective in providing care to underserved areas, and mental health nurses are important members of the team that provides these services. Nurses in outreach programs provide ongoing assessment and intervention to rural residents within their own homes. For some chronically mentally ill individuals, this home treatment may be the only alternative to institutionalization. Not only are these outreach services the "least restrictive" alternative, but they have also been shown to be very efficient and cost-effective without diminishing quality of care.

Bushy (2004) states:

> There are many and varied opportunities for nurses who choose to work in rural settings and for urban-based providers who provide care or outreach services to rural populations. To do this most effectively, nurses must learn what rural Americans prefer relative to their health care needs. Together, as partners, effective solutions can be developed to meet rural America's nursing care needs and to achieve the goals specified in *Health People 2010* in a culturally and linguistically appropriate manner.

SUMMARY

The trend in psychiatric care is shifting from that of inpatient hospitalization to a focus of outpatient care within the community. This trend is largely due to the need for greater cost-effectiveness in the provision of medical care to the masses. The community mental health movement began in the 1960s with the closing of state hospitals and the deinstitutionalization of many individuals with chronic mental illness.

Mental health care within the community targets primary prevention (reducing the incidence of mental disorders within the population), secondary prevention (reducing the prevalence of psychiatric illness by shortening the course of the illness), and tertiary prevention (reducing the residual defects that are associated with severe or chronic mental illness). Primary prevention focuses on identification of populations at risk for mental illness, increasing their ability to cope with stress, and targeting and diminishing harmful forces within the environment. The focus of secondary prevention is accomplished through early identification of problems and prompt initiation of effective treatment. Tertiary prevention focuses on preventing complications of the illness and promoting rehabilitation that is directed toward achievement of the individual's maximum level of functioning.

Registered nurses serve as providers of psychiatric/mental health care in the community setting. Nurses may practice at the basic level or at the advanced practice level, depending on their education, experience, and credentialing. To ensure that a wide range of services are made available as needed, many nurses serve as case managers for persons who are chronically mentally ill. Case management has been shown to enhance the client's functioning by increasing ability to solve problems, improving work and socialization skills, promoting leisure time activities, and endeavoring to diminish dependency on others.

Nurses provide outpatient care for individuals with chronic mental illness in community mental health centers, in day and evening treatment programs, in partial hospitalization programs, in community residential facilities, and with psychiatric home health care (addressed in Chapter 43).

Homeless persons with mental illness provide a special challenge for the community mental health nurse. Care is provided within homeless shelters, at health care centers or store-front clinics, and through mobile outreach programs.

The mental health needs of individuals who live in rural areas are largely underserved. Nurses who choose to work in these areas encounter enormous challenges and abundant opportunities for creating positive change. The rural mental health nurse can be a compelling force for providing quality care at all three levels of prevention to residents of rural areas of our country.

REVIEW QUESTIONS

SELF-EXAMINATION/LEARNING EXERCISE

Select the answer that is *most* appropriate for each of the following questions.

1. Which of the following represents a nursing intervention at the primary level of prevention?
   a. Teaching a class in parent effectiveness training
   b. Leading a group of adolescents in drug rehabilitation
   c. Referring a married couple for sex therapy
   d. Leading a support group for battered women

2. Which of the following represents a nursing intervention at the secondary level of prevention?
   a. Teaching a class about menopause to middle-aged women
   b. Providing support in the emergency room to a rape victim
   c. Leading a support group for women in transition
   d. Making monthly visits to the home of a client with schizophrenia to ensure medication compliance

3. Which of the following represents a nursing intervention at the tertiary level of prevention?
   a. Serving as case manager for a mentally ill homeless client
   b. Leading a support group for newly retired men
   c. Teaching prepared childbirth classes
   d. Caring for a depressed widow in the hospital

4. John, a homeless person, has just come to live in the shelter. The shelter nurse is assigned to his care. Which of the following is a *priority* intervention on the part of the nurse?
   a. Referring John to a social worker
   b. Developing a plan of care for John
   c. Conducting a behavioral and needs assessment on John
   d. Helping John apply for Social Security benefits

5. John has a history of paranoid schizophrenia and noncompliance with medications. Which of the following medications might be the best choice of neuroleptic for John?
   a. Haldol
   b. Navane
   c. Lithium carbonate
   d. Prolixin decanoate

6. Ann is a rural mental health nurse. She has just received an order to begin regular visits to Mrs. W, a 78-year-old widow who lives alone. Mrs. W's primary-care physician has diagnosed her as depressed. Based on knowledge about rural residents, which of the following statements would most likely apply to Mrs. W?
   a. She will most likely have little difficulty establishing trust with the nurse.
   b. She will probably resist therapy for emotional illness.
   c. She will most likely welcome the nurse without question.
   d. She would most likely do better in a group situation than one-to-one with the nurse.

7. Based on a needs assessment, which of the following problems would Ann address during her first visit?
   a. Dysfunctional grieving
   b. Social isolation
   c. Risk for injury
   d. Disturbed sleep pattern

8. Mrs. W. says to Ann, "What's the use? I don't have anything to live for anymore." Which is the best response on the part of the nurse?
   a. "Of course you do, Mrs. W. Why would you say such a thing?"
   b. "You seem so sad. I'm going to do my best to cheer you up."
   c. "Let's talk about why you are feeling this way."
   d. "Have you been thinking about harming yourself in any way?"

9. The physician orders trazodone (Desyrel) for Mrs. W, 150 mg to take at bedtime. Which of the following statements about this medication would be appropriate for Ann to make in teaching Mrs. W. about trazodone?
   a. "You may feel dizzy when you stand up, so go slowly when you get up from sitting or lying down."
   b. "You must be sure and not eat any chocolate while you are taking this medicine."
   c. "We will need to draw a sample of blood to send to the lab every month while you are on this medication."
   d. "If you don't feel better right away with this medicine, the doctor can order a different kind for you."

10. Which of the following statements is true about rural mental health services?
    a. Services are generally adequate to meet the demands.
    b. Rural mental health nurses must be generalists in an era of specialization.
    c. Rural residents are compliant and eager to accept opportunities for change.
    d. Direct reimbursement for services by rural nurses historically has not been a problem.

IMPLICATIONS OF RESEARCH FOR EVIDENCE-BASED PRACTICE

Rew, L., Fouladi, R.T., and Yockey, R.D. (2002). Sexual health practices of homeless youth. *Journal of Nursing Scholarship*, *34*(2), 139–145.

Description of the Study: The purpose of this study was to describe the sexual health practices of homeless adolescents, examine relationships among variables in a conceptual model of sexual health practices, and determine direct and indirect effects of population characteristics, cognitive-perceptual factors, and behavioral factors on sexual health practices among homeless adolescents. A survey was administered to a convenience sample of 414 homeless young men (244) and women (170) aged 16 to 20 years, the majority of whom were Anglo American. Likert-scale questionnaires were administered seeking information regarding sexually-transmitted diseases (STDs), knowledge about AIDS, self-efficacy to use condoms, future time perspective, intentions to use condoms, social support, sexual health practices, assertive communication, and background information.

Results of the Study: Thirty-five percent of the sample reported homosexual or bisexual orientation, and sexual orientation was reported as a reason for leaving home. Over half reported a history of sexual abuse and nearly 1 in 4 had been treated for gonorrhea. Seven percent had been treated for HIV, 8 percent for chlamydia, 3.6 percent for syphilis, and 32 percent had received one or more immunizations to prevent hepatitis B. Future time perspective scores were low, a finding that was not surprising, knowing the daily challenges of living on the street. Perceived social support scores were also low, again being an expected finding, due to lack of socially supportive environments of homes, parents, and schools. The mean safe-sex behavior score was higher than those in a study of university men. The authors speculated that this may indicate that participants were exposed to safe-sex messages more frequently at the street outreach center than were the university men. Those participants who had higher scores in perceived social support and assertive communication also had higher scores in self-efficacy to use condoms.

Implications for Nursing Practice: The authors suggest that the correlation of self-efficacy to use condoms with social support and assertive communication may indicate that an intervention directed at the enhancement of assertive communication skills and social support might result in increased self-efficacy, which could in turn increase safe-sex behaviors. The authors state:

> The relationship of intention to use condoms with future time perspective, social connectedness, and self-efficacy to use condoms, but also with sexual health responsibility indicates yet another domain in which to intervene with homeless adolescents. Interventions that focus on enhancing sexual health responsibility (e.g., seeking health care services if one suspects an STD or refusing to engage in sexual intercourse with someone known to have HIV) could have positive effects on these youth.

This study provides information that can be used by nurses who work with the homeless population, in an effort to change risky behavior and promote positive health care habits under frequently unfavorable conditions.

REFERENCES

American Nurses' Association. (1992). *Case management by nurses*. Washington, DC: American Nurses Publishing.

American Nurses' Association. (2000). Scope and *standards of psychiatric-mental health nursing practice*. Washington, DC: American Nurses Publishing.

American Psychiatric Association. (2000). *Diagnostic and statistical manual of mental disorders* (4th ed.) *Text revision*. Washington, DC: American Psychiatric Association.

Bower, K.A. (1992). *Case management by nurses*. Washington, DC: American Nurses Publishing.

Braun, B. (2005). *Barriers to mental health access for rural residents*. Rural Maryland Council Task Force on Mental Health Services Access. Department of Family Studies. College Park, MD: The University of Maryland.

Bushy, A. (2004). Rural nursing: Practice and issues. *American Nurses Association Continuing Education*. Retrieved December 10, 2004 from http://nursingworld.org/mods/mod700/rurlfull.htm

Case Management Society of America (CMSA). (2002). Retrieved May 29, 2005 from the World Wide Web at http://www.cmsa.org

Harvard Medical School. (2005). The homeless mentally ill. *Harvard Mental Health Letter, 21*(11), 4–7.

Human Resources Administration (HRA). (2002). New York City welfare reform program. Retrieved May 26, 2002 from the World Wide Web at http://www.ci.nyc.ny.us/html/hra/html/serv_welfare-work.html

Lamb, H.R. (1992). Perspectives on effective advocacy for homeless mentally ill persons. *Hospital and Community Psychiatry, 43*(12), 1209–1212.

Langley, C. (2002). Community-based nursing practice: An overview in the United States. In J.M. Sorrell & G.M. Redmond (Eds.). *Community-based nursing practice: Learning through students' stories*. Philadelphia: F.A. Davis.

Mercer, R.T. (2000). Transitions to parenthood. *NurseWeek*. Retrieved May 24, 2002 from http://nurse.cyberchalk.com/nurse/courses/nurseweek/nw1850/menu.html

Miller, M.A., & Rahe, R.H. (1997). Life changes scaling for the 1990s. *Journal of Psychosomatic Research, 43*(3), 279–292.

Murray, R., & Zentner, J. (2001). *Health promotion strategies through the life span* (7th ed.). Upper Saddle River, NJ: Prentice-Hall.

National Alliance for the Mentally Ill (NAMI). (2003). *Assertive Community Treatment (ACT)*. Retrieved May 30, 2005 from the World Wide Web at http://www.nami.org/

National Coalition for the Homeless (NCH). (1999). *HIV/AIDS and homelessness*. Retrieved May 30, 2005 from the World Wide Web at http://www.ari.net/nch/hivaids.html

National Coalition for the Homeless (NCH). (2001). *Homeless families with children*. Retrieved May 30, 2005 from the World Wide Web at http://www.nationalhomeless.org/families.html

National Coalition for the Homeless (NCH). (2002a). *How many people experience homelessness?* Retrieved May 30, 2005 from the World Wide Web at http://www.nationalhomeless.org/numbers.html

National Coalition for the Homeless (NCH). (2002b). *Why are people homeless?* Retrieved May 30, 2005 from the World Wide Web at http://www. nationalhomeless.org/causes.html

National Coalition for the Homeless (NCH). (2004). *Who is homeless?* Retrieved May 30, 2005 from the World Wide Web at http://www.nationalhomeless.org/who.html

Pittman, D.C. (1989). Nursing case management: Holistic care for the deinstitutionalized chronically mentally ill. *Journal of Psychosocial Nursing, 27*(11), 23–27.

President's New Freedom Commission on Mental Health. (2003). *Achieving the Promise: Transforming Mental Health Care in America*. Retrieved May 30, 2005 from the World Wide Web at http://www.mentalhealthcommission.gov/

Raoult, D., Foucault, C., & Brouqui, P. (2001). Infections in the homeless. *The Lancet Infectious Diseases, 1*(2), 77–84.

Sadock, B.J., & Sadock, V.A. (2003). *Synopsis of psychiatry: Behavioral sciences/clinical psychiatry* (9th ed.). Philadelphia: Lippincott Williams & Wilkins.

Scanlon, V.C., & Sanders, T. (2003). *Essentials of anatomy and physiology* (4th ed.). Philadelphia: F.A. Davis.

Spock, B. (2004). *Baby and child care* (8th ed.). New York: Simon & Schuster.

U.S. Conference of Mayors (USCM). (2003). *A status report on hunger and homelessness in America's cities: 2003*. Washington, DC: U.S. Conference of Mayors.

U.S. Conference of Mayors (USCM). (2004). *A status report on hunger and homelessness in America's cities: 2004*. Washington, DC: U.S. Conference of Mayors.

World Health Organization (WHO). (2001). *The World Health Report 2001—Mental Health: New Understanding, New Hope*. Retrieved May 30, 2005 from the World Wide Web at http://www.who.int/whr/

Wright, L.M., & Leahey, M. (2000). *Nurses and families: A guide to family assessment and intervention* (3rd ed.). Philadelphia: F.A. Davis.

CLASSICAL REFERENCES

Caplan, G. (1964). *Principles of preventive psychiatry*. New York: Basic Books.

Erikson, E. (1963). *Childhood and society* (2nd ed.). New York: W.W. Norton.

Mahler, M., Pine, F., & Bergman, A. (1975). *The psychological birth of the human infant*. New York: Basic Books.

Sheehy, G. (1976). *Passages: Predictable crises of adult life*. New York: Bantam Books.

43
CHAPTER

PSYCHIATRIC HOME
NURSING CARE

CHAPTER OUTLINE

OBJECTIVES	APPLICATION OF THE NURSING PROCESS
HISTORICAL ASPECTS	LEGAL AND ETHICAL ISSUES
GENERAL INFORMATION RELATED TO PSYCHIATRIC HOME NURSING CARE	SUMMARY
	REVIEW QUESTIONS
ROLE OF THE NURSE	

KEY TERMS

abandonment	home care	Medicare
Centers for Medicare and Medicaid Services (CMS)	informed consent	psychiatric home care

OBJECTIVES

After reading this chapter, the student will be able to:

1. Define *home care* and *psychiatric home care*.
2. Discuss historical aspects related to the growth in the home health care movement.
3. Identify agencies that provide, and sources of reimbursement for, psychiatric home nursing care.
4. Identify client populations that benefit most from psychiatric home nursing care.
5. Describe advantages and disadvantages

associated with psychiatric home nursing care.
6. Discuss cultural and boundary issues associated with psychiatric home nursing care.
7. Describe the role of the nurse in psychiatric home nursing care.
8. Apply steps of the nursing process to psychiatric home nursing care.
9. Discuss legal and ethical issues that relate to psychiatric home nursing care.

ramatic changes in the health care delivery system and skyrocketing costs have created a need to find a way to provide cost-effective quality care to psychiatric clients. **Home care** has become one of the fastest growing areas in the healthcare system, and is now recognized by many reimbursement agencies as a preferred method of community-based service. More than 20,000 providers deliver home care services to some 7.6 million individuals who require services because of acute illness, long-term health conditions, permanent disability, or terminal illness (National Association for Home Care [NAHC], 2004).

Just what is home health care? The NAHC (1996) has contributed the following definition:

Home care is a simple phrase that encompasses a wide range of health and social services. These services are delivered at home to recovering, disabled, chronically or terminally ill persons in need of medical, nursing, social, or therapeutic treatment and/or assistance with essential activities of daily living.

The psychiatric home care nurse must have knowledge and skills to meet both the physical and psychosocial needs of the homebound client. Serving health care consumers in their home environment charges the nurse with the responsibility of providing holistic care.

This chapter examines some of the issues related to psychiatric home nursing care. Historical aspects and present-day statistics are presented. Strengths and limitations of the concept and role of the nurse are described. Nursing care of the psychiatric home care client is presented in the context of the nursing process. Pertinent legal and ethical issues related to psychiatric home nursing care are examined.

HISTORICAL ASPECTS

The root of home care is found in the practice of visiting nursing, which had its beginnings in the United States in the late 1800s (Domrose, 2002). When physicians began to limit their home visits to clients after World War II, much of this care was relegated to nurses. Visiting nurses associations were established throughout the first half of the 20th century, with much of their services directed toward the poor who could not afford hospital care. In 1965, with the passage of **Medicare** legislation, home nursing care increased dramatically, because it was one of the benefits that Medicare provided for elderly clients who were eligible for the service.

Psychiatric home nursing care did not enjoy the popularity of other types of home care nursing, largely because psychiatric home nursing care was not recognized by the Health Care Financing Administration (HCFA)—now called **Centers for Medicare and Medicaid Services [CMA]**—as a reimbursable service until 1979. Growth through the 1980s was slow, with home care agencies employing psychiatric nurses mainly as consultants to their staff nurses. In recent years this has changed, and psychiatric home nursing care has become available to a large portion of the population.

GENERAL INFORMATION RELATED TO PSYCHIATRIC HOME NURSING CARE

Trends in the movement of psychiatric care into the community setting have increased the demand for in-home services of psychiatric clients. In 1999, 2.7 percent of all clients receiving home care services had a primary psychiatric diagnosis (NAHC, 2004). The increase in psychiatric home care may be related to a number of factors:

● Earlier hospital discharges
● Increased demand for home care as an alternative to institutional care
● Broader third-party payment coverage
● Greater physician acceptance of home care
● The increasing need to contain health care costs, and the growth of managed care

TABLE 43–1	Sources of Payment for Home Care 2003	
SOURCE OF PAYMENT	**PERCENT**
Medicare	31.9
Medicaid	29.0
Private insurance	18.0
Self-pay	18.0
Other	3.1

SOURCE: Centers for Medicare & Medicaid Services (2004).

Psychiatric home nursing care is provided through private home health agencies; private hospitals; public hospitals; government institutions, such as the Veterans Administration; and community mental health centers. Most often, home care is viewed as follow-up care to inpatient, partial, or outpatient hospitalization.

Payment for Home Care

The majority of home health care is paid for by Medicare. Other sources include Medicaid, private insurance, self-pay, and others. The statistics related to sources of payment are presented in Table 43–1. Medicare requires that the following criteria be met in order to qualify for psychiatric home care (Jensen & Miller, 2004):

1. The client is confined to the home
2. The client must receive services under a plan of care established and periodically reviewed by a physician.
3. The client must be in need of skilled nursing care on an intermittent basis.
4. Services must be reasonable and necessary for treating the client's psychiatric diagnosis and/or symptoms.
5. Home health psychiatric care must be provided by a skilled psychiatric nurse

Jensen and Miller (2004) report:

Care can be provided in one's own home or residence, assisted living, adult family homes, or retirement homes, but not in hospitals or skilled nursing facilities. A home health psychiatric care patient is unable to leave the home without considerable difficulty or the assistance of another person. The patient can leave home infrequently or for a short duration, for example, going to church on Sunday. The patient can also go out for medical treatment, partial hospitalization, adult day care, or chemotherapy. A patient can also be homebound for psychiatric reasons, such as depression, agoraphobia, paranoia, or panic disorder.

Although Medicare and Medicaid are the largest reimbursement providers, a growing number of health maintenance organizations (HMOs) and preferred provider organizations (PPOs) are beginning to recognize the cost effectiveness of psychiatric home nursing care and are including it as part of their benefit packages. Most managed care agencies require that treatment, or even a specific number of visits, be preauthorized for psychiatric home nursing care. The plan of treatment and subsequent charting must explain why the client's condition keeps him or her at home and justify the need for services.

Types of Diagnoses

Homebound psychiatric clients most often have diagnoses of depression, dementia, anxiety disorders, bipolar affective disorder, and schizophrenia. Psychiatric nurses also provide consultation for clients with primary medical disorders. Many elderly clients are homebound because of medical conditions that impair mobility and necessitate home care. Psychiatric nurses may provide the following types of home nursing care:

- To clients with primary Axis I psychiatric diagnoses, the symptoms of which are immobilizing, and the client and family require assistance with management of the symptoms.
- To clients who are homebound for medical conditions but have a psychiatric condition for which they have been receiving (and continue to need ongoing) treatment.
- To clients who are homebound with medical conditions and who may develop serious psychiatric symptoms in response to their medical illness.

Table 43–2 identifies some of the conditions for which a psychiatric nursing home care consultation may be sought.

Advantages and Disadvantages of Home Care

Ongoing studies continue to support the cost-effectiveness of psychiatric home nursing care, but there are certain other aspects related to nursing the psychiatric client in his or her home that must be taken into consideration. Being able to observe the client within the context of

---

TABLE 43–2 Conditions that Warrant Psychiatric Nursing Consultation

- When a client has a new psychiatric diagnosis
- When a new psychotropic medication has been added to the regimen
- When the client's mental status exacerbates or causes deterioration in his or her medical condition
- When the client is suspected of abusing alcohol or drugs
- When a client is expressing suicidal ideation
- When a client is noncompliant with psychotropic medication
- When a client develops a fundamental change in mood or a thought disorder
- When a client is immobilized by severe depression or anxiety

SOURCE: Adapted from Schroeder (2001).

---

family and home environment allows for the most comprehensive biopsychosocial assessment. Elderly individuals and individuals with serious and persistent mental illness may feel more comfortable and less threatened in their home environment. In the home, the nurse also may be able to engage significant others, who might be unwilling to participate in an office-based treatment.

A disadvantage of home nursing may be the limitations associated with providing care for a client in an isolated environment without the additional services of other professionals available. If the client has never participated in home care before, he or she, and perhaps also the family, may be distrustful or somewhat confused about what this new form of treatment entails. A nurse may perceive certain constraints to his or her level of authority and autonomy within the personal confines of a client's home. Safety may also be an issue when the position requires visits to neighborhoods where the nurse's security may be at risk. Nurses who plan to practice in psychiatric home care programs need to understand the risks involved and may require additional training in terms of safety issues. Table 43–3 provides some safety tips for home-care practice using the acronym SAFE.

TABLE 43–3 Safety Tips for Home-Care Practice

S—Stay alert.

Be alert and observant of the surroundings. When driving up to the client's home, pay attention to who is on the street around or near the client's home. Observe the condition of the neighborhood. Are there abandoned cars? Are the homes in a good state of repair? Are there any thriving businesses in the area or are the streets deserted? Is litter present on the streets or are they clean and well kept? Pay attention to unusual noises or movement.

A—Announce your arrival in advance.

If the client knows when to expect the nurse, he or she will be watchful for the arrival. Entrance into the residence will be immediate. Home-health nurses are generally viewed as friends of the neighborhood. Neighbors become aware of the schedule and often become protective. Sometimes the informal neighborhood leaders will alert the nurse when something is wrong, such as the presence of drug activity or an increase in crime.

F—Follow your "gut."

Intuition is an excellent warning system. Any situations that create a feeling of discomfort should be taken seriously. If the nurse observes a group of individuals in the distance who instill a feeling of threat or fear, he or she should cross the street, enter the safety of a business, or return to the automobile and drive away. Likewise, when in the client's home, if the nurse feels threatened by family dynamics or a tense situation, he or she should leave immediately. If help is required with the situation, a phone call can be made once the nurse is safely away from danger.

E—Expect the unexpected.

When the nurse expects the unexpected, he or she will be ready for any eventuality. Being mentally prepared to handle an unsafe situation will help the nurse avoid being caught "off guard." With experience and increased confidence, fear usually diminishes; however, the prudent home healthcare nurse is always cautious.

Adapted from Durham (2002).

Cultural and Boundary Issues

Certain cultural and boundary issues exist in psychiatric home nursing care that differ from nursing in the institutional setting. Nurses have always learned that it is never appropriate to accept a gift from a client in the hospital. But what about in the home? Is it appropriate to accept a cup of coffee on a cold day? What about a small token of their appreciation for the care they see the nurse providing? Culturally, would it be an insult if refused by the nurse? It is important for the nurse to be aware of cultural influences that affect boundary issues when he or she enters the private domain of the client. These issues are not completely resolved and warrant further discussion and study.

ROLE OF THE NURSE

The American Nurses Association (ANA) (1999) defines home health nursing as,

> ...the practice of nursing applied to a client with a health condition in the client's place of residence. Clients and their designated caregivers are the focus of home health nursing practice. The goal of care is to initiate, manage, and evaluate the resources needed to promote the patient's optimal level of well-being and function. (p. 3)

Medicare requires that psychiatric home nursing care be provided by "psychiatrically trained nurses," which they define as, "...nurses who have special training and/or experience beyond the standard curriculum required for a registered nurse" (CMS, 2005).

The guidelines that cover psychiatric nursing services are not well defined by CMS. This has presented some reimbursement problems for psychiatric nurses in the past. The CMS statement regarding psychiatric nursing services is presented in Table 43–4.

Preparation for psychiatric home health nursing, in addition to the registered nurse licensure, should include several years of psychiatric inpatient treatment experience. It is also recommended that the nurse have med-

ical–surgical nursing experience, because of common client physical co-morbidity and the holistic nursing perspective. Additional training and experience in psychotherapy is viewed as an asset. However, psychotherapy is not the primary focus of psychiatric home nursing care. In fact, most reimbursement sources do not pay for exclusively insight-oriented therapy. Crisis intervention, client education, and hands-on care are common interventions in psychiatric home nursing care.

Nurses who provide psychiatric home care must have an in-depth knowledge of psychopathology, psychopharmacology, and how medical and physical problems can be influenced by psychiatric impairments. These nurses must be highly adept at performing biopsychosocial assessments. They must be sensitive to changes in behavior that signal that the client is decompensating either psychiatrically or medically so that early intervention may be implemented.

Another important job of the psychiatric home health nurse is monitoring compliance of psychotropic medications. Some clients who are receiving injectable medications remain on home health care only until they can be placed on oral medications. Those clients receiving oral medications require close monitoring for compliance as well as for assistance in tolerating the uncomfortable side effects of some of these drugs. Medication noncompliance is responsible for the majority of psychiatric hospital readmissions. Home health nurses can assist clients with this problem by helping them to see the relationship between control of their psychiatric symptoms and compliance with their medication regimen.

The psychiatric home health nurse provides comprehensive nursing care, incorporating interventions for physical and psychosocial problems into the treatment plan. The interventions are based on the client's mental and physical health status, cultural influences, and available resources. The nurse is accountable to the client at all times during the therapeutic relationship. Nursing interventions are carried out with appropriate knowledge and skill, and referrals are made when the need is outside the scope of nursing practice. Continued collaboration with other members of the health care team (e.g., psychiatrist, social worker, psychologist, occupational therapist, and/or physical therapist) is essential for maintaining continuity of care.

APPLICATION OF THE NURSING PROCESS

Wheeler (1998) identifies the following components of the comprehensive assessment that must be completed during an initial visit or two with the client:

1. Client's perception of the problem and need for assistance

TABLE 43–4	CMS Guidelines for Psychiatric Home Nursing Care

Psychiatric Evaluation, Therapy, and Teaching

The evaluation, psychotherapy, and teaching needed by a patient suffering from a diagnosed psychiatric disorder that requires active treatment by a psychiatrically trained nurse and the costs of the psychiatric nurse's services may be covered as a skilled nursing service. Psychiatrically trained nurses are nurses who have special training and/or experience beyond the standard curriculum required for a registered nurse. The services of the psychiatric nurse are to be provided under a plan of care established and reviewed by a physician.

SOURCE: Centers for Medicare and Medicaid Services (2005).

2. Information regarding client's strengths and personal habits
3. Health history
4. Recent changes
5. Support systems
6. Vital signs
7. Current medications
8. Client's understanding and compliance with medications
9. Nutritional and elimination assessment
10. Activities of daily living (ADLs) assessment
11. Substance use assessment
12. Neurological assessment
13. Mental status examination (See Appendix B)
14. Comprehension of proverbs
15. Global Assessment of Functioning (GAF) scale rating

Other important assessments include information about acute or chronic medical conditions, patterns of sleep and rest, solitude and social interaction, use of leisure time, education and work history, issues related to religion or spirituality, and adequacy of the home environment.

A case study of psychiatric home health care and the nursing process is presented here. A plan of care for Mrs. C (the client in the case study) is presented in Table 43–5. Nursing diagnoses are presented along with outcome criteria, appropriate nursing interventions, and rationales.

CASE STUDY

ASSESSMENT

Mrs. C., aged 76, has been living alone in her small apartment for 6 months since the death of her husband, to whom she had been married for 51 years. Mrs. C. had been an elementary school teacher for 40 years, retiring at age 65 with an adequate pension. She and her husband had no children. A niece looks in on Mrs. C. regularly. It was she who contacted Mrs. C.'s physician when she observed that Mrs. C. was not eating properly, was losing weight, and seemed to be isolating herself more and more. She had not left her apartment in weeks. Her physician referred her to psychiatric home health care.

On her initial visit, Carol, the psychiatric home health nurse, conducted a preliminary assessment revealing the following information about Mrs. C.:

1. Blood pressure 90/60 mm Hg
2. Height 5'5"; weight 102 lb
3. Poor skin turgor; dehydration
4. Subjective report of occasional dizziness
5. Subjective report of loss of 20 lb since the death of husband
6. Oriented to time, place, person, and situation
7. Memory (remote and recent) intact
8. Flat affect
9. Mood is dysphoric and tearful at times, but client is cooperative
10. Denies thoughts to harm self, but states, "I feel so alone; so useless."
11. Subjective report of difficulty sleeping
12. Subjective report of constipation

DIAGNOSIS/OUTCOME IDENTIFICATION

The following nursing diagnoses were formulated for Mrs. C.:

1. Dysfunctional grieving related to death of husband evidenced by symptoms of depression such as withdrawal, anorexia, weight loss, difficulty sleeping, dysphoric/tearful mood.

2. Risk for injury related to dizziness and weakness from lack of activity and low blood pressure, and poor nutritional status.
3. Social isolation related to depressed mood and feelings of worthlessness evidenced by staying home alone, refusing to leave her apartment.

OUTCOME CRITERIA

The following criteria were selected as measurement of outcomes in the care of Mrs. C.:

1. Experiences no physical harm/injury.
2. Is able to discuss feelings about husband's death with nurse.
3. Sets realistic goals for self.
4. Is able to participate in problem solving regarding her future.
5. Eats a well-balanced diet with snacks to restore nutritional status and gain weight.
6. Drinks adequate fluid daily.
7. Sleeps at least 6 hours per night and verbalizes feeling well rested.
8. Shows interest in personal appearance and hygiene. Is able to accomplish self-care independently.
9. Seeks to renew contact with previous friends and acquaintances.
10. Verbalizes interest in participating in social activities.

PLAN/IMPLEMENTATION

A plan of care for Mrs. C. is presented in Table 43–5.

EVALUATION

Mrs. C. was started the second week on trazodone (Desyrel) 150 mg at bedtime. Her sleep was enhanced and within 2 weeks she showed a noticeable improvement in mood. She began to discuss how angry she felt about being all alone in the world. She admitted that she had felt anger toward her husband but experienced guilt and tried to suppress that anger. As she was assured that these feelings were normal, they became easier for her to express.

The nurse arranged for a local teenager to do some weekly grocery shopping for Mrs. C. and contacted the local Meals on Wheels program, which delivered her noon meal to her every day. Mrs. C. began to eat more and slowly to gain a few pounds. She still has an occasional problem with constipation but verbalizes improvement with the addition of vegetables, fruit, and a daily stool softener prescribed by her physician.

Mrs. C. used her walker until she felt she was able to ambulate without assistance. She reports that she no longer experiences dizziness, and her blood pressure has stabilized at around 100/70 mm Hg.

Mrs. C. has joined a senior citizens group and attends activities weekly. She has renewed previous friendships and formed new acquaintances. She sees her physician monthly for medication management and visits a local adult day health center for regular blood pressure and weight checks. Her niece still visits regularly, but her favorite relationship is the one she has formed with her constant canine companion, Molly, whom Mrs. C. rescued from the local animal shelter, and who continually demonstrates her unconditional love and gratitude.

Care for the Caregivers

Another aspect of psychiatric home health care is to provide support and assistance to primary caregivers. When family members are the providers of care on a 7-day-a-week, 24-hour-a-day schedule for a loved one with a chronic mental disorder, it can be very exhausting and very frustrating. A care plan for primary caregivers is presented in Table 43–6.

LEGAL AND ETHICAL ISSUES

Legal Issues

Basic legal concepts for psychiatric nursing in general are discussed in this section as they relate to home psychiatric nursing care. Both national and state laws influence a number of issues that may arise within a home care setting. The psychiatric home health nurse must be familiar

TABLE 43–5	**Care Plan for Psychiatric Home Health Care of Depressed Elderly**

NURSING DIAGNOSIS: DYSFUNCTIONAL GRIEVING
RELATED TO: Death of husband
EVIDENCED BY: Symptoms of depression such as withdrawal, anorexia, weight loss, difficulty sleeping, and dysphoric/tearful mood

OUTCOME CRITERIA	NURSING INTERVENTIONS	RATIONALE
Mrs. C. will demonstrate adaptive grieving behaviors and evidence of progression toward resolution.	1. Assess Mrs. C.'s position in the grief process. 2. Develop a trusting relationship by showing empathy and caring. Be honest and keep all promises. Show genuine positive regard. 3. Explore feelings of anger and help Mrs. C. direct them toward the source. Help her understand it is appropriate and acceptable to have feelings of anger and guilt about her husband's death. 4. Encourage Mrs. C. to review honestly the relationship she had with her husband. With support and sensitivity, point out reality of the situation in areas where misrepresentations may be expressed. 5. Determine if Mrs. C. has spiritual needs that are going unfulfilled. If so, contact spiritual leader for intervention with Mrs. C. 6. Refer Mrs. C. to physician for medication evaluation.	1. Accurate baseline data are required to plan appropriate care for Mrs. C. 2. These interventions provide the basis for a therapeutic relationship 3. Knowledge of acceptability of the feelings associated with normal grieving may help to relieve some of the guilt that these responses generate. 4. Mrs. C. must give up an idealized perception of her husband. Only when she is able to see both positive and negative aspects about the relationship will the grieving process be complete. 5. Recovery may be blocked if spiritual distress is present and care is not provided. 6. Antidepressant therapy may help Mrs. C. to function while confronting the dynamics of her depression.

(Continued on following page)

NURSING DIAGNOSIS: RISK FOR INJURY

RELATED TO: Dizziness and weakness from lack of activity and low blood pressure and poor nutritional status

OUTCOME CRITERIA	NURSING INTERVENTIONS	RATIONALE
Mrs. C. will not experience physical harm or injury.	1. Assess vital signs at every visit. Report to physician should they fall below baseline.	1. Client safety is a nursing priority.
	2. Encourage Mrs. C. to use walker until strength has returned.	2. The walker will assist Mrs. C. from falling.
	3. Visit Mrs. C. during mealtimes and sit with her while she eats. Encourage her niece to do the same. Ensure that easy to prepare, nutritious foods for meals and snacks are available in the house and that they are items that Mrs. C. likes.	3. She is more likely to eat what is convenient and what she enjoys.
	4. Contact local meal delivery service (e.g., Meals on Wheels) to deliver some of Mrs. C.'s meals.	4. This would ensure that she receives at least one complete and nutritious meal each day.
	5. Weigh Mrs. C. each week.	5. Weight gain is a measurable, objective means of assessing whether Mrs. C. is eating.
	6. Ensure that diet contains sufficient fluid and fiber.	6. Adequate dietary fluid and fiber will help to alleviate constipation. She may also benefit from a daily stool softener.

NURSING DIAGNOSIS: SOCIAL ISOLATION

RELATED TO: Depressed mood and feelings of worthlessness

EVIDENCED BY: Staying home alone, refusing to leave apartment

OUTCOME CRITERIA	NURSING INTERVENTIONS	RATIONALE
Mrs. C. will renew contact with friends and participate in social activities.	1. As nutritional status is improving and strength is gained, encourage Mrs. C. to become more active. Take walks with her; help her perform simple tasks around her house.	1. Increased activity enhances both physical and mental status.
	2. Assess lifelong patterns of relationships.	2. Basic personality characteristics will not change. Mrs. C. will very likely keep the same style of relationship development that she had in the past.
	3. Help her identify present relationships that are satisfying and activities that she considers interesting.	3. She is the person who truly knows what she likes, and these personal preferences will facilitate success in reversing social isolation.
	4. Consider the feasibility of a pet.	4. There are many documented studies of the benefits to elderly individuals of companion pets.
	5. Suggest possible alternatives that Mrs. C. may consider as she seeks to participate in social activities. These may include foster grandparent programs, senior citizens centers, church activities, craft groups, and volunteer activities. Help her to locate individuals with whom she may attend some of these activities.	5. She is more likely to attend and participate if she does not have to do so alone.

TABLE 43-6	Care Plan for Primary Caregiver of Client with Chronic Mental Illness

NURSING DIAGNOSIS: CAREGIVER ROLE STRAIN
RELATED TO: Severity and duration of the care receiver's illness and lack of respite and recreation for the caregiver
EVIDENCED BY: Feelings of stress in relationship with care receiver, feelings of depression and anger, family conflict around issues of providing care

OUTCOME CRITERIA	NURSING INTERVENTIONS	RATIONALE
Caregivers will achieve effective problem-solving skills and develop adaptive coping mechanisms to regain equilibrium.	1. Assess prospective caregivers' abilities to anticipate and fulfill client's unmet needs. Provide information to assist caregivers with this responsibility. Ensure that caregivers encourage client to be as independent as possible.	1. Caregivers may be unaware of what the client can realistically accomplish. They may be unaware of the nature of the illness.
	2. Ensure that caregivers are aware of available community support systems from whom they can seek assistance when required. Examples include respite care services, day treatment centers, and adult day-care centers.	2. Caregivers require relief from the pressures and strain of providing 24-hour care for their loved one. Studies have shown that abuse arises out of caregiving situations that place overwhelming stress on the caregivers.
	3. Encourage caregivers to express feelings, particularly anger.	3. Release of these emotions can serve to prevent psychopathology, such as depression or psychophysiological disorders, from occurring.
	4. Encourage participation in support groups comprised of members with similar life situations. Provide information about support groups that may be helpful: a. National Alliance for the Mentally Ill—(800) 950-NAMI b. American Association on Mental Retardation—(800) 424-3688 c. Alzheimer's Association—(800) 272-3900	4. Hearing others who are experiencing the same problems discuss ways in which they have coped may help caregiver adopt more adaptive strategies. Individuals who are experiencing similar life situations provide empathy and support for each other.

with these laws for the protection of both the client and the nurse.

Confidentiality

Client confidentiality is protected by both federal and state statutes. Confidentiality affects all aspects of information that becomes known as a direct result of the agency-client relationship. The only other individuals who should have access to the client's records are other professionals directly involved in the client's care. It is advisable that the agency nurse obtains written permission during the initial contact to share client medical information with these other staff professionals. If this initial permission is not obtained, a release form authorizing release of information should be obtained before medical records are shared with other staff professionals. Third-party payers also require medical information for making payment for services. A release of informa-

tion form for this purpose should be signed during the initial visit.

Clients may also request copies of their medical record, and indeed they have a legal right to the information contained therein. Generally, the original medical record becomes the property of the home health agency, but copies may be provided to the client. Finkelman (1997) presents an issue that may have legal implications for confidentiality. In home health care, does the sharing of medical information with family or significant other (SO) breach the confidentiality of the client? Finkelman (1997) states:

Most psychiatric nurses have confronted this dilemma, and many have crossed the line and shared confidential information without the patient's consent. How often does a nurse obtain an adult patient's permission prior to talking with the patient's family/SO? How does a nurse encourage family/SO participation in the home without sharing information? How does a nurse plan for discharge from home care without the family/SO? (p. 110)

This is an area in which a great deal more discussion is required. An initial consent from the client to share information with family or SO would be in the best interest of all concerned, and the home health nurse should know the policies established by his or her agency.

Another issue concerning confidentiality relates to the documentation of human immunodeficiency virus (HIV) and acquired immune deficiency syndrome (AIDS) status in clients. Legal implications must be taken into account if the documentation will be made accessible to third party payers. Catalano (2003) states:

> Although there is a general requirement to report infection with HIV/AIDS to the Centers for Disease Control and Prevention (CDC), many states have strict laws regarding the confidentiality of the diagnosis. Unauthorized revelation of the diagnosis of HIV/AIDS brings the possibility of a lawsuit against the health-care provider or institution.

Home health care agencies should have policies concerning this type of documentation, and nurses should be aware of these guidelines. In some instances, the agency's policy may be affected by state laws concerning testing and reporting of HIV and AIDS.

Other instances in which states may have statutes that require reporting, regardless of confidentiality include (Ash, 2004; Catalano, A.M.K., 2001; Catalano, J.T., 2003; Finkelman, 1997):

● Child abuse
● Adult abuse
● Possession of illegal substances
● Specific communicable diseases
● Injuries that appear to have been caused by a dangerous weapon
● Deaths of uncertain nature
● Animal bites

It is important for nurses to be knowledgeable about state law, so that required information is reported without breaching client confidentiality.

Informed Consent

Informed consent is an educational process and interpersonal exchange between a client and his or her physician in which information from the physician assists the client to make decisions about health care or treatment. In psychiatry, there has long been conflict about whether or not clients have the competence to make informed decisions about their health care. As was discussed in Chapter 5, there are exceptional instances when procedures may be instituted without client consent. These include situations in which treatment is required to prevent harm to the client or others and emergency situations in which the client is in no condition to exercise

judgment. In regard to psychiatric clients, it must not be assumed that mental illness infers lack of competency to make independent decisions about treatment. Resnick and Noffsinger (2004) state:

> The symptoms of many mental disorders may affect competency. However, a person may exhibit symptoms of a major mental illness and remain competent, as long as the symptoms of the illness do not impair the specific areas of functioning required for competence. Competency is based on an individual's present functioning. (p. 330)

Information about the procedure must be given to the client in language that he or she can understand. Initially, it is presented by the physician, but later can be reinforced by the nurse, who may provide additional information or further explanation. The client's level of comprehension can be assessed by asking the client to paraphrase the information or by questioning the client specifically about the information. Careful documentation of information presented and level of client comprehension is critical for reasons of legal consequence.

Ethical Issues

Right to Refuse Treatment

The right to refuse treatment is closely tied to informed consent. Treatment without consent is allowed in most states only under emergency conditions and circumstances of potential harm to self or others. Clients have the right to make reasoned decisions regarding their treatment. They also have the right to withdraw consent after it has been given. Verbal withdrawal of consent is adequate (Guido, 2001). It should be noted that refusal of treatment should also be based on informed consent. Clients should have sufficient information about the consequences of refusing treatment in order to make a reasoned decision. Careful documentation by the psychiatric home health nurse of the client's decision to refuse treatment is imperative.

Abandonment

The ANA (2000) bases their definition of abandonment on case law, the *Code of Ethics for Nurses*, and definitions used by state boards of nursing. This definition is as follows:

> Patient abandonment is a unilateral severance of the established nurse-patient relationship without giving reasonable notice to the supervisor so that arrangements can be made for continuation of nursing care by others. Refusal to accept an assignment (or a nurse-patient relationship) does not constitute patient abandonment. (p. 13)

Abandonment may occur in home health care when the home health care agency decides it must terminate care while a client may still be in need of service. Home nursing care may be discontinued for any of the following reasons:

● The client refuses to cooperate in the provision of home care.
● Medicare or Medicaid has denied payment for such service, or the client cannot otherwise pay for the service.
● The client is uncooperative, disruptive, or difficult to treat to the point that it is in the best interests of all concerned that the service be discontinued.
● Certain environmental conditions exist that place the nurse in jeopardy (e.g., physical threats, a dangerous dog, or sexual harassment).

To prevent client abandonment, it is important that a reasonable amount of notice be given to the client that services will be discontinued. The amount of time required to be considered reasonable depends on considerations such as the client's condition, the availability of alternative care, and urgency of need to terminate (e.g., danger to the nurse). Agency policies should speak to issues of abandonment. Ongoing communication with the physician and detailed documentation in the agency record is critical.

Least-Restrictive Alternative

Clients have the right to the least-restrictive alternative in treatment, or care in the least restrictive setting. Psychiatric home nursing provides the client with a great deal of control and the least amount of restriction in his or her care. It is important for the nurse to understand this concept of least-restrictive alternative, for indeed there may be times when the client requires more intensive care. The psychiatric homecare nurse has first-line access to the client in a crisis situation. Careful assessment and documentation are important to help determine the appropriate level of care for the client and make recommendations to the physician with the best interests of the client in mind.

SUMMARY

Psychiatric home nursing care has been shown to be a cost-effective way to provide quality care to clients outside the hospital setting. The concept began with the visiting nurses associations that were established in the early 1900s. When Medicare legislation was passed in 1965, home health care was recognized as a benefit, and services escalated. It was not until 1979, however, that psychiatric home nursing care came to be recognized as a reimbursable service.

The majority of home healthcare is paid for by Medicare. Other sources include Medicaid, private insurance, self-pay, and others. Homebound clients most often have diagnoses of schizophrenia, major depression, bipolar disorder, substance abuse, agoraphobia, paranoia, and generalized anxiety.

Besides being cost-effective, home care offers the advantage of observation of the client within the context of family and environment, which allows for the most comprehensive biopsychosocial assessment. Treatment in the home may also be perceived by the client as less threatening than in an institutional environment. Disadvantages to home nursing include lack of professional assistance for the nurse, constraints on the nurse within the client's home environment, and issues related to nursing in potentially unsafe neighborhoods.

Psychiatric home care nurses must have special training is psychiatric mental health nursing. Several years of psychiatric inpatient treatment experience plus 1 year of medical surgical nursing is preferred. Psychiatric nurses are expected to perform hands-on, holistic nursing, not just insight-oriented psychotherapy.

The nursing process is the tool for delivery of nursing care for the psychiatric client in the home care setting. This chapter presented a case study of and care plan for a depressed elderly client receiving psychiatric home nursing care. A care plan for the primary caregiver of a client with a chronic mental illness was also presented.

Legal issues pertaining to home health, such as confidentiality and informed consent, were discussed along with ethical issues, including right to refuse treatment, abandonment, and least restrictive alternative.

IMPLICATIONS OF RESEARCH FOR EVIDENCE-BASED PRACTICE

Neal, L.J. (2001). Public awareness of home care. *Caring, 20*(1), 38–41.

Description of the Study: The purpose of this study was to determine the American public's awareness levels, attitudes, opinions, preferences, and reported behaviors related to home health care. Reports by home care professionals indicate that they often encounter individuals who are unfamiliar with the services available and the eligibility requirements. A survey questionnaire was sent to 76 agency members of the National Association for Home Care (NAHC). Each of these members received an information letter describing the study, two packets of 25 computerized surveys each, 25 self-addressed stamped envelopes, and 2 cover letters addressed to "colleague." The information letter requested that the agency distribute a packet to two sources in their region. Sources included public places and doctors' and dentists' offices where people might be likely to be waiting and inclined to respond to a survey. The letter addressed to "colleague" requested support of the study from the proprietor or manager of the source location at which the surveys would be available. Questions on the survey were related to sample demographics and questions pertaining to attitudes toward and knowledge about services and availability of home health care.

Results of the Study: Most of the participants (89 percent) responded that they were familiar with the terms "home health" and "home care." More individuals in the over-55 age group stated they knew how to obtain services than those in the younger age group. Only about half of the total group stated that they believed services were covered by Medicare, Medicaid, or private insurance. Awareness of home care was less than average for males and those under the age of 65. Awareness of home care was strongest among females, those aged 55–64, and college graduates. Home care had a very positive image (85 percent) among those who had awareness. Hispanics and African-Americans were often less aware of home care services than were others. Thirty-eight percent of the sample could name a home health service they were "aware of," but 61 percent responded "don't know" when asked what types of services they were aware of. Seventy-three percent of the respondents had never used skilled services in the home. Of those who had, most reported positive experiences.

Implications for Nursing Practice: This descriptive study demonstrated that there are many areas related to the subject of home health care of which people are unaware. Participants in the older age groups appeared to have more knowledge of, experience with, and positive perceptions of home care than did participants in the younger age groups. The implications from this study, and from other studies in the literature that the authors reviewed, are that people of all ages require education about many aspects of home care: what it is and is not, who pays for it, and how to access it. Nurses are in a position to provide this kind of information to their clients, and to make referrals for home care, when assessment deems it would be helpful.

TEST YOUR CRITICAL THINKING SKILLS

Sarah is a 71-year-old widow whose husband died 6 years ago. Until recently, Sarah has been very independent and lived in a small apartment in the same town with her daughter and her family. Sarah was active in church and club activities and has many friends and acquaintances.

Six months ago, Sarah began having chest pain and was admitted to the hospital for diagnostic testing. A cardiac catheterization revealed major blockage in three coronary arteries, and Sarah underwent triple coronary artery bypass graft surgery. The surgery was successful and Sarah's physical recovery has been unremarkable. She returned to her apartment and was referred by her cardiologist for home health care by a staff nurse and home health aide who made regular visits to assist Sarah with her postoperative care. She qualified for homebound status because of physical weakness, need for wound care, postoperative pain, and need for assistance with ADLs. Her follow-up medications include digoxin (Lanoxin) and propranolol (Inderal).

As Sarah's physical condition stabilized, the home health staff nurse began to notice Sarah's progressive withdrawal and depressed mood. Instead of increasing her level of activity as her physical strength returned, she became less active and refused to participate in her daily care. She showed no interest in resuming any of the activities in which she had participated prior to her surgery. She began to lose weight. She needed to be reminded to take her medication. She moved in with her daughter, son-in-law, and granddaughter, so that she would not have to be alone at night. The home health staff nurse reported these symptoms to the cardiologist, who referred Sarah's case to a psychiatrist. A computed tomography (CT) scan was ordered to rule out possible neurological disorder, and the results were negative. A psychiatric home nursing care service was enlisted to assess Sarah's condition. Home health aides continued to visit Sarah daily to assist with ADLs and hygiene needs.

During the nurse's first visit, she found Sarah to be very withdrawn. Her daughter reported that Sarah hardly leaves her room and eats very little. Sarah was diagnosed with major depression.

Answer the following questions related to Sarah:

1. Describe initial assessments the psychiatric home care nurse would make in visiting with Sarah.
2. Identify two priority nursing diagnoses for Sarah.
3. What would be the goals of treatment for Sarah?
4. What medical treatment might the psychiatrist prescribe for Sarah based on the psychiatric home health nurse's assessment

REVIEW QUESTIONS

SELF-EXAMINATION/LEARNING EXERCISE

Select the answer that is *most* appropriate for each of the following questions.

1. The primary reason that psychiatric nursing care in the home has experienced slower growth than general home nursing care is that:
   a. Studies have shown that psychiatric home nursing care is not cost effective.
   b. The government did not recognize psychiatric home nursing care as reimbursable until much later than general staff home nursing care.
   c. Most psychiatric clients refuse to accept psychiatric nursing treatment in their homes.
   d. Psychiatric clients must also have a primary medical diagnosis before they can qualify for payment for home psychiatric services.

2. Psychiatric home nursing care has experienced growth in recent years because of all of the following reasons *except*:
   a. Broader third-party payment coverage.
   b. Greater physician acceptance of home care.
   c. Increased demand as an alternative to institutional care.
   d. Lengthier hospital stays for severe and persistently mentally ill clients.

3. The third-party payer responsible for the majority of home health care is:
   a. Medicare.
   b. Medicaid.
   c. Private insurance.
   d. HMOs.

4. Medicare requires that all the following criteria be met in order to qualify for psychiatric home care *except:*
   a. Certification by a physician that the client is homebound.
   b. A physical reason for inability to leave the home.
   c. An acute psychiatric diagnosis or exacerbation of one.
   d. The need for specialized skills of a psychiatric nurse.

5. Which of the following is considered a disadvantage of psychiatric home nursing care?
   a. Family involvement diminishes nurse–client relationship.
   b. Studies have shown it is not cost effective.
   c. The nurse's authority and autonomy may be constrained in the home setting.
   d. Presence of family interferes with comprehensive biopsychosocial assessment.

6. Maria and Tony are part of an Italian family of three generations who live together in one large home. Twyla, a psychiatric home health nurse, was enlisted to make home visits when Maria started to have panic attacks and refused to leave her home. Twyla has been visiting Maria once a week for 6 weeks now, and Maria has improved, and with support and medication is able to leave her home and carry out her activities as required. Two more visits are preauthorized, and Maria and Twyla have been discussing termination. When Twyla arrives for her visit this week, Maria has baked an Italian Easter bread for Twyla. She is very obviously excited to present the gift to Twyla. What is the most appropriate response on Twyla's part?
   a. She explains to Maria that her agency has a policy against accepting gifts from clients.
   b. She refuses the gift, knowing that if she accepts it will interfere with the therapeutic relationship.
   c. She places a call to her supervisor at the home health agency to ask permission to accept the gift.
   d. She accepts the Easter bread knowing that in the Italian culture a refusal would be taken as an insult by Maria.

7. Referrals are an important part of psychiatric home nursing care, and often psychiatric home care nurses refer clients to support groups of individuals with similar types of problems. In the case of Maria, Twyla decides this is not an appropriate intervention. On what might Twyla have based her decision?
   a. Italians are very closely family-oriented and would prefer to care for Maria within the privacy of the family constellation.
   b. There are very few support groups for individuals with panic disorder because treatment of anxiety has been shown to be less than successful in a group situation.
   c. Twyla believes that Maria would be uncomfortable within a group setting, because Italians generally have a large personal distance.
   d. Twyla has decided that Maria is completely well and it is unlikely that she will ever need care or support in the future.

8. Maria asks Twyla what she writes about their visits together. She says to Twyla, "My friend told me that medical record really belongs to me." What is the most appropriate response by Twyla?
   a. "I'm sorry, but I can't share this information with you."
   b. "I'll have to ask my supervisor if I can show you the record."
   c. "The actual record belongs to the agency, but I can get a copy for you."
   d. "I will be happy to tell you what I have written, but I can't show you the record."

9. Following a routine visit to Maria, which of the following situations would Twyla be required to report to the appropriate authority, regardless of confidentiality?
   a. Maria has a small bruise on her arm. She states, "Oh, Tony grabbed me a little too hard. He does that sometimes when he drinks too much."
   b. Maria has a small, open wound on her lower leg. She states, "I accidentally stepped on my neighbor's dog's tail and he bit me."
   c. Maria has itchy blisters on both arms. She states, "I got into the patch of poison ivy behind our house yesterday."
   d. Maria is upset. She is crying. "Tony didn't come home last night. He's done it before."

10. In the instance when a contract for treatment has been made between a client and a psychiatric homecare nurse, if the client decides to withdraw from treatment before the contract expires or before discharge, what must be done?
    a. The client needs only to withdraw consent verbally.
    b. The client must present a written refusal of treatment.
    c. The client must have cosignature of family or significant other to withdraw treatment.
    d. The client does not have the right to refuse treatment until the nurse determines the appropriate time for discharge.

 INTERNET REFERENCES

Additional information related to home health care may be found at:
- http://www.cms.hhs.gov/
- http://www.nahc.org/Consumer/wihc.html
- http://www.nahc.org/Consumer/hcstats.html

REFERENCES

American Nurses Association (ANA). (2000). Support for professional practice. *The American Nurse*, 13,

American Nurses Association (ANA). (1999). *Scope and Standards of Home Health Nursing Practice*. Washington, DC: American Nurses Publishing.

Ash, P. (2004). Children and adolescents. In R.I. Simon & L.H. Gold (Eds.). *Textbook of forensic psychiatry*. Washington, DC: American Psychiatric Publishing.

Catalano, A.M.K. (2001). The nurse-patient relationship. In M.E. O'Keefe (Ed.). *Nursing practice and the law: Avoiding malpractice and other legal risks*. Philadelphia: F.A. Davis.

Catalano, J.T. (2003). *Nursing now: Today's issues, tomorrow's trends* (3rd ed.). Philadelphia: F.A. Davis.

Centers for Medicare & Medicaid Services (CMS). (2004). *Sources of payment for home health care, 2002 & 2003*. Office of the Actuary, National Health Care Expenditures: 1990–2012. Retrieved June 1, 2005 from the World Wide Web at http://www.cms.gov

Centers for Medicare & Medicaid Services (CMS). (2005). *Medicare Benefit Policy Manual*. Baltimore, MD: CMS.

Domrose, C. (2002, December 9). House calls. *NurseWeek* Special Edition: 18–20.

Durham, S.W. (2002). Community-based nursing practice in a home-care setting. In J.M. Sorrell & G.M. Redmond (Eds.). *Community-based nursing practice: Learning through students' stories*. Philadelphia: F.A. Davis.

Finkelman, A.W. (1997). *Psychiatric home care*. Gaithersburg, MD: Aspen Publications.

Guido, G.W. (2001). *Legal issues in nursing* (3rd ed.). Upper Saddle River, NJ: Prentice-Hall.

Jensen, J.E., & Miller, B. (2004). *Home health psychiatric care: A guide to understanding home health psychiatric care as covered under Medicare Part A*. Seattle, WA: The Washington Institute for Mental Illness Research & Training.

National Association for Home Care. (1996). *How to choose a home care provider*. Retrieved June 1, 2005 from the World Wide Web at http://www.nahc.org/Consumer/wihc.html

National Association for Home Care, (2004). *Basic statistics about home care*. Retrieved June 1, 2005 from the World Wide Web at http://www.nahc.org/NAHC/Research/research/04HC_Stats.pdf

Resnick, P.J., & Noffsinger, S. (2004). Competency to stand trial and the insanity defense. In R.I. Simon & L.H. Gold (Eds.). *Textbook of forensic psychiatry*. Washington, DC: American Psychiatric Publishing.

Schroeder, B. (2001). Getting started in home care. *NurseWeek Newsletter* (2002, May, 16). Retrieved May 16, 2002 from the World Wide Web at http://www.nurseweek.com/newsletter/051602

Wheeler, K. (1998). Psychiatric clinical pathways in home care. In P.C. Dykes (Ed.). *Psychiatric clinical pathways: An interdisciplinary approach*. Gaithersburg, MD: Aspen Publishers.

44
C H A P T E R

FORENSIC NURSING

CHAPTER OUTLINE

OBJECTIVES

WHAT IS FORENSIC NURSING?

HISTORICAL PERSPECTIVES

THE CONTEXT OF FORENSIC NURSING
PRACTICE

FORENSIC NURSING SPECIALTIES

APPLICATION OF THE NURSING PROCESS
IN CLINICAL FORENSIC NURSING IN
TRAUMA CARE

APPLICATION OF THE NURSING PROCESS IN
FORENSIC PSYCHIATRIC NURSING IN
CORRECTIONAL FACILITIES

SUMMARY

REVIEW QUESTIONS

KEY TERMS

colposcope
forensic nursing

sexual assault nurse
examiner (SANE)

CORE CONCEPT

forensic

OBJECTIVES

After reading this chapter, the student will be able to:

1. Define the terms *forensic* and *forensic nursing.*
2. Discuss historical perspectives of forensic nursing.
3. Identify areas of nursing within which forensic nurses may practice.
4. Describe forensic nursing specialties.

5. Apply the nursing process within the role of clinical forensic nursing in trauma care.
6. Apply the nursing process within the role of forensic psychiatric nursing in correctional facilities.

 he many roles of nurses continue to increase with the ever-expanding health service delivery system. **Forensic nursing** is an example of a nursing role that is rapidly increasing in its scope of practice. Nurses practicing in this unique specialty may apply their skills to the care of both victims and perpetrators of crime and in a variety of settings, including primary care facilities, hospitals, and correctional institutions. This chapter focuses on defining forensic nursing within varied aspects of the role. A discussion of historical perspectives is included and care of the client is presented within the context of the nursing process.

WHAT IS FORENSIC NURSING?

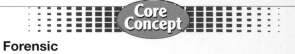

Forensic
Pertaining to the law; legal.

The International Association of Forensic Nurses (IAFN) and the American Nurses Association (ANA) (1997) define forensic nursing as:

The application of forensic science combined with the bio-psychological education of the registered nurse, in the scientific investigation, evidence collection and preservation, analysis, prevention and treatment of trauma and/or death related medical-legal issues. (p. v)

Hufft and Peternelj-Taylor (2003) present the following definition:

A nursing specialty practice that integrates nursing science and forensic science to apply the nursing process to the health and well-being of individual clients, their families, and communities to help bridge the gap between the health-care system and the criminal justice system. (p. 414)

Hancock (2005) suggests that:

Forensic nursing is the application of clinical and scientific knowledge to questions of law, and the civil or criminal investigation for survivors of traumatic injury and/or patient treatment involving court-related issues.

Because this area of nursing is a continuing pioneering effort, roles, definitions, and educational programs are still being formulated.

HISTORICAL PERSPECTIVES

Forensic nursing has its roots in Alberta, Canada, around 1975, where nurses served as investigators for medical examiners in the field of death investigation. They were valued for their biomedical education, their sensitivity in dealing with family members, and their ability to substitute in the role of the medical examiner when required. These are qualities that were often found to be lacking in medically untrained criminal investigative personnel.

The discipline has made great advances since that time. The role of forensic nursing has expanded from concerns solely with death investigation to include the living—the survivors of violent crime—as well as the perpetrators of criminal acts. In 1992, seventy-four nurses, primarily sexual assault nurse examiners, met to form the International Association of Forensic Nurses (Bell, 1999). By 1997, this organization had grown to more than one thousand members.

Violence has reached epidemic proportions in the United States and has been identified as a major public health problem. It is with this in mind that the health care system and the legal system have joined in an attempt to respond to the increasing needs of crime victims. Hufft and Peternelj-Taylor (2003) state, "Forensic nursing is an evolving specialty that has emerged as a dynamic and influential factor in the health care of individuals and communities."

THE CONTEXT OF FORENSIC NURSING PRACTICE

The Forensic Nursing Service (FNS) (1999) has identified a variety of assignments within which the forensic nurse may practice. They include the following:

1. **Interpersonal Violence**
   - Domestic violence/sexual assault
   - Child and elder abuse/neglect
   - Physiological/psychological abuse
   - Drug/alcohol abuse
2. **Public Health and Safety**
   - Environmental hazards
   - Food and drug tampering
   - Holistic health investigation
   - Medically unsupervised abortion practices
   - Epidemiological issues
   - Anatomical gifts (tissue/organ donation)
3. **Emergency/Trauma Nursing**
   - Automobile and pedestrian accidents
   - Traumatic injuries
   - Suicide attempts
   - Work-related injuries
   - Fatal/near-fatal injuries
4. **Patient Care Facilities**
   - Accidents/injuries/neglect
   - Inappropriate treatment/medication administration
5. **Police and Corrections**
   - Custody
   - Abuse

FORENSIC NURSING SPECIALTIES*

Clinical Forensic Nursing Specialty

Clinical forensic nursing is the management of crime victims from trauma to trial. Nurses working in clinical forensics collect evidence through assessment of living victims, survivors of traumatic injury, or those whose death is pronounced in the clinical environment. Clinical forensic nursing involves making judgments related to patient treatment associated with court-related issues. The clinical forensic nurse assesses victims of child and elder abuse and domestic violence. Forensic nurses are asked to differentiate between conditions that simulate accidental injury and those that are purposely inflicted. An essential skill required by the forensic nurse is the ability to assess patterned injury by differentiating marks such as defense wounds, grab marks, and fingernail marks. Clinical forensic nurses focus on observation of the communication and interaction patterns of suspected abuse victims and perpetrators. Many nurses come to forensic nursing from acute-care settings of emergency room nursing, critical care nursing, and perioperative nursing.

In the coroner's office, death notification entails stabilization of the family situation and grief support, skills that are basic to nursing practice. Expert skills in physi-

---

*This section was written by A. Hufft and C. Peternelj-Taylor. Reprinted with permission from J.T. Catalano (Ed.) (2003). *Nursing now! Today's issues, tomorrow's trends* (3rd ed.). Philadelphia: F.A. Davis.

cal assessment, clinical history taking and interviewing, and use of technology have helped advance this nursing role.

Because of their awareness of the effects of violence in society and their ability to assess situations in which potential for violence exists, clinical forensic nurses are often called upon for consultation. By identifying risk factors and cues for violence in health care and workplace settings, these nurses can assist in the development of strategies, policies, and protocols to manage risk and reduce violence and injury. They also assist in the debriefing or resolution of violent events in a workplace or community.

The Sexual Assault Nurse Examiner (SANE)

The **sexual assault nurse examiner (SANE)** is a clinical forensic registered nurse who has received specialized training to provide care to the sexual assault victim. The SANE performs physical and psychosocial examination and collection of physical evidence, therapeutic interactions to minimize the trauma and initiate healing, coordination of referral and collaboration with community-based agencies involved in the rehabilitation of victims, and the judicial processing of sexual assault. The first programs training SANEs were developed in the United States in the late 1970s. SANEs may now earn national certification through the IAFN Forensic Nursing Certification Board and the Center for Nursing Education and Testing.

Forensic Psychiatric Nursing Specialty

Forensic psychiatric nurses integrate psychiatric/mental health nursing philosophy and practice with knowledge of the criminal justice system and assessment of the sociocultural influences on the individual client, the family, and the community, to provide comprehensive psychiatric and mental health nursing. Forensic psychiatric nurses work with mentally ill offenders and with victims of crime. They help victims cope with their emotional wounds and assist in the assessment and care of perpetrators. They focus on identification and change of behaviors that link criminal offenses or reactions to them. These nurses assist perpetrators and victims of crime in dealing with the courts and other aspects of the criminal justice system, minimizing further victimization and promoting functional abilities.

Functional applications of forensic psychiatric nursing include assessment of inmates for physical fitness, criminal responsibility, disposition, and early release. Forensic psychiatric nurses also provide mental health treatment for convicted offenders and those who are not found criminally responsible. In the criminal justice system,

forensic psychiatric nurses deal with destructive, aggressive, and socially unacceptable behavior. These nurses provide interventions that encourage individuals to exercise self-control, foster individual change in behavior, and, in the process, protect other members of society and property.

There has been an increase in the involvement of forensic psychiatric nurses (especially those prepared for advanced practice) in the assessment and treatment of forensic psychiatric patients. These practitioners are involved in the development and refining of clinical roles in forensic psychiatric nursing and are in a position to promote intervention strategies that increase the likelihood of rehabilitation and reintegration of the forensic client into society.

Correctional/Institutional Nursing Specialty

Correctional/institutional nurses work in secure settings, providing treatment, rehabilitation, and health promotion to clients who have been charged with or convicted of crimes. Settings include jails, state and federal prisons, and halfway houses. Prior to the 1960s, most nurses gave little thought to working in the correctional system, even though jails and correctional facilities have always been a part of the community at large. There is a growing awareness of the potential for the correctional population as a target of successful health interventions. Some nurses have created private practices or consultation services in which they identify the health needs and arrange for the care of people detained in custody. This service is provided separate from acute care, which is located in a secured hospital or infirmary section of the institution. Such services are just emerging as health care alternatives and will serve as the model from which community-based care, aimed at decreasing recidivism among those incarcerated, will develop. To guide professional nursing practice, the ANA first published *Standards for Nursing Practice in Correctional Facilities* in 1985; these standards were revised and updated in 1995 and 2001.

Nurses in General Practice

In addition to nurses in specialty practice, nurses in general practice find forensic nursing knowledge of growing importance. Forensic applications in the acute care setting emphasize the use of forensic knowledge and awareness of criminal justice implications for assessment, documentation of care, and reporting of information to police or other law enforcement agencies. Nurses who work in emergency rooms and in critical care units are often in positions to preserve evidence of what might be a criminal offense. Victims of automobile accidents or apparent accidental overdoses are not always what they appear to be. Knowledge of what to look for and how to collect evidence, in addition to knowing whom to call and when, can be valuable in finding out what really happened in such cases. Clients often come into acute care settings with what are first thought to be injuries that are the result of an accident. However, preservation of evidence such as stomach contents, clothing residue, or marks on the skin surface can provide a very different picture—one of injury caused by a self-inflicted wound or violence perpetrated by another.

This chapter focuses on two specialties in forensic nursing: the clinical forensic nurse specialist in trauma care settings and the psychiatric forensic nurse in correctional facilities. The IAFN and ANA (1997) Standards of Care and Standards of Professional Performance for forensic nursing are presented in Table 44–1.

APPLICATION OF THE NURSING PROCESS IN CLINICAL FORENSIC NURSING IN TRAUMA CARE

Assessment

Lynch (1995) states that forensic nurses who work in trauma care settings may "become the designated clinicians who will evaluate and assess surviving victims of rape, drug and alcohol addiction, domestic violence (including abuse of spouse, children, elderly), assaults, automobile/pedestrian accidents, suicide attempts, occupationally related injuries, incest, medical malpractice and the injuries sustained therefrom, and food and drug tampering." All traumatic injuries in which liability is

---

TABLE 44–1   Standards of Care and Standards of Professional Performance for Forensic Nursing

STANDARDS OF CARE

Standard I. Assessment

The forensic nurse shall provide an accurate assessment, based upon data collected, of the physical and/or psychological issues of the client as related to forensic nursing and/or forensic pathology.

Standard II. Diagnosis

The forensic nurse shall analyze the assessment data to determine a diagnosis pertaining to forensic issues in nursing.

Standard III. Outcome Identification

The forensic nurse will identify expected individual outcomes based on the forensic diagnoses of the client.

Standard IV. Planning

The forensic nurse develops a comprehensive plan of action for the forensic client appropriate to forensic interventions to attain expected outcomes.

Standard V. Implementation

The forensic nurse implements a plan of action based on forensic issues derived from assessment data, nursing diagnoses, and medical diagnoses, when applicable, and scientific knowledge.

Standard VI. Evaluation

The forensic nurse evaluates and modifies the plan of action to achieve expected outcomes.

STANDARDS OF PROFESSIONAL PERFORMANCE

Standard I. Quality of Care

The forensic nurse systematically evaluates the quality and effectiveness of forensic nursing practice.

Standard II. Performance Appraisal

The forensic nurse evaluates his/her own forensic nursing practice in relation to professional practice standards and relevant statutes and regulations.

Standard III. Education

The forensic nurse acquires and maintains current knowledge in forensic nursing practice.

Standard IV. Collegiality

The forensic nurse contributes to the professional development of peers, colleagues and others.

Standard V. Ethics

The forensic nurse's decisions and actions are determined in an ethical manner.

Standard VI. Collaboration

The forensic nurse collaborates with the forensic client, family members, significant others and multidisciplinary team members.

Standard VII. Research

The forensic nurse recognizes, values and utilizes research as a method to further forensic nursing practice.

Standard VIII. Resource Utilization

The forensic nurse considers factors related to safety, effectiveness, and cost in planning and delivering forensic services.

SOURCE: International Association of Forensic Nurses and American Nurses Association (1997), with permission.

suspected are considered within the scope of forensic nursing. Reports to legal agencies are required to ensure follow-up investigation; however, the protection of clients' rights remains a nursing priority.

McPeck (2002) reports on the performance of forensic nurses in the aftermath of the September 11, 2001 attack on New York City and Washington, DC. He states:

> [Forensic nurses] worked as mortuary assistants to collect and process biological and evidentiary remains of the victims, many of whom are still missing and probably never will be found. The forensic nurses provided clinical care and support for about 2,000 police officers, firefighters, and emergency workers who were at Ground Zero at any one time. Forensic nurses are trained to intervene in crises and offer that kind of mental support. (p. 25)

With the rise of violence in our society reaching epidemic proportions, the role of the clinical forensic nurse in the care of trauma clients in the emergency department is expanding. The forensic clinical nurse specialist may be the ideal liaison between legal and medical agencies.

Lynch (1995) identifies several areas of assessment in which the clinical forensic nurse specialist may become involved. They include the preservation of evidence, investigation of wound characteristics, and deaths in the emergency department.

Preservation of Evidence

Intentional traumas in the emergency department may be crime related or self-inflicted. Crime-related evidence is essential and must be safeguarded in a manner consistent with the investigation. Brown (2005) identifies common types of evidence as clothing, bullets, gunshot powder on the skin, bloodstains, hairs, fibers, grass, and any other type of debris that is found on the individual, such as fragments of glass, paint, and wood. Often this type of evidence is destroyed in the clinical setting when health care personnel are unaware of its potential value in an investigation. It is important that this type of evidence be saved and documented in all medical or accident instances that have legal implications.

Investigation of Wound Characteristics

When clients present to the emergency department with wounds from undiagnosed trauma, it is important for the clinical forensic nurse specialist to make a detailed documentation of the injuries. Failure to do so may interfere with the administration of justice should legal implications later arise. The following categories of medicolegal injuries are identified (Brown, 2005; Lynch, 1995):

1. Sharp force injuries: includes stab wounds and other wounds resulting from penetration with a sharp object.
2. Blunt force injuries: includes cuts and bruises resulting from the impact of a blunt object against the body.
3. Dicing injuries: multiple, minute cuts and abrasions caused by contact with shattered glass (e.g., often occur in motor vehicle accidents).
4. Patterned injuries: specific injuries that reflect the pattern of the weapon used to inflict the injury.
5. Bite mark injuries: a type of patterned injury inflicted by human or animal.
6. Defense wounds: injuries that reflect the victim's attempt to defend him- or herself from attack.
7. Hesitation wounds: usually superficial, sharp force wounds; often found perpendicular to the lower part of the body and may reflect self-inflicted wounds.
8. Fast-force injuries: usually gunshot wounds; may reflect various patterns of injury.

Nurses managing the client's care in the emergency department must be able to make assessments about the type of wound, the weapon involved, and an estimate of the length of time between the injury and presentation for treatment.

Deaths in the Emergency Department

When deaths occur in the emergency department as a result of abuse or accident, evidence must be retained, the death must be reported to legal authorities, and an investigation is conducted (Lynch, 1995). It is therefore essential that the nurse carefully document the appearance, condition, and behavior of the victim upon arrival at the hospital. The information gathered from the client and family (or others accompanying the client) may serve to facilitate the postmortem investigation and may be used during criminal justice proceedings.

The critical factor is to be able to determine if the cause of death is natural or unnatural. In the emergency department, most deaths are sudden and unexpected. Those that are considered natural most commonly involve the cardiovascular, respiratory, and central nervous systems (Lynch, 1995). Deaths that are considered unnatural include those from trauma, from self-inflicted acts, or from injuries inflicted by another. Legal authorities must be notified of all deaths related to unnatural circumstances.

Nursing Diagnosis

Clinical forensic nurse specialists in the trauma care setting analyze the information gathered during assessment of the client to formulate nursing diagnoses. Common nursing diagnoses relevant to forensic clients in the emergency department include:

1. Risk for posttrauma syndrome
2. Fear

3. Anxiety
4. Risk for self-mutilation
5. Risk for suicide
6. Risk for dysfunctional grieving

Planning/Implementation

Preservation of Evidence

When a trauma victim is admitted to the emergency department, the most obvious priority intervention is medical stabilization. This priority must be balanced against the need to protect rapidly deteriorating physical evidence that can determine if a crime has occurred.

Wounds must be examined to speculate about the type of weapon used and to estimate age of the wound. Clothing must be checked for blood, semen, gunshot residue, or trace materials such as hair, fibers, and other debris. Clothing that is removed from a victim should not be shaken, so any evidence that may be adhering to it is not lost. Each separate item of clothing should be carefully placed in a paper bag, sealed, dated, timed, and signed. Plastic bags should never be used because of the tendency for condensation to occur. This promotes the growth of mold and the decay of biological tissue, which results in contamination of the evidence (Brown, 2005; Lynch, 1995).

When the trauma is sexual assault, a SANE may be called to the emergency department. SANEs usually work on-call, and because most sexual assault victims are women, female nurses are employed as SANEs. Male victims of sexual assault also most often prefer to work with a female SANE, because the perpetrators are usually men and because of the subsequent mistrust of men following the attack.

Ledray (2001) suggests the following essential components of a forensic examination of the sexual assault survivor in the emergency department.

Treatment and Documentation of Injuries

Emergency department (ED) staff typically perform the initial assessments when a sexual assault victim arrives. Vital signs and treatment of serious injuries often occur before the arrival of the SANE. Unless the injuries are life threatening, the forensic examination should occur before medical treatment is administered so as not to destroy physical evidence that is needed to establish that a sexual crime has occurred.

It is often expected that a sexual assault survivor must exhibit cuts and bruises in the genital or nongenital area. It has been estimated that there are no visible physical injuries in 40 to 60 percent of sexual assaults (American Medical Association [AMA], 1999). Absence of physical trauma does not necessarily mean that no force was used and that consent was given. This, however, is the case

often used by defense attorneys in court. The AMA (1999) suggests the use of a traumagram—a diagram of a nude figure on which the locations of visible injuries are made. A written description of the color, size, and location of each wound, abrasion, and laceration is then documented. With the client's permission, photographs of the wounds should be taken for accurate documentation.

The nurse may use a **colposcope** to examine for tears and abrasions inside the vaginal area. A colposcope is an instrument that contains a magnifying lens and to which a 35-mm camera can be attached.

Some states have legally mandated procedures, and some acute care settings also have established protocols, for gathering evidence in cases of sexual assault. In some instances, "rape kits" are available for collecting specimens and lab samples in a competent manner that is consistent with legal requirements and that will not interfere with the victim's option to pursue criminal charges. In addition to the vaginal examination, oral and rectal examinations may be conducted. Fingernail scrapings and body, head, and public hair samples should also be collected. Client hair samples are important to be able to differentiate from those of the assailant. As previously stated, all evidence should be sealed in paper, *not* plastic, bags to prevent the possible growth of mildew from accumulation of moisture inside the plastic container, and the subsequent contamination of the evidence.

Some states may require a urine specimen to test for pregnancy or screen for drugs. It is best, if possible, to wait until the initial internal examination is complete before collecting the urine sample. However, the AMA (1999) states, "Patients needing to urinate before the internal examination should be allowed to do so, with a notation being made in the medical record."

Maintaining the Proper Chain of Evidence

Ledray (2001) states, "Maintaining a proper chain-of-evidence is as important as collecting the proper evidence." Unless the proper chain-of-evidence has been maintained, it cannot be used successfully in a court of law to convict an assailant. The AMA (1999) states,

> To preserve the chain of evidence and the freshness of the samples, check to ensure that they are properly labeled, sealed, refrigerated when necessary, and kept under observation or properly locked until rendered to the proper legal authority.

Treatment and Evaluation of Sexually Transmitted Diseases (STDs)

The AMA (1999) recommends counseling about, and prophylaxis for, STDs to sexual assault victims. Conducted within 72 hours of the attack, several tests and interventions are available. Prophylactic antibiotics may be given to prevent chlamydia, gonorrhea, trichomoniasis, and bacterial vaginosis according to guidelines from the Centers for Disease Control (CDC) (AMA, 1999). They also recommend postexposure prophylaxis using hepatitis B immunoglobulin. Information also should be provided describing symptoms of STDs for which there are no preventive measures. Because incubation periods vary, the importance of follow-up testing must be emphasized.

There is no proven prophylactic intervention for human HIV infection, and this is a growing concern of sexual assault victims. Even though the CDC reports that the risk for acquiring HIV infection through sexual assault is low in most cases, some states mandate testing for HIV as part of the sexual assault protocol. The AMA (1999) states, "Baseline testing can diagnose or rule out preexisting HIV infection, but repeated testing after 6 months and again in 1 year is recommended, particularly when the assailant is known to be HIV positive or the serostatus is unknown."

Pregnancy Risk Evaluation and Prevention

It is important that sexual assault victims receive information related to risks and interventions for prevention of conception as a result of the assault. Evaluation of pregnancy risk is based on the client's ability to relay accurate information about the occurrence of her last menses so that an estimate can be made of time of ovulation. Prophylactic regimens are 97 to 98 percent effective if started within 24 hours of the sexual attack and are generally only recommended within 72 hours (Ledray, 2001). If the client chooses, a regimen of ethinyl estradiol and norgestrel (Ovral) can be administered. Two tablets are taken at the time of treatment and two tablets are taken 12 hours later. An antiemetic, such as trimethobenzamide (Tigan), may be given to prevent nausea and vomiting, the most common side effects of the medication.

Crisis Intervention and Arrangements for Follow-Up Counseling

In the hours immediately following the sexual assault, the rape victim experiences an overwhelming sense of violation and helplessness that began with the powerlessness and intimidation experienced during the rape. Burgess (2004) has identified two emotional response patterns that may occur within hours after a rape and that health care workers may encounter in the emergency department or rape crisis center. In the *expressed response pattern*, the victim expresses feelings of fear, anger, and anxiety through such behaviors as crying, sobbing, smiling, restlessness, and tension. In the *controlled response pattern*, the feelings are masked or hidden, and a calm, composed, or subdued affect is seen. Brown (2005) suggests that helping the victim to regain a sense of control—that is, helping her to make decisions about what she wants to do—can be an effective method of enhancing recovery. Brown (2005) states:

Lack of control during a rape or sexual assault creates special needs in victims. These women need to feel in control [of everything that happens in the ED]. Any hint of lack of control can trigger an uncooperative, difficult, or anxious response, and they may be lost to follow-up. Providing as much control as possible for these women in clinical situations within safety guidelines may greatly increase their comfort level.

This is also an important time to ensure that the victim understands that she is not to blame for what has happened. She may be blaming herself and feeling guilty for certain behaviors, such as drinking or walking alone late at night, that may have placed her in a vulnerable position. It is important to communicate the following to the victim of sexual assault:

● You are safe here.
● I'm sorry that it happened.
● I'm glad you survived.
● It's not your fault. No one deserves to be treated this way.
● You did the best that you could.

Before she leaves the emergency department, the individual should be advised about the importance of returning for follow-up counseling. She should be given the names of individuals to call for support. Often a survivor will not follow up with aftercare because she is too ashamed or is fearful of having to relive the nightmare of the attack by sharing the information in group or individual counseling. For this reason, it may be important for the nurse to get permission from the individual to allow a counselor to call her to make a follow-up appointment.

Deaths in the Emergency Department

The emergency department becomes the scene of legal investigation when death occurs in the trauma care setting. Evidence is preserved and the body is protected until the investigation has been completed. Hufft and Peternelj-Taylor (2003) state:

When investigating a death scene, the clinical forensic nurse interviews witnesses, takes charge of the body, examines the body, photographs the body, secures physical evidence, arranges body transport, and gathers records. The coroner is usually in charge of death investigation. Nurses working in this capacity initiate or assist with death investigation under selected circumstances of homicide, violence, suicide, and suspicious circumstances that indicate a violation of criminal law (e.g., presence of illegal drugs, a body found in water, a fire, explosion). (p. 421)

Anatomical Gifts

When a sudden and unexpected death occurs in the trauma care setting, the clinical forensic nurse may become involved in organ/tissue donation. Some states now require that a request for organ/tissue donation be made of the family when a death occurs under certain circumstances. This is a very painful period for family members, and nurses may feel it is an inappropriate time to present the information associated with an anatomical request. However, most nurses employed in trauma care recognize that organ/tissue recovery for transplantation is a requisite component of their work. Lynch (1995) states:

> As an expert in legal issues and with sensitivity to the deceased's family, a forensic nurse can be used (1) to provide consultation as necessary, (2) to foster staff education, and (3) to perform immediate interventions in the emergency department setting. As a nurse manager, the forensic nurse position can provide an opportunity to create or to advance existing protocol with greater emphasis on the coordination and cooperation between organ/tissue procurement and the medical examiner/coroner system.

Evaluation

Evaluation of the clinical forensic nursing process in the trauma care setting involves ongoing measurement of the diagnostic criteria aimed at resolution of identified real or potential problems. The following types of questions may provide assistance in the evaluation process.

1. Have the physical and psychological needs of the survivors who present themselves to the emergency department been met?
2. Has the evidence in potential criminal investigations been handled such that it can be used in a credible manner?
3. Has the sexual assault survivor received information related to choices pertaining to STDs, pregnancy, and follow-up counseling?
4. In the instance of sudden and unexpected death in the emergency department, have the needs of the grieving family been met?
5. Have the importance of anatomical donations been communicated?

The role of the clinical forensic nurse in trauma care continues to expand. With the level of societal violence at epidemic proportions, clinical forensic nurses potentially may intervene in the examination of victims of all types of abuse situations. The clinical forensic nurse specialist must also strive to be proactive, beginning with educating emergency department staff in the philosophy and interventions of clinical forensic nursing practice. Within the community, proactive responsibilities may include providing information about environmental hazards and issues that may affect public health and safety. Effectiveness of these changes provides measurement for ongoing evaluation.

APPLICATION OF THE NURSING PROCESS IN FORENSIC PSYCHIATRIC NURSING IN CORRECTIONAL FACILITIES

Assessment

Notwithstanding the positive intentions of deinstitutionalization, some negative consequences may have ensued. Raphael (2000) states:

> To the extent that the untreated mentally ill commit crimes and receive prison sentences at a relatively high rate, "deinstitutionalization" of the mentally ill from state and county hospitals may increase prison populations. Indeed, the pronounced increase in the U.S. prison population over the past three decades occurred concurrently with unprecedented declines in the numbers of committed mentally ill. [Trends in continual declines in the mental hospital population] appear to support the contention that deinstitutionalization has shifted the burden of providing services for the mentally ill onto the criminal justice system—i.e., jails and prisons have become de facto mental institutions. (pp. 1–2)

It was believed that deinstitutionalization increased the freedom of mentally ill individuals in accordance with the principle of "least restrictive alternative." Because of inadequate community-based services, however, many of these individuals drifted into poverty and homelessness, increasing their vulnerability to criminalization. Because the bizarre behavior of mentally ill individuals living on the street is sometimes offensive to community standards, law enforcement officials have the authority to protect the welfare of the public and the safety of the individual by initiating emergency hospitalization. Legal criteria for commitment are so stringent in most cases, however, that arrest becomes an easier way of getting the mentally ill person off the street if a criminal statute has been violated. Approximately 16 percent of all inmates have some form of psychological disorder or mental disability (Beck & Maruschak, 2001). Some of these individuals are incarcerated as a result of the increasingly popular "guilty but mentally ill" verdict. With this verdict, the individual is deemed mentally ill, yet is held criminally responsible for his actions. He or she is incarcerated and receives special treatment, if needed, but it is no different from that available for and needed by any prisoner.

The U.S. Department of Justice recently reported that U.S. prisons and jails held more than 2 million inmates in 2004 (U.S. Department of Justice [USDOJ], 2004). The report stated that 46.2 percent of the national jail population was white (including Asian Americans, Native Americans, Alaskan natives, and Pacific Islanders), 38.6 percent were African American, and 15.2 percent were Hispanic. Men accounted for 93 percent of the total.

Care of the mentally ill offender population is a highly specialized area of nursing practice. The rationale of imprisonment for criminal behavior has been identified as:

● Retribution to society
● Deterrence of future crimes
● Rehabilitation and repentance
● Protection of society

If an institution bases its orientation on retribution and deterrence of criminal activity, the prison will reflect a punishment-oriented atmosphere. If rehabilitation and repentance are accepted as a basis for change, mental health programs that encourage reflection and insight may be a part of the correctional setting. Because at times these basic objectives may seem incompatible with each other, nurses who work in correctional facilities may struggle with a cognitive dissonance founded in their basic nursing value system.

Assessing Mental Health Needs of the Incarcerated

Is the provision of mental health care within the custodial environment possible? Or are clinical care concerns incompatible with security issues? What special knowledge and skills must a psychiatric nurse possess to be successful in caring for the mentally ill offender?

Psychiatric diagnoses commonly identified in incarcerated individuals include schizophrenia, bipolar disorder, major depression, substance use disorders, personality disorders, and many have dual diagnoses (Yurkovich & Smyer, 2000). Common psychiatric behaviors include hallucinations, suspiciousness, thought disorders, anger/agitation, and impulsivity. Denial of problems has been found to be the most common behavior among this population. Use of substances and medication noncompliance are common obstacles to rehabilitation. Substance abuse has been shown to have a strong correlation with recidivism among the prison population. Many individuals report that they were under the influence of illegal substances at the time of their criminal actions, and dual diagnoses are common. Detoxification frequency occurs in jails and prisons, and some deaths have occurred from the withdrawal syndrome because of inadequate treatment during this process.

Metzner and Dvoskin (2004) point out that there is a fundamental difference between prisons and jails. They define local jails, which are usually administered by city or county officials, as "facilities that hold inmates beyond arraignment, generally for 48 hours, but less than a year." In contrast, prisons, which are run by state or federal administrations, are correctional facilities that house individuals convicted of major crimes or felonies and who are serving sentences that are usually in excess of a year. A large portion of offenders who are mentally ill, particularly the acutely psychotic, never reach the prison sys-

tem. Frequent arrests for minor offenses may lead to numerous jail incarcerations, a sense of loss of control, and a continual state of crisis. The National Center on Institutions and Alternatives (2002) reports that the suicide rate in county jails is approximately 9 times greater than that of the general population, while the suicide rate in prisons is approximately 1.5 times greater than in the community.

Special Concerns

Overcrowding and Violence

Numerous studies have shown that crowding affects the level of violence in prisons. The prison system is not capable of handling the burden of large numbers of prisoners for which it has become responsible, and many of the infractions by prisoners are violent in nature. The growing number of prisoners is thought to be related to the increasing war on drugs, longer mandatory sentencing, and the "three strikes and you're out" laws. As this population continues to grow, the solution seems to be to continue to construct larger and larger complexes to house the growing numbers of inmates. The unfortunate truth lies in the fact that violent behavior often proves to be resourceful for the individuals who use it in prison.

Inmate violence directed toward prison staff is also a common occurrence. Light (1991) reported the most frequently cited motives as inmate resistance to officer's commands, protest of unjust treatment, resistance to searches and attempt to remove contraband, and staff intervention in fights between inmates. Actual or implied verbal threats and swearing are the common everyday language of most offender clients. Nurses who work in correctional facilities must be able to adjust to the commonality of physical and verbal aggression if they are to prevail in this chosen area of specialization.

Sexual Assault

The number of victims of sexual assault in American prisons is unknown. It is estimated that at least 13 percent of U.S. inmates have been sexually assaulted in prison, with many of them suffering repeated assaults (Pyrek, 2005). The majority of these assaults go unreported because the consequences of "ratting" on fellow prisoners are often far more serious than the rape itself.

Rape in prison is viewed as an act of dominance and power, rather than one that is sexually motivated, and the majority of both victims and victimizers are heterosexuals. Wark (1998) describes the typical victim as "young, white, nonviolent, generally tall and slender with long hair." In other instances, sexual assault is used as a means of punishment and social control when the victim is believed to have violated certain unwritten prison codes. Gang rape is not uncommon, and severe physical injury is often the result if the victim attempts to defend himself.

HIV Infection in the Prison Population

The AIDS rate is six times higher in state and federal prisons than in the general U.S. population (Kantor, 2003). In addition to sexual conduct, other means of HIV transmission among inmates include fights that result in lacerations, bites, or bleeding. Body piercing and tattooing are becoming more popular in prison, and clean instruments for these activities are not available. Intravenous drug use results in sharing of unsterilized injection equipment.

HIV has placed an enormous financial burden on a prison system that was already financially distressed. Some terminally ill prisoners with advanced HIV disease are being granted early compassionate release to family or hospice care and with access to community health services (Kantor, 2003).

The most recent approach to prevention of HIV transmission has shifted from segregation to education. Education of the prison population about HIV is difficult because as many as 50 percent of American prisoners are functionally illiterate, and many do not speak English (Kantor, 2003). Educational programs to meet the communication needs of this special population would be required.

Female Offenders

Women comprise approximately 7 percent of the total population in prisons and jails (USDOJ, 2004). As a minority group, they appear to be discriminated against within the prison system. Their facilities are usually more isolated, making it more difficult for family visits. In some instances, separate institutions do not exist, making it necessary to house male and female offenders in co-correctional facilities. Men are given a greater number of opportunities regarding education and vocational training services. McClellan (2002) states:

My first study of women prisoners uncovered striking disparity: women prisoners were cited more often for disciplinary infractions than were men. Rules scrupulously enforced in women's institutions were routinely ignored in men's. Although their infractions were less serious in nature, women were punished more severely than men. Operating under the same set of court-mandated formal rules, prisons display two gender-differentiated systems of surveillance and control.

Many women are single mothers who are unable to make adequate provision for their children while they serve their time in prison and who often lose custody of their children to the state. Prison health care is mostly inadequate, and the unique health needs of women often go unmet. Many of these women had very little before they were incarcerated, and have come to expect that little is what they deserve. Many report long histories of sexual and emotional abuse throughout their lives. Depression and acting-out behaviors are common in women's prisons.

Nursing Diagnosis

Forensic psychiatric nurse specialists in correctional facilities analyze the information gathered during assessment of the client to formulate nursing diagnoses. Common nursing diagnoses relevant to forensic clients in correctional facilities include:

1. Defensive coping
2. Dysfunctional grieving
3. Anxiety/fear
4. Disturbed thought processes
5. Powerlessness
6. Low self-esteem
7. Risk for self-mutilation
8. Risk for self-directed or other-directed violence
9. Ineffective coping
10. Ineffective sexuality patterns
11. Risk for infection

Planning/Implementation

Psychiatric nurses who work in correctional facilities must be armed with extraordinary psychosocial skills and the knowledge to apply them in the most appropriate manner.

Development of a Therapeutic Relationship

Incarcerated individuals have difficulty trusting anyone associated with authority, including nurses. For most of these individuals, this likely relates back to very early stages of development and lack of nurturing.

Aside from the added difficulty of dealing with this special population, development of a therapeutic relationship in the correctional facility encompasses the same phases of interaction as it does with other clients. Chapter 7 of this text discusses the dynamics of this process at length.

Preinteraction Phase

During this phase the nurse must examine his or her feelings, fears, and anxieties about working with prisoners and in particular violent offenders—perhaps murderers, rapists, or pedophiles. This is the phase in which the nurse must determine whether he or she is able to separate the *person* from the *behavior* and provide the unconditional positive regard that Rogers (1951) believed identified each individual as a worthwhile and unique human being.

Orientation (Introductory) Phase

This is the phase in which the nurse works to establish trust with the client. This is a lengthy and intense process with the prisoner population. The characteristics that have been identified as significant to the development of a therapeutic nurse–client relationship—rapport, trust, and genuineness—are commonly met with suspicion on the part of the offender. Empathy may be used as a tool for manipulating the nurse. It is therefore imperative that limits be established and enforced by all of the nursing staff. Testing of limits is commonplace, so consequences for violation must be consistently administered. Splitting treatment team members against each other is a common ploy among inmates (Schafer, 1999).

Touch and self-disclosure, two elements used in the establishment of trust with clients, are most commonly unacceptable with the prisoner population. A handshake may be appropriate, but any other form of touch between nurse and inmate of the opposite gender is usually restricted in most settings. Self-disclosure is commonly used to convey empathy and to promote trust by helping the client view the nurse as an ordinary human being. With the prisoner population, the client may seek personal information about the nurse in an effort to maintain control of the relationship. Nurses must maintain awareness of the situation and ensure that personal boundaries are not being violated.

Communication within the correctional facility may prove to be a challenge for the nurse. Slang terminology is commonplace and changes rapidly. Some of these terms are presented in Table 44–2.

Working Phase

Nursing skills are implemented during the working phase of the relationship, and promoting behavioral change is the primary goal. This is extremely difficult with offenders who commonly deny problems and resist change. Transference and countertransference issues are more common in working with this population than with other psychiatric clients. Issues are discussed in the treatment team meetings, and ongoing modifications are made as required. Following are some of the interventions associated with psychiatric forensic nursing in correctional institutions.

Counseling and Supportive Psychotherapy. Nurses may work with inmates who are experiencing feelings of powerlessness and grief. Women who have left children behind may fear the permanent loss of custody or of never seeing them again. Helping these individuals work through a period of mourning is an important nursing intervention.

Nurses may also counsel victims of sexual assault. Victims of sexual assault in prison often experience the symptoms associated with rape-trauma syndrome. Feelings of helplessness and vulnerability, coupled with shame, humiliation, and embarrassment are characteristic. Internalized rage can become paralytic. Perception of gender identity may even be compromised.

These individuals often become withdrawn and isolated and are at high risk for suicide. The nurse can recognize these symptoms and intervene as required. All unusual behavior should be shared with the treatment team. Care plans for treating specific behaviors (such as depression and suicide, psychotic behaviors, and antisocial behaviors) are located in Units Three and Four of this text.

Crisis Intervention. Behaviors such as aggression, self-mutilation, suicide attempts, acute psychotic episodes, and posttrauma responses require that the nurse be proficient in crisis intervention. Feelings of helplessness and loss of control are pervasive in the prison population. The chaotic, overburdened prison system lacks the resources to provide the kind of services needed to prevent the continual state of crisis these conditions engender. Suicide risk is higher in jails and prisons than it is in the community. Noncompliance with prison rules, feelings of hopelessness, psychopathology, substance abuse, and overcrowded conditions all contribute to the potential for violence. Threatening behaviors must be reported immediately to all members of the treatment team. A strong foundation in crisis intervention theory and techniques is mandatory for nurses who work in correctional institutions. Techniques of crisis intervention are discussed in Chapter 13 of this text.

Education. Opportunities for teaching abound in the correctional facility. As was mentioned previously, however, because of the level of education of many incarcerated individuals, and because many of them speak little English, the teaching plan must be highly individualized. Many have no desire or motivation to learn and resist cooperating with these efforts. Important educational endeavors with these clients include:

● **Health Teaching.** Most criminals are not in good physical condition when they reach prison. They have lived rough lives of smoking, poor diets, substance abuse, and minimal health care. This is an opportunity for nurses to provide information about ways to achieve optimum wellness.

● **HIV/AIDS Education.** Kantor (2003) states:

   All persons entering prison must be informed in clear, simple terms, *and in their own language*, about how to avoid transmission of HIV and other communicable diseases. Educational programs can reduce fears about HIV and its transmission among the majority of staff and inmates. Individual counseling, peer counseling, support groups, and special programs for women, designed for

TABLE 44–2	Glossary of Prison Slang

Ad-Seg. Administrative segregation. A prisoner placed on ad-seg is being investigated and will go into isolation (the "hole") until the investigation is complete.

Beef. Criminal charges. As, "I caught a burglary beef this time around." Also used to mean a problem. "I have a beef with that guy."

Big Yard. The main recreation yard.

Bit. Prison sentence, usually relatively short. "I got a three-year bit." (opposite of jolt)

Bitch, bitched (v.). To be sentenced as a "habitual offender."

Blocks. Cellhouses.

Books. Administratively controlled account ledger that lists each prisoner's account balance.

Bone Yard. The visiting trailers, used for overnight visits of wives and/or families.

Bum Beef. A false accusation. Also, a wrongful conviction.

Catch a Ride. To ask a friend with drugs to get you high. "Hey man, can I catch a ride?"

The Chain. The bus transports that bring prisoners to prison. One is shackled and chained when transported. As, "I've been riding the chain," or "I just got in on the chain," or "Is there anyone we know on the chain?"

Check-In. Someone who has submitted to pressure, intimidation, debts, etc., and no longer feels secure in population and "checks in" to a protective custody (PC) unit.

Chi-Mo. Child molester, "chester," "baby-raper," "short-eyes," (as "he has short-eyes," meaning he goes after young kids). The worst of the rapo class in the eyes of convicts.

Convict. Guys who count in prison; loyal to the code; aren't stool pigeons; their word is good (opposite of inmate).

C.U.S. Custody unit supervisor/cellhouse supervisor.

De-Seg. Disciplinary segregation. When a person is on de-seg, he is in isolation (the "hole") for an infraction.

Ding. A disrespectful term for a mentally ill prisoner.

Dry Snitching. To inform on someone indirectly by talking loud or performing suspicious actions when officers are in the area.

Dummy Up; Get on the Dummy. To shut up, to pipe down, to be quiet, especially about one's knowledge of a crime.

E.P.R.D. Earliest possible release date.

Fish. A new arrival, a first-timer, a bumpkin, not wise to prison life.

Gate Money. Money the state gives a prisoner upon his release.

Gate Time. At most prisons they yell "gate time," meaning one can get in or out of their cell. See lock-up.

Hacks/Hogs/Pigs/Snouts/Screws/Cops/Bulls. The guards; called "Corrections Officers" by themselves and inmates.

Heat Wave. Being under constant suspicion, thereby bringing attention to those around you.

Hit It. Go away, leave, get lost.

Hold Your Mud. Not tell, even under pressure of punishment.

The Hole. An isolation ("segregation") cell, used as punishment for offenses.

House. Cell.

Hustle. A professional criminal's avocation. Also refers to any scheme to obtain money or drugs while in prison.

I.K. Inmate kitchen.

I.M.U. Intensive Management Unit. Administration's name for "segregation" or "the hole."

Inmate. Derogatory term for prisoners. Used by guards, administrators, other inmates, or new arrivals who don't know the language yet. Opposite of convict.

Jacket. Prison file containing all information on a prisoner. "He's a child molester; it's in his jacket." Also reputation. Prisoners can put false jackets on other prisoners to discredit them.

Jolt. A long sentence. ("I got a life jolt.") Opposite of bit.

Jumping-Out. Turning to crime. "I've been jumping out since I was a kid."

Keister. To hide something in the anal cavity.

Lag. A convict, as in, "He's an old lag, been at it all his life."

Lifer or "All Day." Anyone doing a life sentence. A life jolt.

Lock-Down. When prisoners are confined to their cells.

Lock-Up. Free movement period for prisoners. See also gate time.

Lop. Same as inmate.

Mule. A person who smuggles drugs into the institution.

On the Leg. A prisoner who is always chatting with and befriending guards.

Paper. A small quantity of drugs packaged for selling.

P.C. Protective custody. Also as in "He's a PC case," meaning weak or untrustworthy.

Point/Outfit. Syringe.

Pruno. Homemade wine.

Punk. Derogatory term meaning homosexual or weak individual.

Rapo. Anyone with a sex crime—generally looked down on by convicts.

Rat/Snitch/Stool Pigeon. n., informant. v., to inform.

Stand Point. Watch for "the man" (guard)

Tag/Write-Up. Infraction of institution rules.

The Bag/Sack. Dope.

Tom or George. Meaning "no good" (Tom) or "okay" (George). Used in conversation to indicate if someone or something is okay or no[t]

Turned Out. To be forced into homosexual acts, or to turn someone out to do things for you; to use someone for your own needs.

White Money. Currency within the institution.

Yard-In/Yard-Out. Closing of the recreation yard (yard-in). Recreation yard opens (yard-out).

and by prisoners, have been successful in a number of institutions and seem to be the best educational tools.

Some correctional institutions now provide condoms to inmates, but this remains a point of controversy between legal and public health officials.

● **Stress Management.** Nurses can pr[in]t [information] techniques. and demonstration of stress mana[f]uction of anxi- They can help individuals practi[ce] or substances. ety without resorting to medic[ine] Bureau of Prisons

● **Substance Abuse.** The F[e]

(2005) has established a comprehensive substance abuse treatment strategy in an effort to change inmates' criminal and drug-using behaviors. This strategy begins with drug abuse education and ends with a strong community transition component. The individuals receive information about alcohol and drugs and the physical, social, and psychological impact of abusing these substances. Since its inception, this program has proved highly successful in decreasing recidivism and relapse rates among its participants.

Nurses can participate in substance abuse treatment programs by providing client education (e.g., the effects of substances on the body; the consequences of sharing needles). They can also form support groups for individuals who abuse substances if one does not exist in the institution. A large percentage of the prison population has a history of substance abuse, and many correlate the commission of their crimes with substance use. This is an important area of need for nursing intervention in the correctional system.

Termination Phase

Ideally, the termination phase of the nurse–client relationship ensures therapeutic closure. This is not always possible in the correctional environment. Prisoners are transferred from one institution to another, and from one part of an institution to another, for a variety of reasons, not the least of which are safety and security of self or others. When possible, it is important for nurses to initiate termination with clients so that at least some semblance of closure can be achieved and a review of goal attainment can be accomplished. Community facilities for mentally ill ex-offenders are few, and recidivism is rampant. Johnson and Laffan (2005) state:

> The majority of mentally ill offenders need the basic elements of case management. Psychiatric nurses in correctional settings often act as case managers, beginning prerelease planning upon the initial contact with inmates. Continuation of any treatment and medication from jail and transition to the community-based treatment in a swift manner is critical to success. Unfortunately resources in this area are often lacking. Many inmates may not have predetermined release dates, thereby leading to releases at all hours of the day and night. Prerelease planning and coordination with community-based programs are necessary to promote continuity of care and recidivism. Nurses are vital members of the interdisciplinary team and play significant roles in the assessment, planning, implementation, and evaluation of the case management plan to best meet the needs of patients.

Evaluation

Evaluation of the correctional psychiatric forensic nursing process in the correctional environment involves ongoing measurement of the diagnostic criteria aimed at resolution of identified real or potential problems. The following types of questions may provide assistance in the evaluation process.

1. Has a degree of trust been established in the nurse–client relationship?
2. Has violence by the offender to self or others been prevented?
3. If victimization has occurred, has appropriate care and support been provided to the survivor?
4. Have limits been set on inappropriate behaviors, and has consistency of consequences for violation of the limits been administered by all staff?
5. Have educational programs been established to provide information about health and wellness, HIV/AIDS, stress management, and substance abuse?

Evaluation is an ongoing process and must be assumed by the entire treatment team. Modification of the treatment plan as required is part of the ongoing evaluation process, and positive change within the system is the ultimate outcome. Nurses who work in correctional facilities are "pioneers" within the nursing profession. To share the knowledge gleaned from this specialty area is an important part of the nursing process.

SUMMARY

Forensic nursing, which is a growing area within the profession, is composed of a variety of areas of expertise. Forensic nurses take care of both victims and perpetrators of crime in a variety of settings, including primary care facilities, hospitals, and correctional institutions. The International Association of Forensic Nurses, founded in 1992, now has more than a thousand members.

Forensic nursing specialties include clinical forensic nursing, the sexual assault nurse examiner, forensic psychiatric nursing, and correctional/institutional nursing. Nurses in general practice also find forensic nursing knowledge of importance in their practices, particularly in emergency departments and intensive care units.

This chapter presented discussions of two specialty areas of forensic nursing: clinical forensic nursing in trauma care and forensic psychiatric nursing in correctional facilities. Nursing care of these special populations was presented in the context of the nursing process.

The number of educational offerings pertaining to forensic nursing is growing. Some content is taught in traditional nursing courses, whereas some colleges and universities are establishing forensic nursing courses as electives. Forensic nursing is fertile ground for nursing research, and the complex nature of the specialty lends itself well to those nurses who seek a challenge within the profession.

TEST YOUR CRITICAL THINKING SKILLS

Kim is a 27-year-old woman who recently moved from a small town in Texas to work in the city of Dallas as a reporter for one of the major newspapers. She is 5'6" tall and weighs 115 lb. To keep in shape she likes to jog, which she did regularly in her hometown. She doesn't know anyone in Dallas and has been lonely for her family since arriving. But she has moved into a small apartment in a quiet neighborhood and hopes to meet young people soon through her work and church.

On the first Saturday morning after she moved into her new apartment, Kim decided to get up early and go jogging. It was still dark out, but Kim was not afraid. She had been jogging alone in the dark many times in her hometown. She donned her jogging clothes and headed down the quiet street toward a nearby park. As she entered the park, an individual came out from a dense clump of bushes, put a knife to her throat, and ordered her to the ground. She was raped and beaten unconscious. She remained in that condition until sunrise when she was found by another jogger who called emergency services, and Kim was taken to the closest emergency department. On regaining consciousness, Kim was hysterical, but a sexual assault nurse examiner (SANE) was called to the scene, and Kim was assigned to a quiet area of the hospital, where the post-rape examination was initiated.

Answer the following questions related to Kim.

1. What are the initial nursing interventions for Kim?
2. What treatments must the nurse ensure that Kim is aware are available for her?
3. What nursing diagnosis would the nurse expect to focus on with Kim in follow-up care?

REVIEW QUESTIONS

SELF-EXAMINATION/LEARNING EXERCISE

Identify whether each of the following questions is true or false.

1. All traumatic injuries in which liability is suspected are considered within the scope of forensic nursing.
   a. _____ true   b. _____ false

2. Clinical forensic nursing in the trauma department encompasses preservation of evidence, investigation of wound characteristics, and sudden deaths in the emergency department (ED).
   a. _____ true   b. _____ false

3. Legal authorities must be notified of all deaths that occur in the ED.
   a. _____ true   b. _____ false

4. When a trauma victim is admitted to the ED, the most obvious priority intervention is preservation of evidence.
   a. _____ true   b. _____ false

5. When clothing is removed, it should be shaken to remove any possible evidence that may be adhering to it.
   a. _____ true   b. _____ false

6. Rape victims can be treated prophylactically for sexually transmitted diseases.
   a. _____ true   b. _____ false

7. The most common psychiatric behavior that has been identified among mentally ill offenders is thought disorder.
   a. _____ true   b. _____ false

8. The AIDS rate is higher in state and federal prisons than in the general population.
   a. _____ true   b. _____ false

9. Male offenders receive more educational opportunities in prison than female offenders.
   a. _____ true   b. _____ false

10. Correctional institutions are federally mandated to provide condoms to inmates to prevent the transmission of HIV.
    a. _____ true   b. _____ false

 INTERNET REFERENCES

Additional information related to Forensic Nursing may be found at:
- http://www.forensiceducation.com/
- http://www.forensicnurse.org/

- http://www.amrn.com/
- http://nursing.advanceweb.com/common/Editorial/Editorial.aspx?CC=40302
- http://www.forensicnursemag.com/

IMPLICATIONS OF RESEARCH FOR EVIDENCE-BASED PRACTICE

Yurkovich, E., & Smyer, T. (2000). **Health maintenance behaviors of individuals with severe and persistent mental illness in a state prison.** *Journal of Psychosocial Nursing and Mental Health Services, 38*(6), 20–31.

Description of the Study: The purpose of this study was to define health and health-seeking behaviors of incarcerated individuals experiencing severe and persistent mental illness (SPMI) in a state prison. The researchers conducted a comparative analysis of these findings to two studies that explored the same questions with individuals experiencing SPMI and attending two different community treatment centers. The researchers also examined strategies used by inmates with SPMI to prevent loss of control and maintain health in the prison environment. Information was gathered by in-depth interview using a semistructured interview guide, participant observation, and review of inmates' charts. Nineteen prisoners with SPMI participated. The age range was 21 to 56 and the educational level ranged from 4 to 18 years. Fifteen prisoners had committed crimes against person and 4 had committed crimes against property. Criminal activity was related to substance abuse in 15 of the cases. All interviews were conducted in a room set aside for the researchers in the prison infirmary.

Results of the Study: Individuals in the community are able to define their environment through use of health care providers and the trusted informal system of peers, friends, and relatives. Individuals with SPMI in the corrections facility do not have this connection. Negative response from other inmates to the behavior of inmates with SPMI reduces their ability to seek an appropriate level of assistance and maintain a healthy status. Some comparisons from the study are as follows:

Variable	Community-Based Individuals	Inmates with SPMI
Relationships	Maintains a balance within family	Maintains relationships based on purpose (e.g., to provide protection or prevent abuse)
Feelings	Controls negative feelings and prevents destructive outcome when feeling angry (e.g., leave hostile environment)	Controls negative feelings by self-imposed solitude, lock down, or withdrawal from socialization areas
Attitude	Builds self-esteem through purpose or goal completion	Lack of opportunity for building self-esteem
Functional Behaviors	Performs ADLs and participates in treatment center activities	Lacks opportunities to perform and participate

The prisoners demonstrated a need for education about their illnesses and medications. They demonstrated little insight into how stress and poor physical health affected their mental illness.

Implications for Nursing Practice: The authors state, "This study communicates a message from prisoners with SPMI that tells health care providers how they struggle to maintain a healthy status within a toxic environment and what they need to support this process. Nurses within a correctional setting have a responsibility to assist individuals with SPMI to interpret their environment, define role behaviors, and determine how to maintain wellness within the prison system."

REFERENCES

American Medical Association (AMA). (1999). *Strategies for the treatment and prevention of sexual assault.* Chicago, IL: Science and Public Health Advocacy Programs.

Beck, A.J., & Maruschak, L.M. (2001). *Mental health treatment in state prisons, 2000.* Bureau of Justice Statistics Special Report. Washington, DC: U.S. Department of Justice.

Bell, K. (1999, March). Forensic nursing. Paper presented at the meeting of the Oklahoma Association of Clinical Nurse Specialists, Stroud, Oklahoma.

Brown, K. (2005). Evidence collection and preservation in a healthcare setting. *Nursing Spectrum/Nurseweek CE: Course – CE296b.* Retrieved June 3, 2005 from the World Wide Web at http://www2.nurseweek.com/ce/self-study_modules/

Burgess, A. (2004). Rape violence. *Nurse Spectrum/Nurseweek CE: Course 25.* Retrieved May 23, 2005 from the World Wide Web at http://www2.nursingspectrum.com

Forensic Nursing Service (FNS). (1999). *About forensic nursing.* Retrieved June 4, 2002 from the World Wide Web at http://www.forensicnursing.com/html/about.html/

Hufft, A., & Peternelj-Taylor, C. (2003). Forensic nursing: A specialty for the twenty-first century. In J.T. Catalano (Ed.). *Nursing now! Today's issues, tomorrow's trends* (3rd ed.). Philadelphia: F.A. Davis.

International Association of Forensic Nurses (IAFN) and American Nurses Association (ANA). (1997). *Scope and Standards of Forensic Nursing Practice.* Washington, DC: American Nurses Publishing.

Johnson, J.D., & Laffan, S. (2005). Psychiatric nursing in the correctional setting. *Nursing Spectrum/Nurseweek CE: Course 30Cb.* Retrieved June 5, 2005 from the World Wide Web at http://www2nursingspectrum.com

Kantor, E. (2003). HIV transmission and prevention in prisons. *HIV InSite Knowledge Base.* Retrieved June 5, 2005 from http://hivinsite.ucsf.edu/InSite?page=kb-07&doc=kb-07-04-13

Ledray, L.E. (2001). Evidence collection and care of the sexual assault survivor: The SANE-SART response. *Violence Against Women.* Retrieved June 3, 2005 from The World Wide Web at http://www.vaw.umn.edu/documents/commissioned2forensicevidence/2forensicevidence.html

Light, S. (1991). Assaults on prison officers: Interactional themes. *Justice Quarterly, 8,* 243–261.

Lynch, V.A. (1995, September). Clinical forensic nursing: A new perspective in the management of crime victims from trauma to trial. *Critical Care Nursing Clinics of North America, 7*(3), 489–507.

McClellan, D.S. (2002). Coming to the aid of women in U.S. prisons. *Monthly Review, 54*(2), 33–44.

McPeck, P. (2002). Down to a science. *NurseWeek,* January 21, 2002, 24–25.

Metzner, J.L., & Dvoskin, J.A. (2004). Psychiatry in correctional settings. In R.I. Simon & L.H. Gold (Eds.). *Textbook of Forensic Psychiatry.* Washington, DC: American Psychiatric Publishing.

National Center on Institutions and Alternatives. (2002). *Jail suicide prevention and liability reduction services.* Retrieved June 3, 2002 from the World Wide Web at http://www.igc.org/ncia/suicide.html

Pyrek, K.M. (2003, November/December). Prison-rape elimination act is signed into law. *Forensic Nurse Magazine.* Retrieved June 4, 2005 from the World Wide Web at http://www.forensicnursemag.com/articles/3b1corrections.html

Raphael, S. (2000). The deinstitutionalization of the mentally ill and growth in the U.S. prison populations: 1971 to 1996. Berkeley, CA: The University of California, Goldman School of Public Policy.

Schafer, P. (1999). Working with Dave: Application of Peplau's inter-personal nursing theory in the correctional environment. *Journal of Psychosocial Nursing and Mental Health Services, 37*(9), 18–24.

U.S. Department of Justice (USDOJ). (2004). *Prison and jail inmates at midyear 2004.* Retrieved June 4, 2005 from the World Wide Web at http://www.ojp.usdoj.gov/bjs/pub/pdf/pjim04.pdf

Wark, D. (1998). *Prison violence: Homicide, assault, and rape.* Retrieved April 6, 1999 from http://oak.cats.ohiou.edu/~dw101094/esp/soc4661.html/

Yurkovich, E., & Smyer, T. (2000). Health maintenance behaviors of individuals with severe mental illness in a state prison. *Journal of Psychosocial Nursing and Mental Health Services, 38*(6), 20–31.

C L A S S I C A L   R E F E R E N C E

Rogers, C.R. (1951). *Client centered therapy.* Boston: Houghton Mifflin.

THE BEREAVED INDIVIDUAL

CHAPTER OUTLINE

OBJECTIVES

THEORETICAL PERSPECTIVES ON LOSS AND
BEREAVEMENT

LENGTH OF THE GRIEF PROCESS

ANTICIPATORY GRIEF

MALADAPTIVE RESPONSES TO LOSS

APPLICATION OF THE NURSING PROCESS

ADDITIONAL ASSISTANCE

SUMMARY

REVIEW QUESTIONS

KEY TERMS

advance directives
anticipatory grieving
bereavement overload
delayed grief
hospice

luto
mourning
shiva
velorio

CORE CONCEPTS

grief
loss

OBJECTIVES

After reading this chapter, the student will be able to:

1. Describe various types of loss that trigger the grief response in individuals.
2. Discuss theoretical perspectives of grieving as proposed by Elisabeth Kübler-Ross, John Bowlby, George Engel, and J. William Worden.
3. Differentiate between normal and maladaptive responses to loss.
4. Discuss grieving behaviors common to individuals at various stages across the life span.
5. Describe customs associated with grief in individuals of various cultures.
6. Formulate nursing diagnoses and goals of

care for individuals experiencing the grief response.
7. Describe appropriate nursing interventions for individuals experiencing the grief response.
8. Identify relevant criteria for evaluating nursing care of individuals experiencing the grief response.
9. Describe the concept of hospice care for people who are dying and their families.
10. Discuss the use of advance directives for individuals to provide directions about their future medical care.

oss is anything that is perceived as such by the individual. The separation from loved ones or the giving up of treasured possessions, for whatever reason; the experience of failure, either real or perceived; or life events that create change in a familiar pattern of existence—all can be expe-

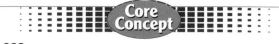

Loss

The experience of separation from something of personal importance.

rienced as loss, and all can trigger behaviors associated with the grieving process. Loss and bereavement are universal events encountered by all beings that experience emotions. Following are examples of some notable forms of loss:

1. A significant other (person or pet), through death, divorce, or separation for any reason.
2. Illness or debilitating conditions. Examples include (but are not limited to) diabetes, stroke, cancer, rheumatoid arthritis, multiple sclerosis, Alzheimer's disease, hearing or vision loss, and spinal cord or head injuries. Some of these conditions not only incur a loss of physical and/or emotional wellness, but may also result in the loss of personal independence.
3. Developmental/maturational changes or situations, such as menopause, andropause, infertility, empty nest, aging, impotence, or hysterectomy.
4. A decrease in self-esteem, if one is unable to meet self-expectations or the expectations of others (even if these expectations are only perceived by the individual as unfulfilled). This includes a loss of potential hopes and dreams.
5. Personal possessions that symbolize familiarity and security in a person's life. Separation from these familiar and personally valued external objects represents a loss of material extensions of the self.

Core Concept

Grief
Deep mental and emotional anguish that is a response to the subjective experience of loss of something significant.

Some texts differentiate the terms **mourning** and grief by describing mourning as the psychological process (or stages) through which the individual passes on the way to successful adaptation to the loss of a valued object. Grief may be viewed as the subjective states that accompany mourning, or the emotional work involved in the mourning process. For purposes of this text, grief work and the process of mourning are collectively referred to as the *grief response*.

This chapter examines human responses to the experience of loss. Care of bereaved individuals is presented in the context of the nursing process.

THEORETICAL PERSPECTIVES ON LOSS AND BEREAVEMENT

Stages of Grief

Behavior patterns associated with the grief response include many individual variations. However, sufficient similarities have been observed to warrant characteriza-tion of grief as a syndrome that has a predictable course with an expected resolution. Early theorists, including Kübler-Ross (1969), Bowlby (1961), and Engel (1964), described behavioral stages through which individuals advance in their progression toward resolution. A number of variables influence one's progression through the grief process. Some individuals may reach acceptance, only to revert back to an earlier stage; some may never complete the sequence; and some may never progress beyond the initial stage. A comparison of the similarities among these three models is presented in Table 45–1.

A more contemporary grief specialist, J. William Worden (2002), offers a set of tasks that must be processed in order to complete the grief response. He suggests that it is possible for a person to accomplish some of these tasks and not others, resulting in an incomplete bereavement, and thus impairing further growth and development.

Elisabeth Kübler-Ross

These well-known stages of the grief process were identified by Kübler-Ross in her extensive work with dying patients. Behaviors associated with each of these stages can be observed in individuals experiencing the loss of any concept of personal value.

Stage I: Denial. In this stage the individual does not acknowledge that the loss has occurred. He or she may say, "No, it can't be true!" or "It's just not possible." This stage may protect the individual against the psychological pain of reality.

Stage II: Anger. This is the stage when reality sets in. Feelings associated with this stage include sadness, guilt, shame, helplessness, and hopelessness. Self-blame or blaming of others may lead to feelings of anger toward the self and others. The anxiety level may be elevated, and the individual may experience confusion and a decreased ability to function independently. He or she may be preoccupied with an idealized image of what has been lost. Numerous somatic complaints are common.

Stage III: Bargaining. At this stage in the grief response, the individual attempts to strike a bargain with God for a second chance, or for more time. The person acknowledges the loss, or impending loss, but holds out hope for additional alternatives, as evidenced by statements such as, "If only I could..." or "If only I had..."

Stage IV: Depression. In this stage, the individual mourns for that which has been or will be lost. This is a very painful stage, during which the individual must confront feelings associated with having lost someone or something of value (called *reactive* depression). An example might be the individual who is mourning a change in body image. Feelings associated with an impending loss (called *preparatory* depression) are also confronted. Examples include permanent lifestyle changes related to

TABLE 45–1	Stages of the Normal Grief Response: A Comparison of Models by Elisabeth Kübler-Ross, John Bowlby, and George Engel

STAGES				
KÜBLER-ROSS	BOWLBY	ENGEL	POSSIBLE TIME DIMENSION	BEHAVIORS
I. Denial	I. Numbness/Protest	I. Shock/Disbelief	Occurs immediately upon experiencing the loss. Usually lasts no more than 2 weeks.	Individual refuses to acknowledge that the loss has occurred.
II. Anger	II. Disequilibrium	II. Developing Awareness	In most cases begins within hours of the loss. Peaks within 2 to 4 weeks.	Anger is directed toward self or others. Ambivalence and guilt may be felt toward the lost object.
III. Bargaining				The individual fervently seeks alternatives to improve current situation.
		III. Restitution		Attends to various rituals associated with the culture in which the loss has occurred.
IV. Depression	III. Disorganization and despair	IV. Resolution of the loss	A year or more.	The actual work of grieving. Preoccupation with the lost object. Feelings of helplessness and loneliness occur in response to realization of the loss. Feelings associated with the loss are confronted.
V. Acceptance	IV. Reorganization	V. Recovery		Resolution is complete. The bereaved person experiences a reinvestment in new relationships and new goals. Terminally ill persons express a readiness to die.

the altered body image or even an impending loss of life itself. Regression, withdrawal, and social isolation may be observed behaviors with this stage. Therapeutic intervention should be available, but not imposed, and with guidelines for implementation based on client readiness.

Stage V: Acceptance. At this time, the individual has worked through the behaviors associated with the other stages and either accepts or is resigned to the loss. Anxiety decreases, and methods for coping with the loss have been established. The client is less preoccupied with what has been lost and increasingly interested in other aspects of the environment. If this is an impending death of self, the individual is ready to die. The person may become very quiet and withdrawn, seemingly devoid of feelings. These behaviors are an attempt to facilitate the passage by slowly disengaging from the environment.

John Bowlby

John Bowlby hypothesized four stages in the grief process. He implies that these behaviors can be observed in all individuals who have experienced the loss of something or someone of value, even in infants as young as 6 months of age.

Stage I: Numbness or Protest. This stage is characterized by a feeling of shock and disbelief that the loss has occurred. Reality of the loss is not acknowledged.

Stage II: Disequilibrium. During this stage, the individual has a profound urge to recover what has been lost. Behaviors associated with this stage include a preoccupation with the loss, intense weeping and expressions of anger toward the self and others, and feelings of ambivalence and guilt associated with the loss.

Stage III: Disorganization and Despair. Feelings of despair occur in response to realization that the loss has occurred. Activities of daily living become increasingly disorganized, and behavior is characterized by restlessness and aimlessness. Efforts to regain productive patterns of behavior are ineffective and the individual experiences fear, helplessness, and hopelessness. Somatic complaints are common. Perceptions of visualizing or being in the presence of that which has been lost may occur. Social isolation is common, and the individual may feel a great deal of loneliness.

Stage IV: Reorganization. The individual accepts or becomes resigned to the loss. New goals and patterns of organization are established. The individual begins a reinvestment in new relationships and indicates a readiness to move forward within the environment. Grief subsides and recedes into valued remembrances.

George Engel

Stage I: Shock and Disbelief. The initial reaction to a loss is a stunned, numb feeling and refusal by the individual to acknowledge the reality of the loss. Engel states that this stage is an attempt by the individual to protect the self "against the effects of the overwhelming stress by raising the threshold against its recognition or against the painful feelings evoked thereby."

Stage II: Developing Awareness. This stage begins within minutes to hours of the loss. Behaviors associated with this stage include excessive crying and regression to a state of helplessness and a childlike manner. Awareness of the loss creates feelings of emptiness, frustration, anguish, and despair. Anger may be directed toward the self or toward others in the environment who are held accountable for the loss.

Stage III: Restitution. In this stage, the various rituals associated with loss within a culture are performed. Examples include funerals, wakes, special attire, a gathering of friends and family, and religious practices customary to the spiritual beliefs of the bereaved. Participation in these rituals is thought to assist the individual to accept the reality of the loss and to facilitate the recovery process.

Stage IV: Resolution of the Loss. This stage is characterized by a preoccupation with the loss. The concept of the loss is idealized, and the individual may even imitate admired qualities of the lost entity. Preoccupation with the loss gradually decreases over a year or more, and the individual eventually begins to reinvest feelings in others.

Stage V: Recovery. Obsession with the loss has ended, and the individual is able to go on with his or her life.

J. William Worden

Worden views the bereaved as active and self-determining rather than passive participants in the grief process. He proposes that bereavement includes a set of tasks that must be reconciled in order to complete the grief process. Worden's four tasks of mourning include the following:

Task I. Accepting the Reality of the Loss. When something of value is lost, it is common for individuals to refuse to believe that the loss has occurred. Behaviors include misidentifying individuals in the environment for their lost loved one, retaining possessions of the lost loved one as though he or she has not died, and removing all reminders of the lost loved one so as not to have to face the reality of the loss. Worden (2002) states:

> Coming to an acceptance of the reality of the loss takes time since it involves not only an intellectual acceptance but also an emotional one. The bereaved person may be intellectually aware of the finality of the loss long before the emotions allow full acceptance of the information as true. (p. 29)

Belief and denial are intermittent while grappling with this task. It is thought that traditional rituals such as the funeral help some individuals move toward acceptance of the loss.

Task II. Working Through the Pain of Grief. Pain associated with a loss includes both physical pain and emotional pain. This pain must be acknowledged and worked through. To avoid or suppress it serves only to delay or prolong the grieving process. People accomplish this by refusing to allow themselves to think painful thoughts, by idealizing or avoiding reminders of that which has been lost, and by using alcohol or drugs. The intensity of the pain and the manner in which it is experienced are different for all individuals. But the commonality is that it *must* be experienced. Failure to do so generally results in some form of depression that commonly requires therapy, which then focuses on working through the pain of grief that the individual failed to work through at the time of the loss. In this very difficult Task II, individuals must "indulge the pain of loss—to feel it and to know that one day it will pass" (Worden, 2002).

Task III. Adjusting to an Environment That Has Changed Because of the Loss. It usually takes a number of months for a bereaved person to realize what his or her world will be like without that which has been lost. In the case of a lost loved one, how the environment changes will depend on the types of roles that person fulfilled in life. In the case of a changed lifestyle, the individual will be required to make adaptations to his or her environment in terms of the change as they are presented in daily life. In addition, those individuals who had defined their identity through that which has been lost will require an adjustment to their own sense of self. Worden (2002) states:

> The coping strategy of redefining the loss in such a way that it can redound to the benefit of the survivor is often part of the successful completion of Task III. (p. 33)

If the bereaved person experiences failures in his or her attempt to adjust in an environment without their valued concept, feelings of low self-esteem may result. Regressed behaviors and feelings of helplessness and inadequacy are not uncommon. Worden (2002) states:

> [Another] area of adjustment may be to one's sense of the world. Loss through death can challenge one's fundamental life values and philosophical beliefs—beliefs that are influenced by our families, peers, education, and religion as well as life experiences. The bereaved person searches for meaning in the loss and its attendant life changes in order to make sense of it and to regain some control of his or her life. (p. 34)

To be successful in Task III, bereaved individuals must develop new skills to cope and adapt to their new environment without the lost concept. Successful achievement of this task determines the outcome of the mourning process—that of continued growth or a state of arrested development.

Task IV. Emotionally Relocating That Which Has Been Lost and Moving on with Life. This task allows for the bereaved person to identify a special place for the lost concept. Individuals need not purge from their history or find a replacement for that which has been lost. Instead, there is a kind of continued presence of the lost concept in the life of the bereaved. The lost concept is *relocated* in the life of the bereaved. Successful completion of Task IV involves letting go of past attachments and forming new ones. There is also the recognition, however, that although the relationship between the bereaved and what has been lost is changed, it is nonetheless still a relationship. Worden (2002) suggests that one never loses memories of a significant relationship. He states:

> For many people, Task IV is the most difficult one to accomplish. They get stuck at this point in their grieving and later realize that their life in some way stopped at the point the loss occurred. (p. 37)

Worden (2002) relates the story of a teenaged girl who had a difficult time adjusting to the death of her father. After two years, when she began to finally fulfill some of the tasks associated with successful grieving, she wrote these words that express rather clearly what bereaved people in Task IV are struggling with: "There are other people to be loved, and it doesn't mean that I love Dad any less."

LENGTH OF THE GRIEF PROCESS

Stages of grief allow bereaved persons an orderly approach to the resolution of mourning. Each stage presents tasks that must be overcome through a painful experiential process. Engel (1964) has stated that successful resolution of the grief response is thought to have occurred when a bereaved individual is able "to remember comfortably and realistically both the pleasures and disappointments of [that which is lost]." The length of the grief process depends on the individual and can last for a number of years without being maladaptive. The acute phase of normal grieving usually lasts 6 to 8 weeks—longer in older adults—but complete resolution of the grief response may take much longer. Sadock and Sadock (2003) state:

> Traditionally, grief lasts about six months to one year, as the grieving person experiences the calendar year at least once without the lost person. Some signs and symptoms of grief may persist much longer than 1 or 2 years, and a survivor may have various grief-related feelings, symptoms, and behavior throughout life. In general, the acute grief symptoms gradually lessen, and within 1 or 2 months the grieving person is able to eat, sleep, and return to functioning. (pp. 62–63)

A number of factors influence the eventual outcome of the grief response. The grief response can be more difficult if:

● The bereaved person was strongly dependent on or perceived that which was lost as an important means of physical and/or emotional support.

● The relationship with that which was lost was highly ambivalent. A love-hate relationship may instill feelings of guilt that can interfere with the grief work.
● The individual has experienced a number of recent losses. Grief tends to be cumulative, and if previous losses have not been resolved, each succeeding grief response becomes more difficult.
● The loss is that of a young person. Grief over loss of a child is often more intense than it is over the loss of an elderly person.
● The state of the person's physical or psychological health is unstable at the time of the loss.
● The bereaved person perceives (whether real or imagined) some responsibility for the loss.

The grief response may be facilitated if:

● The individual has the support of significant others to assist him or her through the mourning process.
● The individual has the opportunity to prepare for the loss. Grief work is more intense when the loss is sudden and unexpected. The experience of *anticipatory grieving* is thought to facilitate the grief response that occurs at the time of the actual loss.

Worden (2002) states:

> There is a sense in which mourning can be finished, when people regain an interest in life, feel more hopeful, experience gratification again, and adapt to new roles. There is also a sense in which mourning is never finished. [People must understand] that mourning is a long-term process, and the culmination [very likely] will not be to a pre-grief state. (pp. 46–47)

ANTICIPATORY GRIEF

Anticipatory grieving is the experiencing of the feelings and emotions associated with the normal grief response before the loss actually occurs. One dissimilar aspect relates to the fact that conventional grief tends to diminish in intensity with the passage of time. Conversely, anticipatory grief may increase in intensity as the expected loss becomes imminent.

Although anticipatory grief is thought to facilitate the actual mourning process following the loss, there may be some problems. In the case of a dying person, difficulties can arise when the family members complete the process of anticipatory grief, and detachment from the dying person occurs prematurely. The person who is dying experiences feelings of loneliness and isolation as the psychological pain of imminent death is faced without family support. Sadock and Sadock (2003) describe another example of difficulty associated with premature completion of the grief response:

> Once anticipatory grief has been expended, the bereaved person may find it difficult to reestablish a previous relationship; this phenomenon is experienced with the return of

persons long gone (for example, to war or confined to concentration camps) and of persons thought to have been dead. (p. 63)

Anticipatory grieving may serve as a defense for some individuals to ease the burden of loss when it actually occurs. It may prove to be less functional for others who, because of interpersonal, psychological, or sociocultural variables, are unable in advance of the actual loss to express the intense feelings that accompany the grief response.

MALADAPTIVE RESPONSES TO LOSS

When, then, is the grieving response considered to be maladaptive? Three types of pathological grief reactions have been described. These include delayed or inhibited grief, an exaggerated or distorted grief response, and chronic or prolonged grief.

Delayed or Inhibited Grief

Delayed or inhibited grief refers to the absence of evidence of grief when it ordinarily would be expected. Many times, cultural influences, such as the expectation to keep a "stiff upper lip," cause the delayed response.

Delayed or inhibited grief is potentially pathological because the person is simply not dealing with the reality of the loss. He or she remains fixed in the denial stage of the grief process, sometimes for many years. When this occurs, the grief response may be triggered, sometimes many years later, when the individual experiences a subsequent loss. Sometimes the grief process is triggered spontaneously or in response to a seemingly insignificant event. Overreaction to another person's loss may be one manifestation of **delayed grief**.

The recognition of delayed grief is critical because, depending on the profoundness of the loss, the failure of the mourning process may prevent assimilation of the loss and thereby delay a return to satisfying living. Delayed grieving most commonly occurs because of ambivalent feelings toward that which has been lost, outside pressure to resume normal function, or perceived lack of internal and external resources to cope with a profound loss.

Distorted (Exaggerated) Grief Response

In the distorted grief reaction, all of the symptoms associated with normal grieving are exaggerated. Feelings of sadness, helplessness, hopelessness, powerlessness, anger, and guilt, as well as numerous somatic complaints, render the individual dysfunctional in terms of management of daily living. Murray and Zentner (2001) describe an exaggerated grief reaction in the following way:

An intensification of grief to the point that the person is overwhelmed, demonstrates prolonged maladaptive behavior, manifests excessive symptoms and extensive interruptions in healing, and does not progress to integration of the loss, finding meaning in the loss, and resolution of the mourning process. (p. 858)

When the exaggerated grief reaction occurs, the individual remains fixed in the anger stage of the grief response. This anger may be directed toward others in the environment to whom the individual may be attributing the loss. However, many times the anger is turned inward on the self. When this occurs, depression is the result. Depressive mood disorder is a type of exaggerated grief reaction.

Chronic or Prolonged Grieving

Some authors have discussed a chronic or prolonged grief response as a type of maladaptive grief response. Care must be taken in making this determination because, as was stated previously, length of the grief response depends on the individual. An adaptive response may take years for some people. A prolonged process may be considered maladaptive when certain behaviors are exhibited. Prolonged grief may be a problem when behaviors such as maintaining personal possessions aimed at keeping a lost loved one alive (as though he or she will eventually reenter the life of the bereaved) or disabling behaviors that prevent the bereaved from adaptively performing activities of daily living are in evidence. Another example is of a widow who refused to participate in family gatherings following the death of her husband. For many years until her own death, she took a sandwich to the cemetery on holidays, sat on the tombstone, and ate her "holiday meal" with her husband. Other bereaved individuals have been known to set a place at the table for the deceased loved one long after the completed mourning process would have been expected.

Normal versus Maladaptive Grieving

Several authors have identified one crucial difference between normal and maladaptive grieving: the loss of self-esteem. Kaplan, Sadock, and Grebb (1994) assert that "marked feelings of worthlessness" are indicative of depression rather than uncomplicated bereavement. Eisendrath and Lichtmacher (2005) affirm:

Grief is usually accompanied by intact self-esteem, whereas depression is marked by a sense of guilt and worthlessness. (p. 1035)

It is thought that this major difference between normal grieving and a maladaptive grieving response (the feeling of worthlessness or low self-esteem) ultimately precipitates depression.

APPLICATION OF THE NURSING PROCESS

Background Assessment Data: Concepts of Death—Developmental Issues

Children

Birth to Age 2. Infants are unable to recognize and understand death, but they can experience the feelings of loss and separation. Infants who are separated from their mothers may become quiet, lose weight, and sleep less. Children at this age will likely sense changes in the atmosphere of the home where a death has occurred. They often react to the emotions of adults by becoming more irritable and crying more.

Ages 3 to 5. Preschoolers and kindergartners have some understanding about death but often have difficulty distinguishing between fantasy and reality. They believe death is reversible, and their thoughts about death may include magical thinking. For example, they may believe that their thoughts or behaviors caused a person to become sick or to die.

Children of this age are capable of understanding at least some of what they see and hear from adult conversations or media reports. They become frightened if they feel a threat to themselves or their loved ones. They are concerned with safety issues and require a great deal of personal reassurance that they will be protected. Regressive behaviors, such as loss of bladder or bowel control, thumb sucking, and temper tantrums are common. Changes in eating and sleeping patterns may also occur.

Ages 6 to 9. Children at this age are beginning to understand the finality of death. They are able to understand a more detailed explanation of why or how the person died, although death is often associated with old age or with accidents. They may believe that death is contagious and avoid association with individuals who have experienced a loss by death. Death is often personified, in the form of a "bogey man" or a monster—someone who takes people away or someone whom they can avoid if they try hard enough. It is difficult for them to perceive their own death. Normal grief reactions at this age include regressive and aggressive behaviors, withdrawal, school phobias, somatic symptoms, and clinging behaviors.

Ages 10 to 12. Preadolescent children are able to understand that death is final and eventually affects everyone, including themselves. They are interested in the physical aspects of dying and the final disposition of the body. They may ask questions about how the death will affect them personally. Feelings of anger, guilt, and depression are common. Peer relationships and school performance may be disrupted. There may be a preoccupation with the loss and a withdrawal into the self. They will require reassurance of their own safety and self-worth.

Adolescents

Adolescents are usually able to view death on an adult level. They understand death to be universal and inevitable; however, they have difficulty tolerating the intense feelings associated with the death of a loved one. They may or may not cry. They may withdraw into themselves or attempt to go about usual activities in an effort to avoid dealing with the pain of the loss. Some teens exhibit acting-out behaviors, such as aggression and defiance. It is often easier for adolescents to discuss their feelings with peers than with their parents or other adults. Some adolescents may show regressive behaviors, whereas others react by trying to take care of their loved ones who are also grieving. In general, individuals of this age group have an attitude of immortality. Although they understand that their own death is inevitable, the concept is so far-reaching as to be imperceptible.

Adults

The adult's concept of death is influenced by cultural and religious backgrounds (Murray & Zentner, 2001). Behaviors associated with grieving in the adult were discussed in the section on "Theoretical Perspectives on Loss and Bereavement."

Elderly Adults

Bateman (1999) states:

> For the older adult, the later years have been described by philosophers and poets as the 'season of loss.' Loss of one's occupational role upon retirement, loss of control and competence, loss in some life experiences, loss of material possessions, and loss of dreams, loved ones, and friends must be understood and accepted if the older adult is to adapt effectively. (p. 144)

By the time individuals reach their 60s and 70s, they have experienced numerous losses, and mourning has become a life-long process. Older persons who were most successful at adapting to losses earlier in life will similarly cope more adaptively with the losses and grief inherent in aging. Unfortunately, with the aging process comes a convergence of losses, the timing of which makes it impossible for the aging individual to complete the grief process in response to one loss before another occurs. Because grief is cumulative, this can result in **bereavement overload**, the person is less able to adapt and reintegrate, and mental and physical health is jeopardized (Halstead, 2005). Bereavement overload has been implicated as a predisposing factor in the development of depressive disorder in the elderly person.

Depression is a common symptom in the grief response to significant losses. It is important to understand the difference between the depression of normal

TABLE 45–2	Normal Grief Reactions versus Symptoms of Clinical Depression	
NORMAL GRIEF	**CLINICAL DEPRESSION**
Self-esteem is intact.	Self-esteem is disturbed.
May openly express anger.	Usually does not directly express anger.
Experiences a mixture of "good and bad days."	Persistent state of dysphoria.
Able to experience moments of pleasure.	Anhedonia is prevalent.
Accepts comfort and support from others.	Does not respond to social interaction and support from others.
Maintains feeling of hope.	Feelings of hopelessness prevail.
May express guilt feelings over some aspect of the loss.	Has generalized feelings of guilt.
Relates feelings of depression to specific loss experienced.	Does not relate feelings to a particular experience.
May experience transient physical symptoms.	Expresses chronic physical complaints.

SOURCE: Adapted from Periyakoil (2001) and Sadock & Sadock (2003).

grieving and the disorder of clinical depression. Some of these differences are presented in Table 45–2.

Background Assessment Data: Concepts of Death—Cultural Issues

As previously stated, bereavement practices are greatly influenced by cultural and religious backgrounds. It is important for health care professionals to have an understanding of these individual differences in order to provide culturally sensitive care to their clients. Clinicians must be able to identify and appreciate what is culturally expected or required, because failure to carry out expected rituals may hinder the grief process and result in unresolved grief for some bereaved individuals. Table 45–3 provides a set of guidelines for assessing culturally specific death rituals. Following is a discussion of selected culturally specific death rituals.

TABLE 45–3	Guidelines for Assessing Culturally Specific Death Rituals

Death Rituals and Expectations
1. Identify culturally specific death rituals and expectations.
2. Explain death rituals and mourning practices.
3. What are specific burial practices, such as cremation?

Responses to Death and Grief
4. Identify cultural responses to death and grief.
5. Explore the meaning of death, dying, and the afterlife.

SOURCE: Purnell & Paulanka (2003). With permission.

African-Americans

Customs of bereaved African-Americans are similar to those of the dominant American culture of the same religion and social class, with a blending of cultural practices from the African heritage. The majority of African-Americans are Protestant, largely Baptist and Methodist (Glanville, 2003). Glanville (2003) states:

One response to hearing about a death of a family member or close member in the African-American culture is *falling-out*, which is manifested by sudden collapse and paralysis and the inability to see or speak. However, the individual's hearing and understanding remain intact. Health-care providers must understand the African-American culture to recognize this condition as a cultural response to the death of a family member or other severe emotional shock, and not a medical condition requiring emergency intervention. (p. 49)

Funeral services may differ from the traditional European-American service with ceremonies and rituals modified by the musical rhythms and patterns of speech and worship that are unique to African-Americans. Feelings are expressed openly and publicly at the funeral, and eulogies are extremely important. Services usually conclude with a viewing of the body and burial at a cemetery. Burial rather than cremation is usually chosen (American Association of Retired Persons [AARP], 2002).

Many African-Americans attempt to maintain a strong connection with their loved ones who have died. This connection may take the form of communication with the deceased's spirit through mediums who are believed to possess this special capability.

Asian-Americans

Chinese-Americans. Death and bereavement in the Chinese tradition are centered on ancestor worship. Chinese people have an intuitive fear of death and avoid references to it. Wang (2003) states:

The purchase of insurance may be avoided because of a fear that it is inviting death. The color white is associated with death and is considered bad luck. Black is also a bad luck color. Red is the ultimate good luck color. (p. 115)

The Chinese often do not express their emotions openly. Mourners are recognized by black armbands and white strips of cloth tied around their heads (Wang, 2003). Traditionally, for a year following a death, a place for the deceased is set at table with a bowl of rice, meat and vegetables, and chopsticks (AARP, 2002).

Japanese-Americans. The dominant religion among the Japanese is Buddhism. On death of a loved one, the body is prepared by close family members. This is followed by a 2-day period of visitation by family and friends, during which there is prayer, burning of incense, and presentation of gifts (AARP, 2002). Funeral ceremonies are held at the Buddhist temple, and cremation is common.

Vietnamese-Americans. Buddhism is the predominant religion among the Vietnamese. Attitudes toward death are influenced by the Buddhist emphasis on cyclic continuity and reincarnation (Nowak, 2003). Many Vietnamese believe that birth and death are predestined (AARP, 2002).

Most Vietnamese people prefer to die at home, and most do not approve of autopsy. Cremation is common. The final moments before the funeral procession are a time of prayer for the immediate family. Individuals in mourning wear white clothing for 14 days. During the following year, men wear black armbands and women wear white headbands (Nowak, 2003). The 1-year anniversary of an individual's death is celebrated. Nowak (2003) states:

> Priests and monks should only be called at the request of the client or family. Clergy visitation is usually associated with last rites by the Vietnamese, especially those influenced by Catholicism, and can actually be upsetting to hospitalized clients. Sending flowers may be startling, as flowers usually are reserved for the rites of the dead. (p. 338)

Filipino-Americans

Following a death in the Filipino community, a wake is held with family and friends. This wake usually takes place in the home of the deceased and lasts up to a week before the funeral. A large proportion of Filipinos are Catholic (AARP, 2002). Pacquiao (2003) states:

> Among Catholics, 9 days of novenas are held in the home or in the church. These special prayers ask God's blessing for the deceased. Depending upon the economic resources of the family, food and refreshments are served after each prayer day. Sometimes the last day of the novena takes on the atmosphere of a *fiesta* or a celebration. Filipino families in the United States follow variations of this ritual according to their social and economic circumstances. (p. 152)

Most follow the traditional custom of wearing dark clothing—black armbands for men and black dresses for women—for 1 year after the death, at which time ritualistic mourning officially ends. Emotional outbursts of uncontrolled crying are common expressions of grief. Fainting as a bereavement practice is not uncommon (Pacquiao, 2003). Burial of the body is most common, but cremation is acceptable.

Jewish-Americans

Traditional Judaism believes in an afterlife, where the soul continues to flourish. However, most Jewish people show little concern about life after death and the focus is concentrated more on how one conducts one's present life (Selekman, 2003). Taking one's own life is forbidden and ultraconservative Jews may deny the person who commits suicide full burial honors; however, the more liberal view is to emphasize the needs of the survivors.

A dying person is never left alone. At death, the face is covered with a cloth, and the body is treated with respect. Autopsy is allowed only if it is required by law, the deceased person has requested it, or it may save the life of another (Selekman, 1998).

For the funeral, the body is wrapped in a shroud and placed in a wooden, unadorned casket. No wake and no viewing take place during a Jewish funeral. Cremation is prohibited. Selekman (1998) states:

> After the funeral, mourners are welcomed to the home of the closest relative. Outside the front door is water to wash one's hands before entering, which is symbolic of cleansing the impurities associated with contact with the dead. The water is not passed from person to person, just as it is hoped that the tragedy is not passed. At the home, a meal is served to all the guests. This "meal of condolence" is traditionally provided by the neighbors and friends. (p. 243)

The 7-day period beginning with the burial is called ***shiva***. During this time, mourners do not work, and no activity is permitted that diverts attention from thinking about the deceased. Mourning lasts 30 days for a relative and 1 year for a parent, at which time a tombstone is erected and a graveside service is held (Selekman, 2003).

Mexican-Americans

Most Mexican-Americans view death as a natural part of life. The predominant religion is Catholic, and many of the death rituals are a reflection of these religious beliefs. A vigil by family members is kept over the sick or dying person. Following the death, large numbers of family and friends gather for a ***velorio***, a festive watch over the body of the deceased person before burial (Zoucha & Purnell, 2003), and a novena of prayers is offered for the soul of the deceased (AARP, 2002).

Mourning is called ***luto*** and is symbolized by wearing black, black and white, or dark clothing and by subdued behavior (AARP, 2002). Often the bereaved refrain from attending movies or social events and from listening to radio or watching television. For middle-aged or elderly Mexican-Americans, the period of bereavement may last for 2 years or more. These mourning behaviors do not indicate a sign of respect for the dead; instead, they demonstrate evidence that the individual is grieving for a loved one. Burial is more common than cremation, and often the body is buried within 24 hours of death, which is required by law in Mexico (Zoucha & Purnell, 2003).

Native-Americans

More than 500 Native-American tribes are now recognized by the U.S. government. Although many of the tribal traditions have been modified throughout the years, some of the traditional Native-American values have been preserved.

The Navajo of the Southwest, the largest Native American tribe in the United States, do not bury the body of a deceased person for 4 days after death. Beliefs require that a cleansing ceremony take place before burial to prevent the spirit of the dead person from trying to assume control of someone else's spirit (Still & Hodgins, 2003). The dead are buried with their shoes on the wrong feet and rings on their index fingers. The Navajo generally do not express their grief openly and are reluctant to touch the body of a dead person. Still and Hodgins (2003) state:

One death taboo involves talking with clients concerning a fatal disease or illness. Effective discussions require that the issue be presented in the third person, as if the illness or disorder occurred with someone else. The healthcare provider must never suggest that the client is dying. To do so would imply that the provider wishes the client dead. If the client does die, it would imply that the provider may have evil powers. (p. 290)

Nursing Diagnosis/Outcome Identification

From analysis of the assessment data, appropriate nursing diagnoses are formulated for the client and family experiencing grief and loss. From these identified diagnoses, accurate planning of nursing care is executed. Possible nursing diagnoses for grieving persons include:

● Risk for dysfunctional grieving related to loss of a valued concept/object; loss of a loved one.
● Risk for spiritual distress related to complicated grief process.

The following criteria may be used for measurement of outcomes in the care of the grieving client:

The client:

1. Acknowledges awareness of the loss.
2. Is able to express feelings about the loss.
3. Verbalizes stages of the grief process and behaviors associated with each.
4. Expresses personal satisfaction and support from spiritual practices.

Planning/Implementation

Table 45–4 provides a plan of care for the grieving person. Selected nursing diagnoses are presented, along with outcome criteria, appropriate nursing interventions, and rationales for each.

TABLE 45–4	Care Plan for the Grieving Person

NURSING DIAGNOSIS: RISK FOR DYSFUNCTIONAL GRIEVING
RELATED TO: Loss of a valued concept/object; loss of a loved one
EVIDENCED BY: Feelings of sadness, anger, guilt, self-reproach, anxiety, loneliness, fatigue, helplessness, shock, yearning, and numbness

OUTCOME CRITERIA	NURSING INTERVENTIONS	RATIONALE
Client will progress through the grief process in a healthful manner toward resolution.	1. Assess client's stage in the grief process.	1. Accurate baseline data are required to provide appropriate assistance.
	2. Develop trust. Show empathy, concern, and unconditional positive regard.	2. Developing trust provides the basis for a therapeutic relationship.
	3. Help the client actualize the loss by talking about it. "When did it happen? How did it happen?" and so forth.	3. Reviewing the events of the loss can help the client come to full awareness of the loss.
	4. Help the client identify and express feelings. Some of the more problematic feelings include: a. Anger. The anger may be directed at the deceased, at God, displaced onto others, or retroflected inward on the self. Encourage the client to examine this anger and validate the appropriateness of this feeling.	4. Until client can recognize and accept personal feelings regarding the loss, grief work cannot progress. a. Many people will not admit to angry feelings, believing it is inappropriate and unjustified. Expression of this emotion is necessary to prevent fixation in this stage of grief.

(Continued on opposite page)

	b. Guilt. The client may feel that he or she did not do enough to prevent the loss. Help the client by reviewing the circumstances of the loss and the reality that it could not be prevented.	b. Feelings of guilt prolong resolution of the grief process.
	c. Anxiety and helplessness. Help the client to recognize the way that life was managed before the loss. Help the client to put the feelings of helplessness into perspective by pointing out ways that he or she managed situations effectively without help from others. Role-play life events and assist with decision-making situations.	c. The client may have fears that he or she may not be able to carry on alone.
	5. Interpret normal behaviors associated with grieving and provide client with adequate time to grieve.	5. Understanding of the grief process will help prevent feelings of guilt generated by these responses. Individuals need adequate time to accommodate to the loss and all its ramifications. This involves getting past birthdays and anniversaries of which the deceased was a part.
	6. Provide continuing support. If this is not possible by the nurse, then offer referrals to support groups. Support groups of individuals going through the same experiences can be very helpful for the grieving individual.	6. The availability of emotional support systems facilitates the grief process.
	7. Identify pathological defenses that the client may be using (e.g., drug/alcohol use, somatic complaints, social isolation). Assist the client in understanding why these are not healthy defenses and how they delay the process of grieving.	7. The bereavement process is impaired by behaviors that mask the pain of the loss.
	8. Encourage the client to make an honest review of the relationship with that which has been lost. Journal keeping is a facilitative tool with this intervention.	8. Only when the client is able to see both positive and negative aspects related to the loss will the grieving process be complete.

NURSING DIAGNOSIS: **RISK FOR SPIRITUAL DISTRESS**

RELATED TO: **Dysfunctional grieving over loss of valued object**

EVIDENCED BY: **Anger toward God, questioning meaning of own existence, inability to participate in usual religious practices**

OUTCOME CRITERIA	NURSING INTERVENTIONS	RATIONALE
Client will express achievement of support and personal satisfaction from spiritual practices.	1. Be accepting and nonjudgmental when client expresses anger and bitterness toward God. Stay with the client.	1. The nurse's presence and nonjudgmental attitude increase the client's feelings of self-worth and promote trust in the relationship.
	2. Encourage the client to ventilate feelings related to meaning of own existence in the face of current loss.	2. Client may believe he or she cannot go on living without lost object. Catharsis can provide relief and put life back into realistic perspective.
	3. Encourage the client as part of grief work to reach out to previously used religious practices for support. Encourage client to discuss these practices and how they provided support in the past.	3. Client may find comfort in religious rituals with which he or she is familiar.
	4. Ensure client that he or she is not alone when feeling inadequate in the search for life's answers.	4. Validation of client's feelings and assurance that they are shared by others offer reassurance and an affirmation of acceptability.
	5. Contact spiritual leader of client's choice, if he or she requests.	5. These individuals serve to provide relief from spiritual distress and often can do so when other support persons cannot.

Evaluation

In the final step of the nursing process, a reassessment is conducted to determine if the nursing actions have been successful in achieving the objectives of care. Evaluation of the nursing actions for the grieving client may be facilitated by gathering information using the following types of questions:

1. Has the client discussed the recent loss with staff and family members?
2. Is the client able to verbalize feelings and behaviors associated with each stage of the grieving process and recognize his or her own position in the process?
3. Has obsession with and idealization of the loss subsided?
4. Is anger toward that which has been lost expressed appropriately?
5. Is the client able to participate in usual religious practices and feel satisfaction and support from them?
6. Is the client seeking out interaction with others in an appropriate manner?
7. Is the client able to verbalize positive aspects about his or her life, past relationships, and prospects for the future?

ADDITIONAL ASSISTANCE

Hospice

Hospice is a program that provides palliative and supportive care to meet the special needs of people who are dying and their families. Hospice care provides physical, psychological, spiritual, and social care for the person for whom aggressive treatment is no longer appropriate. Various models of hospice exist, including freestanding institutions that provide both inpatient and home care; those affiliated with hospitals in which hospice services are provided within the hospital setting; and hospice organizations that provide home care only. Historically, the hospice movement in the United States has evolved mainly as a system of home-based care.

Hospice helps clients achieve physical and emotional comfort so that they can concentrate on living life as fully as possible. Clients are urged to stay active for as long as they are able—to take part in activities they enjoy, and to focus on the quality of life.

The National Hospice and Palliative Care Organization (NHPCO) (2000) has published standards of care based on principles that are directed at the hospice program concept. These principles of care are presented in Table 45–5.

Hospice follows an interdisciplinary team approach to provide care for the terminally ill individual in the familiar surroundings of the home environment. The interdisciplinary team consists of nurses, attendants (homemakers, home health aides), physicians, social workers, volunteers, and other health care workers from other disciplines as required for individual clients.

The hospice approach is based on seven components: the interdisciplinary team, pain and symptom management, emotional support to client and family, pastoral and spiritual care, bereavement counseling, 24-hour on-call nurse/counselor, and staff support. These are the ideal, and not all hospice programs may include all of these services.

Interdisciplinary Team

Nurses. A registered nurse usually acts as case manager for care of hospice clients. The nurse assesses the client's and family's needs, establishes the goals of care, supervises and assists caregivers, evaluates care, serves as client advocate, and provides educational information as needed to client, family, and caregivers. He or she also provides physical care when needed, including IV therapy.

Attendants. These individuals are usually the members of the team who spend the most time with the client. They assist with personal care and all activities of daily living. Without these daily attendants, many individuals would be unable to spend their remaining days in their home. Attendants may be noncertified and provide basic housekeeping services; they may be certified nursing assistants who assist with personal care; or they may be licensed vocational or practical nurses who provide more specialized care, such as dressing changes or tube feedings.

Physicians. The client's primary physician and the hospice medical consultant have input into the care of the hospice client. Orders may continue to come from the primary physician, whereas pain and symptom management may come from the hospice consultant. Ideally, these physicians attend weekly client care conferences and provide in-service education for hospice staff as well as others in the medical community.

Social Workers. The social worker assists the client and family members with psychosocial issues, including those associated with the client's condition, financial issues, legal needs, and bereavement concerns. The social worker provides information on community resources from which client and family may receive support and assistance. Some of the functions of the nurse and social worker may overlap at times.

Trained Volunteers. Volunteers are vital to the hospice concept. They provide services that may otherwise be financially impossible. They are specially selected and extensively trained, and they provide services such as transportation, companionship, respite care, recreational

TABLE 45-5	**Principles of Care—National Hospice and Palliative Care Organization**

Access, Rights, and Ethics

Access: The hospice offers palliative care to terminally ill patients and their families regardless of age, gender, nationality, race, creed, sexual orientation, disability, diagnoses, availability or primary caregiver or ability to pay.
Rights: The hospice respects and honors the rights of each patient and family it serves.
Ethics: The hospice assumes responsibility for ethical decision-making and behavior related to the provision of hospice care.

Bereavement Care and Services

Addressing issues related to loss, grief and bereavement begins at the time of admission to the hospice with the initial assessment and continues throughout the course of care. Bereavement services are provided to help patients, families and caregivers cope with the multitude of losses that occur during the illness and eventual death of the patient. Bereavement services are offered based on a number of factors including the individual assessment, intensity of grief, coping ability of the survivors and their needs, as perceived by each patient, family and caregiver.

Clinical Care and Services

The desired outcomes of hospice intervention are safe and comfortable dying, self-determined life closure and effective grieving, all as determined by the patient and family/caregivers. The interdisciplinary team identifies, assists and respects the desires of the patient and family/caregivers in the facilitation of these outcomes through treatment, prevention and promotion of strategies based on continuous assessment.

Coordination and Continuity of Care

The hospice provides coordinated and uninterrupted service and assures continuity of care across settings from admission through discharge and subsequent bereavement care.

Human Resources

Hospice organizational leaders ensure that the number and qualifications of staff and volunteers are appropriate to the scope of care and services provided by the hospice program.

Interdisciplinary Team

The hospice interdisciplinary team, in collaboration with the patient, family and caregiver, develops and maintains a patient, family and caregiver-directed, individualized, safe and coordinated plan of palliative care.

Leadership and Governance

Hospice has an organizational leadership structure that permits and facilitates action and decision-making by those individuals closest to any issue or process.

Management of Information

The hospice identifies and collects information needed to operate in an efficient manner. Such information is handled in a manner that respects the patient's, family's and hospice's confidentiality.

Performance Improvement and Outcomes Measurement

The hospice defines a systematic, planned approach to improving performance. This approach is authorized and supported by the governing body and leaders.

Safety and Infection Control

The hospice provides for the safety of all staff and promotes the development and maintenance of a safe environment for patients and families served.

Adapted from: National Hospice and Palliative Care Organization. *Standards of practice for hospice programs* (2000). Alexandria, VA: Author. Item No. 711077 available from NHPCO 1–800–646–6460.

activities, light housekeeping, and in general are sensitive to the needs of families in stressful situations.

Rehabilitation Therapists. Physical therapists may assist hospice clients in an effort to minimize physical disability. They may assist with strengthening exercises and provide assistance with special equipment needs. Occupational therapists may help the debilitated client learn to accomplish activities of daily living as independently as possible. Other consultants, such as speech therapists, may be called on for the client with special needs.

Dietitian. A nutritional consultant may be helpful to the hospice client who is experiencing nausea and vomiting, diarrhea, anorexia, and weight loss. A nutritionist can ensure that the client is receiving the proper balance of calories and nutrients.

Counseling Services. The hospice client may require the services of a psychiatrist or psychologist if there is a history of mental illness, or if dementia or depression has become a problem. Other types of counseling services are available to provide assistance in dealing with the special needs of each client.

Pain and Symptom Management

Improved quality of life at all times is a primary goal of hospice care. Thus, a major intervention for all caregivers is to ensure that the client is as comfortable as possible, whether experiencing pain or other types of symptoms common in the terminal stages of an illness.

Emotional Support

Members of the hospice team encourage clients and families to discuss the eventual outcome of the disease process. Some individuals find discussing issues associated with death and dying uncomfortable, and if so, their decision is respected. However, honest discussion of these issues provides a sense of relief for some people, and they are more realistically prepared for the future. It may even draw some clients and families closer together during this stressful time.

Pastoral and Spiritual Care

Hospice philosophy supports the individual's right to seek guidance or comfort in the spiritual practices most suited to that person. The hospice team members help the client obtain the spiritual support and guidance for which he or she expresses a preference.

Bereavement Counseling

Hospice provides a service to surviving family members or significant others after the death of their loved one. This is usually provided by a bereavement counselor, but when one is not available, volunteers with special training in bereavement care may be of service. A grief support group may be helpful for the bereaved and provide a safe place for them to discuss their own fears and concerns about the death of a loved one.

Twenty-Four-Hour On-Call

The standards of care set forth by NHPCO state that care shall be available 24 hours a day, 7 days a week. A nurse or counselor is usually available by phone or for home visits around the clock. The knowledge that emotional or physical support is available at any time, should it be required, provides considerable support and comfort to significant others or family caregivers.

Staff Support

Team members (all who work closely and frequently with the client) often experience emotions similar to those of the client or their family and/or significant others. They may experience anger, frustration, or fears of death and dying—all of which must be addressed through staff support groups, team conferences, time off, and adequate and effective supervision. Burnout is a common problem among hospice staff. Stress can be reduced, trust enhanced, and team functioning more effective if lines of communication are kept open among all members (medical director through volunteer), if information is readily accessible through staff conferences and in-service education, and if staff know they are appreciated and feel good about what they are doing.

Advance Directives

The term **advance directives** refers to either a living will or a durable power of attorney for health care (also called a health care proxy). Either document allows an individual to provide directions about his or her future medical care.

A living will is a written document made by a competent individual that provides instructions that should be used when that individual is no longer able to express his or her wishes for health care treatment. The durable power of attorney for health care is a written form that gives another person legal power to make decisions regarding health care when an individual is no longer capable of making such decisions. Some states have adopted forms that combine the intent of the durable power of attorney for health care (i.e., to have a proxy) and the intent of the living will (i.e., to state choices for end-of-life medical treatment).

Doctors usually follow clearly stated directives. It is important that the physician be informed that an advanced directive exists and what the specific wishes of the client are. In most states, health care professionals are legally bound to honor the client's wishes (Norlander, 2001). In 1990, the U.S. Congress passed legislation requiring that all health care facilities that receive Medicare or Medicaid funds advise clients of their rights to refuse treatment and to make advance directives available to clients on admission (Aiken, 2004). Aiken (2004) states:

> Every state has enacted legislation that allows individuals to execute living wills or durable power of attorney for health care. These directives are binding on healthcare providers. Historically, there were problems between states that had no such legislation and states that did because some states would not accept advance directives from other states. (p. 263)

Catalano (2003) points out that unless a natural death act has been enacted into law by a state, the living will has no mechanism of legal enforcement. These laws have been called "pull the plug" statues and have various names in different states, such as "Removal of Life Support Systems Act" (Connecticut), "Natural Death Act" (Washington), and "Medical Treatment Decision Act" (Arizona) (Mantel, 2005). Catalano (2003) states:

> In some states, a living will is considered only advisory and the physician has the right to comply with the living will or treat the client as the physician deems most appropriate. There is no protection for nurses or other healthcare practitioners against criminal or civil liability in the execution of living wills in states without a natural death act. (p. 147)

Norlander (2001) suggests the following reasons why advance directives sometimes are not honored:

● The advance directive is not available at the time treatment decisions need to be made. This is especially true in emergency situations.
● The advance directive is not clear. Statements such as "no heroic measures" can be interpreted in many different ways.
● The health care proxy is unsure of the client's wishes.

Advance directives allow the client to be in control of decisions at the end of life. It is also a way to spare family and loved ones the burden of making choices without knowing what is most important to the person who is dying.

SUMMARY

Loss is the experience of separation from something of personal importance. Loss is anything that is perceived as such by the individual. Loss of any concept of value to an individual triggers the grief response.

Elisabeth Kübler-Ross identified five stages that individuals pass through on their way to resolution of a loss. These include denial, anger, bargaining, depression, and acceptance. John Bowlby described similar stages that he identified in the following manner: stage I, numbness or protest; stage II, disequilibrium; stage III, disorganization and despair; and stage IV, reorganization. George Engel's stages include shock and disbelief, developing awareness, restitution, resolution of the loss, and recovery. J. William Worden, a more contemporary clinician, has proposed that bereaved individuals must accomplish a set of tasks in order to complete the grief process. These four tasks include accepting the reality of the loss, working through the pain of grief, adjusting to an environment that has changed because of the loss, and emotionally relocating that which has been lost and moving on with life.

The length of the grief process is highly individual, and it can last for a number of years without being maladaptive. The acute stage usually lasts a couple of months, but resolution takes much longer. Kübler-Ross suggests that a calendar year of experiencing significant events and anniversaries without the lost concept may be required.

Anticipatory grieving is the experiencing of the feelings and emotions associated with the normal grief process in response to anticipation of the loss. Anticipatory grieving is thought to facilitate the grief process when the actual loss occurs.

Three types of pathological grief reactions have been described. These include the following:

● Delayed or inhibited grief in which there is absence of evidence of grief when it ordinarily would be expected.
● Distorted or exaggerated grief response in which the individual remains fixed in the anger stage of the grief process and all of the symptoms associated with normal grieving are exaggerated.
● Chronic or prolonged grieving in which the individual is unable to let go of grieving behaviors after an extended period of time and in which behaviors are evident that indicate the bereaved individual is not accepting that the loss has occurred.

Several authors have identified one crucial difference between normal and maladaptive grieving: the loss of self-esteem. Feelings of worthlessness are indicative of depression rather than uncomplicated bereavement.

Grieving behaviors characteristic of children, adolescents, adults, and elderly individuals were described. A discussion of cultural grieving behaviors associated with African-Americans, Asian-Americans, Filipino-Americans, Jewish-Americans, Mexican-Americans, and Native Americans was included. Care of individuals experiencing uncomplicated bereavement was presented in the context of the nursing process. A discussion of hospice care and the use of advance directives was presented.

REVIEW QUESTIONS

SELF-EXAMINATION/LEARNING EXERCISE

Select the answer that is *most* appropriate for each of the following questions.

1. Which of the following is most likely to initiate a grief response in an individual?
   a. Death of the pet dog
   b. Being told by her doctor that she has begun menopause
   c. Failing an exam
   d. a only
   e. All of the above

2. Nancy, who is dying of cancer, says to the nurse, "I just want to see my new grandbaby. If only God will let me live until she is born. Then I'll be ready to go." This is an example of which of Kübler-Ross's stages of grief?
   a. Denial
   b. Anger
   c. Bargaining
   d. Acceptance

3. Gloria, a recent widow, states, "I'm going to have to learn to pay all the bills. Hank always did that. I don't know if I know if I can handle all of that." This is an example of which of the tasks described by Worden?
   a. Task I. Accepting the reality of the loss
   b. Task II. Working through the pain of grief
   c. Task III. Adjusting to an environment that has changed because of the loss
   d. Task IV. Emotionally relocating that which has been lost and moving on with life

4. Engel identifies which of the following as successful resolution of the grief process?
   a. When the bereaved person can talk about the loss without crying
   b. When the bereaved person no longer talks about that which has been lost
   c. When the bereaved person puts all remembrances of the loss out of sight
   d. When the bereaved person can discuss both positive and negative aspects about what has been lost

5. Which of the following is thought to facilitate the grief process?
   a. The ability to grieve in anticipation of the loss
   b. The ability to grieve alone without interference from others
   c. Having recently grieved for another loss
   d. Taking personal responsibility for the loss

6. When Frank's wife of 34 years dies, he is very stoic, handles all the funeral arrangements, doesn't cry or appear sad, and comforts all of the other family members in their grief. Two years later, when Frank's best friend dies, Frank has sleep disturbances, difficulty concentrating, loss of weight, and difficulty performing on his job. This is an example of which of the following maladaptive responses to loss?
   a. Delayed grieving
   b. Distorted grieving
   c. Prolonged grieving
   d. Exaggerated grieving

7. A major difference between normal and maladaptive grieving has been identified by which of the following?
   a. There are no feelings of depression in normal grieving.
   b. There is no loss of self-esteem in normal grieving.
   c. Normal grieving lasts no longer than 1 year.
   d. In normal grief the person does not show anger toward the loss.

8. Which grief reaction can the nurse anticipate in a 10-year-old child?
   a. Statements that the deceased person will soon return
   b. Regressive behaviors, such as loss of bladder control
   c. A preoccupation with that which has been lost
   d. Thinking that they may have done something to cause the death

9. Which of the following is a correct statement when attempting to distinguish normal grief from clinical depression?
   a. In clinical depression, anhedonia is prevalent.
   b. In normal grieving, the person has generalized feelings of guilt.
   c. The person who is clinically depressed relates feelings of depression to a specific loss.
   d. In normal grieving, there is a persistent state of dysphoria.

10. Which of the following is **not** true regarding grieving by an adolescent?
    a. Adolescents may not show their true feelings about the death.
    b. Adolescents tend to have an immortal attitude.
    c. Adolescents do not perceive death as inevitable.
    d. Adolescents may exhibit acting out behaviors as part of their grief.

IMPLICATIONS OF RESEARCH FOR EVIDENCE-BASED PRACTICE

Douglas, R., & Brown, H.N. (2002). Patients' Attitudes Toward Advance Directives. *Journal of Nursing Scholarship, 34*(1), 61–65.

Description of the Study: This study was conducted to investigate hospitalized patients' attitudes toward advanced directives. It explored patients' reasons for completing or not completing advance directive forms, and examined demographic differences between patients who did and did not complete advance directive forms. Subjects consisted of a convenience sample of 30 hospitalized patients. Criteria required that the patients (1) speak English, (2) be at least 18 years of age, (3) be oriented to time and place, and (4) have been approached by an RN regarding advance directives, as documented in the patient chart. Data were collected over a 3-week period in the oncology and medical telemetry units of a teaching hospital in central North Carolina. Interviews were conducted using an adapted advance directive attitude survey (ADAS) in which subjects were asked five general questions regarding perceptions of personal health, whether they had ever received information on advance directives, whether they had ever completed an advance directive, and whether they had ever had a discussion with either their primary physician or family members about end-of-life care. Demographic data were also obtained. The tool was based on a 4-point Likert scale from 1 (strongly disagree) to 4 (strongly agree). Higher scores indicate more favorable attitudes toward advance directives.

Results of the Study: Subjects ranged in age from 24 to 85 years, with a mean age of 57 years. Nineteen were Caucasian, 10 were African-American, and 1 was Hispanic. Ten had completed grade school or junior high, 13 completed high school, 4 completed college, and 3 had master's degrees or beyond. Twelve subjects had been diagnosed with cancer, 5 with respiratory disorders, 4 with sickle cell disease, 3 with cardiac disorders, 2 with vascular disorders, and 1 each with gastrointestinal, musculoskeletal, neurological, and dermatological disorders. Twenty-three subjects had received information on advance directives and 7 said they had received no information. Thirteen of the subjects had completed advance directives and 17 had not.

Participants with the highest mean scores were African-American, female, aged 35 to 49 years, with a high school education. No subject in the 20- to 30-year-old age group had completed an advanced directive, whereas 62 percent of subjects older than age 65 had done so. The two people with the lowest scores both disagreed with the statement that an advance directive would make sure that their family knew what treatment they desired and they would receive the treatment they desired. The 13 participants who had completed advance directives cited the following reasons for doing so: (1) desire not to be placed on life support, (2) desire to name someone to make decisions in event of incapacitation, (3) desire to make decisions easier for spouse or family, (4) failing health, and (5) advancing age. The 17 who had not completed advance directives cited the following reasons: (1) keep putting it off, (2) not necessary at this point in my life, (3) uncomfortable making decisions about life support, (4) never heard of advance directives before, (5) form was too long, (6) trust husband to make those decisions, and (7) advance directives are unnecessary.

Implications for Nursing Practice: The authors suggest that nurses need to explain what advance directives are when asking patients if they have an advance directive. They state: "[Nurses] can explore alternative ways to educate patients about advance directives (e.g., videotape), and follow up with patients who have requested information to see if they have additional questions or need assistance completing an advance directive." They also suggest that nurses need to inform physicians when patients have advance directives. As patient advocates, nurses have the responsibility for making sure that patients understand the purpose of advance directives and what is involved in completing an advance directive, and for ensuring that patients' end-of-life care is executed according to their wishes.

R E F E R E N C E S

Aiken, T.D. (2004). *Legal, ethical, and political issues in nursing* (2nd ed.). Philadelphia: F.A. Davis.

American Association of Retired Persons (AARP). (2002). *Grief and loss: Helping others heal.* Retrieved September 3, 2002 from the World Wide Web at http://www.aarp.org/griefandloss/articles/46_b.html

Bateman, A.L. (1999). Understanding the process of grieving and loss: A critical social thinking perspective. *Journal of the American Psychiatric Nurses Association, 5*(5), 139–147.

Catalano, J.T. (2003). *Nursing now! Today's issues, tomorrow's trends* (3rd ed.). Philadelphia: F.A. Davis.

Eisendrath, S.J., & Lichtmacher, J.E. (2005). Psychiatric disorders. In L.M. Tierney, S.J. McPhee, & M.A. Papadakis (Eds.). *Current medical diagnosis and treatment* (44th ed.). New York: McGraw-Hill.

Glanville, C.L. (2003). People of African-American heritage. In L.D. Purnell & B.J. Paulanka (Eds.). *Transcultural health care* (2nd ed.). Philadelphia: F.A. Davis.

Halstead, H.L. (2005). Spirituality in older adults. In M. Stanley, K.A. Blair, & P.G. Beare (Eds.). *Gerontological nursing: A health promotion/protection approach* (3rd ed.). Philadelphia: F. A. Davis.

Kaplan, H.I., Sadock, B.J., & Grebb, J.A. (1994). *Synopsis of psychiatry: Behavioral sciences, clinical psychiatry* (7th ed.). Baltimore: Williams & Wilkins.

Mantel, D.L. (2005). Laws on death and dying. *Advance for Providers of Post-Acute Care.* Retrieved June 7, 2005 from http://post-acute-care.advanceweb.com/

Murray, R.B., & Zentner, J.P. (2001). *Health promotion strategies through the life span* (7th ed.). Upper Saddle River, NJ: Prentice-Hall.

National Hospice and Palliative Care Organization (NHPCO). (2000). *Standards of Practice for hospice programs.* Alexandria, VA: NHPCO.

Norlander, L. (2001). *To comfort always: A nurse's guide to end of life care.* Washington, DC: American Nurses Publishing.

Nowak, T.T. (2003). Vietnamese-Americans. In L.D. Purnell & B.J. Paulanka (Eds.). *Transcultural health care: A culturally competent approach* (2nd ed.). Philadelphia: F.A. Davis.

Pacquiao, D.F. (2003). People of Filipino Heritage. In L.D. Purnell & B.J. Paulanka (Eds.). *Transcultural health care: A culturally competent approach.* Philadelphia: F.A. Davis.

Periyakoil, V.J. (2001). *Is it grief or depression?* End-of-Life Physician Education Resource Center. Retrieved October 27, 2002 from the World Wide Web at http://www.eperc.mcw.edu/educate/flash/fastfact/226.htm

Purnell, L.D., & Paulanka, B.J. (2003). *Transcultural health care: A culturally competent approach* (2nd ed.). Philadelphia: F.A. Davis.

Sadock, B.J., & Sadock, V.A. (2003). *Synopsis of psychiatry: Behavioral sciences/clinical psychiatry* (9th ed.). Philadelphia: Lippincott Williams & Wilkins

Selekman, J. (2003). People of Jewish heritage. In L.D. Purnell & B.J. Paulanka (Eds.). *Transcultural health care: A culturally competent approach.* Philadelphia: F.A. Davis.

Still, O., & Hodgins, D. (2003). Navajo Indians. In L.D. Purnell & B.J. Paulanka (Eds.). *Transcultural health care: A culturally competent approach* (2nd ed.). Philadelphia: F.A. Davis.

Wang, Y. (2003). People of Chinese heritage. In L.D. Purnell & B.J. Paulanka (Eds.). *Transcultural health care* (2nd ed.). Philadelphia: F.A. Davis.

Worden, J.W. (2002). *Grief counseling and grief therapy: A handbook for the mental health practitioner* (3rd ed.). New York: Springer.

Zoucha, R., & Purnell, L.D. (2003). People of Mexican heritage. In L.D. Purnell & B.J. Paulanka (Eds.). *Transcultural health care: A culturally competent approach.* Philadelphia: F.A. Davis.

C L A S S I C A L   R E F E R E N C E S

Bowlby, J. (1961). Processes of mourning. *International Journal of Psychoanalysis, 42,* 22.

Engel, G. (1964). Grief and grieving. *American Journal of Nursing, 64,* 93.

Kübler-Ross, E. (1969). *On death and dying.* New York: Macmillan.

INTERNET REFERENCES

Additional references related to bereavement may be located at the following Web sites:

- http://www.journeyofhearts.org
- http://www.nhpco.org
- http://www.aarp.org/griefandloss/
- http://www.hospicefoundation.org
- http://www.bereavement.org
- http://www.partnershipforcaring.org/
- http://www.aahpm.org
- http://www.hpna.org

Answers to Chapter Review Questions

CHAPTER 1. THE CONCEPT OF STRESS ADAPTATION

1. b   **2.** d   **3.** a   **4.** b

5.   1. c   2. d   3. b   4. a

6.   1. d   2. a   3. e   4. b   5. c

CHAPTER 2. MENTAL HEALTH/ MENTAL ILLNESS: HISTORICAL AND THEORETICAL CONCEPTS

1. c   **2.** d   **3.** b   **4.** a   **5.** b   **6.** d

7. c   **8.** d   **9.** c   **10.** b

11. compensation = b   rationalization = i
denial = h   reaction formation = f
displacement = a   regression = d
identification = m   repression = o
intellectualization = n   sublimation = g
introjection = c   suppression = j
isolation = k   undoing = l
projection = e

CHAPTER 3. THEORETICAL MODELS OF PERSONALITY DEVELOPMENT

1. b   **2.** c   **3.** d   **4.** b   **5.** b   **6.** b

7. a   **8.** c   **9.** a   **10.** b

CHAPTER 4. CONCEPTS OF PSYCHOBIOLOGY

1. c   **2.** e   **3.** f   **4.** b   **5.** d   **6.** g

7. a   **8.** c   **9.** b   **10.** a   **11.** a   **12.** b

13. d

CHAPTER 5. ETHICAL AND LEGAL ISSUES IN PSYCHIATRIC/MENTAL HEALTH NURSING

1. c   **2.** a   **3.** e   **4.** d   **5.** b   **6.** d

7. b   **8.** e   **9.** a   **10.** c

CHAPTER 6. CULTURAL CONCEPTS RELEVANT TO PSYCHIATRIC/ MENTAL HEALTH NURSING

1. c   **2.** d   **3.** a   **4.** d   **5.** b   **6.** c

7. c   **8.** b   **9.** b   **10.** a

CHAPTER 7. RELATIONSHIP DEVELOPMENT

1. a. The stranger   b. The resource person
     c. The teacher   d. The leader
     e. The surrogate   f. The counselor

2. The counselor

3. It is through establishment of a satisfactory nurse–client relationship that individuals learn to generalize the ability to achieve satisfactory interpersonal relationships to other aspects of their lives.

4. Most often the goal is directed at learning and growth promotion, in an effort to bring about some type of change in the client's life. This is accomplished through use of the problem-solving model.

5. The therapeutic use of self.

6. 1. d   2. a   3. e   4. b   5. c

7. 1. c   2. a   3. d   4. b

CHAPTER 8. THERAPEUTIC COMMUNICATION

1. In the transactional model of communication, both persons are participating simultaneously. They are mutually perceiving each other, simultaneously listening to each other, and mutually and simultaneously engaged in the process of creating meaning in a relationship.

2. a. One's value system
b. Internalized attitudes and beliefs
c. Culture and/or religion
d. Social status
e. Gender
f. Background knowledge and experience
g. Age or developmental level
h. Type of environment in which the communication takes place.

3. Territoriality is the innate tendency to own space. People "mark" space as their own and feel more comfortable in these spaces. Territoriality affects communication in that an interaction can be more successful if it takes place on "neutral" ground rather than in a space "owned" by one or the other of the communicants.

4. Density refers to the number of people within a given environmental space. It may affect communication in that some studies indicate that a correlation exists between prolonged high-density situations and certain behaviors, such as aggression, stress, criminal activity, hostility toward others, and a deterioration of mental and physical health.

5. a. Intimate distance (0–18 inches)—kissing or hugging someone
   b. Personal distance (18–40 inches)—close conversations with friends or colleagues
   c. Social distance (4–12 feet)—conversations with strangers or acquaintances (e.g., at a cocktail party)
   d. Public distance (>12 feet)—speaking in public

6. a. Physical appearance and dress (e.g., young men who have hair down past their shoulders may convey a message of rebellion against the establishment).
   b. Body movement and posture (e.g., a person with hands on hips standing straight and tall in front of someone seated who must look up to them is conveying a message of power over the seated individual).
   c. Touch (e.g., laying one's hand on the shoulder of another may convey a message of friendship and caring).
   d. Facial expressions (e.g., wrinkling up of the nose, raising the upper lip, or raising one side of the upper lip conveys a message of disgust for a situation).
   e. Eye behavior (e.g., direct eye contact, accompanied by a smile and nodding of the head, conveys interest in what the other person is saying).
   f. Vocal cues or paralanguage (e.g., a normally soft-spoken individual whose pitch and rate of speaking increases may be perceived as being anxious or tense).

7. S—Sit squarely facing the client.
   O—Observe an open posture.
   L—Lean forward toward the client.
   E—Establish eye contact.
   R—Relax.

8. a. Nontherapeutic technique: Disagreeing
   b. The correct answer. Therapeutic technique: Voicing doubt

9. a. The correct answer. Therapeutic technique: Giving recognition
   b. Nontherapeutic technique: Complimenting—a judgment on the part of the nurse

10. a. Nontherapeutic: Giving reassurance
    b. Nontherapeutic: Giving disapproval
    c. Nontherapeutic: Introducing an unrelated topic
    d. Nontherapeutic: Indicating an external source of power
    e. The correct answer: Therapeutic technique: Exploring

11. a. Nontherapeutic: Requesting an explanation
    b. Nontherapeutic: Belittling feelings expressed
    c. Nontherapeutic: Rejecting
    d. The correct answer: Therapeutic technique: Formulating a plan of action

12. Therapeutic response: "Do *you* think you should tell him?" Technique: Reflecting
    Nontherapeutic response: "Yes, you must tell your husband about your affair with your boss." Technique: Giving advice

13. a. The correct answer. Therapeutic technique: Reflecting
    b. Nontherapeutic: Requesting an explanation
    c. Nontherapeutic: Indicating an external source of power
    d. Nontherapeutic: Giving advice
    e. Nontherapeutic: Defending
    f. Nontherapeutic: Making stereotyped comments

CHAPTER 9. THE NURSING PROCESS IN PSYCHIATRIC/MENTAL HEALTH NURSING

1. Assessment, diagnosis, outcome identification, planning, implementation, evaluation.

2. a. Implementation
   b. Diagnosis
   c. Evaluation
   d. Assessment
   e. Planning
   f. Outcome identification

3. Nursing diagnoses:
   a. Imbalanced nutrition, less than body requirements
   b. Social isolation
   c. Low self-esteem
   Outcomes:
   a. Client will gain 2 lb/wk in next 3 weeks.
   b. Client will voluntarily spend time with peers and staff in group activities on the unit within 7 days.
   c. Client will verbalize positive aspects about herself (excluding any references to eating or body image) within 2 weeks.

4. Problem-oriented recording (SOAPIE); Focus Charting®; PIE charting.

CHAPTER 10. THERAPEUTIC GROUPS

1. A group is a collection of individuals whose association is founded upon shared commonalities of interest, values, norms, and/or purpose.

2. a. Teaching group
      Laissez-faire leader
   b. Supportive/therapeutic group
      Democratic leader
   c. Task group
      Autocratic leader

3. b	4. i	5. k	6. h	7. e	8. j
9. a	10. d	11. f	12. g	13. c	14. e
15. h	16. f	17. d	18. a	19. c	20. g
21. b					

CHAPTER 11. INTERVENTION WITH FAMILIES

1. e   **2.** a   **3.** f   **4.** c   **5.** b   **6.** d
7. b   **8.** c   **9.** a   **10.** b

CHAPTER 12. MILIEU THERAPY— THE THERAPEUTIC COMMUNITY

1. A scientific structuring of the environment in order to effect behavioral changes and to improve the psychological health and functioning of the individual.
2. The goal of milieu therapy/therapeutic community is for the client to learn adaptive coping, interaction, and relationship skills that can be generalized to other aspects of his or her life.

3. c   **4.** b   **5.** a   **6.** d   **7.** f   **8.** h
9. b   **10.** i   **11.** g   **12.** j   **13.** a   **14.** e
15. c   **16.** k   **17.** m   **18.** l   **19.** d

CHAPTER 13. CRISIS INTERVENTION

1. c   **2.** d   **3.** a   **4.** b   **5.** c   **6.** a
7. d   **8.** b   **9.** b   **10.** d   **11.** c

CHAPTER 14. RELAXATION THERAPY

3a. (1) Anxiety (moderate to severe) related to lack of self-confidence and fear of making errors
(2) Pain (migraine headaches) related to repressed severe anxiety
(3) Disturbed sleep pattern related to anxiety
3b. Some outcome criteria for Linda might be:
(1) Client will be able to perform duties on the job while maintaining anxiety at a manageable level by practicing deep breathing exercises.
(2) Client will verbalize a reduction in headache pain following progressive relaxation techniques.
(3) Client is able to fall asleep within 30 minutes of retiring by listening to soft music and performing mental imagery exercises.
3c. The deep breathing exercises would be especially good for Linda because she could perform them as many times as she needed to during the working day to relieve her anxiety. With practice, progressive relaxation techniques and mental imagery could also provide relief from anxiety attacks for Linda. Any of these relaxation techniques may be beneficial at bedtime to help induce relaxation and sleep. Biofeedback may provide assistance for relief from migraine headaches. Physical exercise, either in the early morning or late afternoon after work, may provide Linda with renewed energy and combat chronic fatigue. It also relieves pent-up tension.

CHAPTER 15. ASSERTIVENESS TRAINING

1. a. AS   b. PA   c. NA   d. AG
2. a. AG   b. NA   c. PA   d. AS
3. a. NA   b. AS   c. PA   d. AG
4. a. PA   b. AG   c. AS   d. NA
5. a. AS   b. NA   c. PA   d. AG
6. a. NA   b. AS   c. AG   d. PA
7. a. AS   b. PA   c. AG   d. NA
8. a. PA   b. NA   c. AG   d. AS
9. a. AG   b. NA   c. AS   d. PA
10. a. AS   b. NA   c. AG   d. PA

CHAPTER 16. PROMOTING SELF-ESTEEM

1. b   **2.** a   **3.** d   **4.** c   **5.** a   **6.** b
7. c   **8.** e   **9.** d   **10.** a

CHAPTER 17. ANGER/ AGGRESSION MANAGEMENT

1. Past history of violence; diagnosis of alcohol abuse/intoxication; current behaviors: abusive and threatening.
2. b   **3.** c   **4.** c   **5.** a
6. Observe at least every 15 minutes; check circulation (temperature, color, pulses); assist with needs related to nutrition, hydration, and elimination; position for comfort and to prevent aspiration.
7. c   **8.** a, b, c   **9.** c   **10.** b

CHAPTER 18. THE SUICIDAL CLIENT

1. b   **2.** a   **3.** c   **4.** a   **5.** d   **6.** c
7. c   **8.** b   **9.** d   **10.** b

CHAPTER 19. BEHAVIOR THERAPY

1. a   **2.** a   **3.** b   **4.** c   **5.** a   **6.** b
7. d   **8.** f, b, d, a, e, c

CHAPTER 20. COGNITIVE THERAPY

1. b   **2.** d   **3.** a   **4.** c   **5.** c   **6.** a
7. d   **8.** a   **9.** b   **10.** c

CHAPTER 21. PSYCHOPHARMACOLOGY

1. a   **2.** c   **3.** d   **4.** b   **5.** c   **6.** b
7. a   **8.** b   **9.** d   **10.** b

CHAPTER 22. ELECTROCONVULSIVE THERAPY

1. c **2.** b **3.** a **4.** c **5.** d **6.** a
7. c **8.** d **9.** b **10.** c

CHAPTER 23. COMPLEMENTARY THERAPIES

1. c **2.** e **3.** f **4.** b **5.** g **6.** a
7. d **8.** c **9.** d **10.** a

CHAPTER 24. CLIENT EDUCATION

1. a **2.** c **3.** d **4.** c **5.** a **6.** b
7. c **8.** d **9.** a **10.** b

CHAPTER 25. DISORDERS USUALLY FIRST DIAGNOSED IN INFANCY, CHILDHOOD, OR ADOLESCENCE

1. b **2.** c **3.** a **4.** b **5.** b **6.** d
7. c **8.** d **9.** a **10.** b

CHAPTER 26. DELIRIUM, DEMENTIA, AND AMNESTIC DISORDERS

1. c **2.** d **3.** b **4.** a **5.** b **6.** c
7. d **8.** a **9.** b **10.** d

CHAPTER 27. SUBSTANCE-RELATED DISORDERS

1. a **2.** c **3.** b **4.** b **5.** a **6.** c
7. a **8.** b **9.** d **10.** a

CHAPTER 28. SCHIZOPHRENIA AND OTHER PSYCHOTIC DISORDERS

1. b **2.** b **3.** c **4.** d **5.** d **6.** a
7. c **8.** b **9.** c **10.** d

CHAPTER 29. MOOD DISORDERS

1. c **2.** b **3.** a **4.** d **5.** c **6.** b
7. c **8.** a **9.** c **10.** b

CHAPTER 30. ANXIETY DISORDERS

1. d **2.** c **3.** d **4.** a **5.** b **6.** c
7. b **8.** c **9.** a **10.** d

CHAPTER 31. SOMATOFORM AND SLEEP DISORDERS

1. b **2.** d **3.** a **4.** d **5.** c **6.** a
7. b **8.** d **9.** b **10.** c

CHAPTER 32. DISSOCIATIVE DISORDERS

1. d **2.** b **3.** a **4.** b **5.** d **6.** c
7. a **8.** c **9.** a **10.** b

CHAPTER 33. SEXUAL AND GENDER IDENTITY DISORDERS

1. b **2.** c **3.** d **4.** a **5.** b **6.** b
7. d **8.** a **9.** e **10.** c

CHAPTER 34. EATING DISORDERS

1. c **2.** a **3.** b **4.** b **5.** c **6.** b
7. c **8.** b **9.** c **10.** a

CHAPTER 35. ADJUSTMENT AND IMPULSE CONTROL DISORDERS

1. b **2.** b **3.** a **4.** c **5.** d **6.** b
7. c **8.** e **9.** a **10.** d

CHAPTER 36. PSYCHOLOGICAL FACTORS AFFECTING MEDICAL CONDITIONS

1. c **2.** g **3.** a **4.** e **5.** h **6.** f
7. d **8.** b **9.** b **10.** d

CHAPTER 37. PERSONALITY DISORDERS

1. d **2.** a **3.** b **4.** d **5.** a **6.** b
7. c **8.** c **9.** d **10.** b

CHAPTER 38. THE AGING INDIVIDUAL

1. c **2.** d **3.** b **4.** a **5.** c **6.** d
7. a **8.** a **9.** c **10.** a

CHAPTER 39. THE INDIVIDUAL WITH HIV DISEASE

1. d **2.** c **3.** a **4.** c **5.** b **6.** d
7. a **8.** a **9.** b **10.** b

CHAPTER 40. PROBLEMS RELATED TO ABUSE OR NEGLECT

1. b   **2.** c   **3.** a   **4.** d   **5.** b   **6.** d
7. a   **8.** b   **9.** b   **10.** d

CHAPTER 41. MEN'S AND WOMEN'S HEALTH ISSUES

1. d   **2.** a   **3.** b   **4.** d   **5.** b   **6.** c
7. a   **8.** c   **9.** d   **10.** a   **11.** d

CHAPTER 42. COMMUNITY MENTAL HEALTH NURSING

1. a   **2.** b   **3.** a   **4.** c   **5.** d   **6.** b
7. c   **8.** d   **9.** a   **10.** b

CHAPTER 43. PSYCHIATRIC HOME NURSING CARE

1. b   **2.** d   **3.** a   **4.** b   **5.** c   **6.** d
7. a   **8.** c   **9.** b   **10.** a

CHAPTER 44. FORENSIC NURSING

1. a   **2.** a   **3.** b   **4.** b   **5.** b   **6.** a
7. b   **8.** a   **9.** a   **10.** b

CHAPTER 45. THE BEREAVED INDIVIDUAL

1. e   **2.** c   **3.** c   **4.** d   **5.** a   **6.** a
7. b   **8.** c   **9.** a   **10.** c

Mental Status Assessment

Gathering the correct information about the client's mental status is essential to the development of an appropriate plan of care. The mental status examination is a description of all the areas of the client's mental functioning. The following are the components that are considered critical in the assessment of a client's mental status.

IDENTIFYING DATA

1. Name
2. Sex
3. Age
4. Race/culture
5. Occupational/financial status
6. Educational level
7. Significant other
8. Living arrangements
9. Religious preference
10. Allergies
11. Special diet considerations
12. Chief complaint
13. Medical diagnosis

GENERAL DESCRIPTION

Appearance

1. Grooming and dress
2. Hygiene
3. Posture
4. Height and weight
5. Level of eye contact
6. Hair color and texture
7. Evidence of scars, tattoos, or other distinguishing skin marks
8. Evaluation of client's appearance compared with chronological age

Motor Activity

1. Tremors
2. Tics or other stereotypical movements
3. Mannerisms and gestures
4. Hyperactivity
5. Restlessness or agitation
6. Aggressiveness
7. Rigidity
8. Gait patterns
9. Echopraxia
10. Psychomotor retardation
11. Freedom of movement (range of motion)

Speech Patterns

1. Slowness or rapidity of speech
2. Pressure of speech
3. Intonation
4. Volume
5. Stuttering or other speech impairments
6. Aphasia

General Attitude

1. Cooperative/uncooperative
2. Friendly/hostile/defensive
3. Uninterested/apathetic
4. Attentive/interested
5. Guarded/suspicious

EMOTIONS

Mood

1. Sad
2. Depressed
3. Despairing
4. Irritable
5. Anxious
6. Elated
7. Euphoric
8. Fearful
9. Guilty
10. Labile

Affect

1. Congruence with mood
2. Constricted or blunted (diminished amount/range and intensity of emotional expression)
3. Flat (absence of emotional expression)

4. Appropriate or inappropriate (defines congruence of affect with the situation or with the client's behavior)

THOUGHT PROCESSES

Form of Thought

1. Flight of ideas
2. Associative looseness
3. Circumstantiality
4. Tangentiality
5. Neologisms
6. Concrete thinking
7. Clang associations
8. Word salad
9. Perseveration
10. Echolalia
11. Mutism
12. Poverty of speech (restriction in the amount of speech)
13. Ability to concentrate
14. Attention span

Content of Thought

1. Delusions
   a. Persecutory
   b. Grandiose
   c. Reference
   d. Control or influence
   e. Somatic
   f. Nihilistic
2. Suicidal or homicidal ideas
3. Obsessions
4. Paranoia/suspiciousness
5. Magical thinking
6. Religiosity
7. Phobias
8. Poverty of content (vague, meaningless responses)

PERCEPTUAL DISTURBANCES

1. Hallucinations
   a. Auditory
   b. Visual
   c. Tactile
   d. Olfactory
   e. Gustatory
2. Illusions
3. Depersonalization (altered perception of the self)
4. Derealization (altered perception of the environment)

SENSORIUM AND COGNITIVE ABILITY

1. Level of alertness/consciousness
2. Orientation
   a. Time
   b. Place
   c. Person
   d. Circumstances
3. Memory
   a. Recent
   b. Remote
   c. Confabulation
4. Capacity for abstract thought

IMPULSE CONTROL

1. Ability to control impulses related to the following:
   a. Aggression
   b. Hostility
   c. Fear
   d. Guilt
   e. Affection
   f. Sexual feelings

JUDGMENT AND INSIGHT

1. Ability to solve problems
2. Ability to make decisions
3. Knowledge about self
   a. Awareness of limitations
   b. Awareness of consequences of actions
   c. Awareness of illness
4. Adaptive/maladaptive use of coping strategies and ego defense mechanisms

DSM-IV-TR Classification: Axes I and II Categories and Codes*

DISORDERS USUALLY FIRST DIAGNOSED IN INFANCY, CHILDHOOD, OR ADOLESCENCE

Mental Retardation

NOTE: *These are coded on Axis II.*

317	Mild Mental Retardation
318.0	Moderate Retardation
318.1	Severe Retardation
318.2	Profound Mental Retardation
319	Mental Retardation, Severity Unspecified

Learning Disorders

315.00	Reading Disorder
315.1	Mathematics Disorder
315.2	Disorder of Written Expression
315.9	Learning Disorder Not Otherwise Specified (NOS)

Motor Skills Disorder

315.4	Developmental Coordination Disorder

Communication Disorders

315.31	Expressive Language Disorder
315.32	Mixed Receptive-Expressive Language Disorder
315.39	Phonological Disorder
307.0	Stuttering
307.9	Communication Disorder NOS

Pervasive Developmental Disorders

299.00	Autistic Disorder
299.80	Rett's Disorder
299.10	Childhood Disintegrative Disorder
299.80	Asperger's Disorder
299.80	Pervasive Developmental Disorder NOS

Attention-Deficit and Disruptive Behavior Disorders

314.xx	Attention-Deficit/Hyperactivity Disorder
314.01	Combined Type
314.00	Predominantly Inattentive Type
314.01	Predominantly Hyperactive-Impulsive Type
314.9	Attention-Deficit/Hyperactivity Disorder NOS
312.xx	Conduct Disorder
.81	Childhood-Onset Type
.82	Adolescent-Onset Type
.89	Unspecified Onset
313.81	Oppositional Defiant Disorder
312.9	Disruptive Behavior Disorder NOS

Feeding and Eating Disorders of Infancy or Early Childhood

307.52	Pica
307.53	Rumination Disorder
307.59	Feeding Disorder of Infancy or Early Childhood

Tic Disorders

307.23	Tourette's Disorder
307.22	Chronic Motor or Vocal Tic Disorder
307.21	Transient Tic Disorder
307.20	Tic Disorder NOS

Elimination Disorders

—	Encopresis
787.6	With Constipation and Overflow Incontinence
307.7	Without Constipation and Overflow Incontinence
307.6	Enuresis (Not Due to a General Medical Condition)

Other Disorders of Infancy, Childhood, or Adolescence

309.21	Separation Anxiety Disorder
313.23	Selective Mutism
313.89	Reactive Attachment Disorder of Infancy or Early Childhood
307.3	Stereotypic Movement Disorder
313.9	Disorder of Infancy, Childhood, or Adolescence NOS

DELIRIUM, DEMENTIA, AND AMNESTIC AND OTHER COGNITIVE DISORDERS

Delirium

293.0	Delirium Due to... (*Indicate the General Medical Condition*)
—	Substance Intoxication Delirium (*refer to Substance-Related Disorders for substance-specific codes*)
—	Substance Withdrawal Delirium (*refer to Substance-Related Disorders for substance-specific codes*)
—	Delirium Due to Multiple Etiologies (*code each of the specific etiologies*)
780.09	Delirium NOS

Dementia

294.xx	Dementia of the Alzheimer's Type, With Early Onset
.10	Without Behavioral Disturbance
.11	With Behavioral Disturbance
294.xx	Dementia of the Alzheimer's Type, With Late Onset
.10	Without Behavioral Disturbance
.11	With Behavioral Disturbance
290.xx	Vascular Dementia
.40	Uncomplicated
.41	With Delirium
.42	With Delusions
.43	With Depressed Mood
294.1x	Dementia Due to HIV Disease
294.1x	Dementia Due to Head Trauma
294.1x	Dementia Due to Parkinson's Disease
294.1x	Dementia Due to Huntington's Disease
294.1x	Dementia Due to Pick's Disease
294.1x	Dementia Due to Creutzfeldt-Jakob Disease
294.1x	Dementia Due to (*Indicate the General Medical Condition not listed above*)
—	Substance-Induced Persisting Dementia (*refer to Substance-Related Disorders for substance-specific codes*)

—	Dementia Due to Multiple Etiologies (*code each of the specific etiologies*)
294.8	Dementia NOS

Amnestic Disorders

294.0	Amnestic Disorder Due to (*Indicate the General Medical Condition*)
—	Substance-Induced Persisting Amnestic Disorder (*refer to Substance-Related Disorders for substance-specific codes*)
294.8	Amnestic Disorder NOS

Other Cognitive Disorders

294.9	Cognitive Disorder NOS

MENTAL DISORDERS DUE TO A GENERAL MEDICAL CONDITION NOT ELSEWHERE CLASSIFIED

293.89	Catatonic Disorder Due to (*Indicate the General Medical Condition*)
310.1	Personality Change Due to (*Indicate the General Medical Condition*)
293.9	Mental Disorder NOS Due to (*Indicate the General Medical Condition*)

SUBSTANCE-RELATED DISORDERS

Alcohol-Related Disorders

Alcohol Use Disorders

303.90	Alcohol Dependence
305.00	Alcohol Abuse

Alcohol-Induced Disorders

303.00	Alcohol Intoxication
291.81	Alcohol Withdrawal
291.0	Alcohol Intoxication Delirium
291.0	Alcohol Withdrawal Delirium
291.2	Alcohol-Induced Persisting Dementia
291.1	Alcohol-Induced Persisting Amnestic Disorder
291.x	Alcohol-Induced Psychotic Disorder
.5	With Delusions
.3	With Hallucinations
291.89	Alcohol-Induced Mood Disorder
291.89	Alcohol-Induced Anxiety Disorder
291.89	Alcohol-Induced Sexual Dysfunction
291.89	Alcohol-Induced Sleep Disorder
291.9	Alcohol Related Disorder NOS

Amphetamine (or Amphetamine-Like)-Related Disorders

Amphetamine Use Disorders

304.40	Amphetamine Dependence
305.70	Amphetamine Abuse

Amphetamine-Induced Disorders

292.89	Amphetamine Intoxication
292.0	Amphetamine Withdrawal
292.81	Amphetamine Intoxication Delirium
292.xx	Amphetamine-Induced Psychotic Disorder
.11	With Delusions
.12	With Hallucinations
292.84	Amphetamine-Induced Mood Disorder
292.89	Amphetamine-Induced Anxiety Disorder
292.89	Amphetamine-Induced Sexual Dysfunction
292.89	Amphetamine-Induced Sleep Disorder
292.9	Amphetamine-Related Disorder NOS

Caffeine-Related Disorders

Caffeine-Induced Disorders

305.90	Caffeine Intoxication
292.89	Caffeine-Induced Anxiety Disorder
292.89	Caffeine-Induced Sleep Disorder
292.9	Caffeine-Related Disorder NOS

Cannabis-Related Disorders

Cannabis Use Disorders

304.30	Cannabis Dependence
305.20	Cannabis Abuse

Cannabis-Induced Disorders

292.89	Cannabis Intoxication
292.81	Cannabis Intoxication Delirium
292.xx	Cannabis-Induced Psychotic Disorder
.11	With Delusions
.12	With Hallucinations
292.89	Cannabis-Induced Anxiety Disorder
292.9	Cannabis-Related Disorder NOS

Cocaine-Related Disorders

Cocaine Use Disorders

304.20	Cocaine Dependence
305.60	Cocaine Abuse

Cocaine-Induced Disorders

292.89	Cocaine Intoxication
292.0	Cocaine Withdrawal
292.81	Cocaine Intoxication Delirium
292.xx	Cocaine-Induced Psychotic Disorder
.11	With Delusions
.12	With Hallucinations
292.84	Cocaine-Induced Mood Disorder
292.89	Cocaine-Induced Anxiety Disorder
292.89	Cocaine-Induced Sexual Dysfunction
292.89	Cocaine-Induced Sleep Disorder
292.9	Cocaine-Related Disorder NOS

Hallucinogen-Related Disorders

Hallucinogen Use Disorders

304.50	Hallucinogen Dependence
305.30	Hallucinogen Abuse

Hallucinogen-Induced Disorders

292.89	Hallucinogen Intoxication
292.89	Hallucinogen Persisting Perception Disorder (Flashbacks)
292.81	Hallucinogen Intoxication Delirium
292.xx	Hallucinogen-Induced Psychotic Disorder
.11	With Delusions
.12	With Hallucinations
292.84	Hallucinogen-Induced Mood Disorder
292.89	Hallucinogen-Induced Anxiety Disorder
292.9	Hallucinogen-Related Disorder NOS

Inhalant-Related Disorders

Inhalant Use Disorders

304.60	Inhalant Dependence
305.90	Inhalant Abuse

Inhalant-Induced Disorders

292.89	Inhalant Intoxication
292.81	Inhalant Intoxication Delirium
292.82	Inhalant-Induced Persisting Dementia
292.xx	Inhalant-Induced Psychotic Disorder
.11	With Delusions
.12	With Hallucinations
292.84	Inhalant-Induced Mood Disorder
292.89	Inhalant-Induced Anxiety Disorder
292.9	Inhalant-Related Disorder NOS

Nicotine-Related Disorders

Nicotine Use Disorders

305.1	Nicotine Dependence

Nicotine-Induced Disorders

292.0	Nicotine Withdrawal
292.9	Nicotine-Related Disorder NOS

Opioid-Related Disorders

Opioid Use Disorders

304.00	Opioid Dependence
305.50	Opioid Abuse

Opioid-Induced Disorders

292.89	Opioid Intoxication
292.0	Opioid Withdrawal
292.81	Opioid Intoxication Delirium
292.xx	Opioid-Induced Psychotic Disorder
.11	With Delusions
.12	With Hallucinations
292.84	Opioid-Induced Mood Disorder
292.89	Opioid-Induced Sexual Dysfunction
292.89	Opioid-Induced Sleep Disorder
292.9	Opioid-Related Disorder NOS

Phencyclidine (or Phencyclidine-Like)-Related Disorders

Phencyclidine Use Disorders

304.60	Phencyclidine Dependence
305.90	Phencyclidine Abuse

Phencyclidine-Induced Disorders

292.89	Phencyclidine Intoxication
292.81	Phencyclidine Intoxication Delirium
292.xx	Phencyclidine-Induced Psychotic Disorder
.11	With Delusions
.12	With Hallucinations
292.84	Phencyclidine-Induced Mood Disorder
292.89	Phencyclidine-Induced Anxiety Disorder
292.9	Phencyclidine-Related Disorder NOS

Sedative-, Hypnotic-, or Anxiolytic-Related Disorders

Sedative, Hypnotic, or Anxiolytic Use Disorders

304.10	Sedative, Hypnotic, or Anxiolytic Dependence
305.40	Sedative, Hypnotic, or Anxiolytic Abuse

Sedative-, Hypnotic-, or Anxiolytic-Induced Disorders

292.89	Sedative, Hypnotic, or Anxiolytic Intoxication
292.0	Sedative, Hypnotic, or Anxiolytic Withdrawal
292.81	Sedative, Hypnotic, or Anxiolytic Intoxication Delirium
292.81	Sedative, Hypnotic, or Anxiolytic Withdrawal Delirium
292.82	Sedative-, Hypnotic-, or Anxiolytic-Induced Persisting Dementia
292.83	Sedative-, Hypnotic-, or Anxiolytic-Induced Persisting Amnestic Disorder
292.xx	Sedative-, Hypnotic-, or Anxiolytic-Induced Psychotic Disorder
.11	With Delusions
.12	With Hallucinations
292.84	Sedative-, Hypnotic-, or Anxiolytic-Induced Mood Disorder
292.89	Sedative-, Hypnotic-, or Anxiolytic-Induced Anxiety Disorder
292.89	Sedative-, Hypnotic-, or Anxiolytic-Induced Sexual Dysfunction
292.89	Sedative-, Hypnotic-, or Anxiolytic-Induced Sleep Disorder
292.9	Sedative-, Hypnotic-, or Anxiolytic-Related Disorder NOS

Polysubstance-Related Disorder

304.80	Polysubstance Dependence

Other (or Unknown) Substance-Related Disorders

Other (or Unknown) Substance Use Disorders

304.90	Other (or Unknown) Substance Dependence
305.90	Other (or Unknown) Substance Abuse

Other (or Unknown) Substance-Induced Disorders

292.89	Other (or Unknown) Substance Intoxication
292.0	Other (or Unknown) Substance Withdrawal
292.81	Other (or Unknown) Substance-Induced Delirium
292.82	Other (or Unknown) Substance-Induced Persisting Dementia
292.83	Other (or Unknown) Substance-Induced Persisting Amnestic Disorder
292.xx	Other (or Unknown) Substance-Induced Psychotic Disorder
.11	With Delusions

.12	With Hallucinations
292.84	Other (or Unknown) Substance-Induced Mood Disorder
292.89	Other (or Unknown) Substance-Induced Anxiety Disorder
292.89	Other (or Unknown) Substance-Induced Sexual Dysfunction
292.89	Other (or Unknown) Substance-Induced Sleep Disorder
292.9	Other (or Unknown) Substance-Related Disorder NOS

SCHIZOPHRENIA AND OTHER PSYCHOTIC DISORDERS

295.xx	Schizophrenia
.30	Paranoid type
.10	Disorganized type
.20	Catatonic type
.90	Undifferentiated type
.60	Residual type
295.40	Schizophreniform Disorder
295.70	Schizoaffective Disorder
297.1	Delusional Disorder
298.8	Brief Psychotic Disorder
297.3	Shared Psychotic Disorder
293.xx	Psychotic Disorder Due to *(Indicate the General Medical Condition)*
.81	With Delusions
.82	With Hallucinations
—	Substance-Induced Psychotic Disorder *(refer to Substance-Related Disorders for substance-specific codes)*
298.9	Psychotic Disorder NOS

MOOD DISORDERS

(Code current state of Major Depressive Disorder or Bipolar I Disorder in fifth digit: 0 = unspecified; 1 = mild; 2 = moderate; 3 = severe, without psychotic features; 4 = severe, with psychotic features; 5 = in partial remission; 6 = in full remission.)

Depressive Disorders

296.xx	Major Depressive Disorder
.2x	Single episode
.3x	Recurrent
300.4	Dysthymic Disorder
311	Depressive Disorder NOS

Bipolar Disorders

296.xx	Bipolar I Disorder
.0x	Single Manic Episode

.40	Most Recent Episode Hypomanic
.4x	Most Recent Episode Manic
.6x	Most Recent Episode Mixed
.5x	Most Recent Episode Depressed
.7	Most Recent Episode Unspecified
296.89	Bipolar II Disorder *(Specify current or most recent episode: Hypomanic or Depressed)*
301.13	Cyclothymic Disorder
296.80	Bipolar Disorder NOS
293.83	Mood Disorder Due to *(Indicate the General Medical Condition)*
—	Substance-Induced Mood Disorder *(refer to Substance-Related Disorders for substance-specific codes)*
296.90	Mood Disorder NOS

ANXIETY DISORDERS

300.01	Panic Disorder Without Agoraphobia
300.21	Panic Disorder With Agoraphobia
300.22	Agoraphobia Without History of Panic Disorder
300.29	Specific Phobia
300.23	Social Phobia
300.3	Obsessive–Compulsive Disorder
309.81	Posttraumatic Stress Disorder
308.3	Acute Stress Disorder
300.02	Generalized Anxiety Disorder
293.89	Anxiety Disorder Due to *(Indicate the General Medical Condition)*
—	Substance-Induced Anxiety Disorder *(refer to Substance-Related Disorders for substance-specific codes)*
300.00	Anxiety Disorder NOS

SOMATOFORM DISORDERS

300.81	Somatization Disorder
300.82	Undifferentiated Somatoform Disorder
300.11	Conversion Disorder
307.xx	Pain Disorder
.80	Associated with Psychological Factors
.89	Associated with Both Psychological Factors and a General Medical Condition
300.7	Hypochondriasis
300.7	Body Dysmorphic Disorder
300.82	Somatoform Disorder NOS

FACTITIOUS DISORDERS

300.xx	Factitious Disorder
.16	With Predominantly Psychological Signs and Symptoms

.19	With Predominantly Physical Signs and Symptoms
.19	With Combined Psychological and Physical Signs and Symptoms
300.19	Factitious Disorder NOS

DISSOCIATIVE DISORDERS

300.12	Dissociative Amnesia
300.13	Dissociative Fugue
300.14	Dissociative Identity Disorder
300.6	Depersonalization Disorder
300.15	Dissociative Disorder NOS

SEXUAL AND GENDER IDENTITY DISORDERS

Sexual Dysfunctions

Sexual Desire Disorders

| 302.71 | Hypoactive Sexual Desire Disorder |
| 302.79 | Sexual Aversion Disorder |

Sexual Arousal Disorders

| 302.72 | Female Sexual Arousal Disorder |
| 302.72 | Male Erectile Disorder |

Orgasmic Disorders

302.73	Female Orgasmic Disorder
302.74	Male Orgasmic Disorder
302.75	Premature Ejaculation

Sexual Pain Disorders

| 302.76 | Dyspareunia (Not Due to a General Medical Condition) |
| 306.51 | Vaginismus (Not Due to a General Medical Condition) |

Sexual Dysfunction Due to a General Medical Condition

625.8	Female Hypoactive Sexual Desire Disorder Due to *(Indicate the General Medical Condition)*
608.89	Male Hypoactive Sexual Desire Disorder Due to *(Indicate the General Medical Condition)*
607.84	Male Erectile Disorder Due to *(Indicate the General Medical Condition)*
625.0	Female Dyspareunia Due to *(Indicate the General Medical Condition)*

608.89	Male Dyspareunia Due to *(Indicate the General Medical Condition)*
625.8	Other Female Sexual Dysfunction Due to *(Indicate the General Medical Condition)*
608.89	Other Male Sexual Dysfunction Due to *(Indicate the General Medical Condition)*
—	Substance-Induced Sexual Dysfunction *(refer to Substance-Related Disorders for substance-specific codes)*
302.70	Sexual Dysfunction NOS

Paraphilias

302.4	Exhibitionism
302.81	Fetishism
302.89	Frotteurism
302.2	Pedophilia
302.83	Sexual Masochism
302.84	Sexual Sadism
302.3	Transvestic Fetishism
302.82	Voyeurism
302.9	Paraphilia NOS

Gender Identity Disorders

302.xx	Gender Identity Disorder
.6	In Children
.85	In Adolescents or Adults
302.6	Gender Identity Disorder NOS
302.9	Sexual Disorder NOS

EATING DISORDERS

307.1	Anorexia Nervosa
307.51	Bulimia Nervosa
307.50	Eating Disorder NOS

SLEEP DISORDERS

Primary Sleep Disorders

Dyssomnias

307.42	Primary Insomnia
307.44	Primary Hypersomnia
347	Narcolepsy
780.59	Breathing-Related Sleep Disorder
307.45	Circadian Rhythm Sleep Disorder
307.47	Dyssomnia NOS

Parasomnias

| 307.47 | Nightmare Disorder |
| 307.46 | Sleep Terror Disorder |

| 307.46 | Sleepwalking Disorder |
| 307.47 | Parasomnia NOS |

Sleep Disorders Related to Another Mental Disorder

| 307.42 | Insomnia Related to *(Indicate the Axis I or Axis II Disorder)* |
| 307.44 | Hypersomnia Related to *(Indicate the Axis I or Axis II Disorder)* |

Other Sleep Disorders

780.xx	Sleep Disorder Due to *(Indicate the General Medical Condition)*
.52	Insomnia type
.54	Hypersomnia type
.59	Parasomnia type
.59	Mixed type
—	Substance-Induced Sleep Disorder *(refer to Substance-Related Disorders for substance-specific codes)*

IMPULSE CONTROL DISORDERS NOT ELSEWHERE CLASSIFIED

312.34	Intermittent Explosive Disorder
312.32	Kleptomania
312.33	Pyromania
312.31	Pathological Gambling
312.39	Trichotillomania
312.30	Impulse Control Disorder NOS

ADJUSTMENT DISORDERS

309.xx	Adjustment Disorder
.0	With Depressed Mood
.24	With Anxiety
.28	With Mixed Anxiety and Depressed Mood
.3	With Disturbance of Conduct
.4	With Mixed Disturbance of Emotions and Conduct
.9	Unspecified

PERSONALITY DISORDERS

NOTE: *These are coded on Axis II.*

301.0	Paranoid Personality Disorder
301.20	Schizoid Personality Disorder
301.22	Schizotypal Personality Disorder
301.7	Antisocial Personality Disorder
301.83	Borderline Personality Disorder
301.50	Histrionic Personality Disorder
301.81	Narcissistic Personality Disorder
301.82	Avoidant Personality Disorder
301.6	Dependent Personality Disorder
301.4	Obsessive-Compulsive Personality Disorder
301.9	Personality Disorder NOS

OTHER CONDITIONS THAT MAY BE A FOCUS OF CLINICAL ATTENTION

Psychological Factors Affecting Medical Condition

316	*Choose name based on nature of factors:*
	Mental Disorder Affecting Medical Condition
	Psychological Symptoms Affecting Medical Condition
	Personality Traits or Coping Style Affecting Medical Condition
	Maladaptive Health Behaviors Affecting Medical Condition
	Stress-Related Physiological Response Affecting Medical Condition
	Other or Unspecified Psychological Factors Affecting Medical Condition

Medication-Induced Movement Disorders

332.1	Neuroleptic-Induced Parkinsonism
333.92	Neuroleptic Malignant Syndrome
333.7	Neuroleptic-Induced Acute Dystonia
333.99	Neuroleptic-Induced Acute Akathisia
333.82	Neuroleptic-Induced Tardive Dyskinesia
333.1	Medication-Induced Postural Tremor
333.90	Medication-Induced Movement Disorder NOS

Other Medication-Induced Disorder

| 995.2 | Adverse Effects of Medication NOS |

Relational Problems

V61.9	Relational Problem Related to a Mental Disorder or General Medical Condition
V61.20	Parent-Child Relational Problem
V61.10	Partner Relational Problem
V61.8	Sibling Relational Problem
V62.81	Relational Problem NOS

Problems Related to Abuse or Neglect

V61.21	Physical Abuse of Child
V61.21	Sexual Abuse of Child
V61.21	Neglect of Child

—	Physical Abuse of Adult
V61.12	(if by partner)
V62.83	(if by person other than partner)
—	Sexual Abuse of Adult
V61.12	(if by partner)
V62.83	(if by person other than partner)

Additional Conditions That May Be a Focus of Clinical Attention

V15.81	Noncompliance with Treatment
V65.2	Malingering
V71.01	Adult Antisocial Behavior
V71.02	Childhood or Adolescent Antisocial Behavior
V62.89	Borderline Intellectual Functioning (coded on Axis II)

780.9	Age-Related Cognitive Decline
V62.82	Bereavement
V62.3	Academic Problem
V62.2	Occupational Problem
313.82	Identity Problem
V62.89	Religious or Spiritual Problem
V62.4	Acculturation Problem
V62.89	Phase of Life Problem

ADDITIONAL CODES

300.9	Unspecified Mental Disorder (nonpsychotic)
V71.09	No Diagnosis or Condition on Axis I
799.9	Diagnosis or Condition Deferred on Axis I
V71.09	No Diagnosis on Axis II
799.9	Diagnosis Deferred on Axis II

NANDA Nursing Diagnoses: Taxonomy II

DOMAINS, CLASSES, AND DIAGNOSES

Domain 1: Health Promotion

Class 1: Health Awareness

Class 2: Health Management

APPROVED DIAGNOSES

Effective therapeutic regimen management
Ineffective therapeutic regimen management
Ineffective family therapeutic regimen management
Ineffective community therapeutic regimen management
Health-seeking behaviors (specify)
Ineffective health maintenance
Impaired home maintenance
Readiness for enhanced therapeutic regimen management
Readiness for enhanced nutrition

Domain 2: Nutrition

Class 1: Ingestion

APPROVED DIAGNOSES

Ineffective infant feeding pattern
Impaired swallowing
Imbalanced nutrition: Less than body requirements
Imbalanced nutrition: More than body requirements
Risk for imbalanced nutrition: More than body requirements

Class 2: Digestion

Class 3: Absorption

Class 4: Metabolism

Class 5: Hydration

APPROVED DIAGNOSES

Deficient fluid volume
Risk for deficient fluid volume
Excess fluid volume
Risk for imbalanced fluid volume
Readiness for enhanced fluid balance

Domain 3: Elimination and Exchange

Class 1: Urinary Function

APPROVED DIAGNOSES

Impaired urinary elimination
Urinary retention
Total urinary incontinence
Functional urinary incontinence
Stress urinary incontinence
Urge urinary incontinence
Reflex urinary incontinence
Risk for urge urinary incontinence
Readiness for enhanced urinary elimination

Class 2: Gastrointestinal Function

APPROVED DIAGNOSES

Bowel incontinence
Diarrhea
Constipation
Risk for constipation
Perceived constipation

Class 3: Integumentary Function

Class 4: Respiratory Function

APPROVED DIAGNOSES

Impaired gas exchange

Domain 4: Activity/Rest

Class 1: Sleep/Rest

APPROVED DIAGNOSES

Disturbed sleep pattern
Sleep deprivation
Readiness for enhanced sleep

Class 2: Activity/Exercise

APPROVED DIAGNOSES

Risk for disuse syndrome
Impaired physical mobility

Impaired bed mobility
Impaired wheelchair mobility
Impaired transfer ability
Impaired walking
Deficient diversional activity
Delayed surgical recovery
Sedentary lifestyle

Class 3: Energy Balance

APPROVED DIAGNOSES

Energy field disturbance
Fatigue

Class 4: Cardiovascular/Pulmonary Responses

APPROVED DIAGNOSES

Decreased cardiac output
Impaired spontaneous ventilation
Ineffective breathing pattern
Activity intolerance
Risk for activity intolerance
Dysfunctional ventilatory weaning response
Ineffective tissue perfusion (specify type: renal, cerebral, cardiopulmonary, gastrointestinal, peripheral)

Class 5: Self-Care

APPROVED DIAGNOSES

Dressing/grooming self-care deficit
Bathing/hygiene self-care deficit
Feeding self-care deficit
Toileting self-care deficit

Domain 5: Perception/Cognition

Class 1: Attention

APPROVED DIAGNOSES

Unilateral neglect

Class 2: Orientation

APPROVED DIAGNOSES

Impaired environmental interpretation syndrome
Wandering

Class 3: Sensation/Perception

APPROVED DIAGNOSES

Disturbed sensory perception (specify: visual, auditory, kinesthetic, gustatory, tactile)

Class 4: Cognition

APPROVED DIAGNOSES

Deficient knowledge (specify)
Readiness for enhanced knowledge (specify)
Acute confusion
Chronic confusion
Impaired memory
Disturbed thought processes

Class 5: Communication

APPROVED DIAGNOSES

Impaired verbal communication
Readiness for enhanced communication

Domain 6: Self-Perception

Class 1: Self-Concept

APPROVED DIAGNOSES

Disturbed personal identity
Powerlessness
Risk for powerlessness
Hopelessness
Risk for loneliness
Readiness for enhanced self-concept

Class 2: Self-Esteem

APPROVED DIAGNOSES

Chronic low self-esteem
Situational low self-esteem
Risk for situational low self-esteem

Class 3: Body Image

APPROVED DIAGNOSES

Disturbed body image

Domain 7: Role Relationships

Class 1: Caregiving Roles

APPROVED DIAGNOSES

Caregiver role strain
Risk for caregiver role strain
Impaired parenting
Risk for impaired parenting
Readiness for enhanced parenting

Class 2: Family Relationships

APPROVED DIAGNOSES

Interrupted family processes
Readiness for enhanced family processes

Dysfunctional family processes: Alcoholism
Risk for impaired parent/infant/child attachment

Class 3: Role Performance

APPROVED DIAGNOSES

Effective breastfeeding
Ineffective breastfeeding
Interrupted breastfeeding
Ineffective role performance
Parental role conflict
Impaired social interaction

Domain 8: Sexuality

Class 1: Sexual Identity

Class 2: Sexual Function

APPROVED DIAGNOSES

Sexual dysfunction
Ineffective sexuality pattern

Class 3: Reproduction

Domain 9: Coping/Stress Tolerance

Class 1: Post-Trauma Responses

APPROVED DIAGNOSES

Relocation stress syndrome
Risk for relocation stress syndrome
Rape-trauma syndrome
Rape-trauma syndrome: Silent reaction
Rape-trauma syndrome: Compound reaction
Post-trauma syndrome
Risk for post-trauma syndrome

Class 2: Coping Responses

APPROVED DIAGNOSES

Fear
Anxiety
Death anxiety
Chronic sorrow
Ineffective denial
Anticipatory grieving
Dysfunctional grieving
Impaired adjustment
Ineffective coping
Disabled family coping
Compromised family coping
Defensive coping
Ineffective community coping

Readiness for enhanced coping (individual)
Readiness for enhanced family coping
Readiness for enhanced community coping
Risk for dysfunctional grieving

Class 3: Neurobehavioral Stress

APPROVED DIAGNOSES

Autonomic dysreflexia
Risk for autonomic dysreflexia
Disorganized infant behavior
Risk for disorganized infant behavior
Readiness for enhanced organized infant behavior
Decreased intracranial adaptive capacity

Domain 10: Life Principles

Class 1: Values

Class 2: Beliefs

APPROVED DIAGNOSES

Readiness for enhanced spiritual well-being

Class 3: Value/Belief/Action Congruence

APPROVED DIAGNOSES

Spiritual distress
Risk for spiritual distress
Decisional conflict (specify)
Noncompliance (specify)
Risk for impaired religiosity
Impaired religiosity
Readiness for enhanced religiosity

Domain 11: Safety/Protection

Class 1: Infection

APPROVED DIAGNOSES

Risk for infection

Class 2: Physical Injury

APPROVED DIAGNOSES

Impaired oral mucous membrane
Risk for injury
Risk for perioperative positioning injury
Risk for falls
Risk for trauma
Impaired skin integrity
Risk for impaired skin integrity
Impaired tissue integrity
Impaired dentition

Risk for suffocation
Risk for aspiration
Ineffective airway clearance
Risk for peripheral neurovascular dysfunction
Ineffective protection
Risk for sudden infant death syndrome

Class 3: Violence

APPROVED DIAGNOSES

Risk for self-mutilation
Self-mutilation
Risk for other-directed violence
Risk for self-directed violence
Risk for suicide

Class 4: Environmental Hazards

APPROVED DIAGNOSES

Risk for poisoning

Class 5: Defensive Processes

APPROVED DIAGNOSES

Latex allergy response
Risk for latex allergy response

Class 6: Thermoregulation

APPROVED DIAGNOSES

Risk for imbalanced body temperature
Ineffective thermoregulation

Hypothermia
Hyperthermia

Domain 12: Comfort

Class 1: Physical Comfort

APPROVED DIAGNOSES

Acute pain
Chronic pain
Nausea

Class 2: Environmental Comfort

Class 3: Social Comfort

APPROVED DIAGNOSES

Social isolation

Domain 13: Growth/Development

Class 1: Growth

APPROVED DIAGNOSES

Delayed growth and development
Risk for disproportionate growth
Adult failure to thrive

Class 2: Development

APPROVED DIAGNOSES

Delayed growth and development
Risk for delayed development

SOURCE: *NANDA Nursing Diagnoses: Definitions & Classification 2005-2006.* (2005). Philadelphia: NANDA International. With permission.

Assigning Nursing Diagnoses to Client Behaviors

Following is a list of client behaviors and the NANDA nursing diagnoses which correspond to the behaviors and which may be used in planning care for the client exhibiting the specific behavioral symptoms.

BEHAVIORS	NANDA NURSING DIAGNOSES
Aggression; hostility	Risk for injury; Risk for other-directed violence
Anorexia or refusal to eat	Imbalanced nutrition: Less than body requirements
Anxious behavior	Anxiety (Specify level)
Confusion; memory loss	Confusion, acute/chronic; Disturbed thought processes
Delusions	Disturbed thought processes
Denial of problems	Ineffective denial
Depressed mood or anger turned inward	Dysfunctional grieving
Detoxification; withdrawal from substances	Risk for injury
Difficulty accepting new diagnosis or recent change in health status	Impaired adjustment
Difficulty making important life decision	Decisional conflict (specify)
Difficulty with interpersonal relationships	Impaired social interaction
Disruption in capability to perform usual responsibilities	Ineffective role performance
Dissociative behaviors (depersonalization; derealization)	Disturbed sensory perception (kinesthetic)
Expresses feelings of disgust about body or body part	Disturbed body image
Expresses lack of control over personal situation	Powerlessness
Fails to follow prescribed therapy	Ineffective therapeutic regimen management
Flashbacks, nightmares, obsession with traumatic experience	Post-trauma syndrome
Hallucinations	Disturbed sensory perception (auditory; visual)
Highly critical of self or others	Low self-esteem (chronic; situational)
HIV positive; altered immunity	Ineffective protection
Inability to meet basic needs	Self-care deficit (feeding; bathing/hygiene; dressing/grooming; toileting)
Insomnia or hypersomnia	Disturbed sleep pattern
Loose associations or flight of ideas	Impaired verbal communication
Loss of a valued entity, recently experienced	Risk for dysfunctional grieving
Manic hyperactivity	Risk for injury
Manipulative behavior	Ineffective coping
Multiple personalities; gender identity disturbance	Disturbed personal identity
Orgasm, problems with; lack of sexual desire	Sexual dysfunction
Overeating, compulsive	Risk for imbalanced nutrition: More than body requirements
Phobias	Fear
Physical symptoms as coping behavior	Ineffective coping
Projection of blame; rationalization of failures; denial of personal responsibility	Defensive coping

Ritualistic behaviors	Anxiety (severe); ineffective coping
Seductive remarks; inappropriate sexual behaviors	Impaired social interaction
Self-mutilative behaviors	Self-mutilation; Risk for self-mutilation
Sexual behaviors (difficulty, limitations, or changes in; reported dissatisfaction)	Ineffective sexuality patterns
Stress from caring for chronically ill person	Caregiver role strain
Stress from locating to new environment	Relocation stress syndrome
Substance use as a coping behavior	Ineffective coping
Substance use (denies use is a problem)	Ineffective denial
Suicidal	Risk for suicide; Risk for self-directed violence
Suspiciousness	Disturbed thought processes; ineffective coping
Vomiting, excessive, self-induced	Risk for deficient fluid volume
Withdrawn behavior	Social isolation

Glossary

A

abandonment. A unilateral severance of the professional relationship between a health care provider and a client without reasonable notice at a time when there is still a need for continuing health care.

abreaction. "Remembering with feeling"; bringing into conscious awareness painful events that have been repressed, and re-experiencing the emotions that were associated with the events.

acquired immunodeficiency syndrome (AIDS). A condition in which the immune system becomes deficient in its efforts to prevent opportunistic infections, malignancies, and neurological disease. It is caused by the human immunodeficiency virus (HIV), which is passed from one individual to another through body fluids.

acupoints. In Chinese medicine, acupoints represent areas along the body that link pathways of healing energy.

acupressure. A technique in which the fingers, thumbs, palms, or elbows are used to apply pressure to certain points along the body. This pressure is thought to dissolve any obstructions in the flow of healing energy and to restore the body to a healthier functioning.

acupuncture. A technique in which hair-thin, sterile, disposable, stainless-steel needles are inserted into points along the body to dissolve obstructions in the flow of healing energy and restore the body to a healthier functioning.

adaptation. Restoration of the body to homeostasis following a physiological and/or psychological response to stress.

adjustment disorder. A maladaptive reaction to an identifiable psychosocial stressor that occurs within 3 months after onset of the stressor. The individual shows impairment in social and occupational functioning, or exhibits symptoms that are in excess of a normal and expectable reaction to the stressor.

advance directives. Legal documents that a competent individual may sign to convey to wishes regarding future healthcare decisions intended for a time when the individual is no longer capable of informed consent. They may include one or both of the following: (1) a living will, in which the individual identifies the type of care that he or she does or does not wish to have performed, and (2) a durable power of attorney for healthcare, in which the individual names another person who is given the right to make healthcare decisions for the individual who is incapable of doing so.

affect. The behavioral expression of emotion; may be appropriate (congruent with the situation); inappropriate (incongruent with the situation); constricted or blunted (diminished range and intensity); or flat (absence of emotional expression).

affective domain. A category of learning that includes attitudes, feelings, and values.

aggression. Harsh physical or verbal actions intended (either consciously or unconsciously) to harm or injure another.

aggressiveness. Behavior that defends an individual's own basic rights by violating the basic rights of others (as contrasted with **assertiveness**).

agoraphobia. The fear of being in places or situations from which escape might be difficult (or embarrassing) or in which help might not be available in the event of a panic attack.

agranulocytosis. Extremely low levels of white blood cells. Symptoms include sore throat, fever, and malaise. This may be a side effect of long-term therapy with some antipsychotic medications.

AIDS. See acquired immunodeficiency syndrome (AIDS).

akathisia. Restlessness; an urgent need for movement. A type of extrapyramidal side effect associated with some antipsychotic medications.

akinesia. Muscular weakness; or a loss or partial loss of muscle movement; a type of extrapyramidal side effect associated with some antipsychotic medications.

Alcoholics Anonymous (AA). A major self-help organization for the treatment of alcoholism. It is based on a 12-step program to help members attain and maintain sobriety. Once individuals have achieved sobriety, they in turn are expected to help other alcoholic persons.

allopathic medicine. Traditional medicine. The type traditionally, and currently, practiced in the United States and taught in U.S. medical schools.

alternative medicine. Practices that differ from usual traditional (allopathic) medicine.

altruism. One curative factor of group therapy (identified by Yalom) in which individuals gain self-esteem through mutual sharing and concern. Providing assistance and support to others creates a positive self-image and promotes self-growth.

altruistic suicide. Suicide based on behavior of a group to which an individual is excessively integrated.

amenorrhea. Cessation of the menses; may be a side effect of some antipsychotic medications.

amnesia. An inability to recall important personal information that is too extensive to be explained by ordinary forgetfulness.

amnesia, continuous. The inability to recall events occurring after a specific time up to and including the present.

amnesia, generalized. The inability to recall anything that has happened during the individual's entire lifetime.

amnesia, localized. The inability to recall all incidents associated with a traumatic event for a specific time period following the event (usually a few hours to a few days).

amnesia, selective. The inability to recall only certain incidents associated with a traumatic event for a specific time period following the event.

amnesia, systematized. The inability to remember events that relate to a specific category of information, such as one's family, a particular person, or an event.

andropause. A term used to identify the male climacteric. Also called *male menopause*. A syndrome of symptoms related to the decline of testosterone levels in men. Some symptoms include depression, weight gain, insomnia, hot flashes, decreased libido, mood swings, decreased strength, and erectile dysfunction.

anger. An emotional response to one's perception of a situation. Anger has both positive and negative functions.

anhedonia. The inability to experience or even imagine any pleasant emotion.

anomic suicide. Suicide that occurs in response to changes that occur in an individual's life that disrupt cohesiveness from a group and cause that person to feel without support from the formerly cohesive group.

anorexia. Loss of appetite.

anorexigenics. Drugs that suppress appetite.

anorgasmia. Inability to achieve orgasm.

anosmia. Inability to smell.

anticipatory grief. A subjective state of emotional, physical, and social responses to an anticipated loss of a valued entity. The grief response is repeated once the loss actually occurs, but it may not be as intense as it might have been if anticipatory grieving has not occurred.

antisocial personality disorder. A pattern of socially irresponsible, exploitative, and guiltless behavior, evident in the tendency to fail to conform to the law, develop stable relationships, or sustain consistent employment; exploitation and manipulation of others for personal gain is common.

anxiety. Vague diffuse apprehension that is associated with feelings of uncertainty and helplessness.

aphasia. Inability to communicate through speech, writing, or signs, caused by dysfunction of brain centers.

aphonia. Inability to speak.

apraxia. Inability to carry out motor activities despite intact motor function.

arbitrary inference. A type of thinking error in which the individual automatically comes to a conclusion about an incident without the facts to support it, or even sometimes despite contradictory evidence to support it.

ascites. Excessive accumulation of serous fluid in the abdominal cavity, occurring in response to portal hypertension caused by cirrhosis of the liver.

assault. An act that results in a person's genuine fear and apprehension that he or she will be touched without consent. Nurses may be guilty of assault for threatening to place an individual in restraints against his or her will.

assertiveness. Behavior that enables individuals to act in their own best interests, to stand up for themselves without undue anxiety, to express their honest feelings comfortably, or to exercise their own rights without denying those of others.

associative looseness. Sometimes called loose associations, a thinking process characterized by speech in which ideas shift from one unrelated subject to another. The individual is unaware that the topics are unconnected.

ataxia. Muscular incoordination.

attachment theory. The hypothesis that individuals who maintain close relationships with others into old age are more likely to remain independent and less likely to be institutionalized than those who do not.

attitude. A frame of reference around which an individual organizes knowledge about his or her world. It includes an emotional element and can have a positive or negative connotation.

autism. A focus inward on a fantasy world, while distorting or excluding the external environment; common in schizophrenia.

autistic disorder. The withdrawal of an infant or child into the self and into a fantasy world of his or her own creation. There is marked impairment in interpersonal functioning and communication and in imaginative play. Activities and interests are restricted and may be considered somewhat bizarre.

autocratic. A leadership style in which the leader makes all decisions for the group. Productivity is very high with this type of leadership, but morale is often low because of the lack of member input and creativity.

autoimmunity. A condition in which the body produces a disordered immunological response against itself. In this situation, the body fails to differentiate between what is normal and what is a foreign substance. When this occurs, the body produces antibodies against normal parts of the body to such an extent as to cause tissue injury.

automatic thoughts. Thoughts that occur rapidly in response to a situation, and without rational analysis. They are often negative and based on erroneous logic.

autonomy. Independence; self-governance. An ethical principle that emphasizes the status of persons as autonomous moral agents whose right to determine their destinies should always be respected.

aversive stimulus. A stimulus that follows a behavioral response and decreases the probability that the behavior will recur; also called punishment.

axon. The cellular process of a neuron that carries impulses away from the cell body.

B

battering. A pattern of repeated physical assault, usually of a woman by her spouse or intimate partner. Men are also battered, although this occurs much less frequently.

battery. The unconsented touching of another person. Nurses may be charged with battery should they participate in the treatment of a client without his or her consent and outside of an emergency situation.

behavior modification. A treatment modality aimed at changing undesirable behaviors, using a system of reinforcement to bring about the modifications desired.

behavioral objectives. Statements that indicate to an individual what is expected of him or her. Behavioral objectives are a way of measuring learning outcomes, and are based on the affective, cognitive, and psychomotor domains of learning.

belief. A belief is an idea that one holds to be true. It can be rational, irrational, taken on faith, or a stereotypical idea.

beneficence. An ethical principle that refers to one's duty to benefit or promote the good of others.

bereavement overload. An accumulation of grief that occurs when an individual experiences many losses over a short period of time and is unable to resolve one before another is experienced. This phenomenon is common among the elderly.

binge and purge. A syndrome associated with eating disorders, especially bulimia, in which an individual consumes thousands of calories of food at one sitting, and then purges through the use of laxatives or self-induced vomiting.

bioethics. The term used with ethical principles that refer to concepts within the scope of medicine, nursing, and allied health.

biofeedback. The use of instrumentation to become aware of processes in the body that usually go unnoticed and to bring them under voluntary control (e.g., the blood pressure or pulse); used as a method of stress reduction.

bipolar disorder. Characterized by mood swings from profound depression to extreme euphoria (mania), with intervening periods of normalcy. Psychotic symptoms may or may not be present.

body image. One's perception of his or her own body. It may also be how one believes others perceive his or her body. (See also **physical self.**)

borderline personality disorder. A disorder characterized by a pattern of intense and chaotic relationships, with affective instability, fluctuating and extreme attitudes regarding other people, impulsivity, direct and indirect self-destructive behavior, and lack of a clear or certain sense of identity, life plan, or values.

boundaries. The level of participation and interaction between individuals and between subsystems. Boundaries denote physical and psychological space individuals identify as their own. They are sometimes referred to as limits. Boundaries are appropriate when they permit appropriate contact with others while preventing excessive interference. Boundaries may be clearly defined (healthy) or rigid or diffuse (unhealthy).

C

cachexia. A state of ill health, malnutrition, and wasting; extreme emaciation.

cannabis. The dried flowering tops of the hemp plant. It produces euphoric effects when ingested or smoked and is commonly used in the form of marijuana or hashish.

carcinogen. Any substance or agent that produces or increases the risk of developing cancer in humans or lower animals.

case management. A health care delivery process, the goals of which are to provide quality health care, decrease fragmentation, enhance the client's quality of life, and contain costs. A case manager coordinates the client's care from admission to discharge and sometimes following discharge. Critical pathways of care are the tools used for the provision of care in a case management system.

case manager. The individual responsible for negotiating with multiple health care providers to obtain a variety of services for a client.

catastrophic thinking. Always thinking that the worst will occur without considering the possibility of more likely, positive outcomes.

catatonia. A type of schizophrenia that is typified by stupor or excitement, stupor characterized by extreme psychomotor retardation, mutism, negativism, and posturing, excitement by psychomotor agitation, in which the movements are frenzied and purposeless.

catharsis. One curative factor of group therapy (identified by Yalom), in which members in a group can express both positive and negative feelings in a nonthreatening atmosphere.

cell body. The part of the neuron that contains the nucleus and is essential for the continued life of the neuron.

Centers for Medicare and Medicaid Services (CMA). The division of the U.S. Department of Health and Human Services responsible for Medicare funding.

child sexual abuse. Any sexual act, such as indecent exposure or improper touching to penetration (sexual intercourse), that is carried out with a child.

chiropractic. A system of alternative medicine based on the premise that the relationship between structure and function in the human body is a significant health factor and that such relationships between the spinal column and the nervous system are important because the normal transmission and expression of nerve energy are essential to the restoration and maintenance of health.

Christian ethics. The ethical philosophy that states one should treat others as moral equals, and recognize the equality of other persons by permitting them to act as we do when they occupy a position similar to ours; sometimes referred to as "the ethic of the golden rule."

circadian rhythm. A 24-hour biological rhythm controlled by a "pacemaker" in the brain that sends messages to other systems in the body. Circadian rhythm influences various regulatory functions, including the sleep-wake cycle, body temperature regulation, patterns of activity such as eating and drinking, and hormonal and neurotransmitter secretion.

circumstantiality. In speaking, the delay of an individual to reach the point of a communication, owing to unnecessary and tedious details.

civil law. Law that protects the private and property rights of individuals and businesses.

clang associations. A pattern of speech in which the choice of words is governed by sounds. Clang associations often take the form of rhyming.

classical conditioning. A type of learning that occurs when an unconditioned stimulus (UCS) that produces an unconditioned response (UCR) is paired with a conditioned stimulus (CS), until the CS alone produces the same response, which is then called a conditioned response (CR). Pavlov's example: food (i.e., UCS) causes salivation (i.e., UCR); ringing bell (i.e., CS) with food (i.e., UCS) causes salivation (i.e., UCR), ringing bell alone (i.e., CS) causes salivation (i.e., CR).

codependency. An exaggerated dependent pattern of learned behaviors, beliefs, and feelings that make life painful. It is a dependence on people and things outside the self, alongwith neglect of the self to the point of having little self-identity.

cognition. Mental operations that relate to logic, awareness, intellect, memory, language, and reasoning powers.

cognitive development. A series of stages described by Piaget through which individuals progress, demonstrating at each successive stage a higher level of logical organization than at each previous stage.

cognitive domain. A category of learning that involves knowledge and thought processes within the individual's intellectual ability. The individual must be able to synthesize information at an intellectual level before the actual behaviors are performed.

cognitive maturity. The capability to perform all mental operations needed for adulthood.

cognitive therapy. A type of therapy in which the individual is taught to control thought distortions that are considered to be a factor in the development and maintenance of emotional disorders.

colposcope. An instrument that contains a magnifying lens and to which a 35-mm camera can be attached. A colposcope is used to examine for tears and abrasions inside the vaginal area of a sexual assault victim.

common law. Laws that are derived from decisions made in previous cases.

community. A group of people living close to and depending to some extent on each other.

compensation. Covering up a real or perceived weakness by emphasizing a trait one considers more desirable.

complementary medicine. Practices that differ from usual traditional (allopathic) medicine, but may in fact supplement it in a positive way.

compounded rape reaction. Symptoms that are in addition to the typical rape response of physical complaints, rage, humiliation, fear, and sleep disturbances. They include depression and suicide, substance abuse, and even psychotic behaviors.

concrete thinking. Thought processes that are focused on specifics rather than on generalities and immediate issues rather than eventual outcomes. Individuals who are experiencing concrete thinking are unable to comprehend abstract terminology.

confidentiality. The right of an individual to the assurance that his or her case will not be discussed outside the boundaries of the health care team.

contextual stimulus. Conditions present in the environment that support a focal stimulus and influence a threat to self-esteem.

contingency contracting. A written contract between individuals used to modify behavior. Benefits and consequences for fulfilling the terms of the contract are delineated.

controlled response pattern. The response to rape in which feelings are masked or hidden, and a calm, composed, or subdued affect is seen.

counselor. One who listens as the client reviews feelings related to difficulties he or she is experiencing in any aspect of life; one of the nursing roles identified by H. Peplau.

covert sensitization. An aversion technique used to modify behavior that relies on the individual's imagination to produce unpleasant symptoms. When the individual is about to succumb to undesirable behavior, he or she visualizes something that is offensive or even nauseating in an effort to block the behavior.

criminal law. Law that provides protection from conduct deemed injurious to the public welfare. It provides for punishment of those found to have engaged in such conduct.

crisis. Psychological disequilibrium in a person who confronts a hazardous circumstance that constitutes an important problem which for the time he or she can neither escape nor solve with usual problem-solving resources.

crisis intervention. An emergency type of assistance in which the intervener becomes a part of the individual's life situation. The focus is to provide guidance and support to help mobilize the resources needed to resolve the crisis and restore or generate an improvement in previous level of functioning. Usually lasts no longer than 6 to 8 weeks.

critical pathways of care. An abbreviated plan of care that provides outcome-based guidelines for goal achievement within a designated length of time.

culture. A particular society's entire way of living, encompassing shared patterns of belief, feeling, and knowledge that guide people's conduct and are passed down from generation to generation.

curandera. A female folk healer in the Latino culture.

curandero. A male folk healer in the Latino culture.

cycle of battering. Three phases of predictable behaviors that are repeated over time in a relationship between a batterer and a victim: tension-building phase; the acute battering incident; and the calm, loving, respite (honeymoon) phase.

cyclothymia. A chronic mood disturbance involving numerous episodes of hypomania and depressed mood, of insufficient severity or duration to meet the criteria for bipolar disorder.

D

date rape. A situation in which the rapist is known to the victim. This may occur during dating or with acquaintances or school mates.

decatastrophizing. In cognitive therapy, with this technique the therapist assists the client to examine the validity of a negative automatic thought. Even if some validity exists, the client is then encouraged to review ways to cope adaptively, moving beyond the current crisis situation.

defamation of character. An individual may be liable for defamation of character by sharing with others information about a person that is detrimental to his or her reputation.

deinstitutionalization. The removal of mentally ill individuals from institutions and the subsequent plan to provide care for these individuals in the community setting.

delirium. A state of mental confusion and excitement characterized by disorientation for time and place, often with hallucinations, incoherent speech, and a continual state of aimless physical activity.

delusions. False personal beliefs, not consistent with a person's intelligence or cultural background. The individual continues to have the belief in spite of obvious proof that it is false and/or irrational.

dementia. Global impairment of cognitive functioning that is progressive and interferes with social and occupational abilities.

dendrites. The cellular processes of a neuron that carry impulses toward the cell body.

denial. Refusal to acknowledge the existence of a real situation and/or the feelings associated with it.

density. The number of people in a given environmental space, influencing interpersonal interaction.

depersonalization. An alteration in the perception or experience of the self so that the feeling of one's own reality is temporarily lost.

derealization. An alteration in the perception or experience of the external world so that it seems strange or unreal.

detoxification. The process of withdrawal from a substance to which one has become dependent.

diagnostically related groups (DRGs). A system used to determine prospective payment rates for reimbursement of hospital care based on the client's diagnosis.

Diagnostic and Statistical Manual of Mental Disorders, 4th ed, Text Revision (DSM-IV-TR). Standard nomenclature of emotional illness published by the American Psychiatric Association (APA) and used by all health care practitioners. It classifies mental illness and presents guidelines and diagnostic criteria for various mental disorders.

dichotomous thinking. In this type of thinking, situations are viewed in all-or-nothing, black-or-white, good-or-bad terms.

directed association. A technique used to help clients bring into consciousness events that have been repressed. Specific thoughts are guided and directed by the psychoanalyst.

discriminative stimulus. A stimulus that precedes a behavioral response and predicts that a particular reinforcement will occur. Individuals learn to discriminate between various stimuli that will produce the responses they desire.

disengagement. In family theory, disengagement refers to extreme separateness among family members. It is promoted by rigid boundaries or lack of communication among family members.

disengagement theory. The hypothesis that there is a process of mutual withdrawal of aging persons and society from each other that is correlated with successful aging. This theory has been challenged by many investigators.

displacement. Feelings are transferred from one target to another that is considered less threatening or neutral.

distraction. In cognitive therapy, when dysfunctional cognitions have been recognized, activities are identified that can be used to distract the client and divert him or her from the intrusive thoughts or depressive ruminations that are contributing to the client's maladaptive responses.

disulfiram. A drug that is administered to individuals who abuse alcohol as a deterrent to drinking. Ingestion of alcohol while disulfiram is in the body results in a syndrome of symptoms that can produce a great deal of discomfort, and can even result in death if the blood alcohol level is high.

domains of learning. Categories in which individuals learn or gain knowledge and demonstrate behavior. There are three domains of learning: affective, cognitive, and psychomotor.

dyspareunia. Pain during sexual intercourse.

dysthymic disorder. A depressive neurosis. The symptoms are similar to, if somewhat milder than, those ascribed to major depression. There is no loss of contact with reality.

dystonia. Involuntary muscular movements (spasms) of the face, arms, legs, and neck; may occur as an extrapyramidal side effect of some antipsychotic medications.

E

echolalia. The parrot-like repetition, by an individual with loose ego boundaries, of the words spoken by another.

echopraxia. An individual with loose ego boundaries attempting to identify with another person by imitating movements that the other person makes.

eclampsia. A toxic condition that can occur late in pregnancy and is manifested by extremely high blood pressure, blurred vision, severe abdominal pain, headaches, and convulsions. The condition is sometimes fatal.

ego. One of the three elements of the personality identified by Freud as the rational self or "reality principle." The ego seeks to maintain harmony between the external world, the id, and the superego.

ego defense mechanisms. Strategies employed by the ego for protection in the face of threat to biological or psychological integrity. (See individual defense mechanisms.)

egoistic suicide. The response of an individual who feels separate and apart from the mainstream of society.

electroconvulsive therapy (ECT). A type of somatic treatment in which electric current is applied to the brain through electrodes placed on the temples. A grand mal seizure produces the desired effect. This is used with severely depressed patients refractory to antidepressant medications.

emaciated. The state of being excessively thin or physically wasted.

emotional injury of a child. A pattern of behavior on the part of the parent or caretaker that results in serious impairment of the child's social, emotional, or intellectual functioning.

emotional neglect of a child. A chronic failure by the parent or caretaker to provide the child with the hope, love, and support necessary for the development of a sound, healthy personality.

empathy. The ability to see beyond outward behavior, and sense accurately another's inner experiencing. With empathy, one can accurately perceive and understand the meaning and relevance in the thoughts and feelings of another.

enmeshment. Exaggerated connectedness among family members. It occurs in response to diffuse boundaries in which there is overinvestment, overinvolvement, and lack of differentiation between individuals or subsystems.

esophageal varices. Veins in the esophagus become distended because of excessive pressure from defective blood flow through a cirrhotic liver.

essential hypertension. Persistent elevation of blood pressure for which there is no apparent cause or associated underlying disease.

ethical dilemma. A situation that arises when on the basis of moral considerations an appeal can be made for taking each of two opposing courses of action.

ethical egoism. An ethical theory espousing that what is "right" and "good" is what is best for the individual making the decision.

ethics. A branch of philosophy dealing with values related to human conduct, to the rightness and wrongness of certain actions, and to the goodness and badness of the motives and ends of such actions.

ethnicity. The concept of people identifying with each other because of a shared heritage.

exhibitionism. A paraphilic disorder characterized by a recurrent urge to expose one's genitals to a stranger.

expressed response pattern. Pattern of behavior in which the victim of rape expresses feelings of fear, anger, and anxiety through such behavior as crying, sobbing, smiling, restlessness, and tenseness; in contrast to the rape victim who withholds feelings in the controlled response pattern.

extinction. The gradual decrease in frequency or disappearance of a response when the positive reinforcement is withheld.

extrapyramidal symptoms (EPS). A variety of responses that originate outside the pyramidal tracts and in the basal ganglion of the brain. Symptoms may include tremors, chorea, dystonia, akinesia, akathisia, and others. May occur as a side effect of some antipsychotic medications.

F

false imprisonment. The deliberate and unauthorized confinement of a person within fixed limits by the use of threat or force. A nurse may be charged with false imprisonment by placing a patient in restraints against his or her will in a nonemergency situation.

family structure. A family system in which the structure is founded on a set of invisible principles that influence the interaction among family members. These principles are established over time and become the "laws" that govern the conduct of various family members.

family system. A system in which the parts of the whole may be the marital dyad, parent-child dyad, or sibling groups. Each of these subsystems are further divided into subsystems of individuals.

family therapy. A type of therapy in which the focus is on relationships within the family. The family is viewed as a system in which the members are interdependent, and a change in one creates change in all.

fetishism. A paraphilic disorder characterized by recurrent sexual urges and sexually arousing fantasies involving the use of non-living objects.

fight or flight. A syndrome of physical symptoms that result from an individual's real or perceived perception that harm or danger is imminent.

flexible boundary. A personal boundary is flexible when, because of unusual circumstances, individuals can alter limits that they have set for themselves. Flexible boundaries are healthy boundaries.

flooding. Sometimes called implosive therapy, this technique is used to desensitize individuals to phobic stimuli. The individual is "flooded" with a continuous presentation (usually through mental imagery) of the phobic stimulus until it no longer elicits anxiety.

focal stimulus. A situation of immediate concern that results in a threat to self-esteem.

focus charting.® A type of documentation that follows a data, action, and response (DAR) format. The main perspective is a client "focus," which can be a nursing diagnosis, a client's concern, change in status, or significant event in the client's therapy. The focus cannot be a medical diagnosis.

folk medicine. A system of health care within various cultures that is provided by a local practitioner, not professionally trained, but who uses techniques specific to that culture in the art of healing.

forensic. Pertaining to the law; legal.

forensic nursing. The application of forensic science combined with the bio-psychological education of the registered nurse, in the scientific investigation, evidence collection and preservation, analysis, prevention and treatment of trauma and/or death related medical-legal issues.

free association. A technique used to help individuals bring to consciousness material that has been repressed. The individual is encouraged to verbalize whatever comes into his or her mind, drifting naturally from one thought to another.

frotteurism. A paraphilic disorder characterized by the recurrent preoccupation with intense sexual urges or fantasies involving touching or rubbing against a nonconsenting person.

fugue. A sudden unexpected travel away from home or customary work locale with the assumption of a new identity and an inability to recall one's previous identity; usually occurring in response to severe psychosocial stress.

G

gains. The reinforcements an individual receives for somaticizing.

gains, primary. The receipt of positive reinforcement for somaticizing through added attention, sympathy, and nurturing.

gains, secondary. The receipt of positive reinforcement for somaticizing by being able to avoid difficult situations because of physical complaint.

gains, tertiary. The receipt of positive reinforcement for somaticizing by causing the focus of the family to switch to him or her and away from conflict that may be occurring within the family.

Gamblers Anonymous (GA). An organization of inspirational group therapy, modeled after Alcoholics Anonymous (AA), for individuals who desire to, but cannot, stop gambling.

gender identity disorder. A sense of discomfort associated with an incongruence between biologically assigned gender and subjectively experienced gender.

generalized anxiety disorder. A disorder characterized by chronic (at least 6 months), unrealistic, and excessive anxiety and worry.

genogram. A graphic representation of a family system. It may cover several generations. Emphasis is on family roles and emotional relatedness among members. Genograms facilitate recognition of areas requiring change.

genotype. The total set of genes present in an individual at the time of conception, and coded in the DNA.

genuineness. The ability to be open, honest, and "real" in interactions with others; the awareness of what one is experiencing internally and the ability to project the quality of this inner experiencing in a relationship.

geriatrics. The branch of clinical medicine specializing in the care of the elderly and concerned with the problems of aging.

gerontology. The study of normal aging.

geropsychiatry. The branch of clinical medicine specializing in psychopathology of the elderly.

gonorrhea. A sexually transmitted disease caused by the bacterium *N. gonorrhoeae* and resulting in inflammation of the genital mucosa. Treatment is through the use of antibiotics, particularly penicillin. Serious complications occur if the disease is left untreated.

"granny-bashing." Media-generated term for abuse of the elderly.

"granny-dumping." Media-generated term for abandoning elderly individuals at emergency departments, nursing homes, or other facilities-literally, leaving them in the hands of others when the strain of caregiving becomes intolerable.

grief. A subjective state of emotional, physical, and social responses to the real or perceived loss of a valued entity. Change and failure can also be perceived as losses. The grief response consists of a set of relatively predictable behaviors that describe the subjective state that accompanies mourning.

grief, exaggerated. A reaction in which all of the symptoms associated with normal grieving are exaggerated out of proportion. Pathological depression is a type of exaggerated grief.

grief, inhibited. The absence of evidence of grief when it ordinarily would be expected.

group therapy. A therapy group, founded in a specific theoretical framework, led by a person with an advanced degree in psychology, social work, nursing, or medicine. The goal is to encourage improvement in interpersonal functioning.

gynecomastia. Enlargement of the breasts in men; may be a side effect of some antipsychotic medications.

H

hallucinations. False sensory perceptions not associated with real external stimuli. Hallucinations may involve any of the five senses.

hepatic encephalopathy. A brain disorder resulting from the inability of the cirrhotic liver to convert ammonia to urea for excretion. The continued rise in serum ammonia results in progressively impaired mental functioning, apathy, euphoria or depression, sleep disturbances, increasing confusion, and progression to coma and eventual death.

histrionic personality disorder. Conscious or unconscious overly dramatic behavior for the purpose of drawing attention to oneself.

HIV associated dementia (HAD). A neuropathological syndrome, possibly caused by chronic HIV encephalitis and myelitis and manifested by cognitive, behavioral, and motor symptoms that become more severe with progression of the disease.

HIV wasting syndrome. An absence of concurrent illness other than HIV infection, and presence of the following: fever, weakness, weight loss, and chronic diarrhea.

home care. A wide range of health and social services that are delivered at home to recovering, disabled, chronically or terminally ill persons in need of medical, nursing, social, or therapeutic treatment and/or assistance with essential activities of daily living.

homocysteine. An amino acid produced by the catabolism of methionine. Elevated levels may be linked to increased risk of cardiovascular disease.

homosexuality. A sexual preference for persons of the same gender.

hormone replacement therapy (HRT). The process of replacing declining hormones— estrogen and progesterone in women, testosterone in men—to prevent symptoms associated with the decline. Female HRT is thought to prevent osteoporosis, hot flashes, and vaginal dryness. Testosterone replacement therapy appears to restore libido and sexual functioning and improves bone mass, muscle mass, and strength in older men.

hospice. A program that provides palliative and supportive care to meet the special needs arising out of the physical, psychosocial, spiritual, social, and economic stresses that are experienced during the final stages of illness and during bereavement.

human immunodeficiency virus (HIV). The virus that is the etiological agent that produces the immunosuppression resulting in AIDS.

humors. The four body fluids described by Hippocrates: blood, black bile, yellow bile, and phlegm. Hippocrates associated insanity and mental illness with these four fluids.

hypersomnia. Excessive sleepiness or seeking excessive amounts of sleep.

hypertensive crisis. A potentially life-threatening syndrome that results when an individual taking MAO inhibitors eats a product high in tyramine. Symptoms include severe occipital headache, palpitations, nausea and vomiting, nuchal rigidity, fever, sweating, marked increase in blood pressure, chest pain, and coma. Foods with tyramine include aged cheeses or other aged, overripe, and fermented foods; broad beans; pickled herring; beef or chicken liver; preserved meats; beer and wine; yeast products; chocolate; caffeinated drinks; canned figs; sour cream; yogurt; soy sauce; and some over-the-counter cold medications and diet pills.

hypnosis. A treatment for disorders brought on by repressed anxiety. The individual is directed into a state of subconsciousness and assisted, through suggestions, to recall certain events that he or she cannot recall while conscious.

hypochondriasis. The unrealistic preoccupation with fear of having a serious illness.

hypomania. A mild form of mania. Symptoms are excessive hyperactivity, but not severe enough to cause marked impairment in social or occupational functioning or to require hospitalization.

hysteria. A polysymptomatic disorder characterized by recurrent, multiple somatic complaints often described dramatically.

I

id. One of the three components of the personality identified by Freud as the "pleasure principle." The id is the locus of instinctual drives; is present at birth; and compels the infant to satisfy needs and seek immediate gratification.

identification. An attempt to increase self-worth by acquiring certain attributes and characteristics of an individual one admires.

illusion. A misperception of a real external stimulus.

implosion therapy. See **flooding**.

incest. Sexual exploitation of a child under 18 years of age by a relative or non-relative who holds a position of trust in the family.

informed consent. Permission granted to a physician by a client to perform a therapeutic procedure, prior to which information about the procedure has been presented to the client with adequate time given for consideration about the pros and cons.

insomnia. Difficulty initiating or maintaining sleep.

insulin coma therapy. The induction of a hypoglycemic coma aimed at alleviating psychotic symptoms; a dangerous procedure, questionably effective, no longer used in psychiatry.

integration. The process used with individuals with dissociative identity disorder in an effort to bring all the personalities together into one; usually achieved through hypnosis.

intellectualization. An attempt to avoid expressing actual emotions associated with a stressful situation by using the intellectual processes of logic, reasoning, and analysis.

interdisciplinary care. A concept of providing care for a client in which members of various disciplines work together with common goals and shared responsibilities for meeting those goals.

intimate distance. The closest distance that individuals will allow between themselves and others. In the United States, this distance is 0 to 18 inches.

introjection. The beliefs and values of another individual are internalized and symbolically become a part of the self, to the extent that the feeling of separateness or distinctness is lost.

isolation. The separation of a thought or a memory from the feeling tone or emotions associated with it (sometimes called emotional isolation).

J

justice. An ethical principle reflecting that all individuals should be treated equally and fairly.

K

Kantianism. The ethical principle espousing that decisions should be made and actions taken out of a sense of duty.

Kaposi's sarcoma. Malignant areas of cell proliferation initially in the skin and eventually in other body sites; thought to be related to the immunocompromised state that accompanies AIDS.

kleptomania. A recurrent failure to resist impulses to steal objects not needed for personal use or monetary value.

Korsakoff's psychosis. A syndrome of confusion, loss of recent memory, and confabulation in alcoholics, caused by a deficiency of thiamine. It often occurs together with Wernicke's encephalopathy and may be termed Wernicke-Korsakoff's syndrome.

L

la belle indifference. A symptom of conversion disorder in which there is a relative lack of concern that is out of keeping with the severity of the impairment.

laissez-faire. A leadership type in which the leader lets group members do as they please. There is no direction from the leader. Member productivity and morale may be low, owing to frustration from lack of direction.

lesbian. A female homosexual.

libel. An action with which an individual may be charged for sharing with another individual, in writing, information that is detrimental to someone's reputation.

libido. Freud's term for the psychic energy used to fulfill basic physiological needs or instinctual drives such as hunger, thirst, and sexuality.

limbic system. The part of the brain that is sometimes called the "emotional brain." It is associated with feelings of fear and anxiety; anger and aggression; love, joy, and hope; and with sexuality and social behavior.

long-term memory. Memory for remote events, or those that occurred many years ago. The type of memory that is preserved in the elderly individual.

luto. In the Mexican-American culture, the period of mourning following the death of a loved one which is symbolized by wearing black, black and white, or dark clothing and by subdued behavior.

M

magical thinking. A primitive form of thinking in which an individual believes that thinking about a possible occurrence can make it happen.

magnification. A type of thinking in which the negative significance of an event is exaggerated.

maladaptation. A failure of the body to return to homeostasis following a physiological and/or psychological response to stress, disrupting the individual's integrity.

malpractice. The failure of one rendering professional services to exercise that degree of skill and learning commonly applied under all the circumstances in the community by the average prudent reputable member of the profession with the result of injury, loss, or damage to the recipient of those services or to those entitled to rely upon them.

managed care. A concept purposefully designed to control the balance between cost and quality of care. Examples of managed care are health maintenance organizations (HMOs) and preferred provider organizations (PPOs). The amount and type of health care that the individual receives is determined by the organization providing the managed care.

mania. A type of bipolar disorder in which the predominant mood is elevated, expansive, or irritable. Motor activity is frenzied and excessive. Psychotic features may or may not be present.

mania, delirious. A grave form of mania characterized by severe clouding of consciousness and representing an intensification of the symptoms associated with mania. The symptoms of delirious mania have become relatively rare since the availability of antipsychotic medications.

marital rape. Sexual violence directed at a marital partner against that person's will.

marital schism. A state of severe chronic disequilibrium and discord within the marital dyad, with recurrent threats of separation.

marital skew. A marital relationship in which there is lack of equal partnership. One partner dominates the relationship and the other partner.

masochism. Sexual stimulation derived from being humiliated, beaten, bound, or otherwise made to suffer.

Medicaid. A system established by the federal government to provide medical care benefits for indigent Americans. Medicaid funds are matched by the states, and coverage varies significantly from state to state.

Medicare. A system established by the federal government to provide medical care benefits for elderly Americans.

meditation. A method of relaxation in which an individual sits in a quiet place and focuses total concentration on an object, word, or thought.

melancholia. A severe form of major depressive episode. Symptoms are exaggerated, and interest or pleasure in virtually all activities is lost.

menopause. The period marking the permanent cessation of menstrual activity; usually occurs at approximately 48 to 51 years of age.

mental health. The successful adaptation to stressors from the internal or external environment, evidenced by thoughts, feelings, and behaviors that are age-appropriate and congruent with local and cultural norms.

mental illness. Maladaptive responses to stressors from the internal or external environment, evidenced by thoughts, feelings, and behaviors that are incongruent with the local and cultural norms, and interfere with the individual's social, occupational, and/or physical functioning.

mental imagery. A method of stress reduction that employs the imagination. The individual focuses imagination on a scenario that is particularly relaxing to him or her (e.g., a scene on a quiet seashore, a mountain atmosphere, or floating through the air on a fluffy white cloud).

meridians. In Chinese medicine, pathways along the body in which the healing energy (qi) flows, and which are links between acupoints.

migraine personality. Personality characteristics that have been attributed to the migraine-prone person. The characteristics include perfectionistic, overly conscientious, somewhat inflexible, neat and tidy, compulsive, hard worker, intelligent, exacting, and places a very high premium on success, setting high (sometimes unrealistic) expectations on self and others.

milieu. French for "middle"; the English translation connotes "surroundings, or environment."

milieu therapy. Also called therapeutic community, or therapeutic environment, this type of therapy consists of a scientific structuring of the environment in order to effect behavioral changes and to improve the individual's psychological health and functioning.

minimization. A type of thinking in which the positive significance of an event is minimized or undervalued.

mobile outreach units. Programs in which volunteers and paid professionals drive or walk around and seek out homeless individuals who need assistance with physical or psychological care.

modeling. Learning new behaviors by imitating the behaviors of others.

mood. An individual's sustained emotional tone, which significantly influences behavior, personality, and perception.

moral behavior. Conduct that results from serious critical thinking about how individuals ought to treat others; reflects respect for human life, freedom, justice, or confidentiality.

moral-ethical self. That aspect of the personal identity that functions as observer, standard setter, dreamer, comparer, and most of all evaluator of who the individual says he or she is. This component of the personal identity makes judgments that influence an individual's self-evaluation.

mourning. The psychological process (or stages) through which the individual passes on the way to successful adaptation to the loss of a valued object.

multidisciplinary care. A concept of providing care for a client in which individual disciplines provide specific services for the client without formal arrangement for interaction between the disciplines.

N

narcissistic personality disorder. A disorder characterized by an exaggerated sense of self-worth. These individuals lack empathy and are hypersensitive to the evaluation of others.

narcolepsy. A disorder in which the characteristic manifestation is sleep attacks. The individual cannot prevent falling asleep, even in the middle of a sentence or performing a task.

natural law theory. The ethical theory that has as its moral precept to "do good and avoid evil" at all costs. Natural law ethics are grounded in a concern for the human good, that is based on man's ability to live according to the dictates of reason.

negative reinforcement. Increasing the probability that a behavior will recur by removal of an undesirable reinforcing stimulus.

negativism. Strong resistance to suggestions or directions; exhibiting behaviors contrary to what is expected.

negligence. The failure to do something which a reasonable person, guided by those considerations which ordinarily regulate human affairs, would do, or doing something which a prudent and reasonable person would not do.

neologism. New words that an individual invents that are meaningless to others, but have symbolic meaning to the psychotic person.

neuroendocrinology. The study of hormones functioning within the neurological system.

neuroleptic. Antipsychotic medication used to prevent or control psychotic symptoms.

neuroleptic malignant syndrome (NMS). A rare but potentially fatal complication of treatment with neuroleptic drugs. Symptoms include severe muscle rigidity, high fever, tachycardia, fluctuations in blood pressure, diaphoresis, and rapid deterioration of mental status to stupor and coma.

neuron. A nerve cell; consists of a cell body, an axon, and dendrites.

neurotic disorder. A psychiatric disturbance, characterized by excessive anxiety and/or depression, disrupted bodily functions, unsatisfying interpersonal relationships, and behaviors that interfere with routine functioning. There is no loss of contact with reality.

neurotransmitter. A chemical that is stored in the axon terminals of the presynaptic neuron. An electrical impulse through the neuron stimulates the release of the neurotransmitter into the synaptic cleft, which in turn determines whether or not another electrical impulse is generated.

nonassertiveness. Individuals who are nonassertive (sometimes called passive) seek to please others at the expense of denying their own basic human rights.

nonmaleficence. The ethical principle that espouses abstaining from negative acts toward another, including acting carefully to avoid harm.

nursing diagnosis. A clinical judgment about individual, family, or community responses to actual and potential health problems/life processes. Nursing diagnoses provide the basis for selection of nursing interventions to achieve outcomes for which the nurse is accountable.

nursing process. A dynamic, systematic process by which nurses assess, diagnose, identify outcomes, plan, implement, and evaluate nursing care. It has been called "nursing's scientific methodology." Nursing process gives order and consistency to nursing intervention.

O

obesity. The state of having a body mass index of 30 or above.

object constancy. The phase in the separation/individuation process when the child learns to relate to objects in an effective, constant manner. A sense of separateness is established, and the child is able to internalize a sustained image of the loved object or person when out of sight.

obsessive–compulsive disorder. Recurrent thoughts or ideas (obsessions) that an individual is unable to put out of his or her mind, and actions that an individual is unable to refrain from performing (compulsions). The obsessions and compulsions are severe enough to interfere with social and occupational functioning.

oculogyric crisis. An attack of involuntary deviation and fixation of the eyeballs, usually in the upward position. It may last for several minutes or hours and may occur as an extrapyramidal side effect of some antipsychotic medications.

operant conditioning. The learning of a particular action or type of behavior that is followed by a reinforcement.

opportunistic infection. Infections with any organism, but especially fungi and bacteria, that occur due to the opportunity afforded by the altered physiological state of the host. Opportunistic infections have long been a defining characteristic of AIDS.

orgasm. A peaking of sexual pleasure, with release of sexual tension and rhythmic contraction of the perineal muscles and pelvic reproductive organs.

osteoporosis. A reduction in the mass of bone per unit of volume which interferes with the mechanical support function of bone. This process occurs because of demineralization of the bones, and is escalated in women about the time of menopause.

overgeneralization. Also called "absolutistic thinking." With overgeneralization, sweeping conclusions are made based on one incident—a type of "all or nothing" kind of thinking.

overt sensitization. A type of aversion therapy that produces unpleasant consequences for undesirable behavior. An example is the use of disulfiram therapy with alcoholics, that induces an undesirable physical response if the individual has consumed any alcohol.

P

palilalia. Repeating one's own sounds or words (a type of vocal tic associated with Tourette's disorder).

panic disorder. A disorder characterized by recurrent panic attacks, the onset of which are unpredictable, and manifested by intense apprehension, fear, or terror, often associated with feelings of impending doom, and accompanied by intense physical discomfort.

paradoxical intervention. In family therapy, "prescribing the symptom." The therapist requests that the family continue to engage in the behavior that they are trying to change. Tension is relieved, and the family is able to view more clearly the possible solutions to their problem.

paralanguage. The gestural component of the spoken word. It consists of pitch, tone, and loudness of spoken messages, the rate of speaking, expressively placed pauses, and emphasis assigned to certain words.

paranoia. A term that implies extreme suspiciousness. Paranoid schizophrenia is characterized by persecutory delusions and hallucinations of a threatening nature.

paraphilias. Repetitive behaviors or fantasies that involve nonhuman objects, real or simulated suffering or humiliation, or nonconsenting partners.

parasomnia. Unusual or undesirable behaviors that occur during sleep (e.g., nightmares, sleep terrors, and sleepwalking).

passive–aggressive behavior. Behavior that defends an individual's own basic rights by expressing resistance to social and occupational demands. Sometimes called indirect aggression, this behavior takes the form of sly, devious, and undermining actions that express the opposite of what they are really feeling.

pathological gambling. A failure to resist impulses to gamble, and gambling behavior that compromises, disrupts, or damages personal, family, or vocational pursuits.

pedophilia. Recurrent urges and sexually arousing fantasies involving sexual activity with a prepubescent child.

peer assistance programs. A program established by the American Nurses' Association to assist impaired nurses. The individuals who administer these efforts are nurse members of the state associations, as well as nurses who are in recovery themselves.

perseveration. Persistent repetition of the same word or idea in response to different questions.

persistent generalized lymphadenopathy (PGL). A condition common in HIV-infected individuals in which there are lymph nodes greater than 1 cm in diameter at two extrainguinal sites persisting for three months or longer, not attributed to other causes, and not associated with other substantial constitutional symptoms.

personal distance. The distance between individuals who are having interactions of a personal nature, such as a close conversation. In the U.S. culture, personal distance is approximately 18 to 40 inches.

personal identity. An individual's self-perception that defines one's functions as observer, standard setter, and self-evaluator. It strives to maintain a stable self-image and relates to what the individual strives to become.

personal self. See **personal identity**.

personality. Deeply ingrained patterns of behavior, which include the way one relates to, perceives, and thinks about the environment and oneself.

personalization. Taking complete responsibility for situations without considering that other circumstances may have contributed to the outcome.

pharmacoconvulsive therapy. The chemical induction of a convulsion used in the past for the reduction of psychotic symptoms, a type of therapy no longer used in psychiatry.

phencyclidine HCl. An anesthetic used in veterinary medicine; used illegally as a hallucinogen, referred to as PCP or angel dust.

phenotype. Characteristics of physical manifestations that identify a particular genotype. Examples of phenotypes include eye color, height, blood type, language, and hairstyle. Phenotypes may be genetic or acquired.

phobia. An irrational fear.

phobia, social. The fear of being humiliated in social situations.

phobia, specific. A persistent fear of a specific object or situation, other than the fear of being unable to escape from a situation (agoraphobia) or the fear of being humiliated in social situations (social phobia).

physical neglect of a child. The failure on the part of the parent or caregiver to provide for a child's basic needs, such as food, clothing, shelter, medical-dental care, and supervision.

physical self. A personal appraisal by an individual of his or her physical being and includes physical attributes, functioning, sexuality, wellness-illness state, and appearance.

PIE charting. More specifically called "APIE," this method of documentation has an assessment, problem, intervention, and evaluation (APIE) format and is a problem-oriented system used to document nursing process.

***Pneumocystis carinii* pneumonia (PCP).** The most common life-threatening opportunistic infection seen in patients with AIDS. Symptoms include fever, exertional dyspnea, and nonproductive cough.

positive reinforcement. A reinforcement stimulus that increases the probability that the behavior will recur.

postpartum depression. Depression that occurs during the postpartum period. It may be related to hormonal changes, tryptophan metabolism, or alterations in membrane transport during the early postpartum period. Other predisposing factors may also be influential.

posttraumatic stress disorder (PTSD). A syndrome of symptoms that develop following a psychologically distressing event that is outside the range of usual human experience (e.g., rape, war). The individual is unable to put the experience out of his or her mind, has nightmares, flashbacks, and panic attacks.

posturing. The voluntary assumption of inappropriate or bizarre postures.

preassaultive tension state. Behaviors predictive of potential violence. They include excessive motor activity, tense posture, defiant affect, clenched teeth and fists, and other arguing, demanding, and threatening behaviors.

precipitating event. A stimulus arising from the internal or external environment that is perceived by an individual as taxing or exceeding his or her resources and endangering his or her well-being.

predisposing factors. A variety of elements that influence how an individual perceives and responds to a stressful event. Types of predisposing factors include genetic influences, past experiences, and existing conditions.

Premack principle. This principle states that a frequently occurring response (R1) can serve as a positive reinforcement for a response (R2) that occurs less frequently. For example, a girl may talk to friends on phone (R2) only if she does her homework (R1).

premature ejaculation. Ejaculation that occurs with minimal sexual stimulation or before, upon, or shortly after penetration and before the person wishes it.

premenstrual dysphoric disorder. A disorder that is characterized by depressed mood, anxiety, mood swings, and decreased interest in activities during the week prior to menses and subsiding shortly after the onset of menstruation.

presenile. Pertaining to premature old age as judged by mental or physical condition. In presenile onset dementia initial symptoms appear at age 65 or younger.

priapism. Prolonged painful penile erection, may occur as an adverse effect of some antidepressant medications, particularly trazodone.

primary dementia. Dementia, such as Alzheimer's disease, in which the dementia itself is the major sign of some organic brain disease not directly related to any other organic illness.

primary prevention. Reduction of the incidence of mental disorders within the population by helping individuals to cope more effectively with stress and by trying to diminish stressors within the environment.

privileged communication. A doctrine common to most states that grants certain privileges under which they may refuse to reveal information about and communications with clients.

problem-oriented recording (POR). A system of documentation that follows a subjective, objective, assessment, plan, implementation, and evaluation (SOAPIE) format. It is based on a list of identified patient problems to which each entry is directed.

progressive relaxation. A method of deep muscle relaxation in which each muscle group is alternately tensed and relaxed in a systematic order with the person concentrating on the contrast of sensations experienced from tensing and relaxing.

projection. Attributing to another person feelings or impulses unacceptable to oneself.

prospective payment. The program of cost containment within the health care profession directed at setting forth preestablished amounts that would be reimbursed for specific diagnoses.

prostatic-specific antigen (PSA). A blood test for the early detection of prostate cancer.

pseudocyesis. A condition in which an individual has nearly all the signs and symptoms of pregnancy but is not pregnant; a conversion reaction.

pseudodementia. Symptoms of depression that mimic those of dementia.

pseudohostility. A family interaction pattern characterized by a state of chronic conflict and alienation among family members. This relationship pattern allows family members to deny underlying fears of tenderness and intimacy.

pseudomutuality. A family interaction pattern characterized by a facade of mutual regard with the purpose of denying underlying fears of separation and hostility.

psychiatric home care. Care provided by psychiatric nurses in the client's home. Psychiatric home care nurses must have physical and psychosocial nursing skills to meet the demands of the client population they serve.

psychodrama. A specialized type of group therapy that employs a dramatic approach in which patients become "actors" in life situation scenarios. The goal is to resolve interpersonal conflicts in a less-threatening atmosphere than the real-life situation would present.

psychodynamic nursing. Being able to understand one's own behavior, to help others identify felt difficulties, and to apply principles of human relations to the problems that arise at all levels of experience.

psychoimmunology. The study of the implications of the immune system in psychiatry.

psychomotor domain. A category of learning in which the behaviors are processed and demonstrated. The information has been intellectually processed, and the individual is displaying motor behaviors.

psychomotor retardation. Extreme slowdown of physical movements. Posture slumps; speech is slowed; digestion becomes sluggish. Common in severe depression.

psychophysiological. Referring to psychological factors contributing to the initiation or exacerbation of a physical condition. Either a demonstrable organic pathology or a known pathophysiological process is involved.

psychosomatic. See **psychophysiological**.

psychotic disorder. A serious psychiatric disorder in which there is a gross disorganization of the personality, a marked disturbance in reality testing, and the impairment of interpersonal functioning and relationship to the external world.

public distance. Appropriate interactional distance for speaking in public or yelling to someone some distance away. U.S. culture defines this distance as 12 feet or more.

pyromania. An inability to resist the impulse to set fires.

Q

qi. In Chinese medicine, the healing energy that flows through pathways in the body called meridians. (Also called "chi.")

R

rape. The expression of power and dominance by means of sexual violence, most commonly by men over women, although men may also be rape victims. Rape is considered an act of aggression, not of passion.

rapport. The development between two people in a relationship of special feelings based on mutual acceptance, warmth, friendliness, common interest, a sense of trust, and a nonjudgmental attitude.

rationalization. Attempting to make excuses or formulate logical reasons to justify unacceptable feelings or behaviors.

reaction formation. Preventing unacceptable or undesirable thoughts or behaviors from being expressed by exaggerating opposite thoughts or types of behaviors.

receptor sites. Molecules that are situated on the cell membrane of the postsynaptic neuron that will accept only molecules with a complementary shape. These complementary molecules are specific to certain neurotransmitters that determine whether an electrical impulse will be excited or inhibited.

reciprocal inhibition. Also called counterconditioning, this technique serves to decrease or eliminate a behavior by introducing a more adaptive behavior, but one that is incompatible with the unacceptable behavior (e.g., introducing relaxation techniques to an anxious person; relaxation and anxiety are incompatible behaviors).

reframing. Changing the conceptual or emotional setting or viewpoint in relation to which a situation is experienced and placing it in another frame that fits the "facts" of the same concrete situation equally well or even better, and thereby changing its entire meaning. The behavior may not actually change, but the consequences of the behavior may change because of a change in the meaning attached to the behavior.

regression. A retreat to an earlier level of development and the comfort measures associated with that level of functioning.

religiosity. Excessive demonstration of or obsession with religious ideas and behavior; common in schizophrenia.

reminiscence therapy. A process of life review by elderly individuals that promotes self-esteem and provides assistance in working through unresolved conflicts from the past.

repression. The involuntary blocking of unpleasant feelings and experiences from one's awareness.

residual stimuli. Certain beliefs, attitudes, experiences, or traits that may contribute to an individual's low self-esteem.

retarded ejaculation. Delayed or absent ejaculation, even though the man has a firm erection and has had more than adequate stimulation.

retrograde ejaculation. Ejaculation of the seminal fluid backwards into the bladder; may occur as a side effect of antipsychotic medications.

right. That which an individual is entitled (by ethical or moral standards) to have, or to do, or to receive from others within the limits of the law.

rigid boundaries. A person with rigid boundaries is "closed" and difficult to bond with. Such a person has a narrow perspective on life, sees things one way, and cannot discuss matters that lie outside his or her perspective.

ritualistic behavior. Purposeless activities that an individual performs repeatedly in an effort to decrease anxiety (e.g., handwashing); common in obsessive compulsive disorder.

S

sadism. Recurrent urges and sexually arousing fantasies involving acts (real, not simulated) in which the psychological or physical suffering (including humiliation) of the victim is sexually exciting.

safe house or shelter. An establishment set up by many cities to provide protection for battered women and their children.

scapegoating. Occurs when hostility exists in a marriage dyad and an innocent third person (usually a child) becomes the target of blame for the problem.

schemas (core beliefs). Cognitive structures that consist of the individual's fundamental beliefs and assumptions, which develop early in life from personal experiences and identification with significant others. These concepts are reinforced by further learning experiences and in turn, influence the formation of other beliefs, values, and attitudes.

schizoid personality disorder. A profound defect in the ability to form personal relationships or to respond to others in any meaningful, emotional way.

schizotypal personality disorder. A disorder characterized by odd and eccentric behavior, not decompensating to the level of schizophrenia.

secondary dementia. Dementia that is caused by or related to another disease or condition, such as HIV disease or a cerebral trauma.

secondary prevention. Health care that is directed at reduction of the prevalence of psychiatric illness by shortening the course (duration) of the illness. This is accomplished through early identification of problems and prompt initiation of treatment.

selective abstraction (sometimes referred to as mental filter). A type of thinking in which a conclusion is drawn based on only a selected portion of the evidence.

self-concept. The composite of beliefs and feelings that one holds about oneself at a given time, formed from perceptions of others' reactions. The self-concept consists of the physical self, or body image; the personal self or identity; and the self-esteem.

self-consistency. The component of the personal identity that strives to maintain a stable self-image.

self-esteem. The degree of regard or respect that individuals have for themselves. It is a measure of worth that they place on their abilities and judgments.

self-expectancy. The component of the personal identity that is the individual's perception of what he or she wants to be, to do, or to become.

self-ideal. See **self-expectancy**.

senile. Pertaining to old age and the mental or physical weakness with which it is sometimes associated. In senile-onset dementia, the first symptoms appear after age 65.

sensate focus. A therapeutic technique used to treat individuals and couples with sexual dysfunction. The technique involves touching and being touched by another and focusing attention on the physical sensations encountered thereby. Clients gradually move through various levels of sensate focus that progress from nongenital touching to touching that includes the breasts and genitals; touching done in a simultaneous, mutual format rather than by one person at a time; and touching that extends to and allows eventually for the possibility of intercourse.

seroconversion. The development of evidence of antibody response to a disease or vaccine. The time at which antibodies may be detected in the blood.

sexual assault nurse examiner (SANE). A clinical forensic registered nurse who has received specialized training to provide care to the sexual assault victim.

sexual exploitation of a child. The inducement or coercion of a child into engaging in sexually explicit conduct for the purpose of promoting any performance (e.g., child pornography).

shaman. The Native American "medicine man" or folk healer.

shaping. In learning, one shapes the behavior of another by giving reinforcements for increasingly closer approximations to the desired behavior.

shelters. A variety of places designed to help the homeless, ranging from converted warehouses that provide cots or floor space on which to sleep overnight to significant operations that provide a multitude of social and health care services.

"ship of fools." The term given during the Middle Ages to sailing boats filled with severely mentally ill people that were sent out to sea with little guidance and in search of their lost rationality.

shiva. In the Jewish-American culture, following the death of a loved one, *shiva* is the 7-day period beginning with the burial. During this time, mourners do not work, and no activity is permitted that diverts attention from thinking about the deceased.

short-term memory. The ability to remember events that occurred very recently. This ability deteriorates with age.

silent rape reaction. The response of a rape victim in which he or she tells no one about the assault.

slander. An action with which an individual may be charged for orally sharing information that is detrimental to a person's reputation.

social distance. The distance considered acceptable in interactions with strangers or acquaintances, such as at a cocktail party or in a public building. U.S. culture defines this distance as 4 to 12 feet.

social skills training. Educational opportunities through role play for the person with schizophrenia to learn appropriate social interaction skills and functional skills that are relevant to daily living.

Socratic questioning (also called guided discovery). When the therapist questions the client with Socratic questioning, the client is asked to describe feelings associated with specific situations. Questions are stated in a way that may stimulate in the client a recognition of possible dysfunctional thinking and produce a dissonance about the validity of the thoughts.

somatization. A method of coping with psychosocial stress by developing physical symptoms.

splitting. A primitive ego defense mechanism in which the person is unable to integrate and accept both positive and negative feelings. In their view, people—including themselves—and life situations are either all good or all bad. This trait is common in borderline personality disorder.

standard precautions. Guidelines established by the Centers for Disease Control (CDC) designed to reduce the risk of transmission of pathogens from moist body substances. Standard precautions apply to blood; all body fluids, secretions, and excretions *except sweat*; nonintact skin; and mucous membranes.

statutory law. A law that has been enacted by legislative bodies, such as a county or city council, state legislature, or the U.S. Congress.

statutory rape. Unlawful intercourse between a man over age 16 and a female under the age of consent. The man can be arrested for statutory rape even when the interaction has occurred between consenting individuals.

stereotyping. The process of classifying all individuals from the same culture or ethnic group as identical.

stimuli. In classical conditioning, that which elicits a response.

stimulus generalization. The process by which a conditioned response is elicited from all stimuli *similar* to the one from which the response was learned.

store-front clinic. Establishments that have been converted into clinics that serve the homeless population.

stress. A state of disequilibrium that occurs when there is a disharmony between demands occurring within an individual's internal or external environment and his or her ability to cope with those demands.

stress management. Various methods used by individuals to reduce tension and other maladaptive responses to stress in their lives; includes relaxation exercises, physical exercise, music, mental imagery or any other technique that is successful for a person.

stressor. A demand from within an individual's internal or external environment that elicits a physiological and/or psychological response.

sublimation. The rechanneling of personally and/or socially unacceptable drives or impulses into activities that are more tolerable and constructive.

subluxation. The term used in chiropractic medicine to describe vertebrae in the spinal column that have become displaced, possibly pressing on nerves and interfering with normal nerve transmission.

substance abuse. Use of psychoactive drugs that poses significant hazards to health and interferes with social, occupational, psychological, or physical functioning.

substance dependence. Physical dependence is identified by the inability to stop using a substance despite attempts to do so; a continual use of the substance despite adverse consequences; a developing tolerance; and the development of withdrawal symptoms upon cessation or decreased intake. Psychological dependence is said to exist when a substance is perceived by the user to be necessary to maintain an optimal state of personal well-being, interpersonal relations, or skill performance.

substitution therapy. The use of various medications to decrease the intensity of symptoms in an individual who is withdrawing from, or experiencing the effects of excessive use of, substances.

subsystems. The smaller units of which a system is composed. In family systems theory, the subsystems are composed of husband-wife, parent-child(ren), or sibling-sibling.

sundowning. A phenomenon in dementia in which the symptoms seem to worsen in the late afternoon and evening.

superego. One of the three elements of the personality identified by Freud that represents the conscience and the culturally determined restrictions that are placed on an individual.

suppression. The voluntary blocking from one's awareness of unpleasant feelings and experiences.

surrogate. One who serves as a substitute figure for another.

symbiotic relationship. A type of "psychic fusion" that occurs between two people; it is unhealthy in that severe anxiety is generated in either or both if separation is indicated. A symbiotic relationship is normal between infant and mother.

sympathy. The actual sharing of another's thoughts and behaviors. Differs from empathy, in that with empathy one experiences an objective understanding of what another is feeling, rather than actually sharing those feelings.

synapse. The junction between two neurons. The small space between the axon terminals of one neuron and the cell body or dendrites of another is called the synaptic cleft.

syphilis. A sexually transmitted disorder caused by the spirochete *T. pallidum* and resulting in a chancre on the skin or mucous membranes of the sexual organs. If left untreated, may go systemic. End-stage disease can have profound effects, such as blindness or insanity.

systematic desensitization. A treatment for phobias in which the individual is taught to relax and then asked to imagine various components of the phobic stimulus on a graded hierarchy, moving from that which produces the least fear to that which produces the most.

T

T-4 lymphocyte. The white blood cell that is the primary target of HIV. These cells are destroyed by the virus, causing the striking depletion of T4 cells associated with HIV infection.

tangentiality. The inability to get to the point of a story. The speaker introduces many unrelated topics, until the original topic of discussion is lost.

tardive dyskinesia. Syndrome of symptoms characterized by bizarre facial and tongue movements, a stiff neck, and difficulty swallowing. It may occur as an adverse effect of long-term therapy with some antipsychotic medications.

technical expert. Peplau's term for one who understands various professional devices and possesses the clinical skills necessary to perform the interventions that are in the best interest of the client.

temperament. A set of inborn personality characteristics that influence an individual's manner of reacting to the environment, and ultimately influences his or her developmental progression.

territoriality. The innate tendency of individuals to own space. Individuals lay claim to areas around them as their own. This phenomenon can have an influence on interpersonal communication.

tertiary prevention. Health care that is directed toward reduction of the residual effects associated with severe or chronic physical or mental illness.

therapeutic group. Differs from group therapy in that there is a lesser degree of theoretical foundation. Focus is on group relations, interactions between group members, and the consideration of a selected issue. Leaders of therapeutic groups do not require the degree of educational preparation required of group therapy leaders.

thought-stopping technique. A self-taught technique that an individual uses each time he or she wishes to eliminate intrusive or negative, unwanted thoughts from awareness.

time out. An aversive stimulus or punishment during which the individual is removed from the environment where the unacceptable behavior is being exhibited.

token economy. In behavior modification, a type of contracting in which the reinforcers for desired behaviors are presented in the form of tokens, which may then be exchanged for designated privileges.

tort. The violation of a civil law in which an individual has been wronged. In a tort action, one party asserts that wrongful conduct on the part of the other has caused harm, and compensation for harm suffered is sought.

Transmission-Based Precautions. Guidelines established by the Centers for Disease Control (CDC) designed for patient documented or suspected to be infected or colonized with highly transmissible or epidemiologically important pathogens for which additional precautions beyond Standard Precautions are needed to interrupt transmission in hospitals. There are three types of Transmission-Based Precautions: Airborne Precautions, Droplet Precautions, and Contact Precautions.

transsexualism. A disorder of gender identity or gender dysphoria (unhappiness or dissatisfaction with one's gender) of the most extreme variety. The individual, despite having the anatomical characteristics of a given gender, has the self-perception of being of the opposite gender, and may seek to have gender changed through surgical intervention.

transvestic fetishism. Recurrent urges and sexually arousing fantasies involving dressing in the clothes of the opposite gender.

triangles. A three-person emotional configuration which is considered the basic building block of the family system. When anxiety becomes too great between two family members, a third person is brought in to form a triangle. Triangles are dysfunctional in that they offer relief from anxiety through diversion rather than through resolution of the issue.

trichotillomania. The recurrent failure to resist impulses to pull out one's own hair.

type A personality. The personality characteristics attributed to individuals prone to coronary heart disease, including excessive competitive drive, chronic sense of time urgency, easy anger, aggressiveness, excessive ambition, and inability to enjoy leisure time.

type B personality. The personality characteristics attributed to individuals who are not prone to coronary heart disease; includes characteristics such as ability to perform even under pressure but without the competitive drive and constant sense of time urgency experienced by the type A personality. Type Bs can enjoy their leisure time without feeling guilty, and they are much less impulsive than type A individuals; that is, they think things through before making decisions.

type C personality. The personality characteristics attributed to the cancer-prone individual. Includes characteristics such as suppression of anger, calm, passive, puts the needs of others before their own, but holds resentment toward others for perceived "wrongs."

type D personality. Personality characteristics attributed to individuals who are at increased risk of cardiovascular morbidity and mortality. The characteristics include a combination of negative emotions and social inhibition.

tyramine. An amino acid found in aged cheeses or other aged, overripe, and fermented foods; broad beans; pickled herring; beef or chicken liver; preserved meats; beer and wine; yeast products; chocolate; caffeinated drinks; canned figs; sour cream; yogurt; soy sauce; and some over-the-counter cold medications and diet pills. If foods high in tyramine content are consumed while an individual is taking MAO inhibitors, a potentially life-threatening syndrome called hypertensive crisis can result.

U

unconditional positive regard. Carl Rogers' term for the respect and dignity of an individual regardless of his or her unacceptable behavior.

undoing. A mechanism used to symbolically negate or cancel out a previous action or experience that one finds intolerable.

universality. One curative factor of groups (identified by Yalom) in which individuals realize that they are not alone in a problem and in the thoughts and feelings they are experiencing. Anxiety is relieved by the support and understanding of others in the group who share similar experiences.

Universal Precautions. Guidelines established by the Centers for Disease Control in which special barrier precautions (e.g., gloves, mask, eye protection) should be used with ALL individuals with whom there is a risk of blood and/or body-fluid exposure.

utilitarianism. The ethical theory that espouses "the greatest happiness for the greatest number." Under this theory, action would be taken based on the end results that will produce the most good (happiness) for the most people.

V

vaginismus. Involuntary constriction of the outer one third of the vagina that prevents penile insertion and intercourse.

values. Personal beliefs about the truth, beauty, or worth of a thought, object, or behavior, that influence an individual's actions.

values clarification. A process of self-discovery by which people identify their personal values and their value rankings. This process increases awareness about why individuals behave in certain ways.

velorio. In the Mexican-American culture, following the death of a loved one, the *velorio* is a festive watch by family and friends over the body of the deceased person before burial.

voyeurism. Recurrent urges and sexually arousing fantasies involving the act of observing unsuspecting people, usually strangers, who are either naked, in the process of disrobing, or engaging in sexual activity.

W

waxy flexibility. A condition by which the individual with schizophrenia passively yields all movable parts of the body to any efforts made at placing them in certain positions.

Wernicke's encephalopathy. A brain disorder caused by thiamine deficiency and characterized by visual disturbances, ataxia, somnolence, stupor, and, without thiamine replacement, death.

word salad. A group of words that are put together in a random fashion without any logical connection.

Y

yin and yang. The fundamental concept of Asian health practices. Yin and yang are opposite forces of energy such as negative/positive, dark/light, cold/hot, hard/soft, and feminine/masculine. Food, medicines, and herbs are classified according to their yin and yang properties and are used to restore a balance, thereby restoring health.

yoga. A system of beliefs and practices, the ultimate goal of which is to unite the human soul with the universal spirit. In Western countries, yoga uses body postures, along with meditation and breathing exercises, to achieve a balanced, disciplined workout that releases muscle tension, tones the internal organs, and energizes the mind, body, and spirit, so that natural healing can occur.

Index

Page numbers followed by f denote figures; those followed by t denote tables.

ADDITIONAL BONUS MATERIAL

To help you in your commitment to psychiatric nursing, we have provided a host of ancillary material. You can find helpful easy-access learning and teaching aids on the **Student CD-ROM** attached to the right and the FREE **Student Online Resource** at www.fadavis.com/townsend.

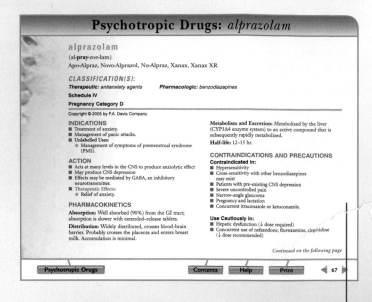

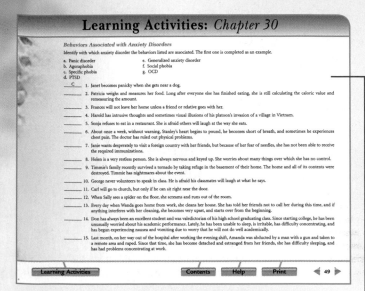

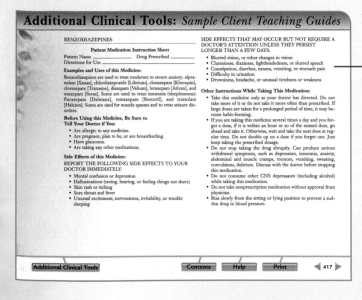

STUDENT CD-ROM

Electronic Test Bank
- **Nearly 300 Questions** to help the student with the course and prepare for the NCLEX® exam
  - **50 alternate item format NCLEX®-style questions**
  - More than **100 NCLEX®-style multiple-choice questions**
  - **135+** multiple-choice review questions
  - **Rationales** for Correct and Incorrect Answers

Electronic Student Workbook
- **More than 400** Helpful Learning Activities
- 55 **Psychotropic Drug Monographs** that can be printed and carried to clinicals
- 23 Sample **Client Education Teaching Guides** that can be reproduced as client/family handouts
- **Care Plans** and **Critical Pathways**
- **Medication Assessment Tool**
- **Levels of Anxiety**
- **Assigning Nursing Diagnoses to Client Behaviors**

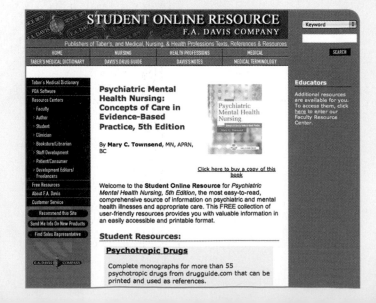

FREE STUDENT ONLINE RESOURCE
www.fadavis.com/townsend

- 5 printable **Concept Map Care Plans** from the text plus 3 preformatted templates for customizing plans of care
- 16 Conventional Nursing **Care Plans**
- **Psychotropic Drug Monographs**
- 5 Schematic **Brain Illustrations**
- Meet the author/Contact the author